Gynecologic Oncology:
Current Diagnosis and Treatment

Gynecologic Oncology: Current Diagnosis and Treatment

Edited by

Hugh M Shingleton MD
J Marion Sims Professor of Gynecology Emeritus, University of Alabama
National Vice President for Cancer Detection and Treatment, American Cancer Society
Clinical Professor of Gynecology, Emory University
Atlanta, Georgia, USA

Wesley C Fowler Jr MD
Leonard Palumbo Professor and Associate Chairman, Department of Obstetrics and Gynecology University of North Carolina at Chapel Hill
School of Medicine, North Carolina, USA

Joseph A Jordan MD, FRCOG
Consultant Gynecologist and Medical Director,
Birmingham and Midland Hospital for Women, Birmingham, UK

W Dwayne Lawrence MD
Chief of Pathology, Hutzel Hospital–The Detroit Medical Center
Professor of Pathology, Wayne State University School of Medicine,
Detroit, Michigan, USA

WB Saunders Company Ltd
London · Philadelphia · Toronto · Sydney · Tokyo

W. B. Saunders Company Ltd 24–28 Oval Road
London NW1 7DX

The Curtis Center
Independence Square West
Philadelphia, PA 19106-3399, USA

Harcourt Brace & Company
55 Horner Avenue
Toronto, Ontario M8Z 4X6, Canada

Harcourt Brace & Company, Australia
30–52 Smidmore Street
Marrickville, NSW 2204, Australia

Harcourt Brace & Company, Japan
Ichibancho Central Building, 22-1 Ichibancho
Chiyoda-ku, Tokyo 102, Japan

This book is printed on acid free paper

A catalogue record for this book is available from the British Library

ISBN 0-7020-1839-2

Typeset by P & R Typesetters Ltd, Wiltshire.
Printed in Great Britain by The Bath Press, Avon.

Dedicated to

Jeanne Louise Shingleton
Louise Pittman Lawrence
Valerie Jordan

for their accomplishments and support

and to the Memory of

Clarence E Ehrlich, MD
Thomas Day Jr., MD
Lynda Lawrence Kemp

Contents

List of Contributors

R D Alvarez MD
Assistant Professor, Gynecologic Oncology
University of Alabama at Birmingham
Department of Obstetrics and Gynecology
618 South 20th Street, Suite 538
Birmingham
Alabama 35233-7333
USA

D Anciaux MD
Fellow, Gynecologic and Obstetrical Pathology
Department of Pathology
Wayne State University School of Medicine
Hutzel Hospital
4707 St Antoine
Detroit
Michigan 48201
USA

M C Anderson FRCOG FRCPath
Reader in Gynecological Pathology
University of Nottingham Medical School
Queens Medical Centre
Nottingham NG7 2UH
UK

V V Baker MD
Chief, Division of Gynecologic Oncology
Professor of Obstetrics and Gynecology
University of Michigan Medical Center
1500 East Medical Center Drive
D2251 Medical Professional Building
Ann Arbor
Michigan 48109-0718
USA

K I Bland MD
J Murray Beardsley Professor and Chairman
Brown University School of Medicine
Rhode Island Hospital
Department of Surgery
593 Eddy Street
Providence
Rhode Island 02903
USA

J R Bosscher MD
Assistant Professor
Department of Obstetrics and Gynecology
Gynecologic Oncology Division
University of Louisville School of Medicine
Louisville
Kentucky 40292
USA

L W Brady MD
Professor and Chairman
Department of Radiation Oncology and Nuclear Medicine
Medical College of Pennsylvania
Hahnemann University
Broad & Vine Streets, MS 200
Philadelphia
Pensylvania 19102-1192
USA

P S Braly MD
Professor and Chief, Gynecologic Oncology
Department of Obstetrics and Gynecology
Louisiana State University Medical Center
1542 Tulane Avenue
New Orleans
Los Angeles 70112-2822
USA

A C Casey MD
Clinical Instructor
Department of Obstetrics and Gynecology
Division of Gynecologic Oncology
UCLA School of Medicine
Room 24-127
Center for the Health Sciences
10833 Le Conte Avenue
Los Angeles
California 90024-1740
USA

K K Chan FRCS FRCOG
Consultant Gynecological Oncologist
Birmingham and Midland Hospital for Women
Showell Green Lane
Sparkhill
Birmingham
B11 4HL
UK

H R Chang MD PhD
Associate Professor of Surgery and Pathobiology
Department of Surgery at Roger Williams Medical Center
825 Chalkstone Avenue
Providence
Rhode Island 02908
USA

J T Comerci Jr, MD
Instructor at Department of Gynecologic Oncology
Director of Division of Gynecologic Oncology

Albert Einstein College of Medicine and Montefiore Medical Center
1695 Eastchester Road, Suite 601
Bronx
New York 10461
USA

M C Comiskey MB BCh MRCP (I)
Senior Registrar in Palliative Medicine
St Oswald's Hospice
Regent Avenue
Gosforth
Newcastle-upon-Tyne NE3 1EE
UK

A F Crawford FRCS MRCOG
Gynecological Oncology Fellow of St Bartholomew's and The Royal Marsden Hospitals
Department of Gynecology
St Bartholomew's Hospital
West Smithfield
London EC1A 7BE
UK

J L Currie MD
Professor and Chair
Department of Obstetrics and Gynecology
Dartmouth-Hitchcock Medical Center
1 Medical Center Drive
Lebanon
New Hampshire 03756
USA

G Deppe MD
Professor at Wayne State University
Director, Division of Gynecologic Oncology
Hutzel Hospital
4707 St Antoine
Detroit
Michigan 48201
USA

P D DePriest MD
Assistant Professor
Department of Obstetrics and Gynecology
Division of Gynecologic Oncology
University of Kentucky Medical Center
800 Rose Street, Room MN 308
Lexington
Kentucky 40536-0084
USA

M Paola Dey MBBS MSc
Lecturer and Honorary Senior Registrar in Public Health Medicine
Centre for Cancer Epidemiology
University of Manchester
Kinnaird Road
Withington
Manchester M20 4QL
UK

M B Dinerman BSc
Information Specialist
American Cancer Society
National Office
1599 Clifton Road NE
Atlanta
Georgia 30329 4251
USA

D L Doering MD
Assistant Professor of Obstetrics and Gynecology
Department of Obstetrics and Gynecology
University of Louisville
PO Box 3086
Louisville
Kentucky 40201
USA

P Doyle BSc MSc PhD
Lecturer at London School of Hygiene and Tropical Medicine
Department of Epidemiology and Population Sciences
London School of Hygiene and Tropical Medicine
Keppel Street
London WC1E 7HT
UK

R Farias-Eisner MD
Department of Obstetrics and Gynecology
Division of Gynecologic Oncology
UCLA School of Medicine
24-127 Center for the Health Sciences
10833 Le Conte Avenue
Los Angeles
California 90024-1740
USA

N J Finkler MD FACOG FACS
Director of Gynecologic Oncology
Assistant Adjunct Professor at Duke University School
Walt Disney Memorial Cancer Institute at Florida Hospital
500 East Rollins Street
Orlando
Florida 32803
USA

H Fox MD FRCPath FRCOG
Emeritus Professor of Reproductive Pathology
Department of Pathology Sciences
University of Manchester
Stopford Building
Oxford Road
Manchester M13 9PT
UK

A Frost MD
Assistant Professor
Department of Radiology
Albert Einstein College of Medicine
1695 Eastchester Road, Suite 601
Bronx
New York 10461
USA

W C Fowler MD
Leonard Palumbo Professor and Associate Chairman
Department of Obstetrics and Gynecology
Division of Gynecologic Oncology
University of North Carolina
Chapel Hill
NC 27599-7570
USA

H H Gallion MD
Associate Professor
Department of Obstetrics and Gynecology
University of Kentucky Medical Center
Room MN 322
800 Rose Street
Lexington
Kentucky 405
USA

R M Giusti MD MSPH
Special Assistant to the Director
Division of Cancer Treatment
National Cancer Institute
Building 31
Room 3A44
31 Center Drive MSC 2440
Bethesda
Maryland 20892-2440
USA

P W Grigsby MD MBA
Professor of Radiation Oncology
Radiation Oncology Center
Mallinckrodt Institute of Radiology
4939 Children's Place, Suite 5500
St. Louis
Missouri 63110
USA

L N Harris MD FRCP(C) FACP
Instructor in Medicine
Department of Hematology and Medical Oncology
Lombardi Cancer Center – Corridor B
Georgetown University Medical Center
3800 Reservoir Road
Washington DC 20007-2197
USA

C W Helm MA FRCSEd FRCS Eng MRCOG FACOG
Director, Division of Gynecologic Oncology
Temple University School of Medicine
3401 N Broad Street
Philadelphia 19140
USA

H D Homesley MD
Professor and Head of Section, Gynecologic Oncology
Department of Obstetrics and Gynecology
Bowman Gray School of Medicine of Wake Forest University
Comprehensive Cancer Center
Medical Center Boulevard
Winston-Salem
North Carolina 27157-1065
USA

A Ilancheran MBBS MMED FRCOG MD FAMS
Consultant in Obstetrics and Gynecology
Gynecology Associates
3 Mount Elizabeth No. 12–18
Mount Elizabeth Medical Center
Singapore 228510

J A Jordan MD FRCOG
Consultant Gynecologist and Medical Director
Birmingham Women's Hospital
Metchley Park Road
Edgbaston
Birmingham
B15 2TC
UK

R L S Jennelle MD
Assistant Professor of Radiation Oncology
Wallace Tumor Institute
UAB Medical Center
619 South 19th Street
Birmingham
Alabama 35233-6832
USA

R Y Kim MD
Professor of Radiation Oncology
UAB Medical Center
619 South 19th Street
Birmingham
Alabama 35233-6832
USA

Y Kim MD
Fellow in Gynecologic Oncology
Department of Obstetrics and Gynecology
Division of Gynecologic Oncology
UCLA School of Medicine
24–127 Center for the Health Sciences
10833 Le Conte Avenue
Los Angeles
California 90024-1740
USA

W D Lawrence MD
Chief of Pathology, Hutzel Hospital
Professor of Pathology, Wayne State University
4707 St Antoine Boulevard
Detroit
Michigan 48201
USA

M E Lippman MD
Director, Lombardi Cancer Center
Professor of Medicine and Pharmacology
Georgetown University Medical School
Lombardi Cancer Center
The Research Building
3970 Reservoir Road
Washington DC 20007
USA

D M Luesley MA MD FRCOG
Honorary Consultant Gynecologist at City Hospital NHS Trust
Reader in Gynecological Oncology
Department of Obstetrics and Gynecology
University of Birmingham
Edgbaston
Birmingham B15 2TG
UK

P J MacKoul MD
Associate Director, Gynecologic Oncology
The Washington Cancer Institute at
Washington Hospital Center
10215 Fernwood Road, Suite 303
Bethesda
Maryland 20817
USA

V K Malviya MD
Associate Professor and Associate Director
Division of Gynecologic Oncology
Hutzel Hospital
Wayne State University
4707 St Antoine
Detroit
Michigan 48201
USA

W J Mann MD FACOG FACS
Director, Gynecologic Oncologist
Riverside Obstetrics and Gynecology Center
314 Main Street
Newport News
Virginia 23601-3813
USA

W A Marston MD
Assistant Professor of Surgery
Division of Vascular Surgery School of Medicine
University of North Carolina at Chapel Hill
Chapel Hill
North Carolina 27599-7212
USA

S Menda MD
Professor of Obstetrics and Gynecology
Department of Obstetrics and Gynecology
Division of Gynecologic Oncology
UCLA School of Medicine
24-127 Center for the Health Sciences
10833 Le Conte Avenue
Los Angeles
California 90024-1740
USA

M Morris MD
Associate Professor of Gynecologic Oncology
Department of Gynecologic Oncology
The University of Texas
M D Anderson Cancer Center
1515 Holcombe Boulevard
Houston
Texas 77030
USA

H B Muss MD
Professor of Medicine
Section of Hematology and Oncology
Comprehensive Cancer Center of Wake Forest University
Bowman Gray School of Medicine
Medical Center Boulevard
Winston-Salem
North Carolina 27157-1082
USA

E S Newlands BA PhD FRCP
Professor of Cancer Medicine
Honorary Consultant at Hammersmith Hospitals NHS Trust
Charing Cross and Westminster Medical School
Fulham Palace Road
London W6 8RF
UK

G A Omura MD
Professor of Medicine and Gynecology
Suite B
2190 Parkway Lake Drive
Birmingham
Alabama 35244
USA

P Papas MD
Assistant Professor of Pathology
Wayne State University
School of Medicine
4707 St Antoine

Detroit
Michigan 48201
USA

C A Perez MD
Professor of Radiology (Radiation Oncology)
Director, Radiation Oncology Center
Mallinckrodt Institute of Radiology
Washington University School of Medicine
Suite 200
4511 Forest Park
St Louis
Missouri 63108
USA

J J Perry MD
Assistant Professor of Medicine
Section of Hematology and Oncology
Comprehensive Cancer Center of Wake Forest University
Bowman Gray Center Boulevard
Winston-Salem
North Carolina 27157-1082
USA

C F B Regnard MBChB BMSc
Honorary Consultant of Palliative Medicine at Royal Victoria Infirmary
Medical Director
St Oswald's Hospice
Regent Avenue
Gosforth
Newcastle-upon-Tyne NE3 1EE
UK

W H Rodgers PhD MD
Associate Professor of Pathology
Head, Section of Cytopathology
Department of Pathology
University of Alabama at Birmingham (UAB)
619 South 19th Street
Kracke Building – Rm 532A
Birmingham
Alabama 35233
USA

P Y Roland MD
Instructor and Fellow in Gynecologic Oncology
Department of Obstetrics and Gynecology
Division of Gynecologic Oncology
University of Alabama of Birmingham
618 South 20th Street
Birmingham
Alabama 35233-7333
USA

T P Rollason MBChE FRCPath
Senior Clinical Lecturer in Pathology at University of Birmingham
Consultant Gynecological Pathologist
Department of Pathology
Birmingham Women's Hospital
Edgbaston
Birmingham B15 2TG
UK

C D Runowicz MD
Associate Professor and Director of Gynecologic Oncology
Albert Einstein College of Medicine and Montefiore Medical Center
1695 Eastchester Road, Suite 601
Bronx
New York 10461
USA

M M Salter MD FACR
Clinical Professor
DCH Cancer Center
801 University Bolvd.
Tuscaloosa
Alabama 35401
USA

R Sands MBChB MRCOG
Clinical Research Fellow
Academic Department of Obstetrics and Gynecology
Chelsea and Westminster Hospital
369 Fulham Road
London SW10 9NH
UK

I dos Santos Silva MD MSc PhD
Clinical Senior Lecturer in Epidemiology
Department of Epidemiology and Population Sciences
London School of Hygiene and Tropical Medicine
Keppel Street
London WC1E 7HT
UK

S M Selvaggi MD
Associate Professor of Pathology
Director Laboratory Cytopathology
Associate Professor of Pathology
Department of Pathology
University of Michigan Hospitals
1500 E. Medical Center Drive
Rm. 2G332/Box 0054
Ann Arbor
Michigan 48109-0054
USA

M I Shafi MBBCh DA MCROG
Senior Lecturer in Obstetrics and Gynecology
City Hospital NHS Trust
Dudley Road

Winson Green
Birmingham B18 7QH
UK

H M Shingleton MD
J Marion Sims Professor of Gynecology,
University of Alabama
National Vice President for Cancer Detection and Treatment at American Cancer Society
Clinical Professor of Gynecology
Emory University
1599 Clifton Road
NE Atlanta
Georgia 30329-4251
USA

D L Shenson
Information Specialist
Department of Obstetrics and Gynecology
Room MN 322
University of Kentucky Medical Center
800 Rose Street
Lexington
Kentucky 405
USA

J H Shepherd DRCS MRCOG FACOG
Consultant Gynecological Surgeon and Oncologist at St Bartholomews and the Royal Marsden Hospitals
Department of Gynecological Oncology
St Bartholomew's Hospital
West Smithfield
London EC1A 7BE
UK

R A Smith PhD
Senior Director, Detection and Treatment
American Cancer Society
1599 Clifton Road
Atlanta
Georgia 30329-4251
USA

M J Solan MD
Clinical Assistant Professor
Radiation Oncologist
Fitzgeral Mercy Hospital
1500 Lansdowne Avenue
Dorby
Pennsylvania 19023
USA

S Soong PhD
Professor and Director of Biostatistics Unit
Department of Biostatics
Comprehensive Cancer Center
University of Alabama at Birmingham
University Station
Birmingham
Alabama 35294
USA

N S A Stuart BM DM MRCP
Honorary Consultant Medical Oncologist at Claterbridge Centre for Oncology
Consultant Medical Oncologist
Department of Oncology and Haematology
Ysbyty Gwynedd
Bangor
Gwynedd LL57 2PW
UK

J Studd DSc MD FRCOG
Consultant Gynecologist
Chelsea and Westminster Hospital
Fulham Road
London SW10 9NH
UK

G P Sutton MD
Mary Fendrich Hulman
Professor and Director of Obstetrics and Gynecology
Department of Obstetrics and Gynecology
Indiana University Medical Center
550 North University Boulevard, Room 2440
Indianapolis
Indiana 46202-5274
USA

G R Tobin MD
Professor and Chair
Division of Surgery
University of Louisville School of Medicine
Louisville
Kentucky 40292
USA

J R van Nagell Jr MD
Professor and Director of Division of Gynecologic Oncology
Department of Obstetrics and Gynecology
University of Kentucky Medical Center
Room MN308
800 Rose Street
Lexington
Kentucky 40536-0084
USA

D W Visscher MD
Associate Professor of Pathology
Department of Pathology
Harper Hospital
Detroit Medical Center
Wayne State University
Michigan 48201
USA

A Warwick MBChB MRCOG
Consultant Obstetrician and Gynecologist
Senior Registrar
Department of Obstetrics and Gynecology
City Hospital NHS Trust
Dudley Road
Birmingham B18 7QH
UK

H Weiss PhD
Research Assistant Professor
Division of Hematology and Oncology
School of Medicine
WTI 153
University of Alabama at Birmingham
Birmingham
Alabama 35294-3300
USA

S D Williams MD
Professor of Medicine
Director at Indiana University Cancer Center
550 North University Boulevard, Room 1640
Indianapolis
Indiana 46254
USA

C B J Woodman MD MRCOG MFPHuM
Professor of Public Health and Epidemiology
Centre for Cancer Epidemiology
University of Manchester
Kinnaird Road
Withington
Manchester M20 4QL
UK

Preface

Gynecological cancer is one of the most interesting and challenging areas of oncology today. Many advances have been made in terms of therapy, diagnosis and prevention. In spite of dramatic improvements in the management of diseases such as teratoma and trophoblastic disease, the situation in other gynecological malignancies is very different. Most women who develop ovarian cancer will die. The mortality from cervix cancer approaches 50% and even in a disease as apparently low grade as endometrial cancer, the five year survival is only 65%.

While significant improvements may depend on sudden serendipitous discoveries, much still remains to be done within our present limitations. Quality of care differs widely in different areas of the world, and the optimal use of resources at our disposal has not yet been established. Within these limitations this book is an attempt to describe good international practice in gynecological cancer and reflects the views of many centers in a number of countries.

Although there are general differences in treatment even among some of these centers of excellence, we have attempted to give a balanced view of gynecologic cancer reflecting state-of-the-art care at this time. The special importance of histopathology and cytopathology in the practice of gynecologic oncology is recognized and considerable emphasis has been placed on these subjects throughout the book.

The book is divided into several sections; in addition to considering the disease sites in considerable detail there are sections on special treatment considerations, special techniques necessary to practice gynecologic oncology at its best, and a section on background topics covering fundamentals of radiation and chemotherapy, biostatistics for the clinician, and staging of cancers.

The book is targeted at the postgraduate textbook level, and in addition to providing established data about each disease, authors have included information about areas of developing interest. While some of these assume varying degrees of importance and will be replaced in time, their inclusion should give the reader insights into the most current approaches to gynecologic oncology as well as providing a flavor of current clinical and basic research.

The book has been made possible only by the help of many important people at all of the major medical centers represented by the editors and authors. The experts in these centers have provided a core of expertise on which it has been possible to draw. To them, their assistants, and to all the other contributors we offer our thanks. Finally, those in our families who have watched occasionally bewildered as this book has come together must be thanked for their patience and support during this endeavor.

Hugh M Shingleton
Wesley C Fowler, Jr.
Joseph A Jordan
W Dwayne Lawrence

Important notice

Every effort has been made to check the drug dosages given in this book. However, as it is possible that dosage schedules have been revised, the reader is strongly urged to consult the drug companies' literature before administrating any of the drugs listed.

1 Epidemiology and Pathogenesis of Cervical Cancer

M P Dey
C B J Woodman

Introduction

Epidemiology is the study of the distribution of diseases and their determinants within human populations. Epidemiologic studies either describe the burden of disease within and between populations (descriptive epidemiology) or investigate potential etiologic factors (analytical epidemiology). Epidemiology can make important contributions to the planning of health services, the formulation of prevention programs and the evaluation of specific interventions.

Cervical cancer is the second most common cause of cancer among women worldwide. In many developed countries there are cervical cytology screening programs, which vary in their degree of organization and intensity, but aim to reduce mortality from cervical cancer by early detection and treatment of 'premalignant' epithelial abnormalities of the cervix. A stream of epidemiologic investigations have suggested consistently that a sexually transmitted agent, probably a virus, may play a major etiologic role in the genesis of this tumor and currently attention is focused on human papillomavirus (HPV).

Descriptive Epidemiology – General Principles

Three main measures are used to describe the impact of cancer: incidence, mortality and survival. Incidence and survival rates can be derived from data sets collected by cancer registries, which include new registrations of cancer within a defined population. Unlike hospital series, this population-based data set is not biased by either case selection or case referral.

Mortality rates are derived from information contained on death certificates. This information is often incomplete or inaccurate. Although this limits the usefulness of mortality as a measure of the burden of disease it is often the most appropriate outcome measure of the effectiveness of specific interventions or preventive programs.

The incidence rate is the number of new primary cases of cancer in a population at risk over a defined period. Mortality rate is the number of deaths from cancer in a population at risk over a defined period. Crude rates are affected by the age structure of the population and this may vary both between and within populations at different points in time. Age-standardized rates allow for variations in population age structures, thereby enabling comparisons between different populations. Directly age-standardized rates are calculated by applying age-specific rates of the population of interest to a notional reference population (e.g. the world standard population).

Population-based survival rates are derived from matching death registrations with cancer registrations. Survival analysis aims to estimate the force of mortality from the cancer under consideration. Its estimation presents two major difficulties: it is not always possible to decide if a patient with cancer has died from the disease or an unrelated cause, and those deaths from other causes will be more frequent in older people. To overcome this problem, it is now usual to estimate a survival rate that allows for deaths from other causes. This is called the relative survival rate and gives a better estimate of the mortality due to the cancer under consideration. It is calculated as the ratio of the crude survival rate to that which would be expected from the general population mortality experience.

International and temporal comparisons of data sets are often hampered by differences in the classification of disease and by variation in the ascertainment of both cases and deaths, and should be interpreted with some caution.

Descriptive Epidemiology of Cervical Cancer

Worldwide cancer of the cervix is an important cause of morbidity and mortality (Parkin *et al.*, 1993). In the majority of developing countries it is the most common cancer in women (Parkin *et al.*, 1992). The highest incidence rates have been observed in South America and India. In contrast, incidence rates are much lower in industrialized countries where cancers of the breast, lung and gastrointestinal system are

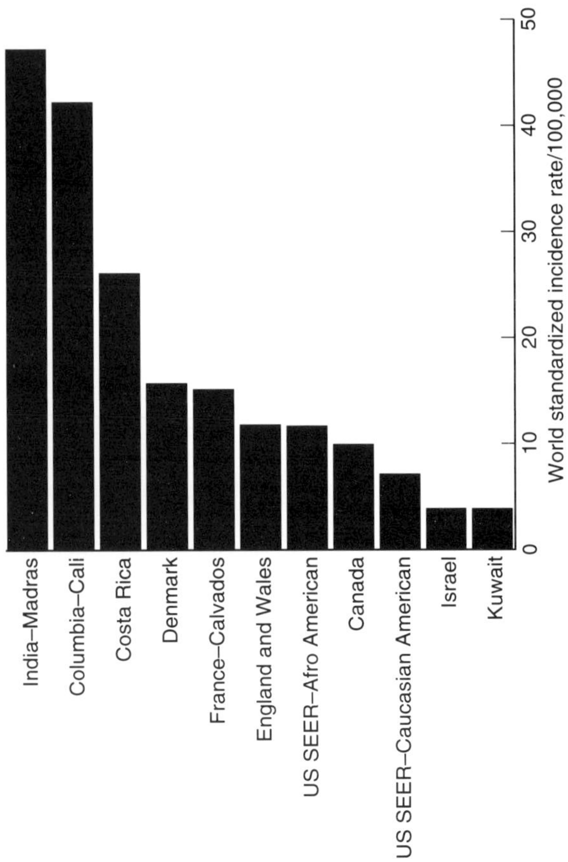

Figure 1.1. International comparison of incidence of cancer of the cervix 1983–1987. (From Cancer Incidence in Five Continents, Vol VI, IARC Scientific Publications.)

more common (*Figure 1.1*). Ethnic differences have also been observed: Afro-Americans have a rate twice that of Caucasian Americans, and particularly low rates have been recorded among Jewish women.

In England and Wales, cancer of the cervix is only the fifth most common cancer in women and the second most common gynecologic cancer after cancer of the ovary. There were 4147 new registrations of cervical cancer in 1989 and the age-standardized incidence rate was 11.8/100,000 (Office of Population Censuses and Surveys, 1989). It is the most common cancer in women under 50 years of age and unlike other gynecologic cancers, the age-specific incidence rate of cervical cancer increases 40-fold between the second and third decade, after which it plateaus before increasing again, albeit less markedly (*Figure 1.2*). There are interregional variations in incidence, with higher rates observed in the north of the country. As with ethnic differences, this variation may in part reflect the inverse correlation observed between lower socioeconomic class and risk of disease, which may in turn be explained by variations in risk factor profile or differences in the uptake of cervical cytology screening.

Population-based estimates of five-year relative survival rates for cervical cancer vary internationally and interregionally (Giles *et al.*, 1987; Woodman *et al.*, 1989; Joslin *et al.*, 1991; Miller *et al.*, 1992; Woodman *et al.*, 1992) (*Figure 1.3*). Recent rates for England and Wales are not available, but the five-year relative survival rate for the north western region of England was 58% for the quinquennium 1985–89. Key independent prognostic variables

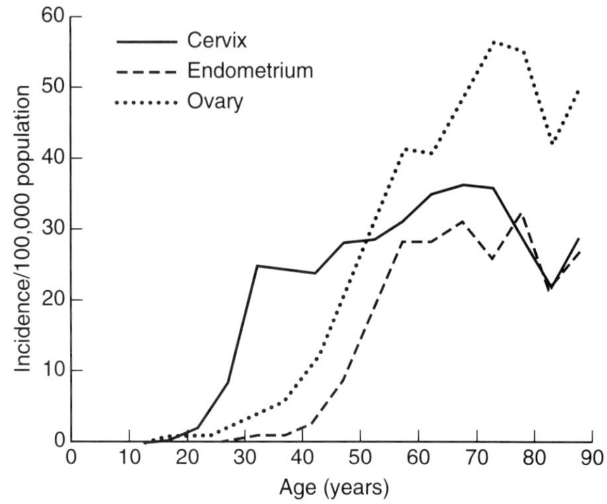

Figure 1.2. Gynecologic cancer age-specific incidence rates in the North West Regional Health Authority, UK, 1985–1989. (From North Western Regional Cancer Registry, UK.)

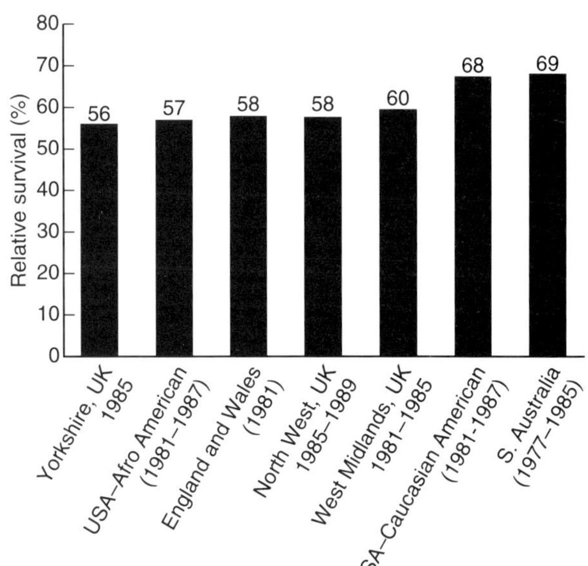

Figure 1.3. Cervical cancer. International comparisons of five-year relative survival.

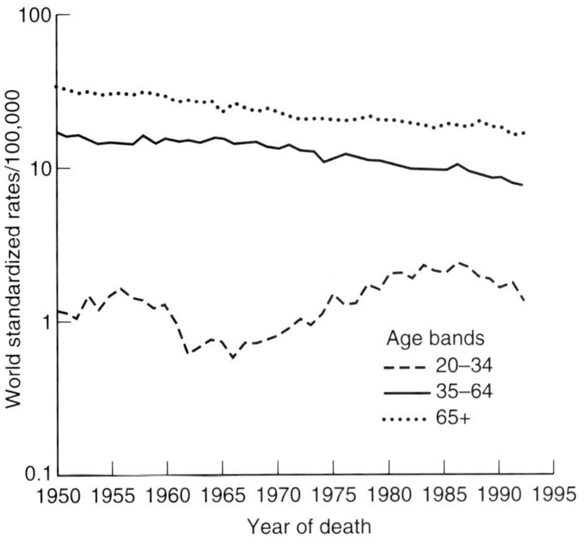

Figure 1.4. Cervical cancer mortality in England and Wales 1950–1992. (From Office of Population of Censuses and Surveys Mortality Statistics, UK.)

include age and stage at presentation: young age is associated with a better prognosis for all stages of disease (Meanwell *et al.*, 1988).

Incidence and mortality from cervical cancer have been decreasing steadily in most developed countries over the last three decades. Marked reductions have been reported from the Nordic Countries (with the exception of Norway), from the USA, from Canada and from Aberdeen in Scotland, all of which have been attributed to well-organized population-based cervical cytology screening programs with high levels of compliance (Ahluwalia *et al.*, 1968; Hakama, 1982; MacGregor *et al.*, 1985; Bjørge *et al.*, 1993; Sigurdsson, 1993). In England and Wales incidence rates have not declined (Office of Population Censuses and Surveys, 1974–1989). This was considered to be due to poor organization of cervical cytology screening and resulted in the initiation of a national call/recall program in 1988 (Day, 1989). However, although incidence rates have remained constant, mortality rates have been declining steadily, even before the reorganization of screening services (*Figure 1.4*).

The majority of cervical cancers are squamous cell. Adenocarcinoma of the cervix is a rare disease accounting for only 5–10% of all cancers of the cervix, but reports from the USA and Norway have shown an increasing incidence in cervical adenocarcinoma, particularly among younger women (Devesa *et al.*, 1989; Bjørge *et al.*, 1993). The rise may be secondary to improved pathologic classification or to increased detection of early asymptomatic lesions by cytological screening, but it is also suggested that it may be attributable to an increased use of oral contraceptives (Devesa *et al.*, 1989).

Risk Factors for Cervical Neoplasia

A stream of epidemiologic inquiries suggest consistently an association between sexually related behaviors and squamous cell carcinoma of the cervix (Brinton, 1992). This has been interpreted as supporting a causal role for a sexually transmitted agent of which HPV is the most recent etiologic agent to come under scrutiny.

The Evidence for a Sexually Transmitted Agent

The earliest evidence implicating sexually related behavior as a risk factor in the etiology of cancer of the cervix came from observations of the low incidence and mortality rates of the disease among religious groups such as nuns and Jewish women. Ecologic studies have demonstrated a positive correlation between the geographic distribution of carcinoma of the cervix and carcinoma of the penis, and higher than expected rates of cancer of the cervix have been found in the wives of men with cancer of the penis and vice versa (Smith *et al.*, 1980; Li *et al.*, 1982).

Numerous case–control studies in different populations have demonstrated consistently two aspects of sexual behavior to be independent risk factors for cancer of the cervix: namely number of lifetime sexual partners and age at first coitus (La Vecchia *et al.*, 1986; Brinton *et al.*, 1987). Women with ten or more lifetime sexual partners have a three times greater risk of developing cervical cancer compared to women with one or less partners, and a two-fold increase in risk of cervical cancer has been observed for women who have sexual intercourse before 16 years of age compared to those who are at least 20 years of age at first coitus (Brinton *et al.*, 1987; Slattery *et al.*, 1989).

In Latin American countries, despite high incidence rates, female sexual monogamy is common and the association between female sexually-related behaviors and cervical cancer is weak. Case–control studies of risk factors for cervical cancer in sexually monogamous women have demonstrated an association between sexual behaviors of the husband and an increased risk of developing cervical cancer in the wife. Such high-risk behaviors include the use of prostitutes, the number of sexual lifetime partners and self-reported genital infections (Brinton *et al.*, 1989).

Oral contraceptives and high multiparity have been shown in some studies to be associated with an increased risk of developing cervical cancer (Brinton *et al.*, 1987; Parazzini *et al.*, 1989). Although these risk factors may be a proxy for other sexual behavior variables, it is also hypothesized that elevated hormone levels induced by both factors may have immunosuppressive effects.

The majority of case–control studies that have included smoking as a risk factor have demonstrated an independent positive association with squamous cell carcinoma of the cervix and a risk 2–4 times that of non-smokers has been reported (Winkelstein, 1990). The relationship is strongest for current smokers, suggesting a late stage effect. Nicotine metabolites have been found in the cervical mucus of smokers (Schiffman *et al.*, 1987), but while some postulate a direct carcinogenic effect of smoking metabolites on the cervix, others argue that a history of smoking may be merely a surrogate for sexual risk factors that have yet to be more precisely defined (Phillips and Davey–Smith, 1994).

Human Papillomavirus

Introduction

The last decade has seen a stream of imaginative and resourceful experimental research that has established an impressive list of oncogenic credentials for HPV. This chapter does not attempt to reprise these developments, but to chronicle the efforts of epidemiologists to define more precisely the role of HPV in the pathogenesis of cancer of the cervix and to illustrate where current scientific uncertainty exists.

Genital HPV infection causes a spectrum of disease including genital warts or condyloma acuminatum, subclinical infections, which can only be identified on colposcopic or light microscopic examination of cytologic or histologic material, and latent infection where the only evidence of HPV infection is the presence of specific HPV DNA sequences in cytologic or histologic specimens (Woodman, 1994).

A reported history of genital warts has been consistently associated with an elevated risk of developing cancer of the cervix in those case–control studies examining this hypothesis. However, it is only following developments in molecular biology enabling the identification of HPV DNA sequences by nucleic acid hybridization that the oncogenic potential of subclinical and latent HPV has begun to be assessed adequately.

Large-scale epidemiologic inquiries have been hampered by uncertainties concerning the robustness of the tests used to detect the presence of HPV DNA sequences. The first generation of investigations used relatively insensitive techniques (e.g. filter *in situ* hybridization) and it has been suggested that this insensitivity may have resulted in an apparent weakening of the association of HPV with cervical cancer (Reeves *et al.*, 1989; Schiffman and Schatzkin, 1994). These difficulties have been overcome by the use of more sensitive techniques (e.g. the polymerase chain reaction, PCR), but confidence in this method was at one time undermined considerably by reports of the ease with which assay procedures could become contaminated (Young *et al.*, 1992.

Approximately 70 types of HPV have been described, and over 20 of these have been found in the genital tract. HPV DNA sequences have been isolated in the nuclei of squamous cells of both premalignant and malignant lesions by PCR. HPV has been reported by different investigators to be present in between 80–100% of cervical intraepithelial neoplasia (CIN3) and cervical cancer tissue samples. The HPV types found most frequently in premalignant and malignant specimens were HPV 16/18/31/33/35 whereas HPV 6/11 are the types most commonly found in genital warts (Walboomers *et al.*, 1994).

Analytic evidence supporting the role of human papillomavirus

Case–control studies

The most impressive evidence of an etiologic role for HPV in cervical cancer comes from the only wholly population-based case–control study so far reported (Munoz *et al.*, 1992). This carefully conducted study was undertaken in Cali, Columbia, and in Spain, two geographic areas with very different incidence rates. Columbia has one of the highest incidence rates for cervical cancer in the world, eight times that of Spain. Central pathologic review of cervical cancer cases and histologic material from women with CIN 3 was performed during the study period in an attempt to reduce misclassification bias. Detection of HPV was undertaken using three different methods: PCR, Southern blot hybridization and ViraPap^{tm}. An imposing positive association with risk estimates of magnitudes rarely seen in epidemiologic investigations was found. This was observed in both countries and with all of the detection methods employed.

Adjusted odds ratios varied between 8.8 (95% confidence intervals (CI) 4.1–19.0) with Southern blot hybridization in Spanish women to 93.2 (95% CI 12.6–687.3) with ViraPap^{tm} in Columbian women. Therefore, although the direction of the association is consistent, there is considerable variation both between countries, and when comparing the two countries, in the detection method employed. While the former is readily explained by the difference in incidence rates between the two countries, the latter is more difficult to interpret. It may be explained partly by the statistical instability introduced by small numbers of HPV-positive controls, reflected in the wide confidence intervals.

The findings of this inquiry have been supported by one other partially population-based case–control study and a number of hospital-based case–control studies (Meanwell *et al.*, 1987; Reeves *et al.*, 1989; Eluf Neto *et al.*, 1994). However, although the risk estimates have been in the same direction they have generally been smaller in magnitude. This may be due to the methodologic flaws inherent in their design: namely the use of less suitable control populations and less sensitive tests to detect the presence of HPV DNA.

Cohort studies

Proof of causality requires evidence that exposure to an etiologic agent has preceded the onset of disease and this cannot be provided by even the most rigorously designed and conducted case–control study. This level of evidence can only be provided by cohort studies in which groups of disease-free women whose exposure status to HPV is known at the start of the study are followed over a period of time to determine the subsequent risk of disease. The major limitation of cohort studies in the investigation of the natural history of cervical cancer is the ethical impossibility of allowing women to develop invasive cancer of the cervix. Therefore these studies are required to use intermediate endpoints (e.g. CIN 3).

'Premalignant' lesions of the cervix, CIN, have been histologically classified into three groups of increasing severity: CIN 1, CIN 2 and CIN 3. While it is generally accepted that CIN 3 has significant invasive potential, it is not as yet possible to predict the likelihood of progression or regression of the lower grades of CIN. This limited understanding of the rate and speed of transition between the various degrees of severity of CIN and between CIN and invasive disease can only be clarified by longitudinal natural history studies in which women with early 'premalignant' cervical lesions are maintained under close observation and only treated when the lesions progress. There have been relatively few of these studies undertaken and the reported rate of progression to CIN 3 has ranged from 16–53%. This marked variation may be explained by differences in the design of the study, including study population, period of follow up, entry criteria and definition of study endpoints (Robertson *et al.*, 1988; Flannelly *et al.*, 1994).

There are also few published cohort studies investigating the role of HPV in the pathogenesis of CIN. Campion *et al.* (1986) followed up 100 women with CIN 1 and reported that 85% of those progressing to more severe lesions had HPV DNA detectable by filter *in situ* hybridization. Koutsky *et al.* (1992) in a cohort study of women attending a sexually transmitted disease (STD) clinic demonstrated an elevated relative risk of 11 (95% CI 4.7–25) of developing CIN 2 or 3 among women with no previous history of cytologic abnormality if they had evidence of HPV 16/18 detected by PCR. The two-year cumulative incidence of severe epithelial abnormality was 28% in women with HPV and 3% in women without HPV. A more recently reported study by Downey *et al.* of 95 women with mildly dyskaryotic smears found on histology to have either CIN 1 or no histologic abnormality failed to demonstrate an association between progression and HPV DNA 16 status detected by PCR (Downey *et al.*, 1994). A surprising finding of this study was that HPV 16-positive women were more likely to have spontaneous regression of epithelial abnormalities.

Again the variable results may be explained by differences in study design, including the study populations, entry criteria, periods of follow up, endpoints and the methods of detection employed. Further definition of the role of HPV in the natural history of cervical cancer requires additional well-conducted cohort studies.

Epidemiology of human papillomavirus

A greater understanding of the epidemiology of genital HPV infection is a necessary prerequisite to a more precise definition of its role in the pathogenesis of cervical neoplasia.

Age and human papillomavirus

The age-specific prevalence of HPV infection decreases with age from a peak in the early twenties, and is markedly different from that observed for women with CIN 3 and cervical cancer (De Villiers *et al.*, 1992; Mugica–Van Herckenrode *et al.*, 1992). This has been interpreted as evidence of the transient nature of HPV infection, with spontaneous resolution of HPV infection occurring in a substantial proportion of cases (Hildesheim *et al.*, 1994). It has been suggested that it is the subgroup of women in whom HPV infection becomes persistent who have an increased risk of subsequent development of cervical cancer.

It must also be remembered that assays based on the detection of DNA sequences can only define 'current infection'. A robust serologic test would provide much useful additional information in that a population of previously exposed individuals could be identified. At present serologic tests are in their infancy and their poor sensitivity and specificity limits their usefulness as an epidemiologic tool. However one population-based seroepidemiologic case–control study has demonstrated an increased risk of developing cervical cancer in women with antibodies to epitopes of high-risk HPV types (Dillner *et al.*, 1994). In this study the prevalence of antibodies of high-risk HPV types was either not age related or only peaked in older age groups (30–39 years) according to the epitope studied. These cross-sectional data provide some limited support for the hypothesis that it is the persistence rather than the acquisition of infection that may be the more important risk factor for cervical cancer. Further studies exploring this hypothesis are urgently required.

Human papillomavirus and sexual behavior

If HPV is the important sexually transmitted etiologic agent in cancer of the cervix then both HPV infection and cervical cancer should share the same sexual behavior risk factor profile. The evidence for a shared risk profile is inconsistent, and indeed, one study has shown an inverse relationship between the number of lifetime partners and the finding of HPV DNA sequences as detected by PCR (Kjaer *et al.*, 1992). Ley *et al.* (1991) carried out a cross-sectional study of women attending a student health clinic and reported that the risk of HPV infection was independently associated with the number of lifetime sexual partners. Further analysis of the population-based case–control study set in Spain and Columbia demonstrated that the presence of HPV DNA detected by PCR was the most important risk factor for cervical cancer and explained the association with sexual risk factors in HPV DNA-positive women. However, in women who were shown to be HPV DNA-negative, the association of sexual risk factors with cancer of the cervix was maintained (Bosch *et al.*, 1992). Koutsky *et al.* found that adjustment for HPV DNA status accounted for the relationship between age at first intercourse and the development of CIN in their cohort of women attending an STD clinic, but the number of sexual partners remained an independent risk factor (Koutsky *et al.*, 1992).

Inconsistency in these various studies may be explained by the complex relationship between sexual risk factors, HPV and cervical cancer, or by the different populations studied. Sexual behavior may be an important determinant of the acquisition of HPV infection in younger women, but it may be more difficult to demonstrate an association with persistent disease in older women.

Non-sexual transmission of genital human papillomavirus

Evidence is accumulating for the non-sexual acquisition of HPV. HPV has been detected in samples taken from both the vulva and the cervix of women claiming not yet to have experienced vaginal intercourse. In addition, low- and high-risk genital HPV types have been found in a variety of non-genital tissues, including laryngeal papillomas, oesophageal tissue, normal oral mucosa and malignant tumours of the oral cavity (Woodman, 1994; Cason *et al.*, 1995).

Support for non-sexual transmission of HPV has been adduced from observations of low concordance between heterosexual partners for the presence of identified HPV types or even the presence of HPV. A study of married couples attending a fertility clinic demonstrated that only nine of 26 couples in whom at least one member was infected, were simultaneously infected with HPV DNA 16 as detected by PCR in cervical scrapes or semen samples (Kyo *et al.*, 1994). In another study of the heterosexual partners of 181 women in whom HPV DNA was detected by *in situ* hybridization in colposcopically-directed biopsy samples, just over one-third of the male partners were found to have HPV detected by *in situ* hybridization or PCR in peniscopically-directed biopsy samples, and only 8% of couples demonstrated concordant HPV types in their specimens (Hippeläinen *et al.*, 1993).

An alternative mode of transmission has been postulated. The finding of HPV DNA sequences in samples taken from the oropharyngeal cavities and external genitalia of newborn babies of HPV DNA-positive mothers suggests that vertical transmission of HPV may be a potential method of acquisition of this infection (Cason *et al.*, 1995).

Further evidence is awaited concerning the frequency and importance of non-sexual transmission. It is conceivable that there may be more serious consequences to exposure to HPV when the infection is acquired for the first time as a result of sexual activity.

Conclusion

It is of course possible that infection with specific HPV types is a necessary, but insufficient, risk factor in the etiology of cervical cancer. A number of other risk factors have been suggested that could interact with HPV, including genetic factors, host immune response, hormonal influences and smoking (Herrington, 1995).

Recent interest has focused on the possibility that concurrent infection with other sexually transmitted diseases may enhance the pathogenecity of HPV. Support for this hypothesis has come from the Spanish/Columbian population-based case–control study where analysis of serum samples obtained from women in the study demonstrated an increased risk of cervical cancer in HPV DNA-negative Spanish women with serum antibodies to *Chlamydia trachomatis* and *Neisseria gonorrhoeae* (De Sanjose *et al.*, 1994). Dillner *et al.* (1994) demonstrated an increased risk of cervical cancer in women with serologic evidence of infection with multiple sexually transmitted disease after adjustment of HPV DNA status. Koutsky *et al.* (1992) also demonstrated an association between antibodies to *C. trachomatis* and an increased risk of CIN, which was maintained even after adjustment for HPV DNA status. These results suggest that an interaction between HPV and other infectious agents cannot be excluded, but studies with larger sample sizes are required to explore this hypothesis further.

Summary of Core Information

- Cancer of the cervix is an important cause of cancer worldwide with the majority of cancers occurring in developing countries. In developed countries it is less common and mortality has been decreasing for some time.
- The weight of epidemiologic evidence continues to point to the likelihood of a sexually transmitted etiologic agent, of which HPV is currently the most attractive candidate.
- An association between HPV and cervical neoplasia and the presence of specific HPV types has been shown consistently in population- and hospital-based case–control studies, but the measures of association derived from cohort studies are less impressive.
- Some have been sufficiently persuaded by the oncogenic credentials of HPV to suggest that a vaccine development program designed to prevent genital HPV infection should be pursued actively. Others have argued that HPV DNA testing could either replace or be used as an adjuvant to cervical screening (Cuzick *et al.*, 1992). Further information on the natural history of cervical HPV infection is necessary before these recommendations can be endorsed.

References

Ahluwalia HS, Path MC & Doll R (1968) Mortality from cancer of the cervix uteri in British Columbia and other parts of Canada. *Brit. J. Prev. Soc. Med.* **22**(3): 61–164.

Bjørge T, Steinar Ø, Thoresen & Gry B Skare (1993) Incidence, survival and mortality in cervical cancer in Norway, 1956–90. *Eur. J. Cancer* **29A**(16): 2291–2297.

Brinton LA, Hamman RF, Huggins GR *et al.* (1987) Sexual and reproductive risk factors for invasive squamous cell cervical cancer. *J. Natl. Cancer Inst.* **79**: 23–30.

Brinton LA, Reeves WC, Brenes MM *et al.* (1989) The male factor in the etiology of cervical cancer among sexually monogamous women. *Int. J. Cancer* **44**: 199–203.

■ Brinton L (1992) Epidemiology of cervical cancer – overview. In: Munoz N, Bosch FX, Shah K & Meheus A (eds) *The Epidemiology of Human Papillomavirus and Cervical Cancer*, pp. 3–23. Lyon: IARC.

Bosch FX, Munoz N, De Sanjose S *et al.* (1992) Risk factors for cervical cancer in Columbia and Spain. *Int. J. Cancer* **52**: 750–758.

Campion MJ, McCance DJ, Cuzick J & Singer A (1986) Progressive potential of mild cervical atypia: prospective cytological colposcopic and virological study. *Lancet* **i**: 237–240.

Cason J, Kaye JN & Best UM (1995) Non sexual acquisition of human genital papillomavirus. *Papillomavirus Report* **6**: 1–7.

Cuzick J, Terry G, Ho L, Hollingworth T & Anderson M (1992) Human papillomavirus type 16 DNA in cervical smears as predictor of high-grade cervical cancer. *Lancet* **339**: 959–960.

Day N (1989) Screening for cancer of the cervix. *J. Epid. Comm. Health* **43**: 103–106.

Devesa S, Young J, Brinton A & Fraumeni J (1989) Recent trends in cervix-uteri cancer. *Cancer* **64**: 2184–2196.

De Villiers E–M, Wagner D, Schneider A *et al.* (1992) Human papillomavirus DNA in women without and with cytological abnormalities: results of a 5-year follow-up study. *Gynaecol. Oncol.* **44**: 33–39.

De Sanjose S, Munoz N, Bosch FX *et al.* (1994) Sexually transmitted agents and cervical neoplasia in Columbia and Spain. *Int. J. Cancer* **56**: 358–367.

Dillner J, Lenner P, Lehtinen M *et al.* (1994) A population based seroepidemiological study of cervical cancer. *Cancer Res.* **54**: 134–141.

Downey G, Bavin PJ & Deery ARS (1994) Relation between human papillomavirus type 16 and potential for progression of minor grade cervical disease. *Lancet* **344**: 432–434.

Eluf Neto J, Booth M, Munoz N. *et al.* (1994) Human papillomavirus and invasive cervical cancer in Brazil. *Br. J. Cancer* **69**: 114–119.

Flannelly G, Anderson D, Kitchener HC *et al.* (1994) Management of women with mild and moderate dyskaryosis. *Br. Med. J.* **308**: 1399–1403.

Giles GG, Armstrong BK & Smith LR (1987) Cancer in Australia 1982. Australasian Association of Cancer Registries and Australian Institute of Health. National Cancer Statistics Publications, No. 1.

Hakama M (1982) Trends in the incidence of cervical cancer in Nordic countries. In: Magnus K (ed.) *Trends in Cancer Incidence, Causes and Practical Implications*, pp. 279–292. Washington DC: Hemisphere Publishing Corporation.

Herrington CS (1995) Human papillomaviruses and cervical neoplasia. II Interaction of HPV with other factors. *J. Clin. Path.* **48**: 1–6.

Hildesheim A, Schiffman MH, Crouitt PE *et al.* (1994) Persistence of type specific human papillomavirus infection among cytologically normal women. *J. Infect. Dis.* **169**: 235–240.

Hippeläinen MI, Yliskoski M, Syrjänen S *et al.* (1993) Low concordance of genital human papillomavirus (HPV) lesions and viral types in HPV infected women and their male sex partners. *J. Sex. Trans. Dis.* **21**(2): 76–82.

Joslin C, Rider L, Round C *et al.* (1991) Yorkshire Cancer Registry Report for the Year 1991 Including Cancer Statistics for 1984–1988. Yorkshire Regional Cancer Organisation.

Kjaer SK, Engholm G, Teisen C *et al.* (1992) Risk factors for cervical human papillomavirus and herpes simplex virus infections in Greenland and Denmark: a population based study. *Am. J. Epidemiol.* **131**: 669–682.

Koutsky LA, Holmes KK, Critchlow SW *et al.* (1992) A

cohort study of the risk of cervical intra-epithelial neoplasia grade 2 or 3 in relation to papillomavirus infection. *New Engl. J. Med.* **327:** 1272–1278.

Kyo S, Inove M, Koyama M *et al.* (1994) Detection of high risk human papillomavirus in the cervix and semen of sex partners. *J. Infect. Dis.* **120:** 682–685.

La Vecchia C, Franceschi S, Decarli A *et al.* (1986) Sexual factors, venereal diseases, and the risk of intraepithelial and invasive cervical neoplasia. *Cancer* **58:** 935–941.

Ley C, Bauer HM, Reingold A *et al.* (1991) Determinants of genital human papillomavirus infection in young women. *J. Natl. Cancer Inst.* **83:** 997–1003.

Li JY, Li FP, Blot WJ, Miller RW & Fraumeni J Jnr (1982) Correlation between cancers of the uterine cervix and penis in China. *J. Natl. Cancer Inst.* **69:** 1063–1065.

MacGregor J, Moss S, Parkin K & Day N (1985) A case-control study of cervical cancer screening in NE Scotland. *Br. Med. J.* **290:** 1543–1546.

Meanwell CA, Blackledge G, Cox MF & Maitland NJ (1987) HPV16 DNA in normal and malignant cervical epithelium: implications for the aetiology and behaviour of cervical neoplasia. *Lancet* **1:** 703–770.

Meanwell CA, Kelly KA, Wilson S *et al.* (1988) Young age as a prognostic factor in cervical cancer: analysis of population based data from 10,022 cases. *Br. Med. J.* **296:** 386–392.

Miller BA, Ries LAG, Hankey BF, Kosary CL & Edwards BIC (1992) Cancer Statistics Review 1973–1989. National Cancer Institute NIH Publ. No. 92–2789.

Mugica–Van Herckenrode C, Malcolm ADB & Coleman DV (1992) Prevalence of human papillomavirus (HPV) infection in Basque country women using slot-blot hybridization: a survey of women at low risk of developing cervical cancer. *Int. J. Cancer* **51:** 581–586.

■ Munoz N, Bosch FX, De Sanjose S *et al.* (1992) The causal link between human papillomavirus and invasive cervical cancer: a population based case-control study in Columbia and Spain. *Int. J. Cancer* **52:** 743–749.

Office of Population Censuses and Surveys. Series MB1, 1974–1989 Cancer Statistics Registrations.

Parazzini F, La Vecchia C, Negri E, Cecchetti G & Fedele L (1989) Reproductive factors and the risk of invasive and intraepithelial cervical neoplasia. *Br. J. Cancer* **59:** 805–809.

Parkin DM, Pisani P & Ferlay J (1993) Estimates of the worldwide incidence of eighteen major cancers in 1985. *Int. J. Cancer* **54:** 594–606.

■ Parkin DM, Muir CS, Whelan SL *et al.* (1992) Cancer incidence in five continents. International Agency for Research on Cancer (WHO) and International Association of Cancer Registries, No. 120, Volume VI.

Phillips AN & Davey–Smith G (1994) Cigarette smoking as a potential cause of cervical cancer: has confounding been controlled. *Int. J. Epidemiol.* **23(1):** 42–49.

Reeves WC, Brinton LA, Garcia M *et al.* (1989) Human papillomavirus infection and cervical cancer in Latin America. *New Engl. J. Med.* **320:** 1437–1441.

Robertson JH, Woodend BE, Crozier EH & Hutchinson J (1988) Risk of cervical cancer associated with mild dyskaryosis. *Br. Med. J.* **297:** 18–21.

Schiffman MH, Haley NJ, Felton JS *et al.* (1987) Biochemical epidemiology of cervical neoplasia: Measuring cigarette smoke constituents in the cervix. *Cancer Res.* **47:** 3886–3888.

Schiffman MH & Schatzkin A (1994) Test reliability is critically important to molecular epidemiology: an example from studies of human papillomavirus infection and cervical neoplasia. *Cancer Res.* **54:** 1944s–1947s.

Sigurdsson K (1993) Effect of organised screening on the risk of cervical cancer. Evaluation of screening activity in Iceland 1964–1993. *Int. J. Cancer* **54:** 563–570.

Slattery ML, Robison LM, Schuman KL *et al.* (1989) Cigarette smoking and exposure to passive smoke are risk factors for cervical cancer. *J. Am. Med. Ass.* **261:** 1593–1598.

Smith PG, Kinlen LJ, White GC, Adelstein AM & Fox AJ (1980) Mortality of wives of men dying with cancer of the penis. *Br. J. Cancer* **41:** 422–428.

Walboomers JMM, De Roda Husman AM, Van den Brule AJC *et al.* (1994) Detection of genital human papillomavirus infections: Critical review of methods and prevalence studies in relation to cervical cancer. In: Stern PL & Stanley MA (eds) *Human Papillomaviruses and Cervical Cancer*, pp. 41–71. Oxford: Oxford University Press.

Winkelstein W Jnr (1990) Smoking and cervical cancer – current status: A review. *Am. J. Epidemiol.* **131:** 945–957.

Woodman C, Wilson S, Prior P *et al.* (1989) Cancer in the West Midlands Region 1981–85. West Midlands Regional Cancer Registry.

Woodman CBJ, Wilson S, Hare L *et al.* (1992) Cancer in the North West. Centre for Cancer Epidemiology, University of Manchester.

■ Woodman CBJ (1994) Epidemiology of HPV and cervical cancer. In: Stern PL & Stanley MA (eds) *Human Papillomaviruses and Cervical Cancer*, pp. 72–91. Oxford: Oxford University Press.

Young LS, Tierney RJ, Ellis JRM, Winter H & Woodman CBJ (1992) PCR for the detection of genital human papillomavirus infection: a mixed blessing. *Ann. Med.* **24:** 215–219.

2 Cytopathology of the Uterine Cervix

S M Selvaggi
W D Lawrence

Introduction

Since the beginning of the nineteenth century, cytology has played an important role in the study of cells as the basic unit in living organisms. Its application to the study of female genital tract disease, however, did not gain wide acceptance either in the USA or in Europe until 1943, when Papanicolaou and Traut (1943) published their monograph on *Diagnosis of Uterine Cancer by the Vaginal Smear*. Subsequently, cytology has become widely used as the initial screening tool in the work-up and management of gynecologic patients.

Diagnostic cytology, as it applies to the uterine cervix, is the study of cells that either exfoliate freely from the cervix into the vaginal cavity or are removed from the cervix by instrumentation. Its main clinical applications are the differentiation of benign from precancerous and malignant cervical lesions, and as a follow-up procedure in patients with a previously treated cervical carcinoma.

This chapter will address the normal and abnormal cytology of the uterine cervix, encompassing the benign cytopathologic aberrations (including inflammatory processes), the effects of therapeutic ionizing radiation on the normal cervical squamous epithelium, the precancerous lesions and their relationship to human papillomavirus (HPV) infection, and the cancerous lesions.

Normal Cytology of the Uterine Cervix

The uterine cervix is composed of the exocervix and the endocervix. The exocervix is the vaginal portion of the cervix, which extends inferiorly from the external os to the reflection of the cervical epithelium onto the vaginal fornix. The endocervical canal is the portion of the uterine cervix that extends superiorly from the external os to the internal os of the uterine isthmus.

Two types of epithelia are present within the uterine cervix: the nonkeratinizing stratified squamous epithelium lining the vaginal face of the exocervix; and the tall, columnar mucus-secreting epithelium lining the endocervix. Since the fullest maturation of the epithelia occurs during a woman's reproductive years, the cellular features described will be those encountered during this time period. Cellular changes occurring in postmenopausal women will be described briefly.

During sexual maturity, the nonkeratinizing stratified squamous epithelium of the exocervix is composed of several layers: the basal cell layer, which is a single row of cells attached to the basal lamina and the source of epithelial cell regeneration; a few layers of parabasal cells, which also contribute to cellular regeneration; the intermediate cell layer, which constitutes the majority of the epithelial thickness; and a superficial layer of squamous cells. Since the cervix is lined by a moist nonkeratinizing squamous epithelium, a granular cell layer similar to that in the skin is not present. On a cytologic smear from such an epithelium, three cell types are generally observed: superficial squamous cells, intermediate squamous cells and parabasal cells (Koss, 1992a).

The superficial cells, which originate from the upper layers of squamous epithelium, range in diameter from 35–45 μm. They are polygonal, thin, flat cells that contain transparent cytoplasm and a small (6 μm diameter) pyknotic nucleus with no discernible chromatin structure (*Figure 2.1*). The cytoplasm usually appears pink on Papanicolaou stain and may contain small, dark keratohyalin granules.

The intermediate squamous cells are similar in size to the superficial cells or slightly smaller. The cells are polygonal and their cytoplasm is usually basophilic on Papanicolaou stain. The major differences between the intermediate and the superficial cells is the nuclear structure; specifically, the round or oval nucleus measures approximately 8 μm in average diameter and exhibits a delicate, evenly-distributed vesicular chromatin pattern (*Figure 2.1*).

Unlike the superficial and intermediate squamous cells, the parabasal cells are small, ranging in size from 12–30 μm in diameter, and are round or oval (*Figure 2.2*). The cytoplasm usually appears dense and basophilic, and the nuclei approximate the size and chromatin pattern of the intermediate cell. Parabasal cells usually constitute no more than 5% of the cells in cervical or vaginal smears from women in their reproductive years. Their numbers increase in women over 35 years of age and they are common in smears from postmenopausal females.

The endocervical canal is lined by a tall,

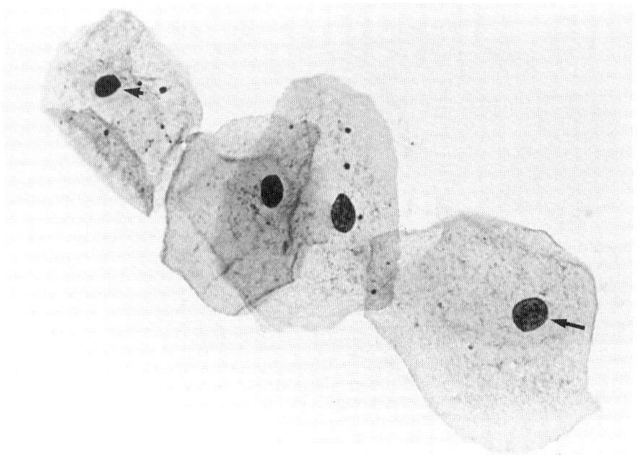

Figure 2.1. A superficial cell containing a small pyknotic nucleus (small arrow). An intermediate cell containing a nucleus with a delicate chromatin pattern (large arrow).

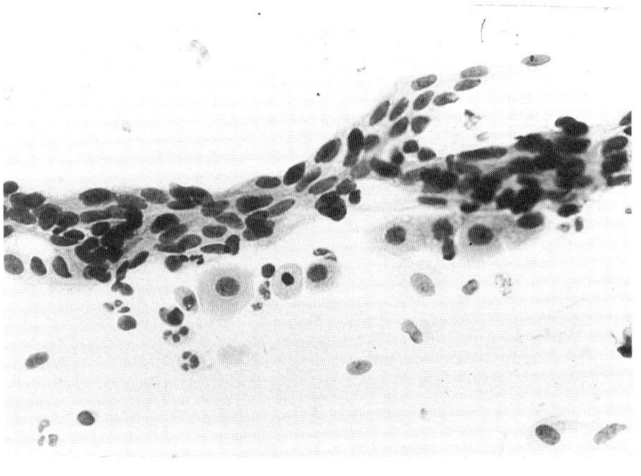

Figure 2.2. An atrophic smear pattern containing parabasal cells.

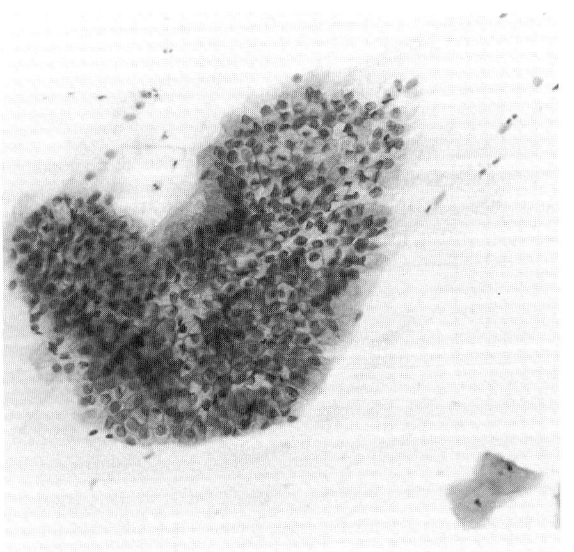

Figure 2.3. A cluster of endocervical cells arranged in a 'honeycomb' pattern.

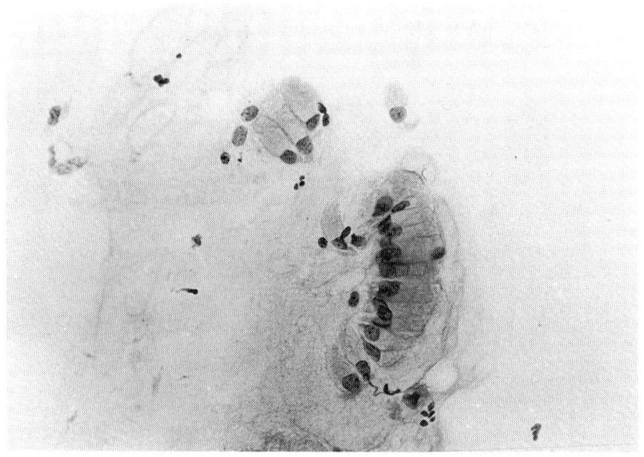

Figure 2.4. Endocervical cells arranged in a 'picket-fence'. Terminal bars and cilia are present.

mucus-secreting, columnar epithelium that forms villous and papillary surface projections. The glandular epithelium of the endocervical canal extends as irregularly branching clefts into the underlying connective tissue; these have been shown not to be true 'glands' by detailed stereoscopic reconstructive studies. Such clefts extend 4–5 mm into the cervical stroma.

In cervical smears (*Figures 2.3 and 2.4*), endocervical cells appear as tall, columnar cells that are usually arranged in either a 'picket-fence' (parallel rows of cells) or a 'honeycomb' pattern. The cell cytoplasm is clear and the nucleus is basal in position. A terminal bar and cilia can occasionally be identified at the apex of the cell. The nucleus is similar to that of an intermediate cell and contains finely granular chromatin. A few small nucleoli may be present.

Nomenclature Systems for Cervical Cytology

As our understanding of cervical cancer and its precursor lesions has evolved, a variety of reporting systems for cervical cytology have emerged over time. When large-scale cervical cytology screening was introduced in the 1950s, Papanicolaou devised a numerical reporting system of five classes, expressed as the roman numerals I to V, with Class I denoting no cytologic abnormality and Class V, cells diagnostic of malignancy. Although the classification system was based on the detection of malignant cells on cervical smears, the issue of precancerous lesions was not addressed.

As the area of cytopathology gained acceptance as a diagnostic field, noted cytopathologists, including Patten and Reagan, advocated replacing the numerical system with readily understandable diagnostic terms (Reagan, 1965). With the emergence of the concept of cervical precursor lesions, Reagan promulgated the use of the term 'dysplasia' to designate these intraepithelial lesions (Reagan *et al.*, 1953). Morphologic criteria were delineated for slight, moderate and severe dysplasia, and carcinoma *in situ* (CIS) (Patten, 1978), as if dysplasia was a separate lesion in behavior and possibly in etiology from CIS. Although some pathologists claim diagnostic success using this system, studies have shown a lack of interobserver reproducibility in subdividing cervical intraepithelial lesions into five separate diagnostic categories including HPV effects, slight, moderate and severe dysplasia, and CIS (Sherman *et al.*, 1991).

As the reporting terminology became more complex, laboratories that were unwilling to abandon the Papanicolaou classification system modified and created their own version of the Papanicolaou numerical classes. Suffice it to say, communication among pathologists was often confusing at best. In December 1988, the National Cancer Institute sponsored a workshop to address this 'diagnostic confusion' and to develop a uniform reporting system for cervicovaginal cytology, which became known as The Bethesda System (TBS) (National Cancer Institute Workshop, 1989; Koss, 1990). Subsequently, modifications were made after a second meeting convened in 1991.

Table 2.1. Descriptive diagnoses of The Bethesda System

I. BENIGN CELLULAR CHANGES
- A. INFECTION
  - Fungal organisms morphologically consistent with *Candida* spp.
  - *Trichomonas vaginalis*
  - Bacteria morphologically consistent with *Actinomyces* spp.
  - Cellular changes associated with herpes simplex virus (HSV)
- B. REACTIVE CHANGES
  - Inflammation (includes typical repair)
  - Intrauterine contraceptive devices
  - Radiation

II. EPITHELIAL CELL ABNORMALITIES
- A. SQUAMOUS CELL
  - Atypical squamous cells of undetermined significance
  - Low-grade squamous intraepithelial lesion (SIL) encompassing slight dysplasia/cervical intraepithelial neoplasia (CIN)1/cellular changes associated with human papillomavirus (HPV)
  - High-grade SIL encompassing moderate dysplasia/CIN 2 and severe dysplasia/carcinoma *in situ* (CIS)/CIN 3
  - Squamous cell carcinoma
- B. GLANDULAR CELL
  - Atypical glandular cells of undetermined significance
  - Endocervical adenocarcinoma

The advantages of TBS include:

- uniform diagnostic terminology to improve communication between the cytopathologist and the health care provider and among cytopathologists;
- the use of terminology that reflects current understanding of the pathogenesis and biology of cervical neoplasia;
- evaluation of specimen adequacy as an integral part of the report;
- the Papanicolaou numerical class system is no longer acceptable for reporting diagnoses.

Table 2.1 summarizes the descriptive diagnoses of TBS for cervical cytology that will be used in this chapter.

Benign/Reactive Cellular Changes of the Uterine Cervix

Benign/reactive cellular changes encompass a spectrum of cytologic changes within the uterine cervix. Cells derived from this type of reaction do not have the features of epithelial cell abnormalities. Rather, the cellular changes in this category are related primarily to slight alterations in nuclear size and morphology. The etiology of such cellular changes of the uterine cervix can often be attributed to inflammation, reparative/regenerative processes, deficiency states, trauma and/or intrauterine contraceptive device (IUD) usage (Bonfiglio and Patten, 1976; Gupta, 1982). Recognition of benign cellular changes associated with these processes is necessary to preclude their misdiagnosis as preneoplastic cervical lesions.

As a response to the aforementioned etiologic insults, the cervical squamous epithelium may respond in a protective fashion by the development of a granular cell layer, which is an abnormal finding as previously mentioned, in nonkeratinizing moist squamous epithelia. Further protection is obtained with the development of a parakeratotic and a hyperkeratotic layer. Cytologically, cellular smears obtained from the surface of a mature stratified squamous epithelium with hyperkeratosis may contain anucleated squames, and if associated with parakeratosis, small cells with pyknotic nuclei and eosinophilic or orangeophilic cytoplasm (*Figure 2.5*).

As a protective mechanism, the columnar ('glandular') epithelium of the cervix, on the other hand, responds to similar insults by undergoing squamous metaplasia and hyperplasia. Squamous metaplasia arises via proliferation of so-called reserve cells to form an immature squamous metaplastic epithelium; final maturation results in a mature stratified squamous epithelium. The nuclei of

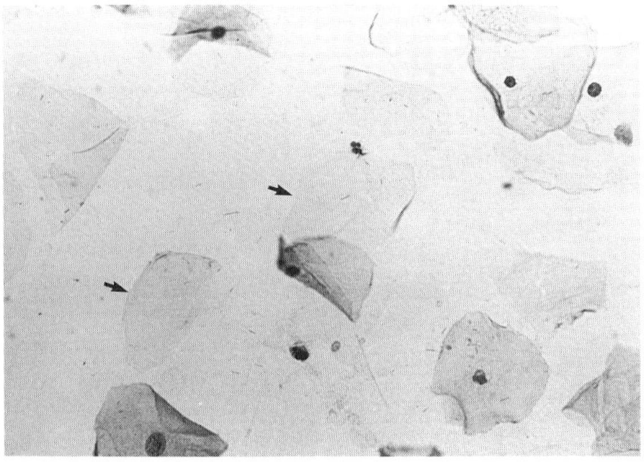

Figure 2.5. Hyperkeratosis containing anucleated squames (arrows).

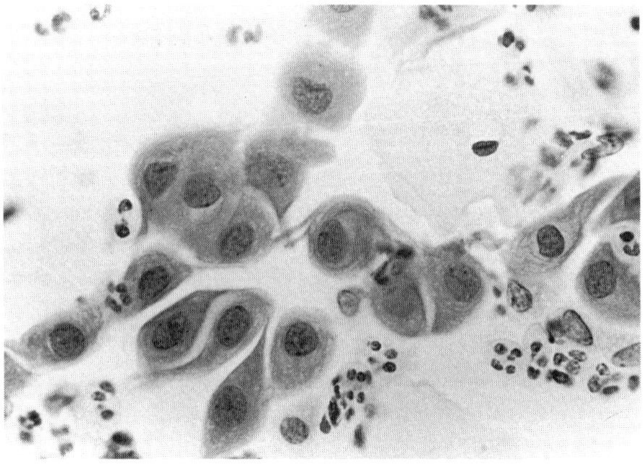

Figure 2.6. Squamous metaplastic cells with round to ovoid nuclei containing finely granular chromatin.

metaplastic squamous cells are generally round to ovoid, with a finely granular, evenly distributed, chromatin pattern (*Figure 2.6*). Small prominent nucleoli may be present (Carmichael and Jeafferson, 1941).

Infectious Processes

Regardless of the cause, infectious processes of the uterine cervix share a variety of epithelial inflammatory reactions and concomitant cellular changes. These inflammatory reactions may represent either the acute or chronic phase of the disease and the resultant cytologic changes may be manifested as alterations in the smear pattern and cellular elements (Bonfiglio and Patten, 1976).

Smear patterns are altered predominantly in acute inflammatory processes, including those caused by specific etiologic agents. An acute inflammatory exudate is the most common finding in such a smear. The smear may show a 'dirty' background because of the cellular exudate and cytolysis. The proportion of parabasal, intermediate and superficial cells is often altered by the inflammatory process.

Cellular changes are best characterized by nuclear alterations, which vary in degree from mild to moderate. A few pathologic processes can induce such specific morphologic changes within the nucleus and/or cytoplasm to permit definitive diagnosis by microscopic examination of the cellular material; such organisms include *Candida albicans, Trichomonas vaginalis, Actinomyces israelii* and herpes simplex virus (HSV).

Specific inflammatory agents

Candida albicans

According to Kearns and Gray (1963), the fungus *C. albicans* causes 80% of the cases of mycotic vulvovaginitis and occurs predominantly in pregnant patients, those with diabetes mellitus, and in those receiving steroids or antibiotic therapy. *Candida* appears in smears as pseudoseptate hyphae and conidiophores or yeast bodies (*Figure 2.7*). Acute inflammation is often prominent. Cellular changes include vacuolization of the cytoplasm, small perinuclear halos, and chromatin clumping in the nuclei of squamous epithelial cells (Heller and Hoyt, 1971).

Trichomonas vaginalis

T. vaginalis is a protozoan that is present in the lower genital tract of up to 20% of sexually active females and is more common in those with promiscuous sexual habits and/or poor genital hygiene. It is more prevalent in gynecologic than obstetric patients, and the former who take oral contraceptives show even higher prevalence rates of this microorganism (Wied *et al.*, 1966). *Trichomonas* is diagnosed in cervical smears by its small

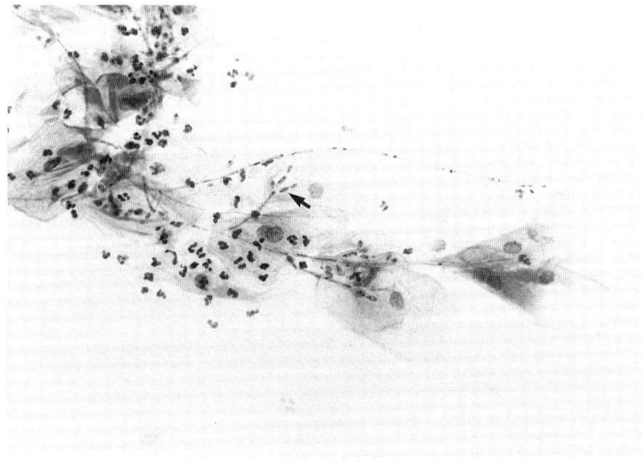

Figure 2.7. Pseudoseptate hyphae and conidiophores (arrow) of *Candida albicans*. Acute inflammatory cells are present in the smear background.

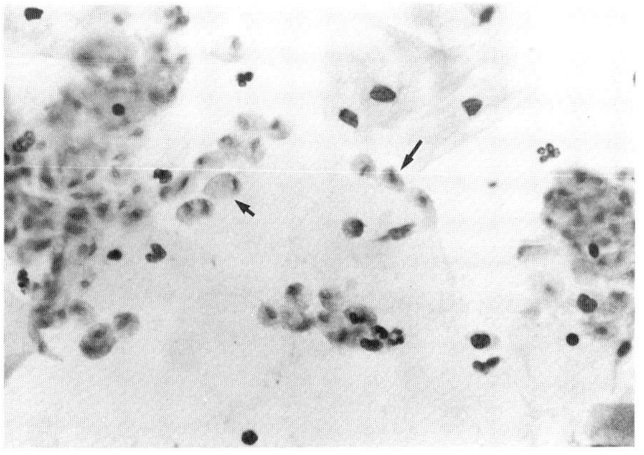

Figure 2.8. Small pear-shaped forms of *Trichomonas vaginalis* containing an eccentric nucleus (small arrow). The protozoa (large arrow) tend to cluster around epithelial cells.

pear-shaped grayish form containing a small ovoid eccentric nucleus (*Figure 2.8*). The surrounding epithelial cells often show enlarged nuclei with small perinuclear halos. Acute inflammation may be present in the background and the protozoan is often accompanied by *Leptothrix*, a bacterium.

Actinomyces israelii

Actinomycosis of the female genital tract is most commonly caused by *A. israelii*, a bacterium composed of branching gram-positive filaments with peripheral clubbing. In Papanicolaou-stained smears containing typical sulfur granules, *Actinomyces* filaments radiate from a central dense core and branch at acute angles; an acute inflammatory exudate is often present (*Figure 2.9*). The organism is noted more commonly in cervicovaginal smears from patients with previous surgical instrumentation, including abortion, and in those using an IUD or pessary (Gupta, 1982). Complications of actinomycosis include pelvic inflammatory disease and consequent infertility problems.

Herpes simplex virus

HSV (usually Type 2) infection is a sexually transmitted disease that results in well-recognized and diagnostic cytologic alterations: these include a 'ground-glass' appearance of the nucleus with margination of the chromatin; intranuclear, eosinophilic, Cowdry Type A inclusions; and multinucleation with nuclear molding (*Figure 2.10*) (Ng, *et al.*, 1970).

The clinical significance of the HSV infection lies in its frequent association with gonorrhea, the risk of spontaneous abortion and neonatal infection, and its role in the development of cervical carcinoma.

Most of the data supporting the association of HSV Type 2 and cervical carcinoma have been collected from seroepidemiologic and immunocytochemical studies (Nahmias *et al.*, 1970; Luthra *et al.*, 1987; Gupta *et al.*, 1988). To date, however, HSV has not been consistently demonstrated in either precancerous or cancerous cervical lesions by more highly specific techniques such as standard Southern blot hybridization (Crum, 1987). Adam *et al.* (1985) and Zur Hausen (1982) have postulated that sequential infections with HSV and HPV may be related to the genesis of cervical carcinoma, thus proposing a cofactor role of HSV in its development.

Figure 2.9. The sulfur granule of *Actinomyces israelii*. Branching filaments radiate from a central core.

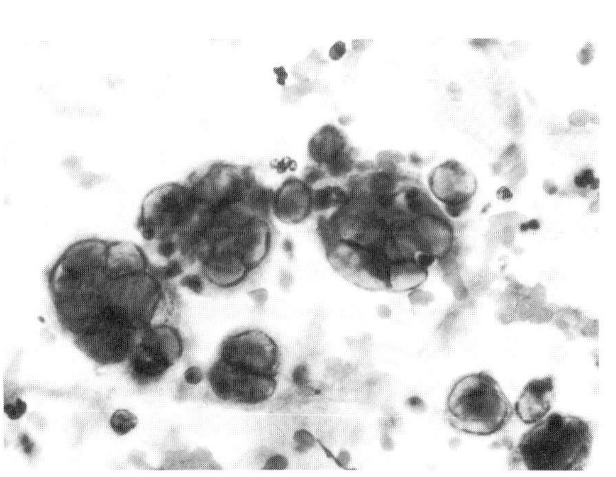

Figure 2.10. Clusters of multinucleated cells with nuclear molding and 'ground-glass' chromatin pattern characteristic of herpes simplex virus (HSV).

Cellular Changes Associated with Repair and Regeneration

Following destruction by inflammation and/or infection, the epithelium of the exocervix and endocervical canal undergoes a repair/regenerative process. In cervical smears, repair cells are typically observed in aggregates with a cohesive sheet-like arrangement (Bibbo *et al.*, 1971; Geirsson *et al.*, 1977; Sugimori, 1982) (*Figure 2.11*). Isolated atypical cells are not present. The nuclei are enlarged and round to oval in configuration with smooth borders. The chromatin is finely granular, and large round nucleoli are present. Proper recognition of the cellular features associated with repair/regenerative processes is important, since some of the cytologic characteristics present are also noted in cancer cells. Unlike malignancy, however, smears associated with repair/regenerative processes lack syncytial cell aggregates, the presence of isolated cells with similar atypical features, a tumor diathesis background, and cells containing nuclei with an irregular, coarsely clumped chromatin pattern.

Cellular Changes Associated with Intrauterine Devices

Although IUDs are no longer widely used as a birth control measure, a significant number of women still retain them and one must be aware of the cytologic changes arising from their use and these can be grouped into two basic categories:

- repair/regenerative changes resulting from inflammation or infections, which often accompany IUD use;
- more specific cellular changes thought to result from IUD use (Gupta, 1982).

Within the first category acute inflammation, which is often severe, is accompanied by atypical

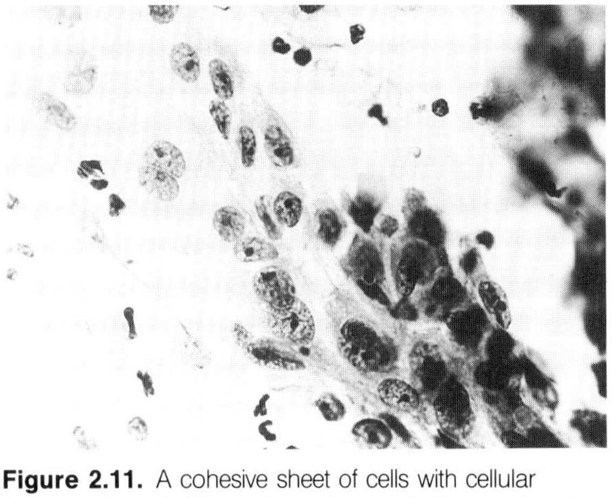

Figure 2.11. A cohesive sheet of cells with cellular features of repair. The cells contain ovoid to round nuclei, granular chromatin and prominent nucleoli.

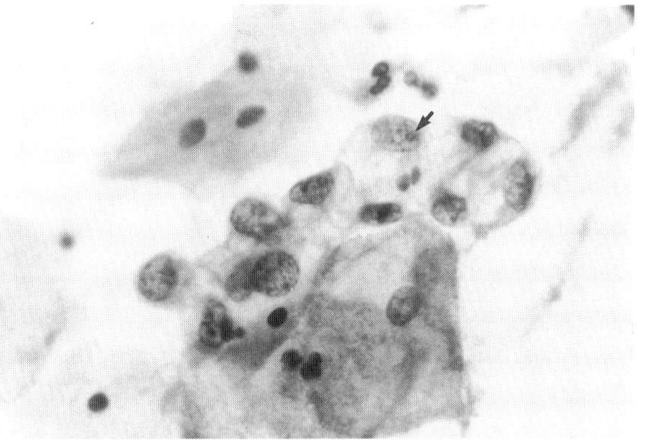

Figure 2.12. A cluster of typical endocervical cells from an intrauterine device (IUD)-user. The cells contain vacuolated cytoplasm and nuclei, some with prominent nucleoli (arrow).

columnar cells containing hyperchromatic nuclei with granular chromatin and prominent nucleoli. Squamous metaplasia and squamous cell atypia are also present. *Actinomyces*, *T. vaginalis* and coccobacillary organisms are often observed.

More specific cellular atypias thought to be induced by the IUD include columnar cell changes and so-called 'IUD cells with a high nuclear/cytoplasmic (N/C) ratio;' the former occur in papillary formations and/or acinar structures. The cells contain abundant foamy or vacuolated cytoplasm (*Figure 2.12*) and hyperchromatic nuclei with coarsely granular cytoplasm and prominent nucleoli. Concomitant squamous metaplasia is often present.

IUD cells with a high N/C ratio contain hyperchromatic nuclei and scanty cytoplasm. The nuclear chromatin is moderately coarse and a variable number of nucleoli are present. Multinucleation is a feature. These highly atypical cells can be difficult to distinguish from a high-grade squamous intraepithelial lesion, in particular, carcinoma *in situ* (CIS). However, unlike CIS, the IUD cells may show multinucleation, and contain clumped chromatin and prominent nucleoli.

Giant cells and psammoma bodies can also be observed in the smears of patients using an IUD.

Cellular Changes Associated with Radiation Therapy

In addition to destroying cells of cervical carcinoma, radiation also affects the benign squamous epithelium of the uterine cervix. Radiation changes may be observed in parabasal, intermediate and superficial squamous epithelial cells. Both nuclear and cytoplasmic enlargement contribute to an increase in cell size. Nuclear changes include macrocytosis, bi- and multinucleation and wavy nuclear envelopes. The chromatin pattern is finely

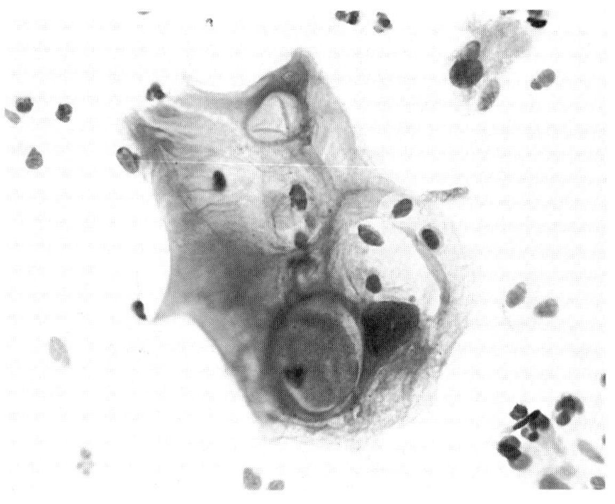

Figure 2.13. Benign radiation changes in a squamous epithelial cell. Large intracytoplasmic vacuoles are present.

granular and hypochromatic, and nucleoli may be found. Cytoplasmic vacuolization is common and phagocytosis and engulfment of neutrophils may be present (*Figure 2.13*). Although cells with bizarre shapes are a product of radiation effect, they can be distinguished from squamous intraepithelial lesions or malignant squamous cells by their normal N/C ratio, finely granular chromatin pattern, and absence of nuclear hyperchromasia, coarse chromatin clumping and irregular macronucleoli (Graham, 1947; Boschann, 1992; Gupta *et al.*, 1987b).

Radiation-induced cellular changes have been reported to persist from 2–20 years after therapy. Some (Wentz and Reagan, 1970) have reported that persistent radiation changes are associated with a better prognosis than the early development of a postradiation squamous intraepithelial lesion; furthermore, they found that the probability of developing recurrent carcinoma was higher for those patients who developed postradiation squamous intraepithelial lesions within three years of treatment than for those with a more delayed onset.

The cytologic features of post-radiation dysplasia are those of classic squamous cell dysplasia. In addition, however, the cells are irregular in configuration and may occur in sheets (Patten *et al.*, 1963).

Cytologic Features of Squamous Epithelial Cell Abnormalities

Atypical Squamous Cells of Undetermined Significance

As early as 1976, Melamed and Flehinger, and Patten (1978) recognized that cellular 'atypias' may antedate the presence of cervical intraepithelial lesions on cervical cytology. The current terminology of TBS (National Cancer Institute Workshop, 1989), which encompasses this group of changes, is 'atypical squamous cells of undetermined significance' or ASCUS. ASCUS is not synonymous with previously used terms such as 'atypia,' 'benign/reactive atypia' or 'inflammatory atypia,' which had included lesions currently classified in TBS as benign/reactive cellular changes. Rather, ASCUS encompasses those cellular abnormalities that are more marked than those attributable to reactive/inflammatory cellular changes, but that quantitatively or qualitatively fall short of a definitive diagnosis of a squamous intraepithelial lesion (SIL). The cytologic criteria used for ASCUS include nuclear enlargement (two or three times that of a normal intermediate squamous cell nucleus), variation in nuclear size and shape, smooth and regular nuclear membranes, and evenly distributed, finely granular, mildly hyperchromatic chromatin (*Figure 2.14*) (Kurman and Solomon, 1994). Binucleation and nucleoli may be present. Included within the ASCUS category are cellular changes suggestive of HPV cytopathic effects, immature or atypical squamous metaplastic cells and non-diagnostic cellular changes that are not attributed to inflammation. ASCUS should be further qualified if possible as to whether a reactive or premalignant process is favored.

Although ASCUS rates may vary for different laboratory settings, a recent National Cancer Institute sponsored workshop to define interim guidelines for the management of abnormal cervical cytology (Kurman *et al.*, 1994) concluded that in most populations a diagnosis of ASCUS may be expected in approximately 5% of smears, and that a greater frequency may represent overuse of the diagnosis. However, in high-risk groups with a

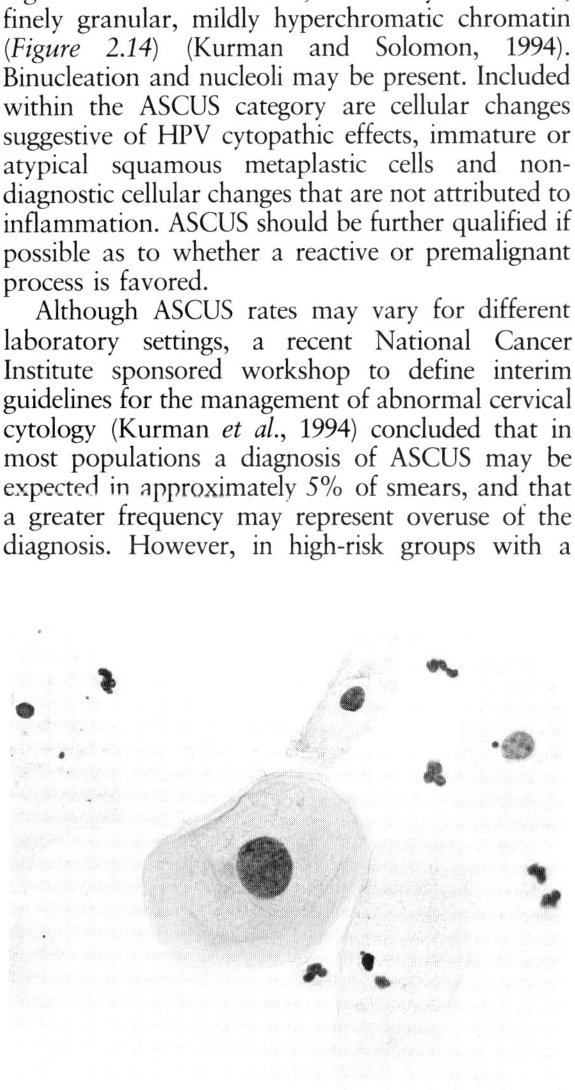

Figure 2.14. An atypical squamous cell of undetermined significance (ASCUS) showing nuclear enlargement. The nuclear membrane is smooth and regular and the chromatin is evenly distributed and finely granular.

higher prevalence of SIL, there will be a correspondingly higher prevalence of ASCUS. Therefore, as a general guide, the rate of ASCUS in a screened population may be 2–3 times the rate of SIL.

Cervical Squamous Intraepithelial Lesions

In TBS, low-grade SIL and high-grade SIL encompass the precursor lesions of squamous cell carcinoma of the cervix. Low-grade SIL includes cellular changes associated with HPV infection and slight dysplasia/cervical intraepithelial neoplasia (CIN)I. High-grade SIL includes moderate dysplasia/ CIN II, severe dysplasia/CIN III and CIS/CIN III.

Use of two-tier SIL terminology is based on our current understanding of the pathogenesis and biology of cervical carcinoma, including:

- current knowledge of the molecular biology of HPV and its association with cervical lesions;
- the clinical behavior and management of cervical lesions;
- low diagnostic interobserver reproducibility in distinguishing cervical lesions and in predicting progression of disease (Kurman, 1991; Kurman *et al.*, 1991).

Although objection has been raised to the inclusion of HPV cytopathic effects (i.e. koilocytosis) in the category of low-grade SIL (Herbst, 1991), HPV molecular analyses have shown a similar heterogeneous distribution of low- and high-risk HPV subtypes in both koilocytosis and slight dysplasia/CIN I lesions (Willett *et al.*, 1989; Nuovo *et al.*, 1991). In addition, long-term follow-up studies of koilocytosis and slight dysplasia/CIN I lesions have shown similar progression rates to CIN III; 14% and 16% respectively (Nasiell *et al.*, 1986; Syrjanen *et al.*, 1988; Kataja *et al.*, 1989). Such data support the premise that koilocytosis and slight dysplasia/CIN I represent the same disease process, further support for the two-tier terminology system.

By comparison, high-grade SILs show a more homogeneous pattern of expression of high-risk HPV subtypes, in particular HPV 16 (Lorincz *et al.*, 1987; Nuovo *et al.*, 1991). If untreated, high-grade SILs have a greater tendency to persist and/or progress than low-grade SILs.

From a practical standpoint, and perhaps most importantly, cytologic and histologic studies have shown a lack of diagnostic reproducibility in subdividing cervical lesions into four or five categories. The most difficult distinction is that between HPV cellular changes and slight dysplasia/ CIN I (Sherman *et al.*, 1991), and between moderate dysplasia/CIN II and severe dysplasia/CIS/CIN III (Robertson *et al.*, 1989; Ismail *et al.*, 1990).

Cytologic features of squamous intraepithelial lesions

In approximately one-third of normal cervices from menstruating females, there is an abrupt transition between the stratified squamous epithelium of the exocervix and the columnar epithelium of the endocervix. In the other two-thirds, the afore-mentioned junction is composed of a zone of immature squamous metaplastic and/or hyperplastic reserve cells. This area is termed the transformation zone and is of considerable importance in the genesis of CIN and subsequent invasive carcinoma of the uterine cervix.

In general, evaluation of the degree of severity of an intraepithelial lesion on a cytologic preparation includes consideration of the arrangement, number and cytologic characteristics of the atypical cells present.

Cells derived from a neoplastic epithelium usually appear in cervicovaginal smears as isolated forms. With increasing degrees of severity, cells occur in syncytial aggregates (*Figure 2.15*). While the number of abnormal cells on a smear varies with the collection technique employed, lower-grade lesions are generally associated with fewer atypical cells than high-grade lesions.

With increasing severity, the cells show an increased N/C ratio and decreased cytoplasmic maturity. The nuclear changes include a progressive increase in nuclear membrane and chromatin abnormalities (Patten, 1978; Koss, 1992b).

The cytologic criteria (Kurman and Solomon, 1994), for low-grade SIL include nuclear enlargement (at least three times that of a normal intermediate squamous cell nucleus) resulting in an increased N/C ratio, moderate variation in nuclear size and shape, smooth to slightly irregular nuclear membranes, and evenly distributed, finely granular, mildly hyper-chromatic nuclear chromatin, which may appear smudged if associated with the cytopathic changes

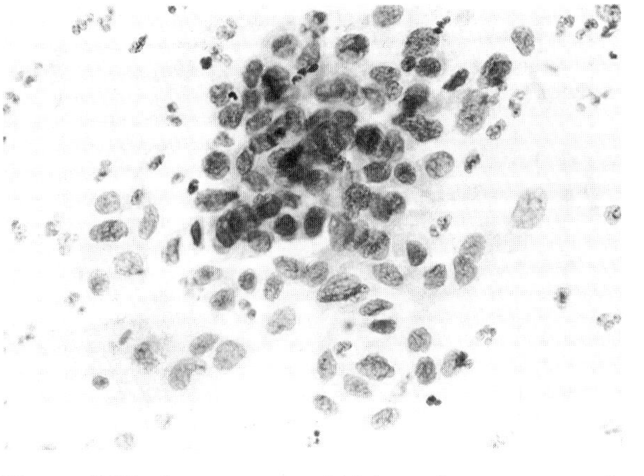

Figure 2.15. An aggregate of high-grade squamous cells in a syncytial arrangement.

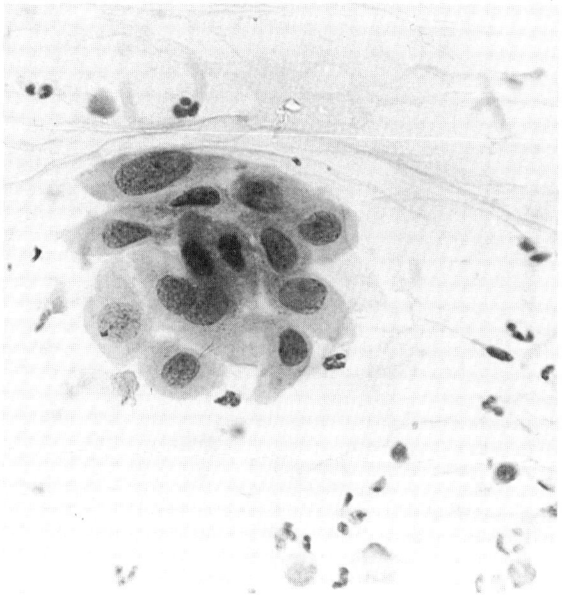

Figure 2.16. Low-grade squamous intraepithelial lesion (SIL). The cell nuclei are regular and the nuclear membranes are smooth. The nuclear chromatin is finely granular.

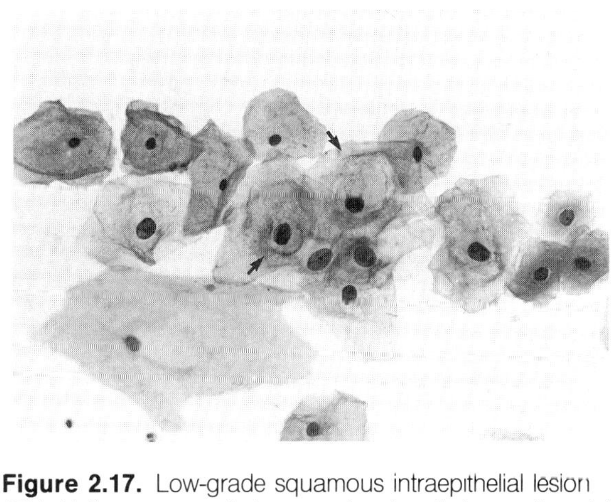

Figure 2.17. Low-grade squamous intraepithelial lesion (SIL). Koilocytes contain large perinuclear halos and nuclei with smudged chromatin (arrows). (Courtesy of SM Selvaggi, Diagnostic Cytopathology, 1988.)

of HPV. The cytoplasm is ample, thin, transparent and eosinophilic on Papanicolaou stain. Distinct cell borders are present (*Figure 2.16*).

In addition to containing the above nuclear abnormalities, cells which demonstrate a large clear perinuclear halo and a peripheral dense rim of cytoplasm are included in the category of low-grade SIL (*Figure 2.17*). This cell has been previously termed a koilocyte and the cellular change as koilocytosis or koilocytotic atypia (Koss and Durfee, 1956; Meisels *et al.*, 1977; Casas–Cordero *et al.*, 1981; Selvaggi, 1986; Selvaggi, 1988).

The cytologic criteria (Kurman and Solomon, 1994) for a high-grade SIL include nuclear enlargement in the range of that present in low-grade SIL, but with an increase in the N/C ratio, moderate to marked variation in nuclear size and shape, and irregular nuclear membranes. Nuclear hyperchromasia is evident and the chromatin may be coarsely granular (*Figure 2.18*).

Although most high-grade SILs consist of cells with a high N/C ratio, some high-grade keratinizing lesions contain ample orangeophilic cytoplasm. Such lesions have been previously termed 'atypical condyloma,' 'keratinizing dysplasia' and 'pleomorphic dysplasia.' In the TBS system they are included in the high-grade SIL category. If, however, marked nuclear changes make the cells difficult to distinguish from an invasive squamous cell carcinoma, this should be mentioned in an explanatory note.

In intraepithelial lesions, a tumor diathesis in the smear background is generally absent.

Human papillomavirus infection and its relationship to cervical intraepithelial neoplasia

The significance of the association between HPV infection and CIN has been an important and controversial issue in recent years. Early cytologic studies showed that the cellular alterations, designated as 'koilocytotic atypia' and thought to be caused by HPV, were present in the cervix of 1% and 2% of all females screened (Meisels *et al.*, 1977; Meisels and Morin, 1981). These findings were later confirmed by electron microscopic studies (Casas Cordero *et al.*, 1981).

Histologic studies have shown that so-called flat

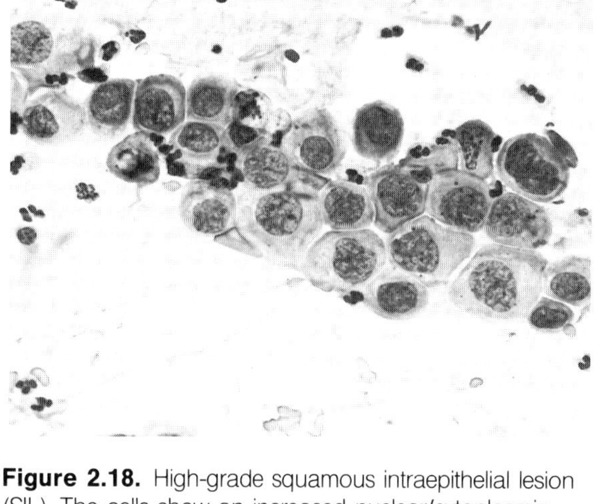

Figure 2.18. High-grade squamous intraepithelial lesion (SIL). The cells show an increased nuclear/cytoplasmic (N/C) ratio. The nuclear membranes are irregular and unevenly thickened. The chromatin is coarse.

cervical condylomas are contiguous with CIN lesions, that at least 25% of CIN II and CIN III lesions have nonadjacent foci of flat condyloma in the same biopsy specimen, and that in many cases cervical lesions have features of both CIN and condyloma (Meisels *et al.*, 1977; Meisels and Morin, 1981; Crum *et al.*, 1983; Selvaggi, 1986).

In support of the histologic (Reid *et al.*, 1982; Reid *et al.*, 1984a,b) and immunocytochemical data (Kurman *et al.*, 1983; Syrjanen, 1983), DNA hybridization and more recently PCR studies (Durst *et al.*, 1983; Boshart *et al.*, 1984; Yee *et al.*, 1985; Lorincz *et al.*, 1986; Reid *et al.*, 1987; Shibata *et al.*, 1988; Nuovo *et al.*, 1991) have shown that the association between HPV infection and CIN is more than would be expected by coincidence.

Statistical studies have shown that patients with coincident CIN and condylomas tend to be younger than patients with CIN alone and their lesions may progress more rapidly to a higher grade CIN; consequently (Meisels and Morin, 1981; Crum *et al.*, 1983; Syrjanen, 1983), early cytologic detection of these lesions may alert the clinician to perform colposcopy and follow-up the patient appropriately.

High-risk HPVs are associated with both low- and high-grade CINs, but are present with significantly greater frequency in the high-grade group as detected by DNA *in situ* hybridization and PCR studies (Durst *et al.*, 1983; Boshart *et al.*, 1984; Yee *et al.*, 1985; Lorincz *et al.*, 1986; Lorincz, 1987; Reid *et al.*, 1987; Gupta *et al.*, 1987a; Nuovo *et al.*, 1991). More than 20 distinct HPV types have been isolated from condylomas and CIN I including HPV serotypes 6, 11, 16, 18, 31, 33 and 35. This heterogeneity is not found in CIN II and CIN III lesions, which contain predominantly HPV serotypes 16, 31, 33 and 35. Therefore, the cytologic and histologic features of HPV-associated cervical lesions are not predictive of biologic behavior.

Multiple epidemiologic studies have implicated the role of other cofactors including herpes simplex virus (Zur Hausen, 1982; LaVecchia *et al.*, 1986; Luthra *et al.*, 1987; Gupta *et al.*, 1988) and cigarette smoking (Slattery *et al.*, 1989) in the development of cervical neoplasia. Among these risk factors, the association between cigarette smoking and cervical carcinoma seems to be the strongest. However, in the absence of HPV infection, the necessary intraepithelial changes that antedate squamous cell carcinoma of the cervix would not be likely to occur.

Cytologic Features Suggestive of Microinvasive Squamous Carcinoma of the Uterine Cervix

As defined by the Society of Gynecologic Oncologists, microinvasive squamous cell carcinoma of the uterine cervix is defined as a lesion that invades the cervical stroma to a depth of 3 mm or less and does not exhibit vascular space invasion. According to Ng *et al.* (1972), the cytologic manifestations of microinvasive carcinoma varied with the depth of stromal invasion; specifically, in cases of microinvasive carcinoma with stromal penetration up to 2 mm, the cells resembled those of CIN III, whereas those lesions 2–3 mm in depth were most characteristic of microinvasive carcinoma. Such cells often occurred in a syncytial arrangement and exhibited a high N/C ratio. Prominent nucleoli in 5–20% of the cells and the presence of a background tumor diathesis aided in distinguishing the cells from high-grade SIL. When the aforementioned cytologic findings are encountered, we and others (Giuntoli *et al.*, 1987), prefer to designate such lesions as 'high-grade SIL, cannot rule out invasion' or 'squamous cell carcinoma with probable invasion.' TBS does not specifically address the issue of microinvasive squamous cell carcinoma.

Cytologic Features of Invasive Squamous Cell Carcinoma

TBS defines squamous cell carcinoma as a malignant tumor composed of squamous cells. For purposes of outlining criteria, the schemes of Wentz and Reagan (1959) will be used and include:

- large cell keratinizing squamous cell carcinoma;
- large cell nonkeratinizing squamous cell carcinoma;
- small cell nonkeratinizing squamous cell carcinoma.

Keratinizing squamous cell carcinoma

The cell population in cases of keratinizing squamous cell carcinoma is composed of a variety of cell forms; there are large cells, which vary in size and shape, hyperkeratosis in the form of anucleate squames, and pleomorphic parakeratosis in the form of small squamous cells with pyknotic nuclei. Approximately 15% of the abnormal cell population is characterized by elongate, tadpole, caudate forms, which are not present in the other types of squamous cell carcinoma. The nuclei have a mean area of approximately 80 μm^2, are often irregular in configuration, and hyperchromatic, with coarsely granular chromatin (Reagan *et al.*, 1957). Macronucleoli are present, but are less frequent than in the other types of squamous cell carcinoma. Cytoplasmic keratinization is present (*Figure 2.19*). Keratinizing squamous cell carcinoma, since it is often an exophytic lesion, may not be associated with a tumor diathesis in the slide background.

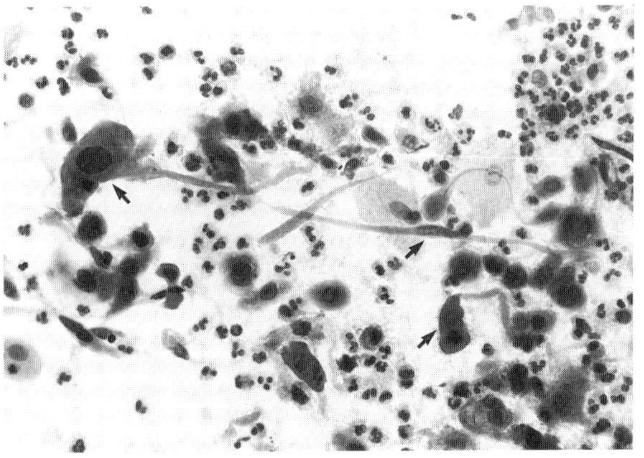

Figure 2.19. Keratinized elongated malignant cells (arrows) containing hyperchromatic nuclei are present. A tumor diathesis is present in the smear background.

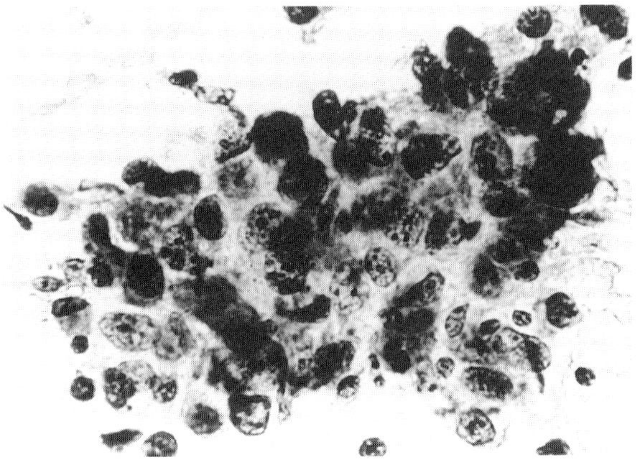

Figure 2.20. An aggregate of pleomorphic nonkeratinizing malignant squamous cells. The cell nuclei contain hyperchromatic coarse chromatin and prominent nucleoli.

Large cell nonkeratinizing squamous cell carcinoma

The cellular sample from nonkeratinizing squamous cell carcinoma is usually characterized by the presence of a tumor diathesis in the smear background. Individual tumor cells are large and are arranged singly and in syncytial aggregates with ill-defined cellular borders. The cytoplasm is cyanophilic. The nuclei are round to oval or irregular in shape and average approximately 90 μm^2 in area (Reagan *et al.*, 1957). The chromatin is hyperchromatic, coarsely granular and irregularly distributed. Macronucleoli are common (*Figure 2.20*).

Small cell (nonkeratinizing) carcinoma

The tumor cells are often present in a tumor diathesis background caused by the destructive process of the invading cancer. The cells are small and occur either singly or in a loose syncytial arrangement. The cytoplasm is scant and cyanophilic. The nuclei, which average 65 μm^2, are round to oval, with hyperchromatic, coarsely granular chromatin (Reagan *et al.*, 1957). Macronucleoli are common.

Adenocarcinoma of the Uterine Cervix

Adenocarcinoma arising primarily from the cervical columnar epithelium constitutes 8–26% of all epithelial malignancies of the uterine cervix. Studies have shown that the relative frequency has been increasing due to an absolute increase in the incidence of cervical adenocarcinoma (Vesterinen *et al.*, 1989; Leminen *et al.*, 1990). An association with previous usage of oral contraceptives, particularly those with a major progestational component has been described (Dallenbach–Hellweg, 1982; Brinton *et al.*, 1987). Adenocarcinoma *in situ* (AIS) represents 9–25% of the cervical adenocarcinomas (Ostor *et al.*, 1984; Boon *et al.*, 1987). It is often associated with CIN and in about one-half of the cases has been associated with CIN III (Maier and Norris, 1980; Wolk *et al.*, 1981).

Cytologic Features of Glandular Epithelial Cell Abnormalities

As defined by TBS (Kurman and Solomon, 1994) atypical glandular cells of undetermined significance (AGUS) show atypical cellular changes beyond those present in benign/reactive processes, but insufficient for a diagnosis of invasive adenocarcinoma. Therefore, lesions in this category include a relatively wide morphologic spectrum from atypical-appearing reactive processes to AIS.

Endocervical adenocarcinoma *in situ*

Cervicovaginal smears from women with AIS usually contain a moderate number of abnormal endocervical cells, the latter occurring predominantly in aggregates and sheets, and less commonly as abnormal single columnar or round cells (Ng and Pacey, 1988; Betsill and Clark, 1986). AIS may be encountered in a variety of growth patterns: these include strips of abnormal columnar cells arranged in a palisading configuration with nuclear pseudostratification, sheets of AIS cells with so-called 'feathered edges,' and abnormal columnar cells in glandular rosettes (*Figure 2.21*). AIS cells contain larger nuclei and less cytoplasm than normal endocervical cells. The cells show slight to moderate nuclear hyperchromasia, the nuclear chromatin is

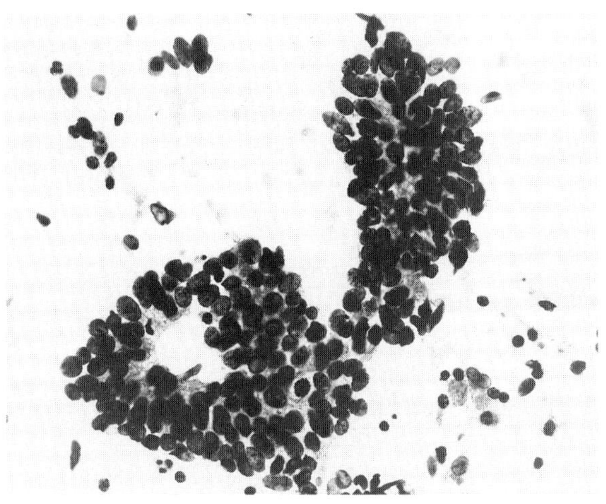

Figure 2.21. A glandular rosette of endocervical adenocarcinoma *in situ* (AIS) cells.

evenly distributed and finely granular, and micronucleoli are present. Macronucleoli, mitotic figures and a tumor diathesis background are not usually evident (Ng and Pacey, 1988; Nguyen and Jeannot, 1984; Betsill and Clark, 1986; Ayer *et al.*, 1987).

Microinvasive endocervical adenocarcinoma

Microinvasive adenocarcinoma is invariably associated with and arises from an *in situ* process; since the distinction between the two may be exceedingly difficult on histopathologic grounds, their delineation purely on a cytologic basis is even more challenging. Cervicovaginal smears from women with microinvasive adenocarcinoma may show essentially the same cellular features as AIS (Ng and Pacey, 1988; Nguyen and Jeannot, 1984; Betsill and Clark, 1986). In an attempt to define cytologic criteria for microinvasion, Ayer *et al.* (1988) analyzed 40 histologically confirmed cases. They noted that cellular dissociation, nuclear pleomorphism with an irregularly clumped chromatin pattern and inconspicuous to prominent nucleoli were frequently present. In a few cases, a tumor diathesis was seen in the smear background. Using these criteria, their diagnostic accuracy rose from 0% to almost 50%. Further studies are needed in order to subclassify microinvasive adenocarcinoma on a cytologic basis. TBS does not specifically address this issue and, to date, there is no uniformly accepted pathologic definition of microinvasive endocervical adenocarcinoma.

Invasive adenocarcinoma

The majority of cervical adenocarcinomas are derived from the endocervical columnar cells and mimic their cells of origin; however, other cell types include endometrioid adenocarcinoma, adenosquamous carcinoma, and clear cell adenocarcinoma.

In endocervical adenocarcinoma the cellular morphology is related to the degree of differentiation of the lesion. As the lesion becomes more poorly differentiated the cells show an increased N/C ratio, the nuclei contain more granular chromatin and prominent nucleoli, and intracytoplasmic vacuoles containing mucin are less frequently present (*Figure 2.22*). The abnormal cells are arranged either singly and/or in clusters and sheets. A tumor diathesis is usually present in the background (Reagan and Ng, 1973, 1988).

Cervical lesions arising from *in utero* exposure to diethylstilbestrol

Between 1943 and 1973 diethylstilbestrol (DES), a synthetic nonsteroidal estrogen, was used widely in an attempt to reduce the threat of spontaneous abortion. After the initial report by Herbst and Scully in 1970 on the association of DES and adenocarcinoma of the vagina in the female offspring of women receiving the drug, the FDA banned the use of DES during pregnancy.

The consequent abnormal structural variations seen within the cervix have been extensively described, but include a partial or complete cervical collar, cervical ridges or folds, a cock's comb appearance of the cervix, and a wide irregular transformation zone extending for variable distances into the cervico-vaginal vault.

DES exposure is associated with several changes visible on cervicovaginal smears. Within the cervix the most common finding is squamous metaplasia

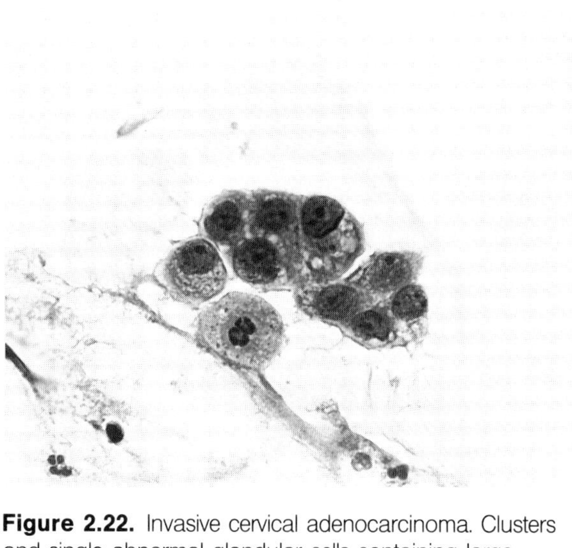

Figure 2.22. Invasive cervical adenocarcinoma. Clusters and single abnormal glandular cells containing large nuclei and prominent nucleoli are present.

and, to a lesser extent, low-grade and high-grade SILs (Fu *et al.*, 1978; Robboy *et al.*, 1979; Welch *et al.*, 1985). No firm link has yet been established between the development of invasive squamous cell carcinoma and prenatal DES exposure (Robboy *et al.*, 1981).

Rarely, intrauterine exposure to DES has been followed several to many years later by clear cell adenocarcinoma of the vagina or cervix in a ratio approximating 7:3 (Scully *et al.*, 1978).

Cytologically, malignant cells arising from clear cell adenocarcinoma are arranged singly and in tight glandular clusters. The nuclei are enlarged and contain prominent large nucleoli and fine to coarsely granular chromatin. The cytoplasm is finely vacuolated and stains positively for glycogen. A tumor diathesis is present in poorly differentiated lesions (Reagan and Ng, 1988).

Summary of Core Information

- Older classifications for reporting cervicovaginal cytology have been replaced by The Bethesda System (TBS), which uses uniform diagnostic terminology that reflects current understanding of the biology of cervical neoplasia.
- Inflammatory or reactive benign cellular changes can be distinguished from true epithelial cell abnormalities and show less cytologic atypia.
- The clinical significance of herpes simplex virus (HSV) lies in its association with gonorrhea, risk of spontaneous abortion and neonatal infection, and its possible co-factor role in the development of cervical cancer.
- Atypical squamous cells of undetermined significance (ASCUS) show more cellular abnormalities than those due to reactive/repair changes, but less than overt squamous intraepithelial lesions (SILs).
- The rate of ASCUS in a screened population may be 2–3 times the rate of SILs.
- If untreated, high-grade SILs have a greater tendency to persist and/or progress than low-grade SILs.
- High-risk HPVs are associated with both low-grade and high-grade cervical intraepithelial neoplasias (CINs), but are present with a greater frequency in the high-grade group.
- The cytologic and histologic features of HPV-associated cervical lesions are not predictive of biologic behavior.
- Cytologic findings suggestive of microinvasive carcinoma are best designated as 'high-grade SIL, cannot rule out invasion.'
- Adenocarcinoma *in situ* (AIS) of the cervix is frequently associated with SIL, which is often high-grade.

References

Adam E, Kaufman RH & Adler-Storthz K (1985) A prospective study of the association of herpes simplex virus and human papillomavirus infection with cervical neoplasia in women exposed to diethylstilbestrol *in utero*. *Int. J. Cancer* **34:** 19–26.

Ayer B, Pacey KF & Greenberg M (1988) The cytologic diagnosis of adenocarcinoma *in situ* of the uterine cervix and related lesions. II. Microinvasive adenocarcinoma. *Acta Cytol.* **32:** 318–324.

Ayer B, Pacey F, Greenberg M & Bousfield L (1987) The cytologic diagnosis of adenocarcinoma *in situ* of the cervix uteri and related lesions. I. Adenocarcinoma *in situ*. *Acta Cytol.* **31:** 397–411.

Betsill W & Clark AH (1986) Early endocervical glandular neoplasia. *Acta Cytol.* **30:** 115–126.

Bibbo M, Keebler CM & Wied GL (1971) The cytologic diagnosis of tissue repair in the female genital tract. *Acta Cytol.* **15:** 133–137.

Bonfiglio TA & Patten SF (1976) Histopathologic spectrum of benign proliferative and intraepithelial neoplastic reactions of the uterine cervix. *J. Repro. Med.* **16:** 253–261.

Boon ME, De Graaf Guilloud JC, Kok LP, Olthof PM & Van Erp EJ (1987) Efficacy of screening for cervical squamous and adenocarcinoma. The Dutch experience. *Cancer* **59:** 862–866.

Boschann HW (1992) Radiation changes in benign cells of the female reproductive tract. In: Wied GL, Keebler CM, Koss LG, Patten SF & Rosenthal DL (eds) *Compendium on Diagnostic Cytology*, pp. 182–190. Chicago: Tutorials of Cytology.

Boshart M, Gissman L, Ikenberg H, Scheurlen W, Kleinheinz A & Zur Hausen H (1984) A new type of papillomavirus DNA, its presence in genital cancer biopsies and in cell lines derived from cervical cancer. *Embo. J.* **3:** 1151–1157.

Brinton LA, Tashima K, Lehman HF *et al.* (1987) Epidemiology of cervical cancer by cell type. *Cancer Res.* **47:** 1706–1711.

Carmichael R & Jeafferson BL (1941) Squamous metaplasia

of the columnar epithelium in the human cervix. *J. Path Bact.* **52:** 173–186.

Casas–Cordero M, Roy M, Fortier M & Meisels A (1981) Origin of the koilocytes in condylomata of the human cervix. Ultrastructural study. *Acta Cytol.* **25:** 383–392.

Crum CP (1987) Vulvar intraepithelial neoplasia. In: Wilkinson EJ (ed.) *Pathology of the Vulva and Vagina*, pp. 79–101. New York: Churchill Livingstone.

Crum CP, Egawa K, Barron B, Fenoglio CM, Levine RU & Richart RM (1983) Human papillomavirus infection (condyloma) of the cervix and cervical intraepithelial neoplasia: A histopathologic statistical analysis. *Gynecol. Oncol.* **15:** 88–94.

Dallenbach–Hellweg G (1982) Occurrence and histologic structure of adenocarcinoma of the endocervix after long-term use of oral contraceptives. *Geburtshilfe Frauenheilkd* **42:** 249–255.

Durst M, Gissman, Ikenberg H & Zur Hausen H (1983) A new type of papillomavirus infection and DNA from a cervical carcinoma and its prevalence in cancer biopsies from different geographic regions. *Proc. Natl. Acad. Sci.* **80:** 3812–3815.

Fu S, Reagan JW, Hawliczek S & Wentz WB (1978) The use of cellular studies in the investigation of the DES-exposed woman. In: Herbst AL (ed.) *Intrauterine Exposure to Diethylstilbestrol in The Human*, pp. 34–44. Chicago: The American College of Obstetricians and Gynecologists.

Geirsson G, Woodworth FE, Patten SF & Bonfiglio TA (1977) Epithelial repair and regeneration in the uterine cervix. I. An analysis of the cells. *Acta Cytol.* **21:** 371–378.

■ Giuntoli RL, Atkinson FB, Ernst CS, Rubin MM & Egan VS (1987) Malignant lesions of the cervix. In: Biello LA, Patterson D & Hoeltzel LE (eds) *Atkinson's Correlative Atlas of Colposcopy, Cytology and Histopathology*, pp. 162–195. Philadelphia: JB Lippincott Company.

Graham RM (1947) Effect of radiation on vaginal cells in cervical carcinoma. I. Description of cellular changes. II. Prognostic significance. *Surg. Gynecol. Obstet.* **84:** 153–165, 166–173.

Gupta PK (1982) Intrauterine contraceptive devices: Vaginal cytology, pathologic changes and clinical implications. *Acta Cytol.* **26:** 571–613.

Gupta JW, Gupta PK, Rosenshein N & Shah KV (1987a) Detection of human papillomavirus in cervical smears. *Acta Cytol.* **31:** 387–396.

Gupta S, Mukherjee K, Gupta YN & Kumar M (1987b) Sequential radiation changes in cytology of vaginal smears in carcinoma of the cervix uteri during radiotherapy. *Int. J. Gynecol. Obstet.* **25:** 303–308.

Gupta MM, Sharma BK, Singh V & Luthra UK (1988) Immunocytological demonstration of HSV-II antigen on exfoliated cells from precancerous lesions of the uterine cervix. *Diag. Cytopathol.* **4:** 48–49.

Heller C & Hoyt V (1971) Squamous cell changes associated with the presence of *Candida* sp. in cervical and vaginal Papanicolaou smears. *Acta Cytol.* **15:** 379–384.

Herbst AL (1991) Concerns regarding the Bethesda System. *Int. J. Gynecol. Pathol.* **10:** 326–328.

Herbst AL & Scully RE (1970) Adenocarcinoma of the vagina in adolescence: a report of seven cases including six clear cell carcinomas (so called mesonephromas). *Cancer* **25:** 745–757.

Ismail SM, Colclough AB, Dinnen JS *et al.* (1990) Reporting cervical intraepithelial neoplasia (CIN): intra- and interpathologist variation and factors associated with disagreement. *Histopathology* **16:** 371–376.

Kataja V, Syrjanen K, Mantyjarvi R *et al.* (1989) Prospective follow-up of cervical HPV infections: Life table analysis of histopathological, cytological and colposcopic data. *Eur. J. Epidemiol.* **5:** 1–7.

Kearns PR & Gray JE (1963) Mycotic vulvovaginitis. *Obstet. Gynecol.* **22:** 621–625.

■ Koss LG (1990) The new Bethesda System for reporting results of smears of the uterine cervix. *J. Natl. Cancer Inst.* **82:** 988–991.

■ Koss LG (1992a) The normal female genital tract. *Diagnostic Cytology and its Histopathologic Basis*, pp. 251–294. Philadelphia: JB Lippincott.

Koss LG (1992b) Epidermoid carcinoma of the uterine cervix and related precancerous lesions. *Diagnostic Cytology and its Histopathologic Basis*, pp. 424–512. Philadelphia: JB Lippincott.

Koss LG & Durfee GR (1956) Unusual patterns of squamous epithelium of the uterine cervix: cytologic and pathologic study of koilocytotic atypia. *Ann. NY Acad. Sci.* **63:** 1245–1261.

Kurman RJ (1991) The Bethesda System: "Pro". *Int. J. Gynecol. Oncol.* **10:** 329–332.

■ Kurman RJ, Henson DE, Herbst AL, Noller KL & Schiffman MH (1994) Interim guideline for management of abnormal cervical cytology. *JAMA* **271:** 1866–1869.

Kurman RJ, Jenson AB & Lancaster WD (1983) Papillomavirus infection of the cervix II. Relationship of intraepithelial neoplasia based on the presence of specific viral structural proteins. *Am. J. Surg. Pathol.* **7:** 39–52.

Kurman GJ, Malkasian GD, Sedlis A & Solomon D (1991) Clinical commentary: From Papanicolaou to Bethesda: The rationale for a new cervical cytologic classification. *Obstet. Gynecol.* **77:** 779–782.

Kurman RJ & Solomon D (1994) *The Bethesda System for Reporting Cervical/Vaginal Cytologic Diagnoses: Definitions, Criteria and Explanatory Notes for Terminology and Specimen Adequacy.* New York: Springer–Verlag.

LaVecchia C, Franceschi S, De Carli A *et al.* (1986) Sexual factors, venereal diseases, and the risk of intraepithelial and invasive cervical neoplasia. *Cancer* **58:** 935–941.

Leminen A, Paavonen J, Forss M, Walhström T & Vesterinen E (1990) Adenocarcinoma of the uterine cervix. *Cancer* **65:** 53–59.

Lorincz AT, Lancaster WD & Temple G (1986) Cloning and characterization of the DNA from a woman with dysplasia of the uterine cervix. *J. Virol.* **58:** 225–230.

Lorincz AT, Temple CG, Kurman RJ, Jensen AB & Lancaster WD (1987) Oncogenic association of specific human papillomavirus types with cervical neoplasia. *J. Natl. Cancer Inst.* **79:** 671–677.

Luthra UK, Pradhakar AK, Seth P *et al.* (1987) Natural history of precancerous and early cancerous lesions of the uterine cervix. *Acta Cytol.* **31:** 226–234.

Maier RC & Norris HJ (1980) Coexistence of cervical intraepithelial neoplasia with primary adenocarcinoma of the endocervix. *Obstet. Gynecol.* **56:** 361–364.

Melamed MR & Flehinger BJ (1976) Nondiagnostic squamous atypia in cervico-vaginal cytology as a risk factor for early neoplasia. *Acta Cytol.* **20:** 108–110.

Meisels A, Fortin R & Roy M (1977) Condylomatous lesions of the cervix II. Cytologic, colposcopic and histologic study. *Acta Cytol.* **21:** 379–390.

Meisels A & Morin C (1981) Human papillomavirus and cancer of the uterine cervix. *Obstet. Gynecol.* **12:** 111–123.

Nahmias AJ, Joseph WE, Naib ZM, Luer CF & Guest A (1970) Antibodies to herpesvirus hominis types 1 and 2 in humans II: women with cervical cancer. *Am. J. Epidemiol.* **9:** 547–552.

Nasiell K, Roger V & Nasiell M (1986) Behavior of mild cervical dysplasia during long-term follow-up. *Obstet. Gynecol.* **67:** 665–669.

National Cancer Institute Workshop (1989) The 1988 Bethesda System for reporting cervical/vaginal cytologic diagnosis. *JAMA* **262:** 931–934.

Ng ABP & Pacey NF (1988) Microinvasive adenocarcinoma and precursors of adenocarcinoma of the uterine cervix. In: Wied GL, Keebler CM, Koss LG & Reagan JW (eds) *Compendium on Diagnostic Cytology*, pp. 39–145. Chicago: Tutorials of Cytology.

Ng ABP, Reagan JW & Linder E (1970) Cellular manifestations of primary and recurrent herpes genitalis. *Acta Cytol.* **14:** 124–129.

Ng ABP, Reagan JW & Linder E (1972) The cellular manifestations of microinvasive squamous cell carcinoma of the uterine cervix. *Acta Cytol.* **16:** 5–13.

Nguyen GK & Jeannot AB (1984) Exfoliative cytology of *in situ* and microinvasive adenocarcinoma of the uterine cervix. *Acta Cytol.* **28:** 461–467.

Nuovo GJ, Darfler MM, Impraim CC *et al.* (1991) Occurrence of multiple types of human papillomavirus in genital tract lesions: Analysis by *in situ* hybridization and the polymerase chain reaction. *Amer. J. Pathol.* **138:** 53–58.

Ostor AG, Pagano R, Davoren RA, Fortune DW, Chanen W & Rome R (1984) Adenocarcinoma *in situ* of the cervix. *Int. J. Gynecol. Pathol.* **3:** 179–190.

Papanicolaou GN & Traut HF (1943) *Diagnosis of Uterine Cancer by the Vaginal Smear.* New York: Commonwealth Fund.

Patten SF (1978) *Diagnostic Cytology of the Uterine Cervix*, 2nd edition. Basel, Switzerland: Karger.

Patten SF, Reagan W, Obenaut M & Ballard LA (1963) Post-irradiation dysplasia of uterine cervix and vagina. An analytical study of cells. *Cancer* **16:** 173–182.

Reagan JW (1965) Presidential address. *Acta Cytol.* **9:** 265–267.

Reagan JW, Hamonic MJ & Wentz WB (1957) Analytical study of cells in cervical squamous-cell cancer. *Lab. Invest.* **6:** 241–250.

Reagan JW & Ng APB (1973) The cells of uterine adenocarcinoma. In: Wied, GL, Koss L & Reagan JW (eds) *Monographs in Clinical Cytology*, pp. 96–112. Basel, Switzerland: Karger.

Reagan JW & Ng ABP (1988) Cellular detection of glandular neoplasms of the uterine cervix. In: Wied GL, Keebler CM, Koss LG & Reagan JW (eds) *Compendium on Diagnostic Cytology*, pp. 146–153. Chicago: Tutorials of Cytology.

Reagan JW, Seidemann IL & Saracusa Y (1953) The cellular morphology of carcinoma *in situ* and dysplasia or atypical hyperplasia of the uterine cervix. *Cancer* **6:** 224–229.

Reid R, Crum CP, Herschman BR *et al.* (1984a) Genital warts and cervical cancer III. Subclinical papillomavirus infection and cervical neoplasia are linked by a spectrum of continuous and biologic change. *Cancer* **53:** 943–953.

Reid R, Greenberg M, Jenson AB *et al.* (1987) Sexually transmitted papillomavirus infections. I. The anatomic distribution and pathologic grade of neoplastic lesions associated with different viral types. *Am. J. Obstet. Gynecol.* **156:** 212–222.

Reid R, Herschman BR, Crum CP *et al.* (1984b) The tissue basis of colposcopic change. *Am. J. Obstet. Gynecol.* **149:** 293–303.

Reid R, Stanhope CR, Herschman BR, Booth E, Phibbs GD & Smith J (1982) I. Evidence of an association between subclinical papillomavirus infection and cervical malignancy. *Cancer* **50:** 377–387.

Robboy SJ, Laufman RH & Prat J (1979) Pathologic findings in young women enrolled in the national cooperative diethylstilbestrol adenosis (DESAD) project. *Obstet. Gynecol.* **53:** 309–317.

Robboy SJ, Truslow GY, Anton J & Richart M (1981) Role of hormones including diethylstilbestrol (DES) in the pathogenesis of cervical and vaginal intraepithelial neoplasia. *Gynecol. Oncol.* **12:** S98–S110.

Robertson AJ, Anderson JM, Swanson BJ *et al.* (1989) Observer variability in histopathologic reporting of cervical biopsy specimens. *J. Clin. Pathol.* **94:** 231–238.

Scully RE, Robboy SJ & Welch WR (1978) Pathology and pathogenesis of diethylstilbestrol-related disorders of the female genital tract. In: Herbst AL (ed.) *Intrauterine Exposure to Diethylstilbestrol in the Human*, pp. 8–21. Chicago, The American College of Obstetricians and Gynecologists.

■ Selvaggi SM (1986) Cytologic detection of condylomas and cervical intraepithelial neoplasia (CIN) of the uterine cervix with histologic correlation. *Cancer* **58:** 2076–2081.

Selvaggi SM (1988) Cytologic indicators of condylomatous lesions of the uterine cervix with histologic correlation: An outpatient laboratory's experience. *Diagn. Cytopathol.* **4:** 277–282.

Sherman ME, Schiffman MH, Kurman RJ, Erozan YS & Wacholder S (1991) The Bethesda System: Interobserver reproducibility of cytologic diagnoses. *The Bethesda System*: Second Conference, Bethesda, MD.

Shibata D, Fu YS, Gupta JW *et al.* (1988) Detection of human papillomavirus in normal and dysplastic tissue by the polymerase chain reaction. *Lab. Invest.* **59:** 555–559.

Slattery ML, Robinson LM, Schuman KL *et al.* (1989) Cigarette smoking and exposure to passive smoke are risk factors for cervical cancer. *JAMA* **261:** 1591–1598.

Sugimori H, Kashimura Y, Kashimura M, Urushima M, Sato A & Takao M (1982) Analytical study of repair cells. *Acta Cytol.* **26:** 439–444.

Syrjanen KJ (1983) Human papillomavirus in association with cervical dysplasia and neoplasia. *Obstet. Gynecol.* **62:** 617–624.

Syrjanen K, Mantyjarvi R, Saarikoski S *et al.* (1988) Factors associated with progression of cervical human papillomavirus (HPV) infection into carcinoma *in situ* during a long-term prospective follow-up. *Br. J. Obstet. Gynaecol.* **95:** 1096–1102.

Vesterinen E, Forss M & Nieminen U (1989) Increase of cervical adenocarcinoma: A report of 520 cases of cervical carcinoma including 112 tumors with glandular elements. *Gynecol. Oncol.* **33:** 49–53.

Welch WR, Robboy SJ, Kaufman RH *et al.* (1985) Pathology of colposcopic findings of 2,635 diethylstilbestrol-exposed young women. *Gynecol. Oncol.* **21:** 277–286.

Wentz WB & Reagan JW (1959) Survival in cervical cancer with respect to cell type. *Cancer* **12:** 384–388.

Wentz WB & Reagan JW (1970) Clinical significance of post-irradiation dysplasia of the uterine cervix. *Am. J. Obstet. Gynecol.* **106:** 812–817.

Wied GL, Davis ME, Frank R, Segan PB, Meir P & Rosenthal EE (1966) Statistical evaluation of the effect of hormonal contraceptives on the cytologic smear pattern. *Obstet. Gynecol.* **27:** 327–334.

Willett GD, Kurman RJ, Reid R, Greenberg M, Jenson AB & Lorincz AT (1989) Correlation of the histologic appearance of intraepithelial neoplasia of the cervix with human papillomavirus types. *Int. J. Gynecol. Pathol.* **8:** 18–25.

Wolk BM, Kime W & Albites V (1981) Simultaneous *in situ* squamous cell carcinoma and microinvasive adenocarcinoma of the cervix. *Int. J. Gynecol. Obstet.* **19:** 69–72.

Yee C, Krishnan–Hewlett I, Baker CC, Schlegal R & Howley PM (1985) Presence and expression of human papillomavirus sequences in human cervical carcinoma cell lines. *Am. J. Pathol.* **119:** 261–366.

Zur Hausen H (1982) Human genital cancer: synergism between two virus infections and synergism between a virus infection and initiating events? *Lancet* **2:** 1370–1372.

3 Histopathology of the Cervix and Vagina

M C Anderson
T P Rollason

Vaginal Tumors

A classification of the tumors of the vagina is given in *Table 3.1*.

Epithelial Tumors

Squamous cell tumors

Although the use of the term vaginal intraepithelial neoplasia (VaIN) is generally accepted, no clear criteria exist for the diagnosis of microinvasive disease at this site. The great majority of carcinomas of the vagina are squamous in type and, in general, the same variants occur as in the vulva and cervix. Adenocarcinomas at this site are most commonly seen in association with intrauterine stilbestrol exposure and are usually of the clear cell (mesonephroid) type.

Vaginal intraepithelial neoplasia

The concept of dividing VaIN (*Figures 3.1 and 3.2*) into three grades on a similar basis to cervical intraepithelial neoplasia (CIN) and vulvar intraepithelial neoplasia (VIN) has much to commend it and has gained general acceptance. This should not, however, be taken to indicate a similar course and outcome to cervical or vulvar disease.

The association between VaIN and CIN and VIN is extremely strong (Aho *et al.*, 1991). Many studies have also demonstrated a relationship between invasive carcinoma of the cervix and VaIN (Hilborne and Fu, 1987). Histologically, VaIN is similar to CIN and VIN, with loss of cellular maturation and polarity, mitoses high in the epithelium, and hyperchromatic nuclei with coarse chromatin clumping. Grading is essentially by level of involvement of the mucosa as for VIN. Associated human papillomavirus (HPV) changes are very frequent and multifocality is not uncommon. Previous irradiation also appears to be associated with the development of VaIN after a variable latent period, sometimes of several years. Histologically, post-irradiation VaIN is said to be characterized by extreme nuclear changes. Wentz and Reagan (1970) found an association between the interval and the development of post-irradiation VaIN and survival after cervical squamous carcinoma.

Microinvasive squamous cell carcinoma

The criteria for the diagnosis of this condition (*Figure 3.3*) are unclear. Drawing a comparison with the cervix, what is illustrated in some cases might better be regarded as 'early stromal invasion' as laid down

Table 3.1. Classification of tumors of the vagina[‡].

Epithelial tumors
Squamous lesions
Vaginal intraepithelial neoplasia (VaIN)*
VaIN 1*
VaIN 2*
VaIN 3*
Squamous cell carcinoma*
Keratinizing*
Nonkeratinizing*
Verrucous*
Warty (condylomatous)
Glandular lesions
Glandular intraepithelial neoplasia (adenocarcinoma *in situ*)*
Adenocarcinoma*
Clear cell adenocarcinoma*
Endometrioid adenocarcinoma
Mucinous adenocarcinoma
Endocervical cell type
Mesenchymal tumors
Leiomyosarcoma*
Embryonal rhabdomyosarcoma (sarcoma botryoides)*
Miscellaneous tumors
Malignant melanoma*
Tumors of germ cell type
Lymphoma
Secondary tumours*

([‡]Benign tumors are not included; *discussed in this chapter.)

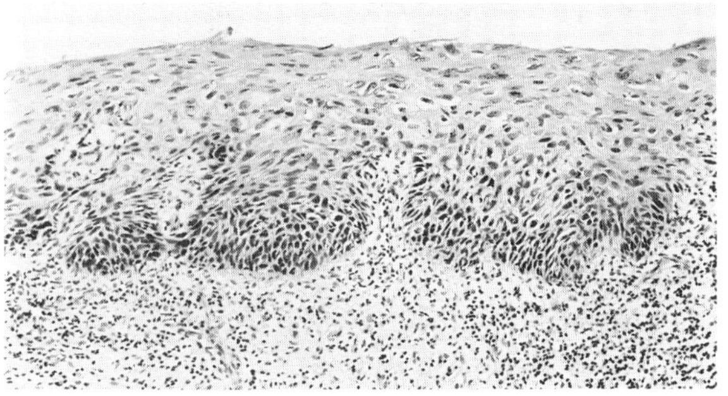

Figure 3.1. Vaginal biopsy showing vaginal intraepithelial neoplasia (VaIN) 1 (undifferentiated cells confined to the lower third of the mucosa) together with human papillomavirus (HPV) effect.

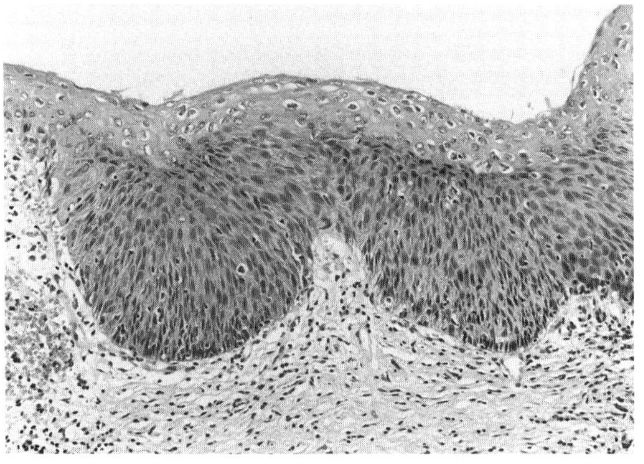

Figure 3.2. Vaginal biopsy showing vaginal intraepithelial neoplasia (VaIN) 2 centrally (undifferentiated cells confined approximately to the lower half of the mucosa) with more severe intraepithelial neoplasia adjacent and superadded human papillomavirus (HPV) effect.

in the Royal College of Obstetricians and Gynaecologists (RCOG) guidelines (Jordan *et al.*, 1982). Until further data are available it is important to document the depth, diameter, differentiation and presence or absence of vessel invasion in all histologic reports on carcinoma of the vagina (Peters *et al.*, 1985).

Invasive squamous cell carcinoma

Vaginal tumors are generally rare and 85–90% of those that do occur are squamous (Hilborne and Fu, 1987). Metastases at this site are 2–9 times as common as primary tumors (Hilborne and Fu, 1987; Schmidt, 1987). In the West Midlands region of England the Regional Cancer Registry figures indicate that vaginal carcinoma makes up only 1.5% of all female genital tract malignancies (Wade–Evans, 1976). Strict rules have been laid down to be followed before acceptance of a tumor as primary vaginal (Kottmeier, 1973), though they appear rather too restrictive both because they must exclude many cases of true multifocal genital tract neoplasia (Schmidt, 1987) and because there would appear to be little embryological or environmental reason for attempting to separate cervical from vaginal vault tumors (Wade–Evans, 1976).

The most important risk factor for the development of vaginal squamous cell carcinoma is a previous history of cervical or, to a lesser extent, vulvar malignancy. This association has led to the concept of lower genital tract neoplasia syndrome (LGTNS).

Three gross patterns of vaginal squamous cell carcinoma are described: nodulo-ulcerative, everting or papillary, and infiltrating or indurated. The nodulo-ulcerative pattern (*Figure 3.4*) is the most common and the infiltrating variant is said to present late.

The World Health Organization (Scully *et al.*, 1994) divides vaginal squamous cell carcinoma into four histological types (keratinizing, nonkeratinizing, verrucous and warty or condylomatous); most cases fall into the moderately differentiated keratinizing group. Spindle cell variants are well described (Branton and Tavassoli, 1993). There appears to be little correlation between grade and type and prognosis except for verrucous carcinoma,

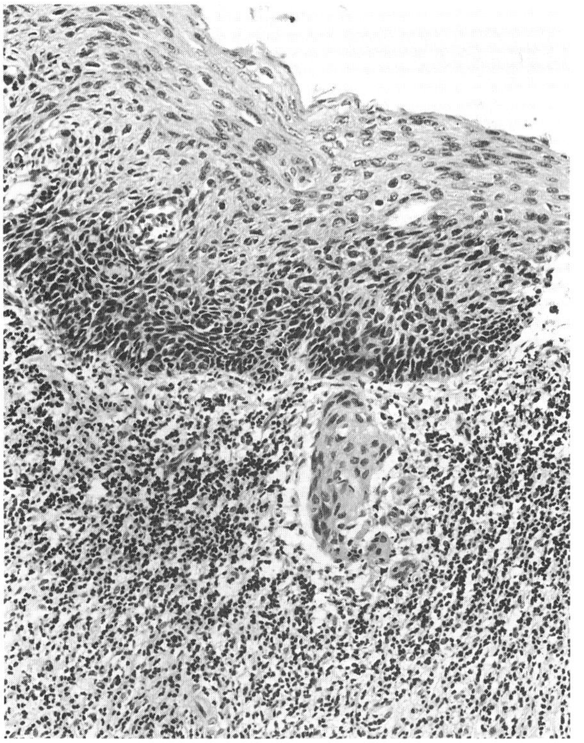

Figure 3.3. Vaginal biopsy showing focus of 'xenoplastic' early invasive squamous cells beneath vaginal mucosa, which does not itself show vaginal intraepithelial neoplasia (VaIN) 3. The pattern of invasion here mimics early cervical stromal invasion.

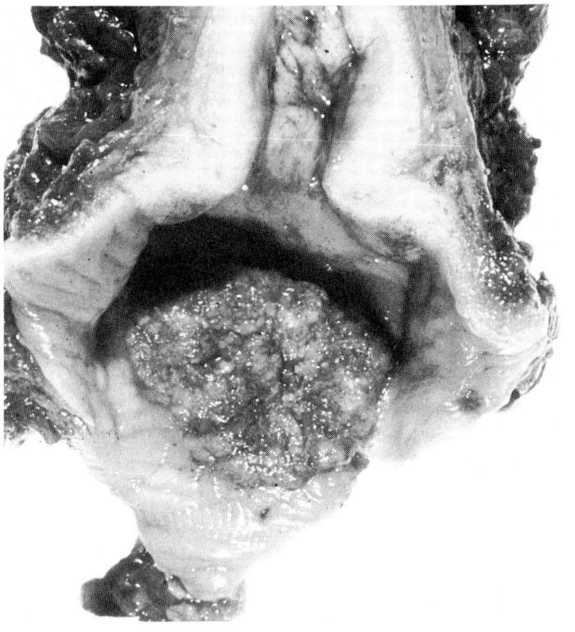

Figure 3.4. Squamous carcinoma of vagina. There is a cauliflower-like 'nodulo-ulcerative' squamous carcinoma in the upper vagina, separate from the cervix.

keratinizing tumors with severe cellular atypia and possibly poorly differentiated carcinomas. The International Federation of Gynecologists and Obstetricians (FIGO) staging provides the best prognostic information.

Squamous cell carcinoma arises most commonly in the upper one-third of the vagina on the posterior wall as does VaIN. The second commonest site is the lower anterior vagina. Approximately 10–20% are multifocal at initial diagnosis. Upper one-third tumors metastasize to the same sites as cervical tumors, whereas lower one-third behave like vulvar tumors metastasizing to the inguinal or occasionally external iliac nodes.

Verrucous carcinoma

Verrucous carcinoma is rare in the vagina, as on the vulva. It is usually seen in postmenopausal women and is large and polypoid. Histologic appearances and behavior are similar to those for the vulvar equivalent (see Chapter 19).

Glandular tumors

Adenocarcinoma of the vagina

Adenocarcinoma of the vagina is usually of clear cell (mesonephroid) type, but other types are recognized, albeit rarely. The frequency of the disease is difficult to assess because some series include diethylstilbestrol (DES)-associated cases, while others do not.

In non-DES-exposed women it appears to be predominantly a disease of the late reproductive years and, as in the DES-exposed, adenosis appears to be a precursor (Sanderberg *et al.*, 1965). Histologically the tumors may show a range of patterns including tubular, solid and papillary areas (*Figure 3.5*) and areas of clear cell differentiation.

Two cases of adenocarcinoma *in situ* of the vagina have been reported (Clement and Benedet, 1979; Cullimore *et al.*, 1989) (*Figure 3.6*). Rare cases of adenocarcinoma arising in endometriosis have been seen (Addison *et al.*, 1979).

Herbst and co-workers (Herbst *et al.*, 1970; Herbst and Scully, 1970; Herbst *et al.*, 1971) established that vaginal clear cell adenocarcinoma had increased in incidence in association with DES exposure *in utero*. Subsequent studies extended these findings to the cervix (Noller *et al.*, 1972). Over 500 cases of clear cell carcinoma are now registered, mainly in the USA. Of these 65% have evidence of *in utero* exposure to DES. The DES-associated

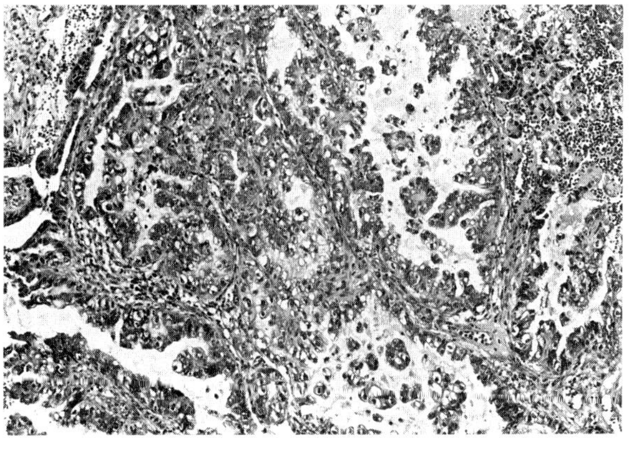

Figure 3.5. Vaginal biopsy – clear cell ('mesonephroid') carcinoma. The common tubulopapillary pattern of 'hobnail' cells is well demonstrated.

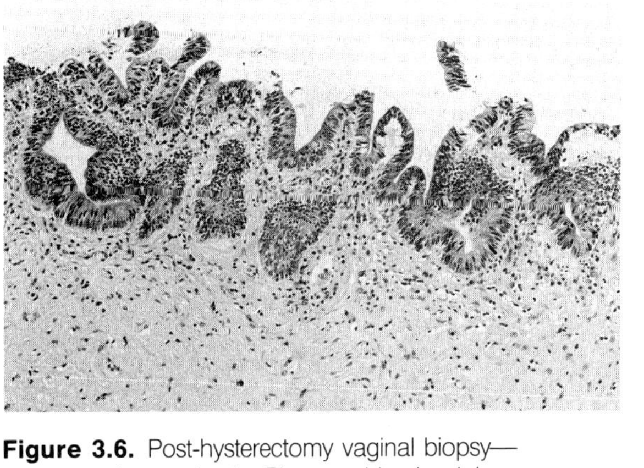

Figure 3.6. Post-hysterectomy vaginal biopsy—adenocarcinoma *in situ*. Pleomorphic glandular epithelium has replaced the surface epithelium of the vagina.

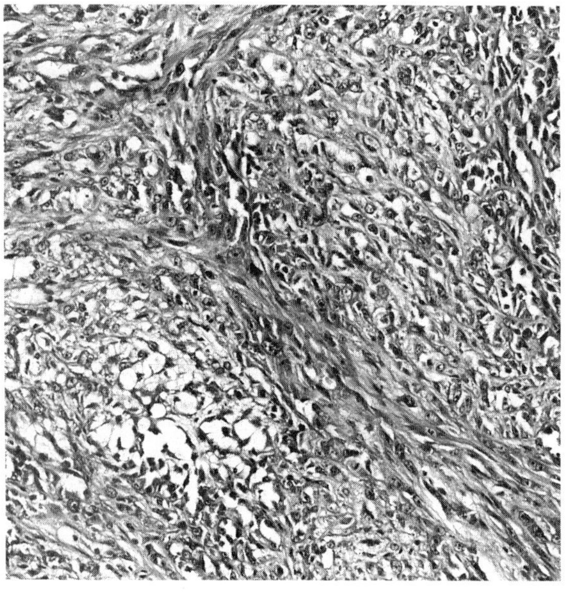

Figure 3.7. Vaginectomy specimen—leiomyosarcoma. The tumor is composed of interweaving bands of pleomorphic spindle cells with blunt nuclei.

tumors reach a peak incidence at 19 years of age (Herbst, 1984).

DES-associated tumors appear to arise equally often in the cervix and vagina and are particularly seen on the ectocervix and upper anterior wall of the vagina (Herbst *et al.*, 1974; Herbst *et al.*, 1979). They may present as nodules or as larger polypoid or ulcerated areas. Histologically the pattern is the same as non-DES-exposed cases (see above). The cells are usually cuboidal, columnar or of 'hobnail' type. No intracellular mucin is evident, but large amounts of glycogen are produced. Approximately 25% recur or metastasize, and metastasis to lungs and other distant sites is more common than in squamous carcinoma; overall, however, prognosis is better than for squamous carcinoma, with a 75% five-year survival (Herbst *et al.*, 1979). Pathologic features associated with a better prognosis are a tubulocystic pattern, a tumor area less than 3 cm^2 and a depth of invasion less than 3 mm (Herbst *et al.*, 1979; Herbst *et al.*, 1974), but the clinical stage is the most important factor.

It is generally accepted that adenosis precedes tumor development, and dysplastic glandular changes have been described (atypical adenosis) in these zones (Robboy *et al.*, 1984). The endometrial/tubal cell type, rather than the endocervical, appears to be the actual precursor cell of malignancy. These tumors should not be confused with the very rare true mesonephric carcinomas arising from mesonephric remnants in the lateral walls of the vagina.

Mesenchymal Tumors

The most important mesenchymal tumor of the vagina is the highly malignant embryonal rhabdomyosarcoma of young children. All other sarcomas are very rare at this site.

Leiomyosarcoma

Leiomyosarcoma appears to be the commonest adult vaginal sarcoma, but is nontheless very rare (Tavassoli and Norris, 1979). The patients are usually middle-aged with a mass, pain or bleeding. The tumor has a soft fleshy appearance. Histologically it is similar to the same tumor elsewhere, with pleomorphic spindle cells arranged in an interweaving pattern (*Figures 3.7 and 3.8*). The major feature indicating malignancy is likely to be a mitotic rate above 5 per 10 high power fields; marked cellular atypia, a size greater than 3 cm, tumor necrosis and an infiltrative margin are also of likely importance.

Embryonal rhabdomyosarcoma (sarcoma botryoides)

Embryonal rhabdomyosarcoma is a rare tumor that usually occurs in the first two years of life. Presentation is usually with bleeding or a mass of oedematous grape-like nodules (*Figure 3.9*). It would appear that the vaginal and cervical tumors are separate entities occurring at different ages, the cervical tumor having a better prognosis (Daya and Scully, 1988).

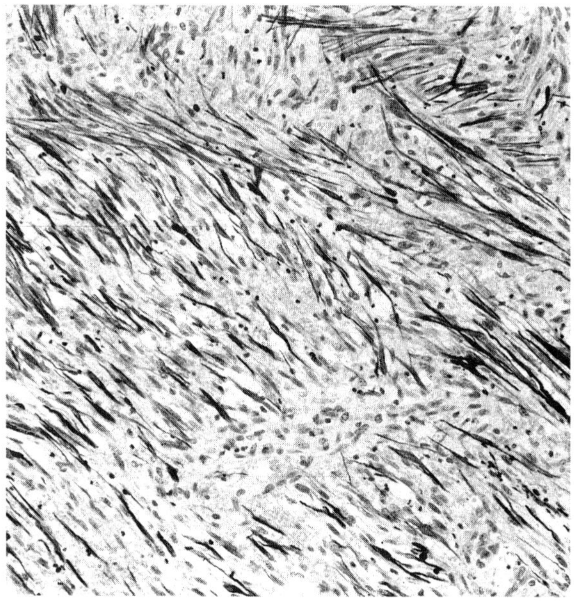

Figure 3.8. Vaginectomy specimen–leiomyosarcoma. Immunocytochemical staining to demonstrate desmin (black strands) indicative of myocyte differentiation.

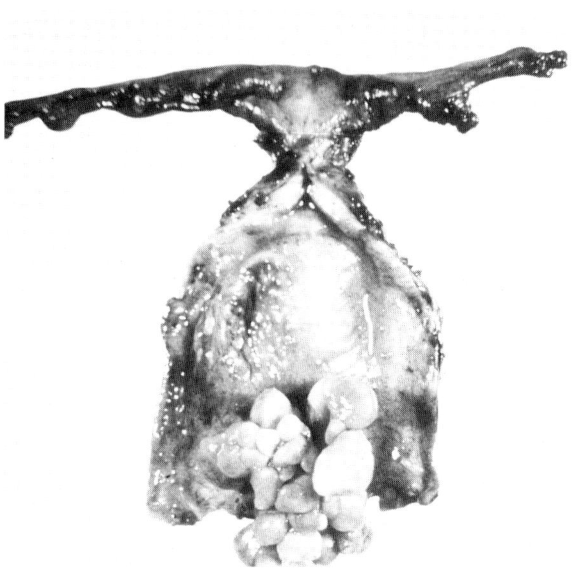

Figure 3.9. There are typical grape-like masses of embryonal rhabdomyosarcoma arising from the lower vagina of an infant.

The tumor is said to arise from the subepithelial zone of the vagina and is composed of deceptively benign-looking hypocellular myxoid tissue with a zone of more cellular tissue beneath the surface mucosa and adjacent to vessels – the so-called cambium zone. Variable numbers of eosinophilic rhabdomyoblasts are seen and striations may be visible. The tumor is locally aggressive and rapidly spreads to adjacent structures. Distant metastases occur late in the disease.

Miscellaneous Tumors

Malignant melanoma

It has been estimated that 3% of vaginal epithelial tumors are malignant melanomas (Chung *et al.*, 1980). Hertig and Gore (1979) found an average of 42 years in their series. The true vaginal primary melanoma presumably arises from junctional melanocytes within the vaginal mucosa, although an origin in included dermal appendages has also been suggested. The lower one-third of the anterior wall, appears to be the commonest site, though melanomas may occur anywhere in the vagina. Attention has been drawn to the occurrence of the acral lentiginous type in the vestibular muco-cutaneous region.

Macroscopically the lesions tend to be raised, often with surface ulceration; the great majority are pigmented. Histologically the tumor is similar to that on the vulvar skin. The prognosis is poor with most patients presenting with large tumors.

Metastatic Tumors

Numerically secondary tumors are the most important vaginal tumors, considerably outnumbering primary vaginal malignant tumors and usually coming from primary carcinomas in the female genital tract.

The commonest primary site is the cervix with involvement of the vagina by direct extension or lymphatic spread. The second most common is the endometrium, which is anecdotally said to favor the suburethral area. Renal carcinoma (*Figures 3.10 and 3.11*) is well described at this site as is metastatic choriocarcinoma, and cases of ovarian carcinoma, transitional cell carcinoma of urothelium, and carcinoma of the bowel, pancreas and breast are also recorded.

Tumors of the Cervix

A classification of tumors of the cervix is given in *Table 3.2*.

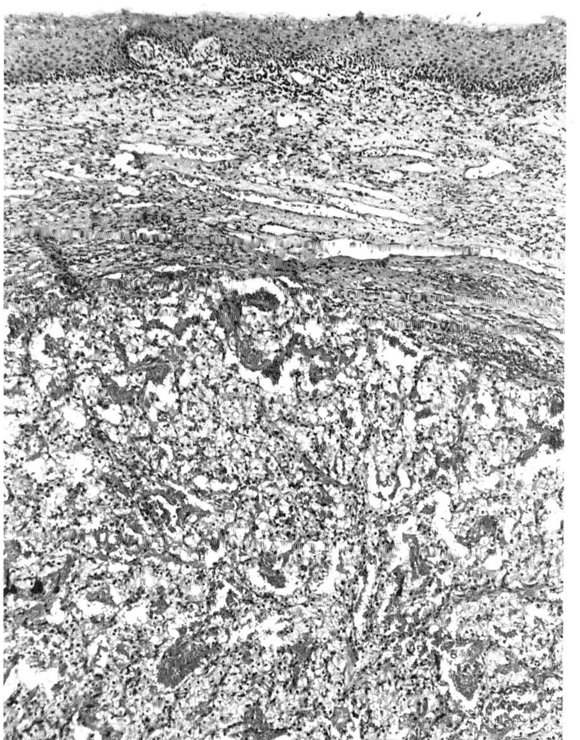

Figure 3.10. Vaginal biopsy – metastatic clear cell carcinoma from kidney. Low-power view to demonstrate replacement of the vaginal wall by metastatic carcinoma.

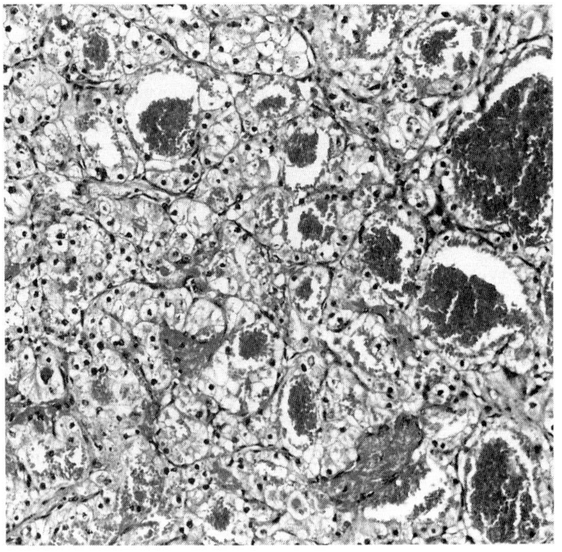

Figure 3.11. Vaginal biopsy – metastatic clear cell carcinoma from kidney. The typical clear cell acinar and trabecular pattern can be appreciated here.

Epithelial Tumors

Squamous cell tumors

Cervical intraepithelial neoplasia

CIN was introduced, both as a system of nomenclature and as a concept, to emphasize that the epithelial abnormalities of the cervix form a continuous spectrum of one disease process: an infinitely variable spectrum in which each degree of abnormality merges imperceptibly into the next. The concept was therefore, in theory, irreconcilable with subdivision, but it has become customary to subdivide CIN into three grades. There is, however, a worrying lack of diagnostic consistency among histopathologists in grading CIN, particularly at the mild end of the disease spectrum (Ismail *et al.*, 1989; Robertson *et al.*, 1989). This has added weight to the concerns first expressed about the consistency of reporting using the dysplasia/carcinoma *in situ* terminology and, later, the CIN terminology. As a result, it has been suggested that the current grading system for CIN should be modified and replaced by a two-tier system (Ismail *et al.*, 1989; Robertson, 1989; Robertson *et al.*, 1989; Richart, 1990).

The Bethesda System (TBS) for reporting cervical and vaginal diseases has adopted a two-tier system for cytological reporting of cervical epithelial abnormalities (Solomon, 1989; Solomon, 1991; Luff *et al.*, 1992). This system divides the epithelial abnormalities into high-grade and low-grade squamous intraepithelial lesions, the high-grade lesions being CIN 2 and CIN 3 and the low-grade lesions CIN 1 and wart virus infection. There has been considerable enthusiasm, particularly in the

Table 3.2. Classification of tumors of the cervix‡.

Epithelial tumors

- *Squamous lesions*
  - Cervical intraepithelial neoplasia (CIN)*
    - CIN 1*
    - CIN 2*
    - CIN 3*
  - Squamous cell carcinoma*
    - Keratinizing*
    - Nonkeratinizing*
    - Verrucous*
    - Warty (condylomatous)*
    - Papillary*
    - Lymphoepithelioma-like*
- *Glandular lesions*
  - Cervical glandular intraepithelial neoplasia (CGIN)*
    - Low-grade CGIN*
    - High-grade CGIN*
  - Adenocarcinoma*
    - Endocervical type*
    - Minimal deviation*
    - Mucinous*
    - Endometrioid*
    - Clear cell*
    - Papillary serous*
- *Other epithelial tumors*
  - Adenosquamous carcinoma*
  - Glassy cell carcinoma
  - Adenoid cystic carcinoma
  - Adenoid basal carcinoma
  - Small cell carcinoma*

Mesenchymal tumors

- Leiomyosarcoma
- Endocervical stromal sarcoma*
- Embryonal rhabdomyosarcoma (sarcoma botryoides)*

Mixed epithelial and mesenchymal tumors

- Adenosarcoma
- Carcinosarcoma (malignant mixed müllerian tumor)*

Miscellaneous tumors

- Malignant melanoma*
- Lymphoma*
- Tumors of germ cell type

Secondary tumors

(‡Benign tumors are not included; *discussed in this chapter.)

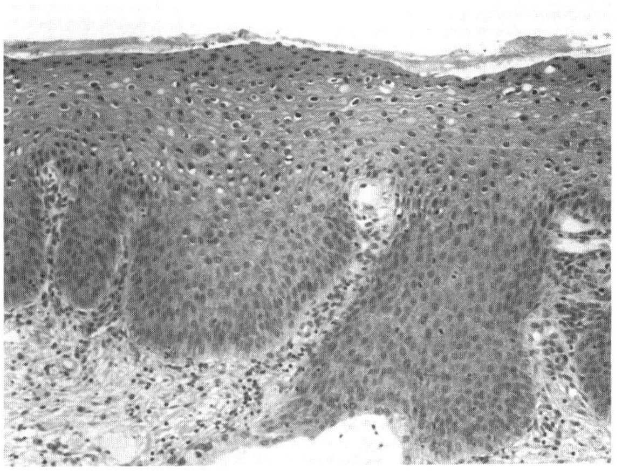

Figure 3.12. Cervical intraepithelial neoplasia (CIN) 1.

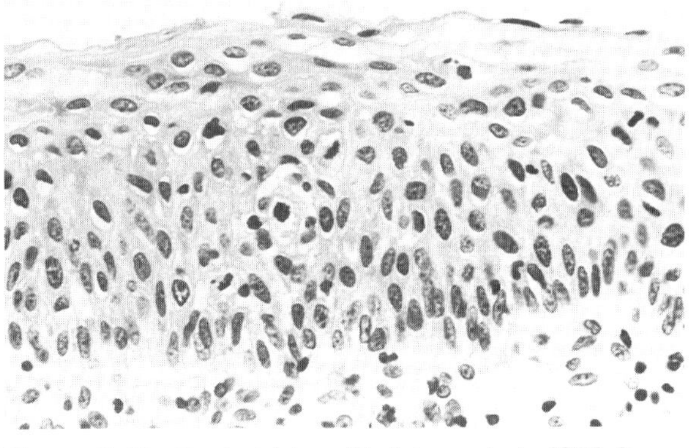

Figure 3.13. Cervical intraepithelial neoplasia (CIN) 2.

USA, for the translation of this system of nomenclature to the histopathological reporting of cervical epithelial abnormalities. The concept of a two-tier system is attractive as it is the most relevant system for patient management because many clinicians already group CIN 2 and CIN 3 together for treatment, and it is simpler to use than the three tier system. However, the most important dividing line, that between CIN 1 and CIN 2, is no better defined in any of the proposed two-tier systems than it is in the established three-tier CIN system. The use of a two-tier grading system will neither eliminate nor reduce errors, though it will have the apparent but illusory effect of increasing the diagnostic consistency of the two categories that have been grouped together (i.e. CIN 2 and CIN 3) (Anderson *et al.*, 1991). The grouping of CIN 1 with epithelium that shows the features of wart virus infection is a point of further concern; it is possible and indeed desirable to distinguish between CIN 1 with wart virus infection and CIN 1 without wart virus infection. Furthermore, the divisions of the two-tier systems are not based on any more scientific data than are the three CIN divisions in terms of prognostic validity as concerns progression to more advanced disease and to invasive carcinoma. Studies looking at the long-term outcome using the divisions of the proposed two-tier systems are needed before the validity of their groupings and points of division can be accepted. The time does not yet seem right for a re-classification of the histopathology of cervical epithelial abnormalities and it is the established three-tier CIN system that will be used in this chapter (Anderson *et al.*, 1991).

Histology The histologic features on which a diagnosis of CIN is based relate to differentiation, nuclear abnormalities and mitotic activity. The grades of CIN may be characterized as follows.

CIN 1 Nuclear abnormalities are mild and are most marked in the basal one-third of the epithelium although some nuclear abnormality persists to the surface; were this no so, a cytologic diagnosis would not be possible. Mitotic figures are present, but are not numerous and are confined to the basal one-third of the epithelium. The upper two-thirds of the epithelium shows good differentiation (*Figure 3.12*).

CIN 2 Nuclear abnormalities are more severe than in CIN 1 and nuclei showing more abnormality are found higher in the epithelium. Mitotic figures, which may be abnormal, are seen in the basal two-thirds of the epithelium (*Figure 3.13*). The upper half of the epithelium shows maturation and differentiation, with some nuclear atypia persisting to the surface.

CIN 3 Marked nuclear abnormalities are present throughout the whole thickness of the epithelium, with mitotic figures found at all levels of the epithelium. Abnormal configurations may be frequent. Maturation and differentiation are either completely absent (*Figure 3.14*) or confined to the superficial one third of the epithelium (*Figure 3.15*).

Attempts have been made to classify CIN, the

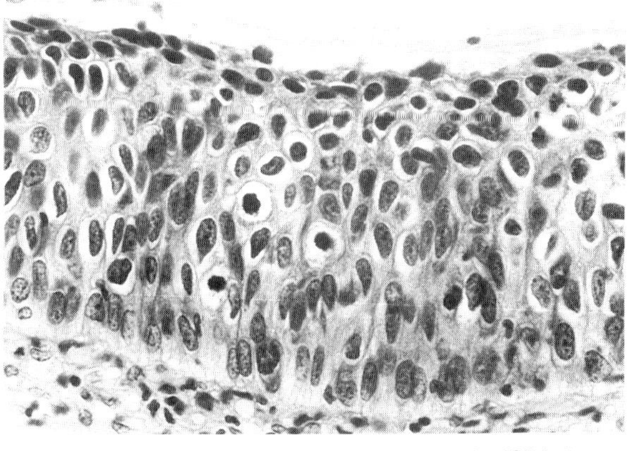

Figure 3.14. Cervical intraepithelial neoplasia (CIN) 3.

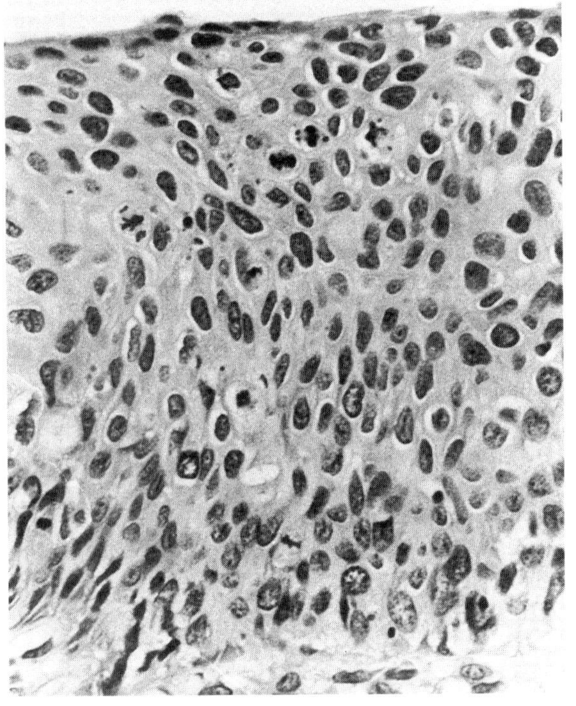

Figure 3.15. Cervical intraepithelial neoplasia (CIN) 3.

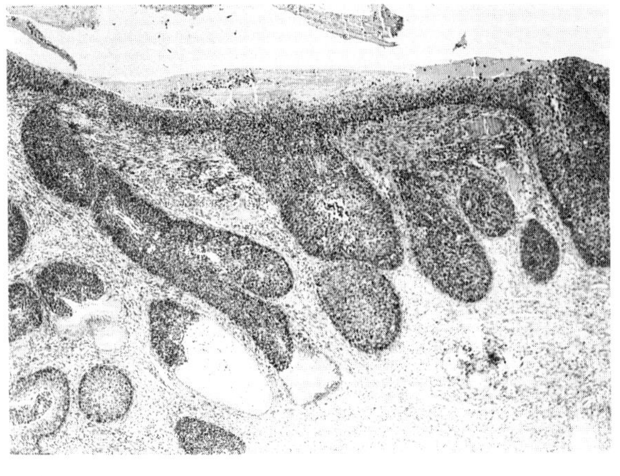

Figure 3.16. Cervical intraepithelial neoplasia (CIN) 3 showing extensive crypt involvement.

most popular distinguishing between small cell nonkeratinizing and large cell nonkeratinizing and keratinizing forms. The histologic appearances of the keratinizing form are quite striking; these result in clinical and colposcopic leukoplakia.

CIN is not solely a surface phenomenon and it must always be remembered that the endocervical crypts may be affected (*Figure 3.16*). Anderson and Hartley (1980) found that 88.6% of 343 conization specimens with CIN 3 had some crypts involved by CIN. The mean depth of involvement was 1.24 mm and the maximum was 5.22 mm. The mean plus three standard deviations (a figure that includes 99.7% of the population) was 3.80 mm. Subsequent work (Abdul–Karim *et al.*, 1982) has shown that the depth of involvement of the crypts becomes more marked as the grade of CIN increases, and that more severe forms of CIN occupy a greater linear dimension on the surface of the cervix than the minor forms.

Microinvasive carcinoma

The concept of microinvasive carcinoma was introduced by Mestwerdt in 1947 and the term was used to describe invasive lesions extending not more than 5 mm into the cervical stroma, in the belief that the small lesions had a much better prognosis than the remainder of Stage I lesions (Mestwerdt, 1951). A diagnosis of microinvasive carcinoma should characterize a tumor that is of measurable size and locally invasive, but nevertheless has negligible potential for metastasis. Unfortunately, information is not available for such a diagnosis to be precisely defined at present.

Histology The earliest stage of invasion is recognizable as a tiny bud of cells pushing into the stroma from an area of CIN (*Figure 3.17*). The invasive tongue of cells is often better differentiated that the CIN from which it has arisen and there is also frequently a pronounced stromal reaction to the infiltrating tumor, expressed either as a localized lymphocytic reaction or a loosening of the stroma; both may be seen together (*Figure 3.18*). These earliest stages of invasive squamous cell carcinoma, shown in *Figures 3.17 and 3.18*, in which invasive

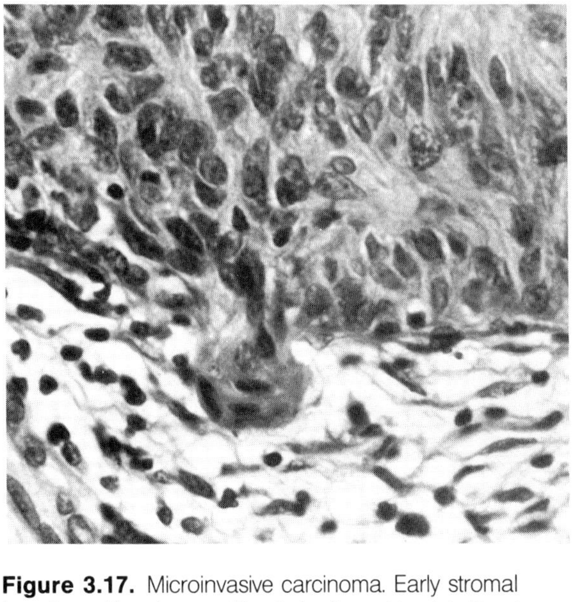

Figure 3.17. Microinvasive carcinoma. Early stromal invasion, with only a small bud of cells pushing into the stroma.

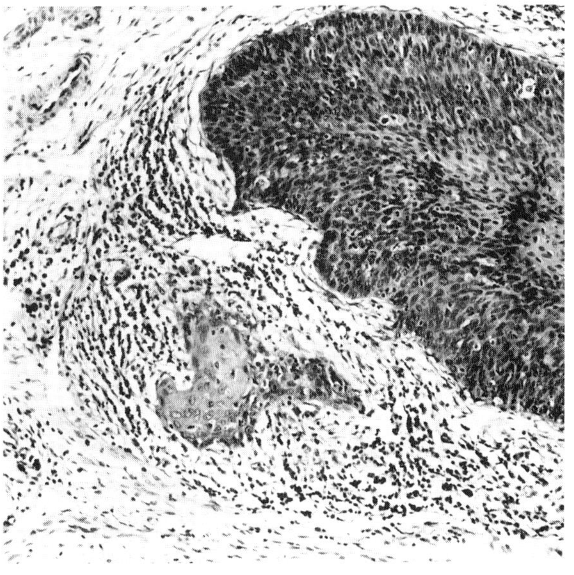

Figure 3.18. Microinvasive carcinoma showing irregularity of the invasive bud with a surrounding stromal reaction.

buds are present either in continuity with an intraepithelial lesion or apparently separated from the nearest surface or crypt basement membrane by not more than 1 mm, are designated early stromal invasion (Stage IA1).

As the invasion becomes more advanced, account is taken of other histological changes: the dimensions of the tumor, lymphatic channel involvement and the pattern of growth.

Tumor dimensions Although there is no general agreement over the maximum depth of invasion that can be included in the category of microinvasive carcinoma, it is accepted that the deeper the invasion, the worse the prognosis and the greater the need for radical treatment. It has been suggested (Burghardt, 1982) that a measurement of tumor volume gives a more reliable indication of the prognosis than measurements in only one or two dimensions. The assessment of volume requires step serial sections: when the distance between the sections is known, the third dimension can be calculated, as well as the two dimensions of depth and width in the section that shows the largest area. Burghardt and Holzer (1977) have shown that there is no risk of metastatic spread until the tumor size reaches 500 mm^3, provided vascular invasion is not seen. Although this method of assessment would probably not be practicable in many busy routine laboratories, it is recommended that measurements of tumor size should be made in two dimensions, assessing depth of invasion and the width of the area over which invasion is occurring.

Vessel space involvement Although it may seem reasonable to argue that an early invasive carcinoma that has vessel space involvement is more likely to have a lymph node metastasis than one in which vessel space involvement is not seen, the information relating to this point in the cervix is conflicting and made all the more difficult by the diversity of lesions that have been accepted as microinvasive. Roche and Norris (1975) examined 30 cervices with microinvasive carcinoma (with invasion of 2–5 mm from the surface epithelium) by step serial sections and found 'capillary-like space' involvement in 57% of patients. These women had all been treated by radical hysterectomy with pelvic lymphadenectomy, but no metastatic deposits were found in the lymph nodes. As a result of this study, it was concluded that the presence of tumor in the vessel spaces surrounding a microinvasive carcinoma was in itself of no value in predicting which patients were likely to have lymph node metastasis. However, Burghardt (1982), Holzer (1982) and Kolstad *et al.* (1982) all suggest that the presence of vessel space involvement is an indicator of an increased risk of metastasis in early invasive carcinoma of the cervix and should therefore be taken into account. Although vessel space involvement may be seen in tumors where the depth of invasion is no greater than 1 mm, it is seen more frequently as the tumor increases in size (Hasumi *et al.*, 1980). These differences of opinion give rise to a dilemma in recommending treatment because if it is believed that vessel space involvement indicates an increased risk of lymph node metastasis, then radical treatment may be necessary, even though the depth of invasion is slight. This problem has not yet been resolved, but it would seem sensible to take account of vessel space involvement in determining whether radical treatment is advisable only in those microinvasive carcinomas in which invasion is to 3 mm or more (Simon *et al.*, 1986). Even so, Maiman *et al.* (1988) reported an overall incidence of pelvic node metastases of 5% in 117 women with invasion of 1–5 mm. The risk when invasion was 3 mm or less was 2%, and one patient with invasion measured at only 2 mm had vessel space involvement and pelvic node metastases.

Growth pattern As shown in *Figures 3.17 and 3.18* the earliest microinvasive tumors have a 'finger-like' pattern of growth. As the tumor becomes larger, the pattern changes to result in a confluent growth pattern, and this confluent growth pattern is therefore more likely to be associated with the presence of metastasis. However, the definition of a confluent growth pattern is not precise and it is likely that the worse prognosis associated with the so-called confluent growth pattern is because these tend to be the larger microinvasive tumors.

Definitions An attempt to improve on the previous definitions of microinvasive carcinoma was made by the Royal College of Obstetricians and Gynaecologists Study Group on preclinical carcinoma of the cervix in 1981 (Jordan *et al.*, 1982). The following proposal was made: carcinoma of the cervix, Stage IA (microinvasive carcinoma) is a histologic diagnosis, which should be made on a large biopsy that removes the whole lesion, preferably a cone biopsy. Two groups should be recognized.

- Early stromal invasion in which invasive buds are present either in continuity with an *in situ* lesion, or apparently separated cells not more than 1 mm from the nearest surface or crypt basement membrane.
- Measurable lesions, which should be measured in two dimensions. The depth should be measured from the base of the epithelium from which it develops and should not exceed 5 mm, and the largest dimension should not exceed 10 mm on the section that shows the greatest extent. When reporting Stage IA lesions, the chosen depth and diameter for including the cases in these statistics should be given. Furthermore, the percentage of confluent lesions in cases with involvement of endothelium-lined spaces (vessels) should be stated.

FIGO has taken account of these recommendations in its most recent staging of cervical carcinoma. However, it should be noted that 7 mm has been recommended as the maximum width of Stage IA2 lesions, rather than 10 mm and that the FIGO definition of Stage IA1 is less precise than that given above. Since the publication of the modified 1985 FIGO staging for cervical cancer there have been several reports retrospectively analyzing the data from series of women with microinvasive carcinoma, most of whom were treated by radical hysterectomy, to determine how this classification of microinvasive carcinoma relates to outcome and whether or not it can be used to guide definitive treatment (Maiman *et al.*, 1988; Kolstad, 1989; Tsukamoto *et al.*, 1989; Burghardt *et al.*, 1991; Sevin *et al.*, 1992). It is generally agreed that Stage IA1 carcinoma (early stromal invasion) behaves in the same way as CIN and that conservative excisional methods of treatment can be used safely if 1 mm is taken as the upper limit for depth of invasion in this category. Stage IA2, however, is a heterogeneous category, with women with larger tumors within the defined measurements having a much higher risk of lymph node metastases and recurrence than those with smaller tumors. Pooled data indicate that a maximum depth of invasion of 3 mm or less is associated with a risk of lymph node metastasis of only 0.3% and a risk of an invasive recurrence of 0.2%. On the other hand, invasion of 3.1–5.0 mm is associated with an overall risk of lymph node metastases of 7.4% and a recurrence rate of 5.4% (Sevin *et al.*, 1992). FIGO Stage IA must therefore **not** be taken as a definition of microinvasion that can be used to determine whether a patient should be treated conservatively or radically; many patients whose tumors fall within this category need radical treatment. All the available evidence indicates that the upper cut-off point for a routine recommendation of conservative treatment should be a maximum depth of invasion of 3 mm and that lymphatic channel involvement should be absent.

Invasive carcinoma

Cervical cancer causes about 1700 deaths each year in England and Wales and is responsible for 4% of all deaths from neoplasia in women. This compares with 14,000 deaths annually from breast cancer, 3900 from ovarian cancer and 1700 from cancer of the uterine corpus. Of the deaths from cervical cancer, 50% occur in the two decades 45–65 with a range from 20 to over 85 years. The peak age incidence for registration of invasive cervical cancer is 60–64 years. It has been estimated that an average woman under 40 years of age has a 2% change of eventually developing cervical cancer.

Squamous cell carcinoma is by far the most common tumor of the cervix, accounting for 85–90% of primary neoplasms, the various types of adenocarcinoma making up a further 5–15% of the total. The remainder are mainly sarcomas, but also include lymphomas and melanoma. The cervix is an unusual site for secondary deposits.

Squamous cell carcinoma

Gross features A squamous cell carcinoma may grow out from the surface of the cervix as a papillary or polypoid excrescence, or its growth may be mainly endophytic, infiltrating into the surrounding structures, without obvious surface growth. If necrosis occurs, ulceration may be conspicuous.

Microscopic features Squamous cell carcinomas may be subdivided histologically according to cell type and histological grade. Keratinizing, non-keratinizing, verrucous, warty (condylomatous), papillary and lymphoepithelioma-like carcinoma are the subdivisions that are recommended by the World Health Organization (Scully *et al.*, 1994).

Keratinizing carcinoma This is composed of islands of squamous cells, the most striking feature of which is the rounded whorls of cells with central nests of brightly eosinophilic keratin (*Figure 3.19*). Cytoplasmic keratinization, keratohyalin granules and intercellular bridges are seen. Although many keratinizing squamous cell carcinomas of the cervix appear by virtue of their keratin production to be well-differentiated tumors, the nuclear grade may sometimes be severe; the term keratinizing does not always equate with low grade.

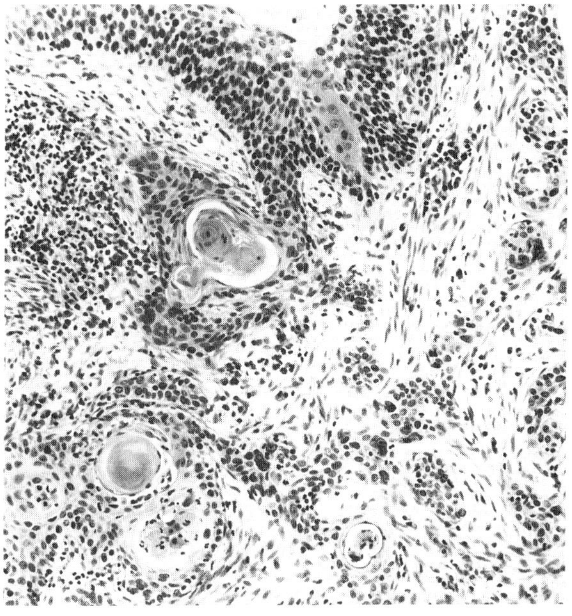

Figure 3.19. Invasive squamous cell carcinoma – keratinizing type.

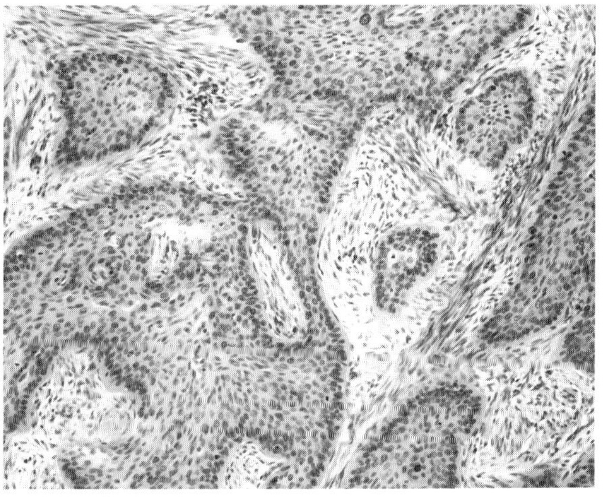

Figure 3.20. Invasive squamous cell carcinoma – nonkeratinizing type.

Nonkeratinizing carcinoma This carcinoma contains cells, which although generally recognizable as being squamous because of their polygonal shape, show little or no keratinization and no keratin pearls (*Figure 3.20*). Occasional tumors in this category are of low nuclear grade, but most are of intermediate or high grade with striking cellular and nuclear pleomorphism. Mitotic figures may be numerous.

Verrucous carcinoma This is a variety of squamous cell carcinoma that is common to many sites including the oral cavity, larynx, foot, anogenital region, vulva, vagina and cervix. It is characterized by an exophytic papillary growth pattern, coupled with deceptively benign cytologic features and painless growth. The tumor grows slowly in size, encroaching gradually on adjoining structures. Much of it is composed histologically of very well-differentiated, benign-looking cells. The papillary fronds are often covered by keratin. The tumor has a well-defined, pushing deep margin, and even adjacent to the basement membrane the degree of atypia may be minimal. Large biopsies are necessary for the diagnosis to be made (Isaac, 1976); the correct diagnosis is not possible if only the surface layers are examined.

Warty (condylomatous) carcinoma This is the name given to a squamous cell carcinoma that has a warty surface and features of HPV infection. It has been suggested that tumors of this type may have a different pathogenesis from most keratinizing carcinomas of the vulva (Kurman *et al.*, 1993), but their establishment as a separate category in the cervix is highly questionable.

Papillary squamous cell carcinomas These have, as their name implies, a papillary architecture and an atypical squamous cell component. Although diagnostic difficulties may arise in determining whether or not invasion is present, the term does not confer a difference in behavior compared with the more usual forms.

Lymphoepithelioma-like carcinoma Lymphoepithelioma-like carcinoma (Walsh *et al.*, 1993; Weinberg *et al.*, 1993) is strikingly similar to the nasopharyngeal tumor of the same name. It is composed of poorly-defined islands of undifferentiated cells in a background intensely infiltrated by lymphocytes. The tumor cells have uniform, vesicular nuclei with prominent nucleoli and moderate amounts of slightly eosinophilic cytoplasm. The cell borders are indistinct, often imparting a syncytial-like appearance to the groups. Immunocytochemistry identifies cytokeratins within the tumor cells and T cell markers in the majority of the lymphocytes.

Outcome The clinical stage of the tumor is the most significant prognostic indicator in cervical cancer, as for most other malignant tumors. Parameters of tumor size that can be assessed in a radical hysterectomy specimen and that have independent statistically significant adverse effects are tumor volume, canal length of tumor, cervical stromal tumor-free rim and parametrial extension (Hale *et al.*, 1991; Smiley *et al.*, 1991). Lymphatic and blood vessel involvement by carcinoma cells are very important risk factors and correlate highly with lymph node metastasis, which is itself a significant prognostic indicator (Hale *et al.*, 1991; Smiley *et al.*, 1991). All the data available on prognostic factors in squamous cell carcinoma of the cervix indicate that tumor grade is of little or no prognostic value.

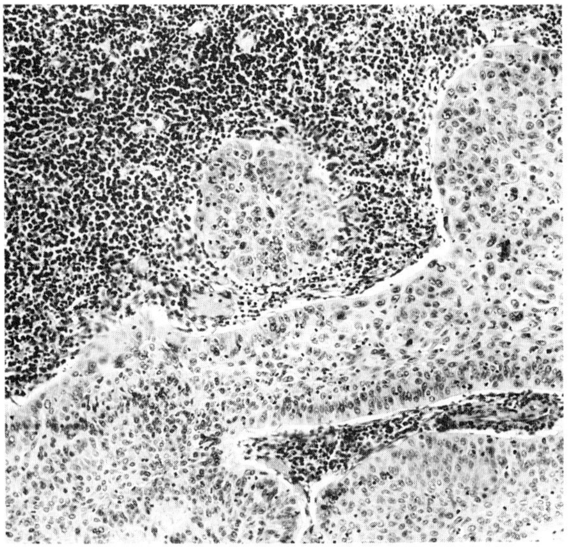

Figure 3.21. Invasive squamous cell carcinoma, showing a dense stromal lymphocytic infiltrate.

It is important to recognize the small cell carcinomas that are not of squamous type because these are associated with a poor prognosis.

All histologic subtypes of squamous cell carcinoma of the cervix grow as rounded or spiked islands of tumor cells pushing through the stroma. The intervening stroma usually contains lymphocytes, presumably representing a host immune response against the tumor antigens, and sometimes this infiltrate is very dense (*Figure 3.21*). It has been demonstrated (Van Nagell *et al.*, 1978) that carcinomas in which there is a very marked lymphocytic and plasma cell reaction in the stroma are associated with a more favorable outcome and lower incidence of metastasis to the lymph nodes than tumors that show little or no stromal reaction. Occasionally, a foreign body reaction is seen in the stroma, and is probably associated with destruction of the keratin-containing tumor cells.

Glandular tumors

Adenocarcinoma

Although the proportion of patients with adenocarcinoma in series of cervical carcinomas is usually quoted as being 5–10%, the figures in individual series range from 4.5–34% (Helper *et al.*, 1952; Davis and Moon, 1975). There has been an apparent increase in the proportion of adenocarcinomas that may be due to the effect of screening and treatment of preinvasive disease on the incidence of squamous cell carcinoma. Even so, Shingleton *et al.* (1981) believe that there is an absolute increase in the proportion of adenocarcinomas in women with cervical cancer.

Cervical glandular intraepithelial neoplasia Adenocarcinoma *in situ* (AIS) of the cervix has been recognized for over 30 years (Friedell and McKay, 1953) and it is being diagnosed with increasing frequency, often in association with squamous CIN (Gloor and Ruzicka, 1982) or at the edge of an invasive adenocarcinoma. The most straightforward microscopical concept of cervical glandular intraepithelial neoplasia (CGIN) is of endocervical crypts showing a normal architectural pattern, but with the epithelium replaced by atypical cells showing a loss of polarity, increased nuclear size, nuclear pleomorphism, anisokaryosis, mitotic activity, reduction in cytoplasmic mucin and stratification (*Figures 3.22 and 3.23*). There is usually a sharp borderline between the normal and abnormal epithelium. The abnormalities may affect surface epithelium and gland crypts either focally, adjacent to the squamocolumnar junction, multifocally or as a widespread field change affecting much of the endocervical columnar crypt field. The glandular abnormalities of the cervix appear to form a spectrum of disease just as squamous intraepithelial

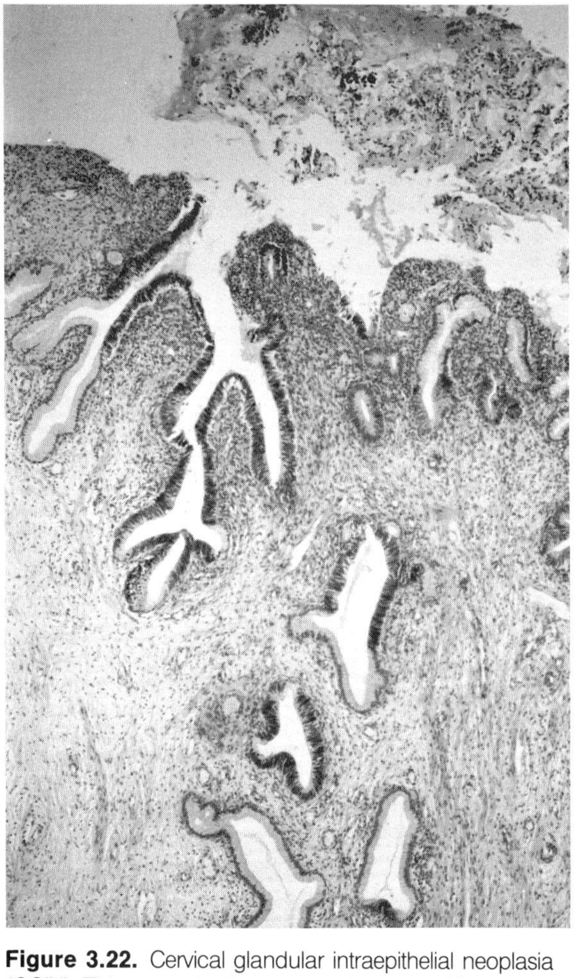

Figure 3.22. Cervical glandular intraepithelial neoplasia (CGIN). This example shows normal crypt architecture.

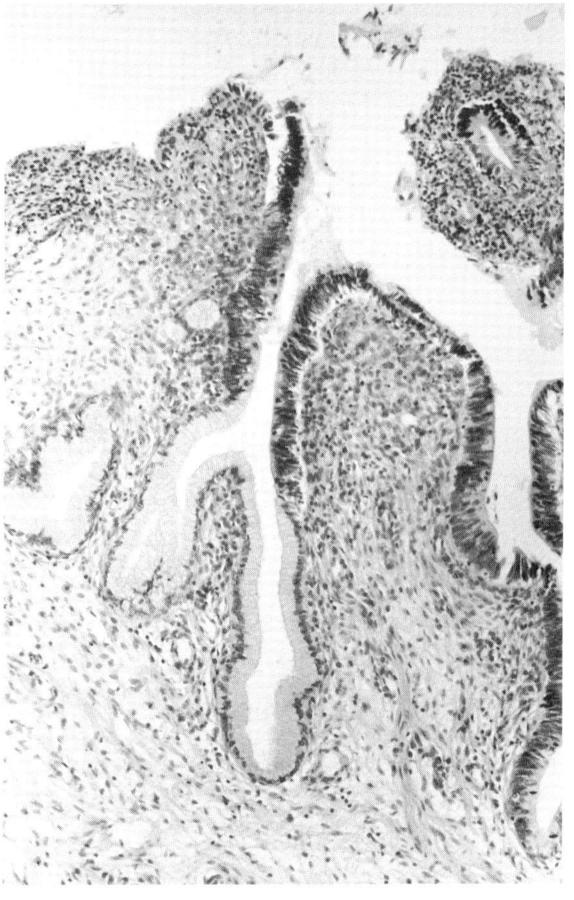

Figure 3.23. High-grade cervical glandular intraepithelial neoplasia (CGIN). At higher magnification the markedly abnormal cell morphology is apparent, with a sharp line of demarcation between normal and abnormal epithelium.

neoplasia does; high-grade CGIN is the term used for the more severe example, and less marked changes are represented by the term low-grade CGIN. Further subdivisions are made according to the histological type of the epithelium into cervical cell, endometrioid-type and intestinal-type (*Figure 3.24*).

Although, as has been implied above, the term CGIN is most appropriately used when the crypt architecture is not appreciably altered, as in *Figure 3.22*, many examples are illustrated (Weisbrot *et al.*, 1972; Ferenczy, 1977) in which there is reduplication and budding of the crypts, sometimes with a back-to-back pattern of the gland (one use of the term 'tunnel clusters'), as seen in *Figures 3.25 and 3.26*. It is not clear to what degree architectural disturbances of this type remain consistent with a diagnosis of CGIN or when the lesion should be considered invasive; there can be no doubt that, if the abnormal glands extend deeper than the deepest extent of the normal crypts, then the tumor must be considered an invasive adenocarcinoma. There seems little value in using the term 'microinvasive adenocarcinoma' (Burghardt, 1973; Qizilbash, 1975); the criteria for making this diagnosis are unclear and likely to be different from those used for squamous cell carcinomas.

CGIN may be present for many years before invasive carcinoma develops. Studies have shown that the average age of women with AIS is 15–18 years less than that of women with invasive carcinoma (Boon *et al.*, 1981; Gloor and Ruzicka, 1982). On reviewing the previous smears of 13

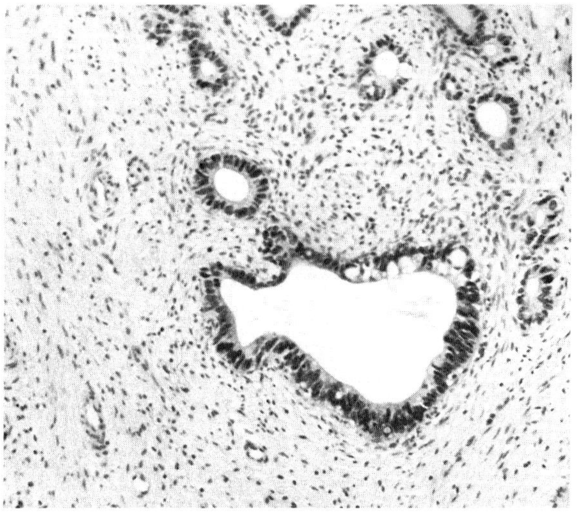

Figure 3.24. Cervical glandular intraepithelial neoplasia (CGIN) of intestinal type.

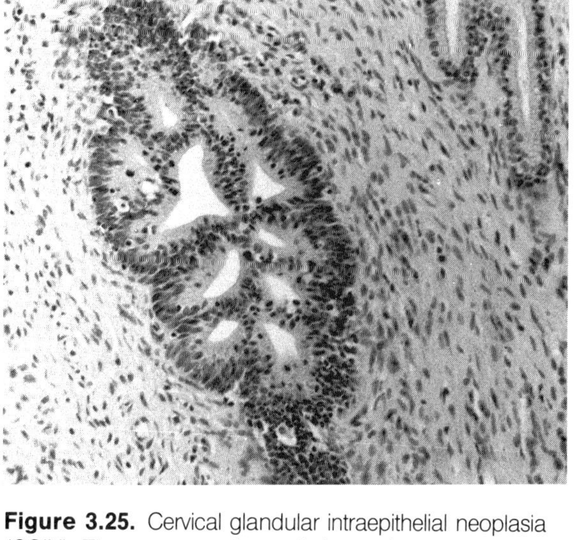

Figure 3.25. Cervical glandular intraepithelial neoplasia (CGIN). The presence of tunnel clusters is not an indication of invasion.

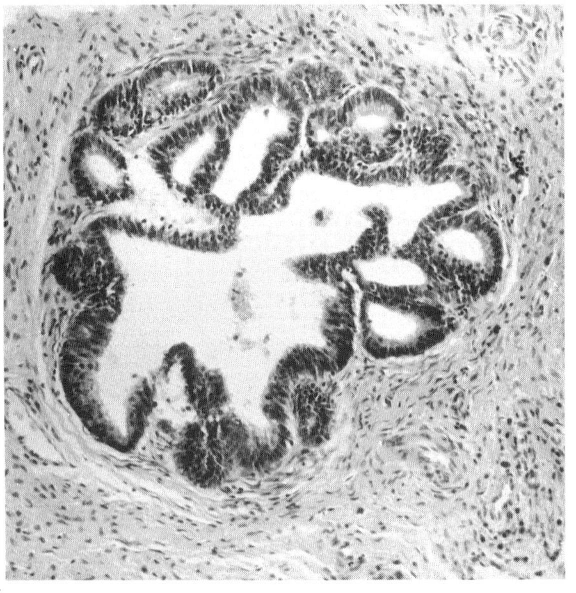

Figure 3.26. Cervical glandular intraepithelial neoplasia (CGIN) showing irregular tunnel clusters, almost amounting to a cribriform pattern.

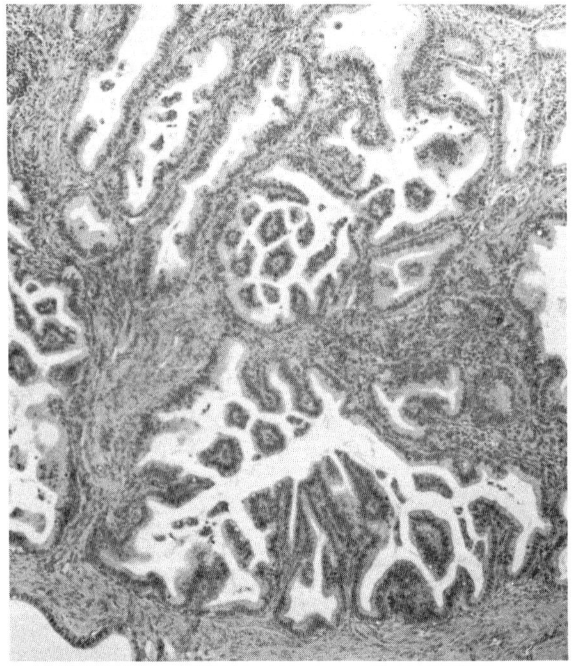

Figure 3.27. Invasive adenocarcinoma – endocervical cell type.

women with invasive adenocarcinoma of the cervix, Boddington *et al.* (1976) found that six had abnormalities for intervals ranging from 2–8 years, indicating a long evolution of the disease.

Invasive adenocarcinomas

Histology Several different patterns of invasive adenocarcinomas of the cervix are found.

Endocervical type The endocervical type of tumor is the commonest, accounting for up to 90% of some series (McKelvey and Goodlin, 1963). The epithelium generally resembles that of the normal endocervical crypts, forming glands of variable size and shape with budding and branching of the epithelium (*Figure 3.27*). The individual cells paradoxically often show less abnormality than is seen in CGIN.

Minimal deviation adenocarcinoma Minimal deviation adenocarcinoma (Kaminski and Norris, 1983; Steeper and Wick, 1986), .previously termed 'adenoma malignum' (Silverberg and Hurt, 1975), describes a carcinoma in which the glandular pattern is very well differentiated and there is virtually no atypia of the epithelial cells (*Figure 3.28*). The correct diagnosis is virtually impossible on a small biopsy because the glandular epithelium shows insufficient atypia to allow distinction from the normal to be made. Nevertheless, the benign appearance of these tumors is misleading and they may be associated with a poor prognosis (Kaku and Enjoji, 1983).

Mucinous tumors Mucinous tumors are composed of cells of enteric type and have abundant, mucin-rich cytoplasm with basal nuclei. The gland lumina are distended by abundant mucin and this may also be present as pools in the stroma (Shingleton *et al.*, 1981).

Endometrioid carcinomas These tumors have a similar appearance to the common type of endometrial carcinoma, so this is a diagnosis that can only be made if the endometrium itself is normal and can really only be made on a complete hysterectomy specimen. The distinction between the endocervical pattern and endometrioid pattern is only possible in a well-differentiated tumor.

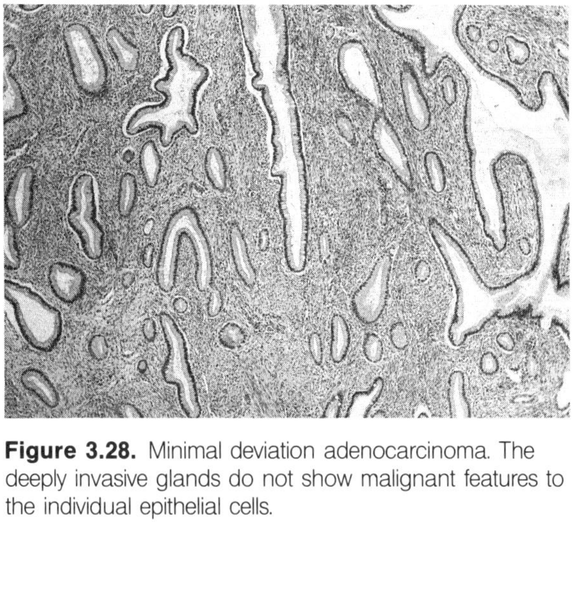

Figure 3.28. Minimal deviation adenocarcinoma. The deeply invasive glands do not show malignant features to the individual epithelial cells.

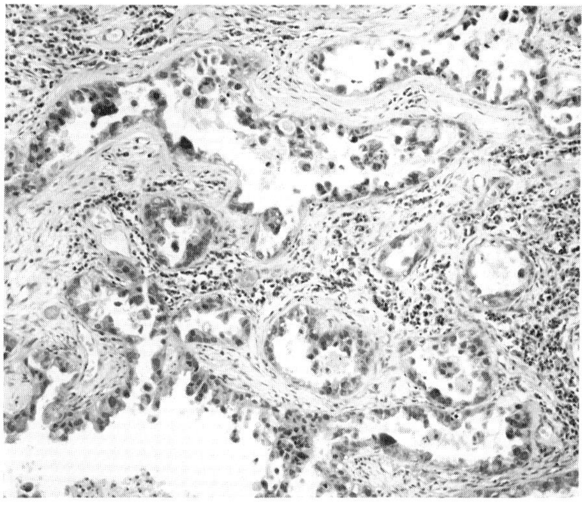

Figure 3.29. Invasive adenocarcinoma – clear cell type. This tubulocystic area shows many cells of 'hobnail' pattern. Paradoxically, clear cells are not prominent.

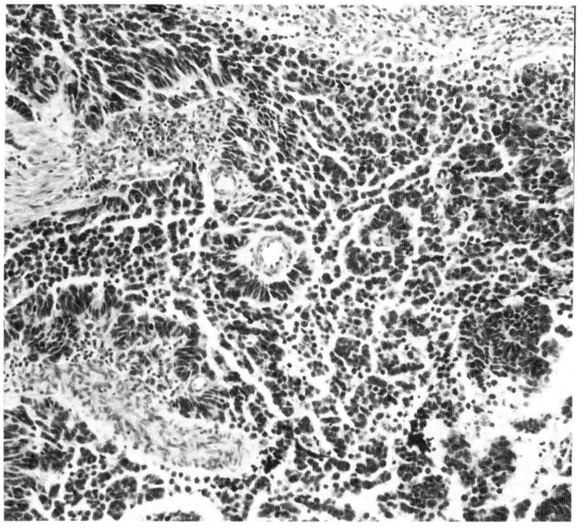

Figure 3.30. Small cell neuroendocrine carcinoma. The appearances are similar to those of a small cell carcinoma of the bronchus.

Clear cell carcinoma There are two types of clear cell carcinoma of the cervix. First, tumors of either endocervical or endometrioid pattern may have small areas of clear cells forming either solid sheets or poorly developed glands. The second type of clear cell tumor is that which has previously been referred to as the mesonephroid (or mesonephric) carcinoma, composed of a variety of patterns: solid, clear cell areas, tubulocystic areas with 'hobnail' epithelium and papillary areas (*Figure 3.29*). This type of tumor, which makes up only about 2% of cervical carcinomas, has been extensively studied because of its development in the daughters of women who were given DES in pregnancy. They are histologically identical to the tumors of the same name found in the ovary, endometrium and vagina. These tumors are of paramesonephric origin rather than meson ephric, as their alternative name might suggest.

Papillary serous carcinoma The papillary tumor is usually seen in conjunction with other patterns and is rare as a pure variant. It is composed of complex papillary fronds supported by a fibrovascular core. The papillary serous carcinoma is a particularly uncommon variant, similar in morphology to the tumor of the same name in the ovary.

Other epithelial tumors

Adenosquamous carcinoma

Adenosquamous carcinoma is composed of a mixture of malignant glandular and squamous epithelial components. Although some authors state that more than a minor component of glandular cells is required to alter the diagnosis from squamous cell carcinoma to adenosquamous carcinoma (Scully *et al.*, 1994), others believe that finding even tiny amounts of mucin in what seems otherwise to be a squamous cell carcinoma puts the tumor into a less favorable outcome group (Buckley *et al.*, 1988; Bethwaite *et al.*, 1992).

Small cell carcinoma

This is composed of small, rounded cells with generally uniform, dark nuclei (*Figure 3.30*) and should be distinguished from small cell non-keratinizing squamous cell carcinomas. These tumors have been shown to have neuroendocrine features and resemble the small cell anaplastic ('oat cell') carcinoma of the bronchus (Tateishi *et al.*, 1975). The prognosis is poor.

Mesenchymal and Miscellaneous Tumors of the Cervix

Embryonal rhabdomyosarcoma (sarcoma botryoides)

Embryonal rhabdomyosarcoma is a tumor usually found in children, presenting as a soft, polypoid, grape-like mass at the introitus and filling the whole vagina. It is a highly malignant tumor arising from the subepithelial müllerian stromal layer, which is present in the cervix and vagina. It is composed of loose, myxoid tissue which contains scattered striated rhabdomyoblasts. The childhood variant is, in the great majority of cases, of vaginal origin and the cervical so-called 'sarcoma botryoides' appears to be a separate entity (Daya and Scully, 1988).

Leiomyosarcoma

This may arise from a leiomyoma of the cervical stroma or from the smooth muscle of the cervical blood vessels.

Sarcomas and carcinosarcomas

Sarcomas and carcinosarcomas containing homologous mesenchymal elements (tissue expected in the cervix) or heterologous mesenchymal elements (tissue not usually found in the cervix), also termed malignant mixed müllerian tumors (MMMT), have been reported (Abell, 1973). Sarcomas of endocervical stromal type are found, arising from the substantia propria of the cervix. The sarcomas and MMMTs behave in a way generally similar to their counterparts in the body of the uterus and are aggressive when poorly differentiated.

Malignant lymphomas

Malignant lymphomas, including Hodgkin's disease, diffuse histiocytic lymphoma and plasmacytoma have all been reported (Neuberg, 1974; Stransky *et al.*, 1953).

Malignant melanoma

This has very rarely been encountered (Jones *et al.*, 1971).

Summary of Core Information

- Vaginal intraepithelial neoplasia (VaIN) is currently divided into three morphologic grades (I, II, and III) similar to cervical intraepithelial neoplasia (CIN) and vulvar intraepithelial neoplasia (VIN); however, its natural history is not necessarily the same.
- VaIN is frequently associated with other examples of lower genital tract squamous intraepithelial neoplasia, including CIN, VIN, and perianal intraepithelial neoplasia.
- Microinvasive squamous carcinoma of the vagina is poorly defined from a clinicopathologic standpoint; until such a definition is accomplished, the pertinent histopathologic parameters should be documented in the report.
- The most common sites of squamous carcinoma of the vagina are the upper one-third of the posterior wall, and the lower one-third of the anterior wall; the former metastasizes like a cervical cancer and the latter like a vulvar cancer.
- Secondary tumors (particularly from the cervix and endometrium) are the most common malignant vaginal tumors and are 2–9 times more common than primary neoplasms.
- Regarding the terminology of CIN, there is considerable controversy over whether the current three-tier (grade) system should be retained or a two-tier system introduced to correspond to that of The Bethesda System (TBS) for cytopathology.
- Although yet controversial, current clinicopathologic data suggest that the criteria for conservative treatment of 'microinvasive' cervical squamous carcinoma are a maximum depth of invasion of 3 mm and no vascular channel involvement.
- Intermediate- to high-grade nonkeratinizing squamous carcinoma is the most common malignant tumor of the cervix and its clinical stage is the most important prognostic parameter.
- Cervical glandular intraepithelial neoplasia (CGIN) may be increasing in frequency and often coexists with squamous intraepithelial neoplasia; consequently, it may be easily overlooked.
- Small cell undifferentiated (neuroendocrine) carcinomas of the cervix tend to occur in younger women and have a poor prognosis.

References

Abdul–Karim FW, Fu YS, Reagan JW & Wentz WB (1982) Morphometric study of intraepithelial neoplasia of uterine cervix. *Obstet. Gynecol.* **60:** 210–214.

Abell MR (1973) *The Uterus*. International Academy of Pathology, Monographs in Pathology. Baltimore: Williams and Wilkins.

Addison WS, Hammond CB & Parker WT (1979) The occurrence of adenocarcinoma in endometriosis of the rectovaginal septum during progestational therapy. *Gynecol. Oncol.* **8:** 193–197.

Aho M, Vesterinen E, Meyer B, Purola E & Paavonen J, (1991) Natural history of vaginal intraepithelial neoplasia. *Cancer* **68:** 195–197.

■ Anderson MC, Brown CL, Buckley CH *et al.* (1991) Current views on cervical intraepithelial neoplasia. *J. Clin. Pathol.* **44:** 969–978.

Anderson MC & Hartley RB (1980) Cervical crypt involvement by intraepithelial neoplasia. *Obstet. Gynecol.* **55:** 546–550.

Bethwaite P, Yeong ML, Holloway L *et al.* (1992) The prognosis of adenosquamous carcinomas of the uterine cervix. *Br. J. Obstet. Gynaecol.* **99:** 745–750.

Boddington MM, Spriggs AI & Cowdell RH (1976) Adenocarcinoma of the uterine cervix: cytological evidence of a long preclinical evolution. *Br. J. Obstet. Gynaecol.* **83:** 900–903.

Boon ME, Baak JPA, Kurver PJH, Overdiep SH & Verdonk GW (1981) Adenocarcinoma *in situ* of the cervix: an underdiagnosed lesion. *Cancer* **48:** 768–773.

Branton PA & Tavassoli FA (1993) Spindle cell epithelioma, the so-called mixed tumor of the vagina. A clinicopathologic, immunohistochemical, and ultrastructural analysis of 28 cases. *Am. J. Surg. Pathol.* **17:** 509–515.

Buckley CH, Beards CS & Fox H (1988) Pathological prognostic indicators in cervical cancer with particular reference to patients under the age of 40 years. *Br. J. Obstet. Gynaecol.* **95:** 47–56.

Burghardt E (1973) Early histological diagnosis of cervical cancer. In: Friedman EA (ed.) *Major Problems in Obstetrics and Gynecology*. Philadelphia: Saunders.

Burghardt E (1982) Diagnostic and prognostic criteria in cervical microcarcinoma. *Clin. Oncol.* **1:** 323–333.

■ Burghardt E, Girardi F, Lahousen M, Pickel H & Tamussino K (1991) Microinvasive carcinoma of the uterine cervix (International Federation of Gynecology and Obstetrics Stage IA). *Cancer* **67:** 1037–1045.

Burghardt E & Holzer E (1977) Diagnosis and treatment of microinvasive carcinoma of the cervix uteri. *Obstet. Gynecol.* **49:** 641–653.

Chung AF, Casey MJ & Flannery JT (1980) Malignant melanoma of the vagina – report of 19 cases. *Obstet. Gynecol.* **55:** 720–727.

Clement PB & Benedet JL (1979) Adenocarcinoma *in-situ* of the vagina: a case report. *Cancer* **43:** 2479–2485.

Cullimore JF, Luesley DM, Rollason TP, Waddell CW & Williams DR (1989) A case of glandular intraepithelial neoplasia involving the cervix and vagina. *Gynecol. Oncol.* **34:** 249–252.

Davis JR & Moon LB (1975) Increased incidence of adenocarcinoma of uterine cervix. *Obstet. Gynecol.* **45:** 79–83.

Daya DA & Scully RE (1988) Sarcoma botryoides of the uterine cervix in young women: A clinicopathological study of 13 cases. *Gynecol. Oncol.* **29:** 290–303.

Ferenczy A (1977) Carcinoma and other malignant diseases of the cervix. In: Blaustein A (ed.) *Pathology of the Female Genital Tract*, pp. 191. New York: Springer–Verlag.

Friedell GH & McKay DG (1953) Adenocarcinoma *in situ* of the endocervix. *Cancer* **6:** 887–897.

Gloor E & Ruzicka J (1982) Morphology of adenocarcinoma *in situ* of the uterine cervix: a study of 14 cases. *Cancer* **49:** 294–302.

■ Hale RJ, Wilcox FL, Buckley CH *et al.* (1991) Prognostic factors in uterine cervical carcinoma: a clinicopathological analysis. *Int. J. Gynecol. Cancer* **1:** 19–23.

Hasumi K, Sakamoto A & Sugano H (1980) Microinvasive carcinoma of the uterine cervix. *Cancer* **45:** 928–931.

Helper TK, Docherty MB & Randall LM (1952) Primary adenocarcinoma of the cervix. *Am. J. Obstet. Gynecol.* **63:** 800–808.

Herbst AL (1984) Diethylstilboestrol exposure – 1984. *N. Engl. J. Med.* **311:** 1433–1435.

Herbst AL, Green THJ & Ulfelder H (1970) Primary carcinoma of the vagina: an analysis of 68 cases. *Am. J. Obstet. Gynecol.* **106:** 210–218.

Herbst AL, Norusis MJ & Rosenow PJ (1979) An analysis of 346 cases of clear cell adenocarcinoma of the vagina and cervix with emphasis on recurrence and survival. *Gynecol. Oncol.* **7:** 111–122.

Herbst AL, Robboy SJ, Scully RE & Poskanzer DC (1974) Clear cell adenocarcinoma of the genital tract in young females. Analysis of 170 registry cases. *Am. J. Obstet. Gynecol.* **119:** 713–724.

Herbst AL & Scully RE (1970) Adenocarcinoma of the vagina in adolescence: a report of 7 cases including 6 clear cell carcinomas (so-called mesonephromas). *Cancer* **25:** 745–757.

Herbst AL, Ulfelder H & Poskanzer DC (1971) Adenocarcinoma of the vagina: association in maternal stilboestrol therapy with tumor appearance in young women. *N. Engl. J. Med.* **284:** 878–881.

Hertig AT & Gore H (1979) Tumors of the female sex organs. In: Hertig AT & Gore H (eds) *Atlas of Tumor Pathology, Tumors of the Vulva, Vagina and Uterus.* Washington DC: Armed Forces Institute of Pathology.

■ Hilborne LH & Fu YS (1987) Intraepithelial, invasive and metastatic neoplasms of the vagina. In: Wilkinson EJ (ed.) *Pathology of the Vagina and Vulva*, pp. 181–207. New York: Churchill Livingstone.

Holzer E (1982) Microinvasive carcinoma of the cervix: clinical aspects, treatment and follow-up. *Clin. Oncol.* **1:** 315–322.

Isaac JH (1976) Verrucous carcinoma of the female genital tract. *Gynecol. Oncol.* **4:** 259–269.

Ismail SM, Colclough AB, Dinnen JS *et al.* (1989) Observer variation in histopathological diagnosis and grading of cervical intraepithelial neoplasia. *Br. Med. J.* **298:** 707–710.

Jones HW, Droegemueller W & Makowski EL (1971) A primary melanocarcinoma of the cervix. *Am. J. Obstet. Gynecol.* **111:** 959–963.

Jordan JA, Sharp F & Singer A (1982) Appendix 1. In: Jordan JA, Sharp F & Singer A (eds) *Pre-clinical Neoplasia of the Cervix*, pp. 301. London: Royal College of Obstetricians and Gynaecologists.

Kaku T & Enjoji M (1983) Extremely well-differentiated adenocarcinoma ('adenoma malignum') of the cervix. *Int. J. Gynecol. Pathol.* **2:** 28–41.

Kaminski PF & Norris HJ (1983) Minimal deviation carcinoma (adenoma malignum) of the cervix. *Int. J. Gynecol. Pathol.* **2:** 141–152.

Kolstad P (1989) Follow-up study of 232 patients with stage Ia1 and 411 patients with stage Ia2 squamous cell carcinoma of the cervix (microinvasive carcinoma). *Gynecol. Oncol.* **33:** 265–272.

Kolstad P, Abeler V, Iversen T & Kjorstad K (1982) Microinvasive carcinoma of the cervix: definition and treatment problems. *Clin. Oncol.* **1:** 335–347.

Kottmeier HL (1973) Carcinoma of the vulva. *Annual Report of Results of Treatment of Carcinoma of the Uterus, Vagina and Ovary*. Stockholm: International Federation of Gynecology and Obstetrics.

Kurman RJ, Toki T & Schiffman MH (1993) Basaloid and warty carcinomas of the vulva – distinctive types of squamous cell carcinoma frequently associated with human papillomaviruses. *Am. J. Surg. Pathol.* **17:** 133–145.

Luff R, Kurman R & Solomon D (1992) The Bethesda system for reporting cervical vaginal cytologic diagnoses

– report of the 1991 Bethesda workshop. *Am. J. Surg. Pathol.* **16:** 914–916.

Maiman MA, Fructer RG, DiMaio TM & Boyce JG (1988) Superficially invasive squamous cell carcinoma of the cervix. *Obstet. Gynecol.* **72:** 399–403.

McKelvey JL & Goodlin RR (1963) Adenoma malignum of the cervix. A cancer of deceptively innocent histological pattern. *Cancer* **16:** 549–557.

Mestwerdt G (1951) Elective therapie des mikrokarzinoms am collum uteri? *Zentralbl. Gynaekol.* **73:** 558–567.

Neuberg R (1974) Immunosuppression and plasmacytoma of the cervix. *J. Obstet. Gynaecol. Br. Commonw.* **81:** 165–167.

Noller KL, Decker DG & Lanier AP (1972) Clear cell adenocarcinoma of the cervix after maternal treatment with synthetic estrogens. *Mayo Clin. Proc.* **47:** 629–630.

Peters WA, Kumar NB & Morley GW (1985) Microinvasive carcinoma of the vagina: A distinct clinical entity? *Am. J. Obstet. Gynecol.* **153:** 505.

Qizilbash AH (1975) *In-situ* and microinvasive adenocarcinoma of the uterine cervix. A clinical, cytological and histological study of 14 cases. *Am. J. Clin. Pathol.* **64:** 155–170.

Richart RM (1990) A modified terminology for cervical intraepithelial neoplasia. *Obstet. Gynecol.* **75:** 131–133.

Robboy SJ, Young RH & Welch WR (1984) Atypical vaginal adenosis and cervical ectropion: association with clear cell adenocarcinoma in diethylstilboestrol exposed offspring. *Cancer* **54:** 869–875.

Robertson AJ (1989) Histopathological grading of cervical intraepithelial neoplasia (CIN) – is there need for a change? *J. Pathol.* **159:** 273–275.

Robertson AJ, Anderson JM, Swanson Beck J *et al.* (1989) Observer variability in histopathological reporting of cervical biopsy specimens. *J. Clin. Pathol.* **42:** 231–238.

Roche WD & Norris HJ (1975) Microinvasive carcinoma of the cervix. The significance of lymphatic invasion and confluent patterns of stromal growth. *Cancer* **36:** 180–186.

Sanderberg EC, Danielson RW, Cauwet RW & Boner BE (1965) Adenosis vaginae. *Am. J. Obstet. Gynecol.* **93:** 209–222.

Schmidt WA (1987) Pathology of the vagina. In: Fox H (ed.) *Haines and Taylor Obstetrical and Gynecological Pathology*, pp. 146–216. London: Churchill Livingstone.

Scully RE, Bonfiglio TA, Kurman RJ, Silverberg SG & Wilkinson EJ (1994) Histological typing of female genital tract tumors. In: *World Health Organization International Histological Classification of Tumors*, pp. 39–63 2nd ed. Berlin: Springer–Verlag.

Sevin BU, Nadji M, Averette HE *et al.* (1992) Microinvasive carcinoma of the cervix. *Cancer* **70:** 2121–2128.

Shingleton HM, Gore H, Bradley DH & Soong SJ (1981) Adenocarcinoma of the cervix 1. Clinical evaluation and pathologic features. *Am. J. Obstet. Gynecol.* **139:** 799–814.

Silverberg SG & Hurt WG (1975) Minimal deviation adenocarcinoma ('adenoma malignum') of the cervix: a reappraisal. *Am. J. Obstet. Gynecol.* **121:** 971–980.

Simon NL, Gore H, Shingleton HM *et al.* (1986) Study of superficially invasive carcinoma of the cervix. *Obstet. Gynecol.* **68:** 19–24.

Smiley LM, Burke TW, Silva EG *et al.* (1991) Prognostic factors in stage IB squamous cervical cancer patients with low risk for recurrence. *Obstet. Gynecol.* **77:** 271–275.

Solomon D (1989) The 1988 Bethesda system for reporting cervical/vaginal cytological diagnoses. *Acta Cytol.* **33:** 567–574.

Solomon D (1991) The Bethesda System for reporting cervical/vaginal cytologic diagnoses: an overview. *Int. J. Gynecol. Pathol.* **10:** 323–325.

Steeper TA & Wick MR (1986) Minimal deviation adenocarcinoma of the uterine cervix ('adenoma malignum'). *Cancer* **58:** 1131–1138.

Stransky GC, Acosta AA, Kaplan AL & Friedman JA (1953) Reticulum cell sarcoma of the cervix. *Obstet. Gynecol.* **41:** 183–187.

Tateishi R, Wade A, Hayakawa K *et al.* (1975) Argyrophil cell carcinomas (apudomas) of the uterine cervix. *Virchows Arch. A Pathol. Anat. Histopathol.* **366:** 260–274.

Tavassoli FA & Norris FJ (1979) Smooth muscle tumors of the vulva. *Obstet. Gynecol.* **53:** 231–224.

Tsukamoto N, Kaku T, Matsukuma K *et al.* (1989) The problem of stage Ia (FIGO, 1985) carcinoma of the uterine cervix. *Gynecol. Oncol.* **34:** 1–6.

Van Nagell JR, Donaldson ES, Wood EG & Parker JC (1978) The significance of vascular invasion and lymphocytic infiltration in invasive cervical cancer. *Cancer* **41:** 228–234.

Wade–Evans T (1976) The aetiology and pathology of cancer of the vagina. *Clin. Obstet. Gynaecol.* **3:** 229–241.

Walsh CB, Kay E, Prendiville W, Turner M & Leader M (1993) Lymphoepithelioma-like carcinoma of the uterine cervix with C-erbB-2, p53 oncoprotein expression and DNA quantification. *Histopathology* **23:** 592–593.

Weinberg E, Hoisington S, Eastman AY *et al.* (1993) Uterine cervical lymphoepithelial-like carcinoma – absence of Epstein–Barr virus genomes. *Am. J. Clin. Pathol.* **99:** 195–199.

Weisbrot IM, Stabinsky C & Davis AM (1972) Adenocarcinoma *in situ* of the uterine cervix. *Cancer* **29:** 1179–1187.

Wentz WB & Reagan JW (1970) Clinical significance of post-irradiation dysplasia of the uterine cervix. *Am. J. Obstet. Gynecol.* **106:** 812–817.

4 Management of Preinvasive Lesions of the Cervix

M I Shafi
J A Jordan

Preinvasive lesions of the cervix have been recognized for over 100 years. In 1886 Sir John Williams presented the Harveian Lectures at which he described eight cases of cervical cancer, one of which was equivalent to carcinoma *in situ* or cervical intraepithelial neoplasia (CIN) 3 (Williams, 1886). In his lecture he stated that "this is the earliest condition of undoubted cancer of the portio vaginalis that I have met with, and it is the earliest condition which is recognizable as cancer. It presented no distinct symptoms, and was discovered accidentally."

After this early description it was not until 1925 that the basic principles of colposcopy were described (Hinselmann, 1925). The system he devised was that of low-power magnification and illumination of the cervix. With this system he hoped to recognize the earliest lesions of the cervix that were invisible to the naked eye. Around this time Schiller described the Schiller iodine test (Schiller, 1929). Normal cervical and vaginal epithelium is characterized by having an abundance of glycogen, whereas glycogen was conspicuously absent in squamous cervical cancer. Schiller's iodine solution applied to the cervix stained normal squamous epithelium rich in glycogen, but failed to stain columnar epithelium and abnormal epithelium, which contained little or no glycogen. The technique of colposcopy did not enjoy favor initially outside the German speaking world and Latin America. In these countries it was used primarily as an initial screen and most of the expertise gained consisted of assessing benign and inflammatory lesions. The technique did not evolve except for the introduction of a green filter, which enhanced recognition of vascular patterns (Kraatz, 1939). The technique further declined when cervical cytology was first described for the screening and detection of premalignant lesions of the cervix (Papanicolaou and Traut, 1941). It was not until it was realized that the disciplines were complementary rather than competitive, that colposcopy mushroomed and is now accepted worldwide.

Carcinoma of the cervix continues to be the second commonest female cancer worldwide, with only breast cancer occurring more commonly. Unlike breast cancer where no obvious preinvasive lesion is easily recognized, the occurrence of preinvasive lesions in cervical cancer is accepted. Whereas breast cancer is typically a disease of the industrialized countries, cervical cancer primarily occurs in developing countries with more than 130,000 cases in China and over 70,000 in India. This compares with approximately 47,000 in Europe, under 16,000 in North America, under 10,000 in Japan and 1200 cases in Australasia. The other important factor is that presentation of disease is late in the developing countries, with 75% presenting with an advanced stage, which is the converse of presentations in the developed countries where 75% present early and cure can be realistically expected. These data have a considerable impact on survival data from this cancer. Women in developed countries both present themselves early because of symptoms and are also part of screening strategies for prevention of cervical cancer. Since its description, the Papanicolaou cervical smear continues to be the only valid way of screening for this disease and adjunctive screening methods remain areas of interest and research.

Within the UK there is a screening strategy of a three-yearly screen from the ages of 20 to 64. In the USA an annual cervical smear is suggested in conjunction with a bimanual examination. In the UK a computerized scheme was commenced in 1988 and since then coverage of the 'at risk' population has increased from 22% to 83%, which is without parallel in the developed world (Farmery and Gray, 1994). This has seen a concomitant fall in mortality from cervical cancer with a 15% decrease between 1985 and 1991 (Imperial Cancer Research Fund, ICRF, 1993). While all age mortality declines, the biggest reduction is in the 55–64 year age group. Encouragingly, the increase in mortality in the under 35-year-olds has also plateaued.

Classification of Precancerous Lesions

The cervical intraepithelial neoplasia (CIN) classification has replaced the World Health Organization classification almost universally; CIN 1, 2 and 3 corresponding to mild, moderate and severe dysplasia/carcinoma *in situ* respectively (Richart, 1967). While categorizing a pathologic spectrum into these three categories was helpful, it has undoubtedly led to overtreatment, and debate centres around the malignant potential of the lesions concerned. There is poor intra- and interobserver agreement between histopathologists at the lower end of the spectrum – CIN 1 and human papillomavirus (HPV) associated changes (Robertson *et al*., 1989; Ismail *et al*., 1990). More recently a revised classification has been suggested with high-grade lesions (CIN 2 and 3), which are likely to behave as cancer precursors, and low-grade lesions (CIN 1 and HPV-associated changes) with unknown, but a probable low progressive potential (Richart, 1990). Previous reports of the progressive potential of CIN refer almost exclusively to CIN 3 lesions that were almost certainly large in nature (McIndoe *et al*., 1984). In this report 948 women with carcinoma *in situ* diagnosed histologically were followed for 5–28 years. Among the 817 women who had normal cytology follow-up, 12 (1.5%) developed invasive carcinoma. A second group of 131 women continued to produce abnormal cytology consistent with cervical neoplasia, and 29 (22%) of them developed invasive carcinoma of the cervix or vaginal vault. Only in 5% did the carcinoma *in situ* disappear in this latter group of women. The progressive potential has been calculated to be 18% at 10 years and 36% at 20 years. Women with continuing abnormal cytology after initial management of carcinoma *in situ* of the cervix were almost 25 times more likely to develop invasive carcinoma than women who had normal follow-up cytology. When compared with the population at large, the chances of women with normal follow-up cytology developing invasive cervical or vaginal vault carcinoma increase three-fold over women who have never had carcinoma *in situ* of the cervix. As a result, there appears to be complete unanimity for the immediate treatment of CIN 3 lesions once diagnosed.

Classification of Cervical Cytology

Reporting of cervical cytology has evolved differently on the two sides of the Atlantic Ocean since the earliest reports (Papanicolaou and Traut, 1941). The British Society for Cervical Cytology (BSCC) has made recommendations for the uniform reporting of cervical cytology (Evans *et al*., 1986). The cytology report should consist of a concise description of cells in precisely defined and generally accepted cytologic terms. This may be followed, if appropriate, by a prediction of the histologic condition based on the overall picture and should include a recommendation for further management of the patient. In North America, the Bethesda reporting system has been advocated (National Cancer Institute Workshop, 1989) and is now required in all nationally accredited cytology laboratories. The classification consists of a statement of adequacy, general categorization (normal vs. other), descriptive diagnoses (infection, miscellaneous), epithelial abnormalities and glandular cells. The classification introduces the term squamous intraepithelial lesion (SIL) to encompass all grades of CIN. SIL is further subdivided into two categories – low-grade, which includes cellular changes associated with HPV infection and CIN 1, and high-grade SIL, which includes CIN 2 and 3. The atypical squamous cells of undetermined significance (ASCUS) category is roughly equivalent to the borderline category used by the BSCC. An enhanced discussion of the Bethesda terminology in cytology is given in Chapter 2.

Management of Abnormal Cervical Smears

A flow diagram illustrating the management of abnormal cervical cytology is shown in *Figure 4.1*. Ideally all women with abnormal cervical cytology

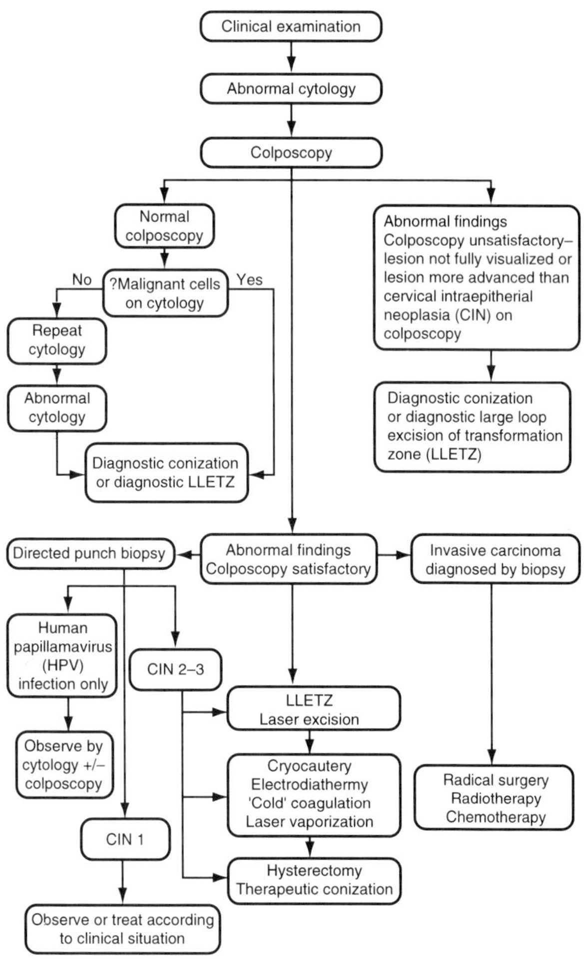

Figure 4.1. Flow diagram for management of abnormal cervical cytology.

should have colposcopic assessment. In those countries where colposcopy is still not available, cone biopsy may need to be performed for those with positive cervical cytology. If the cytologic abnormality is of a minor degree in the presence of a macroscopically normal cervix, the cervical smear may be repeated in 3–6 months and cone biopsy reserved for those in whom the abnormality persists.

Colposcopy is readily accessed in most industrialized countries and allows a more accurate assessment of the cervix. The aim of colposcopy is first to exclude an invasive process and secondarily to identify the extent of the abnormality and its likely grade, which may allow a more conservative approach to management. Colposcopic assessment is deemed to be unsatisfactory if all of the transformation zone is not visualized. This inability to visualize the squamocolumnar junction (SCJ) may be an indication for cone biopsy or other forms of excision of the cervical transformation zone.

Colposcopy

Colposcopy is primarily used to assess women with abnormal cervical cytology and define those women with CIN (*Figure 4.2*). The whole area of the transformation zone needs to be visualized as this area is the site for neoplastic change. Various parameters of the colposcopic assessment are studied including the vascular patterns, the degree of acetowhite epithelium, the border characteristics, the surface pattern and the surface area of the lesion under study. These combine to give a colposcopic opinion as to the likely nature of the lesion. This opinion is often supported by recourse to a directed punch biopsy of the worst area. If significant disease is confirmed, then appropriate treatment is undertaken. If the whole of the transformation zone is not visualized, then colposcopy is deemed to be unsatisfactory, making a colposcopically-directed punch biopsy of the worst area impossible. In this situation, recourse to a cone biopsy or extended diathermy loop procedure is recommended.

If the transformation zone is fully visualized, biopsy of the worst atypical epithelium may be undertaken. Excisional methods such as laser excision or diathermy loop provide considerably more histopathologic material than a punch biopsy. If the colposcopic assessment is entirely normal, management is dependent upon the degree of cytologic abnormality. A diagnostic excision of the transformation zone may be warranted depending on the degree of cytologic abnormality.

If the woman is pregnant at the time of colposcopic assessment, a conservative approach is usually employed and treatment undertaken after delivery. If cancer is suspected, then a large biopsy, usually a wedge biopsy, is taken under general anesthesia because there is a risk for significant hemorrhage.

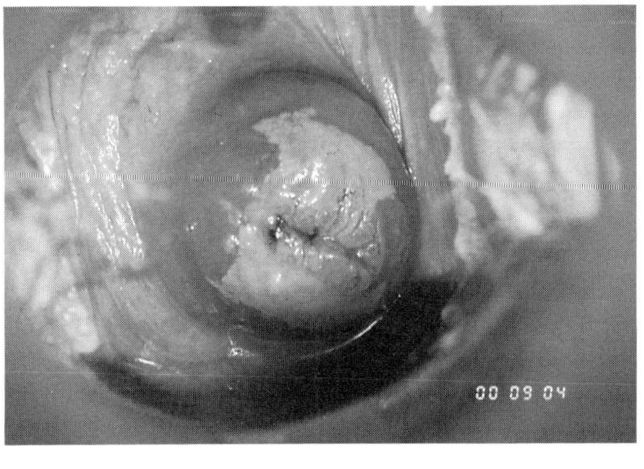

Figure 4.2. Colpophotograph showing area of cervical intraepithelial neoplasia (CIN) following application of acetic acid.

Conservative Methods of Treatment

The methods for treatment are given in *Table 4.1*. Taking into consideration the morbidity of the more radical procedures, a conservative approach can be justified in most women with preinvasive disease. Ideally all women with truly premalignant lesions destined to develop cancer would be selected and treated with a simple, rapid, non-morbid and effective office technique.

Local ablative techniques may be used in specific circumstances. An accurate colposcopic examination is conducted and the lesion visualized in its entirety. Invasive disease is excluded by the colposcopic assessment, cytologic report and a colposcopically-directed punch biopsy or biopsies. The ablative procedure should be undertaken by the colposcopist and there must be provision for good cytologic

Table 4.1. Methods for treatment.

Ablation
Cryocautery
Electrodiathermy
Cold coagulation
Carbon dioxide laser
Excision
Transitional zone excision
Carbon dioxide laser
Large loop excision of transformation zone (LLETZ)/ loop electrosurgical excision procedure (LEEP)
Surgical excision
Cone biopsy
Hysterectomy

and/or colposcopic follow-up. Local ablative techniques may be used to treat all grades of CIN. Destroyed abnormal areas are replaced by normal squamous epithelium.

One important fact is the depth of destruction of any treatment modality. Studies to assess the depth of crypt involvement with CIN suggests that a depth of destruction to 3.8 mm eradicates premalignant disease in 99.7% of cases (Anderson and Hartley, 1980). However, some gland crypts with involvement by CIN to 5 mm in depth were observed, and therefore a destructive depth greater than this is desirable. Ablation to a depth of 5–8 mm has been recommended (Jordan *et al.*, 1985). If depth of destruction is inadequate then this deep-seated component may be a source of residual or recurrent disease.

Cryocautery

Cryocautery destroys tissue by freezing using probes of various shapes and sizes. Large areas of CIN can be treated, but it is probably best reserved for small lesions. Although lesion size is important in determining success or failure using any of the treatment modalities it is especially important when using cryocautery (Richart *et al.*, 1980). The duration of freeze is two minutes from the appearance of the ice ball. The probe is then allowed to defrost and the cervix inspected to ensure that the ice ball has extended beyond the limits of the lesion. With larger lesions, multiple applications may be necessary. Cryoprobes are cheap and widely available. They can be used in the office setting without recourse to analgesia. The depth of destruction is approximately 4 mm and this may be inadequate for some of the CIN lesions with deep gland crypt involvement. Furthermore, depth of destruction cannot be gauged and incomplete eradication of disease may lead to regenerating epithelium covering the residual disease. Despite all this, cryocautery is worthy of consideration as a cheap office procedure, especially for small lesions. Healing after cryocautery is rapid, the endocervical canal is not compromised and fertility is unaffected (Ostergard, 1980).

Electrodiathermy

Although electrodiathermy destroys tissue more effectively than cryocautery, it does require general, regional or local anesthesia. Under colposcopic control, it is possible to destroy up to 1 cm depth using a combination of needle and ball electrodes (Chanen, 1981). The needle is inserted repeatedly at 1–2 mm intervals until the whole transformation zone has been covered. The ball achieves destruction of surface epithelium by a process of fulguration and coagulation. The apparatus is available in most operating theatres, and is cheap and easy to maintain. There may be considerably more thermal necrosis than anticipated, leading to discharge and slough following therapy. Fibrosis is more common than with other forms of ablation, but does not appear to affect subsequent fertility and obstetric outcome (Hammond and Edmonds, 1990). An extension of this technique using a wire loop allows electrodiathermy to be used in an excisional mode.

Cold coagulation

This term was coined by Kurt Semm, the inventor of the instrument in 1966. The apparatus is portable and heat is conveyed to the tissues using a Teflon-coated thermosound. Using overlapping applications of the thermosound for 20 seconds at 100°C, the whole of the transformation zone may be treated. The device is cheap and easily maintained and does not usually require analgesia. Some women may complain of pelvic cramp for the duration of the treatment. Measurement of the depth of destruction is difficult when the surface has been blistered off and the underlying tissue shrivelled by desiccation. The depth of destruction is approximately 2.5–4 mm or more after treatment at 100°C for 30 seconds and always exceeds 4 mm after treatment at 120°C for 30 seconds (De Cristofaro *et al.*, 1988). This technique has been used at the woman's first visit, but with a policy of taking a directed biopsy at the same time for diagnostic purposes. In primary treatment for CIN 3, the success rate was 95% at one year and 92% at five years (Gordon and Duncan, 1991). Repeat cold coagulation for residual or recurrent disease was less successful and is not advised. The outcome for pregnancy was not adversely affected by treatment.

Carbon dioxide laser

Laser is an acronym for 'Light Amplification by Stimulated Emission of Radiation.' The laser converts energy such as heat, light or electricity into radiant energy at a specific wavelength. In gynecologic surgery, the carbon dioxide laser is most widely used and this produces energy at a wavelength of 10.6 μm, which is the infrared portion of the spectrum. Using mirrors and lenses, the laser energy may be focused to a specific spot 0.2–2 mm diameter. The radiation is non-ionizing and its biologic effect is primarily thermal. Tissue at the focal point of the laser is vaporized at the speed of light. The greater the absorptive capacity of the tissue the greater the precision with which the beam may be used, minimizing thermal damage to the surrounding tissue. A micromanipulator attached to the colposcope is used to manipulate the laser and treatment is conducted under direct vision. As the technique is precise, it allows good control of the depth of destruction, good hemostasis and excellent healing because there is minimal thermal damage to the adjacent tissue (Jordan and Jones, 1979). If the destruction is adequate, cure rates are in the region of 94% of selected patients (Jordan *et al.*, 1985). The technique is particularly useful for treating premalignant disease with vaginal involvement. As there are no gland crypts in the vaginal epithelium, destruction to 2–3 mm depth is adequate. The major disadvantage is the initial cost of equipment and maintenance of these machines.

Transformation zone excision

One of the prerequisites of local destructive methods is the exclusion of invasive disease. This depends not only on the skill of the colposcopist, but also on the quality of the diagnostic punch biopsy taken before treatment. An early invasive lesion may not be recognized colposcopically due to its failure to produce alterations in the surface epithelium that can be readily recognized. An increasing catalog of invasive disease following local destructive treatment of CIN points to the fact that errors can be made (Anderson, 1993). Although data on the prevalence/incidence of early invasive cancers are limited, the incidence observed in excisional methods of treatment is increased.

Transformation zone excision has been developed as a conservative excisional technique. Both the laser and diathermy loop have been used for this purpose (Dorsey and Diggs, 1979; Prendiville *et al.*, 1986). Laser excision is technically more demanding than laser vaporization and requires a high-power density beam with a small spot size that can function in a cutting mode. Laser excision is also more time consuming than vaporization. Diathermy loop excision using low-power voltage apparatus is now widely practised. The apparatus can be found in most operating theatres and is relatively cheap. The technique is referred to as 'large loop excision of transformation zone' (LLETZ) in Europe and as 'loop electrosurgical excision procedure' (LEEP) in North America (*Figure 4.3*). Using this technique, a 'see and treat' management strategy for women with abnormal cervical smears can be adopted whereby women are treated at their first visit to the colposcopy clinic. Strict guidelines need to be adhered to because this policy will undoubtedly lead to overtreatment in some women and will also result in an increased histopathologic workload compared to processing punch biopsies. Although histopathology workload is increased, this also results in excisional techniques providing considerably more material for assessment and allowing a more reliable interpretation. Comparing histologic diagnoses from punch biopsies and excisional techniques can show considerable differences (Buxton *et al.*, 1993).

Success rates following local excisional techniques are similar to those quoted for laser ablation and cold coagulation (Luesley *et al.*, 1990). Diathermy loop excision has proven to be a rapid and relatively non-morbid procedure that can be conducted in an office setting and is a cost-effective alternative to other management strategies for CIN. Recent reports also suggest that it has no adverse effect on fertility and the outcome of subsequent pregnancies (Bigrigg *et al.*, 1994).

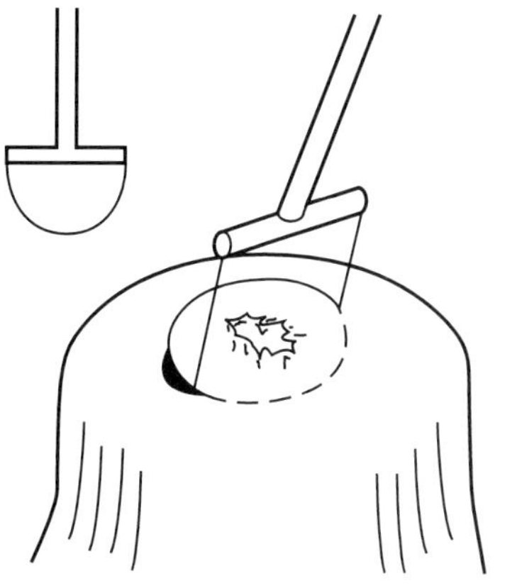

Figure 4.3. Diagrammatic representation of large loop excision of the transformation zone (LLETZ).

Cone Biopsy and Hysterectomy

These traditional excisional techniques still retain a place in the management of CIN. Hysterectomy may need to be contemplated if CIN is present in a woman with other gynecologic conditions such as fibroids, menorrhagia or prolapse. Before operation, colposcopy will identify the extent of the lesion and avoid incomplete excision, which may result in vaginal intraepithelial neoplasia (VaIN). If the lesion is seen to extend onto the vagina, this may be excised as part of the hysterectomy procedure. An alternative is to ablate the vaginal extension of CIN (using laser or diathermy) and then proceed to excision or hysterectomy as indicated.

Cone biopsies performed for therapeutic and diagnostic purposes have a success rate of approximately 93%, even in the absence of colposcopy (McLaren, 1967). With the addition of colposcopy, cone biopsies can be tailored for the individual lesion, leading to smaller cone biopsies, which are associated with significantly less morbidity, but similar success rates, in disease eradication (Jordan, 1976). Schiller's iodine may be used to delineate the extent of abnormality, but colposcopy is preferable. Pooled data suggest that although cone biopsy and hysterectomy are very effective methods of treatment, there is still a 0.3–0.4% incidence of invasive cancer following these procedures (Jordan, 1980).

The size and shape of the cone biopsy is governed by the colposcopic findings. The internal os and as much of the endocervical canal are left intact as is possible within the confines of disease eradication. This limits hemorrhagic morbidity and fertility will be little compromised.

Both hemorrhagic morbidity and postoperative cervical stenosis are dependent upon the length of the cone biopsy performed (Luesley *et al.*, 1985). Cervical stenosis may be entirely asymptomatic or can lead to problems with menstrual dysfunction and dysmenorrhea. Colposcopic and cytologic follow-up is made more difficult and this in turn may delay recognition of residual or recurrent disease. Carbon dioxide laser conization is claimed to avoid the problems of post-cone morbidity, but requires expensive apparatus and considerable operator skill (Fenton *et al.*, 1985).

Histologic incomplete excision at the time of cone biopsy represents a management dilemma. Cervical cytology may in fact be a more useful prognostic guide to residual disease than excision cone margins according to a study looking at hysterectomy after conization (Buxton *et al.*, 1987). In this study no patient had residual disease if the post-cone smear was negative. In those women with severe cervical stenosis, hysterectomy may be contemplated. The risk of invasive disease following incomplete excision is related to the presence of cytologic abnormality following treatment (Woodman *et al.*, 1984). A persistent cytologic abnormality after cone biopsy is a good indicator of residual disease; such women warrant further treatment.

Treatment Failures

The primary objective of treating women with CIN is to prevent invasive cervical cancer. If invasive disease develops or indeed if there is residual CIN, the initial treatment is deemed a failure.

Women who have undergone treatment of CIN remain at higher risk for invasive cervical disease. Those women who have abnormal cervical cytology following treatment have a much higher risk compared to those with normal cytology after treatment (McIndoe *et al.*, 1984). Women who have been treated for CIN therefore need long-term follow-up. With the passage of time, treatment modalities have become more conservative and comparative long-term follow-up is not yet available. Reports of invasive disease after local destructive therapy have been reviewed and many, but not all, of the invasive carcinomas result from inappropriate selection for treatment and a failure to recognize early invasive disease at the time of initial assessment (Anderson, 1993). Invasive disease following transformation zone excision has also been reported (Shafi *et al.*, 1992). It is suggested that the use of excisional procedures should further reduce the small risk of invasive carcinoma developing after treatment for CIN. Cytologic abnormality following treatment, no matter how minor, should be regarded as an indication for colposcopic reassessment.

Colposcopic assessment is technically more difficult in those who have undergone previous treatment. Islands of CIN and indeed invasive disease can be buried under an apparently normal surface epithelium. For failures of initial treatment, it is generally recommended that an excisional method of treatment is used in preference to ablative techniques.

Human Papillomavirus Subtyping

There are many proposals to include HPV subtyping into management protocols for abnormal cervical cytology. Commercially available kits are available that will test for the common oncogenic virus subtypes. Although the use of such techniques has shown considerable promise in cross-sectional studies (Cuzick *et al.*, 1992; Bavin *et al.*, 1993), this has not been translated into any meaningful longitudinal results with regards to progressive potential of those women with oncogenic HPV subtypes because the diagnosis of low-grade disease was a better predictor for progression to high-grade disease than HPV positivity (Downey *et al.*, 1994).

Non-treatment and Serial Colposcopy

The progressive potential of low-grade lesions is unknown and cannot be predicted from cytologic, colposcopic or histologic criteria. Many of these low-grade lesions will regress, but others will persist

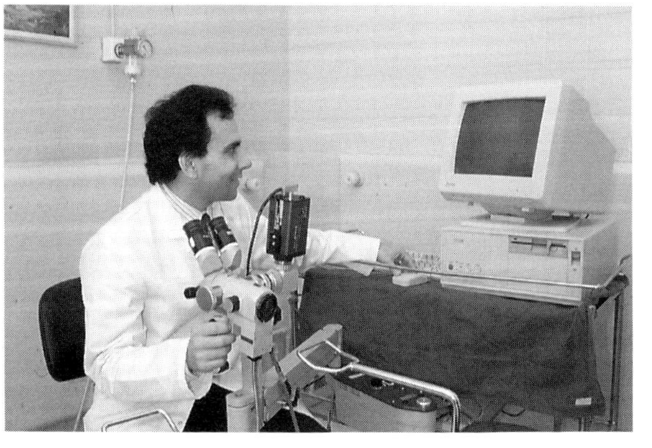

Figure 4.4. Equipment used for digital imaging colposcopy and storage of colposcopic images on computer.

or progress. It has been this importance to predict the behavior of low-grade lesions that has led to the blanket treatment of all grades of CIN (Royal College of Obstetricians and Gynaecologists, 1987). This policy has undoubtedly led to overtreatment for many women who are at negligible risk for invasive disease. National recommendations for the UK have recently been revised to allow CIN 1 lesions to be treated or kept under close surveillance (Duncan, 1992). However, some women are unlikely to accept even a low risk of malignancy and would prefer treatment. Also in a transient population, early intervention may be the preferred option as women are unlikely to adhere to a surveillance program. The introduction of digital imaging colposcopy (*Figure 4.4*) allows scope for close surveillance and will allow serial colposcopies to be performed and easy comparison of the colposcopic images (Shafi *et al.*, 1994).

Summary

The management of CIN has evolved over the last 30 years and has progressively become less radical. Initially cone biopsy showed that hysterectomy was unwarranted in the majority of women with CIN, and more recently even cone biopsy seems like overtreatment for many of these women. Increasingly more young women are seen with cytologic abnormality and this has led to a desire to undertake local ablative or excisional methods of treatment. Cure rates for both ablative and excisional techniques are higher than 90%.

Summary of Management Options

- Colposcopic assessment of women with abnormal cervical cytology should be undertaken before any treatment. This is particularly important if a conservative management approach is to be used.
- Methods used for treatment are either local ablation or local excision or more extensive surgical procedures (i.e. cone biopsy and hysterectomy). Decisions with regards to technique are dependent on locally available techniques, other gynecologic disorders and facilities available for follow-up. Whichever method is used, the depth of destruction should be at least 5–8 mm as gland crypts may be involved with cervical intraepithelial neoplasia (CIN).
- Success rates for local ablative and local excisional techniques are similar after a single treatment episode (90–95%). The advantages of excisional techniques are that the histologic interpretation is enhanced and any early invasive lesion is more likely to be diagnosed correctly.
- After local treatment for CIN, women have a higher risk of developing invasive disease than the general population. Those women that have continuing abnormal cervical cytology following treatment are at greatest risk of developing an invasive lesion.
- For treatment failures it is recommended that an excisional method is used in preference to ablative techniques.
- Non-treatment and serial colposcopic assessment has a role to play in the management of women with cytologic abnormalities and low-grade lesions. If this option is chosen, the woman must avail herself to the surveillance program as default from follow-up is a major concern.

References

Anderson MC (1993) Invasive carcinoma of the cervix following local destructive treatment for cervical intraepithelial neoplasia. *Br. J. Obstet. Gynaecol.* **100:** 657–663.

Anderson MC & Hartley RB (1980) Cervical crypt involvement by intraepithelial neoplasia. *Obstet. Gynecol.* **55:** 546–550.

Bavin PJ, Giles JA, Deery A *et al.* (1993) Use of semi-quantitative PCR for human papillomavirus DNA type 16 to identify women with high grade cervical disease in a population presenting with a mildly dyskaryotic smear report. *Br. J. Cancer* **67:** 602–605.

Bigrigg A, Haffenden DK, Sheehan AL, Codling BW & Read MD (1994) Efficacy and safety of large-loop excision of the transformation zone. *Lancet* **343:** 32–34.

Buxton EJ, Luesley DM, Shafi MI & Rollason T (1993) Colposcopically directed punch biopsy: a potentially misleading investigation. *Br. J. Obstet. Gynaecol.* **100:** 145–148.

Buxton EJ, Luesley DM, Wade-Evans T & Jordan JA (1987) Residual disease after cone biopsy: completeness of excision and follow-up cytology as predictive factors. *Obstet. Gynecol.* **70:** 529–532.

Chanen W (1981) Treatment of CIN by destruction – Electrocoagulation diathermy. *Preclinical Neoplasia of the Cervix*, p. 191. London: RCOG.

Cuzick J, Terry G, Ho L, Hollingworth T & M A (1992) Human papillomavirus type 16 DNA in cervical smears as predictor of high-grade cervical intraepithelial neoplasia. *Lancet* **339:** 959–960.

De Cristofaro D, Fontana P & Pezzoli C (1988) Pathologic study of the cervix after cold coagulation. *Am. J. Obstet. Gynecol.* **159:** 1053–1054.

Dorsey JH & Diggs ES (1979) Microsurgical conization of the cervix by carbon dioxide laser. *Obstet. Gynecol.* **54(5):** 565–570.

Downey GP, Bavin PJ, Deery ARS *et al.* (1994) Relation between human papillomavirus type 16 and potential for progression of minor-grade cervical disease. *Lancet* **344:** 432–435.

■ Duncan ID (1992) NHS cervical screening programme: guidelines for clinical practice and programme management. Oxford: National Co-ordinating Network.

Evans DMD, Hudson E, Brown CL *et al.* (1986) Terminology in gynaecological cytopathology: report of the working party of the British Society for Clinical Cytology. *J. Clin. Pathol.* **39:** 933–944.

Farmery E & Gray M (1994) Report of the first five years of the NHS cervical screening programme. Oxford: National Co-ordinating Network.

Fenton DW, Soutter WP & James CW (1985) A comparison of knife and CO_2 laser excisional cone biopsies. *Gynaecologic Laser Surgery*, p. 77. London: Perinatology Press.

Gordon HK & Duncan ID (1991) Effective destruction of cervical intraepithelial neoplasia (CIN) 3 at 100°C using the Semm cold coagulator: 14 years experience. *Br. J. Obstet. Gynaecol.* **98:** 14–20.

Hammond RH & Edmonds DK (1990) Does treatment for cervical intraepithelial neoplasia affect fertility and pregnancy? *Br. Med. J.* **301:** 1344–1345.

Hinselmann H (1925) Verbesserung der inspektionsmoglichkeit von vulva, vagina und portio. *Munchener medizinische Wochenschrift* **77:** 1733.

Imperial Cancer Research Fund (ICRF) (1993) Cervical cancer research fact sheet: June. London.

Ismail SM, Colclough AB, Dinnen JS *et al.* (1990) Reporting cervical intraepithelial neoplasia (CIN): intra- and interpathologist variation and factors associated with disagreement. *Histopathology* **16:** 371–376.

Jordan JA (1976) The diagnosis and management of premalignant conditions of the cervix. *Clin. Obstet. Gynecol.* **3:** 295–315.

Jordan JA (1980) The modern management of premalignant disease of the cervix. *Controversies in Gynaecological Oncology*, pp. 25–37. London: RCOG.

Jordan JA & Jones HWJ (1979) Laser treatment of cervical intraepithelial neoplasia. *Obstet. Gynecol. Surv.* **34:** 831.

Jordan JA, Woodman CBJ, Mylotte MJ *et al.* (1985) The treatment of cervical intraepithelial neoplasia by laser vaporization. *Br. J. Obstet. Gynaecol.* **92:** 394–398.

Kraatz H (1939) Farbfiltervorshaltung zur leichteren erlernung der kolposkopie. *Zentralblatt für Gynakologie* **63:** 2307–2309.

■ Luesley DM, Cullimore J, Redman CWE *et al.* (1990) Loop diathermy of the cervical transformation zone in patients with abnormal cervical smears. *Br. Med. J.* **300:** 1690–1693.

Luesley DM, McCrum A, Terry PB *et al.* (1985) Complications of cone biopsy related to the dimensions of the cone and the influence of prior colposcopic assessment. *Br. J. Obstet. Gynaecol.* **92:** 158–164.

■ McIndoe WA, McLean MR, Jones RW & Mullins PR (1984) The invasive potential of carcinoma *in situ* of the cervix. *Obstet. Gynecol.* **64:** 451–458.

McLaren HC (1967) Conservative management of cervical precancer. *J. Obstet. Gynaecol. Br. Comm.* **74:** 487–492.

National Cancer Institute Workshop (1989) The 1988 Bethesda system for reporting cervical/vaginal cytologic diagnoses. *JAMA* **262:** 931–934.

Ostergard DR (1980) Cryosurgical treatment of cervical intraepithelial neoplasia. *Obstet. Gynecol.* **56:** 231–233.

Papanicolaou GN & Traut HF (1941) The diagnostic value of vaginal smears in carcinoma of the uterus. *Am. J. Obstet. Gynecol.* **42:** 193–206.

Prendiville W, Davies R & Berry PJ (1986) A low voltage diathermy loop for taking cervical biopsies: a qualitative comparison with punch biopsy forcepts. *Br. J. Obstet. Gynaecol.* **93:** 773–776.

Royal College of Obstetricians and Gynaecologists (1987) *Report of the Intercollegiate Working Party on Cervical Screening*. London.

Richart RM (1967) Natural history of cervical intraepithelial neoplasia. *Obstet. Gynecol.* **56:** 231–233.

■ Richart RM (1990) A modified terminology for cervical intraepithelial neoplasia. *Obstet. Gynecol.* **75:** 131–133.

Richart RM, Townsend DE, Crips W *et al.* (1980) An analysis of long-term follow-up results in patients with cervical intraepithelial neoplasia treated by cryotherapy. *Am. J. Obstet. Gynecol.* **137:** 823–826.

Robertson AJ, Anderson JM, Swanson Beck J *et al.* (1989) Observer variability in histopathological reporting of cervical biopsy specimens. *J. Clin. Pathol.* **42:** 231–238.

Schiller W (1929) Jodpinselung und abschabung des portioepithels. *Zentralblatt für Gynakologie* **53:** 1056–1064.

Shafi MI, Chenoy R, Buxton EJ & Luesley DM (1992) Invasive cervical disease following large loop excision of the transformation zone. *Br. J. Obstet. Gynaecol.* **99:** 614.

■ Shafi MI, Dunn JA, Chenoy R, Buxton EJ, Williams C & Luesley DM (1994) Digital imaging colposcopy, image analysis and quantification of the colposcopic image. *Br. J. Obstet. Gynaecol.* **101:** 234–238.

Williams J (1886) Cancer of the uterus. *Harveian Lectures for 1886*. London: HK Lewis.

Woodman CBJ, Jordan JA & Wade-Evans T (1984) The management of vaginal intraepithelial neoplasia after hysterectomy. *Br. J. Obstet. Gynaecol.* **91:** 707–711.

5 Invasive Cervical Cancer – Primary Surgical Treatment

P Y Roland
H M Shingleton

Historical Overview

Operations to radically excise the cancerous cervix date to as early as 1892, with the development of a radical vaginal hysterectomy by Schauta (1902). The first radical abdominal surgical procedure for cervical carcinoma was performed by Clark in 1895 at the Johns Hopkins Hospital. His work was complemented by the extensive experience of Wertheim of Germany, who in 1912 reported on a series of 500 radical hysterectomy operations begun in 1895. Although Wertheim reported a five-year survival of 70% of patients without nodal metastasis, a procedure-related mortality of 19% prevented widespread acceptance of his operation at that time. Beginning in 1903, radium gained popularity in the treatment of cervical malignancy because of its lower morbidity and mortality. Two contemporaries, Bonney in England (1932) and Meigs in Boston (1951), demonstrated comparable or better survival of 50–80% and lower perioperative mortality for surgery as compared to radiotherapy. This established radical hysterectomy as an appropriate treatment for early stage disease.

The pioneers of radical excision concentrated on wide removal of the primary cancer. Pelvic (and subsequent paraaortic) node dissections came later, when the nodal spread patterns became evident. Neither Clark nor Wertheim appreciated a benefit from pelvic node dissection. While lymphadenectomy has now become a standard part of surgical treatment, the argument over whether it is actually therapeutic or only prognostic continues.

Microinvasion – Definition

A primary goal of cancer staging is to provide prognostic information and guide the physician in the selection of appropriate treatment. The identification of patients with superficially invasive cancer who are at minimal risk for lymph node metastasis and recurrent disease will allow surgical treatment by conservative operations. The 1985 International Federation of Gynecology and Obstetrics (FIGO) definition of early invasion classifies tumors as Stage IA1 when there is 'minimal microscopic invasion' present, and Stage IA2 when tumors demonstrate a depth of invasion of 5 mm or less from the base of the epithelium and 7 mm or less of horizontal spread (Committee, 1986). Numerous studies have reported significant variations in the incidence of pelvic lymph node metastasis when Stage IA2 tumors are examined as a group, ranging from 0–13% (Sevin *et al.*, 1992). This has led some authors to suggest that the contemporary FIGO Stage IA is too broadly defined to provide useful information for the treatment of patients (Burghardt *et al.*, 1991). In contrast, the Society of Gynecologic Oncologists (SGO) in 1974 defined microinvasive carcinoma of the cervix (MIC) as a lesion demonstrating less than or equal to 3 mm invasion below the basement membrane and containing no lymphatic or vascular space invasion. The subset of early cancers fulfilling the SGO definition of MIC rarely if ever metastasize to lymph nodes (van Nagell *et al.*, 1983), and are associated with a low incidence of recurrent disease, less than 5% (Trelford *et al.*, 1992). The occasional recurrence is likely to be intraepithelial neoplasia, and amenable to local therapy (van Nagell *et al.*, 1977).

Treatment of Microinvasion

In reviewing his experience back to 1958, Burghardt and Holzer (1977) suggested that many of these minimally invasive cancers could be treated conservatively with conization or simple hysterectomy. Since that time, many investigators have advocated approaching such lesions with less than radical surgery. Tumors that fulfill the SGO definition of microinvasion have a negligible incidence of lymph node metastasis, and may be treated by vaginal or abdominal hysterectomy. In cases where MIC is diagnosed in the young patient desiring future fertility, cervical conization only may be considered appropriate therapy (Trelford *et al.*, 1992). However, this approach should be limited to select patients with squamous lesions since the clinical behavior of early invasive cervical adenocarcinoma is less well defined. In addition, candidates for conservative therapy should have cone margins that are free of dysplastic or invasive cells, and the patient should be compliant with follow-up recommendations (Morris *et al*., 1993). Patients with 3.1–5.0 mm of invasion, or any Stage IA tumor with lymph–vascular invasion have an increased risk of nodal metastasis and recurrent disease (Simon *et al*., 1986), and might be considered candidates for Class II or modified radical hysterectomy and pelvic lymphadenectomy as described by Piver *et al*. (1974).

Treatment of Larger Volume Tumors

Cervical tumors with greater than 5 mm depth of invasion are classified as Stage IB, and are generally treated by Class III radical hysterectomy with pelvic and paraaortic lymphadenectomy or primary radiation therapy. Of note, some surgeons would suggest that lesions with less than 1 cm stromal invasion can be adequately treated by the Class II operation. Inoue (1984) reported a 92.5% five-year survival in patients with stromal invasion to 1 cm. Alvarez *et al*. (1991) noted a survival greater than 95% in patients with negative pelvic lymph nodes and pathologic tumor diameter less than 1 cm. A low incidence of parametrial tumor involvement in small cervical lesions provides additional evidence supporting less than radical resection. Burghardt *et al*. (1988) demonstrated a 5.2% incidence of parametrial extension in patients with tumor involving less than 20% of the total volume of the cervix. Inoue (1984) noted a 2% incidence of parametrial extension in cases of stromal invasion to 1 cm.

Preoperative Evaluation

Radical hysterectomy is appropriate therapy for patients with invasive cervical cancer confined to the cervix or upper vagina, Stages IB and IIA. Although early reports suggested that very large cervical lesions would be best treated with radiation therapy, contemporary investigators have demonstrated that bulky cervical tumors can be successfully treated primarily by surgery. Alvarez *et al*. (1993) reported on the use of radical hysterectomy and selective adjuvant radiation therapy in patients with cervical lesions equal to or greater than 4 cm, demonstrating a five-year survival of 73.6%. As with any major abdominal–pelvic procedure, the patient should be a good operative candidate free from significant medical conditions that would preclude surgery. Extreme obesity increases the difficulty of the operation such that the morbidly obese patient may be considered a candidate for primary radiation therapy. Many individuals with cervical cancer will be of advanced age, and their fitness for surgery is of prime concern. Chronologic age alone is a poor predictor of operative mortality, and elderly patients without confounding medical conditions may undergo radical surgery with acceptable low mortality (Lichtinger *et al*., 1986; Lawton and Hacker, 1990). In addition to appropriate preoperative testing, radiologic examination of the pulmonary, gastrointestinal and musculoskeletal system may be used in select cases. However, cervical cancer is a clinically staged disease, and results of lymphangiography, computerized tomography (CT) and magnetic resonance imaging (MRI) may not be used to alter clinical stage. The potential role of diagnostic imaging studies on the detection of lymph node metastasis has been evaluated by multiple studies. A review of the literature by Shingleton and Siller (1994) shows that the use of CT scan in the detection of pelvic node metastasis is associated with a sensitivity of 9–26% and a specificity of 89%. CT evaluation of the paraaortic nodes has a sensitivity and specificity of 65% and 89%, respectively. The use of lymphangiography and MRI in this setting lack sensitivity as well. Therefore, the decision to proceed with radical hysterectomy in the newly diagnosed case of cervical cancer must ultimately be based upon clinical and intraoperative findings.

The Surgical Procedure

The operation may be performed using a midline vertical or transverse Maylard skin incision. Upon entering the peritoneal cavity, careful inspection and palpation of pelvic and abdominal organs is conducted. Particular attention is given to the subdiaphragmatic region, retroperitoneal spaces and pelvic and paraaortic lymph node chains. A working knowledge of the types or classes of hysterectomy as described by Piver *et al*. (1974) will allow the surgeon to select the most conservative and appropriate procedure. The Class I or extrafascial hysterectomy is advocated for use in cases of SGO-defined MIC. The goal of the Class II or modified radical hysterectomy is resection of the medial one-third to one-half of the cardinal ligament while maintaining adequate blood supply to the distal ureters and ureterovesical junction. The uterine vessels are ligated medial to the ureter and the uterosacral ligaments are bisected at their midpoint between the uterus and sacrum (*Figure 5.1*). An adequate margin (1–3 cm) of the upper vagina is resected. The Class II procedure is recommended in cases of Stage IA disease with 3–5 mm of invasion or any Stage IA lesion with lymph–vascular space invasion. The Class III procedure of Meigs represents to us the definitive radical hysterectomy in which extensive resection of paracervical and parametrial tissues to the pelvic sidewall occurs (*Figure 5.1*). The anterior and posterior vesicouterine ligaments are divided, completely mobilizing the ureters and

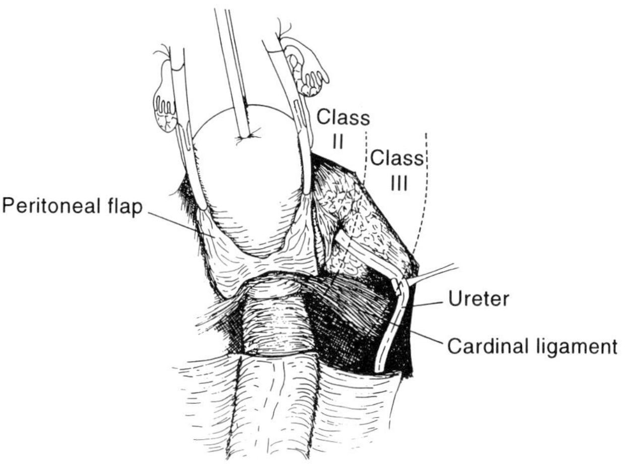

Figure 5.1. Class II and Class III hysterectomies. (From Shingleton and Gusberg, 1988, with permission; redrawn from Piver *et al.*, 1974.)

bladder from the surrounding paracervical tissue. The uterine vessels are ligated at their origin from the hypogastric artery. The uterosacral ligaments are transected at their point of attachment to the sacrum.

Lymphadenectomy

Lymphatic drainage of the cervix, as described by Henriksen (1949), is primarily to the paracervical, parametrial, hypogastric, and external iliac nodes, and then secondarily to the common iliac, inguinal and paraaortic nodal chains. Cumulative studies suggest an incidence of pelvic node involvement in the order of 15% (Martinbeau *et al.*, 1982; Fuller *et al.*, 1989; Alvarez *et al.*, 1991) and a 6% incidence of paraaortic nodal metastasis (Martinbeau *et al.*, 1982; Delgado *et al.*, 1989; Alvarez *et al.*, 1991) in Stage I cervical cancer. The identification of such metastatic disease will distinguish patients with a high risk of treatment failure and allow for the consideration of postoperative adjuvant therapy. Unfortunately reliance on clinical evaluation of nodal status at the time of operation has proven to be inaccurate. Significant numbers of patients with disease apparently confined to the uterus at exploration have pelvic lymph node micrometastasis. Palpation of lymph nodes was demonstrated by Bjornsson *et al.* (1993) to have a sensitivity of 68% and specificity of 100% in detecting metastasis. Welander *et al.* (1981) reported that clinical assessment of the paraaortic nodes missed 10% of biopsy-proved metastasis, and in the case of palpable enlarged nodes had a 20% false positive rate. Therefore, given the potential for error with clinical and radiologic assessment, surgical node sampling and histologic confirmation play an important role in the identification of metastatic disease.

Pelvic and paraaortic lymph node dissections are performed in conjunction with Class II and Class III radical hysterectomy. Nodal tissue superior, lateral, and medial to the common iliac, external iliac, and hypogastric vessels, and in the obturator fossa superior to the obturator nerve is dissected. Paraaortic lymphadenectomy consists primarily of dissection of the node-containing fat pad along the right lateral aspect of the aorta from its bifurcation to the origin of the inferior mesenteric artery. Most American investigators suggest assessment of paraaortic nodes for metastatic disease before proceeding with removal of the uterus. Should metastases be detected, consideration can be given to terminating the procedure in favor of primary radiation therapy with extension of the treatment field to include the paraaortic lymph nodes. Multiple and bilateral pelvic nodal metastases would warrant the same consideration (Potter *et al.*, 1990).

Oophorectomy

Oophorectomy is not an integral part of radical hysterectomy. The incidence of metastasis to the ovaries in Stage IB squamous cell carcinoma is less than 1% (Baltzer *et al.*, 1982; Toki *et al.*, 1991). Reports of ovarian metastasis in adenocarcinoma vary from 0 to 7.7%. In a study of Stage IB adenocarcinoma metastasizing to the ovary, Brown *et al.* (1990) noted that ovarian lesions were only present in patients who were postmenopausal, had positive pelvic nodes, or had obvious ovarian involvement. Therefore, the normal appearing ovaries may be preserved in the premenopausal patient undergoing radical surgery. Some surgeons advocate transposing the preserved ovaries to the paracolic gutter. In this manner, they may be spared the effects of radiation if adjunctive pelvic radiation therapy is used.

Complications of Radical Hysterectomy

The estimated blood loss associated with radical hysterectomy ranges from 1000–1900 ml (Hoskins *et al.*, 1976; Orr *et al.*, 1982). Contemporary experience indicates an operation-associated mortality of approximately 1% (Fuller *et al.*, 1989). Febrile morbidity is one of the most common complications of surgery, affecting one of every three patients (Orr *et al.*, 1982). Fever is commonly caused by atelectasis and urinary tract infection. Less common, but important etiologies of fever in this population include pelvic cellulitis, surgical site wound seroma or infection, and pneumonia. Clarke–Pearson *et al.* (1984) evaluated the incidence of thromboemboli in gynecologic oncology patients, 33% of whom underwent radical hysterectomy and pelvic lymph node dissection, reporting a 17% incidence of thromboemboli and a 4% incidence of pulmonary embolism.

The extensive dissection involved in isolating the ureters and mobilizing the bladder predispose the radical hysterectomy patient to urinary tract dysfunction. Most patients experience early hypertonic bladder dysfunction related to muscle trauma, followed by diminished bladder sensation secondary to denervation. The use of suprapubic bladder catheterization provides symptomatic relief and prevents excessive bladder distension. The patient may be discharged from the hospital with continuous bladder drainage in place and may conduct intermittent voiding trials at home. For such trials, the suprapubic catheter is clamped for brief periods until the urge to void returns. Once post-void residual urine volumes are less than 100 ml the suprapubic catheter is removed, usually within four weeks. Ureteral and vesical fistulae occur with an incidence of approximately 2% and 0.9%, respectively (Shingleton and Orr, 1995b).

Lymph node dissection is associated with the development of lymphocysts, the majority of which are small and asymptomatic. Contemporary studies estimate an incidence of 0.4–2.0% (Mann *et al.*, 1989; Massi *et al.*, 1993). Occasionally, lymphocysts may be symptomatic and associated with abdominal fullness or urinary frequency (Dodd *et al.*, 1970). Indications for drainage include persistent symptoms, recurrent lymphocysts, and progressive ureteral obstruction with associated pyelonephritis (Shingleton and Orr, 1995b). Techniques for management include needle aspiration under local analgesia (Mann *et al.*, 1989), placement of a percutaneous cathether under radiologic guidance (Conte *et al.*, 1990), or operative exploration with the creation of a window for drainage of cyst fluid into the peritoneal cavity (Byron *et al.*, 1966).

Surgical Prognostic Factors

Microinvasive lesions that are properly diagnosed and treated should be considered eminently curable, with a five-year survival of essentially 100% (Simon *et al.*, 1986). Stage IA lesions with 3–5 mm depth of invasion have a small, but significant, risk of lymph node metastasis, and therefore potential for recurrent disease. Considering Stage IB tumors as a whole, treatment by radical hysterectomy is associated with an 85–90% five-year survival (Baltzer *et al.*, 1982; Alvarez *et al.*, 1991). However, certain subsets of patients have a significantly increased risk of recurrent disease and decreased survival. A multitude of studies have been conducted to identify histologic factors identified at the time of surgery that correlate with a poor prognosis. Such surgical prognostic factors can be used in counseling patients as to the prognosis of their disease and allow consideration of adjunctive radiation or chemotherapy (*Table 5.1*).

Cervical lesion size and depth of invasion correlate with poor prognosis. Bulky tumors larger than 4 cm in diameter are associated with an increased rate of nodal metastasis and recurrent disease (*Chung et al.*, 1980; Fuller *et al.*, 1989). Tumor invasion to a depth of two-thirds of the cervical stroma, or greater than 10 mm has a similar effect (Boyce *et al.*, 1981). Tumor cell grade, although highly subjective, is thought by some to be associated with an increased incidence of pelvic node metastasis. For instance, in Stage IB tumors, well-differentiated grade 1 squamous lesions may be associated with a 9% incidence of nodal metastasis versus 25% for poorly-differentiated grade 3 lesions (Fuller *et al.*, 1989). Tumor cell grade may have prognostic significance in adenocarcinoma as well. Contemporary studies of early stage adenocarcinomas by Angel *et al.* (1992) and McLellan *et al.* (1994) have reported a five-year survival for grade 1 lesions of 95–100% versus 50–52% for grade 3 tumors. The finding of tumor within the parametrial tissues correlates with increased risk of pelvic nodal disease (Inoue and Morita, 1990; Delgado *et al.*, 1989). Finally, tumor invasion into lymphatic and vascular channels signifies an increased risk for pelvic nodal involvement (Delgado *et al.*, 1989).

The patient who has developed tumor metastasis to the pelvic lymph nodes experiences a less favorable prognosis, with a five-year survival reported at 55–60% (Baltzer *et al.*, 1982; Burghardt *et al.*, 1987). The location of the highest involved chain may be

Table 5.1. Poor surgical prognostic factors.

Factor	*Supporting Studies*
Cervical lesions >4 cm diameter	Chung *et al.*, 1980 Alvarez *et al.*, 1989 Fuller *et al.*, 1989
Deeply invasive cervical lesion	Boyce *et al.*, 1981 Fuller *et al.*, 1989
Lymphatic or vascular space invasion	Baltzer *et al.*, 1982 Delgado *et al.*, 1989
Advanced tumor cell grade	Kilgore *et al.*, 1988 Fuller *et al.*, 1989
Pelvic lymph node metastasis	Boyce *et al.*, 1981 Burghardt *et al.*, 1987 Inoue and Morita, 1990
Lymph node metastasis at common iliac vessels or above	Hsu *et al.*, 1972 Martinbeau *et al.*, 1982
Positive surgical margins	Creasman *et al.*, 1986 Kim *et al.*, 1988
Parametrial extension of tumor	Delgado *et al.*, 1989 Inoue and Morita, 1990

prognostic, with metastatic disease at the level of the common iliac or paraaortic nodes being associated with decreased survival (Hsu *et al.*, 1972). The actual number of involved lymph nodes may be more informative than the simple existence of metastasis. Inoue and Morita (1990) suggests that the finding of only one involved pelvic node is associated with a survival not significantly different from that of patients with no metastasis (81% versus 89% five-year survival). In addition, several reports have suggested that finding four or more positive lymph nodes is associated with a markedly diminished survival (Hsu *et al.*, 1972; Piver and Chung, 1975).

The identification of one or more of these prognostic factors will signify an individual who has an increased risk of tumor recurrence and resultant decreased survival. For example, Alvarez *et al.* (1989) noted that patients with cervical lesions less than 1 cm in size and having less than two positive lymph nodes had a five-year survival of 92%. In contrast, individuals in the same study population with lesions larger than 4 cm in diameter and having more than two positive lymph nodes experienced an extremely poor five-year survival of 13%. Such patients may be considered for adjunctive chemotherapy or radiation therapy.

Adenocarcinoma

Adenocarcinoma and adenosquamous lesions comprise approximately 15% of cervical malignancies (Kilgore and Helm, 1990; Angel *et al.*, 1992). Although they are evaluated and treated in a manner similar to squamous lesions, their prognosis and treatment is less well defined. A number of reports have suggested that the overall five-year survival of Stage I adenocarcinoma (approximately 80%) is less than that for squamous cell carcinoma (Kilgore *et al.*, 1988; Averette *et al.*, 1993). In addition, adenocarcinoma metastatic to the pelvic lymph nodes appears to have a higher incidence of recurrent disease (Shingleton, 1992). The presence of a mixed adenosquamous cell type is thought by some to predict a particularly poor prognosis. Averette *et al.* (1993) demonstrated significantly reduced survival (63.5%) for surgically treated adenosquamous carcinomas of the cervix over similar-stage squamous and pure adenocarcinomas. In contrast, Helm *et al.* (1992) identified a trend towards a worse prognosis, but found no statistically significant difference in the five-year survival in their series; patients with adenocarcinoma had a 91% five-year survival versus 80% for adenosquamous tumors ($p=0.146$).

In the choice of single modality therapy for early stage adenocarcinoma, surgery may offer a survival advantage over radiation therapy. Kleine *et al.* (1989) noted Stage IB adenocarcinoma patients treated solely with surgery had a survival similar to those with squamous cell carcinoma (85%); however, cases treated by radiation therapy alone demonstrated only a 58.6% five-year survival. Finally, in contrast to the reported successful surgical treatment of squamous cell tumors larger than 3 cm (Alvarez *et al.*, 1993), large volume adenocarcinomas have been associated with a significant recurrence rate in excess of 50% (Shingleton *et al.*, 1981). For these reasons some surgeons advocate the use of combination surgery and radiation therapy for the treatment of the larger lesions (Prempree *et al.*, 1985).

Treatment in Pregnancy

The finding of invasive cervical cancer during pregnancy is quite rare, with an estimated incidence of 0.02% of all gestations. The presence of a gravid state does not worsen the prognosis of a given cancer (Sivanesaratnam *et al.*, 1993) nor does vaginal delivery appear to alter disease course (Lee *et al.*, 1981). The clinical stage at the time of diagnosis influences survival, with pregnant patients demonstrating similar survival to non-pregnant individuals when controlled for stage (Lee *et al.*, 1981; Creasman *et al.*, 1970). Pregnant patients with microinvasion less than or equal to 3 mm as diagnosed by conization may be followed to term without therapy. Treatment by total vaginal hysterectomy can be completed six weeks postpartum. For Stage IA disease with 3–5 mm invasion or any microinvasive lesions with lymph–vascular space invasion, the patient may be followed to term. After delivery, therapy is initiated with modified radical (Class II) hysterectomy and pelvic and paraaortic lymph node dissection. In the case of Stage IB disease a decision must be made weighing desires for expedient maternal therapy versus observation for the development of fetal maturity. Contemporary evidence suggests that modest delays in surgical therapy in the interest of allowing maturation of the fetus can be conducted in the third trimester without obvious detriment to the maternal prognosis (Duggan *et al.*, 1993). One approach to this clinical dilemma is to delay treatment until pulmonary maturity can be documented by amniocentesis. Therapy is then initiated with delivery by cesarean section and immediate radical hysterectomy with pelvic and paraaortic lymphadenectomy.

The pregnant patient with advanced stage cervical cancer is treated with primary radiation therapy. If the fetus is viable, it is delivered by cesarean section before treatment. As in the case of early stage disease, a delay in therapy may be considered to allow for fetal maturation. However, most pregnant patients with cervical cancer present early in the course of their malignancy (Zemlickis *et al.*, 1991) and little is known about the potential adverse effects of delaying treatment with Stage III and IV disease.

Adjuvant Treatment

A number of treatment regimens have been described combining pelvic radiation therapy or chemotherapy with the surgical treatment of cervical cancer. The goal of such treatment is to improve pelvic control of large tumors, decrease the incidence of recurrent disease, and ultimately improve survival. The initial results of combination treatment often appear promising. However, the surgeon must carefully compare the results of combined therapy to those realized by the individual treatments alone to determine if adjunctive therapy offers an advantage to the patient.

Adjuvant Radiotherapy

The use of radiation therapy (whole pelvis teletherapy plus single intracavitary application) followed by extrafascial hysterectomy has been proposed for large-volume or barrel-shaped cervical lesions in the hope of reducing central pelvic recurrence (Nelson *et al.*, 1975). In fact, most recurrent disease in patients treated by this form of combined therapy tends to be in the form of distant metastases (Edinger *et al.*, 1984). However, given a lack of evidence suggesting a survival advantage to pelvic radiation followed by hysterectomy, most American gynecologic oncologists prefer either radiation or surgical therapy alone for a given case and place little emphasis on the use of adjuvant hysterectomy.

Pelvic radiation therapy followed by radical hysterectomy and lymph node dissection for Stage IB disease may have evolved historically at the time radical surgery was re-introduced for a disease process treated almost entirely by radiotherapy (Shingleton and Orr, 1995a). Contemporary studies of squamous cell carcinoma have not demonstrated a survival advantage to the use of radiation followed by radical hysterectomy versus either radiotherapy or radical surgery alone (Gynning *et al.*, 1993; Pearcy, 1988).

Adjunctive radiotherapy following radical hysterectomy and pelvic node dissection is still used today by many for patients felt to have a high risk for pelvic recurrence of the tumor, especially those with pelvic node metastases. Proponents of adjuvant radiation note a reduced incidence of central recurrence and imply that this may translate into improved survival (Monk *et al.*, 1994). Multiple studies have suggested indications for adjuvant treatment, including three or more positive lymph nodes, large tumor size, poor tumor cell grade, lymph–vascular space involvement (Thomas and Dembo, 1991), deep stromal invasion, parametrial involvement (Monk *et al.*, 1994), and close surgical margins (Kim *et al.*, 1988). However, there is little evidence that adjunctive radiotherapy results in improved survival over radical hysterectomy alone. Soisson *et al.* (1990) noted no survival advantage in the combined treatment of 72 patients with high-risk Stage IB and IIA tumors. Kinney *et al.* (1989) reported a matched-control study of 60 patients treated with radical hysterectomy alone versus surgery and adjuvant whole pelvis irradiation. Both groups experienced a similar incidence of recurrence (35%) with adjuvant radiotherapy decreasing the proportion of pelvic recurrence (27% versus 67% in the surgery only group). After controlling for stage, tumor size, and lymph node status there was no significant difference in estimated survival between the two treatment groups. In summary, the desire to provide additional treatment after radical hysterectomy in the patient at risk of recurrent pelvic disease is compelling and understandable. Adjunctive whole pelvis radiotherapy appears to improve pelvic control, if only to provide time for distant metastasis to become evident. Little impact on long-term survival has been realized, however.

Adjuvant Chemotherapy

Recent efforts in the realm of combination therapy have focused on the use of neoadjuvant chemotherapy before pelvic surgery. Sardi (1993) reported interim results on the use of cisplatin (50 mg m^{-2} on day 1), vincristine (1 mg m^{-2} on day 2) and bleomycin (25 mg m^{-2} on days 1, 2 and 3) before radical hysterectomy in Stage IB squamous cell carcinoma of the cervix. A 91.5% response rate (40.5% complete response) in terms of decreasing tumor volume as measured by ultrasound was reported. The authors concluded that tumors with a volume larger than 60 cm^3 ($4 \times 4 \times 4$ cm) benefited from neoadjuvant treatment in terms of improved operability and decreased parametrial extension. Although neoadjuvant chemotherapy may decrease tumor size and make bulky lesions amenable to surgery, further study is needed to determine if this form of treatment affects recurrence or survival patterns (Thomas, 1993).

Post-treatment Surveillance

Physical examination including a careful pelvic examination with a Pap smear of the vaginal cuff should be conducted at three and six months postoperatively, and at six-month intervals for the next 1–2 years. The majority of recurrent disease will present within the first two years of initiating treatment (van Nagell *et al.*, 1979). A routine chest radiograph and intravenous pyelogram as used in the past have low yield for demonstrating occult recurrences and should be reserved for investigating symptoms.

Summary of Management Options

- Patients with microinvasive squamous cell cancer defined as less than or equal to 3 mm invasion below the basement membrane and containing no lymphatic or vascular space invasion may be treated by vaginal or abdominal hysterectomy.
- Cases of microinvasive cervical cancer in young patients desiring future fertility may be treated by cold knife conization. Such treatment should be limited to squamous lesions and have cone margins free of dysplastic or invasive cells.
- Patients with squamous lesions demonstrating 3.1–5.0 mm of invasion, any Stage IA tumor with lymph–vascular space invasion, and cervical adenocarcinoma diagnosed as *in situ* or microinvasion may be considered candidates for Class II, or modified radical hysterectomy and pelvic lymphadenectomy.
- Squamous tumors with greater than 5 mm depth of invasion and invasive adenocarcinomas localized to the cervix are classified as Stage IB and may be treated by Class III radical hysterectomy with pelvic and paraaortic lymphadenectomy.
- Pelvic and paraaortic lymph node dissections may be performed in conjunction with Class II and Class III radical hysterectomy as part of therapy and to provide prognostic information.
- The incidence of metastasis to the ovaries in Stage IB cervical cancer is less than 1%. Therefore, oophorectomy is not an integral part of radical hysterectomy.
- Adjuvant radiotherapy following radical hysterectomy and pelvic node dissection is used today by many practitioners for patients felt to have a high risk for a pelvic recurrence of tumor.

References

Alvarez RD, Potter ME, Soong SJ *et al.* (1991) Rationale for using pathologic tumor dimensions and nodal status to subclassify surgically treated stage IB cervical cancer patients. *Gynecol. Oncol.* **43**(2): 108–112.

■ Alvarez RD, Soong SJ, Kinney WK *et al.* (1989) Identification of prognostic factors and risk groups in patients found to have nodal metastasis at the time of radical hysterectomy for early-stage squamous carcinoma of the cervix. *Gynecol. Oncol.* **35**(2): 130–135.

Alvarez RD, Gelder MS, Gore H & Soong SJ (1993) Radical hysterectomy in the treatment of patients with bulky early stage carcinoma of the cervix uteri. *Surg. Gynecol. Obstet.* **176**(6): 539–542.

Angel C, Dubeshter B & Lin JY (1992) Clinical presentation and management of stage I cervical adenocarcinoma: A 25 year experience. *Gynecol. Oncol.* **44:** 71.

Averette HE, Nguyen HN, Donato DM *et al.* (1993) Radical hysterectomy for invasive cervical cancer: A 25-year prospective experience with the Miami technique. *Cancer* **71:** 1422.

Baltzer J, Lohe KJ, Kopke W & Zander J (1982) Histologic criteria for the prognosis of patients with operated squamous cell carcinoma of the cervix. *Gynecol. Oncol.* **13:** 184–194.

Bjornsson BL, Nelson BE, Reale FR & Rose PG (1993) Accuracy of frozen section for lymph node metastasis in patients undergoing radical hysterectomy for carcinoma of the cervix. *Gynecol. Oncol.* **51**(1): 50–53.

Bonney C (1932) Surgical treatment of carcinoma of cervix. *Br. Med. J.* **2:** 914.

Boyce J, Fruchter R & Nicastri A (1981) Prognostic factors in stage I carcinoma of the cervix. *Gynecol. Oncol.* **12:** 154–165.

Brown JV, Fu YS & Berek JS (1990) Ovarian metastases are rare in stage I adenocarcinoma of the cervix. *Obstet. Gynecol.* **76:** 623.

Burghardt E, Girardi F, Lahousen M *et al.* (1991) Microinvasive carcinoma of the uterine cervix (International Federation of Gynecology and Obstetrics Stage IA). *Cancer* **67**(4): 1037–1045.

Burghardt E & Holzer E (1977) Diagnosis and treatment of microinvasive carcinoma of the cervix uteri. *Obstet. Gynecol.* **49**(6): 641–653.

Burghardt E, Pickelt H, Haas J & Lahousen M (1988) Objective results of the operative treatment of cervical cancer. *Baillière's Clin. Obstet. Gynecol.* 2987.

Burghardt E, Pickel H, Haas J & Lahousen M (1987) Prognostic factors and operative treatment of stages IB to IIB cervical cancer. *Am. J. Obstet. Gynecol.* **156:** 988.

Byron R, Yonemoto R, Davajan V *et al.* (1966) Lymphocysts: Surgical correction and prevention. *Am. J. Obstet. Gynecol.* **94:** 20.

Chung CK, Hannas WA & Stryker JA *et al.* (1980) Analysis of factors contributing to treatment failures in stage IB and IIA carcinoma of the cervix. *Am. J. Obstet. Gynecol.* **138:** 550–556.

Clark J (1895) A more radical method of performing hysterectomy for cancer of the uterus. *Bull. Johns Hopkins Hosp.* **6:** 120.

Clarke–Pearson D, Synan I, Colemen R *et al.* (1984) The natural history of postoperative venous thromboemboli in gynecologic oncology: A prospective study of 382 patients. *Am. J. Obstet. Gynecol.* **148:** 1051–1054.

Committee. Staging Announcement (1986) *Gynecol. Oncol.* **25:** 383–385.

Conte M, Panici P, Guariglia L *et al.* (1990) Pelvic lymphocele following radical paraaortic and pelvic lymphadenectomy for cervical carcinoma: Incidence rate and percutaneous management. *Obstet. Gynecol.* **76:** 268.

Creasman WT, Rutledge FN & Fletcher GH (1970) Carcinoma of the cervix associated with pregnancy. *Obstet. Gynecol.* **36(4):** 495–501.

Creasman W, Soper J and Clarke–Pearson D (1986) Radical hysterectomy as therapy for early carcinoma of the cervix. *Am. J. Obstet. Gynecol.* **155:** 964.

■ Delgado G, Bundy BN, Fowler WC *et al.* (1989) A prospective surgical pathological study of stage 1 squamous carcinoma of the cervix: a gynecologic oncology group study. *Gynecol. Oncol.* **35:** 314.

Dodd GD, Rutledge F & Wallace S (1970) Postoperative pelvic lymphocysts. *Am. J. Roentgen.* **108:** 312.

Duggan B, Muderspach LI, Roman LD *et al.* (1993) Cervical cancer in pregnancy: reporting on planned delay in therapy. (Review). *Obstet. Gynecol.* **82(4 Pt 1):** 598–602.

Edinger D, Watring W, Anderson B & Mitchell G (1984) Residual tumor following radiotherapy for locally advanced carcinomas of the uterine cervix: Prognostic significance. *Eur. J. Gynaecol. Oncol.* **5:** 90.

Fuller AF, Elliott N, Kosloff C *et al.* (1989) Determinants of increased risk for recurrence in patients undergoing radical hysterectomy for stage IB and IIA carcinoma of the cervix. *Gynecol. Oncol.* **33:** 34.

Gynning I, Johnsson JE, Alm PP & Trope C (1983) Age and prognosis in stage IB squamous cell carcinoma of the uterine cervix. *Gynecol. Oncol.* **15:** 18.

Helm CW, Soong SJ, Partridge EE & Shingleton HM (1992) *A Matched Study of Surgically Treated IB Adenosquamous Carcinoma and Adenocarcinoma of the Cervix.* Abstract SGO 1992 Annual Meeting.

Henriksen E (1949) The lymphatic spread of carcinoma of the cervix and of the body of the uterus: A study of 420 necropsies. *Am. J. Obstet. Gynecol.* **58(5):** 924–942.

Hoskins WJ, Ford JH, Lutz MH & Averette HE (1976) Radical hysterectomy and pelvic lymphadenectomy for the management of early invasive cancer of the cervix. *Gynecol. Oncol.* **4:** 278.

Hsu CT, Cheng YS & Su SS (1972) Prognosis of uterine cervical cancer with extensive lymph node metastasis. *Am. J. Obstet. Gynecol.* **114:** 954–962.

Inoue T (1984) Prognostic significance of the depth of invasion relating to nodal metastases, parametrial extension, and cell types. *Cancer* **54:** 3035.

■ Inoue T & Morita K (1990) The prognostic significance of number of positive nodes in cervical carcinoma stages IB, IIA, and IIB. *Cancer* **65:** 1923.

■ Kilgore LC & Helm CW (1990) Adenocarcinoma of the uterine cervix. *Clinical Obstetrics and Gynecology*, pp. 863–871. Philadelphia, PA: JB Lippincott Company.

Kilgore LC, Soong S, Gore H *et al.* (1988) Analysis of prognostic features in adenocarcinoma of the cervix. *Gynecol. Oncol.* **31:** 137.

Kim YR, Salter MM & Shingleton HM (1988) Adjuvant postoperative radiation therapy following radical hysterectomy in stage IB ca of the cervix – Analysis of treatment failure. *Int. J. Radiat. Oncol. Biol. Phys.* **14:** 445–449.

Kinney WK, Alvarez RD, Reid GC *et al.* (1989) Value of adjuvant whole-pelvis irradiation after Wertheim hysterectomy for early-stage squamous carcinoma of the cervix with pelvic nodal metastasis: A matched-control study. *Gynecol. Oncol.* **34:** 258–262.

Kleine W, Rau K, Schwoeorer D & Pfleiderer A (1989) Prognosis of the adenocarcinoma of the cervix: A comparative study. *Gynecol. Oncol.* **35:** 145.

Lawton F & Hacker N (1990) Surgery for invasive gynecologic cancer in the elderly female population. *Obstet. Gynecol.* 76(2): 287–289.

Lee RB, Neglia W & Park RC (1981) Cervical carcinoma in pregnancy. *Obstet. Gynecol.* **58:** 584–589.

Lichtinger M, Averette H, Penalver M & Sevin Bu (1986) Major surgical procedures for gynecologic malignancy in elderly women. *South. Med. J.* **79(12):** 1506–1510.

Mann WJ, Vogel F, Pastner B & Chalas E (1989) Management of lymphocysts after radical gynecologic surgery. *Gynecol. Oncol.* **33:** 248.

Martinbeau PW, Kjorstad KE & Iversen T (1982) Stage IB carcinoma of the cervix. The Norwegian Radium Hospital. Results when pelvic nodes are involved. *Obstet. Gynecol.* **60:** 215–218.

Massi G, Savino L & Susini T (1993) Schauta–Amreich's vaginal hysterectomy and Wertheim–Meigs abdominal hysterectomy in the treatment of cervical cancer: A retrospective analysis. *Am. J. Obstet. Gynecol.* **168:** 928–934.

McLellan R, Dillon MB, Woodruff JD *et al.* (1994) Long-term follow-up of stage I cervical adenocarcinoma treated by radical surgery. *Gynecol. Oncol.* **52:** 253.

Meigs J (1951) Radical hysterectomy with bilateral pelvic lymph node dissections. A report of one hundred patients operated on five or more years ago. *Am. J. Obstet. Gynecol.* **62:** 854.

Monk BJ, Cha DS, Walker JL *et al.* (1994) Extent of disease as an indication for pelvic radiation following radical hysterectomy and bilateral pelvic lymph node dissection in the treatment of stage IB and IIA cervical carcinoma. *Gynecol. Oncol.* **54:** 4–9.

Morris M, Mitchell MF, Silva EG *et al.* (1993) Cervical conization as definitive therapy for early invasive squamous carcinoma of the cervix. *Gynecol. Oncol.* **51(2):** 193–196.

Nelson A, Fletcher G & Wharton J (1975) Indications for adjunctive conservative extrafascial hysterectomy in selected cases of carcinoma of the uterine cervix. *Am. J. Radiol.* **123:** 91.

Orr JW, Shingleton HM, Hatch KD *et al.* (1982) Correlation of perioperative morbidity and conization–radical hysterectomy interval. *Obstet. Gynecol.* **59:** 726.

Pearcy RG, Peel KR, Thorogood J *et al.* (1988) The value of pre-operative intracavitary radiotherapy in patients treated by radical hysterectomy and pelvic lymphadenectomy for invasive carcinoma of the cervix. *Clin. Radiol.* **39:** 95.

Piver MS & Chung SW (1975) Prognostic significance of cervical lesion size and pelvic node metastases in cervical carcinoma. *Obstet. Gynecol.* **46:** 507–510.

■ Piver MS, Rutledge F & Smith PJ (1974) Five classes of extended hysterectomy for women with cervical carcinoma. *Obstet. Gynecol.* **44:** 265–272.

Potter ME, Alvarez RD, Shingleton HM *et al.* (1990) Early invasive cervical cancer with pelvic lymph node involvement: To complete or not to complete radical hysterectomy. *Gynecol. Oncol.* **37(1):** 78–81.

Prempree T, Amornmarn R & Wizenbert MJ (1985) A therapeutic approach to primary adenocarcinoma of the cervix. *Cancer* **56:** 1264.

Sardi J, Sananes C, Giaroli A *et al.* (1993) Results of a prospective randomized trial with neoadjuvant chemotherapy in stage 1B, bulky, squamous carcinoma of the cervix. *Gynecol. Oncol.* **49:** 156–165.

Sevin BU, Nadji M, Avarette HE *et al.* (1992) Microinvasive carcinoma of the cervix. (Review.) *Cancer* **70(8):** 2121–2128.

Schauta F (1902) Die operation des gebarmutterkrebes mittels des Schuchardt'schen paravaginatschmittes. *Monatsschrift Geburtshilfe und Gynakologie* **15:** 133.

Shingleton HM & Orr JW Jr (1995a) Other treatments. In: *Cancer of the Cervix*. Philadelphia: JB Lippincott Company.
Shingleton HM & Orr JW Jr (1995b) Primary surgical treatment of invasive cancer. In: *Cancer of the Cervix*. Philadelphia: JB Lippincott Company.
Shingleton HM, Gore H, Bradley D & Soong SJ (1981) Adenocarcinoma of the cervix: 1. Clinical evaluation and pathologic features. *Am. J. Obstet. Gynecol.* **138:** 799.
Shingleton HM & Gusberg SB (1988) Radical hysterectomy. In: Gusberg SB, Shingleton HM & Deppe G (eds) *Female Genital Cancer*. New York: Churchill Livingstone.
Shingleton HM & Siller BS (1994) The lymphatic system. In: Orr J & Shingleton H, *Complications in Gynecologic Surgery*, pp. 236–259. Philadelphia: JB Lippincott Company.
Shingleton HM (1992) Surgical treatment of cancer of the cervix. *Eur. J. Gynaecol. Oncol.* **13(1):** 45–52.
Simon NL, Gore H, Shingleton HM *et al.* (1986) Study of superficially invasive carcinoma of the cervix. *Obstet. Gynecol.* **68(1):** 19–24.
Sivanesaratnam V, Jayalakshmi P & Loo C (1993) Surgical management of early invasive cancer of the cervix associated with pregnancy. *Gynecol. Oncol.* **48(1):** 68–75.
Soisson AP, Soper JT, Clarke–Pearson DL *et al.* (1990) Adjuvant radiotherapy following radical hysterectomy for patients with stage IB and IIA cervical cancer. *Gynecol. Oncol.* **37:** 390–395.
Thomas GM (1993) Editorial: Is neoadjuvant chemotherapy a useful strategy for the treatment of stage 1B cervix cancer? *Gynecol. Oncol.* **49:** 153–155.
Thomas G & Dembo A (1991) Is there a role for adjuvant pelvic radiotherapy after radical hysterectomy in early stage cervical cancer? *Intern. J. Gynecol. Cancer* **1:** 1.
Toki N, Tsukamoto N, Kaku T *et al.* (1991) Microscopic ovarian metastasis of the uterine cervical cancer. *Gynecol. Oncol.* **41:** 46.
Trelford JD, Tesluk H, Franti CE *et al.* (1992) 20 year follow-up on microinvasive squamous carcinoma of the cervix. *Eur. J. Gynaecol. Oncol.* **13(2):** 155–9.
van Nagell JR, Donaldson ES & Parker JC *et al.* (1977) The prognostic significance of cell type and lesion size in patients with cervical cancer treated by radical surgery. *Gynecol. Oncol.* **5:** 142–151.
van Nagell JR, Greenwell N, Powell DF *et al.* (1983) Microinvasive carcinoma of the cervix. *Am. J. Obstet. Gynecol.* **145:** 981–991.
van Nagell JR, Rayburn WR, Donaldson ES *et al.* (1979) Therapeutic implications of patterns of recurrence in cancer of the uterine cervix. *Cancer* **44:** 2354–2361.
Welander CE, Pierce VK, Nori D *et al.* (1981) Pretreatment laparotomy in carcinoma of the cervix. *Gynecol. Oncol.* **12:** 336–347.
Wertheim E (1912) The extended abdominal operation for carcinoma uteri. *Am. J. Obstet. Dis. Wom. Child.* **66:** 169.
Zemlickis D, Lishner M, Degendorfer P *et al.* (1991) Maternal and fetal outcome after invasive cervical cancer in pregnancy. *J. Clin. Oncol.* **9(11):** 1956–1961.

6 Invasive Cervical Cancer – Primary Radiotherapy

P W Grigsby
C A Perez

Presentation

As invasive lesions become large enough to be visible, they may appear as plaque-like erythematous areas or small areas of superficial ulceration of the ectocervix. With small early invasive lesions, the patient may also be asymptomatic. As these lesions become larger, the first clinical manifestation is usually abnormal bleeding, which occurs as postcoital spotting, intermenstrual bleeding, or more prominent menstrual bleeding. At this stage gross lesions follow a pattern of endophytic growth, exophytic growth, or ulceration. Exophytic lesions tend to bleed frequently. Endophytic and ulcerative lesions often produce a foul-smelling, serosanguinous discharge.

Spread of cervical carcinoma occurs either by direct extension to local structures or via lymph–vascular channels to lymph nodes or other distant sites. Direct extension involves the entire ectocervix. Tumor will then extend to the vaginal fornices, the parametrial tissues, and the endocervix. Extension to the endometrial cavity occurs in about 10–30% of patients according to Mitani *et al.* (1964) and Perez *et al.* (1981). In advanced-stage disease direct extension is most often confined to the parametrial tissues rather than to the vagina. Tumor can compress or encase the ureters to produce hydronephrosis.

Advanced pelvic disease will continue to cause bleeding and discharge. Nonspecific pelvic pain can occur. Urinary frequency and urgency are most often caused by mass effect and pressure rather than direct tumor invasion. Hematuria is uncommon. Mass effect can also cause constipation and tenesmus, but diarrhea and bright red blood are uncommon symptoms. The triad of sciatic pain, leg edema and hydronephrosis occurs in those with large volume paraaortic disease as occurs in recurrent cervical carcinoma (Grigsby *et al.*, 1994) rather than at the time of initial presentation.

Only a small minority of patients present with distant metastatic disease. Lung, liver and bone are frequent sites of metastases. Liver metastases are manifest by right upper quadrant pain and fullness. Lung metastases may present as multiple parenchymal lesions or mediastinal lymph node metastases. These patients often present with a relentless nonproductive cough or hemoptysis. Occasionally patients may have solitary parenchymal lesions that cannot be distinguished from a new primary lesion of the lung. Patients with bone metastases almost always present with bone pain.

Diagnostic Evaluation

The diagnostic evaluation of patients with suspected cervical carcinoma depends on the presumed stage of disease at the time of evaluation.

Following the diagnosis of invasive cervical carcinoma by biopsy, all patients should undergo examination under anesthesia (EUA) to determine extent of disease. Laboratory studies for patients should include a hemogram and complete blood count. Serum chemistries and urinalysis are also performed.

Radiographic evaluation clearly depends on the presumed clinical stage and may vary greatly between institutions and the availability of specific studies. A chest radiograph should be obtained in all patients. Its purpose is primarily as a preoperative (either before hysterectomy or intracavitary implant) test rather than as a screening examination to detect lung metastasis. Lung metastases occur in less than 5% of patients with otherwise known clinical Stages III and IV disease. Pretreatment evaluation of the urinary tract is also mandatory for all stages of disease. It is essential for the surgeon or radiation oncologist to know if a patient has a duplicated collecting system or pelvic kidney. The likelihood of patients having hydronephrosis from tumor is about 6% for Stage I disease, 15% for Stage II, and 35% for Stage III. Evaluation of the urinary tract can be performed by intravenous urogram or computed tomography (CT) with equal accuracy for a duplicated collecting system, pelvic kidney, and hydronephrosis.

A barium enema has been advocated for all patients. However, it is realistic to perform this examination only in symptomatic patients or those with advanced stage disease. Only 6% of patients with otherwise Stage III disease will have Stage IV disease based on barium enema findings.

At the time of EUA, cystoscopy and sigmoidoscopy can be performed. Cystoscopy results (with biopsy) will advance the clinical stage in less than 1% of those with Stage II disease and 18% of those with Stage III. The results of sigmoidoscopy are somewhat similar to those for barium enema; that is, only less than 1% with Stage II and 7% with Stage III tumor on EUA will be found to have Stage IVA disease by sigmoidoscopy findings.

One of the most controversial topics in the diagnostic evaluation of patients with invasive cervical carcinoma is the assessment of pelvic and paraaortic lymph nodes. The probability of patients with Stage IA and small volume IB disease having positive pelvic or paraaortic lymph node metastases is less than 5%. It can then be reasoned that these patients should not undergo any type of lymph node staging procedure.

Surgical lymph node staging has been advocated by some investigators. Most clinical studies of the Gynecologic Oncology Group (GOG) require surgical lymph node staging. In a retrospective review of their data, the GOG found that for patients receiving curative irradiation after a surgical staging procedure the complication rate was 12% if the procedure used a transperitoneal approach compared with only 4% if a retroperitoneal approach was used (Weiser *et al.*, 1989).

Radiographic evaluation of the pelvic and paraaortic lymph nodes can be performed by a number of studies, including ultrasound, lymphangiography, CT and magnetic resonance imaging (MRI). Evaluation of the paraaortic lymph nodes by ultrasound, CT and lymphangiograms was performed in a prospective study by the GOG. Patients at various cooperative group institutions underwent one of these diagnostic studies followed by a surgical staging procedure. The results, reported by Heller *et al.* (1990), demonstrated a sensitivity and specificity of 79% and 73%, respectively for lymphangiography, 34% and 96% for CT, and 19% and 99% for ultrasonography. Similar sensitivity and specificity were also reported by Piver *et al.* (1971). Sensitivity and specificity are similar for CT and MRI (Camilien *et al.*, 1988; Kim *et al.*, 1990; Castellino, 1991).

The status of scalene lymph nodes has been an issue for some investigators (in addition to pelvic and paraaortic lymph status). Routine use of this procedure for patients with Stages II, III, and IV, and recurrent cervical carcinoma has a low yield (Ketcham *et al.*, 1973, 1976; Perez Mesa and Spratt, 1976; Manetta *et al.*, 1989). However, a higher yield has been reported in patients with positive paraaortic lymph nodes. Buschbaum (1979) reported a 35% incidence of positive left scalene lymph node biopsies performed on 23 patients with known positive paraaortic lymph nodes. However, a prospective study by Stehman *et al.*, (1987) found a 7% (4 of 55) incidence of scalene nodes in patients with known positive paraaortic or high common iliac lymph nodes.

EUA is the preferred method for determining local tumor extent. Radiographic evaluation of the cervix for staging purposes has proven to be unreliable. CT has, at best, been reported to be 70–80% accurate in detecting parametrial tumor invasion (Janus *et al.*, 1989; Kim *et al.*, 1990). MRI appears to be more accurate in detecting parametrial invasion with reported accuracies of 86–92% (Janus *et al.*, 1989; Kim *et al.*, 1990). Transected ultrasound appears to give a reliable measurement of tumor size (Magee *et al.*, 1991), but a high false-positive rate for detecting parametrial involvement was reported by Aoki *et al.* (1990).

Staging

The current accepted staging system for carcinoma of the cervix is the 1992 American Joint Committee on Cancer (AJCC) and Federation of International Gynecology and Obstetrics (FIGO) clinical staging system (see *Table 47.1*, page 567) (Beahrs *et al.*, 1992). The staging as shown in *Table 47.1* is accompanied by descriptive notes to the strict definitions that clarify some of the more subtle points for staging. These clarifying notes are summarized below.

Stage IA carcinoma includes minimal microscopically evident stromal invasion as well as small cancerous tumors of measurable size. This stage should be divided into those lesions with minute foci of invasion visible only microscopically as Stage IA1 and macroscopically measurable microcarcinomas as Stage IA2. The term 'IB occult' should be omitted. The diagnosis of both stages IA1 and IA2 should be based on microscopic examination of removed tissue, preferably a conization of the cervix that must include the entire lesion. The lower limit of Stage IA2 should be measurable macroscopically, and the upper limit is given by the measurement of the two largest dimensions in any given section. The depth of invasion should not be more than 5 mm taken from the base of the epithelium, either surface or glandular, from which it originates. The second dimension, the horizontal spread, must not exceed 7 mm. Vascular space involvement, either venous or lymphatic, should not alter the staging, but should be recorded. Lesions of greater size should be classified as Stage IB.

As a rule, it is impossible to estimate clinically whether cancer of the cervix has extended to the uterine corpus or not. Extension to the uterine corpus should therefore be disregarded for clinical staging.

A patient with a growth fixed to the pelvic wall by a short and indurated, but not nodular, parametrium should be allotted to Stage IIB. On occasion it is impossible, at clinical examination to decide whether a smooth and indurated parametrium is truly cancerous or only inflammatory. Therefore, the tumor should be classified as Stage III only if the parametrium is nodular on the pelvic wall or if the growth itself extends to the pelvic wall.

The presence of hydronephrosis or nonfunctioning kidney due to stenosis of the ureter by cancer permits a case to be classified as Stage III even if according to the other findings the case should be allotted to Stage I or II.

The presence of bullous edema does not permit a tumor to be designated as Stage IV. Ridges and furrows in the bladder wall should be interpreted as signs of submucous involvement of the bladder if they remain fixed to the growth during palpation (i.e. examination of the vagina or rectum during cystoscopy). A finding of malignant cells in cytologic washings from the urinary bladder requires further examination and a biopsy from the wall of the bladder.

Clinical procedures and their results that are allowed by FIGO for defining clinical stage include physical examination, pelvic EUA cystoscopy, and proctoscopy. Radiologic examinations that can alter staging include chest and skeletal radiographs and intravenous urography. Lymphangiography and laparoscopy do not alter stage.

FIGO clinical staging has several deficiencies in that several important prognostic factors are not taken into account. FIGO does not allow for the inclusion of findings of CT, MRI, lymphangiogram or surgical staging. Findings not explicitly accounted for in the staging system include the presence of tumor emboli in vascular spaces, endometrial extension, positive lymph nodes and tumor size (Perez *et al.*, 1992).

Radiation Therapy

For many years controversy has existed between advocates of radical surgery or radiation therapy for the treatment of various groups of patients with carcinoma of the uterine cervix. Regardless of personal preferences, treatment should be closely coordinated between the gynecologist and radiation oncologist, and an integrated team approach should be vigorously pursued.

A direct comparison of the results obtained with these two modalities is not feasible because of the well-defined selection of patients: younger patients with a better general condition and smaller tumors are treated surgically and less favorable groups receive radiation therapy. In addition, surgical exploration eliminates patients with more advanced disease from the surgical group (Hoskins *et al.*, 1976), except those with selected Stage IVA lesions. It is critical that the results of surgical series are reported based on the initial clinical staging to enable meaningful comparison with irradiated patients.

Treating carcinoma *in situ* with various surgical approaches is well established. However, irradiation may be useful for the treatment of some of these lesions, particularly in postmenopausal patients with strong medical contraindications for surgery or when there is extension of the lesion to the vaginal wall or multifocal carcinoma *in situ* in both the cervix and the vagina (DelRegato and Cox, 1965; Creasman and Rutledge, 1972; Kolstad and Klem, 1976; Grigsby and Perez, 1991b).

Stage IA

The definition of microinvasive (Stage IA) carcinoma of the cervix lacks uniform diagnostic criteria; to arrive at a definition of Stage IA, volume of tumor in the stroma may be a more reliable criterion than depth of invasion (Burghardt and Holzer, 1977). Depth of invasion and tumor confluence have been identified as prognostic factors that should be taken into consideration in the planning of therapy (Benson and Norris, 1977; Hasumi *et al.*, 1980). When depth of penetration of the stroma by tumor is less than 3 mm the incidence of lymph node metastasis is 1% or less and a lymph node dissection or external pelvic irradiation is not warranted (Nelson *et al.*, 1975a; Seski *et al.*, 1977; Fennell, 1978). Early carcinoma of the cervix (Stage IA) can be treated with intracavitary radioactive sources alone (6000–8000 mgh—5500–7000 cGy to point A in one or two insertions) or with a total abdominal or modified radical hysterectomy. With more extensive lesions a Wertheim's radical hysterectomy with pelvic lymphadenectomy or external pelvic and intracavitary irradiation similar to that used for Stage IB are the preferred treatments. Tumor control with all treatment methods is close to 100%, and most patients eventually die of intercurrent disease (Creasman and Parker, 1973; Ruch *et al.*, 1976).

Stages IB and IIA

The selection of definitive irradiation or radical surgery for Stage IB and IIA carcinoma of the cervix is controversial, and the preference of one procedure over the other depends on the institution, the gynecologist or radiation oncologist involved, the general condition of the patient, and the prognostic features of the lesion (Perez, 1987). Radical hysterectomy has been preferred by some for young women because of the desire to preserve the ovaries (Webb, 1975) and the possibility of a more pliable vagina after surgery; according to some gynecologists, treatment with radical pelvic surgery may influence sexual function to a lesser degree than radiation therapy (Abitbol and Davenport, 1974; Seibel *et al.*, 1979). However, Vincent *et al.* (1975) found no difference in sexual functioning of patients following surgery or irradiation. Also, ovarian function can be diminished or absent in 15–40% of patients undergoing radical hysterectomy with ovarian preservation without irradiation (Hodel *et al.*, 1982; Belinson *et al.*, 1984; Husseinzadeh *et al.*, 1984).

Another important alleged advantage of surgery is the opportunity to carry out a thorough pelvic and upper abdominal evaluation because at times there is a discrepancy between the clinical and surgical pathologic stage. However, surgical staging has not been shown to improve overall patient survival (Nelson *et al.*, 1974; Wharton *et al.*, 1977; Potter *et al.*, 1993).

Despite a slower regression after irradiation, reflecting the cellular kinetics and a slow growth, no difference in tumor control or survival has been observed in adenocarcinoma compared with epidermoid carcinoma (Sala *et al.*, 1962; Ubinas and Marcial, 1966; Rutledge *et al.*, 1968; Weiner and Wizenberg, 1975; Grigsby *et al.*, 1988). Because of the predeliction for endocervical involvement in adenocarcinoma, a combination of irradiation and conservative hysterectomy has been advocated by some authors (Rutledge *et al.*, 1968, 1975), although survival is comparable to that seen with irradiation alone (Grigsby *et al.*, 1988; Eifel *et al.*, 1990).

Bulky endocervical carcinoma (so-called barrel-shaped cervix) has a higher incidence of central recurrence, pelvic and paraaortic lymph node metastases, and distant dissemination (Lu *et al.*, 1976; Fletcher, 1983). Because of the inability of the intracavitary sources to encompass all of the tumor in a high dose volume, larger doses of external irradiation to the whole pelvis or extrafascial hysterectomy or both have been advocated to improve therapeutic results (Durrance *et al.*, 1969; O'Quinn *et al.*, 1980). Durrance *et al.* (1969) and Nelson *et al.* (1975b) recommended an extrafascial conservative hysterectomy six weeks after completion of high-dose preoperative irradiation (2000 cGy whole pelvis, 3000 cGy additional dose to parametria with midline shielding and intracavitary insertion of 6000 mgh). Similar results were reported by Perez and Kao (1985) in an analysis of 128 patients with barrel-shaped Stage IB, IIA and IIB carcinoma of the cervix treated with the combined approach or using higher intracavitary doses (8500 mgh—8000 cGy to point A) in addition to external therapy.

Mendenhall *et al.* (1991) reviewed the outcome of 150 patients with Stage IB, IIA or IIB disease greater than 6 cm diameter. Although not a randomized study, 50% of patients received irradiation alone and 50% received irradiation and hysterectomy. Their review demonstrated a local control of 74% for irradiation alone and 76% for combined therapy. Absolute and cause-specific survivals were also equivalent. Similar results have also been reported by Thoms *et al.* (1992) for Stage IB patients with 6–8 cm tumors. A recently closed GOG prospective study randomized patients with Stage IB or IIA disease greater than 4 cm diameter to irradiation alone or preoperative irradiation and hysterectomy. Results of the study are currently pending. The major cause of treatment failure is distant metastases, which are significantly more common than in the non-barrel-shaped tumors (*Figure 6.1*).

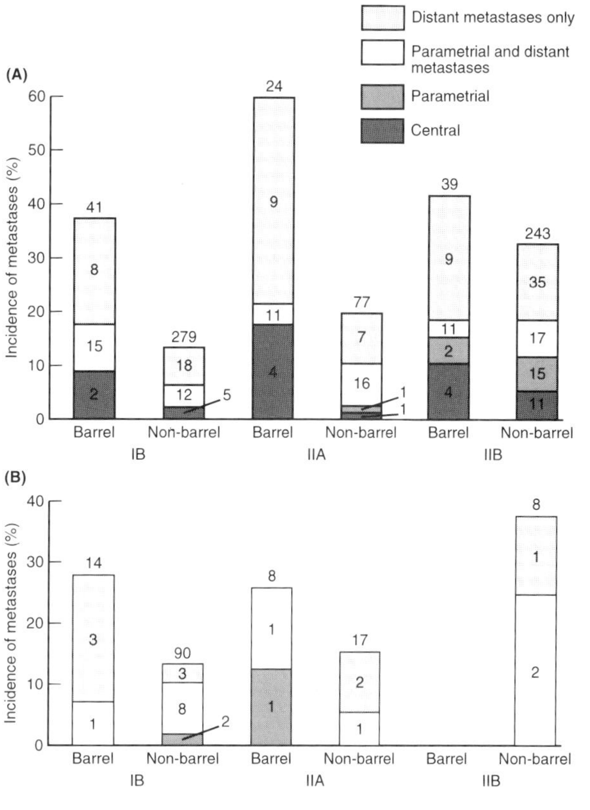

Figure 6.1. Patterns of failure in patients (1959–1980) with Stages IB, IIA and IIB carcinoma of the uterine cervix, comparing barrel- or non-barrel-shaped cervix. A higher incidence of distant metastases is noted in the barrel-shaped cervix patients, treated with either irradiation alone (**A**) or irradiation combined with surgery (**B**). (From Perez *et al.*, 1985a.)

Stages IIB, III and IVA

Patients with Stage IIB and III disease are treated with irradiation alone. Patients with Stage IVA tumors (bladder or rectal invasion) can be treated with either high doses of whole pelvis external irradiation, intracavitary sources and additional parametrial irradiation, or pelvic exenteration (Bricker and Modlin, 1951; Brunschwig and Daniel, 1960; Kiselow *et al.*, 1967; Ulfelder, 1967; Barber, 1969; Deckers *et al.*, 1971; Fletcher, 1971).

At the present time, there is no definitive evidence that chemotherapeutic agents have proven effectiveness in the adjuvant treatment of patients with advanced disease who have a higher incidence of pelvic failures and distant metastasis. Several preliminary reports (John *et al.*, 1978; Thomas *et al.*, 1984; Potish *et al.*, 1986; Twiggs *et al.*, 1986; Kuske *et al.*, 1989) suggest that morbidity from combinations of chemotherapy—usually cisplatin and 5-fluorouracil (5-FU)—concomitant with definitive irradiation is acceptable and may improve tumor control; data on long-term survival are not available.

Postoperative Radiation Therapy Following Radical Hysterectomy

Patients who have undergone radical hysterectomy without preoperative radiation therapy are considered for postoperative irradiation if they have any of the following:

- positive pelvic lymph nodes;
- microscopic positive margins of resection in the cervix; or
- deep stromal invasion or lymphatic permeation.

Treatment consists of 5000 cGy to the whole pelvis when metastatic pelvic lymph nodes or deep stromal invasion is present. Patients with positive common iliac or paraaortic node metastases should receive 5000 cGy to the paraaortic region as well (Perez, 1987).

At our institution, patients with microscopically positive margins in the cervical area are usually treated with external irradiation consisting of 2000 cGy to the whole pelvis followed by 3000 cGy with a midline block in combination with an intracavitary insertion for 6500 cGy surface dose (1800–2000 mgh) to the upper vagina with Fletcher–Suit afterloading colpostats.

There are no controlled studies showing improved survival with postoperative pelvic irradiation following radical surgery in the presence of positive pelvic nodes. Guttman (1970) reported on 50 patients receiving postoperative pelvic irradiation (4000–5000 cGy) 4–5 weeks after radical hysterectomy. The overall 5- and 10-year survival rates for the entire group were 76% and 50%, respectively. Complications were uncommon (two hydronephroses, one vesicovaginal fistula, and one leg edema).

Fuller *et al.* (1982) found that 71 of 431 patients with Stage IB and IIA carcinoma of the uterine cervix had pelvic lymph node metastases at radical hysterectomy. Postoperative irradiation (4000 cGy in four weeks) was given. Among 32 patients with one or two positive nodes survival in the irradiated group was slightly higher than in the non-irradiated group (about 60% versus 40% at five years). Lower survival was observed in seven patients with three or more nodes who received postoperative irradiation. Nahhas *et al.* (1983) reported two of nine recurrences with postoperative irradiation compared with two of four after radical hysterectomy and lymphadenectomy alone. However, a panel summarized the anecdotal experience at several institutions in the USA, and a review of available literature (Morrow, 1980) showed:

- a lack of controlled studies to evaluate the efficacy of postradical hysterectomy irradiation in patients with early carcinoma of the cervix having metastatic pelvic lymph nodes;
- no difference in survival in irradiated or non-irradiated patients (50–83% 5–7-year survival);
- higher incidence of pelvic failures in non-irradiated (84% in 57 recurrent cases) compared with irradiated patients (50% in 18 recurrent cases).

Tattersall *et al.* (1992) performed a prospective randomized study of patients with positive pelvic lymph nodes following completion of radical hysterectomy and lymph node dissection. Postoperatively all patients received pelvic irradiation and were randomized to receive chemotherapy or not. The chemotherapy regimen consisted of cisplatin, vinblastine and bleomycin. No difference was observed in overall or disease-free survivals. A similar study is being conducted through the combined efforts of the Radiation Therapy Oncology Group, (RTOG), Southwest Oncology Group, and GOG. In this study the patient population is identical to that of the Tattersall study, all patients receive postoperative pelvic irradiation and are randomized to receive chemotherapy (cisplatin and 5-FU) or not. This is an ongoing study.

Another ongoing study being performed by the GOG in the postoperative setting randomizes patients with negative lymph nodes but other poor prognostic factors such as capillary space invasion, large tumor size or deep stromal invasion by tumor to receive pelvic irradiation or not. Chemotherapy is not a component of this study.

Carcinoma of the Cervix Inadvertently Treated with a Simple Hysterectomy

Occasionally, because of inadequate preoperative workup, a simple or total abdominal hysterectomy is performed, and invasive carcinoma of the cervix is incidentally found in the surgical specimen. When carcinoma is detected following an abdominal or vaginal hysterectomy, the prognosis is worse if postoperative irradiation is not administered. It is

Table 6.1. Treatment policies for invasive epidermoid carcinoma of the cervix after inadvertent simple (total) hysterectomy (from Perez, 1992).

Group	Tumor extent	Treatment (cGy) Whole pelvis	Split fields	Intracavitary ovoids: surface dose (cGy)
I	Microinvasion (≤3 mm invasion) margins clear	0	0	6500–7000
II	Fully invasive or occult (>3 mm) margins clear	2000	3000	6500
III	Microscopic residual (+margins) or lymphatic permeation in HI	3000	2000	7500–8000
IV	Gross residual 'cut across tumor'	4000	1000–2000	7500
V	Recurrent tumor	4000	1000–2000	8000+ interstitial radiation

critical that these patients receive radiation therapy as soon as their postoperative status allows it. Durrance (1968) and Andras *et al.* (1973) have reported survival rates similar to those of the intact uterus when these patients are treated appropriately.

If only microinvasive carcinoma is found and an extrafascial hysterectomy with wide cuff is performed, no additional therapy is necessary. If a less-comprehensive dissection is carried out, an intracavitary insertion with vaginal colpostats should be performed to deliver 6000 cGy mucosal dose to the vault. The usual therapy in patients with microscopic residual invasive tumor consists of 2000 cGy whole pelvis and 3000 cGy to the parametria combined with an intracavitary insertion to the vaginal vault for 6000 cGy mucosal dose. If there is a residual tumor present in the vaginal vault, the whole pelvis dose should be increased to 4000 cGy and the parametrial dose increased by an additional 1000–2000 cGy. An intracavitary insertion as outlined above should be carried out. If there is residual tumor at completion of therapy, interstitial implants with needles should be carried out to increase the dose to this volume (*Table 6.1*).

Durrance (1968) pointed out that patients with tumor at the margin of resection or gross residual tumor have a less favorable prognosis than those without residual tumor.

Green and Morse (1969) reported nine of 30 patients (30%) surviving five years after definitive irradiation for treatment of invasive cervical carcinoma after inadvertent simple hysterectomy. The same authors noted that 14 of 32 patients treated with a surgical procedure, usually a Wertheim's hysterectomy, died within five years. Eight of nine patients with negative nodes survived, and one died of postoperative complications. The same authors observed that the five-year cure rate was 30% for patients treated within one year of hysterectomy in contrast to 16% for those treated after one year. The time at which the patient is treated, in addition to the bulk of tumor, is therefore an important prognostic factor.

Radiation Therapy Techniques

At the present time the two main modalities of irradiation are external photon beam and brachytherapy. External irradiation is used to treat the whole pelvis and the parametria including the common iliac lymph nodes, while the central disease (cervix, vagina, and medial parametria) is primarily irradiated with intracavitary sources.

Table 6.2 summarizes the policies of irradiation for carcinoma of the uterine cervix at the Mallinckrodt Institute of Radiology.

External Irradiation

External pelvic irradiation is delivered before intracavitary insertions to patients with bulky cervical lesions in order to improve the geometry of the intracavitary application, exophytic easily bleeding tumors, or tumors with necrosis or infection.

When invasive carcinoma of the uterine cervix is irradiated, it is important to deliver adequate doses to the pelvic lymph nodes. For Stages IB and IIA, 16.5 × 16.5 cm portals at the midplane are sufficient. For patients with Stages IIB, III, and IVA, somewhat larger portals, 16.5 × 20 cm, are used to cover all of the common iliac nodes in addition to the cephalad half of the vagina (*Figures 6.2 and 6.3*). A 2 cm margin lateral to the bony pelvis is adequate. If there is no vaginal extension, the lower margin of the port is at the inferior border of the obturator foramen. When there is vaginal involvement, the entire length of the vagina should be treated down to the introitus (*Figure 6.3*). The distal extension of the tumor may be identified by placing a radiopaque clip or bead on the vaginal wall or by inserting a small rod with an opaque marker in the vagina at the time of simulation. In these patients the portals should be modified to cover the inguinal lymph nodes (*Figure 6.4*) because of the increased probability of metastases.

Table 6.2. Carcinoma of the uterine cervix: Mallinckrodt Institute of Radiology policies of treatment with irradiation (from Perez, 1992).

		External irradiation (cGy)*		**Brachytherapy**		
Tumor stage	*Tumor extent*	*Whole pelvis*	*Additional parametrial dose (midline shield)*	*Two insertions (mgh RaEq)*†	*Dose to point A*	*Total dose to point A (cGy)*
IA		0	0	6500–8000	7000	6000–7500
IB (small)	Superficial ulceration; less than 2 cm in diameter or involving fewer than two quadrants	0	4500	8000	7000	6500–7000
IB (2–4 cm)	Four quadrant involvement; no endocervical component or significant expansion	1000	4000	7000	6500–7500	7500–8500
IIA, IIB	Non-barrel-shaped type	2000	3000	8000	7000	8500
IB–IIA (bulky)‡ IIB, IIIA	Barrel-shaped cervix; parametrial extension	2000	3000	8000	7000	8500–9000
IIIB	Parametrial involvement	2000	4000	8000	7000	8500–9500
IIB, IIIB, IV	Poor pelvic anatomy; patients not readily treated with intracavitary insertions (barrel-shaped cervix not regressing; inability to locate external os)	4000	2000	6500	6000	8500–9500

*180 cGy/day, five weekly fractions, using 15 or higher MV photon beams, two portals treated daily.
†60–80 cGy/h at point A. In patients over 65 years or with history of previous pelvic inflammatory disease or pelvic surgery, reduce doses by 10%.
‡In Stage IB and IIA, if complete regression is not obtained, perform extrafascial conservative hysterectomy (reduce brachytherapy dose to 6000 mgh).

When there is persistent parametrial tumor after 5000–6000 cGy has been delivered to the parametria, an additional 1000 cGy in five or six fractions may be delivered with reduced port (8 × 12 cm portal for unilateral and 12 × 12 cm portal for bilateral parametrial coverage) (*Figure 6.5*). The midline shield should be in place to protect the bladder and rectosigmoid (*Figure 6.6*).

If metastatic paraaortic lymph nodes are suspected or confirmed, the retroperitoneal tissues need to be irradiated with a field that includes both the paraaortic nodes and the pelvic tissues (*Figures 6.7 and 6.8*).

Because of the thickness of the pelvis, high-energy beams are particularly suited for this treatment. They decrease the dose of radiation delivered to the peripheral normal tissues and provide a more homogeneous dose distribution in the central pelvis. With lower-energy photon (4–6 MV) beams, higher maximum doses must be given to accomplish the prescribed tumor dose, and more complex field arrangements should be used (three-field or four-field pelvic box or rotational techniques) to minimize the dose to the bladder and rectum and to avoid subcutaneous fibrosis while delivering an adequate dose to the cervix and parametria (*Figure 6.9*). With lower-energy photons, the whole pelvis dose should be limited to 4500–5000 cGy.

Doses of Irradiation

Stage IA (microinvasive) tumors are treated with intracavitary therapy only (6000 cGy in one insertion or 7000–7500 cGy in two insertions to point A).

The optimal dose for invasive carcinoma of the cervix is delivered with a combination of whole pelvis, intracavitary, and, at times, interstitial therapy. Some institutions use lower doses of whole pelvis external irradiation (1000 cGy for Stage 1B and 2000 cGy for Stages IIA, IIB, and III) in addition to parametrial doses (with midline 5 half-value layer (HVL) block) to complete 5000 cGy in Stages IB and IIA or 6000 cGy to the involved parametrial tissues for more advanced stages.

At Washington University an assortment of step-wedges designed in accordance with the isodose curves of the intracavitary applications is used to block the midline (*Figure 6.10*). The intracavitary insertions, usually two, deliver 7000–7500 mgh (6500–7000 cGy to point A) in Stage IB tumors and 7500–8000 mgh (7000–7500 cGy) for Stage IIA, IIB,

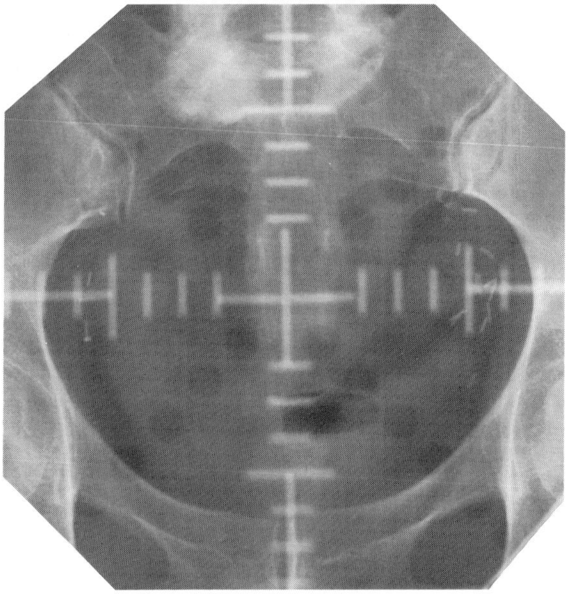

Figure 6.2. Anterior–posterior simulation film of the pelvis illustrating portals used for external irradiation for Stages IB and IIA. The field size is 16.5 × 16.5 cm at the midplane of the pelvis. The lower portal margin is usually placed at the bottom of the obturator foramen, the upper border is at the sacroiliac joints, and the lateral borders are 2 cm beyond the bony pelvis.

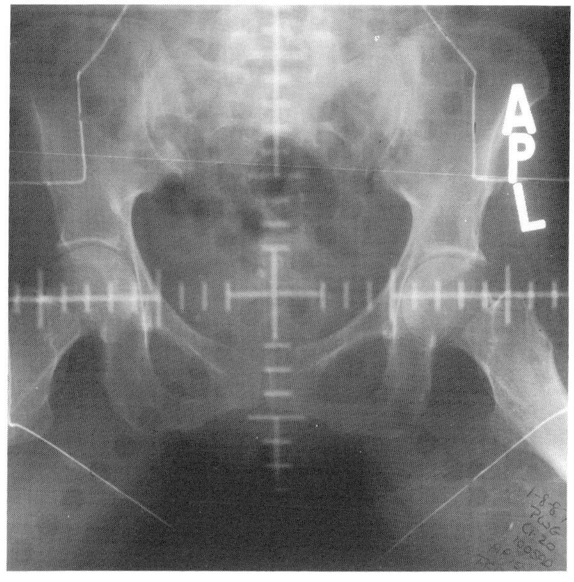

Figure 6.4. Anterior–posterior simulation film of the pelvis and groins illustrating portals used for external irradiation. The portals are expanded laterally to cover the groin lymph nodes in patients with tumor present in the distal one-third of the vagina.

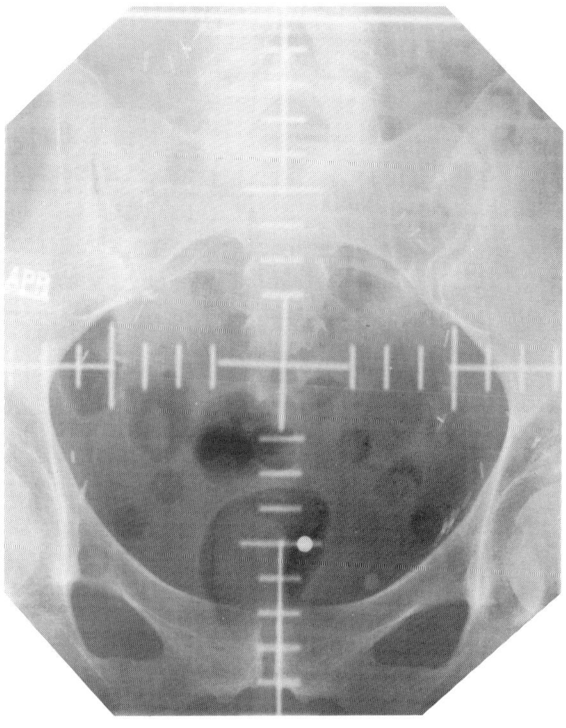

Figure 6.3. Anterior–posterior simulation film of the pelvis illustrating portals used for external irradiation for Stages IIB, III and IV. The field size is 16.5 × 20 cm at the midplane of the pelvis. The lower border is usually placed at the bottom of the ischial tuberosities, the upper border is at the L4–5 interspace, and the lateral borders are 2 cm beyond the bony pelvis.

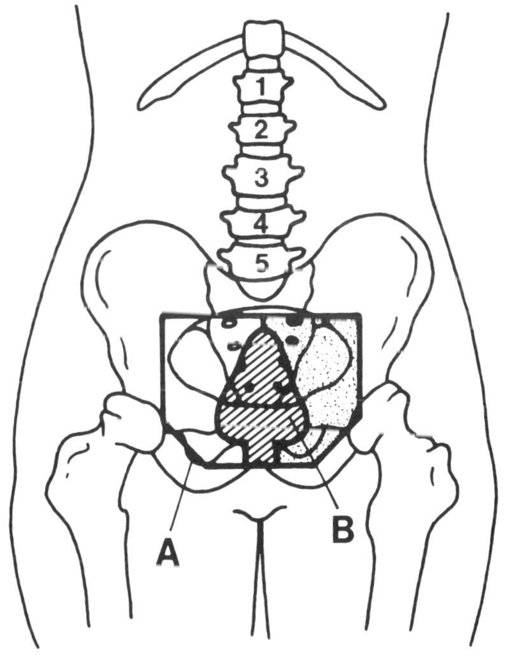

Figure 6.5. Diagram of the reduced portals used for parametrial boost in patients with Stages IIB and III after completion of whole pelvis irradiation. If residual bilateral parametrial involvement is present 12 × 12 cm ports are used (**A**). If there is unilateral parametrial involvment only half of the pelvis is treated with an 8 × 12 cm field. Midline wedge or rectangular block is used to shield volume treated with brachytherapy.

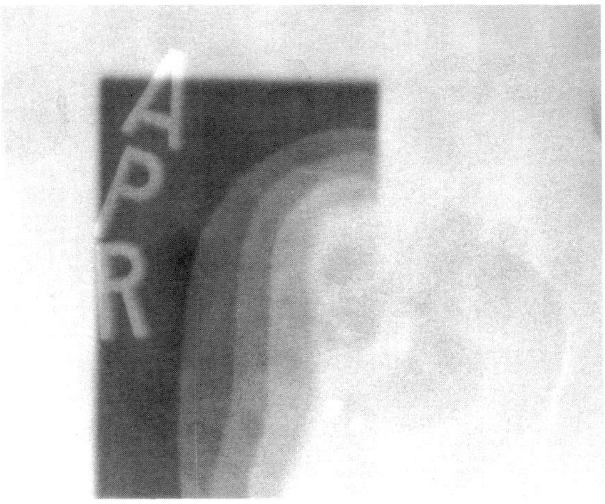

Figure 6.6. Portal localization film demonstrating reduced unilateral parametrial boost showing the position of the midline shield.

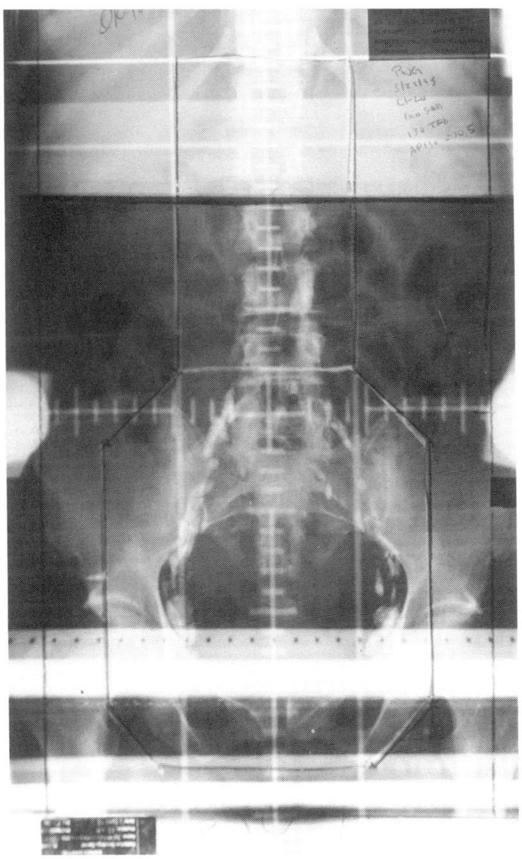

Figure 6.7. Anterior–posterior simulation film of the pelvis and paraaortic lymph nodes illustrating portals used for external irradiation. The top border of the portal is at the T12–L1 interspace and is about 8 cm wide.

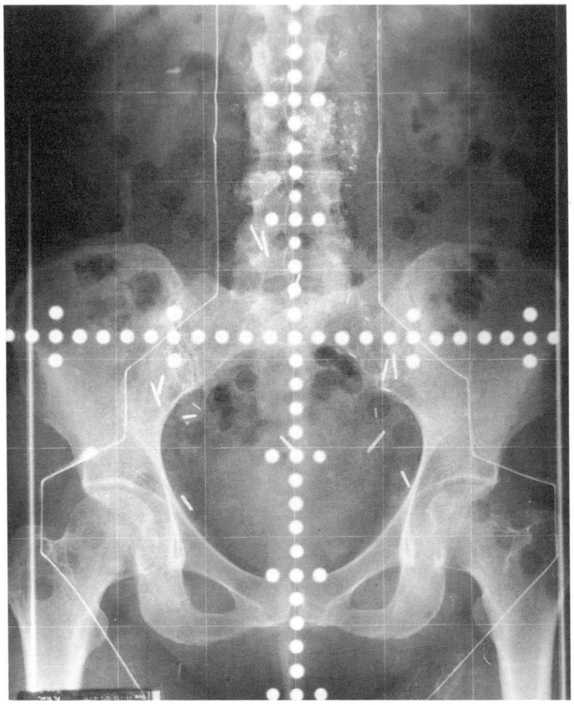

Figure 6.8. Simulation film illustrating the portal used for a patient with carcinoma of the uterine cervix with pelvic, periaortic and inguinal lymph nodes. (From Perez, 1987.)

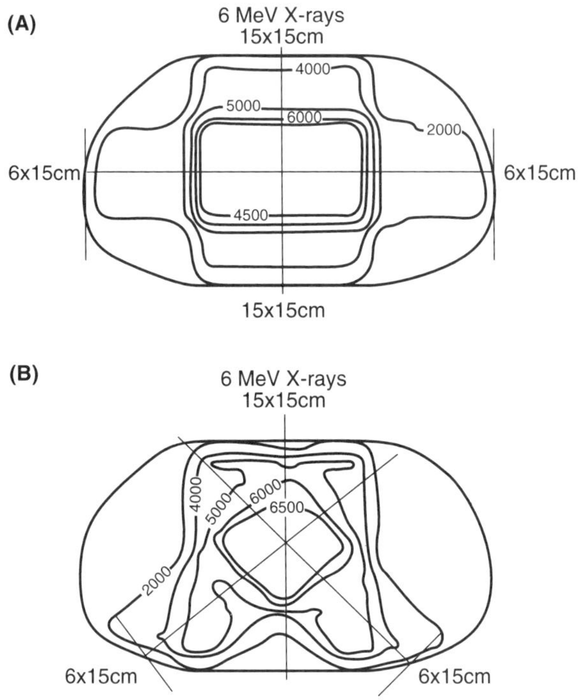

Figure 6.9. Examples of isodose curves for 'box' (**A**) and three-field (posterior oblique fields) (**B**) for irradiation of the pelvis with low-energy photons. (From Perez *et al.*, 1985a.)

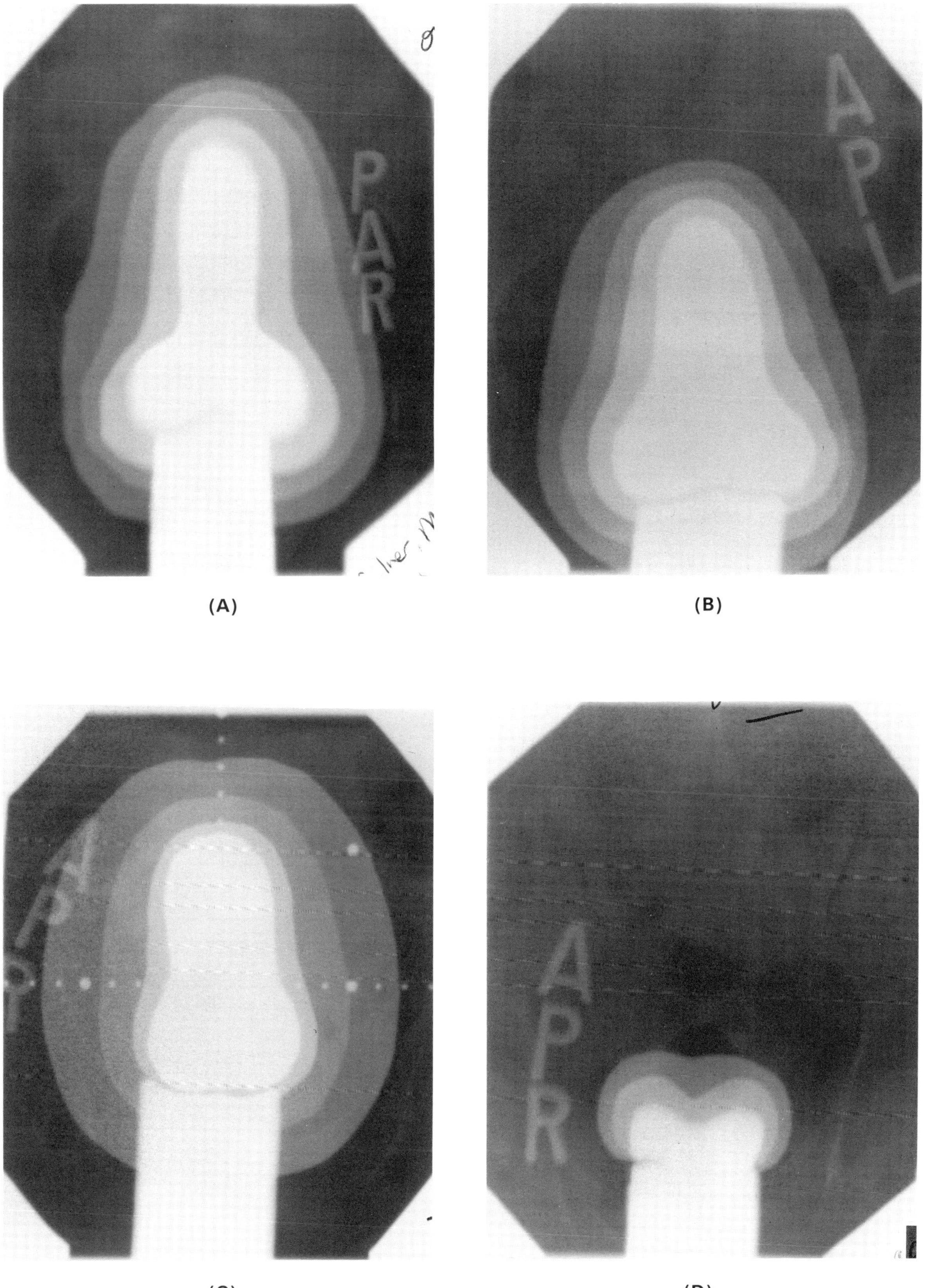

Figure 6.10. Localization films of examples of different stepwedges used to shield the midline during external irradiation. Stepwedges are designed according to the dose distribution from the intracavitary brachytherapy sources.

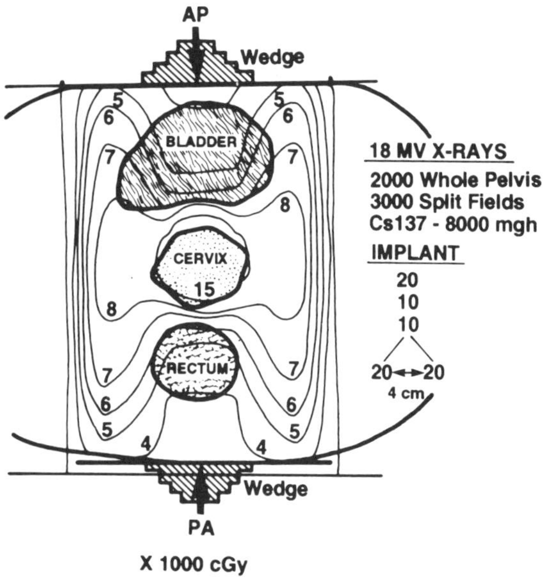

Figure 6.11. Composite isodose curves for a patient with Stage IB carcinoma of the uterine cervix treated with external irradiation and two intracavitary insertions. The doses and source arrangement are shown.

and III lesions. This technique affords a high central dose to the cervix, paracervical tissues, and parametria as well as a moderate homogeneous dose to the external iliac lymph nodes without exceeding the bladder and rectal tolerance doses (*Figure 6.11*).

Other institutions prefer higher doses of whole pelvis external irradiation (usually 4000 cGy) with an additional parametrial dose shielding the midline to complete 5000 cGy in patients with Stages IB and IIA and 5500–6000 cGy for patients with Stage IIB, III, or IVA tumors. This is usually combined with one or two intracavitary insertions for approximately 5000–6000 mgh (4500–5500 cGy to point A) (Perez, 1987).

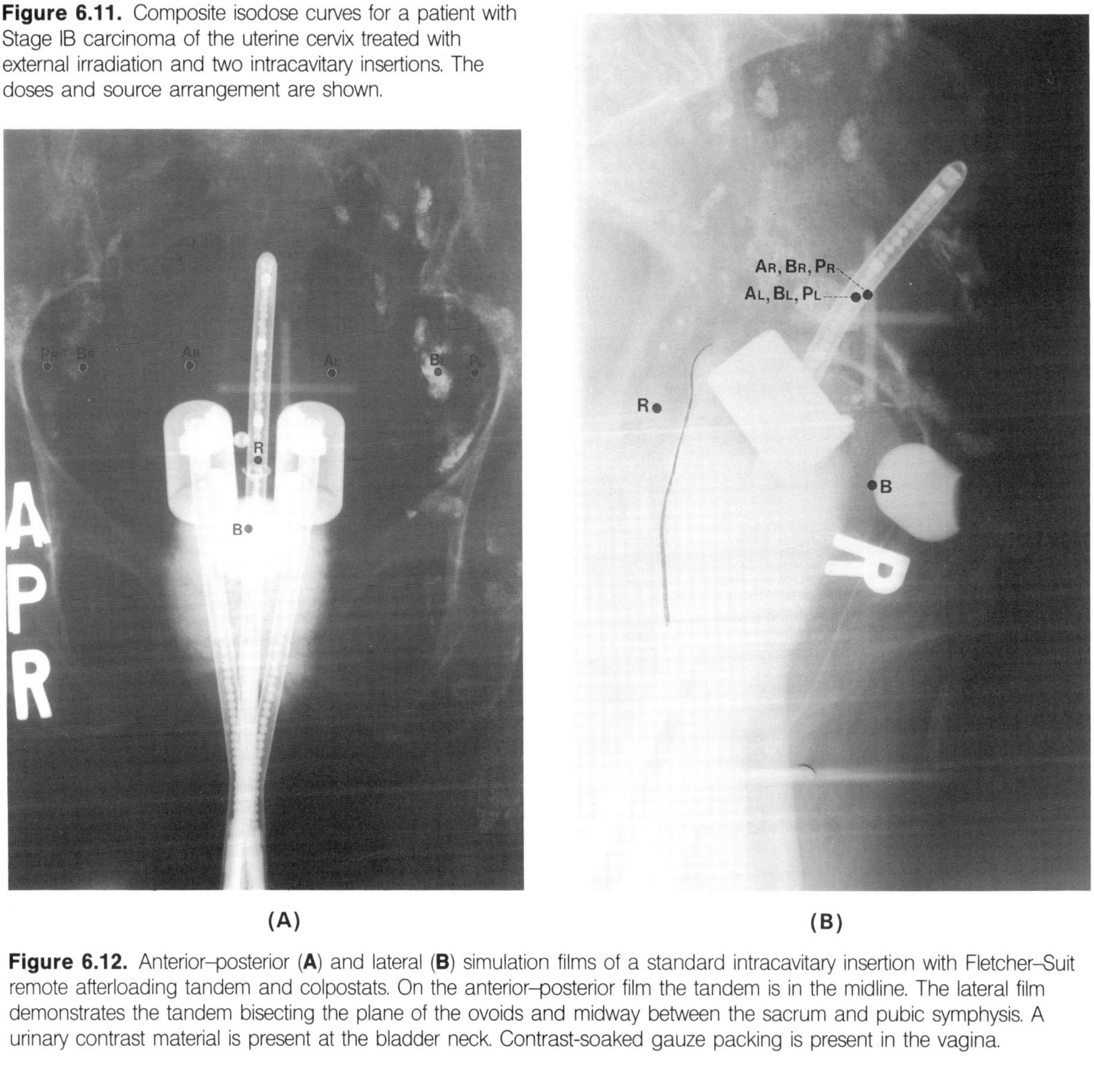

(A) (B)

Figure 6.12. Anterior–posterior (**A**) and lateral (**B**) simulation films of a standard intracavitary insertion with Fletcher–Suit remote afterloading tandem and colpostats. On the anterior–posterior film the tandem is in the midline. The lateral film demonstrates the tandem bisecting the plane of the ovoids and midway between the sacrum and pubic symphysis. A urinary contrast material is present at the bladder neck. Contrast-soaked gauze packing is present in the vagina.

Brachytherapy

There are several isotopes available although at the present time, cesium 137 is the most popular. Brachytherapy can be delivered with intracavitary techniques using applicators consisting of an intrauterine tandem and vaginal colpostats (*Figure 6.12*). There are a variety of applicators used for intracavitary therapy, the majority being after-loading. Recently remote afterloading devices using conventional or high-dose rate exposures have been introduced in clinical practice (Utley *et al.*, 1984). The intracavitary therapy, with its rapid dose fall-off as a function of distance, yields a high dose to the uterus and paracervical tissues, but it is inadequate to treat the pelvic lymph nodes, and external irradiation is necessary to supplement the dose. Also, interstitial implants with needles (*Figure 6.13*) in limited tumor volumes are helpful in specific clinical situations (i.e. localized residual tumor). Appropriate adjustment of total dose prescribed needs to be carried out. Radiographs of the application are

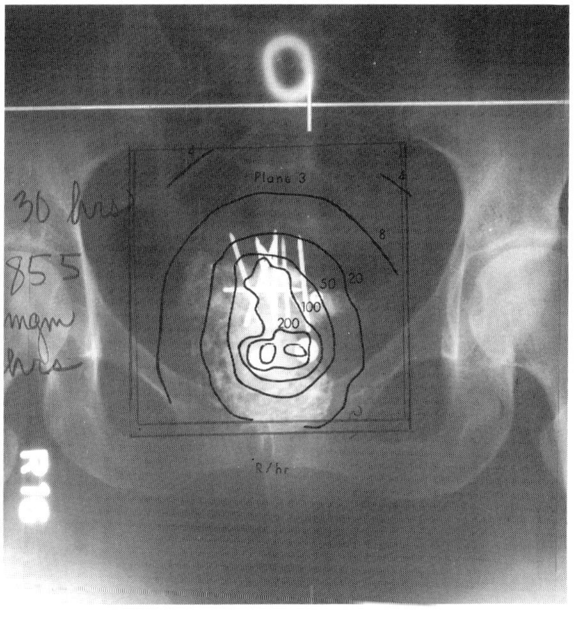

(A)

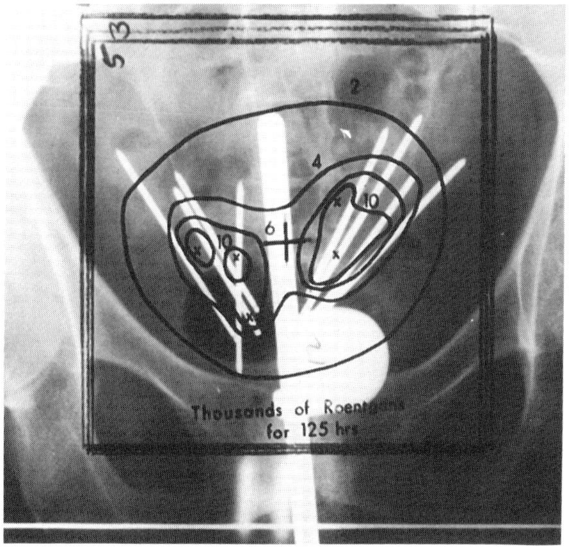

(B)

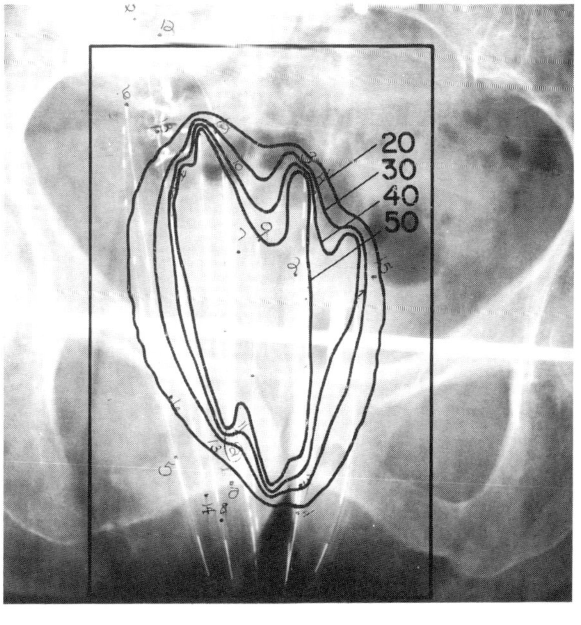

(C)

Figure 6.13. (**A**) Radiograph of the pelvic illustrating interstitial implant in the cervix in a patient with Stage IB on whom the cervical os could not be identified. A dose of 7000 cGy was delivered in combination with external irradiation. (**B**) Example of bilateral parametrial implant used to boost the dose in a patient on whom only an afterloading tandem was placed in combination with whole pelvis and parametrial irradiation for treatment of Stage IIB carcinoma. (**C**) Example of afterloading iridium interstitial implant used to boost the dose in the right paravaginal and parametrial tissues in a patient with Stage IIB carcinoma of the cervix. (From Perez, 1987.)

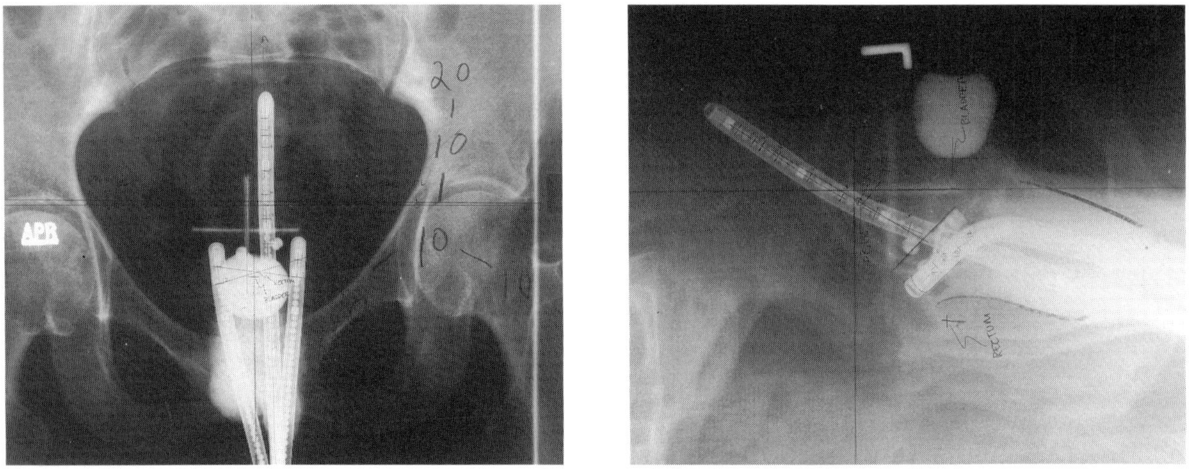

(A) (B)

Figure 6.14. Anterior–posterior (**A**) and lateral (**B**) simulation films of an intracavitary insertion with Fletcher–Suit remote afterloading tandem and minicolpostats.

always obtained using dummy sources, and the active sources can be inserted after the films have been reviewed and the position of the applicators is judged to be satisfactory.

There are some technical problems in achieving satisfactory intracavitary insertions because of the configuration of the tumor or the vagina. If the vaginal vault is narrow, it may be impossible to insert regular-size colpostats successfully, in which case miniovoids should be used (*Figure 6.14*). When miniovoids cannot be inserted, it is better to use a protruding source in the vaginal vault and cervix (usually 20–30 mg) with a plastic sleeve around the afterloading tandem (*Figure 6.15*).

In general, the first intracavitary insertion is scheduled after 1000–2000 cGy of external irradiation if an adequate geometry exists in the pelvis. Otherwise, 3000–4000 cGy is delivered before the first application to decrease the size of the lesion and to improve the relationship of the applicators to the cervix and vagina. The second application is performed 1–2 weeks later after external therapy.

Combination of Irradiation and Surgery

At some institutions the combination of preoperative irradiation and a radical hysterectomy has been used in the treatment of patients with Stage IB and IIA disease (Christensen *et al.*, 1964; Morton *et al.*, 1964; Rampone *et al.*, 1973; Quigley *et al.*, 1975). Sometimes an intracavitary insertion alone is used (5000–6000 mgh). The rationale for the use of an operation has been the alleged inability of irradiation to eradicate completely the metastatic tumor in the pelvic lymph nodes (Leveuf and Godord, 1934; Taussig, 1934; Morton *et al.*, 1964).

When metastatic pelvic lymph nodes or positive surgical margins are found after a hysterectomy, postoperative irradiation is delivered. If only intracavitary therapy was given preoperatively, 2000 cGy whole pelvis and 3000 cGy to the parametria are administered while shielding the midline. If some external therapy is delivered preoperatively, an additional parametrial dose to complete 5000–5500 cGy should be given, again shielding the midline with an appropriate block. In patients not irradiated preoperatively on whom postoperative irradiation is indicated, we administer a combination of external irradiation (2000 cGy whole pelvis and 3000 cGy to the parametria with a small midline block) and an intracavitary insertion for 6000 cGy to the vaginal mucosa (1800 mgh) with two colpostats. In other patients external irradiation alone (5000 cGy to the midplane of the pelvis) has been used. In these patients great care should be exercised in designing treatment techniques, including intracavitary insertions, since because of the surgical extirpation of the uterus, the bladder and the rectosigmoid may be in closer proximity to the radioactive sources than in the patient with intact uterus (*Figure 6.16*). Furthermore, the vascular supply may be affected by the surgical procedure and adhesions may cause fixation of small bowel loops in the pelvis.

Results of Treatment

Patients with Stage IA disease are effectively treated with intracavitary ^{137}Cs insertions only. In patients with microinvasive carcinoma treated at Washington University, no local or regional failures were noted

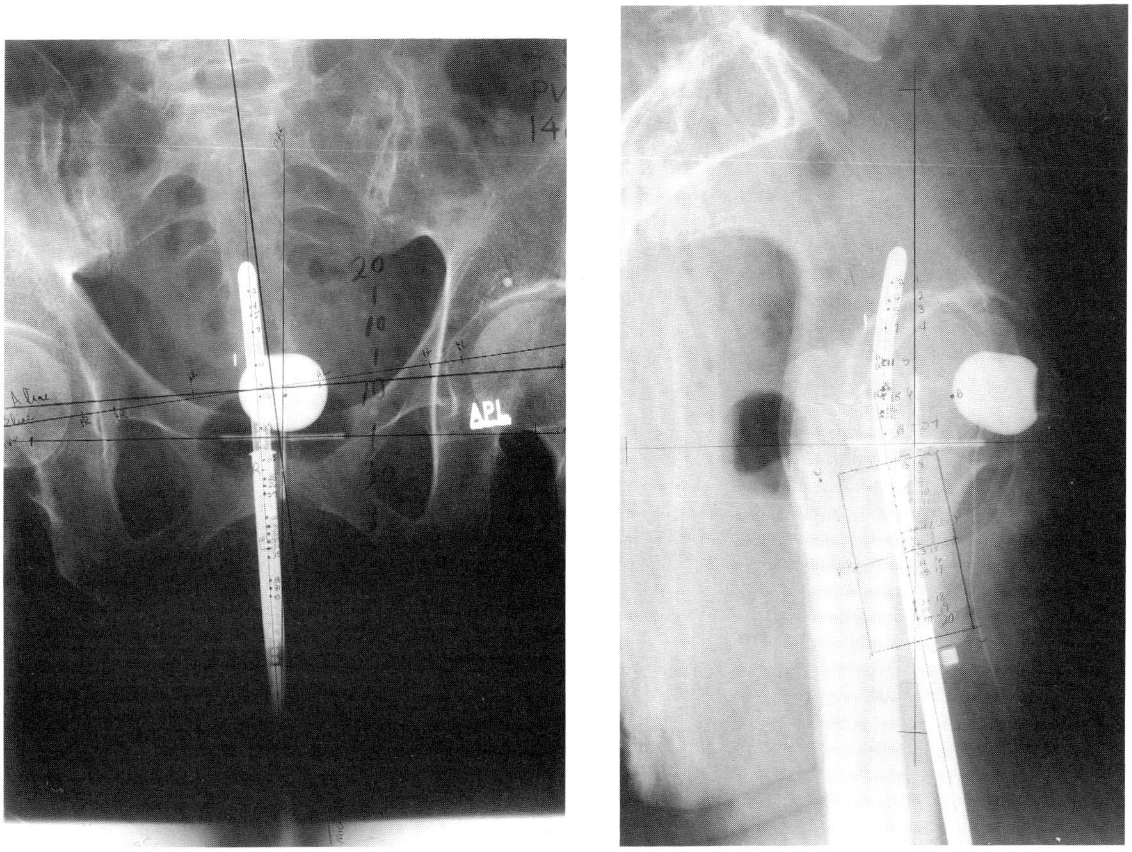

(A) (B)

Figure 6.15. Anterior–posterior (**A**) and lateral (**B**) simulation films of an intracavitary implant demonstrating the use of a Fletcher–Suit remote afterloading tandem without colpostats in a narrow vaginal vault. A Delclos vaginal cylinder is placed over the tandem in the cervix to create a 'protruding source.'

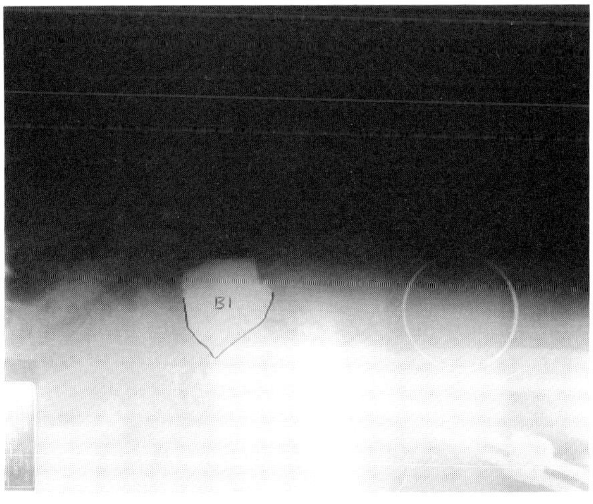

Figure 6.16. Lateral simulation film of colpostats in the vaginal vault of a patient following hysterectomy. Note the proximity of the bladder (contains contrast) and the rectum to the colpostats.

and the corrected five-year survival (for intercurrent disease) was 100% (Grigsby and Perez, 1991b).

Hamberger *et al.* (1978) reported on 151 patients with Stage IA or IB lesions less than 1 cm in diameter treated with intracavitary therapy alone. No failures were noted in 41 patients with Stage IA and only four of 93 patients (4%) with Stage IB, small volume. Of 17 patients with more advanced Stage IB lesions, three (18%) treated with intracavitary therapy only had regional failures. The doses of irradiation were relatively high (8640–1360 mgh). Only three patients (2%) developed Grade 3 complications (one hemorrhagic cystitis, one ureteral stricture with hydronephrosis and one rectovaginal fistula).

Volterrani and Lombardi (1980) reported a fve-year survival rate of 82.6% in 23 patients with occult Stage IB carcinoma of the cervix treated with intracavitary radium only (^{226}Ra application using derivation from Paris method to deliver 7500 mgh). However, the five-year survival rates were only 64.8% in Stage IB disease, 50% in Stage II, and

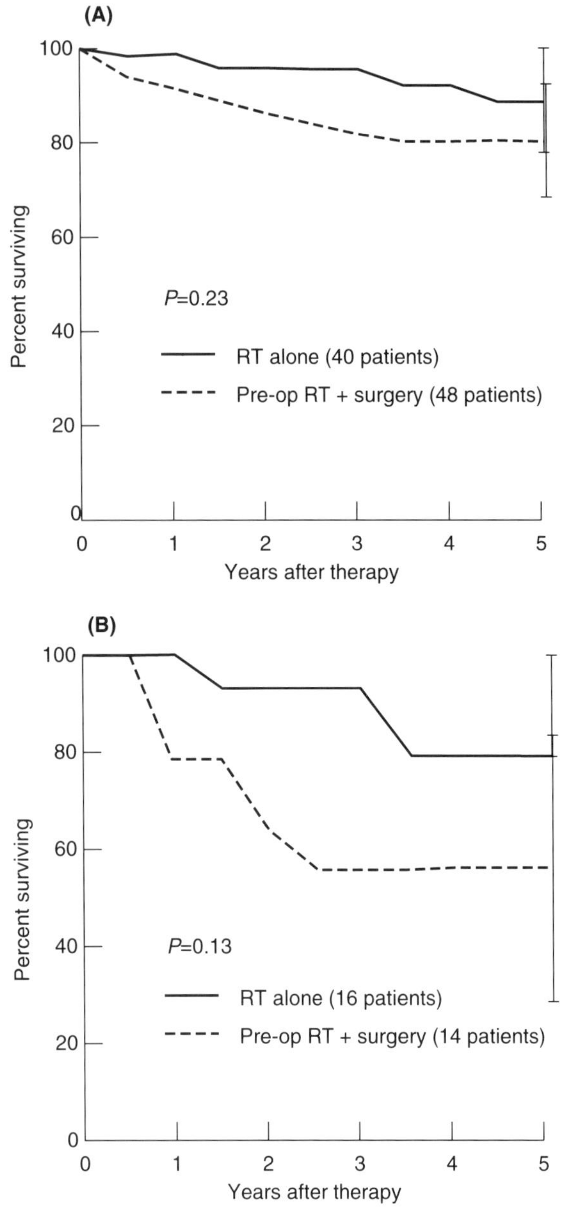

Figure 6.17. Survival curves (actuarial disease-free survival by treatment) of patients with Stage IB (**A**) and IIA (**B**) carcinoma of the uterine cervix treated with irradiation alone (RT) or combined with surgery in a randomized study from 1966–1979. (From Perez *et al.*, 1987.)

29.8% in Stage III. The results are substantially inferior to those obtained with a combination of intracavitary and external irradiation. It is obvious that intracavitary therapy alone is grossly inadequate to irradiate effectively larger primary tumors, including barrel-shaped lesions as well as any parametrial extension. Unfortunately, the authors did not report the exact location of the failures.

The usual five-year survival rate for Stage IB is 86–92% and for Stage IIA, about 75%. Either surgery or adequate irradiation is equally effective in the treatment of Stage IB and IIA carcinoma of the cervix (*Figure 6.17*). Numerous non-controlled studies support the merits of either modality (Parker *et al.*, 1967; Brunschwig, 1968; Pilleron *et al.*, 1972; Park *et al.*, 1973; Surwit *et al.*, 1976; Sall *et al.*, 1979). In prospectively randomized studies Newton (1975) and Roddick and Greenlaw (1971) reported comparable survival and pelvic recurrences in patients with Stage IB and IIA carcinoma of the uterine cervix treated with a radical hysterectomy or irradiation alone. Other reports show no significant difference in survival or pelvic tumor control with either modality (*Tables 6.3 and 6.4*). Kielbinska *et al.* (1973), in a long-term follow-up of 792 women treated by irradiation and 789 women treated with hysterectomy and irradiation for Stage I cervical carcinoma, found no difference in survival, general health, incidence of recurrent carcinoma, or appearance of second primary malignancy.

Einhorn *et al.* (1980), in a non-randomized study, observed better survival in 49 patients with Stage IB disease receiving combined therapy (100% at five years) in comparison with 64 patients treated with irradiation alone (81% at five years). No difference was observed in 25 patients with Stage IIA treated with combined therapy and 40 treated with irradiation alone (about 75% five-year survival). Patients with metastatic lymph nodes have survival rates that are approximately 50% of those with negative nodes (Pilleron *et al.*, 1974; Morley and Seski, 1976).

Perez *et al.* (1987) reported on a prospectively randomized study of 118 selected patients with Stage IB and IIA carcinoma of the uterine cervix in which patients were randomly assigned to be treated with irradiation alone (as described previously) or irradiation and surgery (2000 cGy whole pelvis, one intracavitary insertion for 5000–6000 mgh, followed by a radical hysterectomy with pelvic lymphadenectomy 26 weeks later). The actuarial tumor-free five-year survival was 80% for 40 Stage IB patients treated with irradiation alone and 82% for 48 patients treated with preoperative irradiation and surgery ($p=0.23$) (*Figure 6.17a*). In 16 patients with Stage IIA disease, actuarial tumor-free survival was 56% with irradiation alone and 79% in 14 patients treated with irradiation and surgery ($p=0.13$) (*Figure 6.17b*). In patients with Stage IB treated with irradiation alone, the pelvic failure rate was 2.5% and distant metastases, 7.5%. In the group receiving preoperative irradiation and surgery, the pelvic failure rate was 12.5% and distant metastases 4.2%. In Stage IIA patients receiving irradiation alone the pelvic failure rate was 6.3%, combined pelvic recurrence with distant metastases, 18.8%, and distant metastases alone, 12.5%. The incidence of grade 2–3 complications with radiation therapy alone was 13.8% and with preoperative irradiation and surgery, 11%.

When combined therapy is used, the dose of

Table 6.3. Survival rates for Stages I and II carcinoma of the cervix treated by radical hysterectomy and pelvic lymphadenectomy (from Hoskins *et al.*, 1976).

Authors	*Stage*	*Number of patients*	*Survivors**	*Percentage survival*
Blaikley *et al.* (1969)	IB	98	64	65.5
	IB & IIA	161	96	50.8
Brunschwig and Barber (1966)	IB (A)[†]	173	141	81.5
	IB & IIA (B)[†]	308	231	76.0
Christensen *et al.* (1964)	IB	168	137	82.7
	IB & IIA	219	168	77.0
Ketcham *et al.* (1971)	IB	28	Actuarial	86.0
	IB & IIA	42		87.0
Liu and Meigs (1955)	IB	116	91	78.4
	IB & IIA	165	119	72.1
Masterson (1967)	IB	120	105	87.5
	IB & IIA	150	124	82.5
Park *et al.* (1973)	IB	126	Actuarial	91.0
Average	IB			81.9
	IB & IIA			74.2

*Patients dead of intercurrent disease were included with survivors when data were available.
[†]Surgical and pathologic classification.

Table 6.4. Five-year survival of patients with Stages I and II carcinoma of the cervix treated by radiotherapy (from Hoskins *et al.*, 1976).

Authors	*Stage*	*Number of patients*	*Survivors**	*Percentage Survival*
Blaikley *et al.* (1969)	I	183	123	67.2
	I & II	551	296	53.7
Dickson (1972)	IB	348	249	71.6
	IB & IIA	983	509	60.0
Fletcher (1971)	IB	549	Actuarial	91.5
	IB & IIA	973		83.5
Kline *et al.* (1969)	IB	45	37	81.4
	IB & IIA	64	47	70.5
Kottmeier (1964)	IB	611	547	89.5
	IB & IIA	1576	1244	78.9
Muirhead and Green (1968)	I	194	152	78.0
	I & II	306	208	68.0
Perez *et al.* (1980)	IB	312	Actuarial	87.0
	IIA	98	NED	73.0
Wall *et al.* (1966)	I	101	87	86.4
	I & II	208	153	
Average	I			83.5
	I & II			75.6

*Patients dead of intercurrent disease were included with survivors when data were available.
NED, No evidence of disease.

Table 6.5. Carcinoma of the uterine cervix, Stages IB and IIA; numbers and percentages (in parentheses) of metastatic pelvic lymph nodes and dose of irradiation delivered to lymph nodes (from Perez *et al.*, 1979).

	Stage IB		**Stage IIA**		
Authors	*Surgery alone*	*Preoperative X-ray therapy*	*Surgery alone*	*Preoperative X-ray therapy*	*Estimated dose (cGy) to nodes*
Christensen *et al.* (1964)	29/167 (17.4)	—	27/104 (26.0)	—	0
Morley and Seski (1976)	18/143 (12.6)	—	—	—	0
Morton *et al.* (1964)	9/38 (23.7)	4/32 (12.5)	—	—	1800
Sweeney and Douglas (1962)	—	5/39 (12.8)	—	9/54 (16.6)	3500
Rampone *et al.* (1973)	—	81/537 (15.0)	—	—	2000
Decker *et al.* (1965)	—	5/38 (13.1)	—	11/45 (24.4)	4000
Quigley *et al.* (1975)	—	13/136 (9.6)	—	—	1800
Parker *et al.* (1967)	15/95 (16.0)	6/73 (8.2)	7/16 (44.0)	20/71 (28.0)	Not stated
Gray *et al.* (1958)	5/44 (11.4)	3/58 (5.2)	6/17 (35.3)	Included in I	4500
Perez *et al.* (1980)	—	2/43 (4.6)	—	2/24 (8.3)	3000–4000
Perez *et al.* (1980)	—	0/32 (0.0)	—	—	4001–5000
Rutledge *et al.* (1965)	—	1/30 (3.3)	—	4/39 (10.3)	5000

irradiation delivered to the lymph nodes (*Table 6.5*), the time of the operation and the pathologic examination of the specimen are critical in determining the presence of post-irradiation residual tumor.

Rutledge *et al.* (1965) reported a 3% incidence of metastatic lymph nodes in 30 patients with Stage I, 10% in 39 patients with Stage IIA, and 18% in 73 patients with Stage IIB or III carcinoma of the uterine cervix who underwent a bilateral pelvic lymphadenectomy six weeks after completion of definitive radiation therapy as part of a randomized study. The dose of irradiation to the lymph nodes ranged from 5000–6000 cGy delivered with megavoltage external photon beam and intracavitary radium insertions. The survival rate in these patients was comparable to that observed with irradiation alone (*Figure 6.18*). Complications were somewhat higher in the patients treated with the combination of the two modalities.

Perez *et al.* (1975) noted that in patients with primary carcinoma of the uterine cervix who have endometrial stromal invasion or tumor only in the curettement, the addition of a hysterectomy did not improve survival since most of the patients failed because of distant dissemination. Pelvic and distant recurrences were approximately the same whether radiation therapy was used alone or in combination with surgery.

van Nagell *et al.* (1979) found that the recurrence rate was 5% for tumors less than 2 cm in diameter treated with either radical hysterectomy or irradiation for Stage IB disease. These authors recommend radical surgery for patients with tumors of 2 cm or less. For lesions 2–5 cm in diameter, the failure rate was 24% for surgery, but only 11% for irradiation.

Almost all patients with Stage IIB disease are treated with irradiation alone, and the five-year survival rate is 60–65%. Occasionally a conservative hysterectomy is performed after high-dose preoperative irradiation in patients with barrel-shaped cervix and limited medial parametrial infiltration that regresses completely 4–6 weeks after completion of the irradiation. Before 1965 a pelvic lymphadenectomy was carried out in some patients after full-course radiation therapy, but this procedure did not improve the survival over that with irradiation alone. For Stage IIIB disease the five-year survival rate ranges from 30–48%. This may be related to the socioeconomic status of the patients, extent of the disease, techniques of irradiation, and dose delivered to the parametrium. Allt (1969) and, in an update of the same randomized study, Johns (1976) reported better pelvic tumor control and survival and fewer complications in a group of 65 patients with Stage IIB and III cervical carcinoma treated with 22 MV photons in comparison with 61 patients treated with cobalt-60 (^{60}Co) external irradiation and intracavitary insertions (*Figure 6.19*).

Interstitial parametrial implants have been used to supplement standard external and intracavitary techniques. Prempree (1983) reported a 96% local tumor control rate and 61% five-year disease-free survival in 23 patients with intact uterus, Stage IIIB carcinoma of the cervix, treated with a combination of external irradiation and intracavitary and interstitial implant to the parametrium. Likewise, he described a 23% local failure rate and 69% five-year survival in 26 patients with similar stage carcinoma of the cervix treated in the same manner but in whom the uterine cavity could not be probed or was absent. Overall, major complications were noted in 8% of the 49 patients.

Aristizabal *et al.* (1983) described the treatment

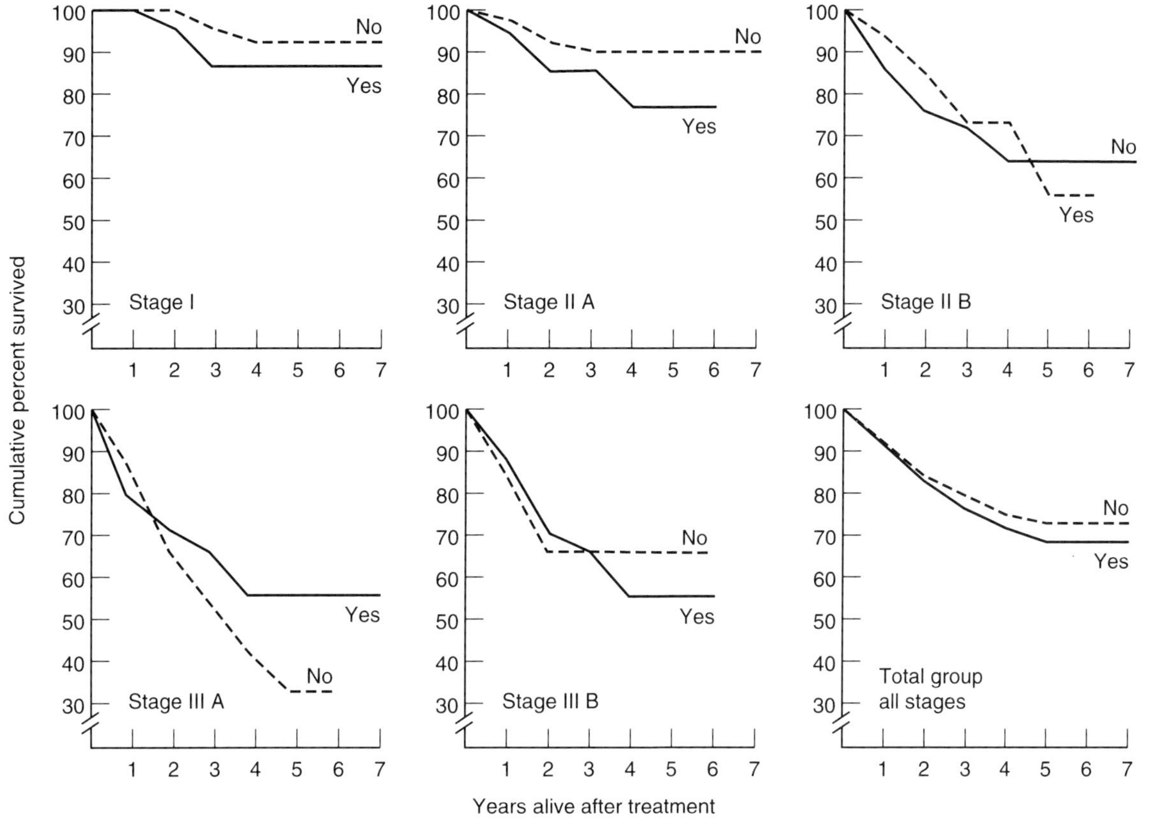

Figure 6.18. Survival curves of patients treated for squamous cell carcinoma of the cervix. Curves for Stages I, IIA, IIB, IIIA and IIIB and all stages combined are shown. Patients who had lymphadenectomy added to their treatment are represented by solid curves. The broken curves are for patients who had radiation treatment only. (From Rutledge *et al.*, 1965.)

of 21 patients with locally advanced invasive carcinoma of the uterine cervix treated with transperineal interstitial implants using a specially designed plastic template with predrilled holes in a concentric pattern for insertion of plastic or steel needles. A central opening in the template could be used to insert the plastic vaginal cylinder. With a mean follow-up of 26 months, local tumor control was reported in 18 of the patients (85%). Seven patients (33%) developed grade 2 or 3 complications. The loading of the obturator needles or the use of the central cylinder sources probably contributed to the relatively high incidence of complications. The authors have discontinued the use of the obturator surface needles except when there is gross residual tumor in the central area.

Martinez *et al.* (1985) using a special applicator consisting of two acrylic cylinders, a template with an array of holes that serve as guides to localize the trocars, and a cover plate, have treated 37 patients with advanced or recurrent carcinoma of the cervix and 26 with vaginal–urethral tumors. Doses of approximately 3500 cGy were given in addition to external irradiation (3600 cGy whole pelvis and 1400 cGy to pelvic side wall). They reported six local failures in the patients with cervical lesions and five

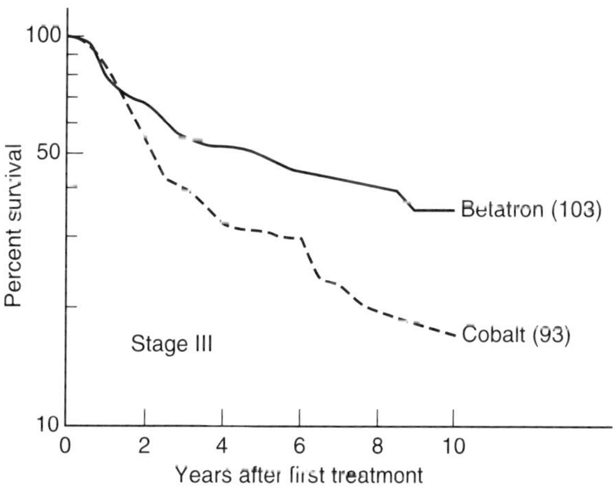

Figure 6.19. Actuarial survival of patients with Stage III carcinoma of the uterine cervix randomized to receive comparable doses of external irradiation with either 22 MV photons (betatron) or ^{60}Co. (From Johns, 1976.)

in the group with vaginal–urethral tumors. The overall complication rate was 5.1%.

Maruyama and Muir (1984) have used californium-252 (^{252}Cf) neutron brachytherapy in conjunction with fractionated external photon irradiation to treat carcinoma of the uterine cervix. A relative biologic effectiveness (RBE) of six was assumed for the ^{252}Cf relative to the ^{137}Cs. Nearly total tumor clearance was achieved at completion of therapy in over 90% of 41 patients. Tumor regression was more rapid in the ^{252}Cf group than in similar patients treated with ^{137}Cs and the same dose of external irradiation.

Occasionally brachytherapy procedures cannot be performed because of medical reasons or an unusual anatomic configuration of the pelvis or the tumor (i.e. extensive lesion and inability to identify the cervical canal). These patients may be treated with higher doses of external irradiation alone.

Castro *et al.* (1970) reported results in 118 patients with invasive cervical carcinoma treated with 5000–6000 cGy to the whole pelvis (four-field box technique) and additional doses to residual tumor with reduced anterior–posterior–posterior–anterior (AP–PA) portals to complete 7000 cGy tumor dose. With doses below 5000 cGy no pelvic tumor control was obtained in 32 patients, but disease control and survival were significantly enhanced with higher doses (*Table 6.6*). Complications increased with higher doses; for instance, severe sigmoiditis was noted in none of 32 patients treated with 5000 cGy, one of 28 receiving 6000 cGy, and four of 44 in the 7000 cGy group.

The anatomic sites of failure for carcinoma of the uterine cervix after irradiation are closely correlated with the stage of the tumor. Cervical or vaginal vault (central) recurrences should always be confirmed by biopsy. When possible, parametrial recurrences should be documented by needle biopsy. However, a clinical diagnosis can be made in the presence of a 'triad' consisting of sciatic pain, leg edema and hydronephrosis. CT or lymphangiography is useful in outlining the tumor in the regional lymph nodes. Extrapelvic metastases are documented by clinical examination, radiographic and/or radionuclide studies, and biopsy when indicated.

The incidence of pelvic recurrence or distant metastasis in 1178 patients treated with definitive irradiation at Washington University is shown in *Table 6.7* (Perez *et al.*, 1991). *Table 6.8* shows the incidence of pelvic failures with various treatment techniques. Despite the fact that the patients treated with interstitial implant were in a high-risk group, the local control is comparable to that of patients treated with standard techniques.

Jampolis *et al.* (1975) analyzed post-irradiation recurrences in 1178 patients with squamous cell carcinoma of the intact uterus treated at MD Anderson Cancer Center and reported similar figures. These authors pointed out that central recurrences were extremely rare in Stage IB and IIA

Table 6.6. Carcinoma of the cervix: external radiotherapy only. NED (no evidence of disease) rates and rates of control within irradiated area at 36 months (1954–1966) (from Castro *et al.*, 1970).

	Whole pelvis dose (cGy)* ≥5000		*6000*		≤7000†	
Stage	*NED*	*Control*	*NED*	*Control*	*NED*	*Control*
I, II, IIIA	0/2	0/2	1/8	3/8	7/14‡	12/14
IIIB, IV	0/30	0/30	6/20	9/20	5/34‡	11/34

*To nearest 1000 cGy tumor dose/week.
†7500 cGy (6 patients); 8000 cGy (1 patient).
‡Intercurrent disease (3 patients).

Table 6.7. Incidence of tumor recurrence in patients treated with definitive irradiation (from Perez *et al.*, 1991).

			Site of recurrence							
			Pelvic		*Pelvic +DM*		*Total pelvic failures*		*DM only*	
Stage	*No. of patients*	*Five-year disease-free survival (%)*	*No.*	*(%)*	*No.*	*(%)*	*No.*	*(%)*	*No.*	*(%)*
IB	384	85	6	(2)	31	(8)	37	(10)	36	(9)
IIA	128	70	4	(3)	20	(16)	24	(19)	24	(19)
IIB	353	72	38	(11)	43	(12)	81	(23)	54	(15)
III	293	52	48	(16)	73	(25)	121	(41)	54	(18)
IVA	20	0	3	(15)	12	(60)	15	(75)	4	(20)

DM, distant metastasis.

Table 6.8. Carcinoma of the uterine cervix: pelvic recurrences and type of brachytherapy insertions (from Perez *et al.*, 1985b). (Figures in parentheses are percentages.)

	Stage				
Type of insertions	*IB*	*IIA*	*IIB*	*III*	*IVA*
Tandem and ovoids	20/267 (7.5)	11/73 (15.1)	30/171 (17.5)	35/110 (31.8)	4/5 (80.0)
Tandem with protruding vaginal source	0/30	1/14 (7.1)	4/30 (13.3)	17/43 (39.5)	2/2 (100.0)
Interstitial (combined with other)	0/3	0/7	6/30 (20.0)	15/37 (41.0)	0/1
Combination of applicators (excluding interstitial)	3/23 (13.0)	1/11 (9.1)	7/49 (14.3)	14/37 (37.8)	4/5 (80.0)
Ovoids only	0	0	0/4	1/5	0
No implant	1/1 (100.0)	0	1/2 (50.0)	7/12 (58.3)	4/5 (80.0)

(2%) and that in most instances they could be attributed to improper placement of the vaginal colpostats, which could produce low doses of irradiation in the cervix. Parametrial recurrences in Stage I, IIA, and IIB disease were correlated with lateral deviation of the radium system without compensation from the external irradiation in about 75% of the patients. The overwhelming cause of failure in patients with Stage IIIB tumors was massive parametrial infiltration that could not be controlled with doses of 7000 cGy.

In a review of 849 patients treated with irradiation alone (external and intracavitary), Perez *et al.* (1983) illustrated a correlation of doses delivered to the medial parametrium and pelvic failures. There was no significant improvement in tumor control with increasing doses of irradiation in Stage IB. However, with Stages IIA, IIB and III, improved tumor control was noted with total doses over 8000–9000 cGy to point A (Perez *et al.*, 1991) (*Figure 6.20*). Moreover, higher doses delivered to the lateral parametrium were correlated with greater tumor control in Stages IIB and III (*Figure 6.21*).

Periaortic lymph node metastases are frequently combined with distant dissemination but are clinically apparent in only 10–20% of the patients who have recurrences. It is important to stress the high incidence of distant metastasis in patients with Stage III and IV carcinoma of the cervix, which makes imperative the development of adequate adjuvant therapy to improve the prognosis of these patients. The most common metastatic sites are the lungs, mediastinal lymph nodes, liver and bones. Radiation therapy can salvage about 50% of patients with localized pelvic recurrences after surgery alone (Deutsch and Parsons, 1974; Fuller *et al.*, 1982).

Sequelae of Treatment

Major complications of radiation therapy for Stages I and IIA carcinoma of the cervix range from 3–5% and for Stages IIB and III from 10–15%. The most frequent major complications for the various stages are listed in *Tables 6.9 and 6.10*. Perez *et al.* (1984), Kottmeier (1964) and Pourquier *et al.* (1982) have noted a greater incidence of complications with higher doses of irradiation. Pourquier *et al.* (1982) and Perez *et al.* (1984) have reported that with doses below 7500–8000 cGy delivered to limited volumes, Grade 2 and 3 complications in the urinary tract and rectosigmoid were approximately 5%. However, these increased to over 10% with higher doses of irradiation to these organs (*Figure 6.22*). Likewise, doses over 6000 cGy were correlated with a greater incidence of small bowel injury (*Figure 6.23*). The same analysis showed that patients who developed sequelae of therapy had a slightly better survival than patients who did not develop any complications. This was related to improved tumor control with higher doses of irradiation (Perez *et al.*, 1991).

Higher doses of external irradiation to the whole pelvis have also been associated with a greater number of complications (Strockbine *et al.*, 1970). Injury to the gastrointestinal tract usually appears within the first two years after radiation therapy, whereas complications of the urinary tract are seen more frequently 3–4 years after treatment (Kottmeier, 1964).

When preoperative irradiation is combined with surgery, the complication rate tends to be somewhat higher (5–10%), particularly because of injury to the ureter or the bladder (ureteral stricture or uretero- or vesicovaginal fistula). The dose and

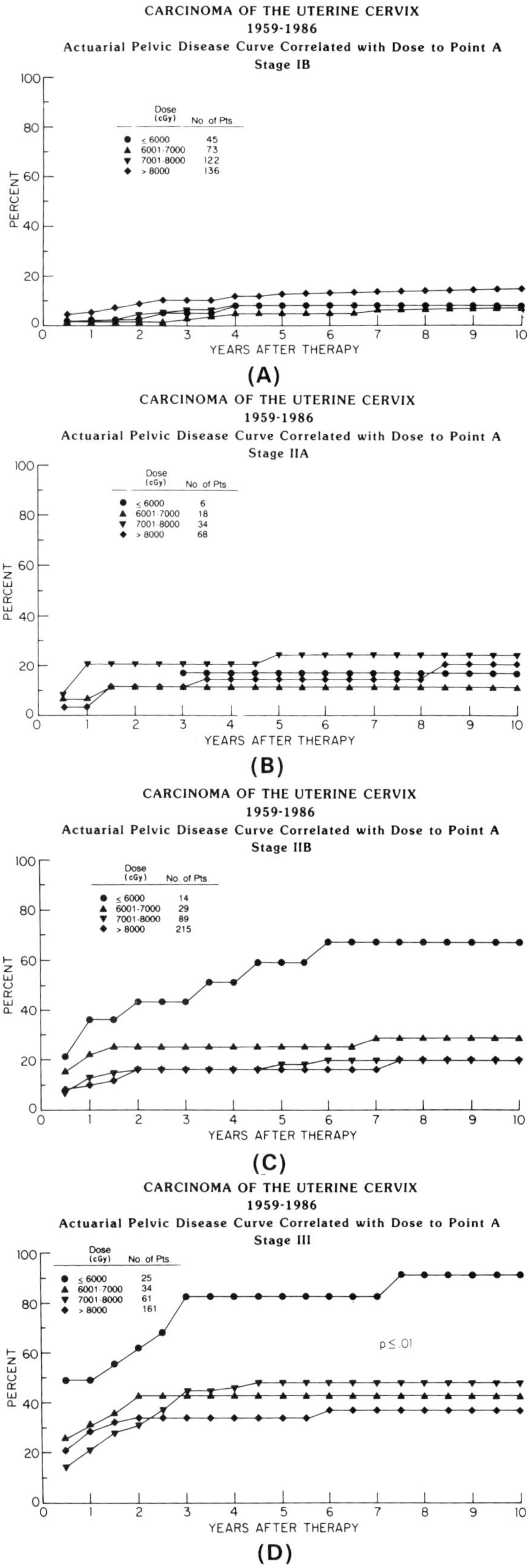

Figure 6.20. Actuarial rate of pelvic recurrence correlated with dose to point A. (**A**) Stage IB; (**B**) Stage IIA; (**C**) Stage IIB; (**D**) Stage III. (From Perez *et al.*, 1991.)

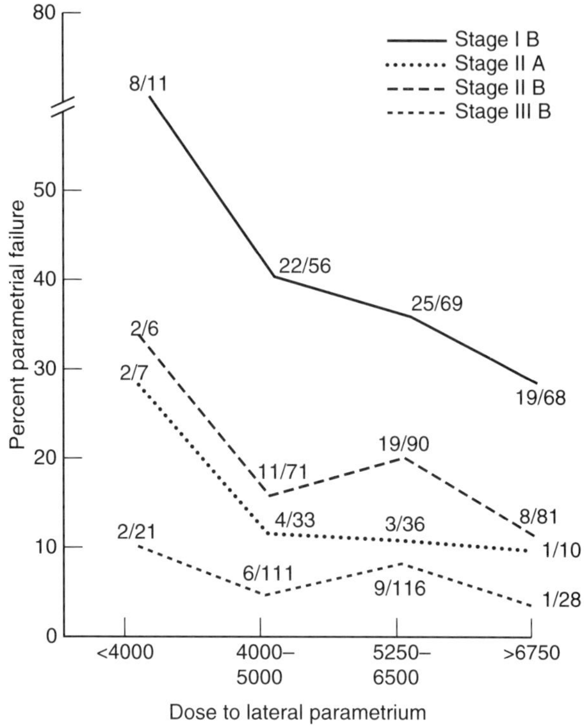

Figure 6.21. Local/marginal parametrial recurrences correlated with dose to the lateral parametrium in patients with various stages of carcinoma of the uterine cervix. Better tumor control was observed in Stages II and III with higher doses of irradiation. (From Perez *et al.*, 1983.)

techniques of irradiation and the type of surgical procedures performed are important in determining the morbidity of combined therapy. Nelson *et al.* (1975b) reported a 17.5% incidence of severe complications in 80 patients treated with radiation and radical hysterectomy in contrast to 7.4% major complications in 95 patients treated with high-dose preoperative irradiation and conservative extrafascial hysterectomy. For 12 patients with invasive cervical carcinoma treated at Washington University with low-dose preoperative irradiation and a radical hysterectomy with lymphadenectomy or high-dose preoperative irradiation and a conservative extrafascial hysterectomy, Jacobs *et al.* (1985) noted a major complication rate of 5%. The survival was comparable in patients with or without complications.

The pre-therapy staging laparotomy is fraught with a significant number of complications, particularly if irradiation (over 5000–5500 cGy) is given when metastatic paraaortic lymph nodes are found. The usual operative complications may be noted such as pneumonia, thrombophlebitis, cardiovascular accident, hepatitis, or evisceration. Late complications include those of combined surgery and irradiation in the abdomen and pelvis. The incidence of complications has been 5–20% depending on the

Table 6.9. Carcinoma of the uterine cervix Mallinckrodt Institute of Radiology (1959–1986): Grade 2 sequelae (from Perez *et al.*, 1991).

	Stage				
	IB	*IIA*	*IIB*	*III*	*IVA*
Total no. of patients treated	384	128	353	293	20
No. of patients with sequelae	40 (10.4%)	12 (9.4%)	47 (13.3%)	29 (9.9%)	0
No. of complications	46 (12%)	17 (13.3%)	65 (18.4%)	32 (10.9%)	0
Rectum–rectosigmoid					
Rectal stricture		1	3	1	
Proctitis	6	1	13	6	
Rectal ulcer	1			2	
Diverticulitis			1		
Small bowel					
Small bowel obstruction	2		4	4	
Malabsorption syndrome	3		1	1	
Urinary					
Cystitis	2	2	9	3	
Bladder ulcer	2	1	3		
Ureteral stricture		1			
Urethral stricture			1		
Extensive cystocele	1				
Incontinence			1		
Other					
Vaginal stenosis	21	4	9	6	
Vault necrosis	6	4	2	4	
Post-op pelvic abscess*			1	1	
Lymphocyst*			2	1	
Pulmonary embolus			1		
Subcutaneous fibrosis	1				
Leg edema			5	1	
Hemorrhage			1		
Thrombosis of pelvic blood vessels		1			
Arteriosclerosis	1		5	2	
Thrombophebitis			3		
Pelvic fibrosis		1			
Acute pelvic cellulitis		1			

*Patients underwent post-irradiation pelvic lymphadenectomy.

extent of the paraaortic lymph node dissection, a transperitoneal or retroperitoneal approach for the operation, and the dose of irradiation given (Lepanto *et al.*, 1975; Wharton *et al.*, 1977; Piver *et al.*, 1978).

Palliation of Locally Advanced Cervix Carcinoma

Frequently the radiation oncologist is faced with the dilemma of treating a patient with Stage IV or recurrent carcinoma who requires palliation of pelvic pain or bleeding and in whom the general condition does not warrant a prolonged course of external irradiation with conventional fractionation. If vaginal bleeding is the main concern, a single intracavitary insertion with tandem and colpostats for about 6000 mgh (5500 cGy to point A) will suffice. If previous irradiation was delivered, lower intracavitary doses should be prescribed (4500–5000 mgh).

Several high-dose fractionation schedules have been used, and Meoz *et al.* (1983) described satisfactory palliation with single doses of 1000 cGy

Table 6.10. Carcinoma of the uterine cervix Mallinckrodt Institute of Radiology (1959–1986): Grade 3 sequelae (from Perez *et al.*, 1991).

	Stage				
	IB	*IIA*	*IIB*	*III*	*IVA*
Total no. of patients treated	384	128	353	293	20
No. of patients with sequelae	18 (4.7%)	13 (10.2%)	33 (9.3%)	24 (8.2%)	1 (5%)
No. of sequelae	22 (5.7%)	20 (15.6%)	44 (12.5%)	35 (11.9%)	1 (5%)
Rectum–rectosigmoid					
Rectovaginal fistula	2	1	7	9	
Rectouterine fistula	1				
Colon–vaginal fistula			1		
Rectal stricture	3	4	2	2	
Proctitis	2	2	5	2	
Rectal ulcer			1		
Sigmoid performation	1		3		
Small bowel					
Small bowel obstruction	2	5	9	7	
Small bowel perforation			2		
Enterocolic fistula	1				
Enterocutaneous fistula		1		1	
Enterovaginal fistula			1		
Enteritis/cachexia				1	
Urinary					
Vesico–vaginal fistula	1		4	6	1
Uretero–vaginal fistula				1	
Cystitis	2				
Bladder ulcer				1	
Ureteral stricture	5	5	6	4	
Other					
Post-op pelvic abscess*			1		
Pulmonary embolus				1	
Hemorrhage			1		
Pelvic infection	1		1		
Neuritis		1			
Thrombosis of pelvic blood vessels		1			
Neuropathy radiation myelitis	1				

*Patients underwent post-irradiation pelvic lymphadenectomy.

combined with misonidazole, delivered every 3–6 weeks for a total of 3000 cGy. Complications in the long-term survivors were relatively high (15%). We have used two fractions in two consecutive days to administer 750 cGy in each, repeating every 2–3 weeks, for a total of 3000 cGy. With smaller fields (12 × 12 cm) additional 1500 cGy in two daily fractions can be given to residual tumor 2–3 weeks later. Occasionally this regimen is combined with an intracavitary insertion (4500 mgh), blocking the midline for the last 1500 cGy external dose.

The RTOG conducted a phase I/II trial using multiple (twice-daily) fractions of 370 cGy each to deliver 740 cGy in two consecutive days, repeated

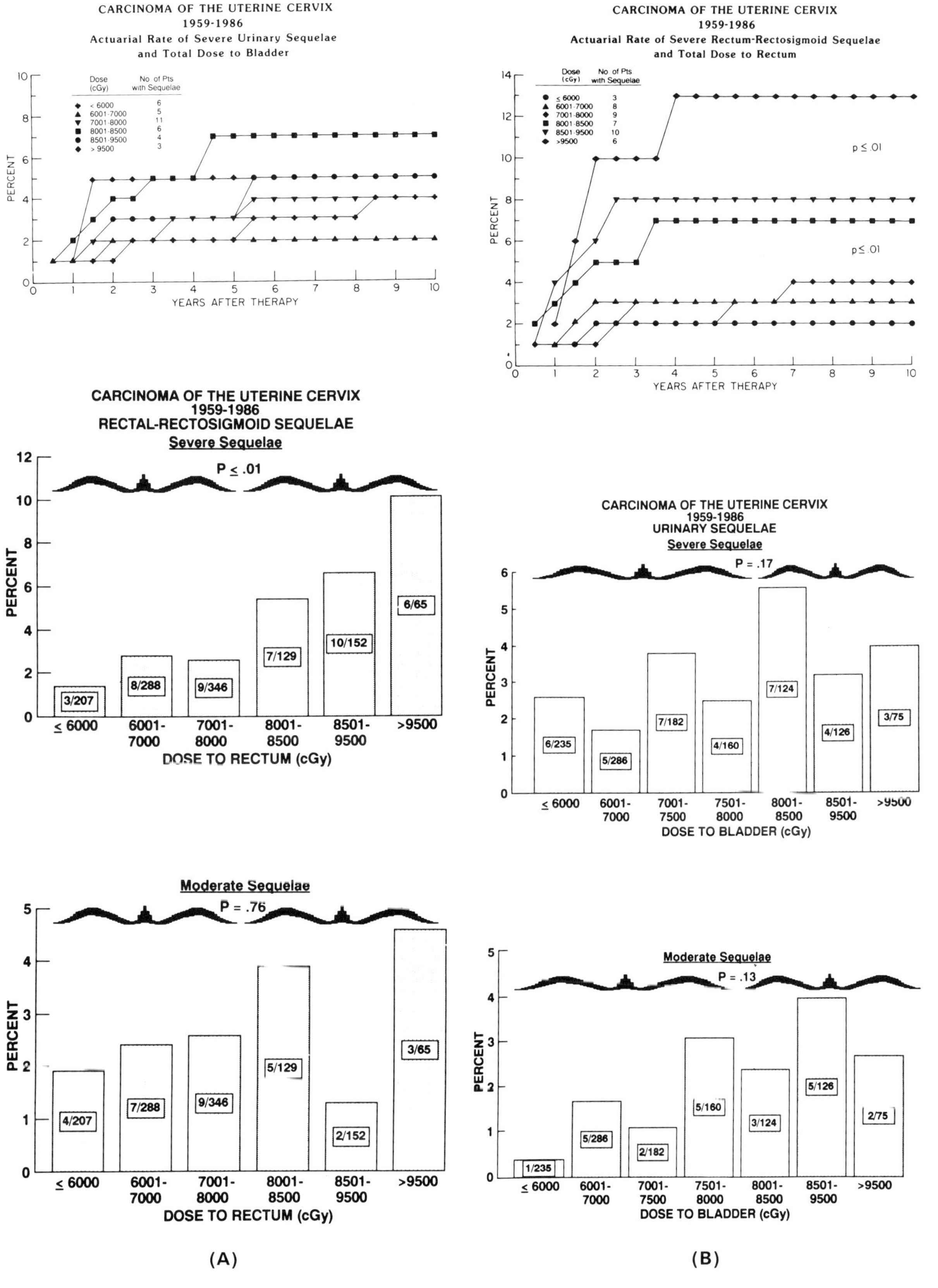

Figure 6.22. Rectosigmoid (**A**) and urinary (**B**) sequelae correlated with dose to rectum and actuarial rates of severe sequelae correlated with total dose to rectum for each. (From Perez *et al.*, 1991.)

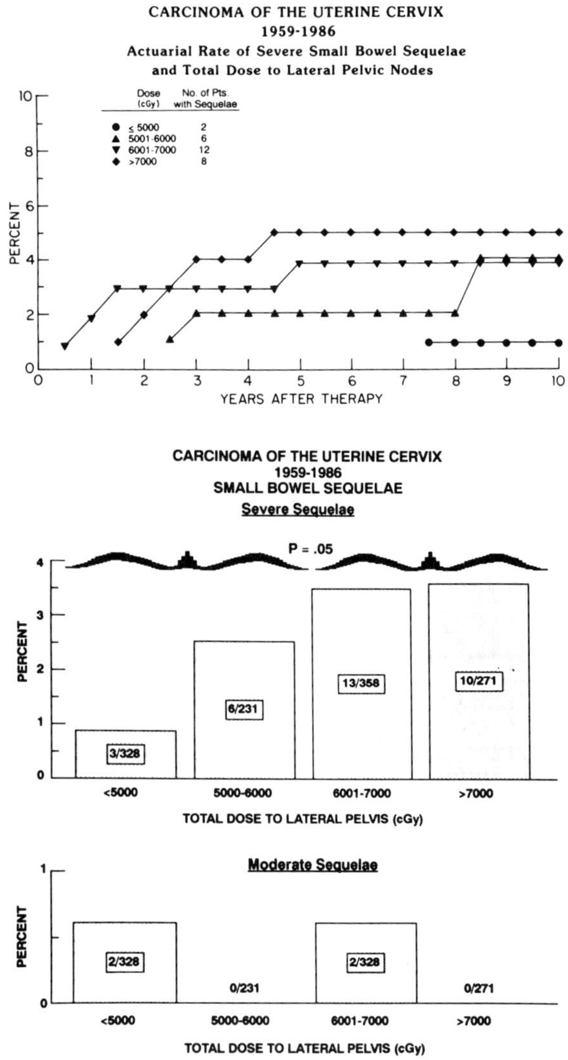

Figure 6.23. Small bowel sequelae and actuarial rate of severe small bowel sequelae correlated with total dose to lateral pelvic nodes. (From Perez *et al.*, 1991.)

every 3–6 weeks for a total of 4440 cGy. Significant sequelae of therapy were less than 5% (Spanos *et al.*, 1989).

Treatment of Recurrent Carcinoma of the Cervix

After Definitive Irradiation

Irradiation of previously irradiated patients must be undertaken with extreme caution. It is very important to analyze the techniques used in the initial treatment (beam energy, volume, doses delivered with external or intracavitary irradiation). Also, the period of time between the two treatments must be taken into consideration since it is postulated that some repair of the initial damage may take place in the interval. However, it is foolhardy to assume that previously irradiated tissues will have the same tolerance as newly irradiated tissues. In general, we give external irradiation to limited volumes (4000–4500 cGy, 180 cGy tumor dose (TD) per fraction), preferentially using lateral portals. Occasionally, intracavitary or interstitial irradiation can be used to treat relatively circumscribed recurrences.

Puthawala *et al.* (1982) treated 14 patients who had carcinoma of the uterine cervix recurring in the pelvis with interstitial implants. Seven exhibited tumor control (50%). All patients had received definitive radiation therapy at the time of initial treatment with whole pelvis doses ranging from 5000–6500 cGy delivered in 5–8 weeks and intracavitary irradiation varying from 4000–5000 mgh. Palliation of symptoms after re-irradiation was obtained in about 80% of patients. The authors described no postoperative mortality. Of the patients, 30% experienced mild to moderate symptoms of proctitis and cystitis shortly after the interstitial implant, but in most the symptoms resolved within three months. Severe complications occurred in 15% of the patients (soft tissue necrosis and one instance each of rectovaginal fistula, vesicovaginal fistula, enterovaginal fistula and rectal stricture).

Prasasvinichai *et al.* (1978) noted a 17.6% five-year survival among 51 patients with recurrent tumor limited to the pelvis, treated with irradiation alone, pelvic exenteration (10 patients), or a combination of exploratory laparotomy, debulking, and irradiation (10 patients). Prempree *et al.* (1979) treated eight patients with late invasive cervical carcinoma recurrent after primary irradiation: three survived tumor free more than five years after retreatment.

After Previous Surgery

It is substantially easier to treat surgical recurrences with irradiation. We believe that a combination of external irradiation (2000–4000 cGy TD), depending on the volume of tumor, and additional parametrial dose with midline shielding for a total of 5000–6000 cGy is needed. In addition, an intracavitary insertion, which may cover the vaginal vault or the entire vagina depending on tumor volume, should be delivered. The total mucosal dose from the external and intracavitary therapy can approach 12000 cGy without a high risk. It is extremely useful to combine these techniques with interstitial irradiation to boost the dose to the vaginal vault or the parametrium or paravaginal tissues, when the volume of disease requires it. Doses of 2000–3000 cGy are administered

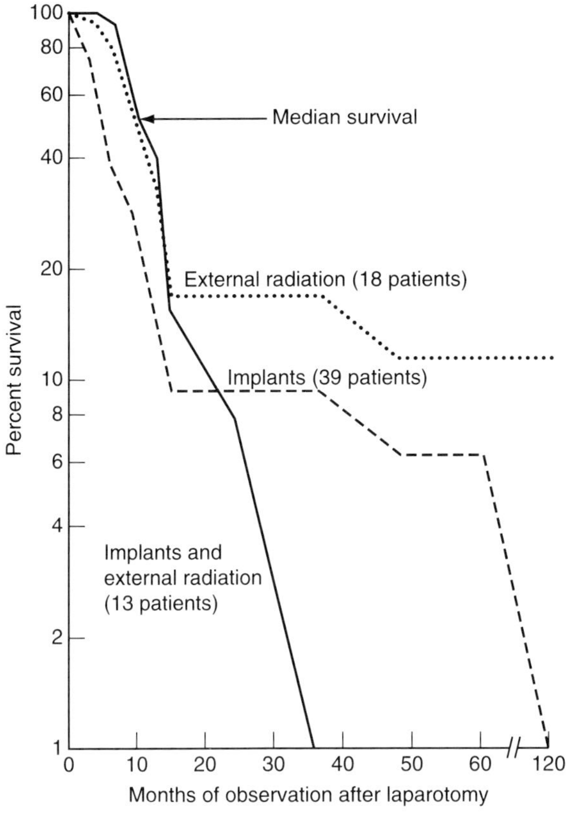

Figure 6.24. Survival of 70 patients in a non-randomized study of recurrent carcinoma of the uterine cervix treated with radiation therapy (external, brachytherapy or a combination). (From Evans *et al.*, 1971.)

with single, double or volume implants, depending on the extent of the tumor.

Friedman and Pearlman (1965) reported a 42% tumor-free survival in 38 patients treated with irradiation after primary surgical therapy (seven were irradiated electively for close or positive margins, lymphatic permeation, pelvic lymph node involvement, etc.). Six of the seven patients were tumor free for 2–5 years. Of 14 patients with limited central recurrence, eight were tumor free from 3.5–9 years. The worst results were noted with persistent or recurrent peripheral pelvic tumor (three of 11 patients survived tumor free more than five years) or with massive pelvic recurrences (palliation was achieved in only six patients). Evans *et al.* (1971) reported on 114 patients found to have unresectable carcinoma of the cervix after primary irradiation or surgical treatment. Of seventy patients treated with irradiation (external, interstitial, or combination), 10% lived 15 months or longer, and 5% survived five years or more (*Figure 6.24*). Satisfactory palliation was observed in a large proportion of patients.

Extended Field Irradiation

Extended field irradiation to electively treat the paraaortic lymph nodes is an interesting hypothesis. In a multivariate analysis of multiple prognostic factors in a group of 626 surgically-staged patients by Stehman *et al.* (1991), the most significant prognostic factor for tumor recurrence and death was the presence of histologically positive paraaortic lymph nodes.

Elective treatment of the paraaortic lymph nodes has been evaluated in two independent prospective randomized studies. The European Organization of Radiation Therapy Community (EORTC) performed a study of 441 patients with Stage IB, IIB, and III disease. Patients with Stages IB and early IIB (medial parametrium) were known to have positive pelvic lymph nodes. Those with late Stage IIB (lateral parametrium) and Stage III had positive or negative pelvic lymph nodes. Patients with known positive paraaortic lymph nodes were not eligible for the study. Randomization was between pelvic irradiation and pelvic and paraaortic irradiation. Analysis of all patients did not demonstrate a survival advantage to either arm of the study. However, the rate of the development of paraaortic lymph node metastasis was greater by a factor of 2.8 in the pelvic irradiation only arm.

The RTOG performed a study of elective paraaortic irradiation for patients with Stage IB (greater than 4 cm), IIA, and IIB disease. The paraaortic lymph node status was not evaluated in all patients. The study included 330 patients (Rotman *et al.*, 1990) and the results demonstrated an improved survival rate and a decreased rate of metastatic disease for the arm that included paraaortic irradiation ($p=0.04$). The RTOG is currently performing a study of pelvic and paraaortic irradiation compared with pelvic irradiation plus concomitant chemotherapy with cisplatin and 5-FU (RTOG, 90-01).

Chemotherapy and Irradiation

Chemotherapy agents have been combined with irradiation for primary treatment of cervical cancer in a number of settings. Several non-randomized studies with small numbers of patients (Grigsby and Perez, 1991a), and some prospective randomized studies have been performed. The chemotherapeutic agents that have been used have, for the most part, been radiation sensitizers. The prospective randomized phase III studies that have been performed are outlined below in chronological order.

The GOG performed a study of Stage IIIB and IVA patients who were randomized to pelvic irradiation alone or pelvic irradiation plus weekly hydroxyurea. Only 104 of the 190 patients accrued to the study were evaluable. The three-year disease-free survival rates were 13% for the irradiation alone arm and 26% for the irradiation plus hydroxyurea arm (Hreshchyshyn *et al.*, 1979). Following completion of this study, the GOG performed a study randomizing patients with Stages IIB–IVA to irradiation plus hydroxyurea versus irradiation plus misonidazole (Stehman *et al.*, 1993). The results of this study revealed a five-year survival rate of 53% for the hydroxyurea arm and a five-year rate of 44% for the misonidazole arm ($p=0.066$). Severe leukopenia was more frequent in the hydroxyurea arm than in the misonidazole arm.

The RTOG performed a randomized study of irradiation alone versus irradiation plus misonidazole for patients with Stage IIIB and IVA disease (Leibel *et al.*, 1987). Of 119 patients, the median survival was 1.9 years for irradiation alone and 1.6 years for irradiation plus misonidazole. Overgaard *et al.* (1989) randomized 331 patients to receive irradiation alone or irradiation plus misonidazole for Stage IIB, III, and IVA disease. This study also showed no difference in local tumor control, disease-free survival, or crude survival in the two arms. A final study used a new hypoxic cell sensitizer, pimonidazole in a randomized study (Dische *et al.*, 1993). Their study randomized patients with Stage II or III cervical cancer to irradiation alone or irradiation plus pimonidazole. The hazard ratios for local control and survival were 2.10 and 1.58, respectively, indicating a worse outcome for those receiving pimonidazole.

Investigators at the University of Hong Kong (Wong *et al.*, 1989) randomized 64 patients with Stages IIB and III disease to radiation therapy alone, irradiation plus weekly cisplatin, or irradiation plus twice-weekly cisplatin. Local control and survival were identical for the three treatment arms.

Recent randomized studies by the GOG include study #85, which randomized patients with Stages IIB to IVA disease to either irradiation plus hydroxyurea or irradiation plus cisplatin and 5-FU. Results of that study are pending. The current chemotherapy trial by this group also includes patients with Stages IIB to IVA disease. Their study randomized patients to one of the following three treatment arms:

- irradiation plus hydroxyurea;
- irradiation plus weekly cisplatin;
- irradiation plus hydroxyurea, cisplatin and 5-FU.

Patients are currently being accrued to this study.

A prospective study performed by the National Cancer Institute of Brazil compared irradiation alone to neoadjuvant chemotherapy with bleomycin, vincristine, mitomycin and cisplatin followed by pelvic irradiation. The trial included 107 patients with Stage IIIB disease. The overall survival rates were 39% for the irradiation alone arm and 23% for the neoadjuvant chemotherapy arm ($p=0.02$). Locoregional and distant failures were similar for both arms. Severe toxicity from the chemotherapy attributed to the decreased overall survival of that group.

The RTOG is currently conducting a study of patients with Stages IB (bulky >4 cm)–IVA disease. The study randomizes patients to either pelvic and paraaortic irradiation or pelvic irradiation and concomitant chemotherapy with three cycles of cisplatin and continuous infusion 5-FU.

Hyperbaric Oxygen, Hypoxic Sensitizers, and Hyperthermia Combined with Irradiation

No definite conclusions can be drawn concerning the use of hyperbaric oxygen for carcinoma of the cervix, but it seems to increase the effect of irradiation both in the tumor and the normal tissues. The results of one study indicated an increase in five-year survival and a significant decrease in local recurrence with hyperbaric oxygen (Volterrani and Lombardi, 1980). However, several reports also showed increased morbidity with hyperbaric oxygen (Glassburn *et al.*, 1974; Fletcher *et al.*, 1977; Watson *et al.*, 1978). It is possible that hyperbaric oxygen administered with fewer high-dose fractions may be more efficacious than when combined with conventional dose and fractionation schemes (Dische, 1979). The trials reported have not shown an increased incidence of distant metastasis, which has been reported in a clinical study and in some animal experiments (Johnson and Walton, 1974).

Dische (1980) reported preliminary observations on the use of misonidazole in the treatment of advanced carcinoma of the cervix in ten patients. The morbidity of this therapy is comparable to that observed with irradiation alone except for some misonidazole neurotoxicity. All ten patients had over 50% tumor regression, results felt to be very promising. A randomized study by the RTOG comparing the sensitizing effects of misonidazole in Stages III and IVA carcinoma of the cervix (daily dose of $400\ \text{mg m}^{-2}$ for a total of $12\ \text{g m}^{-2}$) treated with conventional fractionation showed no significant difference in tumor control or survival (Leibel *et al.*, 1987).

Because of technologic limitations to the delivery of adequate heat to large parts of the body such as the pelvis, the evaluation of hyperthermia in the treatment of carcinoma of the uterine cervix has been sparse. Hornback *et al.* (1986) reported on a non-randomized study in which the combination of microwave hyperthermia (433 MHz) and irradiation resulted in improved pelvic tumor control and survival in a group of 79 patients in comparison with previously irradiated historic controls.

Carcinoma of the Cervix and Pregnancy

In patients with invasive carcinoma the lesion is usually clinically apparent. Multiple punch biopsies are adequate to confirm the diagnosis.

Since there is a greater need to institute therapy as soon as possible, the accepted method of treatment for patients in the first six months of pregnancy is to carry out definitive surgery or radiation therapy, as indicated by the stage of the disease (Dudan *et al.*, 1973; Thompson *et al.*, 1975). In the third trimester of pregnancy when the fetus may be salvaged, a cesarean section is preferred followed by definitive treatment. However, several authors report that vaginal delivery does not affect the prognosis deleteriously. Creasman *et al.* (1970) reported on 98 patients, 48 treated by irradiation, 45 by irradiation followed by surgery, and five with a radical hysterectomy alone. The survival was comparable to that of non-pregnant patients for similar stages. The survival for patients with Stage I was comparable whether the patients were allowed to deliver vaginally or a cesarean section was performed (about 85% in Stage I and 50–64% in Stage II). Also, the percentage of infants surviving (over 80%) was the same in both groups.

If it is decided to terminate the pregnancy, the patient is initially treated with external irradiation to the whole pelvis (4000 cGy in four weeks). Usually an abortion will occur, and there will be some involution of the uterus. After this dose of irradiation an evacuation of the uterus and an intracavitary insertion can be performed under general anesthesia. If surgery is to be performed, approximately 5000 mgh is given. If not, two intracavitary insertions for a total of 8000 mgh and an additional 1000–2000 cGy is delivered to the parametria with a midline block. The usual surgical procedure is a radical hysterectomy with lymphadenectomy except in the case of microinvasive carcinoma, in which case the lymphadenectomy is not performed.

Kinch (1961), Symmonds (1966), Creasman *et al.* (1970), and others have reported similar 5- to 7-year survival in pregnant and non-pregnant patients; the stage of the disease at the time of diagnosis was the only determining prognostic factor (*Figure 6.25*).

If a radical hysterectomy is performed and positive pelvic lymph nodes are found, the usual postoperative radiation including external beam and intracavitary insertion should be carried out.

Survival is the same regardless of the trimester of the pregnancy in which definitive treatment is instituted (Symmonds, 1966; Creasman *et al.*, 1970).

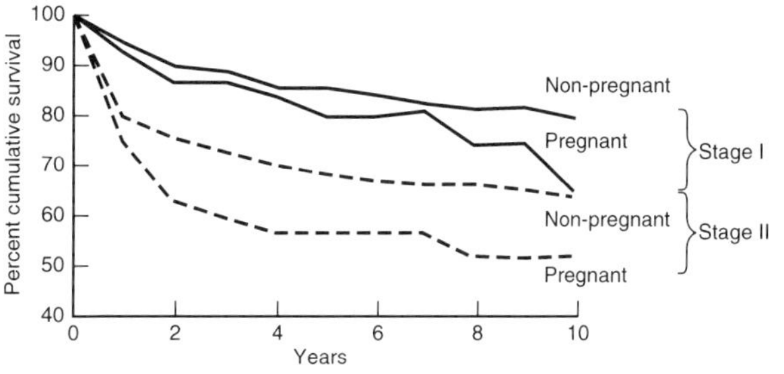

Figure 6.25. Actuarial survival rates for pregnant and non-pregnant women with carcinoma of the cervix. (From Creasman *et al.*, 1970.)

The practice popularized 30 years ago of administering a 'restraining dose of radium' and deferring definitive radiation therapy until delivery is carried out should be strongly discouraged. Strauss (1940) reported that two of 11 babies were born with microcephaly in addition to other complications such as alopecia, facial deformity, eye damage, and chromosomal abnormalities.

Hopkins and Morley (1992) reviewed the treatment results of 53 pregnant patients with Stage IB cervical cancer. The authors concluded that the incidence of cervical cancer occurring with pregnancy has decreased at their institution over the past 30 years and that the survival is not altered because of the pregnancy. Duggan *et al.* (1993) evaluated 27 patients with Stage IB cervical cancer who were pregnant. Their population included patients who chose immediate treatment at the time of diagnosis of cervical cancer and those who chose to delay cancer treatment until after delivery of the fetus. The mean time from diagnosis to treatment for the delayed treatment group was 144 days compared with 17 days for the immediate treatment group. They reported good fetal outcome for the delayed treatment group, obvious fetal deaths for the immediate treatment group, and an identical survival for both treatment groups with a median post-treatment follow-up of 23 months.

Carcinoma of the Cervical Stump

Subtotal hysterectomy, a relatively popular procedure for benign conditions of the uterus in past years, is rarely performed today. These patients are, of course, at risk of developing carcinoma of the uterine cervix.

It is important to divide patients with carcinoma of the cervical stump into either:

- true, when the first symptom occurs three or more years after subtotal hysterectomy;

- coincidental, when the symptoms are noticed before the third postoperative year (Sala and DeLeon, 1963).

Moss *et al.* (1973) recommend two years' elapse after hysterectomy as the time for the classification of these lesions. This distribution is important because the prognosis for carcinoma of the true stump is significantly better than for coincidental lesions, which probably means that carcinoma was present at the time the hysterectomy was performed.

When surgery is performed for Stage I tumors, it is somewhat more difficult because of the previous surgical procedures and the presence of adhesions in the pelvis. When irradiation is administered, the lack of a uterine cavity into which to insert a tandem containing three or more sources makes intracavitary therapy more difficult. Whenever possible, sources should be inserted in the remaining cervical canal. Occasionally, transvaginal irradiation may be used to boost the dose delivered to central disease in the stump. It is important to deliver more whole pelvis irradiation.

In general, patients with Stage I disease are treated with a combination of 2000 cGy to the whole pelvis and 3000 cGy to the parametria with midline shielding combined with two intracavitary insertions. The dose of intracavitary therapy depends on the number of sources that can be placed in the cervical canal (1000–3000 mgh for 1–3 sources). The vaginal vault should receive about 7000 cGy mucosal dose (approximately 2000 mgh). More advanced stages should be treated with 4000 cGy whole pelvis and 2000 cGy to the parametria with midline shielding, combined with the same intracavitary doses. If there is bulky disease present in the cervix, parametrium or vagina, then interstitial therapy with needles is advisable. When there is no opportunity to insert any sources in the cervical canal, the whole pelvis dose must be increased to 6000 cGy. When intravaginal cones are used, 3000–5000 cGy air-dose is delivered in 2–4 weeks, 3–5 fractions weekly. Moss *et al.* (1973) limit the dose to the vaginal vault for transvaginal irradiation to 3000 cGy in 10 days.

The five-year survival, anatomic sites of failure and incidence of recurrences for carcinoma of the cervical stump treated with irradiation are similar to those reported for patients with carcinoma of the intact uterus (Creadick, 1958; Sala and DeLeon, 1963; Wimbush and Fletcher, 1969; Wolff *et al.*, 1972).

Because of the close proximity of the bladder, rectum and small intestine to the intracavitary sources and because of the often higher doses of whole pelvis external beam irradiation given, complications are somewhat more frequent than for carcinoma of the cervix with an intact uterus. Wimbush and Fletcher (1969) reported five fistulas, six cases of severe proctosigmoiditis and 12 cases of vault necrosis in 238 patients treated with definitive irradiation.

Kovalic *et al.* (1991) reviewed 70 patients with clinical stages 0–IIIB carcinoma of the cervical stump treated with irradiation. The ten-year progression-free survivals by clinical stages were as follows: 0, 100%; IA, 100%; IB, 79%; IIA, 100%; IIB, 66%; and IIIB, 39%. These results compare favorably with treatment results obtained for those treated with irradiation alone for carcinoma of the intact uterine cervix.

High Dose Rate Brachytherapy

High dose rate (HDR) brachytherapy has replaced traditional low dose rate (LDR) brachytherapy for carcinoma of the cervix at many institutions throughout the world. The transition from HDR to LDR has occurred for several reasons despite a lack of prospective randomized trials comparing treatment outcome and toxicity for these two brachytherapy dose rates. However, a significant body of clinical experience has developed so that one can safely and effectively perform brachytherapy for patients with cervical carcinoma with either HDR or LDR remote afterloading technology.

Examples of the various HDR brachytherapy dose fractionation schedules are shown in *Table 6.11*. A summary of several non-randomized clinical experiences for the use of HDR brachytherapy for Stages I–IV cervical cancer is given in *Table 6.12*.

Teshima *et al.* (1993) performed a randomized study of LDR versus HDR brachytherapy for 430 patients with Stages I–III cervical cancer. The five-year cause-specific survival results for Stages I, II and III were 85%, 73% and 53%, respectively, for patients treated with HDR brachytherapy and 93%, 78% and 47%, respectively, for LDR brachytherapy. The external beam irradiation schedule was identical in the two groups of patients. None received chemotherapy. Moderate and severe complications occurred in 4% of those treated with LDR brachytherapy and in 10% of those treated with HDR brachytherapy ($p = 0.023$). The authors conclude that LDR and HDR brachytherapy have equivalent survival results, but that their specific dose schedule for HDR brachytherapy should be altered to reduce the moderate and severe complication rate.

An additional study of LDR versus HDR brachytherapy was performed by Patel *et al.* (1993). In this study, 482 patients with Stage I, II and III cervical cancer were randomized to either LDR or HDR brachytherapy. The five-year disease-free survivals were 81%, 66% and 72%, respectively, for

Table 6.11. HDR brachytherapy for carinoma of the cervix: dose fractionation schedule (from Fu and Phillips, 1990).

Authors	Dose/Fx at point A (Gy)	No. Fxs	No. Fx/wk	External beam Dose (Gy)	External beam Timing
Glaser (1988)	6–7	5–6	1	40–50	A
Vahrson and Romer (1988)	6–14*	3–7	0.5–1	45–46	C
Cikaric (1988)	9–10	4	1	35–46	C
Akine *et al.* (1988)	3–5	5–6	2–3	29–67	B
Himmelmann *et al.* (1985)	8.5†	5	1	40–50	A
Kuipers (1988)	8.5	2	2	46	B
Sato *et al.* (1984)	6.1	5	1	50–60	B
Shigematsu *et al.* (1983)	8–10	3	1	40	C
Taina and Gronroos (1981)	7.5–10	3–5	1	50	A
Aria *et al.* (1980)	3–7	4–13	1–3	45–65	C

A = after; B = before; C = concurrent with brachytherapy; Fx = fraction.
*Dose-maximum on the A-line (or A-plane) 2 cm lateral from the central axis of the applicator.
†Dose at the surface of the target volume.

Table 6.12. HDR versus LDR brachytherapy for carcinoma of the cervix: survival (from Fu and Phillips, 1990).

Authors	Stage	No. of patients HDR/LDR	Five-year survival (%) HDR	Five-year survival (%) LDR
Glaser (1988)	I–III	493/288	59*	33* ($p = 0.001$)
Vahrson and Romer (1988)	I	24/206	71	74
	II	37/213	76	53 ($p < 0.05$)
	III	29/138	62	24 ($p < 0.001$)
Cikaric (1988)	II	85/66	54	70
	III	52/120	37	43
Akine *et al.* (1988)	IIB	20/83	60	56
	IIIB	37/212	54	38
Kuipers (1988)	I	21/32	76	80
	II	54/71	74	68
	III	36/42	36	48
Sato *et al.* (1984)	II	31/40	55	55
	III	44/85	57	49
Shigematsu *et al.* (1983)	IIB & III	143/106	55	55
Taina and Gronroos (1981)	I & II	40/30	90†	73†
Rotte (1980)	I	42/28	83	89
Aria *et al.* (1980)	I	86/31	83	87
	II	173/125	71	75
	III	212/253	51	49
	IV	46/80	24	16

*Relapse-free survival.
†Three-year survival.

Stages I, II and III treated with LDR brachytherapy, and 85%, 71% and 82, respectively, for Stages I, II and III treated with HDR brachytherapy. Severe Grade 3 and 4 complications were not significantly different between the two groups: 2.4% for LDR and 0.4% for HDR brachytherapy. The authors conclude that HDR and LDR brachytherapy produce equivalent survival and toxicity results.

Summary of Management Options

- Stage IA (microinvasive) tumors are treated with intracavity therapy only (6000 cGy in one insertion or 7000–7500 cGy in two insertions to point A).
- The selection of definitive irradiation or radical surgery for Stage IB and IIA carcinoma of the cervix is controversial, and the preference of one procedure over the other depends on the institution, the gynecologist or irradiation oncologist involved, the general condition of the patient, and the prognostic features of the lesion.
- Despite a slower regression after irradiation, no difference in tumor control or survival has been observed for adenocarcinoma compared with epidermoid carcinoma.
- Bulky endocervical carcinoma (so-called barrel-shaped cervix) has a higher incidence of central recurrence, pelvic and paraaortic lymph node metastases, and distant dissemination. The benefits of combined irradiation and extrafascial hysterectomy for this lesion are unclear with regard to local control.
- Patients with Stage IIB and III disease are treated with irradiation alone. Patients with Stage IVA tumors (bladder or rectal invasion) can be treated with high doses of whole pelvis external irradiation, intracavity sources and addition parametrial irradiation.
- At the present time, there is no definitive evidence that chemotherapeutic agents have proven effectiveness in the adjuvant treatment of patients with advanced disease.
- No controlled studies have been performed showing improved survival with postoperative pelvic irradiation following radical surgery in the presence of positive pelvic nodes.
- If metastatic paraaortic lymph nodes are suspected or confirmed, the retroperitoneal tissues may be irradiated with a field that includes both the paraaortic nodes and the pelvic tissues. High-energy beams are especially suited for this treatment.
- Elective treatment of the paraaortic lymph nodes has been evaluated in independent prospective randomized studies. Analysis of patients in one study did not demonstrate a survival advantage in either arm. In the other, the results demonstrated an improved survival rate and a decreased rate of metastatic disease for the arm that included paraaortic irradiation ($p = 0.04$).
- The optimal dose for invasive carcinoma of the cervix is delivered with a combination of whole pelvis, intracavity, and, at times, interstitial therapy: 5000 cGy for Stages IB and IIA or 6000 cGy to the involved parametrial tissues for more advanced stages.
- When carcinoma is detected following an abdominal or vaginal hysterectomy, the prognosis is worse if postoperative irradiation is not administered.
- When metastatic pelvic lymph nodes or positive surgical margins are found after a hysterectomy, we administer a combination of external irradiation (2000 cGy whole pelvis and 3000 cGy to the parametria with a small midline block) and an intracavity insertion for 6000 cGy to the vaginal mucosa (1800 mgh) with two colpostats.
- Major complications of radiation therapy for Stages I and IIA carcinoma of the cervix range from 3–5% and for Stages IIB and III from 10% to 15%.
- Injury to the gastrointestinal tract usually appears within the first two years after irradiation therapy, whereas complications of the urinary tract are seen more frequently 3–4 years after treatment.
- For palliation: if vaginal bleeding is the main concern, a single intracavity insertion with tandem and colpostats for about 6000 mgh (5500 cGy to point A) will suffice.
- Irradiation of previously irradiated patients must be undertaken with extreme caution.
- Chemotherapeutic agents have been combined with irradiation for primary treatment of cervical cancer in a number of settings. The chemotherapeutic agents that have been employed have, for the most part, been radiation sensitizers.
- No definitive conclusions can be drawn concerning the use of hyperbaric oxygen in carcinoma of the cervix.
- Since there is a greater need to institute therapy as soon as possible, the accepted method of treatment for patients in the first six months of pregnancy is to carry out definitive surgery or radiation therapy, as indicated by the stage of the disease.
- The five-year survival, anatomic sites of failure and incidence of recurrences for carcinoma of the cervical stump treated with irradiation are similar to those reported for patients with carcinoma of the intact uterus.
- High dose rate (HDR) brachytherapy has replaced traditional low dose rate (LDR) brachytherapy for carcinoma of the cervix at many institutions.

References

Abitbol MM & Davenport JH (1974) Sexual dysfunction after therapy for cervical carcinoma. *Am. J. Obstet. Gynecol.* **119:** 181–189.

Akine Y, Arimoto H, Ogino T *et al.* (1988) High dose-rate intracavitary irradiation in the treatment of carcinoma of the uterine cervix: early experience with 84 patients. *Int. J. Radiat. Oncol. Biol. Phys.* **4:** 893–898.

Allt W (1969) Supervoltage radiation treatment in advanced cancer of the uterine cervix. *Can. Med. Assoc. J.* **100:** 792–797.

Andras E, Fletcher G & Rutledge F (1973) Radiotherapy of carcinoma of the cervix following simple hysterectomy. *Am. J. Obstet. Gynecol.* **115:** 647–655.

Aoki S, Hata T, Senoh D *et al.* (1990) Parametrial invasion of uterine cervical cancer assessed by transrectal ultrasonography: preliminary report. *Gynecol. Oncol.* **36:** 82–89.

Aria T, Morita S, Kutsutani Y *et al.* (1980) Relationship between total iso-effect dose and number of fractions for the treatment of uterine cervical carcinoma by high dose rate intracavitary irradiation. In: Bates T & Berry R (eds) *High Dose Rate Afterloading in the Treatment of Cancer of the Uterus,* pp. 75–79. London: British Journal Radiology Special Report 17.

Aristizabal SA, Surwit EA, Hevezi JM *et al.* (1983) Treatment of advanced cancer of the cervix with transperineal interstitial irradiation. *Int. J. Radiat. Oncol. Biol. Phys.* **9:** 1013–1017.

Barber H (1969) Relative prognostic significance of preoperative and operative findings in pelvic exenteration. *Surg. Clin. North Am.* **49:** 431–447.

Beahrs O, Henson D, Hutter R & Myers M (eds) (1992) *Manual for Staging of Cancer,* 4th edition, pp. 155–157. Philadelphia: JB Lippincott

Belinson JL, Doherty M & McDay JB (1984) A new technique for ovarian transposition. *Surg. Gynecol. Obstet.* **159:** 157–160.

Benson W & Norris H (1977) A critical review of the frequency of lymph node metastasis and death from microinvasive carcinoma of the cervix. *Obstet. Gynecol.* **19:** 632–638

Blaikley JB, Lederman M & Pollard W (1969) Carcinoma of the cervix at Chelsea Hospital for Women, 1935–1965. Five year and 10-year results of treatment. *J. Obstet. Gynecol. Br. Commwth.* **76:** 729–740.

Bricker E & Modlin J (1951) The role of pelvic evisceration in surgery. *Surgery* **30:** 76–94.

Brunschwig A (1968) The surgical treatment of cancer of the cervix stage I and II. *Am. J. Roentgenol. Rad. Ther. Nucl. Med.* **102:** 147–151.

Brunschwig A & Barber HRK (1966) Surgical treatment of carcinoma of the cervix. *Obstet. Gynecol.* **27:** 21–29.

Brunschwig A & Daniel W (1960) Pelvic exenteration operations. *Ann. Surg.* **151:** 571–576.

Burghardt E & Holzer E (1977) Diagnosis and treatment of microinvasive carcinoma of the cervix uteri. *Obstet. Gynecol.* **49:** 641–653.

Buschbaum H (1979) Extrapelvic lymph node metastases in cervical carcinoma. *Am. J. Obstet. Gynecol.* **133:** 814–824.

Camilien L, Fordon D, Fruchter R *et al.* (1988) Predictive value of computerized tomography in the presurgical evaluation of primary carcinoma of the cervix. *Gynecol. Oncol.* **30:** 209–215.

Castellino R (1991) Retroperitoneal and pelvic lymph node imaging. *Cancer* **67:** 1219–1222.

Castro JR, Issa P & Fletcher GH (1970) Carcinoma of the cervix treated by external irradiation alone. *Radiology* **95:** 163–166.

Christensen A, Lange P & Neilsen E (1964) Surgery and radiotherapy for invasive cancer of the cervix: Surgical treatment. *Acta Obstet. Gynecol.* **43:** 59–87.

Cikaric S (1988) Radiation therapy of cervical carcinoma using either HDR or LDR afterloading: comparison of 5-year results and complications. *Strahlenther. Onkol.* 82 (suppl): 119–122.

Creadick RN (1958) Carcinoma of the cervical stump. *Am. J. Obstet. Gynecol.* 75: 565–574.

Creasman W & Parker R (1973) Microinvasive carcinoma of the cervix. *Clin. Obstet. Gynecol.* **16:** 261–275.

Creasman W & Rutledge F (1972) Carcinoma *in situ* of the cervix. *Obstet. Gynecol.* **3:** 373–380.

Creasman WT, Rutledge FN & Fletcher GH (1970) Carcinoma of the cervix associated with pregnancy. *Obstet. Gynecol.* **36:** 495–501.

Decker DG, Aaro LA, Hunt AB *et al.* (1965) Sequential radiation and operation in carcinoma of the uterine cervix. *Am. J. Obstet. Gynecol.* **92:** 35–42.

Deckers P, Ketcham A, Sugarbaker E *et al.* (1971) Pelvic exenteration for primary carcinoma of the uterine cervix. *Obstet. Gynecol.* **37:** 647–659.

DelRegato J & Cox J (1965) Transvaginal roentgentherapy in the conservative management of carcinoma *in situ* of the uterine cervix. *Radiology* **84:** 1090–1095.

Deutsch M & Parsons JA (1974) Radiotherapy for carcinoma of the cervix recurrent after surgery. *Cancer* **34:** 2051–2055.

Dickson RJ (1972) Late results of radium treatment of carcinoma of the cervix. *Clin. Radiol.* **23:** 528–535.

Dische S (1979) Hyperbaric oxygen: The Medical Research Council Trials and their clinical significance. *Br. J. Radiol.* **51:** 888–894.

Dische S (1980) Misonidazole in the clinic at Mount Vernon. *Cancer Clin. Trials* **3:** 175–178.

Dische S, Chassagne D, Hope-Stone HF *et al.* (1993) A trial of Ro 03-8799 (pimonidazole) in carcinoma of the uterine cervix: an interim report from the Medical Research Council Working Party on advanced carcinoma of the cervix. *Radiother. Oncol.* **26:** 93–103.

Dudan RC, Yon JL Jr, Ford JH Jr *et al.* (1973) Carcinoma of the cervix and pregnancy. *Gynecol. Oncol.* **1:** 283–289.

Duggan B, Muderspach L, Roman L *et al.* (1993) Cervical cancer in pregnancy: reporting on planned delay in therapy. *Obstet. Gynecol.* **82:** 598–602.

■ Durrance F (1968) Radiotherapy following simple hysterectomy in patients with stage I and II carcinoma of the cervix. *Am. J. Roentgenol. Rad. Ther. Nucl. Med.* **102:** 165–169.

Durrance F, Fletcher G & Rutledge F (1969) Analysis of central recurrent disease in stages I and II squamous cell carcinomas of the cervix on intact uterus. *Am. J. Roentgenol. Rad. Ther. Nucl. Med.* **106:** 831–838.

■ Eifel P, Morris M, Oswald M *et al.* (1990) Adenocarcinoma of the uterine cervix. Prognosis and patterns of failure in 367 cases. *Cancer* **65:** 2507–2514.

Einhorn N, Bygdeman M & Sjoberg B (1980) Combined radiation and surgical treatment for carcinoma of the uterine cervix. *Cancer* **45:** 720–723.

Evans SR Jr, Hilaris BS & Barber HRK (1971) External vs interstitial irradiation in unresectable recurrent cancer of the cervix. *Cancer* **28:** 1284–1288.

Fennell R (1978) Microinvasive carcinoma of the uterine cervix. *Obstet. Gynecol. Surv.* **33:** 406–411.

■ Fletcher G (1971) Cancer of the uterine cervix: Janeway Lecture. *Am. J. Roentgenol. Rad. Ther. Nucl. Med.* **111:** 225–242.

Fletcher G (1983) *Textbook of Radiotherapy*, 3rd edition, pp. 620–665 Philadelphia: Lea & Febiger.

Fletcher GH, Lindberg RD, Caderao JB *et al.* (1977) Hyperbaric oxygen as a radiotherapeutic adjuvant in advanced carcinoma of the uterine cervix. Preliminary results of a randomized trial. *Cancer* **39:** 617–623.

Friedman M & Pearlman AW (1965) Carcinoma of the cervix: Radiation salvage of surgical failures. *Radiology* **84:** 801–811.

■ Fu K & Phillips T (1990) High-dose-rate versus low-dose-rate intracavitary brachytherapy for carcinoma of the cervix. *Int. J. Radiat. Oncol. Biol. Phys.* **19:** 791–796.

Fuller A, Elliott N, Kosloff C *et al.* (1982) Lymph node metastases from carcinoma of the cervix, stages IB and IIA: Implications for prognosis and treatment. *Gynecol. Oncol.* **13:** 165–174.

Glaser FH (1988) Comparison of HDR afterloading with ^{192}IR versus conventional radium therapy in cervix cancer: 5-year results and complications. *Strahlenther. Onkol.* **82** (suppl): 106–113.

Glassburn JR, Damsker JI, Brady LW *et al.* (1974) Hyperbaric oxygen and radiation in the treatment of advanced cervical carcinoma. In: Trapp W (ed.) *Fifth International Hyperbaric Congress Proceedings II*, pp. 813–819. Burnaby, Canada: Simon Fraser University.

Gray MJ, Gusberg SB & Guttman R (1958) Pelvic lymph node dissection following radiotherapy. *Am. J. Obstet. Gynecol.* **76:** 629–633.

Green T & Morse W (1969) Management of invasive cervical cancer following inadvertent simple hysterectomy. *Obstet. Gynecol.* **33:** 763–769.

Grigsby P, Perez C, Kuske R *et al*. (1988) Adenocarcinoma of the uterine cervix: lack of evidence for a poor prognosis. *Radiother. Oncol.* **12:** 289–296.

Grigsby P, Vest M & Perez C (1994) Recurrent carcinoma of the cervix exclusively in the paraaortic nodes following radiation therapy. *Int. J. Radiat. Oncol. Biol. Phys.* **28:** 451–455.

Grigsby PW & Perez CA (1991a) Efficacy of 5-fluorouracil by continuous infusion and other agents as radiapotentiators for gynecological malignancies. In: Rotman M & Rosenthal CJ (eds) *Medical Radiology: Concomitant Continuous Infusion Chemotherapy and Radiation*, pp. 259–267. Heidelberg: Springer–Verlag.

■ Grigsby PW & Perez CA (1991b) Radiotherapy alone for medically inoperable carcinoma of the cervix: Stage IA and carcinoma *in situ*. *Int. J. Radiat. Oncol. Biol. Phys.* **21:** 375–378.

Guttman R (1970) Significance of postoperative irradiation in carcinoma of the cervix: a ten-year study. *Am. J. Roentgenol. Rad. Ther. Nucl. Med.* **108:** 102– 108.

Hamberger AD, Fletcher GH & Wharton JT (1978) Results of treatment of early stage I carcinoma of the uterine cervix with intracavitary radium alone. *Cancer* **41:** 980–985.

Hasumi K, Sakamoto A & Sugano H (1980) Microinvasive carcinoma of the uterine cervix. *Cancer* **45:** 928–931.

■ Heller PB, Malfetano JH & Bundy BN (1990) Clinical-pathologic study of stage IIB, III, and IVA carcinoma of the cervix: Extended diagnostic evaluation for paraaortic node metastasis—A Gynecologic Oncology Group study. *Gynecol. Oncol.* **38:** 425–430.

Himmelmann A, Holmberg E, Oden A & Skogsberg K (1985) Intracavitary irradiation of carcinoma of the cervix stage IB and IIA: a clinical comparison between a remote high dose-rate afterloading system and a low dose-rate manual system. *Acta Radiol. Oncol.* **24:** 139–144.

Hodel K, Rich WM, Austin P & DiSaia PJ (1982) The role of ovarian transposition in conservation of ovarian function in radical hysterectomy followed by pelvic radiation. *Gynecol. Oncol.* **13:** 195–202.

Hopkins M & Morley G (1992) The prognosis and management of cervical cancer associated with pregnancy. *Obstet. Gynecol.* **80:** 9–13.

Hornback NB, Shidnia H, Shupe RE *et al.* (1986) Advanced stage IIIB cancer of the cervix treatment by hyperthermia and radiation. *Gynecol. Oncol.* **3:** 160–167

■ Hoskins W, Ford J, Lutz M et al. (1976) Radical hysterectomy and pelvic lymphadenectomy for the management of early invasive cancer of the cervix. *Gynecol. Oncol.* **4:** 278–290.

Hreshchyshyn M, Aron B, Boronow R *et al.* (1979) Hydroxyurea or placebo combined with radiation to treat stages IIIB and IV cervical cancer confined to the pelvis. *Int. J. Radiat. Oncol. Biol. Phys.* **5:** 317–322.

Husseinzadeh N, Nahhas WA, Velkly DE *et al.* (1984) The preservation of ovarian function in young women undergoing pelvic radiation therapy. *Gynecol. Oncol.* **18:** 373–379.

Jacobs AJ, Perez CA, Camel HM *et al.* (1985) Complications in patients receiving both irradiation and radical hysterectomy for carcinoma of the uterine cervix. *Gynecol. Oncol.* **22:** 273–280

Jampolis S, Andras J & Fletcher GH (1975) Analysis of sites and causes of failure of irradiation in invasive squamous cell carcinoma of the intact uterine cervix. *Radiology* **115:** 681–685.

Janus C, Mendelson D, Moore S *et al.* (1989) Staging of cervical carcinoma: accuracy of magnetic resonance imaging and computed tomography. *Clin. Imaging* **13:** 114–116.

John M, Cooke K, Flam M *et al.* (1978) Preliminary results of concomitant radiotherapy and chemotherapy in advanced cervical carcinoma. *Gynecol. Oncol.* **28:** 101–110.

Johns H (1976) Optimization of energy and equipment. In: Kramer S, Suntharalingam N & Zinninger GF (eds) *High-Energy Photons and Electrons, Clinical Applications in Cancer Management*, pp. 333–345. New York: John Wiley & Sons.

Johnson RJR & Walton RJ (1974) Sequential study on the effect of the addition of hyperbaric oxygen on the 5 year survival rates of carcinoma of the cervix treated with conventional fractional irradiations. *Am. J. Roentgenol. Rad. Ther. Nucl. Med.* **120:** 111–117.

Ketcham A, Chretien P, Hoye R *et al.* (1973) Occult metastases to the scalene lymph nodes in patients with clinically operable carcinoma of the cervix. *Cancer* **31:** 180–182.

Ketcham A, Sindelar W, Felix E & Bagley D (1976) Diagnostic scalene node biopsy in the preoperative evaluation of the surgical cancer patient. *Cancer* **38:** 948–952.

Ketcham AS, Hoye RC, Taylor PT *et al.* (1971) Radical hysterectomy and lymphadenectomy for carcinoma of the uterine cervix. *Cancer* **28:** 1272–1277.

Kielbinska S, Ludwika T & Fraczek O (1973) Studies of mortality and health status in women cured of cancer of the cervix uteri; comparison of long-term results of radiotherapy and combined surgery and radiotherapy. *Cancer* **32:** 245–252.

Kim S, Choi B, Lee H *et al.* (1990) Uterine cervical carcinoma: comparison of CT and MR findings. *Radiology* **175:** 45–51.

Kinch RAH (1961) Factors affecting the prognosis of the cervix in pregnancy. *Am. J. Obstet. Gynecol.* **82:** 45–51.

Kiselow M, Butcher H & Bricker E (1967) Results of the radical surgery treatment of advanced pelvic cancer. A 15-year study. *Ann. Surg.* **166:** 428–436.

Kline JC, Schultz AE, Vermund H *et al.* (1969) High dose radiotherapy for carcinoma of the cervix. Method and results. *Am. J. Obstet. Gynecol.* **104:** 479–484.

Kolstad P & Klem V (1976) Long-term follow-up of 1121 cases of carcinoma *in situ*. *Obstet. Gynecol.* **48:** 125–129.

Kottmeier HL (1964) Complications following radiation therapy in carcinoma of the cervix and their treatment. *Am. J. Obstet. Gynecol.* **88:** 854–866.

Kovalic J, Grigsby P, Perez C & Locket M (1991) Cervical stump carcinoma. *Int. J. Radiat. Oncol. Biol. Phys.* **20:** 933–938.

Kuipers T (1988) Dosimetry and complication rate in the treatment of cervix carcinoma with external irradiation and brachytherapy. *Strahlenther. Onkol.* **82** (suppl): 1127–1131.

Kuske RR, Perez CA, Grigsby PW *et al.* (1989) Phase I/II study of definitive radiotherapy and chemotherapy (cisplatin and 5-fluorouracil) for advanced or recurrent gynecologic malignancies. *Am. J. Clin. Oncol. (CCT)* **12:** 467–473.

Leibel S, Bauer M, Wasserman T *et al.* (1987) Radiotherapy with or without misonidazole for patients with stage IIIB or stage IVA squamous cell carcinoma of the uterine cervix: Preliminary report of a Radiation Therapy Oncology Group randomized trial. *Int. J. Radiat. Oncol. Biol. Phys.* **13:** 541–549.

Lepanto P, Littman P, Mikuta J *et al.* (1975) Treatment of paraaortic nodes in carcinoma of the cervix. *Cancer* **35:** 1510–1513.

Leveuf J & Godord H (1934) L'exerese chirugicale des ganglions pelviens complement de la curtherapie des cancers du col d'uterus. *J. Chir.* **43:** 177–187.

Liu W & Meigs JV (1955) Radical hysterectomy and pelvic lymphadenectomy. A review of 473 cases including 244 for primary invasive carcinoma of the cervix. *Am. J. Obstet. Gynecol.* **69:** 1–32.

Lu T, Macasaet M & Nelson J (1976) The barrel shape cervix. *Am. J. Obstet. Gynecol.* **124:** 596–600.

Magee B, Logue J, Swindell R *et al.* (1991) Tumor size as a prognostic factor in carcinoma of the cervix: assessment by transrectal ultrasound. *Br. J. Radiol.* **64:** 812–815.

Manetta A, Podczaski E, Larson J *et al.* (1989) Scalene lymph node biopsy in the preoperative evaluation of patients with recurrent cervical cancer. *Gynecol. Oncol.* **33:** 332–334.

Martinez A, Edmundson G, Cox RS *et al.* (1985) Combination of external beam irradiation and multiple-site perineal applicator (MUPIT) for treatment of locally advanced or recurrent prostatic, anorectal, and gynecologic malignancies. *Int. J. Radiat. Oncol. Biol. Phys.* **11:** 391–398.

Maruyama Y & Muir W (1984) Human cervical cancer clearance after ^{252}Cf neutron brachytherapy versus conventional photon brachytherapy. *Am. J. Clin. Oncol. (CCT)* **7:** 347–352.

Masterson JG (1967) The role of surgery in the treatment of early carcinoma of the cervix. *Clin. Obstet. Gynecol.* **10:** 922–939.

Mendenhall W, McCarty P, Morgan L *et al.* (1991) Stage IB or IIA–B carcinoma of the intact uterine cervix >6 cm in diameter: is adjuvant extrafascial hysterectomy beneficial? *Int. J. Radiat. Oncol. Biol. Phys.* **21:** 899–904.

Meoz RT, Spanos WJ, Doss L *et al.* (1983) Misonidazole combined with large-fraction pelvic irradiation in the treatment of patients with advanced pelvic malignancies. Preliminary report of an ongoing RTOG phase I-II study. *Am. J. Clin. Oncol. (CCT)* **6:** 417–422.

Mitani Y, Yukinari S, Jimi S & Iwasaki H (1964) Carcinomatous infiltration into the uterine body in carcinoma of the uterine cervix. *Am. J. Obstet. Gynecol.* **89:** 984–989.

Morley GW & Seski JC (1976) Radical pelvic surgery versus radiation therapy for stage I carcinoma of the cervix (exclusive of microinvasion). *Am. J. Obstet. Gynecol.* **126:** 785–798.

Morrow C (1980) Panel Report: Is pelvic radiation beneficial in the postoperative management of Stage IB squamous cell carcinoma of the cervix with pelvic node metastasis treated by radical hysterectomy and pelvic lymphadenectomy? *Gynecol. Oncol.* **10:** 105–110.

Morton D, Lagasse L, Moore J *et al.* (1964) Pelvic lymphadenectomy following radiation in cervical carcinoma. *Am. J. Obstet. Gynecol.* **88:** 932–938.

Moss WT, Brand WN & Battifora H (1973) *Radiation Oncology: Rationale, Technique, Results*, pp. 408–453. St. Louis: CV Mosby.

Muirhead W & Green LS (1968) Carcinoma of the cervix. Five year results and sequelae of treatment. *Am. J. Obstet. Gynecol.* **101:** 744–749.

Nahhas W, Sharkey F, Whitney C *et al.* (1983) The prognostic significance of vascular channel involvement and deep stromal penetration in early cervical carcinoma. *Am. J. Clin. Oncol. (CCT)* **6:** 259–264.

Nelson A, Averette H & Richart R (1975a) Detection, diagnostic evaluation and treatment of dysplasia and early carcinoma of the cervix. *CA* **25:** 134–151.

Nelson A, Fletcher G & Wharton T (1975b) Indications for adjunctive conservative extrafascial hysterectomy in selected cases of carcinoma of the uterine cervix. *Am. J. Roentgenol. Rad. Ther. Nucl. Med.* **123:** 91–99.

Nelson J, Macasaet M, Lu T *et al.* (1974) The incidence and significance of paraaortic lymph node metastases in late invasive carcinoma of the cervix. *Am. J. Obstet. Gynecol.* **118:** 749–756.

Newton M (1975) Radical hysterectomy or radiotherapy for stage I cervical cancer. *Am. J. Obstet. Gynecol.* **123:** 535–542.

O'Quinn A, Fletcher G & Wharton J (1980) Guidelines for conservative hysterectomy after irradiation. *Gynecol. Oncol.* **9:** 68–79.

Overgaard J, Bentzen S, Kolstad P *et al.* (1989) Misonidazole combined with radiotherapy in the treatment of carcinoma of the uterine cervix. *Int. J. Radiat. Oncol. Biol. Phys.* **16:** 1069–1072.

Park RC, Patow WE, Rodgers RR *et al.* (1973) Treatment for stage I carcinoma of the cervix. *Obstet. Gynecol.* **41:** 117–122.

Parker RT, Wilbanks GD, Yowell RK *et al.* (1967) Radical hysterectomy with and without preoperative radiotherapy for cervical cancer. *Am. J. Obstet. Gynecol.* **99:** 933–943.

Patel F, Sharma S, Negi P *et al.* (1993) Low dose rate vs high dose rate brachytherapy in the treatment of carcinoma of the uterine cervix: a clinical trial. *Int. J. Radiat. Oncol. Biol. Phys.* **28:** 335–341.

Perez C (1987) Carcinoma of the uterine cervix. In: Perez C & Brady L (eds) *Principles and Practice of Radiation Oncology*, pp. 919–965. Philadelphia: JB Lippincott.

Perez C (1992) Uterine cervix. In: Perez C & Brady L (eds) *Principles and Practice of Radiation Oncology*, 2nd edition, pp. 1143–1202. Philadelphia: JB Lippincott.

Perez C, Camel H, Askin F & Breaux S (1981) Endometrial extension of carcinoma of the uterine cervix: A prognostic factor that may modify staging. *Cancer* **48:** 170–180.

Perez C, Camel H & Kao M (1987) Randomized study of preoperative radiation and surgery or irradiation alone in the treatment of stage IB and IIA carcinoma of the uterine cervix: final report. *Gynecol. Oncol.* **27:** 129–140.

■ Perez C, Grigsby P, Nene S *et al.* (1992) Effect of tumor size on prognosis of carcinoma of uterine cervix treated with irradiation alone. *Cancer* **69:** 2796–2806.

Perez C & Kao M (1985) Radiation therapy alone or combined with surgery in barrel-shaped carcinoma of the uterine cervix (stages IB, IIA IIB). *Int. J. Radiat. Oncol. Biol. Phys.* **11:** 1903–1909.

Perez CA, Breaux S, Askin F *et al.* (1979) Irradiation alone or in combination with surgery in stage IB and IIA carcinoma of the uterine cervix. A non-randomized comparison. *Cancer* **43:** 1062–1072.

Perez CA, Breaux S, Bedwinek JM *et al.* (1984) Radiation therapy alone in treatment of the uterine cervix. II. Analysis of complications. *Cancer* **54:** 235–246.

Perez CA, Breaux S, Madoc–Jones H *et al.* (1983) Radiation therapy alone in the treatment of carcinoma of the uterine cervix. I. Analysis of tumor recurrence. *Cancer* **51:** 1393–1402.

Perez CA, Camel HM, Kao MS *et al.* (1980) Randomized study of preoperative radiation and surgery or irradiation alone in the treatment of stage IB and IIA carcinoma of the uterine cervix. Preliminary analysis of failures and complications. *Cancer* **45:** 2759–2768.

Perez CA, DiSaia PJ, Knapp RC *et al.* (1985a) Gynecologic tumors. In: DeVita VT, Hellman S & Rosenberg SA (eds) *Cancer, Principles and Practice of Oncology*, 2nd edition, pp. 1013–1081. Philadelphia: JB Lippincott.

Perez CA, Fox S, Lockett MA *et al.* (1991) Impact of dose in outcome of irradiation alone in carcinoma of the uterine cervix: Analysis of two different methods. *Int. J. Radiat. Oncol. Biol. Phys.* **21:** 885–898.

Perez CA, Kuske R & Glasgow GP (1985b) Review of brachytherapy techniques for gynecologic tumors. *Endocurie Hypertherm. Oncol.* **1:** 153–175.

Perez CA, Zivnuska F, Askin F *et al.* (1975) Prognostic significance of endometrial extension from primary carcinoma of the uterine cervix. *Cancer* **35:** 1493–1504.

Perez Mesa C & Spratt J (1976) Scalene node biopsy in the pretreatment staging of carcinoma of the cervix uteri. *Am. J. Obstet. Gynecol.* **125:** 93–95.

Pilleron JP, Durand JC & Hamelin JP (1974) Prognostic value of node metastasis in cancer of the uterine cervix. *Am. J. Obstet. Gynecol.* **119:** 458–462.

Pilleron JP, Durand JC & Lenoble JC (1972) Carcinoma of the uterine cervix, stages I and II, treated by radiation therapy and extensive surgery (1000 cases). *Cancer* **29:** 593–596.

Piver MS, Vongtama V & Barlow JJ (1978) Para-aortic lymph node irradiation for carcinoma of the uterine cervix using split-course technique. *Gynecol. Oncol.* **3:** 168–175.

Piver MS, Wallace S & Castro J (1971) The accuracy of lymphangiography in carcinoma of the uterine cervix. *Am. J. Roentgenol. Rad. Ther. Nucl. Med.* **111:** 278–283.

Potish R, Twiggs L, Adcock L et al. (1986) Effect of cisplatinum on tolerance to radiation therapy in advanced cervical cancer. *Am. J. Clin. Oncol. (CCT)* **9:** 387–391.

Potter ME, Spencer S, Soong SJ & Hatch KD (1993) The influence of staging laparotomy for cervical cancer on patterns of recurrence and survival. *Int. J. Gynecol. Can.* **3:** 169–174.

Pourquier H, Dubois JB & Deland R (1982) Cancer of the uterine cervix. Dosimetric guidelines for prevention of late rectal and rectosigmoid complications as a result of radiotherapeutic treatment. *Int. J. Radiat. Oncol. Biol. Phys.* **8:** 1887-1895.

Prasasvinichai S, Glassburn JR & Brady LW (1978) Treatment of recurrent carcinoma of the cervix. *Int. J. Radiat. Oncol. Biol. Phys.* **4:** 957–961.

Prempree T (1983) Parametrial implant in stage IIIB cancer of the cervix. III. A 5-year study. *Cancer* **52:** 748–750.

■ Prempree T, Kwon T, VillaSanta U *et al.* (1979) Management of late second or late recurrent squamous cell carcinoma of the cervix uteri after successful initial radiation treatment. *Int J. Radiat. Oncol. Biol. Phys.* **5:** 2053–2057.

Puthawala AA, Syed AM, Fleming PA *et al.* (1982) Re-irradiation with interstitial implant for recurrent pelvic malignancies. *Cancer* **50:** 2810–2814.

Quigley M, Knab D & McMaha E (1975) Carcinoma of the cervix. A third treatment. *Obstet. Gynecol.* **45:** 650–655.

Rampone J, Klem V & Kolstad P (1973) Combined treatment of stage IB carcinoma of the cervix. *Obstet. Gynecol.* **41:** 163–167.

Roddick JW Jr & Greenlaw RH (1971) Treatment of cervical cancer. *Am. J. Obstet. Gynecol.* **19:** 754–764.

Rotman M, Choi K, Guze C *et al.* (1990) Prophylactic irradiation of the paraaortic lymph node chain in stage IIB and bulky stage IB carcinoma of the cervix, initial treatment results of RTOG 7920. *Int. J. Radiat. Oncol. Biol. Phys.* **19:** 513–521.

Rotte K (1980) A randomized clinical trial comparing a high dose-rate with a conventional dose-rate technique. In: Bates T & Berry R (eds) *High Dose Rate Afterloading in the Treatment of Cancer of the Uterus*, pp. 75–79. London: British Journal Radiology Special Report 17.

Ruch R, Pitcock J & Ruch W (1976) Microinvasive carcinoma of the cervix. *Am. J. Obstet. Gynecol.* **125:** 87–92.

Rutledge F, Galakatos A, Wharton J *et al.* (1975) Adenocarcinoma of the uterine cervix. *Am. J. Obstet. Gynecol.* **122:** 236–245.

Rutledge F, Gutierrez A & Fletcher G (1968) Management of Stage I and II of the uterine cervix on the intact uterus. *Am. J. Roentgenol. Rad. Ther. Nucl. Med.* **102:** 161–164.

Rutledge FN, Fletcher GH & MacDonald EJ Pelvic (1965) lymphadenectomy as an adjunct to radiation therapy in treatment for cancer of the cervix. *Am. J. Roentgenol. Rad. Ther. Nucl. Med.* **93:** 607–614.

Sala J, Gleason J & Spratt J (1962) Adenocarcinoma of the cervix uteri. Report of 104 cases. *Mo. Med.* **59:** 1168–1173.

Sala JM & DeLeon AD (1963) Treatment of carcinoma of the cervical stump. *Radiology* **81:** 300–306.

Sall S, Pineda AA, Calanog A *et al.* (1979) Surgical treatment of stages IB and IIA invasive carcinoma of the cervix by radical abdominal hysterectomy. *Am. J. Obstet. Gynecol.* **135:** 422–446.

Sato S, Yajima A & Suzuki M (1984) Therapeutic results using high-dose rate intracavitary irradiation in cases of cervical cancer. *Gynecology Oncology* **19:** 143–147.

Seibel M, Freeman M & Graves W (1979) Carcinoma of the cervix and sexual function. *Obstet. Gynecol.* **55:** 484–487.

Seski J, Abell M & Morley G (1977) Microinvasive squamous carcinoma of the cervix. Definition, histologic analysis, late results of treatment. *Obstet. Gynecol.* **50:** 410–414.

Shigematsu Y, Ozeki S, Kawamura Y & Kurachi K (1983)

Treatment of carcinoma of the uterine cervix by remotely controlled afterloading intracavitary radiotherapy with high-dose rate: a comparative study with a low-dose rate system. *Int. J. Radiat. Oncol. Biol. Phys.* **9:** 351–356.

■ Spanos W, Guse C, Perez C *et al.* (1989) Phase II study of multiple daily fractionations in the palliation of advanced pelvic malignancies: Preliminary report of RTOG 8502. *Int. J. Radiat. Oncol. Biol. Phys.* **17:** 659–661.

Stehman F, Bundy B, DiSaia P *et al.* (1991) Carcinoma of the cervix treated with irradiation therapy. I. A multivariate analysis of prognostic variables in the Gynecologic Oncology Group. *Cancer* **67:** 2776–2785.

■ Stehman F, Bundy B, Hanjani P *et al.* (1987) Biopsy of the scalene fat pad in carcinoma of the cervix uteri metastatic to the paraaortic lymph nodes. *Surg. Gynecol. Obstet.* **165:** 503–506.

Stehman FB, Bundy BN, Thomas G *et al.* (1993) Hydroxyurea versus misonidazole with radiation in cervical carcinoma: long-term follow-up of a Gynecologic Oncology Group trial. *J. Clin. Oncol.* **11:** 1523–1528.

Strauss A (1940) Irradiation of carcinoma of the cervix uteri in pregnancy. *Am. J. Roentgenol. Rad. Ther. Nucl. Med.* **43:** 552–566.

Strockbine MF, Hancock JE & Fletcher GH (1970) Complications in 831 patients with squamous cell carcinoma of the intact uterine cervix treated with 3000 rads or more whole pelvis irradiation. *Am. J. Roentgenol. Rad. Ther. Nucl. Med.* **108:** 293–304.

Surwit E, Fowler WC, Palumob L *et al.* (1976) Radical hysterectomy with or without preoperative radium for stage IB squamous cell carcinoma of the cervix. *Obstet. Gynecol.* **48:** 130–133.

Sweeney WJ III & Douglas RG (1962) Treatment of carcinoma of the cervix with combined radiation and extensive surgery. *Am. J. Obstet. Gynecol.* **84:** 981–991.

Symmonds RE (1981) Carcinoma of the cervix associated with pregnancy. In: Lewis (ed.) *Synopsis of Gynecology*, pp. 181–192.

Taina E & Gronroos M (1981) A comparison of clinical results following high dose rate intracavitary afterloading irradiation with Co^{60} (cathetron) and conventional radium therapy for stage I–II cervical carcinoma. *Acta Obstet. Gynecol. Scand. Suppl.* **103:** 31–38.

■ Tattersall M, Ramirez C & Coppleson M (1992) A randomized trial of adjuvant chemotherapy after radical hysterectomy in stage IB–IIA cervical cancer patients with lymph node metastasis. *Gynecol. Oncol.* **46:** 176–181.

Taussig F (1934) Iliac lymphadenectomy with irradiation in the treatment of cancer of the cervix. *Am. J. Obstet. Gynecol.* **28:** 650–667.

Teshima T, Inoue T, Ikeda H *et al.* (1993) High-dose rate and low-dose rate intracavitary therapy for carcinoma of the uterine cervix. *Cancer* **72:** 2409–2414.

Thomas G, Dembo A, Beal F *et al.* (1984) Concurrent radiation, mitomycin-C and 5-fluorouracil in poor prognosis carcinoma of cervix: preliminary results of a phase I–II study. *Int. J. Radiat. Oncol. Biol. Phys.* **10:** 1785–1790.

Thompson JD, Caputo TA, Franklin EW *et al.* (1975) The surgical management of invasive cancer of the cervix in pregnancy. *Am. J. Obstet. Gynecol.* **121:** 853–863.

Thoms W, Eifel P, Smith T *et al.* (1992) Bulky endocervical carcinoma: a 23-year experience. *Int. J. Radiat. Oncol. Biol. Phys.* **23:** 491–499.

Twiggs L, Potish R, McIntyre R *et al.* (1986) Concurrent weekly cis-platinum and radiotherapy in advanced cervical cancer: A preliminary dose escalating toxicity study. *Gynecol. Oncol.* **24:** 143–148.

Ubinas J & Marcial V (1966) Adenocarcinoma of the cervix: A review of cases; Dr I. Gonzalez–Martinez Oncologic Hospital. *J. Am. Med. Wom. Assoc.* **21:** 571–574.

Ulfelder H (1967) Extended radical surgery for recurrent and advanced cervical cancer. *Clin. Obstet. Gynecol.* **10:** 940–957.

Utley JF, Von Essen CF, Horn RA *et al.* (1984) High dose rate afterloading brachytherapy in carcinoma of the uterine cervix. *Int. J. Radiat. Oncol. Biol. Phys.* **10:** 2259–2264.

Vahrson G & Romer G (1988) 5-year results with HDR afterloading in cervix cancer: dependence on fractionation and dose. *Strahlenther. Onkol.* **82** (suppl): 139–146.

Van Nagell JR, Rayburn W, Donaldson ES *et al.* (1979) Therapeutic implications of patterns of recurrence in cancer of the uterine cervix. *Cancer* **44:** 2354–2361.

Vincent CE, Vincent B & Greiss FC (1975) Some marital–sexual concomitants of carcinoma of the cervix. *South. Med. J.* **68:** 552–558.

Volterrani F & Lombardi F (1980) Long term results of radium therapy in cervical cancer. *Int. J. Radiat. Oncol. Biol. Phys.* **6:** 565–570.

Wall JA, Collins VP, Hudgins PT *et al.* (1966) Carcinoma of the cervix. Review of clinical experience during a 20-year period. *Am. J. Obstet. Gynecol.* **96:** 57–63.

Watson ER, Halnan KE, Dische S *et al.* (1978) Hyperbaric oxygen and radiotherapy: A Medical Research Council trial in carcinoma of the cervix. *Br. J. Radiol.* **51:** 879–887.

Webb G (1975) The role of ovarian conservation in the treatment of carcinoma of the cervix with radical surgery. *Am. J. Obstet. Gynecol.* **122:** 476–484.

Weiner S & Wizenberg M (1975) Treatment of primary adenocarcinoma of the cervix. *Cancer* **35:** 1514– 1516.

■ Weiser EB, Bundy BN, Hoskins WJ *et al.* (1989) Extraperitoneal versus transperitoneal selective para-aortic lymphadenectomy in the pretreatment surgical staging of advanced cervical carcinoma (A Gynecologic Oncology Group study). *Gynecol. Oncol.* **33:** 283–289.

Wharton J, Jones H & Day T (1977) Preirradiation celiotomy and extended field irradiation for invasive carcinoma of the cervix. *Obstet. Gynecol.* **49:** 333–338.

Wimbush PR & Fletcher GH (1969) Radiation therapy of carcinoma of the cervical stump. *Radiology* **93:** 655–658.

Wolff JP, Lacour J, Chassagne D *et al.* (1972) Cancer of the cervical stump. A study of 173 patients. *Obstet. Gynecol.* **39:** 10–16.

Wong L, Choo Y, Choy D *et al.* (1989) Long-term follow-up of potentiation of radiotherapy by cis-platinum in advanced cervical cancer. *Gynecol. Oncol.* **35:** 159–163.

7 Treatment of Locally Advanced and Recurrent Cervical Cancer

R Y Kim
H M Shingleton

Introduction

Despite the frequent success of surgery and irradiation in curing cancer of the uterine cervix, there remain a number of women who are not cured by standard therapy. The incidence of pelvic recurrence for Stage I and IIA disease ranges from 10–15% after irradiation or radical surgery alone (Piver and Chung, 1975; Montana *et al.*, 1983). The recurrence rate for Stage IIB and III ranges from 30–50% after definitive radiation therapy (Jampolis *et al.*, 1975; Kim *et al.*, 1989; Coia *et al.*, 1990). The most common site of recurrence is in the pelvis, followed by the paraaortic nodes, lungs, lower vagina, and the axial skeleton.

The clinical presentation of recurrent cervical cancer is variable and often insidious, although the usual symptoms of central pelvic recurrence are vaginal discharge and bleeding. Pelvic sidewall recurrence may be silent or cause pelvic pain and swelling of lower extremities.

The most common method of diagnosis in patients who develop pelvic recurrent disease is the bimanual pelvic examination. However, the pelvic fibrosis following radiation therapy makes this examination for early detection of recurrence difficult. Nodularity within the fibrosis is a hallmark of recurrence. Few recurrences are detected by Pap smear alone except for central recurrences involving the upper vagina. Pap smears after radiation treatment can be very difficult to interpret and difficult to perform due to a fibrotic upper vagina. When recurrent cancer is suspected in the pelvis clinically, cervical, upper vaginal and parametrial needle biopsy may be necessary to confirm its presence. Diagnostic evaluation for those with recurrent cancer should include a chest film, computed tomography (CT) of pelvis and abdomen, complete blood count, and tests of renal and liver function. CT is established as a valuable method for assessing pelvic malignancy, but a few reports focus on its use in detecting and evaluating recurrent carcinoma (Christine *et al.*, 1988).

It is as important to make an early diagnosis of recurrent cancer as it is to make a primary diagnosis of invasive disease. Prognosis mainly depends on the extent of recurrent disease. Because the majority of recurrences appear within the first two years after treatment, follow-up visits should be most frequent during this time interval.

The treatment of recurrent cervical cancer depends on the mode of previous therapy and the site of recurrence. Patients who were treated initially with surgery should be considered for radiation therapy, and those who had radiation therapy initially should be considered for surgical treatment. Chemotherapy is investigational or palliative only and reserved for women not considered curable by the other modalities.

Definitive Radiotherapeutic Approaches for Recurrent Cervix Cancer

Recurrence after Previous Surgery

Although the frequency of cervical cancer recurrence after primary surgery is somewhat varied in the literature, the distribution of recurrences in the central pelvis, pelvic sidewall and extrapelvic sites is approximately the same (Webb & Symmonds, 1980; Krebs *et al.*, 1982; Burke *et al.*, 1987). The incidence of central pelvic recurrence alone is low, ranging from 1.5–6% (Krebs *et al.*, 1982; Shingleton *et al.*, 1983). The site of recurrence may influence the time of diagnosis and prognosis. Central pelvic recurrences are easy to detect early by pelvic examination and have a better prognosis than pelvic sidewall recurrences. Patients who can be cured by radiotherapy include those with central and/or pelvic sidewall recurrence without extrapelvic spread.

Pelvic recurrences in surgical patients who have not previously had irradiation can be successfully treated by radiation therapy. The results of radiation therapy are varied in different institutions, and depend on the site of the recurrence, tumor volume and aggressiveness of the radiation treatment (*Table 7.1*). The long-term survival rate for central recurrence is better (30–80%) than for pelvic sidewall recurrence (5–30%). Major complication rates range from 6–11% (Tan *et al.*, 1991).

After external pelvic radiation therapy ranging

Table 7.1. Results of radiotherapy for postsurgical recurrent cervical cancer.

Authors	*No. of patients*	*Long-term survival (%)*		*Comments*
		Central	*Pelvic wall*	
Deutsch and Parson (1974)	31	30	5	External/brachy At least 30 months FU
Ciatto *et al.* (1980)	115	81	30	Mainly external 5 yrs FU
Krebs *et al.* (1982)	26	27	13	No detail RT At least 24 months FU
Larson *et al.* (1988)	17	83	30	External/brachy Median 48 months FU
Potter *et al.* (1990)	28	30	33	External/brachy Median 74 months FU
Tan *et al.* (1991)	100	42	15	External/brachy 5 yrs FU

External = external radiotherapy; brachy = brachytherapy; RT = radiation therapy; FU = follow-up.

Table 7.2. Interstitial brachytherapy in advanced cervical carcinoma. (Modified from Kim, 1993.)

Author	*No. of patients*	*Stage*	*CR (%)*	*Major complication (%)*
Prempree *et al.* (1978)	18	IIIB	78	11.0
Aristizabal *et al.* (1983)	106	IIB–IVA	76	18.0
Ampuero *et al.* (1983)	24	IIB–IVA	62	37.5
Martinez *et al.* (1985)	37	IIB–IIIB	83	5.4
Syed *et al.* (1987)	135	IB–IVA	78	10.4

CR = complete response.

from 4000–4500 cGy, an appropriate choice of brachytherapy is the most important consideration to ensure that the tumor is encompassed by the technique used. Transvaginal cone or vaginal mold/ovoids should be limited to isolated small residual tumors. Patients with bulky central recurrence may require interstitial implantation using a template for adequate tumor coverage, in addition to the external beam. Doses of 2000–3000 cGy are given as a boost dose, depending on the extent of the tumor. If an interstitial implant is not feasible, external beam can be given with reduced portals.

Interstitial Implant

The efforts to improve local control by delivering a high-dose of radiation with conventional methods (intrauterine tandem and vaginal ovoids) have been disappointing in advanced or recurrent carcinoma of the cervix. Interstitial radiation therapy allows the delivery of high dose radiation to a precisely determined tumor volume. Because of the rapid fall-off outside the treatment volume, a smaller area of normal tissue is exposed. The properties of interstitial brachytherapy make it the most promising treatment modality for advanced and recurrent disease.

Implants can be done at the time of exploratory laparotomy using either iodine-125 (^{125}I) as a permanent implant or iridium-192 (^{192}Ir) as a temporarily removable afterloading implant. The tumor dose of 2000–3000 cGy in 2–3 days calculated at 0.5 cm outside the implant volume for ^{192}Ir in addition to the external pelvic irradiation (4000–4500 cGy) and 13,000–16,000 cGy in a one-year period at the periphery of an ^{125}I implant has been used. Homogeneous irradiation of afterloading interstitial radiation is possible with the development of modern templates by Syed and Puthawala (1987) and Martinez *et al.* (1985), both of which are fashioned after the parametrial radium distribution suggested by Corscaden *et al.* (1948) (*Figure 7.1*). Several authors have published encouraging results from the use of interstitial implants in patients with distorted vaginal anatomy or large tumors not treatable with conventional intracavitary radiation (*Table 7.2*).

Severe complications can occur in up to 21% of patients. Most are caused by loading of needles under the surface of the vaginal cylinder in addition to the uterine tandem, resulting in a high dose to the

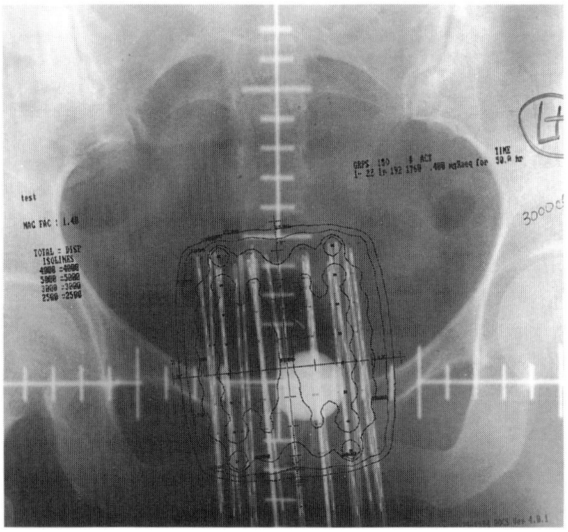

Figure 7.1. Anterior–posterior view of the pelvis showing parametrial interstitial afterloading needles superimposed with isodose lines for centrally recurrent cervical cancer.

anterior and posterior wall. A dose rate of more than 100 cGy hr should be avoided. Although morbidity has been minimized due to modification of the technique, high complications related to interstitial implants are still a concern. In the case of previous radical hysterectomy, bladder and small bowel became attached to the vaginal apex, making interstitial implants undesirable. Patient selection and laparoscopy- or laparotomy-controlled implants should minimize the complication rate.

Lateral extension of large central disease is difficult to cover completely with the transperineal template technique because of the pubic arch. This limitation is overcome by placing the transperineal needles obliquely. Recurrence outside the true pelvis, but below the bifurcation of the abdominal aorta, is not amenable to the transperineal implant technique, whether removable or permanent. These lesions might be approached transperitoneally for possible resection or permanent ^{125}I implants.

Recurrence after Previous Radiotherapy

Due to improved pelvic radiotherapy, recurrences confined to the central portion of the pelvis alone and potentially amenable to radical surgery are limited in number. Perez *et al.* (1983) reported that central pelvic failure alone was observed in only 7% of patients (less than 2% in Stage IB and IIA, 8.7% in Stage IIB, and 14.6% in Stage III). Therefore, the majority of patients with recurrent disease after previous radiotherapy do not have resectable disease. Those patients who cannot be treated with an exenteration pose a difficult management problem. In the past, discouraging cancer control and high complication rates have tempered enthusiasm for radical reirradiation. Those patients who benefitted from reirradiation in general were those who received far less than optimal radiation during their initial therapy.

The outcome of reirradiation with curative intent varies considerably in the literature (*Table 7.3*). These are very selected patients; the modalities of treatments and follow-up periods are varied. In general, reports of reirradiation with the more favorable outcomes have included cervical cancer patients as well as some with endometrial and vaginal cancer. Overall five-year survivals for recurrent cervical cancer alone range from 5–15% (Jones *et al.*, 1970; Evans *et al.*, 1971; Nori *et al.*, 1981; Sommers *et al.*, 1989). Although it is difficult to compare different series of reirradiation directly, clearly the use of additional external beam radiotherapy is hazardous. In patients requiring reirradiation with external beam, precautions must be observed to minimize the volume of normal tissue exposed to radiation. Contrast visualization of the small bowel is used to assess the amount of tissue within the treatment volume and extensively-shaped secondary collimation is required to shield critical structures.

Interstitial implants using various isotopes such as ^{125}I and ^{192}Ir have been used in the past for the treatment of recurrent malignancy. For reirradiation, interstitial irradiation has a distinct advantage over external irradiation because it can deliver a cancerocidal dose directly to the tumor mass while sparing surrounding normal tissue. However, the complication rates are still high and must be seriously considered before embarking on interstitial therapy. Exploratory laparotomy becomes an integral part of treatment and unresectable or residual tumor can be readily implanted with permanent ^{125}I and/or removable ^{192}Ir during this procedure. Puthawala *et al.* (1982) reported on the results of reirradiation with interstitial brachytherapy alone in 40 patients with recurrent pelvic malignancy; 26 of these patients had exploratory laparotomy at the time of implants. Of the 40 patients, 13 (33%) remained alive and disease-free to a minimum follow-up period of two years. Serious complications such as soft tissue necrosis and fistulae were observed in 15% of these patients. For local control, high doses (6000–7000 cGy) are needed, much as one would use for initial treatment.

Radical reirradiation should be selected only for those with localized, small-volume, centrally-located tumor masses. However, the most important factor relative to reirradiation is disease-free interval (Jones *et al.*, 1970; Sommers *et al.*, 1989). Prempree *et al.* (1984) reported that patients with small central disease that recurred more than five years after initial radiation treatment can achieve a 40% long-term survival with treatment compared to no long-term survival in patients with earlier recurrence.

Table 7.3. Results of reirradiation for postradiation recurrent cervical cancer.

Authors	No. of patients	Long-term survival (%)	Major complication (%)	Comments
Jones *et al.* (1970)	53	10	34	External/brachy 5 yrs FU
Evans *et al.* (1971)	70	6.2		Mainly brachy 5 yrs FU
Nori *et al.* (1981)	75	10*	12	Brachy 5 yrs FU
Puthawala *et al.* (1982)	40	33+	15	Brachy 24 months FU
Prempree *et al.* (1984)	8	37.5	12.5	Late/central lesion Mainly brachy, 5 yrs FU
Russell *et al.* (1987)	25	56+	28	External/brachy 10–61 months FU
Sommers (1989)	71	4*		External, 5 yrs FU
	10	15		External/brachy, 5 years FU
Randall *et al.* (1993)	13	46+	7.6	Brachy 24–71 months FU

External = external radiotherapy; brachy = brachytherapy; FU = follow-up.
+Other recurrent gynecological cancers as well as cervical cancer.
*Paraaortic metastases in some recurrent cervical cancers.

Combined Chemotherapy/ Radiation Therapy

The use of chemotherapy as a radiation sensitizer (concurrent chemotherapy) is an attractive approach for improving local control rates. The concept of concurrent radiation and chemotherapy offers a number of theoretical advantages compared with the use of chemotherapy before irradiation.

The chemotherapy of advanced or recurrent cancer of the cervix has been associated with variable response rates. Single-agent cisplatin remains the more widely used antineoplastic drug in this disease. Cisplatin has also been shown to be an effective radiosensitizer. The bases for this combined approach in patients with recurrent cancer are several. First, improved results for squamous cell carcinoma of other sites has been reported, such as head and neck, esophagus and anus. Second, the use of chemotherapeutic agents as radiation sensitizers in the treatment of advanced cancer of the cervix has been shown to be beneficial in studies using hydroxyurea, cisplatin, 5-fluorouracil (5-FU), mitomycin-C or combinations. Thomas *et al.* (1987) reported the results of salvage therapy in 17 patients with cancer of the cervix recurrent after primary surgery using 5-FU with or without mitomycin-C and radiation therapy. Eight of the 17 patients (47%) were alive and disease-free at 21–58 months, which is an improved result compared to that quoted for radiation alone. Because of the small numbers and non-randomized nature of this study, it is hard to say at the present time how much chemotherapy as sensitizer contributes to disease-free survival. However, such a study can provide a guide to future research directions.

Pelvic Arterial Infusion/ Radiation Therapy

The use of pelvic arterial infusion with a variety of chemotherapeutic agents has been reported for over 20 years for the treatment of advanced or recurrent disease (Scarabelli *et al.*, 1987). Unfortunately, the responses have been limited and of short duration. Previous data reveal that most studies were carried out in patients with recurrent disease after surgery and/or radiotherapy. This could be an unfavorable factor because the vascular supply to the tumor site after surgery and especially radiation therapy may be compromised. Recently, the technical difficulties of intraarterial drug administration have been overcome by an implantable delivery system that minimizes the risk of infection and the requirement for multiple invasive procedures to secure vascular access (Rettenmaier *et al.*, 1988). Further study is warranted with this combination method as a part of a sequential therapeutic plan with surgery and/or radiotherapy.

Hyperthermia/Radiation Therapy

Hyperthermia at temperatures of 42.5°C or above as an adjuvant to radiotherapy raises the response rates in treatment of superficial measurable tumors from 30% to 70% (Perez *et al.*, 1991). Heat in itself kills cells under hypoxic conditions and cells in S-phase. As these cells are more resistant to radiation therapy, heat ideally complements radiation. Externally applied methods include microwaves, radiofrequency, capacitive heating or ultrasound. However, the technical problem of heating a deep-seated tumor such as cancer of the cervix has prevented a universally accepted method of administering the therapy in a consistent fashion. External hyperthermia for heating a deep-seated cancer is under investigation, but has encountered significant problems. To date, intracavitary hyperthermia (Li *et al.*, 1991) has been the simplest means for highly localized heating of tumors located near natural body orifices. However, major disadvantages of intracavitary hyperthermia include difficulty of obtaining intratumoral temperature measurements in most treated patients and inhomogeneous temperature distribution.

The difficulties and limitations of using a non-invasive technique for inducing homogeneous local hyperthermia have lead to renewed interest in interstitial hyperthermia for various types of primary tumors including those of the cervix. The use of afterloading interstitial implants provides an opportunity to use interstitial radiotherapy and hyperthermia together. Recently, Bloss *et al.* (1992) compared tumor response and complications of 16 patients receiving the combination of external and interstitial radiotherapy with nine patients receiving the same treatment plus interstitial hyperthermia (Stages II/IIIB). Despite a bias toward more advanced disease in the group treated with hyperthermia, no difference was detected between the two groups in tumor response rate and disease-free survival. Most reports are based on the treatment of small numbers of patients with recurrent tumors and do not provide sufficient data on important clinical parameters. Phase III, site-specific, prospective randomized trials need to be developed for recurrences as well as for patients with previously untreated tumors in order to provide data about the effectiveness of hyperthermia for cervical cancer.

Altered Fractionation of Radiation Therapy

Attempts to relate physical dose factors to a biologic effect have been numerous; examples are strandquist plot, NSD (normal standard dose), TDF (time, dose, fractionation), and most recently, the linear–quadratic equation. The most useful aspect of the linear–quadratic model is the recognition of early- and late-reacting tissues. The fraction size is the dominant factor in determining late tissue toxicity, while overall treatment time has little effect. By contrast, fraction size and overall treatment time both determine the response of early-reacting tissue such as normal mucosa and most tumors.

Although there is no pure form, altered fractionation can be divided into hyperfractionation and accelerated fractionation. The basic aim of hyperfractionation is to further separate early and late effect by using small fraction size (115–120 cGy) and almost the same overall treatment time. It is hoped that this allows the slowly-responding tissue to tolerate a higher radiation dose, which increases the probability of tumor control. While many phase II trials using hyperfractionation in a number of sites including lung, head and neck cancer have been available with encouraging results, there have been few clinical trials for cancer of the cervix. Recently, phase II Radiation Therapy Oncology Group (RTOG) and Gynecologic Oncology Group (GOG) trials with a twice daily fractionation schedule of external irradiation along with brachytherapy in advanced cancer of the cervix was completed. The results of both studies are still pending. Varghese *et al.* (1992) reported preliminary data showing that a 20% increase in the total dose with the hyperfractionation schedule is feasible with an acceptable normal tissue toxicity for cancer of the cervix.

Accelerated fractionation is the use of conventional fraction size (200 cGy) and markedly shortened overall treatment time to defeat the tumor-proliferating and accelerated repopulation for rapidly growing tumors. Unfortunately, this approach is limited due to acute toxicity to rapidly proliferating normal tissues.

Recently, a hybrid referred to as accelerated hyperfractionation, using a moderately shortened overall treatment time and a twice daily dose with a decrease in dose per fraction (150–160 cGy), has been tested for head and neck cancer. The limitation of this approach is again acute toxicity of early responding tissues requiring a break of approximately ten days to two weeks or reduced fields and a concomitant boost dose at the end of the treatment program. Wang (1987) reported that accelerated hyperfractionation was well tolerated and produced rapid shrinkage of gross tumor in 38 patients with carcinoma of the cervix. Phase III randomized trials of altered fractionation are necessary to confirm this finding before its routine use for advanced or recurrent cancer of the cervix.

Intraoperative Radiation Therapy (IORT)

Intraoperative radiation therapy (IORT) combines localized high-dose irradiation with the ability to shield or temporarily remove radiation-sensitive structures. The radiation is given in a single dose of 1500–2500 cGy with a 6–15 MeV electron beam of a dedicated linear accelerator during the surgical procedure. Although there are indications of benefit from IORT in a number of tumor sites such as the pancreas, rectum and stomach, the use of this modality for gynecologic tumors has been only minimally explored. Gynecologic tumors often adhere to the pelvic sidewall where the use of IORT with surgical resection may be of substantial benefit. Monge *et al.* (1993) investigated the use of IORT in 26 patients with recurrent gynecologic cancer. Two groups – previous radiation therapy (group I) and previous surgery (group II) – were treated with a combination of surgical resection, IORT (1000–2500 cGy) and external beam irradiation (if not previously irradiated). Local control rate was 33% and 77% respectively in group I and group II. The ability to control local disease in a given neoplasm with radiation therapy is known to depend on both the tumor burden and the total dose administered. Therefore, the inability to achieve a full dose of radiation therapy because of previous treatment with radiotherapy or because of gross residual disease is a compromising factor.

Although IORT seems to offer some advantages, the use of single large fractions causes a predictably high complication rate, especially in previously irradiated patients. Shaw *et al.* (1987) reported that a peripheral lower extremity neuropathy was the most common IORT-associated toxicity (32%), characterized by unilateral pain (100%), numbness/tingling (69%), or weakness (50%).

Combined Operative and Radiotherapeutic Treatment (CORT)

The combined operative and radiotherapeutic treatment (CORT) is a new radiosurgical treatment concept for patients with recurrent gynecologic malignancy infiltrating the pelvic wall.

Extension of the tumor to the pelvic sidewall has been considered a contraindication for exenteration. This may be difficult to determine clinically for even the most experienced surgeon because of radiation fibrosis. CT or magnetic resonance imaging (MRI) scans may help in predicting adequate margins of resectability, but in any instance where resectability is questionable, the patient should be offered exploratory laparotomy to definitely resolve the issue. As with surgery for any solid tumor, the problem of surgical margins with exenteration is also a key issue.

To improve local control in patients with close or positive margins, IORT or CORT can be used. In CORT, the low-dose rate ^{192}Ir or fractionated high-dose rate brachytherapy is used. CORT is more biologically sound than one large single fraction of radiation that is delivered intraoperatively (IORT). Fourquet *et al.* (1985) used this approach for 51 patients with advanced and recurrent colorectal cancer. The local control rate at 12 months was 64%, and only 6% developed severe complication.

Recently, Hockel and Knapstein (1992) reported preliminary results with CORT for recurrent cervical tumors infiltrating the pelvic sidewall. This combined treatment consisted of five parts including:

- staging laparotomy;
- maximum debulking of tumor from the pelvic wall and exenteration of infiltrating central pelvic organs;
- implantation of afterloading tubes for brachytherapy;
- pelvic wall plasty with muscle and omental flap to create a protective distance between the tubes and the remaining pelvic organs;
- postoperative remote afterloading high-dose brachytherapy of the tumor bed.

Of the 18 patients evaluated, recurrent tumor was reduced to microscopic levels in three of them. Tumor debulking to less than 5% of the original tumor volume was carried out in six patients. In the remaining cases, the residual tumor volume after debulking ranged from 5–20%. Of the 18 patients evaluated for local control after treatment by CORT, 11 patients (61%) had no evidence of disease at follow-up of 6–32 months. The residual tumor volume after debulking strongly correlated with disease-free survival. One patient had a fatal thromboembolism and three patients with previous radiation of more than 7500 cGy developed gastrointestinal fistulae. This combined approach potentially could improve the prognosis of more patients with recurrent gynecologic cancer with less morbidity than that associated with some other therapies. However, further experience is needed.

Palliative Radiotherapy

Radiation Therapy for Locally Advanced or Recurrent Cervix Cancer

The radiation oncologist is often faced with the challenge of treating a patient with a Stage IVB or recurrent carcinoma that requires palliation and in whom the general condition does not warrant a prolonged course of external irradiation with conventional fractionation. If vaginal bleeding is the main concern, a single intracavitary insertion with tandem and colpostats for 5000–5500 cGy to point A should be sufficient. Also, transvaginal electron or orthovoltage beam therapy in a dose of 1000–1500 cGy in 2–3 fractions directed at the bulk of the central disease can be beneficial.

Meoz *et al.* (1983) described satisfactory palliation with a single dose of 1000 cGy to the pelvis, delivered every 3–6 weeks for a total dose of 3000 cGy.

Complications were relatively high (approximately 15%). Spanos *et al.* (1987) reported a Phase II study of a twice a day split course of irradiation in 142 patients. Irradiation consisted of 370 cGy fractions given twice daily for two consecutive days, repeated at 3–6 week intervals for a total of three courses, aiming at a total dose of 4440 cGy. Of the 142 evaluable patients, 83 (59%) received three courses of irradiation; 29 patients (20%) received two courses; and an additional 29 (20%) received only one course. For patients completing three courses of irradiation, the complete plus partial response rate was 45%. Also, there was a significant decreased incidence of complications compared with a single dose of 1000 cGy given for a total of 3000 cGy. Multiple daily fractionation appears to be a safer way to deliver palliative irradiation.

Radiation for Symptomatic Metastases

Metastases from cancer of the cervix are rather predictably to the pelvis, paraaortic nodes and the lungs. *Table 7.4* shows the pattern of distant metastases. The lung was the most common site for single organ metastases. The lymph nodes were the most common site for multiple organ metastases, especially in the area of the supraclavicular and paraaortic lymph nodes.

Table 7.4. Sites of distant metastases in 2220 patients with squamous cell carcinoma of the cervix. (Modified from Carlson *et al.*, 1967.)

Site	*Single organ metastases (No. of patients)*	*Multiple organ metastases (No. of patients)*
Nodes	33 (30.0%)	157 (67.9%)
Supraclavicular	9	57
Paraaortic	12	54
Inguinal	8	43
Mediastinal	1	37
Iliac	1	28
Cervical	1	16
Axillary	0	12
Other	1	38
Lung	40 (36.3%)	86 (37.0%)
Bone	18 (16.3%)	67 (29.0%)
Abdomen	8 (7.2%)	97 (41.9%)
Generalized	0	37
Peritoneum	2	11
Liver	6	42
Gastrointestinal	0	24
Other	0	54
Miscellaneous	11	101

Bone metastases are infrequent, occurring in 3–4% of patients (Barmeir *et al.*, 1985). Though metastases can occur in any bone, the vertebral spine, especially the lumbar spine, is the most common site. Bony involvement can arise either hematogenously or direct extension from metastatic lymph nodes; however, the most common pattern of lumbar spine involvement is direct extension from paraaortic nodal metastatic tumor, and is characteristic of bone metastases from the cancer of the cervix (Kim *et al.*, 1987). Symptoms suggesting spinal cord compression necessitate an evaluation with an MRI scan and expedient palliative radiotherapy. Metastases to the skull or long bones are uncommon and imply systematic hematogenous dissemination of the cancer. External irradiation to bone metastases is often effective in relieving pain. Palliative irradiation treatment at doses of 3000 cGy in ten fractions is the generally accepted treatment. Brain metastases causing distressing CNS symptoms and symptomatic growing nodal metastases can be effectively palliated with a 3000 cGy in ten fractions.

Surgical Approaches

Surgery for Primary Treatment of Advanced Cervical Cancer

Surgical staging data have proven the inaccuracy of clinical staging (Lagasse *et al.*, 1980) and some individuals with clinical Stage IIIB disease are technically resectable by radical hysterectomy and pelvic node dissection. American gynecologic oncologists have, however, dismissed them as candidates for primary surgical treatment since the sheer volume of pelvic disease in these individuals predicts close or tumor-involved surgical margins and regional nodal metastases. An occasional patient with Stage IIIB or Stage IVA is a candidate for urinary or fecal diversion at the time of their primary treatment by radiation therapy; however, such diversions are only indicated if fistulae exist at the time of presentation.

Primary exenteration has been advocated by some individuals as initial treatment for individuals with Stage IVA cervical cancer. For instance, Ketcham *et al.* (1970) used this approach quite often. One rationale for primary surgery is that radiation may produce fistulae of the bladder or rectum in individuals if tumor involves the anterior and posterior vaginal walls. In actual experience, however, such fistulae occur in only 4–5% of cases (Upadhyay *et al.*, 1988). At the University of Alabama, the gynecologic oncologists did not need to perform a primary exenteration for cervical cancer in many years, electing to use pelvic irradiation as the first line of treatment instead. It is tempting to use primary exenteration occasionally, however, especially in young women with advanced disease at presentation if the cancer is confined to the central pelvis. Too often, however, staging reveals metastases to regional or distant lymph nodes and one abandons the ultraradical resection in favor of radiation therapy.

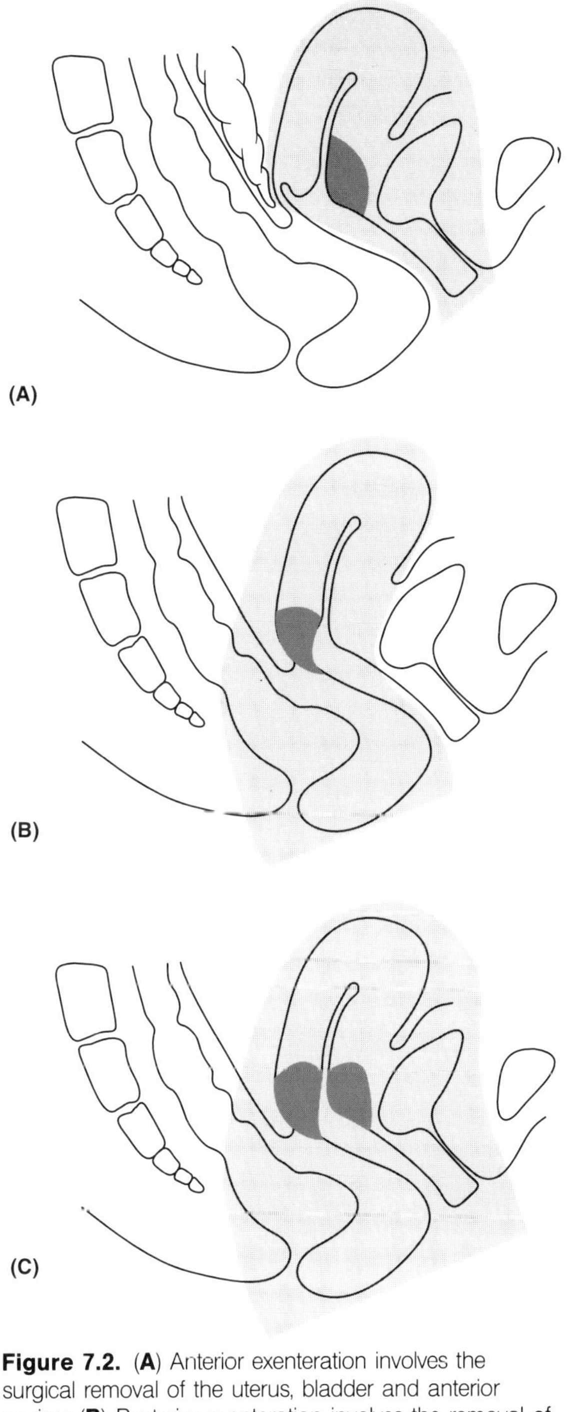

Figure 7.2. (**A**) Anterior exenteration involves the surgical removal of the uterus, bladder and anterior vagina: (**B**) Posterior exenteration involves the removal of the rectum, uterus and posterior vagina: (**C**) Total exenteration involves the removal of the bladder, urethra, uterus, the entire vagina and the rectum. (Courtesy of Shingleton and Orr, 1987.)

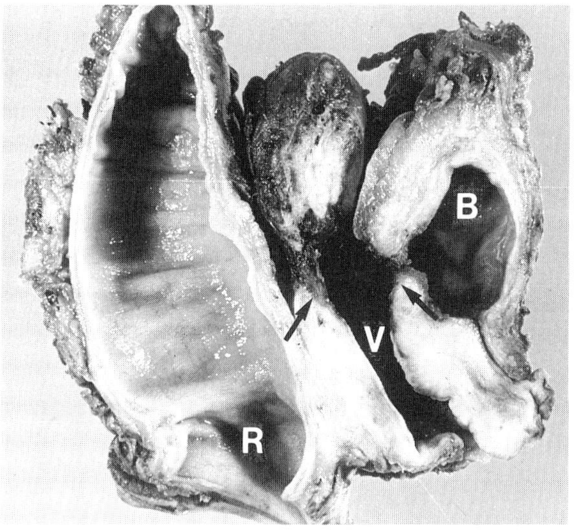

Figure 7.3. Total exenteration specimen (B, bladder; V, vagina; R, rectum). Note the malignant ulcer involving the cervix and adjacent anterior and posterior vaginal walls (arrows).

Surgery for Recurrent Cancer

Pelvic exenteration is an operation used as a last chance of cure in women with recurrent cancer limited to the central pelvis. Since Perez *et al.* (1983) and others have shown that recurrences (all clinical stages combined) are confined to the central pelvis following curative irradiation therapy in less than 10% of the cases, one can understand the relative rarity of this operation. Indeed, as radiation therapy techniques have improved in the past quarter century, pelvic exenterative surgery is becoming a rarity even in major medical centers in the USA, with an estimated performance rate of about 40–50/year nationally (Shingleton *et al.*, 1995). Absolute and relative contraindications for the operation have been summarized recently by Barber (1988); some advocate total exenteration for recurrent cervical cancer, while selective use of partial exenteration is advocated by others (*Figure 7.2*). Important considerations are the general health of the patient and her ability to withstand such a major operation, as well as the availability of experienced surgeons capable of performing all parts of the procedure including fecal and urinary diversions and pelvic and vaginal reconstruction. Patients fare better when one surgeon or team of surgeons performs all phases of the surgery including intraoperative assessment of tumor spread, specimen removal (*Figure 7.3*), urinary and fecal diversions, and the reconstructive phase. While it is true that these operations can be viewed as an aggregate of several operations often performed individually (cystectomy, radical hysterectomy, pelvic lymphadenectomy, colostomy, urinary diversion, abdomino–perineal resection, rectal anastomosis), one cannot assume that those who have mastered the individual operations will be expert in performing the larger operation or in providing postoperative care of the exenteration patient. The best results are achieved by oncology services with sufficient patients to allow the surgical team to become proficient in the perioperative care of such individuals, and this is currently available in only a handful of centers.

Operative mortality rates and long-term survival of these women reflect the above considerations (*Table* 7.5). The improved survival in modern series reflects improved techniques of intraoperative monitoring, the judicious use of antibiotics, and the use of total parenteral nutrition during the perioperative period. Improvements in operative techniques (i.e. better pelvic floor closures and the use of omental or myocutaneous flaps to obliterate the pelvic 'dead space' and bring in additional blood supply) are also factors. Better survival is associated with partial rather than with total exenteration (*Table* 7.6), and is also age-related, older women tolerating the operation less well than younger ones (*Table* 7.7). As the safety of the operations has improved, an era of reconstruction has also begun; a variety of techniques is available for vaginal reconstruction (Hatch and Shingleton, 1988). Considerable experience has accumulated concerning the use of rectal re-anastomosis to avoid a permanent colostomy. There has been a move away from ileal and sigmoid urinary conduits (using irradiated segments of bowel) toward use of a non-irradiated segment such as transverse colon (Baker and Shingleton, 1988). Continent urinary conduits have been suggested by Kock *et al.* (1982) and as yet have not gained widespread use in pelvic exenteration for gynecologic cancer due to the disadvantages of using irradiated bowel segments for such conduits, as well as other drawbacks in perfecting such a technique.

It has been suggested by some that there is a place for palliative exenterations (Stanhope and Symmonds, 1985). The likelihood of cure in situations in which the disease has spread beyond

Table 7.5. Operative mortality rates and five-year survival for recent series of pelvic exenterations. (From Shingleton *et al.*, 1988. Reprinted with permission from The American College of Obstetricians and Gynecologists (Obstetrics and Gynecology, 1988, **73**, 1027–1034.)

Authors	*No. of patients*	*Operative mortality (%)*	*Five-year survivors (%)*
Ketcham *et al.* (1970)	162	7	38.0
Brunschwig (1970)	581⁺	8°	19.9
Symmonds (1975)	198	8.1*	33.0
Rutledge (1977)	296	13.5	42.1
Averette (1984)	92	23.9**	37.0
Shingleton *et al.* (1988)	143⁺	6.3	50.0

⁺Cervical cancer cases only.
*3.0% in last 102 operations.
**10.4% in last 33 operations.
°165 cases in 1962–1966.

Table 7.6. Survival related to the type of exenteration in patients with recurrent cervical cancer. (Modified from Shingleton and Orr, 1987.)

		Anterior exenteration[1]			*Total exenteration*		
Authors	*Year*	*No. of patients*	*Surgical mortality (%)*	*Five-year survival (%)*	*No. of patients*	*Surgical mortality (%)*	*Five-year survival (%)*
Ingeroll & Ulfelder	1966	18	—	11.1	53	—	26.4
Brunschwig	1967	95	10.5	18.9	217	20.3	17.1
Inguilla & Cosmil	1967	32	25.0	21.9	51	49.0	5.9
Ketcham *et al.*	1970	9	—	44.0	81	—	25.0
Creasman & Rutledge	1974	271	—	33.3	59	—	20.3
Symmonds	1975	59	—	42.0	36	—	41.0
Shingleton *et al.*	1988	63	1.6	58.0	78	10.3	42.0

[1]Partial exenteration.

Table 7.7. Pelvic exenteration for cancer of the cervix University of Alabama at Birmingham: age-related operative mortality. (Modified from Shingleton and Orr, 1987, p. 227.)

		Type of exenteration				
Age group	*No. of patients*	*Anterior*	*Posterior*	*Total*	*Deaths/ age group (%)*	*Deaths cum. (%)*
<40	33	19	0	14	0	0
41–50	40	11	2	27 (2)	5.0	2.7
51–60	45	24 (1)	0	21 (3)	8.8	5.1
>60	25	14	0	11 (3)	12.0	6.3

(1), (2), (3) – deaths by type of operation.

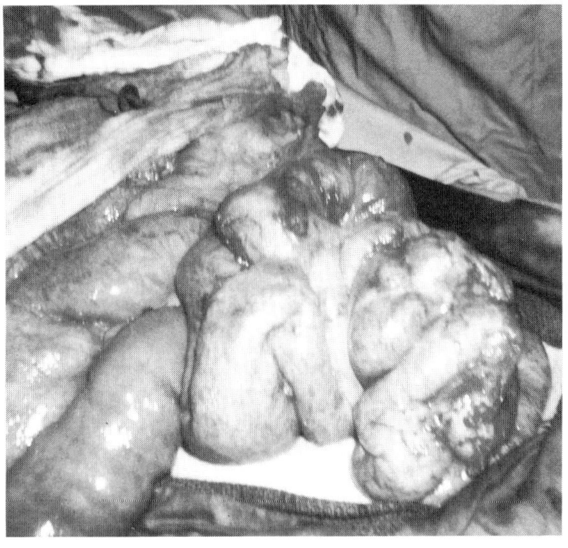

Figure 7.4. Marked radiation damage to small bowel in a patient given postoperative whole-pelvis radiotherapy (50 Gy) following radical hysterectomy.

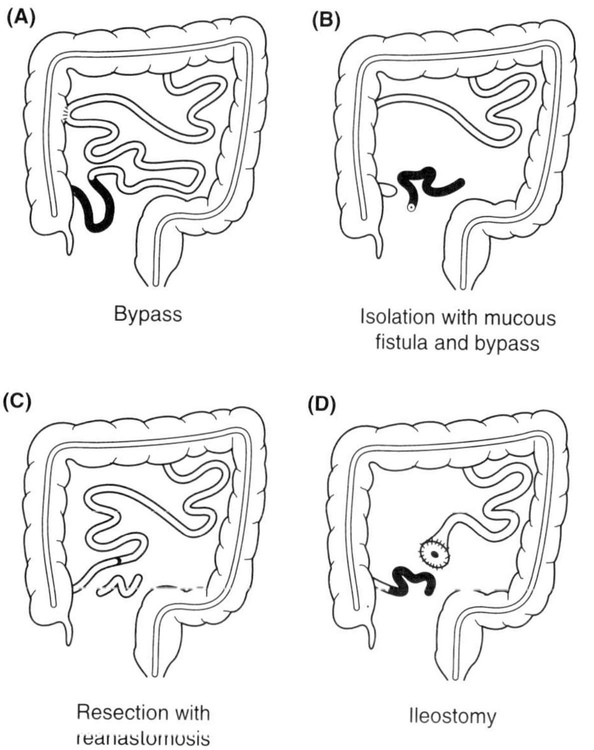

Figure 7.5. Operations for radiation injuries of the ileum. (**A**) A simple bypass of the damaged area of intestine: (**B**) A bypass of the damaged area of intestine with isolation of this segment from the intestinal tract. (**C**) Resection of the injured area of intestine. (**D**) Diversion of the intestinal tract proximal and distal to the injured area of intestine. (Courtesy of Delgado and Smith, 1982, p. 103.)

the central pelvis is small and would not seem to justify the morbidity and potential mortality of these operations (i.e. the risk of this surgery is great enough that it should be applied only when there is a chance of cure that exceeds the operative mortality rate).

Surgery for Radiotherapy Complications

Irradiation injury to the urinary or gastrointestinal tract may occur at any time following radiation therapy; however, it usually occurs in the first two years following the therapy (Smith, 1982). The presentation is ordinarily partial or complete intestinal obstruction, which often requires surgery for correction (*Figure 7.4*). Other injuries less frequently encountered are peritonitis secondary to bowel perforation and enteric fistulae. Operations advocated for correcting radiation injuries to the ileum are bypass, bypass associated with isolation of the damaged segment and mucous fistula, resection with re-anastomosis (*Figure 7.5*), or ileostomy. Large bowel injuries include rectovaginal fistula, proctosigmoiditis, or large bowel obstruction. In addition to these, a few patients will develop perforation of the viscus or other more complex fistulae. Diverting colostomies are the most commonly used procedure for the above complications. Rectovaginal fistulae due to radiation damage are difficult to repair; the 'fold over'

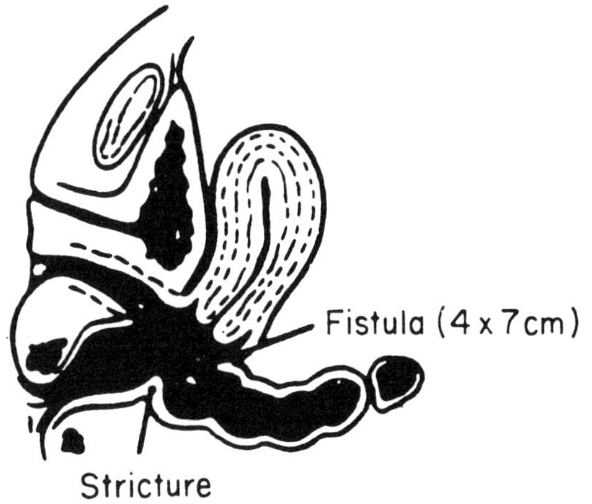

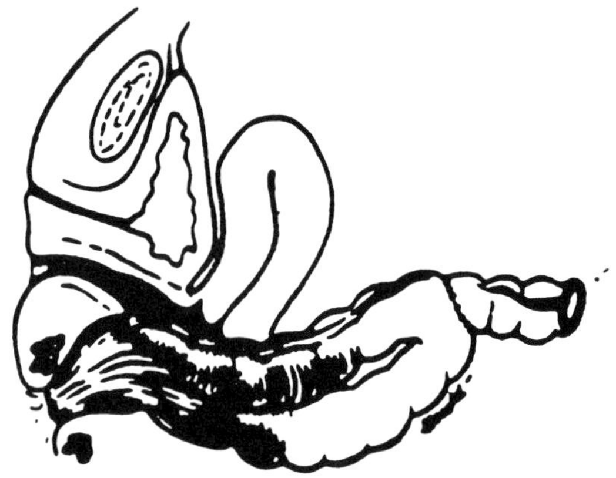

Figure 7.6. The Bricker technique for repair of a large rectovaginal fistula. (From Bricker and Johnston, 1979, p. 499, by permission.) (Reprinted in and use approved by Delgado and Smith, 1982, p. 221.)

procedure such as advocated by Bricker and Johnston (1979; *Figure 7.6*) or other techniques bringing in new blood supply by means of myocutaneous or omental flaps are necessary for successful closure.

Ureteral obstruction as a manifestation of radiation damage is uncommon compared to tumor recurrence as the basis for the obstruction. A few individuals in the first few years following radiation are candidates for urinary diversion if radiation fibrosis is proven to be the basis for the obstruction. If the finding is unilateral, transureteroureterostomy might be considered. Vesicovaginal fistula secondary to radiation damage to the bladder is another indication for urinary diversion. Should the bladder fistula be closed successfully (usually requiring bringing in a new blood supply by techniques such as the Martius bulbocavernosus flap) then an 'undiversion' may be possible, usually in the form of converting the ileal conduit to an ileocystostomy. The subject is well discussed by Boronow (1982).

Severe radiation necrosis has been considered by some as an indication for pelvic exenteration. These patients typically present with pain, fistula of the bowel or bladder, chronic vaginal bleeding or foul vaginal discharge. Exenterations in women with severe pelvic radiation damage are fraught with high complication rates and therefore may or may not improve their quality of life. Often urinary or fecal diversion alone will relieve many of the symptoms with less morbidity than that associated with pelvic exenteration.

Summary of Management Options

- It is important to make an early diagnosis of recurrent cancer because additional treatment offers some chance of cure.
- Exenterative surgery is rarely, if ever, indicated as primary treatment.
- In general, women with recurrent cancer following primary surgery should be considered for radiation therapy, and those who recur following primary radiation therapy should be considered for salvage surgical treatment.
- For women with primary surgical failure, an appropriate choice for brachytherapy is the most important consideration as a boost technique following external pelvic radiation therapy.
- When resectability is in question for pelvic recurrence after radiotherapy, the patient should be offered exploratory laparotomy to resolve the issue.
- To improve local control in women with close or positive pelvic tumor margins at the time of exenteration, intraoperative radiotherapy (IORT) or combined operative and radiotherapeutic treatment (CORT) may be beneficial.
- If a tumor is not resectable after previous radiotherapy, radical reirradiation in the form of interstitial implants may be considered for localized small-volume disease.
- A short course of palliative radiotherapy can be effective treatment for women with locally advanced symptomatic cervical cancer or with symptomatic local metastatic disease.

References

Ampuero F, Doss LL, Khan M, Skipper B & Hilgers RD (1983) The Syed-Neblett interstitial template in locally advanced gynecological malignancy. *Int. J. Radiat. Oncol. Biol. Phys.* **9:** 1897–1903.

Aristizabal SA, Valencia A, O'Campo G & Surwit E (1985) Interstitial parametrical irradiation in cancer of the cervix, Stage IIB–IIIB. *Endocuriether Hyperthermia* **1:** 41–48.

Baker VV & Shingleton HM (1988) Urinary diversion. In: Gusberg SB, Shingleton HM & Deppe G (eds) *Female Genital Cancer*, pp. 573–588. New York: Churchill Livingstone.

■ Barber HRK (1988) Pelvic exenteration. In: Gusberg SB, Shingleton HM & Deppe G (eds) *Female Genital Cancer*, pp. 567–569. New York: Churchill Livingstone.

Barmeir E, Langer O, Levy JL *et al.* (1985) Unusual metastases in carcinoma of the cervix. *Gynecol. Oncol.* **20:** 307–316.

Bloss JD, Berman ML, Syed N *et al.* (1992) Treatment of advanced carcinoma of the uterine cervix with interstitial radiotherapy and hyperthermia. *Endocurietherapy/Hyperthermia Oncol.* **8:** 145–150.

Boronow R (1982) Urologic complications secondary to radiation alone or radiation and surgery. In: Delgado G & Smith JP (eds) *Management of Complications in Gynecologic Surgery*, pp. 163–197. New York: John Wiley & Sons.

Bricker EM & Johnston WD (1979) Repair of post-irradiation rectovaginal fistula and stricture. *Surg. Gynecol. Obstet.* **148:** 499–506.

Burke TW, Hoskins WJ, Heller PB *et al.* (1987) Prognostic factors associated with radical hysterectomy failure. *Gynecol. Oncol.* **26:** 153–159.

Carlson V, Delclos L & Fletcher GH (1967) Distant metastases in squamous cell carcinoma of the uterine cervix. *Radiology* **88:** 961–966.

Christine WH, Husband JE, William MP, Dobbs HJ & Cosgrove DO (1988) The value of CT in the diagnosis of recurrent carcinoma of the cervix. *Clin. Radiol.* **39:** 496–501.

Ciatto S, Pirtoli L & Cionini L (1980) Radiotherapy for postoperative failures for carcinoma of the cervix. *Surg. Gynecol. Obstet.* **151:** 621–624.

Coia L, Won M, Lanciano R *et al.* (1990) The pattern of care outcome study for cancer of the uterine cervix. Results of the second practice survey. *Cancer* **66:** 2451–2456.

Corscaden JA, Gusberg SB & Donlan CP (1948) Precision dosage in interstitial irradiation of cancer of the cervix uteri. *Am. J. Roentgenol.* **60:** 522–524.

■ Delgado G & Smith JP (1982) *Management of Complications in Gynecologic Surgery*, p. 103. New York: John Wiley & Sons.

Deutsch M & Parson JA (1974) Radiotherapy for carcinoma of the cervix recurrent after surgery. *Cancer* **34:** 2051–2055.

Evans SR, Hilaris BS & Barber HRK (1971) External vs interstitial irradiation in unresectable recurrent cancer of the cervix. *Cancer* **28:** 1284–1288.

Fourquet A, Enker WE, Shank B *et al.* (1985) The value of interstitial radiation in advanced and recurrent colorectal cancer. *Endocurietherapy/Hyperthermia* **1:** 113–117.

Hatch KD & Shingleton HM (1988) Reconstructive surgery of the vulva and vagina. In: Gusberg SB, Shingleton HM & Deppe G (eds) *Female Genital Cancer*, pp. 621–644. New York: Churchill Livingstone.

Hockel M & Knapstein PG (1992) The combined operative and radiotherapeutic treatment (CORT) of recurrent tumors infiltrating the pelvic wall: First experience with 18 patients. *Gynecol. Oncol.* **46:** 20–28.

Jampolis S, Andras GJ & Fetcher GH (1975) Analysis of sites and causes of failures of irradiation in invasive squamous cell carcinoma of the intact uterine cervix. *Radiol.* **115:** 681–685.

Jones TK, Levitt SH & King ER (1970) Retreatment of persistent and recurrent carcinoma of the cervix with irradiation. *Radiol.* **95:** 167–174.

Ketcham AS, Deckers PJ, Sugerbaker EV, Hoye RC, Thomas LB & Smith RR (1970) Pelvic exenteration for carcinoma of the uterine cervix, a 15-year experience. *Cancer* **26:** 513–521.

Kim RY (1993) Radiotherapeutic management in carcinoma of the uterine cervix: Current status. *Int. J. Gynecol. Cancer* **3:** 337–348.

Kim RY, Wepplemann B, Salter MM & Brascho DJ (1987) Skeletal metastases from cancer of the uterine cervix: Frequency, patterns, and radiotherapeutic significance. *Int. J. Radiat. Oncol. Biol. Phys.* **13:** 705–708.

Kim RY, Trotti A, Wu CJ, Song SJ & Salter MM (1989) Radiation alone in the treatment of uterine cervix; analysis of pelvic failure and dose response relationships. *Int. J. Rad. Oncol. Biol. Phys.* **17:** 973–978.

Kock NG *et al.* (1982) Urinary diversion via a continent ileal reservoir: clinical results in 12 patients. *J. Urol.* **128:** 469–475.

Krebs HB, Helmkamp BF, Sevin BU *et al.* (1982) Recurrent cancer of the cervix following radial hysterectomy and pelvic node dissection. *Obstet. Gynecol.* **59:** 422–427.

Lagasse L *et al.* (1980) Results and complications of operative staging in cervical cancer: experience of the Gynecologic Oncology Group. *Gynecol. Oncol.* **9:** 90–98.

■ Larson DM, Copeland LJ, Stringer CA *et al.* (1988) Recurrent cervical carcinoma after radical hysterectomy. *Gynecol. Oncol.* **30:** 381–387.

Li DJ, Chou CK, Luk KH *et al.* (1991) Design of intracavitary microwave applicators for the treatment of uterine cervix carcinoma. *Int. J. Hyperthermia* **7:** 693–701.

Martinez A, Edmundson GK, Cox RS, Gunderson LL & Howes AE (1985) Combination of external beam irradiation and multiple site perineal applicator (MUPIT) for treatment of locally advanced or recurrent prostate, anorectal, gynecologic malignancies. *Int. J. Radiat. Oncol. Biol. Phys.* **11:** 391–398.

Meoz RT, Spanos WJ, Doss L *et al.* (1983) Misonidazole combined with large-fraction pelvic irradiation in the treatment of patients with advanced pelvic malignancies: preliminary report of an ongoing RTOG Phase I–II study. *Am. J. Clin. Oncol.* **6:** 417–422.

Monge RM, Jurado M, Azinovic I *et al.* (1993) Intraoperative radiotherapy in recurrent gynecological cancer. *Radioth. Oncol.* **28:** 127–133.

Montana GS, Fowler WC, Varia MA, Walton LA & Mack Y (1983) Carcinoma of the cervix Stage IB. Results of treatment with radiation therapy. *Int. J. Radiat. Oncol. Biol. Phys.* **9:** 45–49.

Nori D, Hilaris BS, Kim HS *et al.* (1981) Interstitial irradiation in recurrent gynecologic cancer. *Int. J. Radiat. Oncol. Biol. Phys.* **7:** 1513–1517.

Perez CA, Breaux S, Madoc-Jones H *et al.* (1983) Radiation therapy alone in the treatment of carcinoma of uterine cervix. Analysis of tumor recurrence. *Cancer* **51:** 1393–1402.

Perez CA, Pajak T, Emami B *et al.* (1991) Randomized

Phase III study comparing irradiation and hyperthermia with irradiation alone in superficial measurable tumors. *Am. J. Clin. Oncol.* **14:** 133–141.

Piver S & Chung WS (1975) Prognostic significance of cervical lesion size and pelvic node metastases in cervical cancer. *Obstet. Gynecol.* **46:** 507–510.

■ Potter ME, Alvarez RD, Gay FL & Shingleton HM (1990) Optimal therapy for pelvic recurrence after radical hysterectomy for early-stage cervical cancer. *Gynecol. Oncol.* **37:** 74–77.

Prempree T, Arornmarin R, Villasanta U, Kwon T & Scott RM (1984) Retreatment of very late recurrent invasive squamous cell carcinoma of the cervix with irradiation. *Cancer* **54:** 1950–1955.

Prempree T & Scott RM (1978) Treatment of Stage IIIB carcinoma of the cervix: improvement in local by radium needle to implant to supplement the dose to the parametrium. *Cancer* **42:** 1105–1113.

Puthawala AA, Syed AMN, Fleming PA & Disaia PJ (1982) Re-irradiation with interstitial implant for recurrent pelvic malignancies. *Cancer* **50:** 2810–2814.

Randall ME, Evans L, Greven KM, McCunniff AJ & Doline RM (1993) Interstitial reirradiation for recurrent gynecologic malignancies. Results and analysis of prognostic factors. *Gynecol. Oncol.* **48:** 23–31.

Rettenmaier MA, Morgan MF, Ramsinghani NF *et al.* (1988) Treatment of advanced and recurrent squamous carcinoma of the uterine cervix with constant intraarterial infusion of Cisplatin. *Cancer* **61:** 1301–1303.

Russell AH, Koh WJ, Markette K *et al.* (1987) Radical reirradiation for recurrent or second primary carcinoma of the female reproductive tract. *Gynecol. Oncol.* **27:** 226–232.

Scarabelli C, Tumolo S, DePaoli A *et al.* (1987) Intermittent pelvic arterial infusion with peptichemio, doxorubicin, and cisplatin for locally advanced and recurrent carcinoma of the uterine cervix. *Cancer* **60:** 25–30.

Shaw EG, Gunderson LL, Martin JK, Beart RW & Podratz KC (1987) Toxicity and results of intraoperative radiation therapy for primary unresectable and recurrent pelvic malignancies. Processing of the American Radium Society. *Am. J. Clin. Oncol.* **10:** 105.

Shingleton HM & Orr JW Jr (1987) *Cancer of the Cervix: Diagnosis and Treatment.* New York: Churchill Livingstone.

Shingleton HM, Hatch KD, Gore H *et al.* (1983) Tumor recurrence and survival in Stage IB cancer of the cervix. *Am. J. Clin. Oncol.* **6:** 265–272.

■ Shingleton HM, Soong S-J, Gelder MS, Hatch KD, Baker VV & Austin JM Jr (1988) Clinical and histopathologic factors predicting recurrence and survival after pelvic exenteration for cancer of the cervix. *Obstet. Gynecol.* **73:** 1027–1034.

Shingleton HM *et al.* (1995) PCE Data: American College of Surgeons. *Gynecol. Oncol,* In press.

Smith JP (1982) Complications related to radiated gastrointestinal tract. In: Delgado G & Smith JP (eds) *Management of Complications in Gynecologic Oncology*, p. 102. New York: John Wiley & Sons.

Sommers GM, Grigsby PW, Perez CA *et al.* (1989) Outcome of recurrent cervical carcinoma following definitive irradiation. *Gynecol. Oncol.* **35:** 150–155.

Spanos WJ Jr, Wassermann T, Meoz R *et al.* (1987) Palliation of advanced pelvic malignant disease with large fraction pelvic radiation and misonidazole: Final report of RTOG Phase I/II study. *Int. J. Radiat. Oncol. Biol. Phys.* **13:** 1479–1482.

Stanhope CR & Symmonds RE (1985) Palliative exenteration: what, when and why? *Am. J. Obstet. Gynecol.* **152:** 12–16.

Syed AM & Puthawala AA (1987) Interstitial–intracavitary 'Syed–Neblett' applicator in the treatment of carcinoma of the cervix. In: Nori D & Hilaris BS (eds) *Radiation Therapy of Gynecological Cancer*, pp. 297–307. New York: Alan R. Liss.

Tan R, Chung CH, Liu MT, Lai YL & Chang KH (1991) Radiotherapy for postoperative recurrent uterine cervical carcinoma. *Acta Oncolog.* **30:** 353–356.

Thomas GM, Dembo AJ, Black B *et al.* (1987) Concurrent radiation and chemotherapy for carcinoma of the cervix recurrent after radical surgery. *Gynecol. Oncol.* **27:** 254–260.

Upadhyay SK, Symonds RP, Haelterman N & Watson ER (1988) The treatment of Stage IV carcinoma of cervix by radical dose radiotherapy. *Radiother. Oncol.* **11:** 15–19.

Varghese C, NB D, Rangad F *et al.* (1992) Hyperfractionation in advanced carcinoma of the uterine cervix: a preliminary report. *Int. J. Radiat. Oncol. Biol. Phys.* **23:** 393–396.

Wang CC (1987) Altered fractionation radiation therapy for gynecologic cancers. *Cancer* **60:** 2064–2067.

Webb MJ & Symmonds RE (1980) Site of recurrence of cervical cancer after radical hysterectomy. *Am. J. Obstet. Gynecol.* **138:** 813–817.

8 Vaginal Cancer

C W Helm
K K Chan

Introduction

Primary carcinoma of the vagina represents less than 2% of all gynecologic malignancies. Secondary spread from sites such as the cervix, vulva, endometrium, ovary and rectum occurs more frequently than primary disease. The relative rarity of primary carcinoma of the vagina is exaggerated by its definition which excludes tumors of the vagina which also involve either the cervix or vulva.

Squamous cell carcinoma of the vagina (SCC) represents approximately 85% of all histologic types, followed by adenocarcinoma (8%), sarcoma and melanoma (3%), and more rarely undifferentiated, small cell and endodermal sinus tumor.

Progress in understanding the disease and improving treatment has been slow and outcome of treatment has not improved in recent years (Davis *et al.*, 1991; FIGO, 1989).

This chapter will concentrate on SCC and adenocarcinoma.

Squamous Cell Carcinoma

The mean age at presentation is in the seventh decade of life (Al-Kurdi and Monaghan, 1981; Benedet *et al.*, 1983; Manetta *et al.*, 1990; Davis *et al.*, 1991; Kucera and Vavra, 1991). However, it occurs in younger women and many series report its occurrence in the third decade. Most commonly it involves the upper one-third of the vagina (Rutledge, 1967; Benedet *et al.*, 1983, Gallup *et al.*, 1987).

Etiology

There is an association with long-term vaginal pessary use (Way, 1948; Rutledge, 1967; Herbst *et al.*, 1970; Al-Kurdi and Monaghan, 1981; Macnaught *et al.*, 1986), previous cervical disease, both intraepithelial and invasive carcinoma (Kanbour *et al.*, 1974; Benedet *et al.*, 1983; Peters *et al.*, 1985a) and radiotherapy to the pelvis (Rutledge, 1967; Pride and Buchler, 1977; Peters *et al.*, 1985a). Although not all agree with this view (Perez and Camel, 1982), evidence suggests a relative risk of 2.7 of developing vaginal cancer after radiotherapy for carcinoma of the cervix and that the most pronounced risk occurs in women less than 45 years of age at the time of radiotherapy.

A relationship between hysterectomy for benign conditions and the development of vaginal carcinoma and intraepithelial neoplasia has been reported (Gallup *et al.*, 1987), but not confirmed (Herman *et al.*, 1986; Brinton *et al.*, 1990).

A case–control study showed limited education, low family income and a history of genital warts and abnormal cervical smears as risk factors. Smoking and sexual behavior, which are strongly associated with cervical carcinoma, were not implicated (Brinton *et al.*, 1990).

Pre-malignant Phase

Vaginal intraepithelial neoplasia (VaIN) may act as a precursor of invasive carcinoma of the vagina (Scokel *et al.*, 1961; Graham and Meigs, 1962; Rutledge, 1967; Hummer *et al.*, 1970; Geelhoed *et al.*, 1976; Lee and Symmonds, 1976). Invasive carcinoma can develop from untreated VaIN 3 (Geelhoed *et al.*, 1976), and areas of VaIN 3 may be associated with unsuspected microinvasive or invasive disease (Ireland and Monaghan, 1988; Hoffman *et al.*, 1992); invasive carcinoma may develop following treatment for VaIN.

Treatment of VaIN 3 should potentially reduce the chance of a patient developing invasive carcinoma of the vagina although this remains unproven.

VaIN occurs at a lower mean age (i.e. 50 years) than invasive carcinoma, with a range from the late teens to the eighties (Cramer and Cutler, 1974; Gallup and Morley, 1975; Hernandez-Linares *et al.*, 1980; Benedet and Sanders, 1984; Woodman and Jordan, 1984; Hoffman *et al.*, 1991), and most commonly affects the upper part of the vagina (Rutledge, 1967; Benedet *et al.*, 1983; Gallup *et al.*, 1987). It may be multifocal.

Presentation

The majority of patients present with post-menopausal vaginal bleeding or discharge (Al-Kurdi and Monaghan, 1981; Ball and Berman, 1982; Benedet *et al.*, 1983; Manetta *et al.*, 1990; Kucera and Vavra, 1991). The cancer may cause pain and discomfort depending on size and site, urinary symptoms such as dysuria, frequency and retention, and problems with defecation including tenesmus. It may present as a mass if present at the lower end of the vagina. As with vulvar carcinoma there may be a considerable delay before presentation (Manetta *et al.*, 1990). A significant minority of women are asymptomatic, diagnosis being made at a routine examination or cytologic screening.

Spread

Carcinoma of the vagina spreads by local infiltration into the surrounding tissues, distantly via the lymphatic system and, at a later stage, the blood stream.

The bladder, anorectum, urethra, vulva and cervix are most at risk by local spread. Lateral spread is to the paracolpium and thence out to the pelvic sidewall.

There is a fine capillary network throughout the mucosa and the muscularis in which lymphatic channels anastomose freely before draining into regular defined channels (Plentl and Friedman, 1971).

Although different regions of the vagina drain principally to particular nodal groups in the pelvis and groin the intercommunicating lymphatics give the potential for drainage to any pelvic nodal group from any region of the vagina.

Staging

The FIGO (International Federation of Gynecology and Obstetrics) staging is based on clinical examination and investigations, which may include cystoscopy, proctoscopy, chest radiography, intravenous urography and barium enema (FIGO, 1989). Additional investigations such as computed tomography (CT) and magnetic resonance imaging (MRI) scans cannot be used for official staging of the disease. A commentary regarding the clinical staging of vaginal cancer as well as the current FIGO staging is included in *Chapter 47* and *Table 47.2*.

Diagnosis

A definitive diagnosis can only be made by histologic examination. It is important to send the pathologist a specimen that allows accurate assessment. This may require total excision of small lesions or full-thickness incisional biopsies including areas of normal mucosa in others. Almost always such biopsies need to be taken under general or regional anesthesia.

Some patients present with abnormal cytologic smears and in the absence of an obvious lesion will require colposcopic assessment. Often this will need to be performed under general or regional anesthesia to allow both an adequate examination and adequate biopsies to be taken. It is particularly important to be able to examine the corners at the vault of the vagina in patients who have undergone hysterectomy.

Previous radiotherapy may lead to abnormal cells on cytology and work-up to evaluation of such women may be difficult due to severe radiation changes in the vagina including vaginitis and stenosis.

Pre-treatment Assessment

Once a diagnosis has been made the principle aim must be to determine the extent of spread of the tumor, both local and distant, from the history, physical examination and special investigations. Local examination often needs to be performed under general anesthetic because of patient discomfort or inaccessibility of the vagina. Ideally the examination should be carried out jointly by radiation and gynecologic oncologists and should include examination of the lower genital tract and groins for nodal enlargement. Vaginoscopy will allow assessment of possible adjacent VaIN, vulvar intraepithelial neoplasia (VIN) or cervical intraepithial neoplasia (CIN). Severe atrophic changes in the vagina will make assessment very difficult and a course of estrogen cream may be helpful.

All patients require a chest radiograph. Cystoscopy, sigmoidoscopy and MRI/CT scan of the abdomen and pelvis may be performed to assess local spread as well as paraaortic, pelvic and inguinal lymph node enlargement, which may require further evaluation.

Treatment

Treatment of vaginal carcinoma is best planned with cooperation between radiation and gynecologic oncologists and depends on the stage of disease (*Table 8.1*).

Radiation therapy

Radiation therapy is the most widely used treatment modality for all stages of disease. It can potentially spare the patient major destructive surgery, but may have significant complications. The general principles are to give an adequate tumoricidal dose to the primary site and the major sites of spread in the pelvis and groins.

Small Stage I lesions ($\leqslant$2 cm) are treated using a vaginal cylinder or an interstitial implant. Because of the inverse square law vaginal cylinders can deliver only a low dose to submucosal tissues beneath the

Table 8.1. Vaginal carcinoma: management for primary disease by stage.

Stage	*Radiation therapy**	*Surgery***
I		
Lesion <2 cm No LVS, grade ≤2	Intracavitary/interstitial implant	Depth of invasion <3 mm: wide excision/vaginectomy
Lesion >2 cm or <2 cm with LVS, grade 3	Intracavitary/interstitial implant External beam to vagina, pelvis	Radical vaginectomy/hysterectomy Pelvic and paraaortic node dissection (NB Difficult to differentiate Stage I and II)
Lesion in lower one-third vagina and suspicious or positive groin nodes	Include external beam to groins	Include radical vulvectomy/groin node dissection
II and III		
Lesion in upper two-thirds of vagina	Intracavitary/interstitial implant External beam to pelvis, vagina	Lesion at vault and no or early parametrial involvement. Radical vaginectomy/hysterectomy, pelvic and paraaortic node dissection Lesion adjacent to bladder/rectum and no or early parametrial involvement. Anterior, posterior or total exenteration
Lesion in lower one-third vagina and suspicious or positive groin nodes	Include external beam to groins	Include radical vulvectomy/groin node dissection
IV	Intracavitary/interstitial implant External beam to pelvis, vagina, groins plus chemotherapy	Lesion involves bladder or rectum without distant spread or pelvic sidewall involvement. Anterior, posterior or total exenteration

*Radiation also indicated for poor prognostic features following surgery (i.e. positive nodes, close or involved margins). Radiation for more advanced disease may be given in conjunction with radiosensitizers such as cisplatin and 5-fluorouracil.
**The role of surgery in the management of vaginal carcinoma is limited. Vaginal reconstruction should be considered when vaginectomy is performed. Exenterative surgery has a role in the treatment of radiation failures.
LVS, lymph vascular space involvement.

tumor whereas interstitial implants allow higher doses. A dose of 6000–7000 cGy to the whole vaginal mucosa inclusive of the tumor bed is required. Stage I lesions >2 cm or those with adverse features such as poor grade or lymph–vascular space invasion require external beam therapy to control disease spread to the paracolpium and whole pelvis (4000–5000 cGy) in addition to treatment of the primary site using brachytherapy. Where tumor involves the upper vagina and the uterus is present it may be possible to use a uterine tandem and vaginal ovoids as for cervical cancer. External beam therapy should include the entire vagina down to the introitus, and pelvic lymph nodes to the level of the upper common iliac chain (*Figure 8.1*).

With Stage IIA lesions that do not have extensive paravaginal/parametrial infiltration, Perez (1992) uses interstitial and intracavitary only to 4500–5500 cGy at 0.5 cm beyond the deep margin of the tumor. For Stages IIB, III and IV, external beam 4000 cGy is given to the whole pelvis, with an additional 1500 cGy parametrial boost by midline shielding of the bladder and rectum. Interstitial (*Figure 8.2*) and intracavitary brachytherapy deliver total doses of 7500 cGy to the tumor and 6500 cGy to the parametrium and paracolpium (Perez, 1992). The groins are irradiated to 5000 cGy in patients with disease affecting the lower one-third of the vagina and those with suspicious or positive nodes.

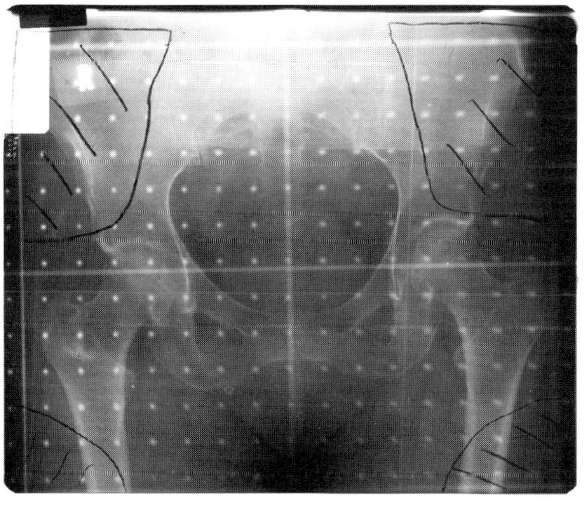

Figure 8.1. Treatment planning radiograph for patient with carcinoma of the vagina. The hatched areas represent areas blocked out. (Courtesy of Dr Glenda Smith, Radiation Oncology, Temple University Hospital, Philadelphia PA.)

In advanced disease radiosensitizers such as cisplatin, carboplatin, 5-fluorouracil (5-FU) and

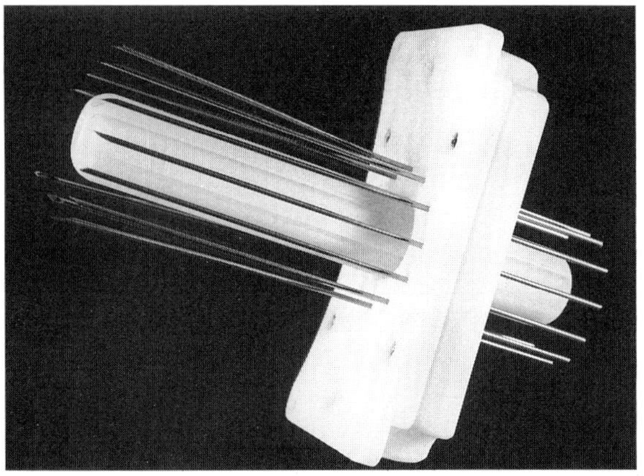

Figure 8.2. Syed–Neblett applicator for interstitial radiation delivery. (Courtesy of Dr Glenda Smith, Radiation Oncology, Temple University Hospital, Philadelphia PA.)

hydroxyurea may be used to enhance the tumoricidal effects of the radiation.

Radiotherapy may also be given following surgery in circumstances where there is a high chance of recurrence, typically for positive lymph nodes or close margins. It also has a role in the palliation of advanced disease.

When there is tumor at the vaginal vault following a previous hysterectomy a laparotomy will allow adherent bowel to be freed and positioning of interstitial needle implants to be made under direct vision. An omental flap may be fashioned and brought down onto the vault to reduce the potential for radiotherapy damage to adjacent structures. In addition, when the tumor involves the lower vagina the inguinal nodes may be dissected before radiation whether or not they are clinically involved.

Complications of radiotherapy

Serious side-effects are reported in approximately 5% of patients treated for Stage I and 15% treated for Stage II (Perez *et al.*, 1988) and are particularly devastating to young women. Acute problems including desquamation of groin and vulvar skin, vaginitis, dysuria and proctitis are common, but generally short-lived. More serious later problems include rectovaginal and enterocutaneous fistula, rectal ulceration and stricture, and small bowel obstruction. Bladder problems include vesicovaginal fistula, bladder neck contracture and urethral stricture, which may lead to permanent and debilitating problems with micturition (Perez *et al.*, 1988). The vagina may become stenosed and ulcerated and this may be prevented by the use of vaginal dilators.

Surgery

The role of surgery is very limited because local anatomy mandates that to be curative surgery has to be radical for all but a select group of early lesions. It is often impossible to determine the exact extent of disease before surgery (particularly Stage I confined to the mucosa from Stage II with submucosal infiltration), and this, together with the rich submucosal network of lymphatics and the proximity of the bowel and bladder, makes it easy to perform less than optimal 'conservative' surgery.

Lesions early enough to be treated solely by wide local excision (including partial or total vaginectomy) are often found incidentally after excision of lesions containing VaIN. Such conservative surgery may be sufficient for lesions with a depth of invasion <3 mm from the surface without lymph–vascular space invasion or confluence (Peters *et al.*, 1985b; Eddy *et al.*, 1990; Hoffman *et al.*, 1992; Morley and Peters, 1992). However, such cases have been known to recur.

Adequate surgical treatment of most cases of Stage I disease requires a radical excision of all or part of the vagina and paracolpium. Lesions in the upper two-thirds of the vagina require radical vaginectomy and bilateral pelvic node dissection. If the uterus is still present then dissection of the ureters mandates that a radical hysterectomy is performed. If the patient has previously undergone a hysterectomy, radical vaginectomy is technically more difficult. The incidence of pelvic lymph node involvement in Stage I disease is 6–14%, and in Stage II, 26–32% (Al-Kurdi and Monaghan, 1981; Davis *et al.*, 1991). Paraaortic node dissection may be considered in the case of large tumors.

Lesions in the lower one-third of the vagina need more extensive surgery. In addition to radical excision of the vagina and pelvic lymphadenectomy they require a modified radical vulvectomy and bilateral inguinal node dissection. Al-Kurdi and Monaghan (1981) reported that 38% of patients with carcinoma Stage I, II and IV involving the lower one-third of the vagina had positive inguinal nodes. Of 13 patients with lesions in the lower vagina, three (23%) had positive pelvic nodes and negative inguinal nodes.

Radical surgery as for Stage I disease is an option for early Stage II disease particularly in a young patient without parametrial involvement where the tumor is at the vaginal vault. Where the tumor lies close to the bladder or rectum or actually involves these structures, but where there is not extensive parametrial involvement, a primary exenteration alone may be curative.

Vaginal reconstruction will be necessary in young patients using one of several techniques including gracilis or rectus abdominis myocutaneous flaps, sigmoid colon interposition or by split-thickness

Table 8.2. Carcinoma of the vagina: survival[1] for Stages I and II.

				Stage I			Stage II			
Authors	*Year*	*Years of accrual*	*Histology*[2]	*No.*	*Treatment*	*Survival (%)*	*No.*	*Treatment*	*Survival (%)*	*Follow-up details*
Al-Kurdi *et al.*	1981	1947–1979	Mixed	14	R,S,C	71				5 yrs min. (5–32 yrs)
Ball & Berman	1982	1947–1978	Mixed	27	R8S19	76	17	R957C1	37	1 yr min. 80% 5 yrs
Perez & Camel	1982	1950–1977	Mixed	39	R	90	60	R	IIa 58 IIb 38	3 yrs min.
Prempree *et al.*	1982	1957–1970	Mixed				31	R	65	5 yrs min.
Benedet *et al.*	1983	1950–1980	Mixed	32	R,S	75	31	R,S	68	2 yrs min.
Puthawala *et al.*	1983	1976–1979	Mixed				16	R	75	40 months min. (40–84 months)
Rubin *et al.*	1985	1958–1980	SCC	14	R7S5C2	78	29	R21S3C5	52	3 yrs min.
MacNaught *et al.*	1986	1962–1982	SCC	14	R	68	22	R	34	*
Gallup *et al.*	1987	1971–1984	SCC				12	R11S1	75	2 yrs
Manetta *et al.*	1988	1976–1986	Mixed				15	R	60	2 yrs min. (26–126 months)
Andersen	1989	1976–1985	Mixed	12	R10S2	58				*
Manetta *et al.*	1990	1976–1988	Mixed	15	R9S6	87	17	R15S1C1	70	2 yrs min. (24–153 months)
Davis *et al.*	1991	1960–1987	Mixed	44	R14S25C5	88	45	R9S27C9	53	Median 4.4 yrs SI; 3.2 yrs SII
Eddy *et al.*	1991	1970–1989	Mixed	25	R10S5C10	73	39	R26S2C8[3]	39	<2 yrs min.
Kucera & Vavra	1991	1952–1984	Mixed	73	R	77	110	R	45	5 yrs min.

[1]Detail from studies with ⩾10 cases in any one stage.
[2]Mixed is generally squamous cell and adenocarcinomas +/− clear-cell adenocarcinoma.
[3]One patient had chemotherapy alone and two had no treatment.
*Information not given.
(R, radiotherapy; S, surgery; C, surgery and radiotherapy. Given with numbers if stated.)

Table 8.3. Carcinoma of the vagina: survival[1] for Stages III and IV.

				Stage III			Stage IV			
Authors	*Year*	*Years of accrual*	*Histology*	*No.*	*Treatment*	*Survival (%)*	*No.*	*Treatment*	*Survival (%)*	*Follow-up*
Al-Kurdi *et al.*	1981	1947–1979	Mixed				9	R2S7	22	5 yrs min. (5–32 yrs)
Perez & Camel	1982	1950–1977	Mixed	12	R	40	8	R	0	3 yrs min.
Prempree *et al.*	1982	1957–1970	Mixed	20	R	40				5 yrs min.
Benedet *et al.*	1983	1950–1980	Mixed	12	R,S	42	14	R,S	21	2 yrs min.
Rubin *et al.*	1985	1958–1980	SCC	13	R11S2	54	9	R8S1	0	3 yrs min.
MacNaught *et al.*	1986	1962–1982	SCC	18	R	29	7	R	14	*
Gallup *et al.*	1987	1971–1984	SCC				6	R3S3	17	2 yrs
Manetta *et al.*	1990	1976–1988	Mixed				6	R5S1	17	2 yrs min. (24–153 months)
Eddy *et al.*	1991	1970–1989	Mixed	15	R	38	11	R5S1C5	25	<2 yrs min.
Kucera & Vavra	1991	1952–1984	Mixed	174	R	31	77	R	18	5 yrs min.

[1]Stage III data from series with ⩾10 patients, stage IV with series ⩾5 patients.
[2]Mixed is generally squamous cell and adenocarcinomas +/− clear-cell adenocarcinoma.
*Information not given.
(R, radiotherapy; S, surgery; C, surgery and radiotherapy. Given with numbers if stated.)

skin graft. Such patients will require extensive preoperative counselling and follow-up.

Patients developing carcinoma in the vagina following previous radiation treatment for carcinoma of cervix pose a real problem and surgery may be the only option.

Complications of surgery

The complications of surgery include the major complications of radical hysterectomy and surgery on the vulva and groins. The major specific problems with regard to vaginectomy are urinary and rectal fistula, and chronic bladder and rectal dysfunction. Radical vaginal surgery may cause major alterations in body image perception and severe physical and psychosexual problems.

Chemotherapy

The encouraging response of SCC of the anus and vulva to chemotherapy agents (Nigro *et al.*, 1974; Levin *et al.*, 1986), has stimulated the use of chemotherapeutic agents given with radiotherapy before surgery. 5-FU and cisplatin are the most popular, but mitomycin C has also been used (Thomas *et al.*, 1989).

Survival after Treatment

Results of treatment are given in *Tables 8.2 and 8.3.* Most studies report the results of mainly radiotherapy treatment and include the results for adenocarcinoma and SCC together. For Stage IVA there are long-term survivors (32–50%) whereas survivors of Stage IVB are negligible (Eddy *et al.*, 1991; Kucera and Vavra, 1991).

Recurrence

Recurrent disease is common following radiotherapy and is difficult to treat (Perez *et al.*, 1988). Localized recurrence in the central pelvis may be suitable for exenteration.

Adenocarcinoma

Adenocarcinoma of the vagina is much rarer than SCC and no series contain more than a handful of cases other than those focusing on clear-cell adenocarcinoma.

Definitive data on the relative survival in relation to SCC are not available. Some investigators report a worse outcome for SCC (Al–Kurdi and Monaghan, 1981), while others report no significant difference (Davis *et al.*, 1991; Eddy *et al.*, 1991). In general, adenocarcinoma is treated in the same way as SCC.

Clear-cell Adenocarcinoma

An association between clear-cell carcinoma of the vagina (CCCA) and exposure to diethylstilbestrol (DES) *in utero* was reported by Herbst *et al.* (1971). Over 500 cases of clear-cell carcinoma of vagina and cervix have been registered, 25% having no history of exposure to DES.

The risk of cancer developing in females exposed to DES *in utero* is estimated at 1:1000 up to 35 years of age (Melnick *et al.*, 1987) and is highest if the hormone was taken before 12 weeks' gestation (Herbst *et al.*, 1986); 91% occur between the ages of 15–27 (median age 19 years) (Melnick *et al.*, 1987). It most commonly arises on the anterior wall of the upper vagina. At diagnosis 59% are Stage I, 33% Stage II, 7% Stage III and 1% Stage IV (Herbst *et al.*, 1979).

Surgical treatment has been commonly used because the young age of the patients heightens the need to preserve sexual function. It has included radical hysterectomy with pelvic lymph node dissection and partial or complete vaginectomy and vaginal reconstruction. Local excision in the form of vaginectomy or wide excision is associated with a higher recurrence rate (Senekjian *et al.*, 1987). Radiotherapy is usually given for patients with adverse prognostic features following surgery and for advanced disease.

Prognostic factors include the size of the tumor, the depth of invasion, lymph node metastasis and close resection margins (Robboy *et al.*, 1974). Patients with the tubulocystic subtype do better and those aged 19 and over do significantly better than those under 15 years of age (Herbst *et al.*, 1979). Stage I survival in clear cell carcinoma of the vagina is over 90% (Senekjian *et al.*, 1987). Stage II survival is 76%, Stage III 30%, and Stage IV 0% (Herbst *et al.*, 1979).

Clear-cell carcinoma has a greater tendency to recur late and develop metastases in distant sites more frequently than SCC (Robboy *et al.*, 1974; Herbst *et al.*, 1979), particularly the lungs and supraclavicular nodes.

Summary of Management Options

- Stage I lesions <2 cm in dimension with no lymph–vascular space involvement and grade 1–2 may be treated with brachytherapy alone or wide local excision provided the depth of invasion is <3 mm.
- Other cases of cancer of the vagina require external beam therapy to the vagina, paracolpium and pelvis in addition to brachytherapy. Cases involving the lower one-third of the vagina or with suspicious or positive groin nodes require the addition of external beam therapy to the groins.
- In more advanced disease chemotherapy should be considered with radiation therapy.
- Radiation is indicated post-surgery when poor prognostic features such as positive nodes are present or where there are close/involved margins.
- Radical surgery may be considered for primary treatment for lesions other than in paragraph 1. Stage I and II small lesions involving only the vault of the vagina with no or early parametrial involvement may be treated with radical vaginectomy/hysterectomy and pelvic and paraaortic node dissection. For lesions which lie adjacent to the bladder or rectum, radiation therapy should be considered; however, some may require exenteration. Where the lower one-third of the vagina is involved or there are suspicious or positive groin nodes then radical vulvectomy and groin node dissection may be considered.
- Local recurrence in the vagina or central pelvis following radiotherapy may be treated by exenteration.

References

Al-Kurdi M & Monaghan JM (1981) Thirty-two years experience in management of primary tumours of the vagina. *Brit. J. Obstet. Gynaecol.* **88:** 1145–1150.

Andersen ES (1989) Primary carcinoma of the vagina: A study of 29 cases. *Gynecol. Oncol.* **33:** 317–320.

Ball HG & Berman ML (1982) Management of primary vaginal carcinoma. *Gynecol. Oncol.* **14:** 154–163.

Benedet JL, Murphy KJ, Fairey RN & Boyes DA (1983) Primary invasive carcinoma of the vagina. *Obstet. Gynecol.* **62:** 715–719.

Benedet JL & Sanders BH (1984) Carcinoma *in situ* of the vagina. *Am. J. Obstet. Gynecol.* **148:** 695–700.

Brinton LA, Nasca PC, Mallin K *et al.* (1990) Case-control study of *in situ* and invasive carcinoma of the vagina. *Gynecol. Oncol.* **38:** 49–54.

Cramer D & Cutler S (1974) Incidence and histopathology of malignancies of the female genital organs in the United States. *Am. J. Obstet. Gynecol.* **118:** 443–460.

Davis KP, Stanhope CR, Garton GR *et al.* (1991) Invasive vaginal carcinoma: analysis of early-stage disease. *Gynecol. Oncol.* **42:** 131–136.

Eddy GL, Marks RD, Miller MC & Underwood PB (1991) Primary invasive vaginal carcinoma. *Am. J. Obstet. Gynecol.* **165:** 292–298.

Eddy GL, Singh KP & Gansler TS (1990) Superficially invasive carcinoma of the vagina following treatment for cervical carcinoma: a report of 6 cases. *Gynecol. Oncol.* **36:** 376–379.

FIGO (1989) Carcinoma of the vagina. In: Petterson F (ed.) *Annual Reports on the Results of Treatment in Gynecological Cancer*, vol. 20, p. 175. Stockholm: FIGO.

Gallup DG & Morley G (1975) Carcinoma *in situ* of the vagina. *Obstet. Gynecol.* **46:** 334–340.

Gallup DG, Talledo OE, Shah KJ & Hayes C (1987) Invasive squamous cell carcinoma of the vagina. *Obstet. Gynecol.* **69:** 782–785.

Geelhoed GW, Henson DE, Taylor PT & Ketcham AS (1976) Carcinoma *in-situ* of the vagina following treatment for carcinoma of the cervix: A distinctive clinical entity. *Am. J. Obstet. Gynecol.* **124:** 510–516.

Graham JB & Meigs JV (1962) Recurrence of tumor after total hysterectomy for carcinoma *in situ*. *Am. J. Obstet. Gynecol.* **64:** 1159–1162.

Herbst AL, Anderson S, Hubby MM *et al.* (1986) Risk factors for the development of diethylstilbestrol-associated clear cell adenocarcinoma: A case-control study. *Am. J. Obstet. Gynecol.* **154:** 814–822.

Herbst AL, Green TH & Ulfelder H (1970) Primary carcinoma of the vagina. *Am. J. Obstet. Gynecol.* **106:** 210–218.

Herbst AL, Ulfelder H & Poskanzer DC (1971) Aderocarcinoma of the vagina. *New Eng. J. Med.* **204:** 878–881.

■ Herbst AL, Norusis MJ, Rosenow PJ *et al.* (1979) An analysis of 346 cases of clear cell adenocarcinoma of the vagina and cervix with emphasis on recurrence and survival. *Gynecol. Oncol.* **7:** 111–122.

Herman JM, Homesley HD & Dignan MB (1986) Is hysterectomy a risk factor for vaginal cancer? *JAMA* **256:** 601–603.

Hernandez-Linares W, Puthawala A & Nolan JF (1980) Carcinoma in situ of the vagina: past and present managment. *Obstet. Gynecol.* **56:** 356–360.

■ Hoffman MS, DeCesare SL, Roberts WS *et al.* (1992) Upper vaginectomy for *in situ* and occult, superficially invasive carcinoma of the vagina. *Am. J. Obstet. Gynecol.* **166:** 30–33.

Hoffman MS, Roberts WS, LaPolla JP *et al.* (1991) Laser vaporization of grade 3 vaginal intra-epithelial neoplasia. *Am. J. Obstet. Gynecol.* **165:** 1342–1344.

Hummer WK, Mussey E, Decker DG & Dockerty MB (1970) Carcinoma *in situ* of the vagina. *Am. J. Obstet. Gynecol.* **108:** 1109–1116.

Ireland D & Monaghan JM (1988) The management of the patient with abnormal vaginal cytology following hysterectomy. *Brit. J. Obstet. Gynaecol.* **95:** 973–975.

Kanbour AI, Klionsky B & Murphy AI (1974) Carcinoma of the vagina following cervical cancer. *Cancer* **34:** 1838–1841.

■ Kucera H & Vavra N (1991) Radiation management of primary carcinoma of the vagina: clinical and histopathological variables associated with survival. *Gynecol. Oncol.* **40:** 12–16.

Lee RA & Symmonds RE (1976) Recurrent carcinoma *in situ* of the vagina in patients previously treated for *in situ* carcinoma of the cervix. *Obstet. Gynecol.* **48:** 61–64.

Levin W, Goldberg G, Altaras M *et al.* (1986) The use of concomitant chemotherapy and radiotherapy prior to surgery in advanced stage carcinoma of the vulva. *Gynecol. Oncol.* **25:** 20–25.

Macnaught R, Symonds RP, Hole D & Watson ER (1986) Improved control of primary vaginal tumours by combined external beam and interstitial radiotherapy. *Clin. Radiol.* **37:** 29–32.

Manetta A, Gutrecht EL & Berman ML (1990) Primary invasive carcinoma of the vagina. *Obstet. Gynecol.* **76:** 639–642.

Manetta A, Pinto JL, Larson JE *et al.* (1988) Primary invasive carcinoma of the vagina. *Obstet. Gynecol.* **72:** 77–81.

Melnick S, Cole P, Anderson D & Herbst AL (1987) Rates and risks of diethylstilbestrol-related clear cell adenocarcinoma of the vagina and cervix. *N. Eng. J. Med.* **316:** 514–516.

Morley GW and Peters WA (1992) Microinvasive carcinoma of the vagina. In: Coppleson M (ed.) *Gynecologic Oncology,* pp. 501–504. New York: Churchill Livingstone.

Nigro ND, Vaitkevicius VK & Considine B (1974) Combined therapy for cancer of the anal canal: a preliminary report. *Dis. Col. Rect.* **17:** 354–356.

Perez CA (1992) Vagina. In: Perez CA & Brady LW (eds) *Principles and Practice of Radiation Oncology,* pp. 1258–1272. Philadelphia: J.P. Lippincott.

Perez CA & Camel HM (1982) Long term follow-up in radiation therapy of carcinoma of the vagina. *Cancer* **49:** 1308–1315.

■ Perez CA, Camel HM & Galakatos AE (1988) Definitive irradiation in carcinoma of the vagina: long-term evaluation of results. *Int. J. Radiat. Oncol. Biol. Phys.* **15:** 1283–1290.

Peters WA, Kumar NB & Morley GW (1985a) Carcinoma of the vagina. Factors influencing treatment outcome. *Cancer* **55:** 892–897.

■ Peters WA, Kumar NB & Morley GW (1985b) Microinvasive carcinoma of the vagina: A distinct clinical entity? *Am. J. Obstet. Gynecol.* **153:** 505–507.

Pettersson F (1989) Carcinoma of the vagina *Annual Report on The Results of Treatment in Gynecological Cancer.* **20:** 174.

■ Plentl AA & Friedman EA (1971) *Lymphatic System of the Female Genitalia,* pp. 51–55. Philadelphia: Saunders.

Prempree T, Viravathana T, Slawson RG *et al.* (1982) Role of radiation therapy in the management of primary carcinoma of the vagina. *Acta Radiat. Oncol.* **21:** 195–201.

Pride GC & Buchler DA (1977) Carcinoma of the vagina 10 or more years following pelvic irradiation therapy. *Am. J. Obstet. Gynecol.* **127:** 513–517.

Puthawala A, Syed AMN, Nalick R *et al.* (1983) Integrated external and interstitial radiation therapy for primary carcinoma of the vagina. *Obstet. Gynecol.* **62:** 367–372.

Robboy SJ, Herbst AL & Scully RE (1974) Clear cell adenocarcinoma of the vagina and cervix in young females: Analysis of 37 tumors that persisted or recurred after primary therapy. *Cancer* **34:** 606–614.

Rubin SC, Young J & Mikuta JJ (1985) Squamous carcinoma of the vagina. *Gynecol. Oncol.* **20:** 346–353.

Rutledge F (1967) Cancer of the vagina. *Obstet. Gynecol.* **97:** 635–655.

Scokel PW, Collier RC, Jones WN *et al.* (1961) Relation of carcinoma *in situ* of the vagina to the early diagnosis of vaginal cancer. *Am. J. Obstet. Gynecol.* **82:** 397–400.

Senekjian EK, Frey KW, Anderson D & Herbst AL (1987) Local therapy in Stage 1 clear cell adenocarcinoma of the vagina. *Cancer* **60:** 1319–1324.

Thomas G, Dembo A & DePetrillo A (1989) Concurrent radiation and chemotherapy in vulvar carcinoma. *Gynecol. Oncol.* **34:** 263–267.

Way S (1948) Primary carcinoma of the vagina. *J. Obstet. Gynecol. Br. Emp.* **LV:** 739–745.

Woodman CBJ & Jordan JA (1984) The management of vaginal intraepithelial neoplasia after hysterectomy. *Br. J. Obstet. Gynaecol.* **91:** 707–711.

9 The Etiology and Epidemiology of Uterine Tumors

W J Mann

Introduction

The most common malignancy of the uterine corpus is endometrioid adenocarcinoma, accounting for nearly 80% of all cancers reported. Frequently microscopic examination reveals areas of squamous epithelium, and if this comprises at least 10% of the tumor, the malignancy may be designated adenosquamous carcinoma, or adenocarcinoma with squamous elements. Considerable attention and time may be spent on grading the squamous component, or debating whether it is benign or malignant, but the grade of the glandular component and histologic evidence of myometrial invasion or extrauterine spread are probably of more prognostic importance. Recently a serous papillary adenocarcinoma variant has been described that may appear structurally deceptively well differentiated, but that has marked cellular atypia and acts very aggressively. This is clearly separated from papillary, well-differentiated endometrioid carcinoma. Other rare tumor types include mucinous and clear cell adenocarcinoma, pure squamous carcinoma, undifferentiated carcinoma and other bizarre cell types, represented by case reports. These uncommon malignancies may carry a worse prognosis and possibly occur in older patients, but their infrequency makes efforts at understanding their etiology or epidemiology fruitless at this time. Consequently our discussion will focus on endometrioid adenocarcinoma.

Premalignant Precursor Lesion

Historically, descriptions of endometrial carcinoma were accompanied by the recognition of lesions felt to precede or develop into cancer. These associated endometrial lesions appeared to constitute a premalignant phase of this disease, more recently suggested to be analogous to the relationship of cervical intraepithelial neoplasia (CIN) to invasive cervical cancer. It has even been suggested that they should be referred to as EIN, endometrial intraepithelial neoplasia. Traditionally, cystic or 'Swiss cheese' hyperplasia was felt to precede adenomatous hyperplasia, which when accompanied by atypia of glandular cells, becomes atypical adenomatous hyperplasia. This could progress to carcinoma *in situ* and ultimately endometrial carcinoma. In theory, the further along the progression the lesion, the more likely it would develop into cancer. So-called cystic hyperplasia progresses to cancer over 2–15 years in 1–10% of patients (Kurman *et al.*, 1985). In women with adenomatous hyperplasia, cancer develops in 1–14 years in 12–22% of patients (Kurman *et al.*, 1985). When structural abnormalities of glands are combined with epithelial atypia, 29–100% develop cancer over 1–5 years (Kurman *et al.*, 1985). However, considerable difference exists in the definitions of these precursor lesions, so understandably the rate of progression according to different authors varies from 1–100%. In addition, some studies include patients with previous radiation to the uterus, which confuses the picture further. The evidence lending credibility to the premalignant nature of these hyperplastic endometria is threefold:

- a review of prior curettings in patients who subsequently develop carcinoma reveals previous hyperplasia (Petterson *et al.*, 1985);
- uteri containing cancer simultaneously contain the hyperplasia (Ritzmann and Hillemanns, 1977),
- histologically the hyperplasias resemble the cancer.

To a clinician, these precursor lesions are important in that those associated with a low risk of progression afford time for hormonal or other therapy, while those with a high likelihood of progression or of possible confusion with actual invasive carcinoma are best handled by extirpative surgery. However, hormonal therapy can reverse endometrial pathology, but will not remove the underlying cause. The target end organ (the endometrium) has been protected, but the endogenous source of the carcinogenic change has not been removed or neutralized, and will persist. Therefore, if therapy is stopped, endometrial lesions may recur and progress. This author's personal bias, based on clinical experience and a review of the literature on hyperplasias and neoplastic progression, is that only complex hyperplasia (that is gland structural abnormality and an increased number of glands relative to stroma, in association with marked cellular atypicality of the epithelium) has a significant risk of progressing to or being associated with invasive carcinoma (*Figures 9.1 and 9.2*). Silverberg (1988) in a detailed and thoughtful review of endometrial changes suggests that the differences in the results of retrospective studies of hyerplasias are not easily resolved and only close communication between the gynecologist and pathologist can lead to a meaningful pathologic diagnosis that will aid clinical management. He also, more importantly, emphasizes that all the information relative to the hyperplasias and their natural history probably bears on a minority of patients with endometrial cancer. While some authors might argue that these lesions account for a majority of any given clinical series, a more thoughtful assessment is that while some endometrial cancers can clearly be placed in the context of representing one end of the spectrum of progressive endometrial abnormalities, other carcinomas clearly do not fit into this neat conceptual framework.

For example, Koss *et al.* (1984) sampled the endometrium of 2586 asymptomatic women and found 6.9 occult cancers per 1000 women. He did

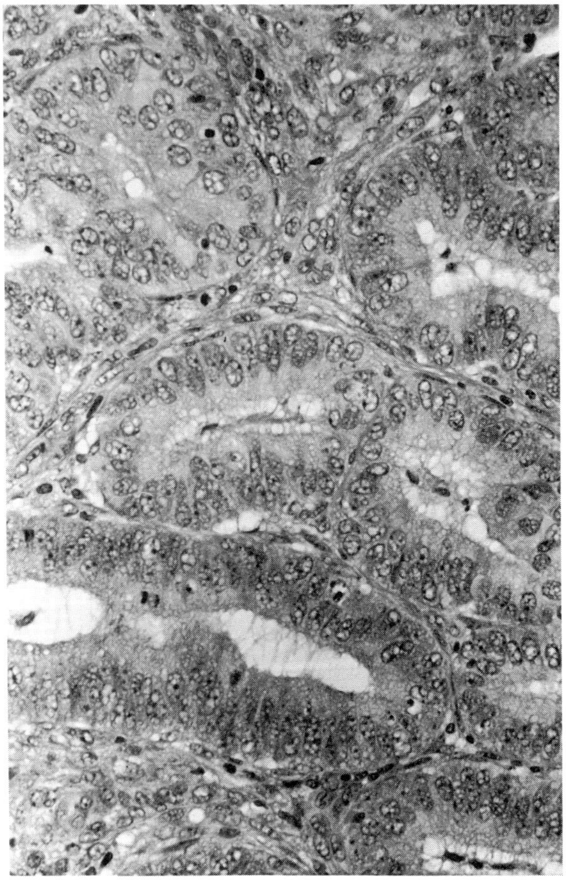

Figure 9.1. Atypical hyperplasia.

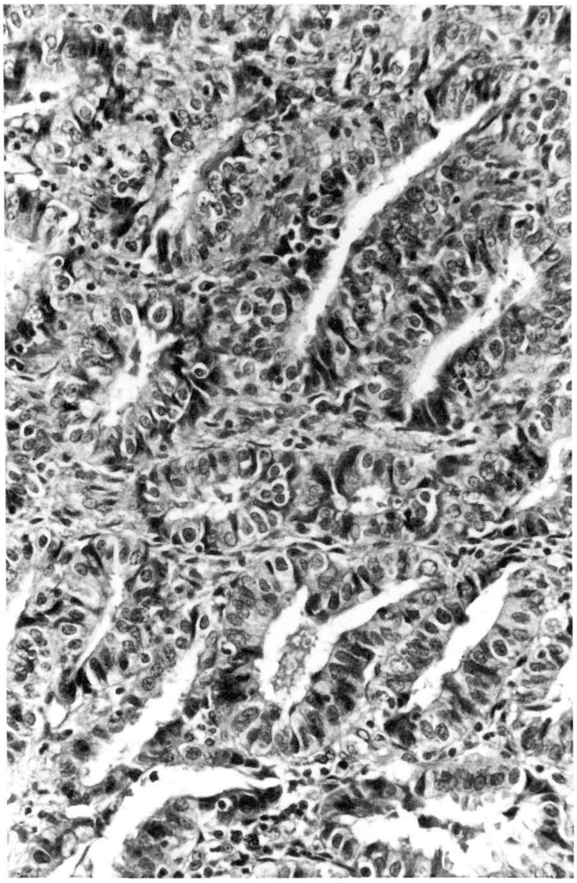

Figure 9.2. Well-differentiated carcinoma. Histologic examination of atypical hyperplasia (see *Figure 9.1*) and well-differentiated carcinoma shows similarities.

not find hyperplasia to be more frequent, as you would expect of a precursor, nor did he find it concurrently. There seems to be a clear dichotomy in endometrial cancers – the one group being well-differentiated adenocarcinoma, resulting from a gradual endometrial degeneration from atypical complex hyerplasia and having a generally good prognosis, and the other, perhaps arising without a recognizable precursor, being moderate to poorly differentiated with a more aggressive nature and a poorer prognosis.

Recognition of these two subsets of patients is important to any discussion of etiologic factors since nearly all studies focus on the well-differentiated lesions, often emphasizing the similarities between these patients with 'favorable' cancers and those with hyperplasia.

Age Distribution

Endometrial adenocarcinoma is predominantly a disease of elderly postmenopausal woman, occurring most frequently in those aged 55–65 years. However, it has been reported in a 10-year-old girl, with larger series usually reporting 20–25% of patients as premenopausal and 2–5% under the age of 40 (Kjellgren, 1979; Gallagher and Elwood, 1982). It is of interest to note that this age distribution differs minimally for large series from Japan, Sweden, British Columbia, Canada, Australia, Britain and the USA. As modern society ages and life expectancy gradually increases, more women will be at risk. However, at extreme old age (over 80–85 years), there appears to be a declining incidence (Bond, 1986).

Incidence and Mortality

The incidence of endometrial carcinoma varies from one nation to another, with the highest being in the USA (45.8/100,000) and the Federal Republic of Germany (33.8/100,000), and the lowest in India (1.8/100,000) and Japan (1.7) (Mahboubi *et al.*, 1982). There appears, at least in the USA, to be a higher incidence in white females (45.8/100,000) than in blacks (19.3/100,000). However, the accuracy of such figures is somewhat in question due to concern over misdiagnosis of hyperplasia, failure to correct for the proportion of females who have no uterus, and inaccuracies in data collection (i.e. separating out cervical cancer and uterine sarcomas).

Another concern over assessing the incidence of endometrial cancer is that there may be significant changes over 5–7 years noted in some nations, but not in others. In addition, these changes are not unidirectional and may only affect certain subgroups of a population or certain age ranges within a subgroup. This will be discussed in more detail when the data relating to exogenous estrogen therapy are presented.

Among gynecologic malignancies, endometrial carcinoma is more common than cervical or ovarian carcinoma. Relative to cancer of the cervix, this reflects an apparent decrease in cases of invasive cervical disease as well as an actual increase in endometrial cancer (Cramer *et al.*, 1974; Dunn, 1974). The American Cancer Society predicts 15,800 new cases of cervical cancer in 1995 compared to 32,800 endometrial cancers and 26,600 ovarian cancers. In that same year, 4800 deaths are expected due to cervical cancer, 14,500 due to ovarian cancer and 5900 due to endometrial cancer (Wingo *et al.*, 1995). Some authors (Gallagher and Elwood, 1982; King *et al.*, 1982), but not all (Lyon and Gardner, 1977), who do note an increased incidence of endometrial cancer do not detect a parallel increase in mortality. A review of these cases revealed a number of misdiagnosed hyperplasias, but still indicated an increase in cancers. The failure to see an increase in mortality probably reflects earlier diagnosis of well-differentiated Stage I International Federation of Gynecology and Obstetrics (FIGO) disease, which has a favorable prognosis. But one must also recognize that listed causes of death are notoriously inaccurate and that elderly cancer patients are likely to succumb to concurrent cardiovascular disease.

Risk Factors for Endometrial Cancer

Reviews from institutions testing large numbers of patients with endometrial cancer have identified several clinical characteristics of these women. These stigmata are prevalent in patients with the precursor hyperplasias, adding further credence to viewing these lesions as prodromal (Garnett, 1958).

Obesity

When compared with healthy gynecologic patients, patients with cervical cancer, or ideal weight charts, 20–75% of women with endometrial cancer are found to be overweight or obese (Jensen, 1985). The variation depends on whether the patients are considered overweight based on an excess above predicted ideal weight or above an arbitrary weight. Kjellergren (1977) found that endometrial cancer patients tended to be overweight when younger compared to controls and to have an increasing risk of cancer as their weight increased. If 21–50 pounds overweight, they had three times the risk of their counterpart controls. Banders–van Halewijn and Poortman (1982) found a stepwise increased risk with every 10 kg over 60 kg, rising to a risk of 5.8 if over 98 kg. Wynder *et al.* (1966) also found greater risk associated with obesity, and, with others, noted that taller patients seemed to have an enhanced risk (Jensen, 1986; Tretle and Magnus, 1990). Brinton *et al.* (1992) found weight but not height was associated with increased risk.

Blitzer *et al.* (1976) reviewed historical data on 56,111 females with obesity and found that there was no excess of malignancies over the general population with the single exception of endometrial cancer. Obese women had an increased relative risk of 1.6 over controls (*Figure 9.3*). Shapira *et al.* (1991) found that the increased risk of obesity was associated with upper body fat localization.

Fox and Sen (1970) found no association between endometrial cancer and obesity in their 300 cases, and Koss *et al.* (1984) also found none in his screening of 2586 asymptomatic patients. These two studies stand out because there are so many which do link obesity to endometrial cancer. However, it must be recognized that 30–80% of patients with endometrial cancer are not obese, and the percentage of obese patients who develop this cancer is quite small.

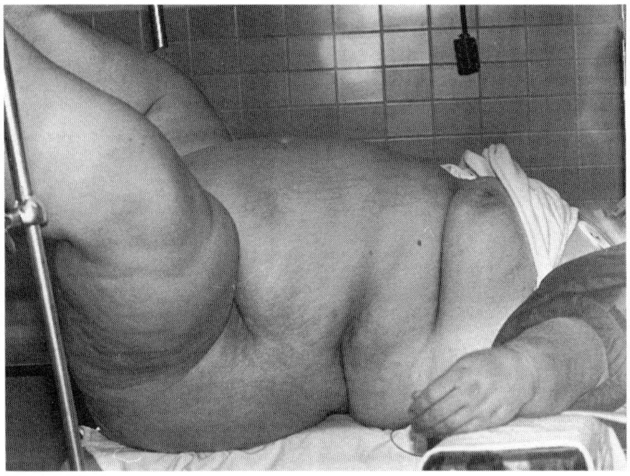

Figure 9.3. Typical obese patient with endometrial carcinoma.

Physical Activity

Zheng *et al.* (1993) found that women in Shangai with occupations with a low level of physical activity (professionals, government officials, clerical workers) had an increased incidence of cancer of the endometrium. The incidence was reduced in women with high activity jobs (service workers, craftsmen). A Swiss and Italian cooperative study suggested that increased activity was associated with a lower risk of endometrial cancer (Levi *et al.*, 1993). Physical activity was divided into four levels, and based only on patients' evaluation and report.

Menstrual Abnormalities and Parity

Reports of patients with endometrial cancer have long noted that these women commonly have histories of irregular menses and are of low parity. Large series have documented that 18–40% of patients are nulliparous (Randall and Goddard, 1956; Kjellgren, 1979). This is true both for countries with a high incidence of endometrial cancer, such as the USA (Elwood *et al.*, 1977), and also in countries with a low incidence, such as Japan (Masubuchi and Nemoto, 1972). Parazzini *et al.* (1991) in a Milan study found that nulliparity and other reproductive factors, such as age of first and last childbirth, induced and spontaneous abortions, decreased the relative risk of developing endometrial cancer more for premenopausal women than postmenopausal women.

In addition, an increased cancer risk is also associated with early menarche and late menopause (Jensen, 1985). Looking at registry data on 1270 patients with chronic anovulation, Coulam *et al.* (1983) found an increased risk of 3.1 for endometrial carcinoma, but for no other malignancies.

These observations are best synthesized in a Swedish study of Petterson *et al.* (1986), who define 'menstruation span' as a numerical means of quantifying age at menarche, age at menopause and parity (*Figure 9.4*). When compared with age-matched controls, endometrial cancer patients had a statistically significant longer menstruation span, and a span greater than 39 carried 4.2 times the risk of a span of 25 or less. While nulliparity and late menopause increased risk, each full term pregnancy was shown to decrease risk. Furthermore, the increased risk associated with late menopause stopped after 67 years of age, suggesting that the influence of the presumed endocrine factors associated with anovulation, nulliparity and late menopause are limited in time, and cancer developing after 70 years of age may be etiologically different.

Endometrial Carcinoma in Young Women

As mentioned previously, endometrial cancer is a disease of elderly postmenopausal women. However, there are a small number of young women who develop this disease, and they are of special interest since they could potentially serve to highlight risk factors for the overall population.

Jeffrey *et al.* (1987) reviewed 27 women under 45 years of age, and found five were incorrectly diagnosed and actually had hyperplasia. Of the remaining 22, four were obese, nine were nulliparous and one had chronic anovulation. Of these 22 patients, 15 had concurrent adenomatous hyperplasia. Other authors looking at young endometrial cancer patients have confirmed a high incidence of obesity, menstrual irregularity and nulliparity (Henderson *et al.*, 1983), and also found cases of hyperplasia mistaken for cancer (Kempson and Pokorney, 1968).

It is interesting to note that several authors, in admittedly small series ranging from 10–32 patients, have found polycystic ovaries (PCO) or Stein–Leventhal syndrome in 10–70% (Peterson, 1978). In a review of young women with hyperplasia, Chamlian and Taylor (1970) found 24 of 97 patients had this syndrome. While other case reports note this association of endometrial cancer with PCO, it is difficult to know whether other risk factors, such as obesity, can be singled out. The magnitude of the risk of PCO is also unclear. Jackson and Dockerty

MENSTRUATION SPAN:
- age at menopause
- age at menarche
- number of births × 1.5

Figure 9.4. Menstruation span: age at menopause – age at menarche – number of births × 1.5.

(1957) analyzed 43 cases of Stein–Leventhal syndrome and found 17 with endometrial cancer. This may be an artificially high estimate based on a small series and without strict histologic definition of criteria for malignancy, but it does suggest an increased risk for patients with PCO.

It should be noted that a large majority, but not all, of the cancers described were superficial and well differentiated (Farhi *et al.*, 1986). While most were surgically removed, a few apparently resolved with only progestational treatment. The only study of young women that found a high incidence of myometrial invasion (66%), had limited material for pathology review, and included only 10.3% of women under 40 years of age (Quinn *et al.*, 1985).

Functional Ovarian Tumors

Case reports and small review series have suggested an association of estrogen-secreting tumors of the ovary with endometrial hyperplasia and/or cancer. However, the rarity of these cases leads to a potential exaggeration of their significance in reports from regional centers (Emge, 1953; Koller, 1966).

The endometrial lesions described, when invasive, appear to be well differentiated and superficial, which again raises questions as to their actual virulence. It may be that patients with these rare ovarian lesions, notably granulosa and theca cell tumors, have a risk for endometrial disease; however, the overwhelming majority of endometrial cancer patients do not have these lesions.

Abnormal Glucose Metabolism

In reviewing their patients with endometrial cancer, Lynch *et al.* (1952) found abnormal serum glucose levels in 42% of their patients, while other authors in the USA also found an increased, but less quantified, risk (Van Nagell *et al.*, 1972; Elwood *et al.*, 1977). Studies in Malta and Poland also found an increased risk of endometrial cancer in patients with abnormal glucose metabolism.

Since obesity is associated with endometrial carcinoma and also with disturbances in glucose metabolism, it is difficult to separate these two factors. However, Damon (1960) found a 19% incidence of diabetes in patients who were no more obese than nondiabetics, and Wynder *et al.* (1966) found that obesity alone would not explain a greater than expected incidence of diabetes in their data. Benjamin and Romney (1964) compared results in cancer patients from New York and South Africa, and found a similar incidence of diabetes (13% in the USA and 15% in South Africa), and also abnormal glucose metabolism in an additional 5–9%. When focusing on premenopausal or young women, abnormal glucose metabolism was again associated with an increased risk of endometrial cancer (Geisler *et al.*, 1969).

However, others (Villani *et al.*, 1986; Shenker *et al.*, 1983) have found no increased risk for endometrial cancer in their patients with abnormal glucose metabolism.

No uniformity exists in defining what constitutes abnormal glucose metabolism. Some studies rely on random glucose levels, while others require abnormal glucose tolerance tests. Kessler (1971) makes the interesting point that all of the studies relating diabetes to endometrial cancer are clinical reviews of patient material. No one has demonstrated diabetic changes at autopsy.

A group of Finnish investigators carried out mass screening using endometrial biopsies, of 597 asymptomatic women with diabetes and/or hypertension, aged 45–69 years (Gronoos *et al.*, 1993). They found histologic precursors of endometrial cancer in 6.3% of women with diabetes, but only 1.3% with hypertension. Obesity did not explain the observed results. This study suggests a potential role for screening to detect precursors and possibly prevent the development of invasive disease.

Previous Pelvic Irradiation

Several of the original articles developing the argument that hyperplastic endometrial lesions develop into invasive endometrial adenocarcinoma included patients who had received previous irradiation. Hertig and Sommers (1949) reviewed 32 cases of endometrial cancer in patients who had previous endometrial biopsies: 20 had previous pelvic radiation. In defining the entity 'carcinoma *in situ*' of the endometrium, Hertig *et al.* (1949) reviewed 64 cases, ten of whom had pelvic radiation. All of these patients were irradiated for benign disease, and Palmer and Spratt, (1956) reported an additional 31 cases after irradiation for leiomyoma. Fortunately, radiation is no longer used for benign disease.

However, therapeutic radiation for cervical cancer may also carry a risk of a second endometrial primary (Gallion *et al.*, 1987). Fehr and Prem (1974) reviewed 2294 patients irradiated for squamous cell carcinoma of the cervix and found 12 endometrial cancers (0.52%). Petterson *et al.* (1985) looked at second malignancies in women treated from 1914–1965 and found an excess of second primaries in the endometrium. None of these data consider the potential interactions with other risk factors.

Hypertension

In reviewing young women with endometrial cancer, approximately 19% were found to be hypertensive (Geisler *et al.*, 1969; Peterson, 1978). In the postmenopausal age group, 27–65% were found to be hypertensive (Obrink *et al.*, 1981; Wharton *et al.*, 1986; Zemla, 1986). There is a suggestion that this is a higher incidence than would be expected based on obesity alone (Wynder *et al.*, 1966), but most studies do not provide age and weight controls.

Hepatic Dysfunction

Zemla (1986) found an increased risk of endometrial cancer associated with jaundice in his series of 173 patients. Speert (1949) observed cirrhosis during autopsies of endometrial cancer patients, and in an extensive review of 504 patients found cirrhosis in 0.8%.

Pituitary Function

Benjamin (1974) measured growth hormone (HGH) levels in endometrial cancer patients and controls. Both groups were all obese and had abnormal glucose tolerance curves. He found HGH levels were higher in patients than in controls for prolonged times and postulated that this might be related to higher estrogen levels. However, Brown (1974) found no difference in levels of HGH, TSH and ACTH in cancer patients, but diminished luteinizing hormone (LH). Again, elevated estrogen was postulated as the cause.

Estrogen levels have not been consistently shown to be elevated in endometrial cancer patients. Benjamin and Deutsch (1976) found no measurable estriol (E3) and higher estrone (E1) and estradiol (E2), but acknowledged patient obesity may affect E2 levels in their study. They also found low follicle stimulating hormone (FSH) levels.

Geisler *et al.* (1969) and Kennedy *et al.* (1982) noted a 13.7% incidence of thyroid disease in a series of 61 premenopausal patients with endometrial cancer, and Zemla (1986) found an increased risk associated with thyroid disease. Van Nagell *et al.* (1972) found no association or risk with thyroid disease.

All of the above suggests hypothalamic or pituitary dysfunction, but lacks evidence in weight-controlled studies.

Effect of Cigarette Smoking

While clearly related to a horrible loss of life from lung cancer and cardiovascular disease, cigarette smoking may be protective against endometrial cancer. Smith *et al.* (1984) found an increased risk of endometrial cancer of 1.27 in premenopausal women who smoked, but a markedly decreased risk of 0.44 in postmenopausal women. This is consistent with Jeffrey *et al.* (1987) who found that eight of 22 young women with endometrial cancer were smokers, and with Stockwell and Hymen (1987) who found a clear reduction in risk for women over 50 years of age who smoked at least 20 cigarettes a day. It appears smoking may reduce the increased risk associated with obesity (Lawrence *et al.*, 1987) and may also reduce the potential risk associated with estrogen therapy. If the woman stops smoking, the benefit disappears (Lesko *et al.*, 1985). It is unclear how smoking reduces the risk of endometrial cancer. It has been proposed that cigarette smoking lowers estrogen production, or possibly increases metabolism, perhaps because the metabolism of cigarette byproducts induces enzyme systems involved in estrogen metabolism. Lower levels of E1, E2 and E3 have been found in the urine of smokers (MacMahon *et al.*, 1982). Smoking may also induce an earlier menopause, or ovarian atrophy. Tyler *et al.* (1985) suggested that the protective effect of smoking does not occur in women under 55 years of age. A Shanghai study, in contrast, found that smokers had an increased risk of endometrial cancer; this study agreed about other factors identified in other studies as increasing risk, such as nulliparity, exogenous estrogens and late menopause (Shu *et al.*, 1991).

The potential risk reduction is obviously outweighed by lung cancer and cardiovascular morbidity and mortality.

Dietary Considerations

Zemla *et al.* (1986) reviewed the dietary habits of 173 patients in Poland, each compared with two age-matched controls. There was no apparent risk associated with rural or urban living, industrial or non-industrial work, or exposure to metallurgy, coal or coke. However, risk increased with the consumption of fried meats. If eaten daily, the relative risk was 4.9. Boiled meat was not associated with an increased risk, and a lowered risk was associated with the consumption of raw vegetables. In Italian studies, LaVecchia *et al.* (1984) and Villani *et al.* (1986) both found an increased cancer risk with increasing consumption of lipids, fats and oils, and less risk with green vegetables, fruit, liver and fish.

However, it is difficult to evaluate the above findings, since all the increase in risk may be related more to caloric excess than any specific food entity.

Shu *et al.* (1993) found in Shanghai that high caloric intake from fat and protein was associated with an increased cancer risk, but not if the calories came from carbohydrates. A high consumption of meat, eggs and fresh fish was associated with an increased risk, but not consumption of fruit or vegetables. Barbone *et al.* (1993) in the USA used logistic regression to evaluate for dietary risk, controlling for total calories, and multiple other known or presumed risk factors. He found an inverse association between endometrial cancer and protein intake, and no association with total intake of animal and vegetable fat. Frequent consumption of several vegetables and dairy products was associated with a statistically significant decreased risk. Carotene and nitrate consumption were protective.

Relation to Breast and Other Cancers

Both cancer of the breast and endometrium are associated with low parity and obesity. Schwartz *et al.* (1985) found an excess of ovarian, colon, and breast cancers in Israeli endometrial carcinoma patients; Adami *et al.* (1987) reviewed 60,065 breast cancer patients in Sweden and found 260 endometrial cancers instead of an expected 151, giving a relative risk of 1.72. This risk was greater in older women and the second cancers appeared predominantly in the first five years of follow-up. Kennedy *et al.* (1982) and Baitor (1963) found similar data for increased breast primaries in endometrial cancer patients in the USA.

Hakala *et al.* (1991) emphasized that endometrial cancer is the second most common malignancy in the recognized inherited cancer family syndromes (nonpolyposis colorectal carcinoma), more specifically the Lynch syndrome II. These patients present most often with abnormal bleeding and are diagnosed at an earlier age (48.3 years). Endometrial biopsies may be helpful in following patients with known colorectal cancer syndromes, and prophylactic hysterectomy at the time of bowel resection may be appropriate.

Exogenous Estrogen Administration

It has been recognized for over 40 years that in any series of endometrial cancer patients there is a significant number who have received exogenous estrogens. Hertig *et al.* (1949) in defining carcinoma *in situ* of the endometrium noted that four of his 64 patients had been treated with estrogen. Cutler *et al.* (1972) reported adenocarcinoma occurring in patients with gonadal dysgenesis treated with stilbesterol, while Jensen and Ostergaard (1959) had shown that estrogen usage was increased in endometrial cancer patients when compared to a control population.

However, this relationship received little attention until the mid 1970s, when both the medical literature, and more importantly, the American lay press, emphasized several studies showing an increased risk of endometrial cancer in patients taking estrogen replacement therapy (Astedt, 1982). Smith *et al.* (1975) reported a 4.54 increased risk of endometrial cancer in estrogen users, with a less obvious risk if other known risks were present. Ziehl and Finkle (1975) found 57% of their 94 patients had used estrogen, which when compared to controls, 15% of whom had used estrogen, gave a risk of 7.6. Furthermore, if used for 1–4.9 years, the risk was 5.6, but increased to 13.9 if used for seven years or more.

Quint (1975) compared surgeries for endometrial cancer in 1960–1966 and 1967–1973, and found an increase in the number of cases with no increase in the incidence of nulliparity or obesity, but a parallel increase in estrogen therapy. Mack *et al.* (1976) found an eight-fold risk for estrogen users, similar to a 7.4 risk found by Ziehl and Finkle (1976). A pathology review of the latter study confirmed the diagnoses were indeed correct (Gordon *et al.*, 1977). This study of Ziehl and Finkle (1976), as well as others (Kelsey, 1982), showed an increased risk with an increased duration of exposure to estrogens. The risk was also shown to increase with dosage. Jick *et al.* (1979) suggested a 1–3% yearly risk for estrogen users over non-users, and when the incidence of endometrial cancer was compared over time with estrogen use, increasing incidence paralleled increased use (Austin and Rose, 1982). When publicity led to less acceptance of replacement therapy, the number of prescriptions written fell as did the incidence. Estrogen use did not seem to increase the risk associated with obesity, diabetes or hypertension, and the risk was primarily in women over 50 years of age (Austin and Rose, 1979; Walker and Jick, 1979; Ewertz and Jensen, 1984). Estrogen use increased a patient's risk even if no other known risk factors were present (Weiss *et al.*, 1980). Estrogen users who smoked had the same risk as non-users (Franks *et al.*, 1987).

The tumors found in estrogen users are predominantly well differentiated and superficially invasive (Underwood *et al.*, 1979; Elwood and Boyes, 1980; Hulka *et al.*, 1980; Obrink *et al.*, 1981), and often accompanied by hyperplasia. Not surprisingly, therefore, they are associated with better survival than those found in non-estrogen users (Collin *et al.*, 1980). In the USA Jick *et al.* (1980) estimated that 15,000 cases of endometrial cancer could be attributed to estrogen use from 1971–1975.

These reports linking estrogen use with an increased risk of endometrial cancer were criticized and challenged on many fronts. MacRae (1980) pointed out that the problem with epidemiologic studies is that they are not double-blind, so an unknown bias may be present. One criticism is that estrogen may simply increase detection, not actually cause new cancers (Greenland and Neutra, 1981). Horwitz *et al.* (1981a) argue that while a review of estrogen-related cancers confirms the diagnosis in 84–98% of cases, the estrogen may only be causing bleeding from benign proliferative endometrium associated with the cancers, which leads to diagnosis. Feinstein and Horowitz (1978) argued that if case controls were selected based on diagnostic procedure, there would be no increased risk. Klopper (1980) found an increase in the incidence of attributable deaths to endometrial cancer in the UK, and suggested a relative increase in elderly nulliparous females would increase the disease incidence. Salmi (1980) found no increase in endometrial cancer in Finland, where E3 and E2 are used as opposed to conjugated estrogens. Koss *et al.* (1980) noted an increased incidence of endometrial cancer in Norway, Czechoslovakia and the Soviet Union, where estrogen had not been used.

It has also been argued that endometrial cancer can be asymptomatic and estrogen would 'unmask' these lesions. This runs counter to current teaching, which is that early abnormal bleeding heralds this cancer. However, Horowitz *et al.* (1981a) reviewed all necropsies from 1918–1978 at Yale University and from 1952–1978 at Massachusetts General Hospital in Boston, and found 24 undiagnosed cancers in 8998 women, which they argue is much higher than the yearly expected incidence. However, their figures represent the results of an entire lifetime of risk for their study cases and such a comparison with incidence rates is meaningless. It does show that asymptomatic endometrial cancers do exist, and this author has personally cared for a number of women found to have advanced endometrial cancer, and no postmenopausal bleeding.

To a thoughtful person, the extremely large number of studies using different methodologies that reach the same statistical conclusion, the dose effect, the increase of risk with the length of exposure, the decrease of risk with cessation of administration, and the increase of risk for women with no other known factors are compelling arguments to accept that estrogen replacement therapy increases a postmenopausal woman's risk of developing endometrial cancer.

However, given the tremendous benefits of preventing osteoporosis, cardiovascular disease and the genitourinary symptoms of estrogen deficiency, it is pertinent to note that cyclic progestin therapy lowers the risk of estrogen replacement (Gambrell, 1984).

Because of the health benefits of estrogen replacement therapy, even patients who have been diagnosed and treated for endometrial cancer are considered candidates for estrogen replacement (Lee *et al.*, 1990; Creasman *et al.*, 1986). Estrogen should have no deleterious effect on patients with tumors having a good prognosis, while there is a theoretical risk to patients likely to have recurrent or persistent cancer of promoting cancer growth (ACOG Committee, 1991).

Oral contraceptives constitute a second form of exogenous estrogen therapy. Kelly *et al.* (1976) reported endometrial carcinoma in three patients on sequential contraceptives, Lyon and Frisch (1976) added a case report, and Silverburg and Makowski (1975) reported 21 patients aged 21–39 years who developed endometrial cancer while on oral contraceptives. In this latter series, 13 cases were on sequential agents and seven on combined formulations. Six were obese and two nulliparous. Silverburg *et al.* (1977) studied 30 endometrial cancer patients under 40 years of age; 20 were on sequentials. The pill users had lesions that histologically appeared to have a good prognosis and had only a 6% incidence of obesity, a 15% incidence of nulliparity and no hypertension. Lyon and Frisch (1976) sampled the endometrium of 12 women on sequential pills from 13–93 months, finding both hyperplasia and carcinoma *in situ*. These agents were subsequently taken off the market.

Weiss and Sayretz (1980) found sequential pills were associated with an increased risk of 7.3 for endometrial cancer, but that combination pills were associated with a protective effect. Several other studies confirmed that patients taking combination oral contraceptives had one-half the risk of non-users of developing endometrial cancer (Kaugman *et al.*, 1980; Hulka *et al.*, 1982; Centers for Disease Control Cancer and Steroid Hormone Study, 1983). The use of oral contraceptives is protective despite similar histories regarding smoking, age of menarche and parity for users and non-users, and the protective effect of oral contraceptive use exists regardless of how long they are taken, or how long ago (Jick *et al.*, 1983). The protective effect of oral contraceptives may be related to the relative strength of the estrogen and progestin in the pill, with stronger progestins being more protective (Rosenblatt *et al.*, 1991).

Interestingly, the use of intrauterine contraceptives is also associated with a markedly decreased risk of endometrial cancer, presumably through local structural and biochemical changes in the endometrium (Castellsague *et al.*, 1993).

Tamoxifen is a nonsteroidal anti-estrogen used to prevent or delay recurrence of breast cancer. However, it acts by competing for estradiol binding sites and may in fact be considered as a 'weak' estrogen. There have been case reports of endometrial cancer developing in patients on tamoxifen as well as in patients developing endometrial polyps and hyperplasia (DeMuylder *et al.*, 1991). Not all authors agree that tamoxifen causes endometrial cancer (Andersson *et al.*, 1991), but there is a growing literature suggesting that as many as 30% of women taking this drug will develop some type of endometrial abnormality, the majority of which are benign. The recognized increased risk of endometrial cancer in breast cancer patients, and the possibility of bias introduced by extensively screening cancer patients, clouds the issue. Tamoxifen also has beneficial effects on a woman's risk of coronary heart disease and osteoporosis (Spicer *et al.*, 1991). It is prudent to balance the potential risks and benefits of tamoxifen therapy, just as when providing estrogen replacement therapy to menopausal women. At this time, it would seem advisable to follow women on tamoxifen closely, with endometrial biopsies for abnormal bleeding, or possibly on a routine basis. Vaginal ultrasound may also be useful in detecting endometrial lesions and suggesting when office hysteroscopy or endometrial biopsy are appropriate.

The Estrone Hypothesis

Because of the risks associated with low parity and menstrual irregularity, estrogen-secreting ovarian tumors, sequential contraceptives and estrogen replacement therapy, considerable emphasis has been placed on attempts to find a measurable hormonal imbalance in endometrial cancer patients. Estriol (E3) is absent in postmenopausal females, and while some authors report an elevation in serum E1 and E2 (Benjamin and Deutsch, 1976), most report no difference between patients and controls (Judd *et al.*, 1976; Lucas and Yen, 1979). Estrogen in post-menopausal women comes from peripheral aromatization of adrenal androstenedione into E1, occuring primarily in adipose cells (Gambrell, 1979). Obesity increases aromatization, but obese cancer patients cannot be distinguished from obese controls (Herschapf and Bradlow, 1987). In the nucleus, E1 is converted to E2, a potent endometrial growth promoter (Tseng and Gurpide, 1973). Obesity also correlates with decreased levels of steroid hormone binding globulin (SHBG), which leads to increased circulating free hormone and increases metabolic clearance rate (Siiteri, 1985).

This extragenital peripheral conversion of adrenal precursors leads to endogenous estrone production and prolonged unopposed stimulation of the endometrium, which increases the risk of endometrial cancer. This is the 'estrone hypothesis' (Siiteri *et al.*, 1976) and provides a working model to understand how several risk factors can be understood. Exogenous estrogen or estrogen-secreting tumors directly stimulate the endometrium, while PCO increases androstenedione levels.

Current thinking is that cancer is a two-step process requiring an initiating event and a promoter. Certainly estrogen may serve as the promoter, but the initiation or cause remains unknown.

It must be recognized, though, that endometrial cancer has arisen in ovulatory patients, and that not all tumors show hormonal receptors. In fact, all that has been said may only apply to one subset of patients with endometrial cancer. Bokham (1985) found 65% of his patients had obesity and hyperestrogenism, and their cancers were well differentiated, superficially invasive and associated with an 85.6% five-year survival. The other 35% of his patients had no hormonal abnormalities and 62.5% had poorly differentiated cancers with 65.7% deep myometrial invasion and a 58.5% five-year survival.

Table 9.1. Risk factors associated with endometrial cancer.

Endogenous
Obesity
Amenorrhea
Nulliparity
Diabetes
Hypertension
Polycystic ovary syndrome
Estrogen-secreting tumors
Liver dysfunction
High fat diet
White race
Previous breast cancer
Low physical activity level
Exogenous
Pelvic irradiation
Estrogen replacement therapy (non-cyclic)
Sequential oral contraception
Tamoxifen

Finally, MacMahon (1974) emphasizes that nearly half of all patients found to have endometrial cancer have no identifiable risk factors, making attempts at screening of limited value (*Table 9.1*).

Tumors of the Uterine Muscle

Benign leiomyomas of the uterus are extremely common, occurring in up to 30% of all women over 30 years of age, but their etiology has received little attention. They appear to be more common in black women than in white. Exogenous estrogen or pregnancy stimulate their growth, while they often shrink in size after the menopause. Parazzini *et al.* (1988) found that current smoking and multiparity decrease the risk of uterine leiomyomas, while risk was increased with an earlier age of menarche and last birth, and more commonly these women were better educated, and used intrauterine devices and oral contraceptives. They found no associations with body mass, history of spontaneous or induced abortions, and age at first birth.

Sarcomas of the uterus are extremely rare, and quite lethal. Their histologic classification is complex, and not uniform. Hence, their epidemiology has received little attention. Typically sarcomas occur in postmenopausal women, but they have been reported at all ages. It has been estimated that uterine sarcomas comprise 2–5% of all uterine malignancies, with studies suggesting a range of 1 to 8 to 1 to 143 endometrial carcinomas (Ali and Wells, 1993).

The risk of sarcoma may be lower in parous women, while late menarche and early menopause increase risk (Schwartz *et al.*, 1989). These authors found no association with a history of infertility, use of oral contraceptive or sexual activity. Previous pelvic irradiation may increase the risk of subsequent uterine sarcoma (Meredith *et al.*, 1986).

Summary of Core Information

- Cancer of the endometrium is the most common gynecologic malignancy. It occurs primarily in postmenopausal women, but 20–25% of patients are premenopausal.
- Obesity, low levels of physical activity, low parity, late menopause, diabetes, hypertension, estrogen-secreting ovarian tumors, breast cancer, and exogenous estrogen therapy are among recognized risk factors.
- Up to 50% of patients developing endometrial cancer do not have identifiable risk factors.
- Histologic precursor lesions in the endometrium have been identified.
- It has been estimated that uterine sarcoma comprises 2–5% of all uterine malignancies, with studies suggesting a range of 1 to 8, to 1 to 143 endometrial carcinomas. Typically, sarcomas occur in postmenopausal women, but they have been reported at all ages.
- Previous pelvic irradiation may increase the risk of subsequent uterine sarcoma.

References

■ ACOG Committee on Gynecologic Practice (1991) Estrogen replacement therapy and endometrial cancer. *Int. Gynecol. Obstet.* **36:** 76.

Adami HO, Krissemo UB & Bergkvist E (1987) On the age-dependent association between cancer of the breast and of the endometrium. A nationwide cohort study. *Br. J. Cancer* **55:** 77–80.

Ali S & Wells M (1993) Mixed mullerian tumors of the uterine corpus: a review. *Int. J. Gynecol. Cancer* **3:** 1–11.

Andersson M, Storm HH & Mouridsen HT (1991) Incidence of new primary cancers after adjuvant tamoxifen therapy and radiotherapy for early breast cancer. *J. Nat. Cancer Inst.* **83:** 1013–1017.

Antune CM, Stolley PD, Rosenstein NB *et al.* (1979) Endometrial cancer and estrogen use. *New Eng. J. Med.* **300:** 9–13.

Astedt B (1982) On the role of estrogens in endometrial carcinogenesis. *Acta Obstet. Gynecol. Scand. Suppl.* **106:** 33–35.

Austin DF & Rose KM (1979) Increase in cancer of the corpus uteri in the San Francisco–Oakland standard metropolitan statistical area, 1960–1975. *J. Nat. Cancer Institute* **62:** 13–16.

Austin DF & Rose KM (1982) The decreasing incidence of endometrial cancer: Public health implications. *Am. J. Public Health* **72:** 65–68.

Baanders–van Halewijn EA & Poortman J (1982) A case-controlled study of endometrial cancer within a cohort. *Maturitas* **7:** 69–76.

Baitor JC (1963) The incidence of independent tumors among uterine cancer patients. *Cancer* **16:** 842–853.

Barbone F, Austin H & Partridge EE (1993) Diet and endometrial cancer: A case-control study. *Am. J. Epidemiol.* **137:** 393–403.

Benjamin F & Romney SL (1964) Disturbed carbohydrate metabolism in endometrial cancer. *Cancer* **17:** 386–390.

Benjamin F (1974) Growth hormone response to insulin hypoglycemia in endometrial cancer. *Obstet. Gynecol.* **43:** 257–261.

Benjamin F & Deutsch S (1976) Plasma levels of fractionated estrogens and pituitary hormones in endometrial carcinoma. *Am. J. Obstet. Gynecol.* **126:** 638–647.

Blitzer PH, Blitzer EC & Rimm AA (1976) Association between teenage obesity and cancer in 56,111 women: all cancers and endometrial cancer. *Prevent. Med.* **5:** 20–31.

■ Bokhman JV (1983) Two pathogenetic types of endometrial carcinoma. *Gynecol. Oncol.* **15:** 10–17.

Bond AP (1986) Carcinoma of the endometrium – changing trends in aetiology and management. *Br. J. Clin. Pract.* **40:** 157–164.

Brinton LA, Berman ML, Mortel R *et al.* (1992) Reproductive, menstrual, and medical risk factors for endometrial cancer: Results from a case-control study. *Am. J. Obstet. Gynecol.* **167:** 1317–1325.

Brown R (1974) Anterior pituitary function and its significance in the aetiology of endometrial cancer. *J. Obstet. Gynaecol. Br. Common.* **81:** 947–951.

Castellsague X, Thompson WD & Dubrow R (1993) Intra-uterine contraception and the risk of endometrial cancer. *Int. J. Cancer.* **54:** 911–916.

Centers for Disease Control Cancer and Steroid Hormone Study (1983) Oral contraceptive use and the risk of endometrial cancer. *JAMA* **249:** 1600–1604.

Chamlian DL & Taylor HB (1970) Endometrial hyperplasia in young women. *Obstet. Gynecol.* **36:** 659–666.

Christopherson WM, Mendez WM, Parker JE, Lundin FE & Ahuja EM (1971) Carcinoma of the endometrium: A study of changing rates over a 15 year period. *Cancer* **27:** 1005–1008.

Collin J, Allen LH, Donner A & Adams O (1980) Oestrogen use and survival in endometrial cancer. *Lancet* **2:** 961–963.

■ Corscaden JA & Gusberg SB (1974) The background of cancer of the corpus. *Am. J. Obstet. Gynecol.* **53:** 419–431.

Coulam CB, Anneyers JF & Krang JS (1983) Chronic anovulation syndrome and associated neoplasms. *Obstet. Gynecol.* **61:** 403–407.

Cramer DW, Cutler SJ & Christine B (1974) Trends in the incidence of endometrial cancer in the United States. *Gynecol. Oncol.* **2:** 130–143.

Creasman WJ, Henderson D, Hinshaw W & Clarke–Pearson DL (1986) Estrogen replacement therapy in the patient treated for endometrial cancer. *Obstet. Gynecol.* **67:** 326–330.

Cutler BS, Forbes AP, Ingersoll FM & Scully RE (1972) Endometrial carcinoma after stilbestrol therapy in gonadal dysgenesis. *New Eng. J. Med.* **287:** 628–631.

Damon A (1960) Host factors in cancer of the breast and uterine cervix and corpus. *J. Nat. Cancer Inst.* **24:** 485–516.

De Muylder X, Neven P, DeSomer M, Van Belle Y, Vanderick G & De Muylder E (1991) Endometrial lesions in patients undergoing tamoxifen therapy. *Int. J. Gynecol. Obstet.* **36:** 127–130.

DeVere RD & Dempster KR (1953) A case of Stein–Leventhal syndrome associated with carcinoma of the endometrium. *J. Obstet. Gynaecol. Br. Empire* **60,** 865–867.

Dunn JE (1974) Geographic considerations of endometrial cancer. *Gynecol. Oncol.* **2:** 114–121.

Elwood JM, Cole P, Rothman KJ & Kaplan SD (1977) Epidemiology of endometrial cancer. *J. Nat. Cancer Inst.* **59:** 1055–1060.

Elwood JM & Boyes DA (1980) Clinical and pathological features and survival of endometrial cancer patients in relation to prior use of estrogens. *Gynecol. Oncol.* **10:** 173–187.

Emge LA (1953) Endometrial cancer and feminizing tumors of the ovaries. *Obstet. Gynecol.* **1:** 511–515.

Ewertz M & Jensen OM (1984) Trends in the incidence of cancer of the corpus uteri in Denmark 1943 1980. *Am. J. Epidem.* **119:** 725–732.

Farhi DC, Nosanchuk J & Silverberg SG (1986) Endometrial adenocarcinoma in women under 25 years of age. *Obstet. Gynecol.* **68:** 741–745.

Fehr PE & Prem KA (1974) Malignancy of the uterine corpus following irradiation therapy for squamous cell carcinoma of the cervix. *Am. J. Obstet. Gynecol.* **119:** 685–692.

■ Feinstein AR & Horowitz RI (1978) A critique of the statistical evidence associating estrogen with endometrial cancer. *Cancer Res.* **38:** 4001–4003.

Fox H & Sen DK (1970) A controlled study of the constitutional stigmata of endometrial adenocarcinoma. *Br. J. Cancer* **24:** 30–36.

Franks AL, Kendricks JS & Tyler CW (1987) Post-menopausal smoking, estrogen replacement therapy and the risk of endometrial cancer. *Am. J. Obstet. Gynecol.* **156:** 20–23.

Gallagher RP & Elwood JM (1982) Recent trends in recorded incidence and mortality from uterine cancer. *NCI Monograph* **62:** 83–87.

Gallion HH, Van Nagell JR, Donaldson ES & Powell DE (1987) Endometrial cancer following radiation therapy for cervical cancer. *Gynecol. Oncol.* **27:** 76–83.

Gambrell RD (1979) The role of hormones in the etiology of breast and endometrial cancer. *Acta Obstet. Gynecol. Scand. Suppl.* **88:** 73–81.

Gambrell RD (1984) Hormones in the etiology and prevention of breast and endometrial cancer. *South. Med. J.* **77:** 1509–1515.

Garnett JD (1958) Constitutional stigmas associated with endometrial carcinoma. *Am. J. Obstet. Gynecol.* **76:** 11–19.

Geisler HE, Huber CP & Rogers S (1969) Carcinoma of the endometrium in premenopausal women. *Am. J. Obstet. Gynecol.* **104:** 657–663.

Gordon J, Reagan JW, Finkle W & Ziel HK (1977) Estrogen and endometrial carcinoma. *New Eng. J. Med.* **297:** 570–571.

Greenland S & Neutra R (1981) An analysis of detection bias and proposed corrections in the study of estrogens and endometrial cancer. *J. Chron. Dis.* **34:** 433–438.

Gronoos M, Salmi TA, Vuento MH *et al.* (1993) Mass screening for endometrial cancer directed in risk groups of patients with diabetes and patients with hypertension. *Cancer* **71:** 1279–1282.

Hakala T, Mecklin J–P, Forss M, Jarvinen H & Lehtovirta P (1991) Endometrial carcinoma in the cancer family syndrome. *Cancer* **68:** 1656–1659.

Henderson BE, Casagrande MC, Pike T, Mack T, Rosario I & Duke A (1983) The epidemiology of endometrial cancer in young women. *Br. J. Cancer* **47:** 749–756.

Herschopf RJ & Bradlow HL (1987) Obesity, diet, endogenous estrogen, and the risk of hormone sensitive cancers. *Am. J. Clin. Nat.* **45:** 283–289.

Hertig AT & Sommers SC (1949) Genesis of endometrial cancer. 1. Study of prior biopsies. *Cancer* **2:** 946–956.

Hertig AT, Sommers SC & Bergloff H (1949) Genesis of endometrial cancer. III. Carcinoma *in situ*. *Cancer* **2:** 964–971.

Hoogerland DL, Buchler DA, Crowley JJ & Carr WF (1978) Estrogen use – risk of endometrial cancer. *Gynecol. Oncol.* **6:** 451–458.

Horowitz RI, Horwitz SM, Feinstein AR & Robboy ST (1981a) Necropsy diagnosis of endometrial cancer and detection-bias in case/control studies. *Lancet* **2:** 66–68.

Horowitz RI, Feinstein AR, Vidone RA, Sommers SC & Robboy SJ (1981b) Histopathologic distinctions in the relationship of estrogens and endometrial cancer. *JAMA* **246:** 1425–1427.

Hulka BS, Kaufman DG, Fowler WC, Grimson RC & Greenberg BG (1980) Predominance of early endometrial cancers after long-term estrogen use. *JAMA* **244:** 2419–2422.

Hulka BS, Chambless LE, Kaufman DG, Fowler WC & Greenberg BG (1982) Protection against endometrial carcinoma by combination-product oral contraceptives. *JAMA* **247:** 475–477.

Jackson RL & Dockerty MB (1957) The Stein–Leventhal syndrome: Analysis of 43 cases with special reference to association with endometrial carcinoma. *Am. J. Obstet. Gynecol.* **73:** 161–173.

Jeffrey JD, Taylor R, Robertson DI & Stuart GCE (1987) Endometrial carcinoma occurring in patients under the age of 45 years. *Am. J. Obstet. Gynecol.* **156:** 366–370.

Jensen EI & Ostergaard E (1959) Clinical studies concerning the relationships of estrogens to the development of cancer of the corpus uteri. *Am. J. Obstet. Gynecol.* **67:** 1094–1102.

Jensen H (1985) Endometrial cancer: A retrospective epidemiological study. *Dan. Med. Bull.* **32:** 219–229.

Jensen H (1986) Relationship of premorbid state of nutrition to endometrial carcinoma. *Acta Obstet. Gynecol. Scand.* **65:** 301–306.

Jick H, Watkins RN, Hunter JR *et al.* (1979) Replacement estrogens and endometrial cancer. *New Eng. J. Med.* **300:** 218–222.

Jick H, Walker AM & Rothman KJ (1980) The epidemic of endometrial cancer: A commentary. *Am. J. Pub. Health* **70:** 264–267.

Jick SS, Walker AM & Jick H (1993) Oral contraceptives and endometrial cancer. *Obstet. Gynecol.* **82:** 931–935.

Judd HL, Lucas WE & Yen SSC (1976) Serum 17B-estradiol and estrone levels in postmenopausal women with and without endometrial cancer. *J. Clin. Endocrin. Metab.* **43:** 272–278.

Kaufman DW, Shapiro S, Slone D *et al.* (1980) Decreased risk of endometrial cancer among oral contraceptive users. *New Eng. J. Med.* **303:** 1045–1047.

Kelly HW, Milers PA, Buster JE & Seragg WH (1979) Adenocarcinoma of the endometrium in women taking sequential oral contraceptives. *Obstet. Gynecol.* **47:** 200–202.

Kelsey JL, Livolsi VA, Holford TR *et al.* (1982) A case-control study of cancer of the endometrium. *Am. J. Epidem.* **116:** 333–342.

Kempson RL & Pokorney GE (1968) Adenocarcinoma of the endometrium in women aged forty and younger. *Cancer* **21:** 650–662.

Kennedy AW, Casey MJ, Gondos B & Mehuscas EGH (1982) Carcinoma of the endometrium: Review of experience at a community hospital, 1971–1977. *Gynecol. Oncol.* **14:** 164–174.

Kessler II (1971) Cancer and diabetes mellitus: A review of the literature. *J. Chron. Dis.* **23:** 579–600.

King HS, Wigle DT, Hill GB & Selins J (1982) Uterine cancers in Alberta: trends of incidence and mortality. *Canad. Med. Assoc. J.* **127:** 591–594.

Kjellgren O (1979) Epidemiology and pathophysiology of corpus carcinoma. *Acta Obstet. Gynecol. Scand. Suppl.* **65:** 78–82.

Klopper A (1980) The risk of endometrial carcinoma from oestrogen therapy of the menopause. *Acta Endocrin. Suppl.* **233:** 29–35.

Koller O (1966) Granulosa- and theca-cell tumors of genital cancers. *Acta Obstet. Gynecol. Scand.* **45:** 114–120.

Koss LG, Cramer D, Ferenczy A *et al.* (1980) Recent advances in endometrial neoplasia. *Acta Cytol.* **24:** 478–493.

Koss LG, Schreiber K, Oberlander SG, Moussouris HF & Lesser M (1984) Detection of endometrial carcinoma and hyperplasia in asymptomatic women. *Obstet. Gynecol.* **64:** 1–11.

Kurman RT, Kominski PF & Norris HJ (1985) The behavior of endometrial hyperplasia. *Cancer* **56:** 403–412.

La Vecchia C, Franceschi S, Gallus G *et al.* (1982) Prognostic features of endometrial cancer in estrogen users and obese women. *Am. J. Obstet. Gynecol.* **144:** 387–392.

Lawrence C, Tessaro I, Durgerian S *et al.* (1987) Smoking, body weight and early stage endometrial cancer. *Cancer* **59:** 1665–1669.

Lee RB, Burke TW & Park RC (1990) Estrogen replacement therapy following treatment for stage I endometrial carcinoma. *Gynecol. Oncol.* **36:** 189–191.

Lesko SM, Rosenburg L, Kaufman DW *et al.* (1985) Cigarette smoking and the risk of endometrial cancer. *New Eng. J. Med.* **313:** 593–596.

Levi F, La Vecchia C, Negri E & Franceschi S (1993) Selected physical activities and the risk of endometrial cancer. *Br. J. Cancer* **67:** 846–851.

Lucas WE & Yen SC (1979) A study of endocrine and metabolic variables in postmenopausal women with endometrial carcinoma. *Am. J. Obstet. Gynecol.* **134:** 180–186.

Lynch HT, Krush AJ, Larsen AL & Magnuson CW (1952) Endometrial carcinoma: Multiple primary malignancies, constitutional factors and heredity. *Am. J. Med. Sciences* **252**, 381–390.

Lyon FA & Frisch MJ (1976) Endometrial abnormalities occurring in young women on long term sequential oral contraception. *Obstet. Gynecol.* **47:** 639–643.

Lyon JL & Gardner JW (1977) The rising frequency of hysterectomy: its effect on uterine cancer rates. *Am. J. Epidem.* **105:** 439–443.

Mack TM, Alce MC, Henderson BE *et al.* (1976) Estrogens and endometrial cancer in a retirement community. *New Eng. J. Med.* **294:** 1262–1267.

MacMahon B (1979) Risk factors for endometrial cancer. *Gynecol. Oncol.* **2:** 122–129.

MacMahon B, Trichopoulos D, Cole P & Brown J (1982) Cigarette smoking and urinary estrogens. *New Eng. J. Med.* **307:** 1062–1065.

MacRae KD (1980) Health risks of oestrogen therapy. *J. Endocr.* **89:** 1458–1488.

Mahboubi E, Eyler N & Wynder EL (1982) Epidemiology of cancer of the endometrium. *Clin. Obstet. Gynecol.* **25:** 5–18.

Masubuchi K & Nemoto H (1972) Epidemiologic studies on uterine cancer at Cancer Institute Hospital, Tokyo, Japan. *Cancer* **30:** 268–275.

Meredith RF, Eisert DR, Kaka Z, Hodgson SE, Johnston GA & Boutselis JG (1986) An excess of uterine sarcomas after pelvic irradiation. *Cancer* **58:** 2003–2007.

Obrink A, Burne G, Collen J & Tjernberg B (1981) Estrogen regimen of women with endometrial carcinoma. *Acta Obstet. Gynecol. Scand. Suppl.* **60:** 191–197.

Palmer JP and Spratt DW (1956) Pelvic carcinoma following irradiation for benign gynecological disease. *Am. J. Obstet. Gynecol.* **92:** 497–505.

Parazzini F, La Vecchia C, Negri E, Cecchetti G & Fedele L (1988) Epidemiologic characteristics of women with uterine fibroids: A case-control study. *Obstet. Gynecol.* **72:** 853–857.

Parazzini F, La Vecchia C, Negri E, Fedele L & Balotta F (1991) Reproductive factors and risk of endometrial cancer. *Am. J. Obstet. Gynecol.* **164:** 522–527.

Peterson EP (1978) Endometrial carcinoma in young women. *Am. J. Obstet. Gynecol.* **31:** 702–707.

Petterson B, Adami H, Lindgren A & Hesselius I (1985) Endometrial polyps and hyperplasia as risk factors for endometrial carcinoma. *Acta Obstet. Gynecol. Scand. Suppl.* **64:** 653–659.

Petterson B, Adami H, Bergshom R & Johanson E (1986) Menstruation span – a time-limited risk factor for endometrial carcinoma. *Acta Obstet. Gynecol. Scand. Suppl.* **65:** 247–255.

Petterson F, Fotiou S, Einhorn N & Silfversward C (1985) Cohort study of the long term effect of irradiation for carcinoma of the uterine cervix. *Acta Radiologica Onc.* **24:** 145–151.

Quinn BC, Kneale BJ & Fortune DW (1985) Endometrial cancer in premenopausal women: a clinicopathological study. *Gynecol. Onc.* **20:** 298–306.

Quint BC (1975) Changing patterns in endometrial carcinoma. *Obstet. Gynecol.* **22:** 498–501.

Randall JH & Goddard WB (1956) A study of 531 cases of endometrial carcinoma. *Surg. Gynecol. Obstet.* **103:** 221–226.

Ritzmann H & Hillemanns HG (1977) Die hyperplasieformen des endometriums und ihre beziehungen zum endometriumkarzinom. *Archiv. fur Gynakologie* **223:** 345–356.

Rosenblatt KA, Thomas DB & The WHO Collaborative Study of Neoplasia and Steroid Contraceptives (1991) Hormonal content of combined oral contraceptives in relation to the reduced risk of endometrial carcinoma. *Int. J. Cancer* **49:** 870–874.

Salmi T (1980) Endometrial carcinoma risk factors, with special reference to the use of oestrogens. *Acta Endocrin. Suppl.* **233:** 37–43.

Schapira DV, Kumar NB, Lyman GH, Cavanagh D, Roberts WS & LaPolla J (1991) Upper-body fat distribution and endometrial cancer risk. *JAMA* **266:** 1808–1811.

Schenker JG, Birchenfeld A & Schwartz S (1983) Endometrial cancer in Israel 1969–1975. *Int. J. Gynaecol. Obst.* **20:** 455–461.

Schwartz SM, Thomas DB & The World Health Organization Collaborative Study of Neoplasia and Steroid Contraceptives (1989) A case–control study of risk factors for sarcomas of the uterus. *Cancer* **64:** 2487–2492.

Schwartz Z, Ohel G, Birchenfeld A, Anteby SO & Schenken JG (1985) Second primary malignancy in endometrial carcinoma patients. *Gynecol. Oncol.* **22:** 40–45.

Shu, X–O, Brinton LA, Zheng W, Gao YT, Fan J & Fraumeni JF (1991) A population-based case–control study of endometrial cancer in Shangai, China. *Int. J. Cancer* **49:** 38–43.

Shu X–O, Zhen W, Potischman N *et al.* (1993) A population-based case–control study of dietary factors and endometrial cancer in Shanghai, People's Republic of China. *Am. J. Epidemiol.* **137:** 155–165.

Siiteri PK, William JE & Tahaki NK (1976) Steroid abnormalities in endometrial and breast carcinoma: A unifying hypotheses. *J. Steroid Biochem.* **7:** 897–903.

Siiteri PK (1985) Adipose tissue as a source of hormones. *Am. J. Clin. Nutrition* **45:** 277–282.

■ Silverberg SG (1988) Hyperplasia and carcinoma of the endometrium. *Sem. Diag. Path.* **5:** 135–153.

Silverberg SG & Makowski EL (1975) Endometrial carcinoma in young women taking oral contraceptive agents. *Am. J. Obstet. Gynecol.* **46:** 503–506.

Silverberg SG, Makowski EL & Roche WD (1977) Endometrial cancer in women under 40 years of age. *Cancer* **29:** 592–598.

Smith DC, Rentie R, Thompson DT & Herrman WL (1975) Association of exogenous estrogen and endometrial cancer. *New Eng. J. Med.* **293:** 1164–1167.

Smith EM, Somers MF & Burns TL (1984) Effects of smoking on the development of female reproductive cancers. *J. Nat. Cancer Inst.* **73:** 371–376.

Speert H (1949) Carcinoma of the endometrium in young women. *Surg. Gynecol. Obstet.* **88:** 332–336.

Spicer DV, Pike MC, Henderson BE & Groshen S (1991) Correspondence – tamoxifen and estrogen replacement therapy as agents of disease prevention. *J. Nat. Cancer Inst.* **83:** 63.

Stockwell HG & Lyman GH (1987) Cigarette smoking and the risk of female reproductive cancer. *Am. J. Obstet. Gynecol.* **157:** 35–40.

Tretle S & Magnus K (1990) Height and weight in relation to uterine corpus cancer morbidity and mortality. A follow-up study of 570,000 women in Norway. *Int. J. Cancer* **46:** 165–172.

Tseng L & Gurpide E (1973) Effect of estrone and progesterone on the nuclear uptake of estradiol by slices of human endometrium. *Endocrin.* **93:** 245–248.

Tyler CW, Webster LA, Ory HW & Rubin GL (1985) Endometrial cancer: How does cigarette smoking influence the risk of women under age 55 years having this tumor? *Am. J. Obstet. Gynecol.* **151:** 899–905.

Underwood PB, Miller MC, Kreutner A, Johner CA & Lutz MH (1979) Endometrial carcinoma: The effect of estrogen. *Gynecol. Oncol.* **8:** 60–73.

Van Nagell JR, Roddick JW & Wallace JO (1972) Clinical correlations of endometrial carcinoma. *Am. J. Obstet. Gynecol.* **112:** 935–937.

Villani C, Picci G, Pietrangeli D, Pace S & Tomao S (1986) Role of diet in endometrial cancer patients. *Eur. J. Gynaecol. Onc.* **7:** 139–143.

Walker AM & Jick H (1980) Declining rates of endometrial cancer. *Obstet. Gynecol.* **56:** 733–736.

Walker AM & Jick H (1979) Cancer of the corpus uteri: Increasing incidence in the United States, 1970–1975. *Am. J. Epidem.* **110:** 47–51.

Weiss NS, Farewell VT, Szekely DR, English DR & Kiviat N (1980) Oestrogens and endometrial cancer: Effect of other risk factors on the association. *Maturitas* **2:** 185–190.

Weiss NS & Sayvetz TA (1980) Incidence of endometrial cancer in relation to the use of oral contraceptives. *New Eng. J. Med.* **302:** 551–554.

Wharton JT, Mikuta JJ, Mettlin C *et al.* (1986) Risk factors and current management of carcinoma of the endometrium. *Surg. Gynecol. Obstet.* **162:** 515–520.

Wingo PA, Tong T & Bolden S (1995) Cancer statistics. *Ca – A Cancer Journal for Clinicians* **45:** 8–30.

Wynder EL, Escher GC & Mantel N (1966) An epidemiological investigation of cancer of the endometrium. *Cancer* **19:** 489–520.

Zemla B (1986) Study of risk factors in invasive cancer of the corpus uteri. *Neoplasma* **33:** 621–629.

Zheng W, Shu X–O, McLaughlin JK, Chow W–H, Gao YT & Blot WJ (1993) Occupational physical activity and the incidence of cancer of the breast, corpus uteri, and ovary in Shanghai. *Cancer* **71:** 3620–3624.

Ziehl HK & Finkle WD (1976) Association of estrone with the development of endometrial carcinoma. *Am. J. Obstet. Gynecol.* **124:** 735–740.

10 Malignant Uterine Tumors

D Anciaux
W D Lawrence

Introduction

Malignant uterine tumors are comprised of epithelial or mesenchymal elements, or combinations thereof; the first two categories are designated as carcinomas and sarcomas, respectively, and the latter are regarded as biphasic, or mixed carcinosarcomas; rare variants include those with sex cord-like and germ cell elements. Although malignant uterine tumors represent 10–15% of all cancers in females, approximately 90% of them are represented by endometrial carcinomas.

Uterine Carcinomas

Incidence

Endometrial carcinoma has become the most common female genital tract malignancy in North America and Northern Europe. Indeed, the National Cancer Institute's Surveillance, Epidemiology, and End Results (SEER) program, which regularly tracks site-specific cancer frequencies and incidence rates in the USA, reported that 48.2% of histologically confirmed invasive female genital tract cancers arose in the uterine corpus; of that group, 94% were comprised of purely epithelial elements. Cancers of the uterine cervix contributed to approximately a fifth and those arising in the ovary to a quarter of invasive female genital tumors. This large proportion of uterine corpus cancer is due, at least in part, to the continuing decline in the incidence of squamous cell carcinoma of the uterine cervix consequent to the early detection of its precursors. Actually, however, the incidence of endometrial carcinoma has varied during the last few decades, a manifestation not only of an overall increase in longevity, but also of changes in patterns of exogenous hormone use. In the decade from 1970–1980, an increased incidence of endometrial carcinoma occurred in developed countries; however, subsequently the trend appears to have been reversed (Austin and Rose, 1982; Cancer and Steroid Hormone Study, 1987). Although an increase in the incidence of endometrial adenocarcinoma has recently been noted in Africa and Asia, it is still 4–5 times less frequent than in the developed world (Doll *et al.*, 1970). Moreover, in low risk populations unusual histologic variants predominate over the typical endometrioid type of adenocarcinoma.

Predisposing Factors

The role of hyperestrinism (Ziehl and Finkle, 1975; Gray *et al.*, 1977) in the pathogenesis of ordinary endometrial carcinoma is now well documented and supported by a 2–3-fold increased risk of the latter in women receiving unopposed estrogens for two years or more (Harlap, 1992). The same pathophysiologic mechanism explains the higher risk of endometrial cancer associated with nulliparity, late menopause, estrogen-producing tumors, the polycystic ovary syndrome (PCO) and obesity (MacMahon, 1974). In several relatively recent studies, a significant percentage of endometrial carcinomas has also been reported in women treated with tamoxifen for breast cancer (Malfetano, 1990; Silva *et al.*, 1994). Oral contraceptives, on the other hand, appear to have a protective effect; indeed, one year of their use has been purported to decrease the risk of endometrial cancer by virtually one-half for a period of 15 years (Thomas, 1991).

Other less well understood predisposing factors include diabetes mellitus, hypertension, a high fat diet and previous radiation therapy for other malignant conditions. Several studies also suggest a predisposing genetic factor by demonstrating a higher incidence of both endometrial and breast cancer in the direct relatives of individuals diagnosed with endometrial carcinoma.

Role of Endometrial Hyperplasia in the Genesis of Carcinoma

The aforementioned same risk factors that are implicated in the development of endometrial carcinoma can be applied to the genesis of endometrial hyperplasia, reinforcing the latter's role as a precursor to malignancy. The classification of endometrial hyperplasia has been revised recently to emphasize the prognostic importance of glandular cytologic atypia (Ausems *et al.*, 1985; Lawrence, 1995) (*Table 10.1*). Indeed, the progression rate to carcinoma is only 2% in hyperplasia without atypia, but as high as 25% or more in endometrial hyperplasia accompanied by cytologic atypia (Kurman *et al.*, 1985). The microscopic features used to differentiate between a focus of well-differentiated adenocarcinoma and atypical endometrial hyperplasia, complex type, are the presence of stromal

Table 10.1. Histologic classification of (tumors and) related lesions of the uterine corpus (modified from classification and nomenclature as developed under the auspices of the International Society of Gynecological Pathologists and adopted by the World Health Organization).

- **1.** Epithelial (tumors and) related lesions
  - **1.1.** Endometrial hyperplasia
    - **1.1.1.** Simple
    - **1.1.2.** Complex (adenomatous)
  - **1.2.** Atypical endometrial hyperplasia
    - **1.2.1.** Simple
    - **1.2.2.** Complex (adenomatous with atypia)

invasion (ideally accompanied by a desmoplastic stromal response), glands arranged back to back with no intervening stroma (a cribriform pattern), or stromal necrosis (Silverberg, 1988; Hendrickson *et al.*, 1983). Finally, the importance of extensive sampling of the endometrium in the uterus must be emphasized as 17–25% of carcinomas are found in cases previously diagnosed as hyperplasia by endometrial curettage. The presence of concomitant hyperplasia in the endometrium adjacent to an adenocarcinoma should be mentioned in the surgical pathology report because of its prognostic implication. Indeed, carcinomas arising in a background of endometrial hyperplasia more often tend to be hormone dependent, affect premenopausal women and have a better prognosis than those developing in an atrophic endometrium, usually in older postmenopausal women (Nyholm *et al.*, 1993). Tumors in the latter group of patients are frequently poorly differentiated, tend to be hormonally nonresponsive and exhibit an aggressive clinical course (Bokhman, 1983).

Clinical Features

The typical case of endometrial carcinoma occurs in a perimenopausal or postmenopausal woman with a mean age of 59 years. The most common presenting symptom is vaginal bleeding. In fact, an endometrial carcinoma is found in 14% of cases of post-menopausal bleeding (Procope, 1971). However, the tumor can occasionally be asymptomatic and even discovered incidentally (Koss *et al.*, 1984). The complaint of pelvic pain is a poor prognostic indicator since it tends to occur late in the course of the disease.

Diagnosis and Sampling Methods

Endometrial carcinoma can occasionally be detected by cervical cytology, but the yield of this method is low. Direct endometrial cytologic sampling has been tested as a detection tool and the reported results have been variable with the diagnostic accuracy ranging from 57–92% (Creasman and Weld, 1976; Cramer and Osborne, 1981). Although this technique may be useful in experienced hands (Bistoletti and Hjerpe, 1993), it is probably best regarded as inappropriate for routine screening or diagnostic purposes. Whether the best method for detection is an endometrial biopsy or curettage remains a controversial issue and discrepancies have been found with both techniques. Importantly, whatever the sampling method used, a definitive diagnosis of either endometrial hyperplasia or adenocarcinoma requires histologic confirmation.

Staging

The International Federation of Gynecology and Obstetrics (FIGO) staging system was revised in 1988 and changed to one based on surgical rather than clinical staging (*Table 10.2*). Clinical staging is now used only in patients who are not candidates for surgery. Currently, emphasis is placed on features derived from microscopic examination of the uterus such as histologic grade, the depth of myometrial invasion, and involvement of the cervix. These histopathologic parameters are useful in the prediction of lymph node involvement and hence must be assessed intraoperatively in order to determine the necessity for lymph node dissection. Several studies have proved frozen section assessment of the aforementioned parameters to be superior to

Table 10.2. The surgical staging system for uterine corpus carcinoma. (From FIGO stages – 1988 Revision.)

Stage I	Confined to the uterine corpus
IA	Tumor limited to endometrium
IB	Invasion of less than one-half of the myometrium
IC	Invasion of more than one-half of the myometrium
Stage II	Uterine cervix involved
IIA	Endocervical glandular involvement only
IIB	Cervical stromal invasion
Stage III	Pelvic extension
IIIA	Tumor invades serosa and/or adnexa and/or positive peritoneal cytology
IIIB	Vaginal metastasis
IIIC	Metastases to pelvic and/or paraaortic lymph nodes
Stage IV	Extrapelvic extension
IVA	Tumor invasion of bladder and/or bowel mucosa
IVB	Distant metastases including intraabdominal and/or inguinal lymph nodes

gross examination alone (Malviya *et al.*, 1989; Fanning *et al.*, 1990). In some cases, however, the determination of depth of myometrial invasion, or whether 'true' invasion is even present, may require deferral of the frozen section diagnosis. Indeed, the differentiation between 'true' myometrial invasion and involvement of adenomyosis by cancer may sometimes be difficult or virtually impossible, even on permanent sections.

Natural History

Endometrioid adenocarcinoma, the most common type of uterine corpus carcinoma, generally has a good prognosis since it usually remains confined to the endometrium for long periods before invasion of the myometrium ensues. When local extrauterine extension occurs, the vagina, bladder, rectum, parametria and ovaries are frequently involved. In the case of concomitant endometrial and ovarian tumors that exhibit similar histologic characteristics, it may be impossible to determine their origin. However, current thinking indicates that approximately one-quarter of uterine endometrioid adenocarcinomas are accompanied by synchronous ovarian endometrioid tumors, often of identical grade and histopathologic appearance (Eisner *et al.*, 1989). The probability of synchronous primaries is especially enhanced when the ovarian tumor is small and unilateral and the uterine tumor is well differentiated and noninvasive.

Lymph node metastases usually spread first to the hypogastric and iliac chains, followed then by periaortic involvement. In the rare cases where the tumor is located in the isthmus, the inguinal nodes may be affected. Hematogenous dissemination, most often to the lungs, liver and bones, usually occurs late in the course of the disease. Peritoneal involvement is rare and occurs mainly in cases of uterine serous papillary carcinoma. The five-year survival of endometrial carcinoma, all histologic types and stages considered, is 78% although the prognosis is worse for the histologic subtypes comprised of uterine serous papillary, clear cell poorly differentiated adenocarcinoma with squamous differentiation ('adenosquamous carcinoma'), and pure squamous carcinomas. *Table 10.3* shows the five-year survival of uterine endometrioid adenocarcinoma broken down by stage at presentation.

Table 10.3. Five-year survival by stage for uterine endometrioid carcinoma (from Abeler *et al.*, 1992).

Stage	*Five-year survival (%)*
I	83
II	71
III	39
IV	27

Table 10.4. Five-year survival by grade (International Federation of Gynecology and Obstetrics (FIGO)/ISGP* grade) for endometrial carcinoma (endometrioid type); all stages considered (from Abeler *et al.*, 1992).

Grade	*Five-year survival*
I	86.8
II	75.0
III	58.3

*ISGP: International Society of Gynecological Pathologists

Prognostic Factors

The depth of myometrial invasion is the most important prognostic factor and predictor of lymph node metastasis, and hence, of overall survival. Historically, pathologists have been instructed to indicate the depth of invasion as to whether the tumor penetrates to the inner, mid, or outer third of the myometrium; however, the new FIGO staging system requires that such should now be expressed as the deepest point of invasion within the inner or outer half of the myometrium. Involvement of adenomyosis by adenocarcinoma is not considered as 'true' invasion; it does not affect the prognosis, even in those instances where the mid and outer levels of the myometrium are involved as long as the tumor is confined to adenomyotic foci (Jacques and Lawrence, 1990).

In general, but not invariably, more poorly differentiated endometrioid cancers are more likely to invade the myometrium, to have a higher frequency of lymph node involvement and to show poor survival. A large population-based study from a Norwegian hospital shows a significant difference in survival depending on the grade of the tumor (*Table 10.4*) (Abeler *et al.*, 1992). Deep myometrial invasion was present in 8.7% of FIGO Grade I and 43.3% of FIGO Grade III tumors. Pelvic and paraaortic lymph node metastases are present in 1–5% of patients with well-differentiated carcinomas compared to 17–26% of patients with poorly-differentiated tumors (Creasman *et al.*, 1987).

However, the depth of myometrial invasion is a good predictor of lymph node metastasis, recurrence and survival, independent of the histologic grade of the tumor. The rate of paraaortic lymph node involvement increases from 5% for tumors with no or superficial myometrial invasion to 46% for deep invasion (Piver *et al.*, 1982; Boronow *et al.*, 1984; Doering *et al.*, 1989). According to Abeler *et al.* (1992), the five-year survival is affected in an equally dramatic fashion, dropping from 88.7% for tumors limited to the endometrium to 63% for tumors with deep myometrial invasion.

Invasion of the cervical stroma by endometrial

adenocarcinoma, warranting the designation of a Stage II adenocarcinoma, is usually associated with higher grade tumors and deep myometrial invasion. A relatively recent Gynecologic Oncology Group (GOG) study reports an overall recurrence rate of 32.6% when the tumor involves the cervix compared to 14.5% when the tumor is limited to the corpus (Morrow *et al.*, 1991). The extent of invasive disease in the cervix, whether limited to the mucosa or involving the stroma, also appears to have prognostic significance (Kadar *et al.*, 1992).

The presence of vascular invasion is usually associated with poorly-differentiated cancers and deep myometrial invasion, but is also a good independent predictor of recurrence. Lymph node metastases are four times more frequent in the presence of vascular space invasion (Creasman *et al.*, 1987; Ambros and Kurman, 1992).

The finding of malignant cells in pelvic washings taken at the time of surgery for endometrial carcinoma is associated with a higher risk of subsequent abdominal or distant recurrence of disease. Positive peritoneal cytology is found in approximately 10% of FIGO Stage I tumors. A study by Creasman *et al.* (1981) reports a recurrence rate of 34% in cases with positive peritoneal cytology and 10% in those with negative cytology. Such adenocarcinoma cells apparently seed the peritoneal cavity either by the transtubal route or by lymph node metastasis; they must be distinguished from reactive mesothelial cells, which can appear extremely atypical and result in 'false positive' peritoneal cytology.

Gross Features

Most endometrial adenocarcinomas arise in the corpus and have a similar gross appearance; rarely, however, they originate in the uterine isthmus. They arise most frequently on the posterior wall, and present either as an exophytic mass or as a diffuse thickening of the endometrium. The tumor is often friable, gray-white and focally ulcerated. If it is invasive, one may appreciate on cut section either pushing or infiltrating borders in the myometrium. Areas of hemorrhage and necrosis may be seen, and involvement of the cervix may be discerned on gross examination of the specimen.

Microscopic Features

Endometrioid adenocarcinoma

This is the histologic prototype of endometrial adenocarcinomas and represents 75% of them. It is composed of round to tubular-shaped, relatively uniform glands with variable degrees of atypia and mitotic activity; proliferation of malignant glandular cells in a solid growth pattern is present in variable proportions, varying from none to virtually all of the tumor. Endometrioid carcinomas are graded according to their architectural and cytologic (primarily nuclear) features. The FIGO and International Society of Gynecological Pathology (ISGP) histologic grading systems are based primarily on architectural features, evaluating the amount of the tumor comprised of recognizable glandular structures as opposed to the amount of nonsquamous (nonmorular) tumor growing in a solid pattern. A solid proliferation as defined above occupying 5% or less of the tumor represents a Grade I (*Figures 10.1 and 10.2*), 6–50% is a Grade II and more than 50% of solid growth, a Grade III (*Figure 10.3*). If the degree of nuclear atypia appears inappropriate for, or out of proportion to, the architectural pattern

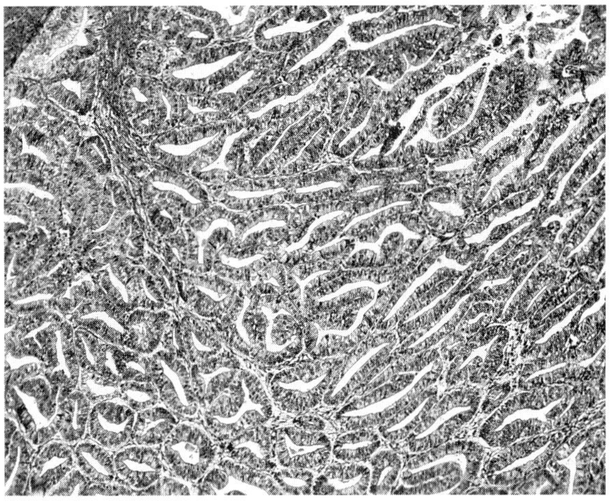

Figure 10.1. FIGO Grade I endometrioid adenocarcinoma; low magnification. The tumor is composed entirely of well-differentiated tubular type glands.

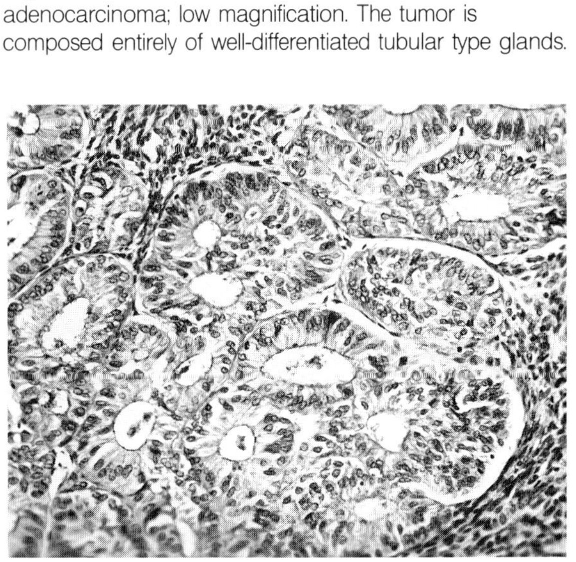

Figure 10.2. FIGO Grade I endometrioid adenocarcinoma; higher magnification. The glands are 'back to back' with no intervening stroma; the nuclei show mild pleomorphism.

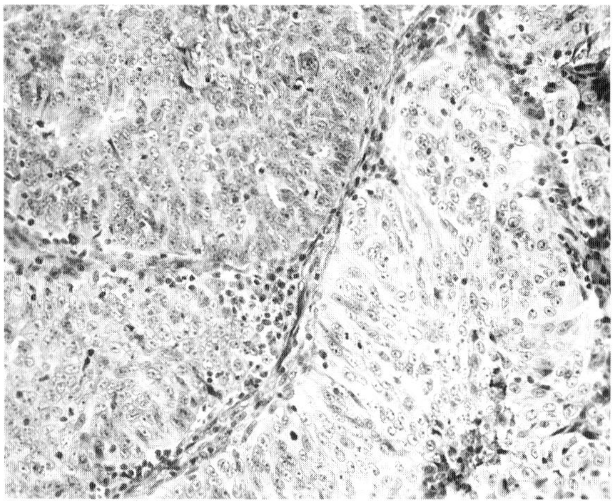

Figure 10.3. FIGO Grade III adenocarcinoma showing a predominantly solid pattern and marked nuclear atypia.

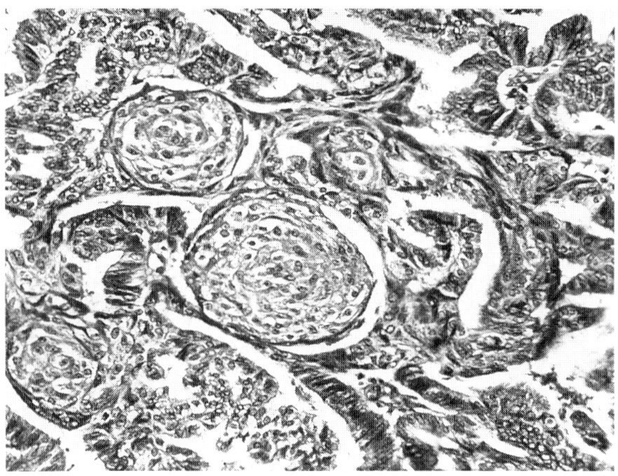

Figure 10.4. Adenocarcinoma with squamous differentiation (adenoacanthoma). The squamous component shows minimal atypia and is present in well-differentiated glands.

both the FIGO and ISGP systems permit raising Grade I and II tumors by one point. Certain subtypes of endometrial carcinoma such as the clear cell carcinoma and the uterine serous papillary carcinoma are generally not graded according to the criteria espoused by the FIGO or the ISGP, but rather by their nuclear grade.

Confusion may arise in the distinction of solid growth of the glandular component from areas of squamous differentiation, a finding which may be encountered in up to 50% of endometrioid carcinomas. Strict criteria, such as the notation of keratinization when present, the presence of intercellular bridges, sharp cellular margins and an eosinophilic or glassy cytoplasm, should be applied to ensure the accurate identification of squamous differentiation. The previously used terms of adenoacanthoma and adenosquamous carcinoma have now been replaced by the more general designation of adenocarcinoma with squamous differentiation. Historically, the term adenoacanthoma was applied to low-grade endometrial adenocarcinomas in which the squamous element was present in the form of cytologically bland, rounded, 'mulberry-like' nodules of immature, metaplastic-appearing squamous cells, often in glandular lumens (*Figure 10.4*); the term adenosquamous carcinoma was restricted to higher-grade tumors in which the squamous component was found either in the form of a well- to moderately-differentiated keratinizing squamous carcinoma or as intimately admixed squamous and glandular elements, not infrequently in a spindled growth pattern (*Figure 10.5*).

The use of the terms adenoacanthoma and adenosquamous carcinoma is currently eschewed. This is because:

- there is usually a good and parallel correlation between the degree of differentiation of both components;
- the prognosis appears to be determined mainly by the glandular elements;
- although adenosquamous carcinoma was previously believed to carry a worse prognosis (Alberhasky *et al.*, 1982), some now argue that the presence of squamous differentiation does not appear to affect the prognosis of endometrioid carcinoma (Zaino *et al.*, 1991). Others, however, dispute this premise.

Mesenchymal types of benign metaplasia, such as osseous or cartilaginous varieties, are rarely encountered and should not be mistaken for the mesenchymal component of a carcinosarcoma (malignant mixed müllerian tumor).

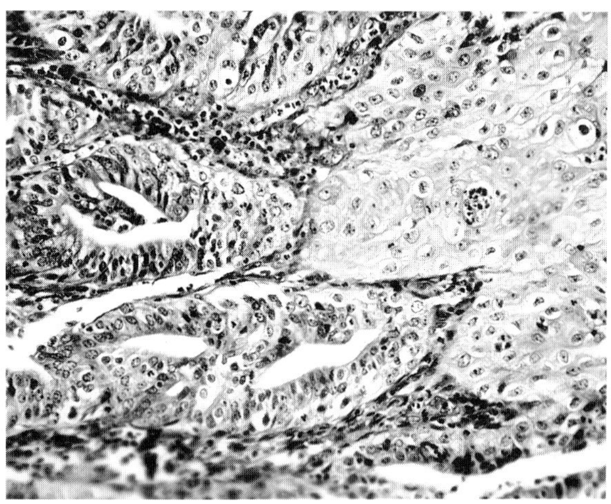

Figure 10.5. Adenocarcinoma with squamous differentiation (adenosquamous carcinoma). The squamous component is similar to a well-differentiated squamous carcinoma, with atypia that parallels the glandular component.

Non-endometrioid types of endometrial carcinoma

Uterine serous papillary carcinoma

So-called uterine serous papillary carcinoma represents 5–10% of all endometrial carcinomas, tends to occur in older women than the usual endometrioid type, and usually arises in a background of endometrial atrophy (Dunton *et al.*, 1991). Microscopically, it closely resembles its ovarian counterpart and may represent one component of a multicentric or 'field effect' type of neoplasia in the müllerian-derived glandular epithelium of the female genital tract. It shows broad fibrovascular cores lined by a budding epithelium with exfoliating clusters (*Figure 10.6*). The cells are small and round, the nuclei are pleomorphic with macronucleoli, and multinucleated giant cells are often present. Mitotic figures and necrosis are frequent and psammoma bodies are seen in about one-third of the cases (*Figure 10.7*).

Uterine serous papillary carcinoma carries a dismal prognosis with a five-year survival of only 40% for Stage I tumors (Hendrickson *et al.*, 1982; Carcangiu and Chambers, 1992); the latter is due, at least in part, to its propensity for deep myometrial and vascular invasion, sometimes accompanied by transtubal spread to involve the tissues of the pelvic peritoneum. The differential diagnosis includes not only the villoglandular variant of endometrioid carcinoma, but also clear cell carcinoma, which frequently coexists with uterine serous papillary carcinoma.

Clear cell carcinoma

Clear cell carcinoma accounts for approximately 5% of all endometrial carcinomas and tends to afflict

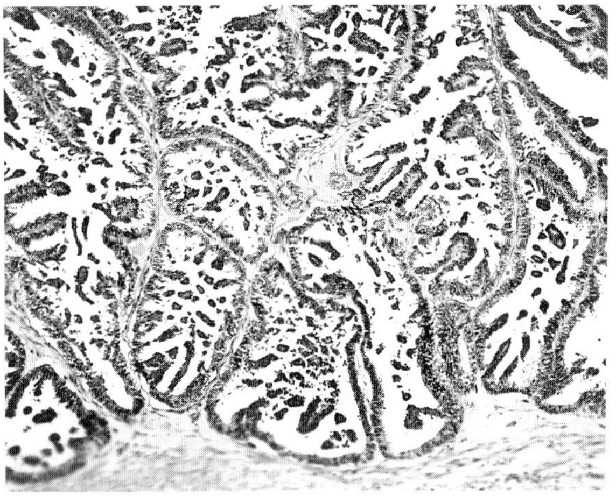

Figure 10.6. Uterine serous papillary carcinoma; low magnification. A complex papillary pattern is accompanied by exfoliated 'pinched off' clusters of malignant cells.

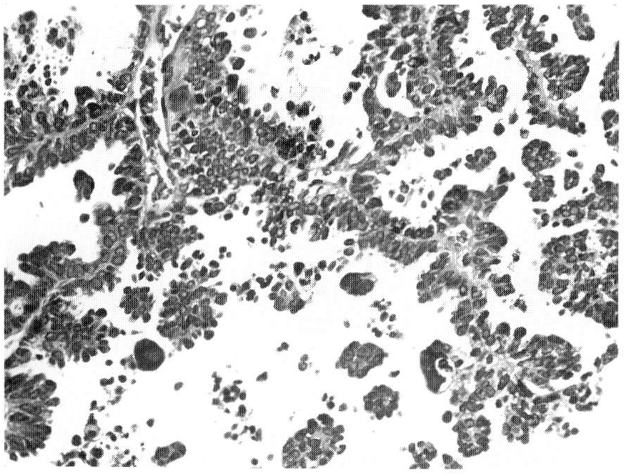

Figure 10.7. Uterine serous papillary carcinoma; high magnification. The cells lining the fibrovascular papillae show marked nuclear atypia. Psammoma bodies are present in the mid and lower portion of the photomicrograph.

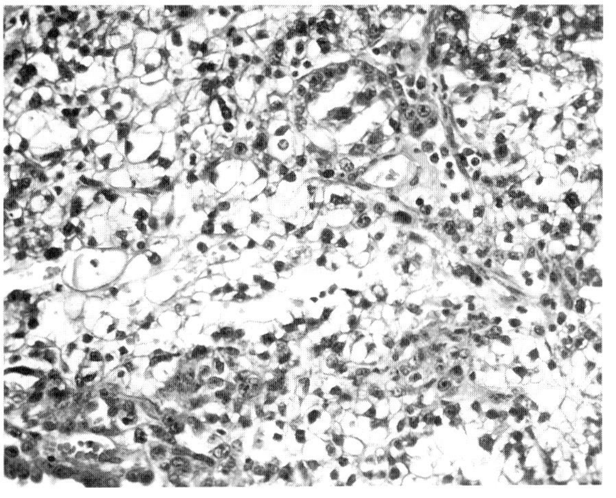

Figure 10.8. Clear cell carcinoma. The tumor is composed of sheets of clear cells that contained glycogen washed out in processing. Nuclei appear relatively bland.

older women. Microscopically, it displays a solid, papillary, tubular or mixed pattern (*Figure 10.8*). It is often composed predominantly of 'hobnail' cells (*Figure 10.9*), admixed with clear cells containing abundant cytoplasmic glycogen; the latter is 'washed out' during processing of the tissue leaving a clear space in the cytoplasm and giving the tumor its characteristic appearance. The nuclei are generally pleomorphic and mitotic figures may be abundant. A dense hyalinized stroma is a frequent finding and is quite a good marker for clear cell carcinoma. Some tumors contain intraluminal rather than intracytoplasmic mucin (Webb and Lagios, 1987).

The differential diagnosis of clear cell carcinoma includes the Arias–Stella reaction of pregnancy, yolk sac tumors and the uterine serous papillary

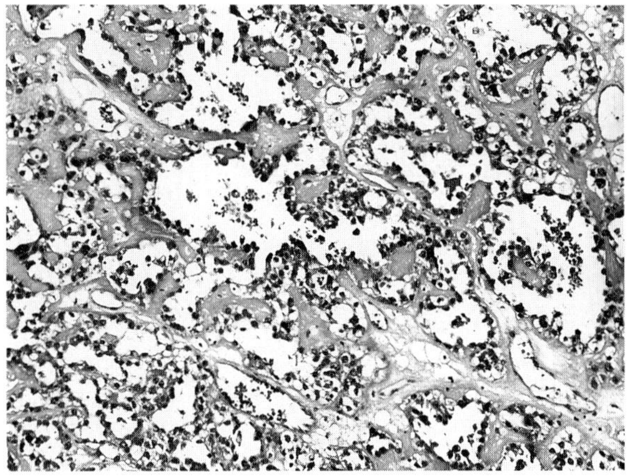

Figure 10.9. Clear cell carcinoma. The papillae in this tumor are lined by 'hobnail' cells and there is prominent stromal hyalinization.

carcinoma. As previously mentioned, the histologic grade of both clear cell and serous papillary carcinomas is based primarily on their nuclear features, obviating a FIGO/ISGP system grade. Both, however, have an equally poor prognosis, the five-year survival of clear cell carcinoma being 44% when all stages are considered (Christopherson *et al.*, 1982). On the other hand, the rare endometrial yolk sac tumors usually affect younger women, contain Schiller–Duval bodies and result in an elevated serum alpha-fetoprotein.

Undifferentiated carcinoma

Undifferentiated carcinomas constitute probably less than 5% of all endometrial carcinomas. The mean age of occurrence is in the mid-sixties. Undifferentiated carcinomas, by definition, display no evidence of glandular or squamous differentiation. Some workers divide them into large and small/intermediate cell types (Abeler *et al.*, 1991). Virtually all undifferentiated carcinomas are positive for cytokeratin, although half of them stain with vimentin and about half of the 'small cell' tumors show positivity for the ubiquitous neural marker neuron-specific enolase. The prognosis for all varieties of undifferentiated carcinomas of the endometrium is comparatively poor with a five-year survival of 58%.

Miscellaneous types of endometrial carcinoma

Pure mucinous carcinoma is a rare, well-differentiated tumor resembling endocervical adenocarcinoma. The periodic acid–Schiff-positive, diastase-resistant intracytoplasmic mucin has a variable distribution in the tumor and in the cytoplasm itself. Stains for mucicarmine and immunostains for carcinoembryonic antigen, however, are strongly positive (Cohen *et al.*, 1982). The differential diagnosis includes mucinous metaplasia arising in a benign endometrium, primary endocervical carcinoma and focal mucinous differentiation in an otherwise typical endometrioid carcinoma. Mucinous carcinoma of the endometrium has a good prognosis because it is usually discovered early; however, stage for stage the behavior is similar to that of the usual endometrioid carcinoma (Ross *et al.*, 1983).

Squamous carcinoma is exceedingly rare in its pure form and to date less than 30 cases have been reported. Before making the diagnosis, a cervical primary obviously has to be excluded. Additionally, the absence of a glandular component, to exclude the more common endometrioid adenocarcinoma with squamous differentiation, has to be proven by extensive tumor sampling. Pure squamous carcinomas can, at times, be very well differentiated and difficult to recognize in an endometrial curetting. Squamous carcinoma of the endometrium is commonly associated with chronic inflammation, cervical stenosis and pyometra. An established precursor is ichthyosis uteri; the latter, now a rare condition, often arose secondary to either instillation of steam or formalin as a means of treatment of chronic endometritis and is manifested by replacement of the endometrium by metaplastic squamous epithelium. Pure squamous carcinoma carries a poor prognosis (Bibro *et al.*, 1980).

Secretory carcinoma is usually encountered as a very well-differentiated adenocarcinoma that resembles the normal secretory endometrium because of the presence of numerous subnuclear glycogen vacuoles (*Figure 10.10*). It is rarely seen in its pure form and carries a good prognosis. Ciliated cell carcinoma is very uncommon, has a good prognosis and is composed predominantly of ciliated cells (Hendrickson and Kempson, 1983). Villo-

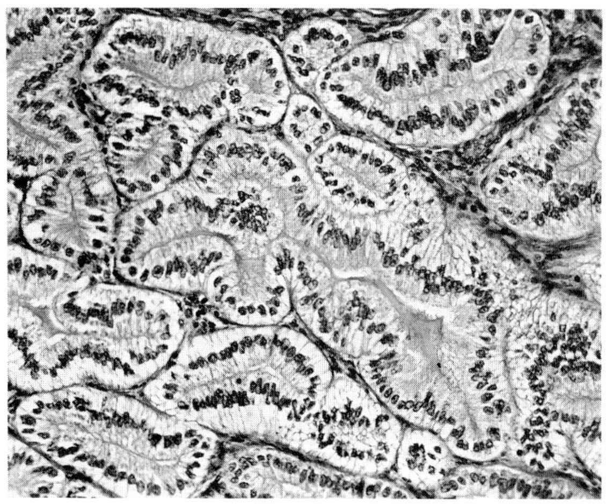

Figure 10.10. Secretory carcinoma. A variant of well-differentiated endometrioid carcinoma that resembles a day 17 secretory endometrium.

glandular or papillary carcinoma is composed of either short blunt papillae or long, finger-like filigree-type fibrovascular cores, usually lined by cells showing a minimal degree of cytologic atypia. It is important to distinguish this variant, which carries a good prognosis, from the much more aggressive uterine serous papillary carcinoma (Chen *et al.*, 1985), although a recent study (Ambros *et al.*, 1994) suggests that the behavior may be intermediate between the classic endometrioid type and the serous papillary type.

So-called glassy cell carcinoma is currently thought to be a poorly differentiated variant of adenosquamous carcinoma; although usually found in the cervix, it may very rarely arise in the endometrium. The cells have copious eosinophilic or amphophilic cytoplasm with a pronounced glassy or 'ground glass' appearance with refractile cell borders. As in the cervix, endometrial glassy cell carcinoma is a poorly-differentiated neoplasm that carries a poor prognosis (Hachisuga *et al.*, 1990).

Choriocarcinoma has been rarely found as a primary tumor of the endometrium in postmenopausal women. Current thinking supports its origin from extragonadal germ cell differentiation within somatic cells rather than from residual gestational trophoblastic disease or from aberrant germ cells misplaced in embryogenesis. The tumor exhibits the typical biphasic appearance of choriocarcinoma elsewhere and serum human chorionic gonadotropin is usually elevated. In contrast to gestational choriocarcinoma, this tumor does not respond well to chemotherapeutic intervention and behaves aggressively. Yolk sac tumors may also arise by a similar mechanism from the endometrium.

Uterine Sarcomas

Introduction

Malignant mesenchymal tumors of the uterine corpus may be either pure monophasic neoplasms or biphasic when admixed with epithelial elements. They are rare and represent less than 5% of all malignant tumors of the uterine corpus. In general, malignant mesenchymal tumors tend to occur in older women. Their clinical presentation is similar to that of endometrial carcinoma; however, no clear relationship has been found with the risk factors usually associated with the latter.

Leiomyosarcoma and Atypical Smooth Muscle Tumors

Leiomyosarcoma is the most frequently encountered type of pure uterine sarcoma; although representing about one-third of them, it still accounts for only slightly more than 1% of all uterine malignancies. Virtually all leiomyosarcomas arise *de novo* and only very rarely have been proved to originate in a preexisting leiomyoma.

Clinical Features

Leiomyosarcomas occur at a mean age of 52 years, at least a decade later than their benign counterpart, the leiomyoma. In a postmenopausal woman, a rapid increase in the size of a presumed leiomyoma should at least raise the suspicion of leiomyosarcoma. The most common presenting symptoms are vaginal bleeding, lower abdominal pain and/or an abdominal mass. Most often, however, the diagnosis is made after hysterectomy.

Gross Features

In 50–75% of cases, a leiomyosarcoma presents as a solitary, intramural mass, occasionally bulging into the endometrial cavity and often involving the cervix. The tumor is soft, fleshy and gray-yellow to pink, with areas of hemorrhage and necrosis. In contrast to the associated leiomyomas, which are frequently present, the margins of a leiomyosarcoma are poorly defined.

Microscopic Features

Leiomyosarcomas are highly cellular tumors made of whorls and interlacing bundles of spindle cells with elongated hyperchromatic nuclei displaying prominent nucleoli (*Figure 10.11*). Multinucleated and osteoclast-like giant cells are seen in about

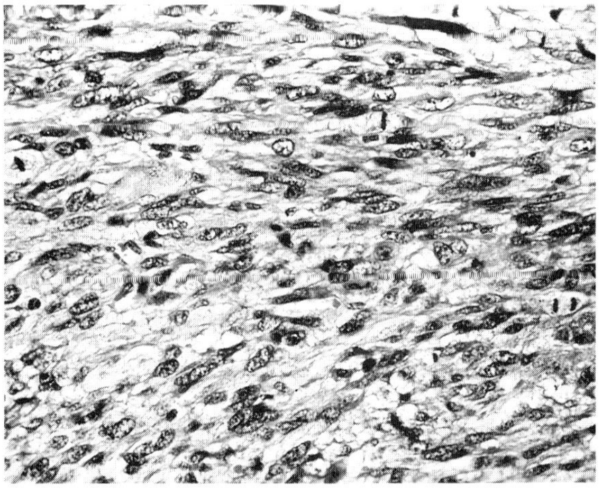

Figure 10.11. Leiomyosarcoma. There is significant nuclear atypia along with numerous mitotic figures and hypercellularity.

one-half of them. Invasion of the surrounding myometrium is common and extension beyond the uterus is determinant of malignancy. Although most workers would agree that the usual leiomyosarcoma does not present a diagnostic dilemma, there has been considerable controversy engendered over the past two decades concerning the histopathologic criteria (particularly the mitotic index) that are required for the diagnosis of malignancy in atypical uterine smooth muscle tumors. In regard to the latter, the pathologist should use caution in his/her pathologic examination and count only indisputable mitotic figures on thinly-sectioned, well-fixed and well-stained slides. The clinical setting must also be taken into account; for example, the pathologist should be wary of making a diagnosis of leiomyosarcoma in a grossly unremarkable and particularly small, well-circumscribed uterine tumor.

Most typical leiomyosarcomas exhibit an increased mitotic rate and the numerical definition of a malignant mitotic index has sparked considerable discussion. Some favor the diagnosis of leiomyosarcoma for any atypical smooth tumor exhibiting more than five mitoses per ten high power fields (HPF), whereas most others argue for a figure of ten mitoses or greater per ten HPF to define malignancy. Although the latter mitotic index as well as the aforementioned marked cellularity and nuclear atypia are present in about three-quarters of leiomyosarcomas, the remainder of them may be more problematic to classify. The problem with using mitotic index alone is exemplified by a type of smooth muscle neoplasm that often occurs in younger women and has been designated as a 'mitotically active leiomyoma,' or 'leiomyoma with increased mitotic index'; such tumors are well circumscribed, show minimal to no nuclear atypia and necrosis, but have a prodigious mitotic rate, sometimes up to 20 mitoses per ten HPF (Perrone and Dehner, 1988). Abnormal mitotic figures, a feature commonly seen in malignant smooth muscle tumors, are not seen. Virtually all of the mitotically active leiomyomas manifest a benign biologic behavior.

Table 10.5. Smooth muscle tumors of uncertain malignant potential (from Kempson and Hendrickson, 1988).

Usual histologic appearance with
- Cytologic atypia and 2–5 MF/10 HPF
- Hypercellularity, no atypia and 5–10 MF/10 HPF
- 10–15 MF/10 HPF without hypercellularity or atypia
- Infiltrating margins and 5–9 MF/10 HPF
- Any abnormal mitotic figure or necrosis

Epithelioid or bizarre pattern with 2–5 MF/10 HPF
Intravenous leiomyomatosis with 2–5 MF/10 HPF
Parasitic leiomyoma with 5–9 MF/10 HPF

MF, mitotic figure; HPF, high power field.

Recently, Bell *et al.* (1994) have studied a large series of problematic smooth muscle tumors with clinical follow-up and have suggested that the following morphologic features be evaluated in such tumors: the degree of cytologic atypia (mild, moderate, severe); the mitotic index; and the presence or absence of coagulative tumor cell necrosis. Evaluating the aforementioned microscopic features, they divided uterine smooth muscle neoplasms into:

- ordinary leiomyoma;
- leiomyomas with increased mitotic index;
- atypical leiomyoma with low risk of recurrence;
- smooth muscle tumor of low malignant potential;
- leiomyosarcoma.

Bell *et al.* (1994) emphasized the importance of coagulative tumor cell necrosis as an important predictor of clinical outcome. They placed those tumors with less than ten mitotic figures per ten HPF and either no or only mild cytologic atypia, but with coagulative cell necrosis, into the low malignant potential category.

Some unusual variants should be kept in mind, such as myxoid leiomyosarcoma, which can be easily misdiagnosed. Indeed, because of the myxoid background, the tumor is less cellular and therefore the mitotic count is often artificially decreased (King *et al.*, 1982). Metastasizing leiomyoma is a rarely described entity that usually presents many years after operative procedures (Abell and Little, 1975). It occurs in the lungs, pelvic soft tissues, lymph nodes, mesentery and mediastinum. The tumors have a bland appearance and some think that they could in fact be low-grade leiomyosarcomas that were originally misdiagnosed (Peters *et al.*, 1994).

Prognosis

Stage is the most important prognostic factor and, at the time of diagnosis, most leiomyosarcomas have spread beyond the uterus. Poor prognosis is also associated with vascular invasion, postmenopausal status, anaplasia and a high mitotic index, although the latter two are not unanimously agreed upon. The five-year survival varies from 25–40% and reaches 40–70% when only Stage I and II tumors are considered. Most recurrences occur within two years of the initial diagnosis. Metastases are most common in the pelvis, and later in the course of the disease, in the lungs, liver and bones.

Endometrial Stromal Sarcoma

This tumor was first described in 1908 and better characterized in 1965 by Norris and Taylor. It is the rarest primary neoplasm of the uterine cavity and in most large series represents less than 10% of uterine sarcomas. Endometrial stromal tumors in general are divided into benign and malignant variants, the former represented by so called endometrial stromal nodules and the latter by low-grade endometrial stromal sarcomas and high-grade stromal sarcomas.

Clinical features

Endometrial stromal tumors in general affect younger women than other uterine malignancies; studies have demonstrated the mean age to range from 42–53 years and approximately half occur in premenopausal patients (Chang *et al.*, 1990). Symptoms include vaginal bleeding or worsening menorrhagia accompanied by abdominal pain. On palpation, the uterus is enlarged with irregular contours. Occasionally, the tumor may be polypoid and protrude through the cervical os. Rarely, the presentation is that of a pelvic or pulmonary metastasis or, in cases of high-grade sarcoma, the tumor may be rarely detected by a cervicovaginal Pap smear. Commonly, however, the lesion is first detected on an endometrial curettage. Although the differential diagnosis in such cases is between an endometrial stromal nodule and a low-grade stromal sarcoma, the final diagnosis in most cases can only be made on hysterectomy following examination of the margins with the surrounding endomyometrium.

Gross features

Endometrial stromal nodules appear well circumscribed whereas low-grade stromal sarcomas have infiltrative margins with the surrounding endomyometrium. Although the latter sometimes may appear grossly to be well circumscribed, half of them will show diffuse myometrial invasion by worm-like masses or nodules and roughly one-third will have gross extrauterine extension. Another pattern of intramural growth is that of diffuse myometrial thickening.

The component of the tumor found within the endometrium is tan, soft, smooth-surfaced and polypoid, and on cut section shows areas of hemorrhage, necrosis and cystic degeneration.

High-grade stromal sarcomas are usually large fleshy masses bulging into the endometrial cavity accompanied by multiple masses infiltrating the myometrium.

Microscopic features

Endometrial stromal nodules and low-grade endometrial stromal sarcomas have an identical histologic appearance and closely resemble normal proliferative endometrial stroma. Cytologic atypia is minimal. Mitotic figures are usually less than three per ten HPF although counts of more than ten per ten HPF have been reported (Fekete and Vellios, 1984), and abnormal mitotic figures and necrosis are absent. The sole difference between these two entities is, as already mentioned, the presence of myometrial invasion in the sarcoma. A characteristic histologic feature of the latter is the prominence of small blood vessels resembling spiral arterioles (*Figure 10.12*). Areas of hyalinization and thick collagen bands are also common.

Vascular invasion is frequent in low-grade stromal sarcoma and is responsible for its previous designation as endolymphatic stromal myosis (*Figure 10.13*). Approximately 20% of them show epithelial-type differentiation in the form of trabeculae, mesothelial-like structures or glands. Smooth muscle differentiation may also be present.

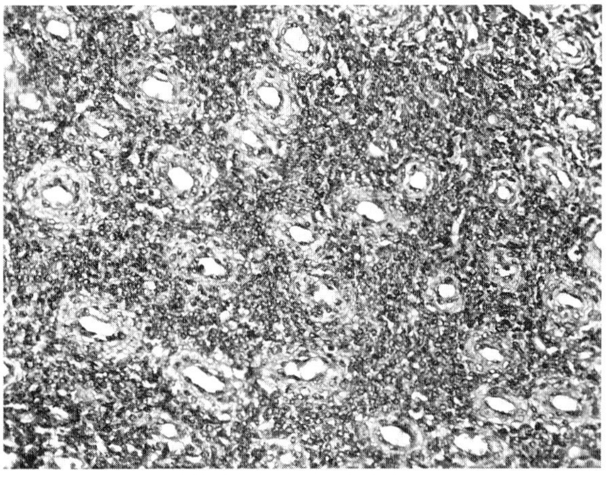

Figure 10.12. Low-grade endometrial stromal sarcoma; high magnification. Characteristic 'spiral arteriole-like' blood vessels are present.

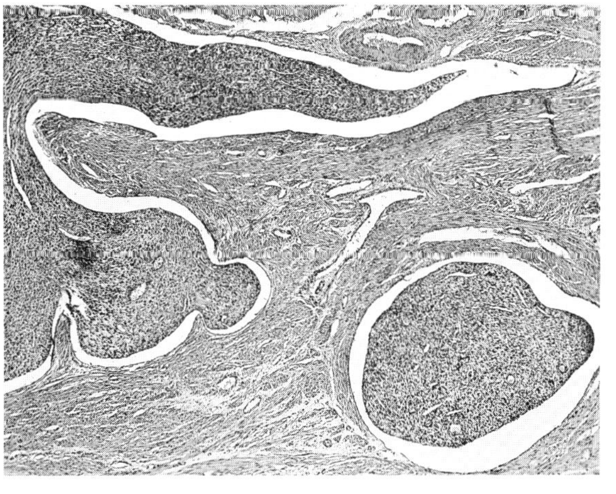

Figure 10.13. Low-grade stromal sarcoma. Prominent ectatic lymphatic vessels are full of sarcoma that grows in an invasive 'worm-like' fashion.

High-grade stromal sarcoma may resemble endometrial stroma to some extent, but displays a much higher degree of cytologic atypia than the low-grade variant; the mitotic index is typically more than 20 mitotic figures per ten HPF in the most active areas. The cells have abundant cytoplasm, vesicular nuclei with clumped chromatin and prominent nucleoli. Bizarre multinucleated cells and abnormal mitotic figures may be seen. Other features that separate it from the low-grade stromal sarcoma are the less prominent vasculature and a more destructive pattern of myometrial invasion.

Histopathologic classification of some endometrial stromal tumors may be difficult. In these cases, flow cytometry or hormone receptor assays may prove of some help in the future (Dunton *et al.*, 1990; El–Naggar *et al.*, 1991). Even though only a few cases have been examined, low-grade tumors have almost always been diploid, whereas flow cytometric results have been variable in high-grade stromal neoplasms. Estrogen and progesterone receptors are often positive in the former and almost always negative in the latter.

Immunohistochemistry may be used to exclude other types of neoplasms. Stains for vimentin in low-grade stromal sarcomas are usually positive and those for epithelial membrane antigen to date have always been negative. Other stains including those for desmin and cytokeratin, however, show variable results and are of little help (Farhood and Abrams, 1991; Binder *et al.*, 1991).

Prognosis

Stage appears to be the most significant prognostic factor. The long-term survival is greater than 80% for Stage I low-grade stromal sarcoma, but drops to 40–50% in more advanced stages; in high-grade stromal sarcoma long-term survival ranges from 0–50% (Fekete and Vellios, 1984; Chang *et al.*, 1990). Overall, low-grade sarcomas tend to have an indolent course marked by local recurrences or metastases appearing many years after diagnosis whereas high-grade stromal neoplasms are rapidly progressive with early recurrence and death.

Controversial viewpoints regarding the classification and prognostic factors of endometrial stromal sarcomas have recently emerged. Evans (1982) divides stromal tumors in two groups: one includes the tumors closely resembling endometrial stroma, the second group comprises less well-differentiated neoplasms similar to the stromal component of carcinosarcoma. Chang *et al.* (1990) agrees with this point of view and is also of the opinion that, at least for Stage I tumors, mitotic activity and cytologic atypicality are not reliably predictive of recurrence. Others prefer to classify these tumors into three categories: low-grade, high-grade and undifferentiated endometrial stromal neoplasms, the latter two being more likely to recur and behave aggressively.

Combined Smooth Muscle–Stromal Tumors

In these tumors, both smooth muscle and stromal components are equally represented. Their biologic behavior is poorly documented, but is likely to be malignant if the stromal element predominates and if the margin is infiltrative. According to Hendrickson and Kempson (1983), they should be regarded as of stromal origin and treated as such if their histogenesis is in any doubt.

Mixed Epithelial–Mesenchymal Tumors

Adenosarcoma

Adenosarcoma was first described in 1974 by Clement and Scully. It is considerably more frequent than its benign counterpart, the adenofibroma. The mean age of occurrence is lower than that for carcinosarcomas. Although adenosarcoma more commonly arises in the endometrium, it can also originate in the cervix, the fallopian tube, the ovary and paraovarian tissues. Extrauterine primaries appear to affect younger patients and behave more aggressively (Clement and Scully, 1978, 1990).

Gross features

Adenosarcomas present as solitary, polypoid, fleshy masses, usually arising from the fundus of the uterus. On cut section the presence of the dilated cystic glands that are characteristically present within the tumor may sometimes be appreciated.

Microscopic features

Adenosarcomas are comprised of intimately admixed malignant stromal elements, and benign, but atypical, epithelial elements. They exhibit an architecture reminiscent of the phyllodes tumor of the breast, characterized by broad leaf-like papillary processes projecting onto the surface. The epithelial component is typically represented by either inactive or proliferative-type glands; however, they sometimes display secretory changes or exhibit mucinous, squamous, serous or clear cell metaplasia. A mild to moderate degree of cytologic atypia is commonly seen; however, in some cases the glands may become severely atypical. The latter is more frequently seen as a focal phenomenon and the overall appearance is nowhere near that of the carcinosarcoma in which the glands and stroma are both clearly and diffusely malignant.

The mesenchymal element is generally homologous, composed of cell types indigenous to the endomyometrium (fibrosarcoma, stromal sarcoma or leiomyosarcoma). The stroma tends to form concentric hypercellular rings around the glands ('periglandular cuffing') (*Figure 10.14*). Cellular atypia of both the glandular and stromal elements may be variable and extensive sampling of the tumor may be necessary to ensure that the most atypical areas are represented. In the most mitotically active foci, there are often more than four mitotic figures per ten HPF (*Figure 10.15*). Hemorrhage, necrosis, fibrosis, hyalinization and foam cells may be seen. Sex cord-like epithelial formations have been described within adenosarcomas and about one-quarter of them contain heterologous elements, most commonly in the form of striated muscle, but also of cartilage or fat (Clement and Scully, 1989a).

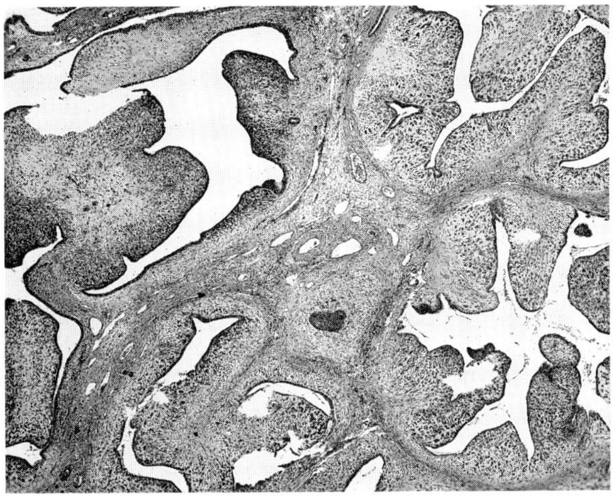

Figure 10.14. Adenosarcoma; low magnification. The appearance is reminscent of phyllodes tumor of the breast. The cleft-like spaces show characteristic periglandular cuffing by hypercellular stroma.

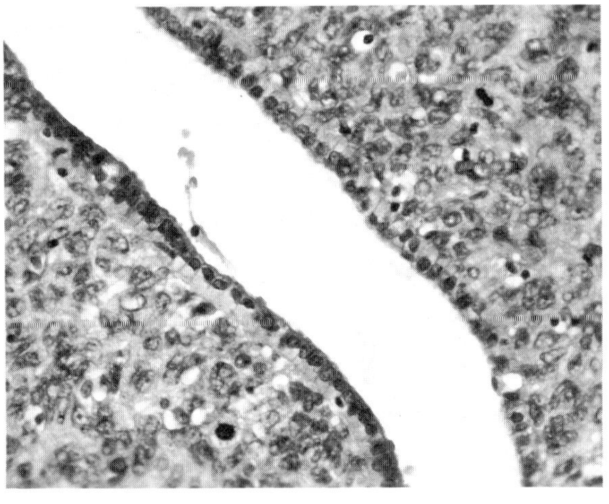

Figure 10.15. Adenosarcoma; high magnification. The atypical, but benign, glandular epithelium is surrounded by hypercellular and mitotically active low-grade sarcomatous stroma.

Some adenosarcomas may undergo sarcomatous overgrowth; the latter is characterized by having at least one-quarter of the tumor composed solely of sarcoma (Clement and Scully, 1989b).

Prognosis

Adenosarcoma tends to be less aggressive than carcinosarcoma. Recurrences often occur at an interval of more than five years, predominantly in the vagina, pelvis and abdominal cavity. Only 5% will eventually metastasize, and then usually the mesenchymal component. Clinicopathologic indicators of poor prognosis are the presence of myometrial invasion, seen in about one-quarter of cases; extrauterine spread; necrosis; a high mitotic count; and sarcomatous overgrowth (Kaku *et al.*, 1992). The last feature clearly has an adverse effect on prognosis, with recurrence rates reaching 44–70% in comparison to 14–25% in its absence. The presence of heterologous elements has a yet undetermined prognostic significance.

Carcinosarcoma

The term carcinosarcoma was used previously to designate only homologous tumors but has now been expanded to include those biphasic tumors with heterologous elements. Although it is the most common uterine sarcoma, it still represents only 2–3% of all malignancies of the uterine corpus.

Clinical features

Carcinosarcoma predominantly affects older and usually perimenopausal women, with a mean age of 65 years. Its symptoms include vaginal bleeding, abdominal pain and distension, and urinary symptoms due to extrauterine spread. On inspection of the vaginal vault, the tumor commonly protrudes through the cervical os. As is true with pure uterine sarcomas, there appears to be no clear relationship with the risk factors implicated in endometrial carcinoma. There is, however, a well-documented association with a history of previous radiation in the case of carcinosarcoma (Norris and Taylor, 1965).

Gross features

Carcinosarcoma usually presents as a large, solitary, polypoid mass that may be sessile or pedunculated. It expands into the endometrial cavity and may eventually extend through the endocervical canal to protrude through the external cervical os. The cut surface of a carcinosarcoma is firm to fleshy and has a variegated appearance secondary to the presence of hemorrhage and necrosis. On cut section, hard gritty areas may reflect the presence of heterologous elements such as cartilage or bone.

Microscopic features

A carcinosarcoma is characterized by an intimate admixture of malignant epithelial and mesenchymal components. One should keep in mind, however, that the two components are not necessarily present in endometrial curettings. The epithelial component is typically of the endometrioid type and moderately to poorly differentiated; it can, however, show all the varied histopathologic patterns encountered in endometrial carcinoma, including serous papillary, clear cell and squamous differentiation. The mesenchymal element is generally a high-grade sarcoma of no specific histologic type, but fibrous, stromal and smooth muscle differentiation may be recognized (*Figure 10.16*). Heterologous elements are present in about half of the cases, usually found in the less well-differentiated part of the tumor. In decreasing order of frequency, they are represented by malignant striated muscle (*Figure 10.17*), cartilage, bone or fat (*Figures 10.17 and 10.18*). Since the benign counterpart of such elements can very rarely be seen in endometrial carcinoma, that possibility should be excluded before making the diagnosis of carcinosarcoma.

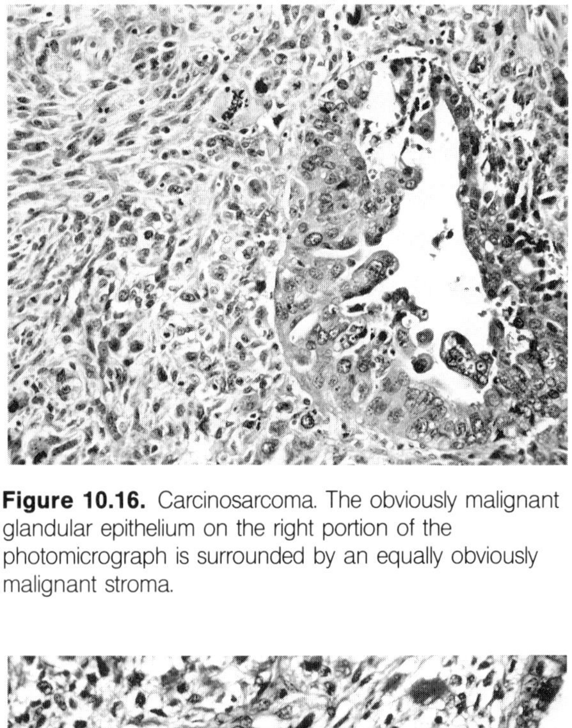

Figure 10.16. Carcinosarcoma. The obviously malignant glandular epithelium on the right portion of the photomicrograph is surrounded by an equally obviously malignant stroma.

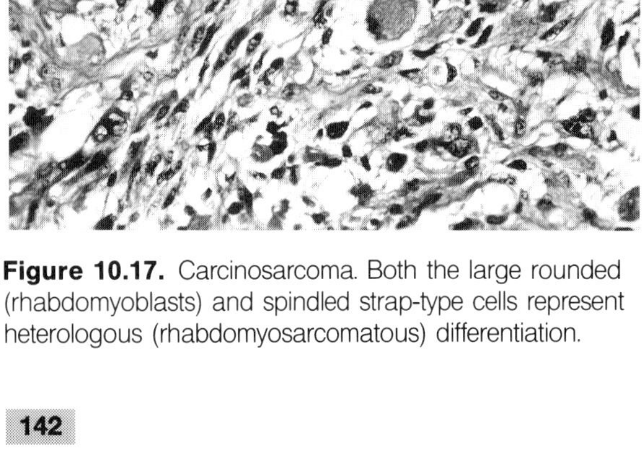

Figure 10.17. Carcinosarcoma. Both the large rounded (rhabdomyoblasts) and spindled strap-type cells represent heterologous (rhabdomyosarcomatous) differentiation.

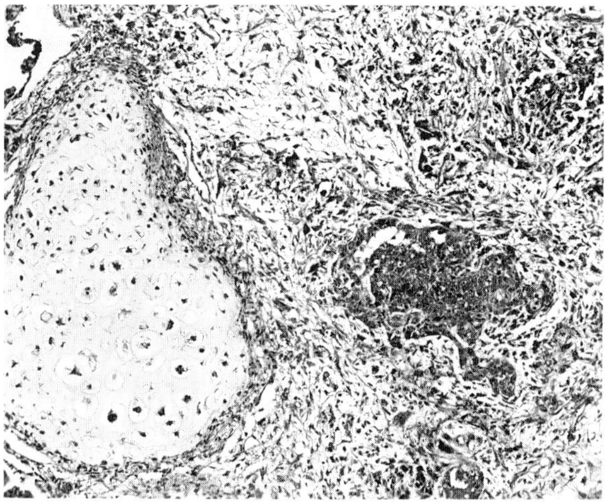

Figure 10.18. Carcinosarcoma with heterologous elements ('malignant mixed müllerian tumor'). Malignant cartilage in the left portion of the photomicrograph merges with surrounding spindled sarcoma and an island of poorly-differentiated carcinoma.

About one-quarter of carcinosarcomas are limited to the endometrium and rarely are confined to an endometrial polyp. Vascular invasion by the epithelial component is common and is often reflected in the histologic appearance of metastases (Silverberg *et al.*, 1990).

Pathogenesis

Several different theories have been advanced to explain the pathogenesis of carcinosarcoma. Such have included the possibility of a 'collision tumor' in which the epithelial and mesenchymal malignancies develop separately, but intermingle in a random growth pattern. Other workers have favored a 'composition tumor' in which the neoplastic component is a carcinoma and the mesenchymal one is atypical, but benign and reactive, mesenchyme. Some workers favor the theory of a 'combination tumor' in which both the epithelial and mesenchymal elements derive from a common stem cell (Silverberg *et al.*, 1990). Most recent studies favor the latter, which is supported by the fact that immunohistochemical stains for cytokeratin and epithelial membrane antigen are frequently positive in the mesenchymal component (DeBrito *et al.*, 1993). For that reason, some current investigators prefer to classify most carcinosarcomas as a type of metaplastic carcinoma.

Prognosis

The most important clinicopathologic factors in the prediction of biologic behavior are the stage of the tumor and the depth of myometrial invasion. The five-year survival in early stage disease is 40–50% compared to 25–30% for patients with more advanced disease (Schweizer *et al.*, 1990). Pelvic lymph node metastases are present in 17% of patients with carcinosarcoma that grossly appears to be confined to the uterus (Silverberg *et al.*, 1990). Other poor risk factors are the finding of vascular space invasion, extension to the cervix and positive peritoneal cytology.

The biologic behavior of the tumor appears to depend largely, if not solely, on the histologic type and grade of the carcinomatous component of the tumor; the histologic appearance of the mesenchymal component does not apparently influence the risk of metastasis or survival. An increased risk of metastasis or recurrence is also associated with factors such as large size, deep myometrial invasion, extrauterine spread or extension to the cervix and vascular space invasion (Schweizer *et al.*, 1990).

Miscellaneous Mesenchymal Tumors

Pure homologous and heterologous sarcomas, which lack the epithelial component of carcinosarcoma, occur rarely in the uterus (even in the endometrium, in which case they often have no resemblance to endometrial stroma). Among pure heterologous sarcomas, rhabdomyosarcoma is the most frequently encountered (Podczaski *et al.*, 1990), followed by chondrosarcoma, osteosarcoma and liposarcoma. Some tumors are comprised of an admixture of several of these.

Primitive neuroectodermal tumors are rare tumors that may affect all ages, but tend to occur predominantly in postmenopausal women (Daya *et al.*, 1992). They are soft, fleshy, gray-white, polypoid masses that originate in the endometrium and invade the myometrium. On microscopic examination, they are composed of small round cells with oval to round hyperchromatic nuclei. Foci of glial differentiation, Homer–Wright pseudorosettes and perivascular ependymal-type rosettes may be seen. The tumor often exhibits positive staining for such neural markers as neuron-specific enolase, glial fibrillary acidic protein, chromogranin and S100. Their natural history has not been well studied due to their rarity and the few numbers of them that have been reported; however, in other organ sites such neoplasms tend to have an aggressive biologic behavior.

Other rare tumors such as angiosarcomas (Quinones *et al.*, 1991) and primary lymphomas (Ferry and Young, 1991) can also occur in the uterus.

Summary of Core Information

- According to the new WHO classification, approximately one-quarter to one-third of women with atypical hyperplasia, complex type, progresses to adenocarcinoma.
- There are two broad types of endometrial carcinomas: one associated with hyperestrinism, endometrial hyperplasia, young age and good prognosis; the other, non-hormonally influenced, is associated with endometrial atrophy, older age and poor prognosis.
- The three main prognostically important and pathologically determined features in endometrial carcinoma are the FIGO histologic grade of the tumor, the depth of myometrial invasion and the presence of endocervical invasion.
- For adenocarcinomas with squamous differentiation, the prognosis appears to be related to the degree of differentiation of the glandular element rather than to that of the squamous element.
- Matched stage for stage and grade for grade, younger women with endometrial adenocarcinoma have a better prognosis than older women.
- Uterine serous papillary carcinoma is a high-grade tumor with a poor prognosis, probably related to its propensity for deep myometrial and vascular invasion and transtubal spread to the peritoneal surfaces.
- Multiple histopathologic criteria including the mitotic index, the degree of cytologic atypia, and the presence of tumor cell necrosis, are evaluated in determining the benign or malignant categorization of smooth muscle tumors.
- Most smooth muscle tumors are readily categorized as overtly benign or malignant; however, some are in the borderline arena and are best classified as of uncertain malignant potential.
- Adenosarcomas tend to occur in younger women than carcinosarcomas and are less aggressive with a much better prognosis.
- Carcinosarcomas are the most common uterine sarcoma and often present as a polypoid mass protruding from the cervical os.
- The biologic behavior of carcinosarcomas appears to depend largely on the depth of myometrial invasion and the stage of the tumor.

References

■ Abeler VM, Kjorstad KE & Berle E (1992) Carcinoma of the endometrium in Norway: a histopathological and prognostic survey of a total population. *Int. J. Gynecol. Cancer* **2:** 9–22.

Abeler VM, Kjorstad KE & Nesland JM (1991) Undifferentiated carcinoma of the endometrium. *Cancer* **68:** 98–105.

Abell MR & Little ER (1975) Benign metastasizing uterine leiomyoma: multiple lymph nodal metastases. *Cancer* **36:** 2206–2213.

Alberhasky RC, Connelly PJ & Christopherson WM (1982) Carcinoma of the endometrium. Mixed adenosquamous carcinoma. A clinicopathological study of 68 cases with long term follow-up. *Am. J. Clin. Pathol.* **77:** 655–664.

Ambros RA, Ballouk F, Maljetano HJ *et al.* (1994) Significance of papillary (villoglandular) differentiation in endometrioid carcinoma of the uterus. *Am. J. Surg. Pathol.* **18(6):** 569–575.

Ambros RA & Kurman RJ (1992) Combined assessment of vascular and myometrial invasion as a model to predict prognosis in Stage I endometrioid adenocarcinoma of the uterine corpus. *Cancer* **69:** 1424–1431.

Ausems WE, VanderKamp JK & Baak JAP (1985) Nuclear morphometry in the determination of the prognosis of marked atypical endometrial hyperplasia. *Int. J. Gynecol. Pathol.* **4:** 180–185.

Austin DF & Rose KM (1982) The decreasing incidence of endometrial cancer: public health implications. *Am. J. Public Health* **72:** 65–68.

■ Bell WS, Kempson LR & Hendrickson RM (1994) Problematic uterine smooth muscle neoplasms. *Am. J. Surg. Pathol.* **18(6):** 535–558.

Bibro MC, Kapp DS, LiVolsi VA *et al.* (1980) Squamous carcinoma of the endometrium with ultrastructural observations and review of the literature. *Gynecol. Oncol.* **10:** 217–223.

Binder SW, Neiberg RK, Cheng L *et al.* (1991) Histologic and immunohistochemical analysis of nine endometrial stromal tumors: an unexpected high frequency of keratin protein positivity. *Int. J. Gynecol. Pathol.* **10:** 191–197.

Bistoletti P & Hjerpe A (1993) Routine use of endometrial cytology in clinical practice. *Acta Cytol.* **37(6):** 867–870.

Bokhman J (1983) Two pathogenetic types of endometrial carcinoma. *Gynecol. Oncol.* **15:** 10–17.

Boronow RC, Morrow CP, Creasman WT *et al.* (1984) Surgical staging in endometrial cancer and clinical pathologic findings of a prospective study. *Obstet. Gynecol.* **63:** 825–832.

Cancer and Steroid Hormone Study of the Centers for Disease Control and the National Institute of Child Health and Human Development (1987) Combination oral contraceptive use and the risk of endometrial cancer. *JAMA* **257:** 796–800.

Carcangiu ML & Chambers JT (1992) Uterine papillary serous carcinoma: a study of 108 cases with emphasis on the prognostic significance of associated endometrioid carcinoma, absence of invasion and concomitant ovarian carcinoma. *Gynecol. Oncol.* **47:** 298–305.

Chang LK, Crabtree SG, Lim–Tan KS *et al.* (1990) Primary uterine endometrial stromal neoplasms. *Am. J. Surg. Pathol.* **14(5):** 415–438.

Chen J, Trost DC & Wilkinson EG (1985) Endometrial papillary adenocarcinomas: two clinicopathologic types. *Int. J. Gynecol. Pathol.* **4:** 279–285.

Christopherson WM, Alberhasky RC & Connelly PJ (1982) Carcinoma of the endometrium I. A clinicopathologic study of clear-cell carcinoma and secretory carcinoma. *Cancer* **49:** 1511–1523.

Clement PB & Scully RE (1974) Müllerian adenosarcoma of the uterus. A clinicopathologic analysis of ten cases of a distinctive type of müllerian mixed tumor. *Cancer* **34:** 1138–1149.

Clement PB & Scully RE (1978) Extrauterine mesodermal (müllerian) adenosarcoma: a clinicopathologic analysis of five cases. *Am. J. Clin. Pathol.* **69:** 276–283.

Clement PB & Scully RE (1989a) Müllerian adenosarcomas of the uterus with sex cord-like elements: a clinicopathologic analysis of eight cases. *Am. J. Clin. Pathol.* **91:** 664–672.

Clement PB & Scully RE (1989b) Müllerian adenosarcoma of the uterus with sarcomatous overgrowth: a clinicopathologic analysis of 10 cases. *Am. J. Surg. Pathol.* **13:** 28–38.

Clement PB & Scully RE (1990) Müllerian adenosarcoma of the uterus: a clinicopathologic analysis of 100 cases with a review of the literature. *Hum. Pathol.* **21:** 363–381.

Cohen C, Shulman G & Budgeon LR (1982) Endocervical and endometrial adenocarcinoma, an immunoperoxidase and histochemical study. *Am. J. Surg. Pathol.* **6:** 151.

Cramer GH & Osborne RJ (1981) Endometrial neoplasia: screening the high risk patient. *Am. J. Obstet. Gynecol.* **139:** 285–288.

Creasman WT, DiSaiai PJ, Blessing JA *et al.* (1981) Prognostic significance of peritoneal cytology in patients with endometrial cancer and preliminary data concerning therapy with intraperitoneal radiopharmaceuticals. *Am. J. Obstet. Gynecol.* **141:** 921–927.

Creasman WT, Morrow PC, Bundy NB *et al.* (1987) Surgical pathologic spread patterns of endometrial cancer. *Cancer* **60:** 2035–2041.

Creasman WT & Weld JC (1976) Screening techniques in endometrial carcinoma. *Cancer* **38:** 936–940.

Daya D, Lukka H & Clement PB (1992) Primitive neuroectodermal tumors of the uterus: a report of four cases. *Hum. Pathol.* **23:** 1120–1129.

DeBrito PA, Silverberg SG & Orenstein JM (1993) Carcinosarcoma (malignant mixed müllerian [mesodermal] tumor) of the female genital tract: immunohistochemical and ultrastructural analysis of 28 cases. *Hum. Pathol.* **24:** 132–142.

Doering LD, Barnhill RD, Weiser BE *et al.* (1989) Intraoperative evaluation of depth of myometrial invasion in Stage I endometrial adenocarcinoma. *Obstet. Gynecol.* **74:** 930–933.

Doll R, Muir C & Waterhouse J (1970) *Cancer Incidence in 5 Continents.* International Union against Cancer, 2, p. 44. Berlin: Springer–Verlag.

Dunton CJ, Balsara G, McFarland M *et al.* (1991) Uterine papillary serous carcinoma: a review. *Obstet. Gynecol. Surv.* **46:** 97–102.

Dunton CJ, Kelsten ML, Brooks SE *et al.* (1990) Low grade stromal sarcoma: DNA flow cytometric analysis and estrogen progesterone receptor data. *Gynecol. Oncol.* **37:** 268–275.

Eisner RF, Nieberg RK & Berek JS (1989) Synchronous primary neoplasms of the female reproductive tract. *Gynecol. Oncol.* **33:** 335–339.

El–Naggar AK, Abdul–Karim FW, Silva EG *et al.* (1991) Uterine stromal neoplasms: a clinicopathologic and DNA flow cytometric correlation. *Hum. Pathol.* **22:** 897–903.

Evans HL (1982) Endometrial stromal sarcoma and poorly differentiated endometrial sarcoma. *Cancer* **50:** 2170–2182.

Fanning J, Tsukada Y & Piver S (1990) Intraoperative frozen section diagnosis of depth of myometrial invasion in endometrial adenocarcinoma. *Gynecol. Oncol.* **37:** 47–50.

Farhood IA & Abrams J (1991) Immunohistochemistry of endometrial stromal sarcomas. *Hum. Pathol.* **22:** 224–230.

Fekete PS & Vellios F (1984) The clinical and histologic spectrum of endometrial stromal neoplasms: a report of 41 cases. *Int. J. Gynecol. Pathol.* **3:** 198–212.

Ferry JA & Young RH (1991) Malignant lymphoma pseudolymphoma and hematopoietic disorders of the female genital tract. *Pathol. Annual.* **26(Part 1):** 227–263.

FIGO stages – 1988 Revision. *Gynecol. Oncol.* (1989), **35:** 125–127.

Gray LA, Christopherson WM & Hoover RN (1977) Estrogens and endometrial carcinoma. *Obstet. Gynecol.* **49(4):** 385–389.

Hachisuga T, Sugimori H, Kaku T *et al.* (1990) Glassy cell carcinoma of the endometrium. *Gynecol. Oncol.* **36:** 134–138.

Harlap S (1992) The benefits and risks of hormone replacement therapy: an epidemiologic overview. *Am. J. Obstet. Gynecol.* **166:** 1986–1992.

Hendrickson M, Ross J, Eifel P, Martines A & Kempson R (1982) Uterine papillary serous carcinoma. A highly malignant form of endometrial adenocarcinoma. *Am. J. Surg. Pathol.* **6:** 93–108.

Hendrickson MR & Kempson RL (1983) Ciliated carcinoma – a variant of endometrial adenocarcinoma: a report of 10 cases. *Int. J. Gynecol. Pathol.* **2:** 1–12.

Hendrickson MR, Ross JC & Kempson RL (1983) Toward the development of morphologic criteria for well differentiated adenocarcinoma of the endometrium. *Am. J. Surg. Pathol.* **7:** 819–838.

Jacques SM & Lawrence WD (1990) Endometrial adenocarcinoma with variable-level myometrial involvement limited to adenomyosis: a clinicopathologic study of 23 cases. *Gynecol. Oncol.* **37:** 401–407.

Kadar N, Maljetano HJ & Homesley DH (1992) Determinants of survival of surgically staged patients with endometrial carcinoma histologically confined to the uterus: implications for therapy. *Obstet. Gynecol.* **80:** 655–659.

Kaku T, Silverberg SG, Major FJ *et al.* (1992) Adenosarcoma of the uterus: a Gynecologic Oncology Group clinico-pathologic study of 31 cases. *Int. J. Gynecol. Pathol.* **11:** 75–88.

Kempson RL & Hendrickson MR (1988) Pure mesenchymal neoplasms of the uterine corpus: selected problems. *Semin. Diagn. Pathol.* **5:** 172–198.

King ME, Dickersin GR & Scully RE (1982) Myxoid leiomyosarcoma of the uterus: a report of six cases. *Am. J. Surg. Pathol.* **6:** 589–598.

Koss LG, Schreiber K, Oberlander SG *et al.* (1984) Detection of endometrial cancer and hyperplasia in asymptomatic women. *Obstet. Gynecol.* **64:** 1–11.

■ Kurman RJ, Kaminski PF & Norris HJ (1985) The behavior of endometrial hyperplasia. A long term study of 'untreated' hyperplasia in 170 patients. *Cancer* **56:** 403–412.

Lawrence WD (1995) The histopathologic diagnosis of endometrial hyperplasia and atypical endometrial hyperplasia. *Am. Soc. Clin. Pathol. Tumor Diagnosis and Treatment.* **22(5):** 57–82.

MacMahon B (1974) Risk factors for endometrial cancer. *Gynecol. Oncol.* **2:** 122–129.

Malfetano JH (1990) Tamoxifen associated endometrial carcinoma in post-menopausal breast cancer patients. *Gynecol. Oncol.* **39:** 82–84.

Malviya VK, Deppe G, Malone JM, Sundareson AS & Lawrence WD (1989) Reliability of frozen section examination in identifying poor prognostic indicators in stage I endometrial adenocarcinoma. *Gynecol. Oncol.* **34:** 299–304.

Morrow CP, Bundy BN, Kurman RJ *et al.* (1991) Relationship between surgical-pathological risk factors and outcome in clinical Stage I and II carcinoma of the endometrium: a Gynecologic Oncology Group Study. *Gynecol. Oncol.* **40:** 55–65.

Norris HJ & Taylor HB (1965) Post-irradiation sarcomas of the uterus. *Obstet. Gynecol.* **26:** 689–694.

Nyholm HCJ, Nielsen AL & Norup P (1993) Endometrial cancer in postmenopausal women with and without previous estrogen replacement treatment. Comparison of clinical and histopathological characteristics. *Gynecol. Oncol.* **49:** 229–235.

Perrone T & Dehner PL (1988) Prognostically favorable 'mitotically active' smooth muscle tumors of the uterus. *Am. J. Surg. Pathol.* **12(1):** 1–8.

Peters AW, Howard RD, Andersen AW *et al.* (1994) Uterine smooth muscle tumors of uncertain malignant potential. *Obstet. Gynecol.* **83:** 1015–1020.

Piver MS, Lele SB & Barlow JJ (1982) Para-aortic node evaluation in Stage I endometrial carcinoma. *Obstet. Gynecol.* **59:** 97–100.

Podczaski E, Sees J, Kaminski P *et al.* (1990) Rhabdomyosarcoma of the uterus in a postmenopausal patient. *Gynecol. Oncol.* **37:** 439–442.

Procope BJ (1971) Etiology of post menopausal bleeding. *Obstet. Gynecol. Scand.* **50:** 311.

Quinones GE, Paraskevas MP, Diocee MS *et al.* (1991) Angiosarcoma of the uterus: a case report. *Am. J. Obstet. Gynecol.* **164:** 90–92.

Ross J, Eifel PH, Cox RS *et al.* (1983) Primary mucinous adenocarcinoma of the endometrium. A clinicopathologic and histochemical study. *Am. J. Surg. Pathol.* **7:** 715–729.

Schweizer W, Demopoulos R, Beller V *et al.* (1990) Prognostic factors for malignant mixed müllerian tumors of the uterus. *Int. J. Gynecol. Pathol.* **9:** 129–136.

Silva EG, Tornos CS & Follen-Mitchell M (1994) Malignant neoplasms of the uterine corpus in patients treated for breast carcinoma: the effects of tamoxifen. *Int. J. Gynecol. Pathol.* **13:** 248–258.

Silverberg SG (1988) Hyperplasia and carcinoma of the endometrium. *Semin. Diagn. Pathol.* **5:** 135–153.

■ Silverberg SG, Major FJ, Blessing JA *et al.* (1990) Carcinosarcoma (malignant mixed mesodermal tumor) of the uterus: a Gynecologic Oncology Group pathologic study of 203 cases. *Int. J. Gynecol. Pathol.* **9:** 1–19.

■ Thomas DB (1991) The WHO collaborative study of neoplasia and steroid contraceptives: the influence of combined oral contraceptives on risk of neoplasms in developing and developed countries. *Contraception* **43:** 695–710.

Webb GA & Lagios MD (1987) Clear cell carcinoma of the endometrium. *Am. J. Obstet. Gynecol.* **156:** 1486–1491.

Zaino RJ, Kurman RJ, Herbold D *et al.* (1991) The significance of squamous differentiation in endometrial carcinoma: data from a Gynecologic Oncology Group Study. *Cancer* **68:** 2293–3202.

Ziel HK & Finkle WD (1975) Increased risk of endometrial carcinoma among users of conjugated estrogens. *N. Engl. J. Med.* **293:** 1167–1170.

11 Epithelial Uterine Tumors

H D Homesley

Introduction

A myriad of clinically significant recent findings in endometrial carcinoma contribute to current approaches. An understanding of the presentation and diagnosis of disease is key because screening techniques are not currently used. Fortunately, abnormal vaginal bleeding leads to early detection and treatment.

There are a variety of treatment approaches employed at this time, primarily based upon surgical findings. The use of radiation therapy has evolved over time in that two decades ago most patients received preoperative intrauterine radium implants. At least in the USA, few patients now receive preoperative radiation. The role of postoperative radiation is unclear as this awaits prospective randomized trials.

The treatment options are based upon surgical findings. Follow-up of patients with endometrial cancer is fairly standard with the recognition that the cancer commonly recurs in the pelvis and distantly. Recurrence is primarily related to the extent of disease at initial surgical exploration.

Presentation

Overall ten-year corrected survival is 72% for white patients and 40% for black patients (Aziz *et al.*, 1993). Low socioeconomic status does not explain the poor survival in black patients. Although there are similar percentages of patients with Stage I and II, more blacks have Stage III disease. Likewise, blacks have a higher percentage of Grade 3, positive lymph nodes, positive cytology, and are more likely to have deep invasion.

When the length of time between the onset of vaginal bleeding and the initial visit to a physician is compared, there is no difference in the times between those presenting with early versus advanced disease (Shipley and Nelson, 1993). Patients with advanced endometrial carcinoma do not necessarily delay seeking medical attention when compared to patients with early disease.

Endometrial carcinoma in premenopausal women is generally associated with a favorable histologic type. Serous or clear cell carcinomas are rare. Often the young patient is recognized at an early stage and has an excellent prognosis. Adenocarcinoma of the endometrium in patients 45 years or younger accounts for 3–8% of all endometrial cancers and presents with the usual symptoms of abnormal vaginal bleeding. Endometrial carcinoma can develop years after endometrial ablation (Copperman *et al.*, 1993). Careful postoperative surveillance is warranted because cryptic endometrial adenocarcinoma does occur after ablation. Endometrial carcinoma can develop while taking estrogen and progestin hormone replacement therapy in about 5% of the patients with a median of over five years after onset of use. Inadequate progestin suppression is suspected as the etiology of the endometrial carcinoma.

Several reports have linked tamoxifen administration with endometrial carcinoma (Magriples *et al.*, 1993). From 1980–1990, 53 patients with a history of breast carcinoma who subsequently developed a malignant tumor of the corpus were identified. Of these patients, 15 received tamoxifen for breast carcinoma and 38 did not. The mean interval between detection of the breast and endometrial cancers was five years in the tamoxifen group and 12 years in the 'no tamoxifen' group. Of the patients in the tamoxifen group, 67% had poorly differentiated endometrial carcinoma associated with a poor outcome compared with 24% in the 'no tamoxifen' group. Patients in the tamoxifen group were much more likely to die of endometrial cancer (33% versus 3%).

The recommendation is that patients with cancer of the breast who have been on tamoxifen for over two years should be screened with endovaginal sonograms for the thickness of the endometrium; thickness over 5 mm should be investigated with hysteroscopy and fractional uterine curettage.

Diagnosis

While cervical cytology can predict the presence of malignancy for a small proportion of women with endometrial cancer, cervical cancer screening does not have a major impact on reducing the morbidity and mortality from endometrial cancer. Currently, endometrial cytology has no generally accepted definition for malignancy. There is considerable interobserver variation in the classification of abnormal endometrial cytology. Endometrial cytology does not identify atypical endometrial cells in the precursor state.

Because endometrial carcinoma is a common tumor, primary care physicians should maintain a high index of suspicion. Endometrial aspiration biopsy is considered a simple office-based procedure with a low risk and a good yield, although this is not recommended for general screening because of the associated discomfort. Any perimenopausal or postmenopausal woman with abnormal bleeding patterns should be evaluated. A positive biopsy can save a patient the time, cost, and inconvenience of dilatation and curettage; a negative finding should be interpreted with caution. In patients with known endometrial carcinoma, preoperative endometrial sampling can fail up to 33% of the time to demonstrate the correct diagnosis (Ferry *et al.*, 1993). Poor results are associated with well-differentiated, low-volume, minimally-invasive tumors; early tumors may therefore be overlooked with endometrial sampling.

Transvaginal Ultrasound

Dilatation and curettage been the method of choice for diagnosing endometrial cancer in postmenopausal women for many years. Less than 10% of women with postmenopausal bleeding have endometrial cancer. Vaginal sonography for measuring endometrial thickness has proven to be a sensitive diagnostic method for diagnosing endometrial pathology. An endometrial thickness of 4 mm or less, including both endometrial layers, indicates a very low risk for endometrial carcinoma as well as any other major endometrial pathology in women with postmenopausal bleeding. Since vaginal sonography is such a simple and noninvasive diagnostic test, vaginal sonographic assessment of the endometrium should be the primary method for excluding any endometrial abnormality in women with postmenopausal bleeding. Irregular echodensity or a clear alignment between endometrium and myometrium has little value in the diagnosis of premalignant lesions of the endometrium (Brolmann *et al.*, 1993). However, patients with an endometrial thickness less than 3 mm do not need any endometrial curettage. As much as one-third of endometrial samplings might be avoided. Vaginal sonography can be used as a prebioptic examination for screening of endometrial carcinoma in postmenopausal high-risk patients with diabetes mellitus, hypertension, and obesity, but without a history of vaginal bleeding (Maly *et al.*, 1992). About 3% of asymptomatic patients can be discovered to have endometrial carcinoma.

The ten-day progesterone challenge test has been advocated to detect endometrial pathology in asymptomatic women not taking hormonal treatment (Macia *et al.*, 1993). The ten-day test is more sensitive than the five-day test. A positive correlation between the amount of bleeding after the progesterone challenge test and the endometrial thickness by transvaginal ultrasonography has been found. There is a significant correlation between the length of bleeding and endometrial thickness. The combined use of these two techniques may be effective screening for normal postmenopausal women.

If vaginal sonographic assessment of the endometrium with regard to its thickness and structure (homogeneity, echogeneity and median echo) is recommended for noninvasive screening, a saline infusion through a flexible catheter during transvaginal sonography can provide visual contrast and uterine expansion for better visualization (Parsons and Lense, 1993). Hyperplasia and neoplasia are not distinguishable, but the approach for biopsy and therapy is validated by this simple and well-tolerated technique.

Transvaginal ultrasound has been found to be highly accurate and a convenient method for preoperatively evaluating myometrial invasion (Sahakian *et al.*, 1991). Potentially this evaluation could influence the selection of therapy for poor-risk candidates or direct appropriate management of patients with deep invasion. When histologic invasion is at least 33%, transvaginal ultrasound has been reported to be 100% accurate with no false-negatives although adenomyosis and leiomyomas may lead to inaccurate interpretation.

The use of transvaginal color Doppler sonography in the early detection of endometrial cancer has also been investigated (Kubesik–Urek *et al.*, 1993). There was a significantly lower resistance index of 0.37 ± 0.07 in endometrial cancer than in patients with benign uterine lesions. Central vessels within endometrial carcinoma tend to have lower velocity and impedance than peripheral vessels.

Magnetic Resonance Imaging

When transvaginal sonography is compared with magnetic resonance imaging (MRI) in detecting the depth of myoinvasion, no difference is demonstrated (Del Maschio *et al.*, 1993). Histologic examination revealed findings concordant with the two imaging techniques in 76% of the patients. Among the discordant, there were instances of understaging and overstaging.

Non-enhanced T2-weighted and contrast material-enhanced T1-weighted MRI were compared in assessing myometrial invasion in patients with proven endometrial cancer (Sironi *et al.*, 1992). The sensitivity and specificity of contrast-enhanced T1-weighted MRI was higher than that of non-enhanced T2-weighted MRI. The overall sensitivity of enhanced T1-weighted MRI was 88% whereas that of non-enhanced T2-weighted MRI was 71%.

An effort to evaluate the capability of ultra-low field MRI for staging endometrial carcinoma revealed more accurate detection of cervical extension, and MRI was better than computed tomography (CT) in detecting tumor invasion to the outer half of the myometrium (Varpula and Klemi, 1993). The sensitivity of CT and MRI for deep myometrial invasion was 67% versus 83%, respectively. MRI at 0.02 Tesla (T) was not able to differentiate tumors with superficial myometrial invasion from those confined entirely to the endometrium. The detection of metastatic lymphadenopathy is difficult by all examination methods.

Tumor Markers

CA-125, CA-19.9, CA-50, carcinoembryonic antigen (CEA), tissue plasminogen activator (TPA), and alfa-fetoproteins were assessed in 24 women with endometrial carcinoma and 28 healthy women (Indraccolo *et al.*, 1991). These markers were not useful for screening of endometrial carcinoma.

Staging

In 1988, the International Federation of Gynecology and Obstetrics (FIGO) Cancer Committee changed the staging (*see Table 47.3*) of endometrial cancer from clinical to surgicopathologic (Homesley, 1992). The major changes in staging are the use of the depth of myometrial invasion, identification of tumor cells in peritoneal cytologic examination, and spread to the retroperitoneal lymph nodes. Preoperative endocervical curettage is no longer necessary. Currently the high level of operability of patients with endometrial carcinoma makes this staging system a viable one providing information about the need for additional treatment (Mangioni *et al.*, 1993). There is still controversy concerning the need and type of pelvic lymph node resection to detect nodal metastasis.

Prognostic Factors

From the Gynecologic Oncology Group (GOG) surgical–pathologic staging trial, the frequency, relative risk, and associated survival of independent risk factors (*Tables 11.1 and 11.2*) were delineated (Morrow *et al.*, 1991). These findings have directed the design and analysis of GOG trials in endometrial cancer.

The number of tumor-related risk factors present may be the best predictor of survival of patients with endometrial carcinoma confined to the uterus and may provide the optimal basis for individualization of treatment (Homesley and Zaino, 1994). The determinant factors that influence the survival of patients with endometrial cancer histologically confined to the uterus were reviewed in 262 patients to assign risk of recurrence (Kadar *et al.*, 1992). After excluding patients with clear cell and serous tumors, survival was adversely affected by increasing stage, tumor grade and depth of myometrial invasion, cervical stromal and vascular space invasion and increasing age. The greatest effect on survival was obtained by dichotomizing grade as Grade 3 versus Grade 1 or 2, myometrial invasion as invasion of more versus less than the inner third of the myometrium, and the cervical spread as the presence or absence of stromal invasion. The joint effect of the tumor-related prognostic factors was best expressed by constructing three risk groups

Table 11.1. Frequency of risk factors (Gynecologic Oncology Group #33): endometrial cancer (n=895) (from Morrow *et al.*, 1991).

	Frequency (%)	*Relative risk*
Uterine (n=675=75%)		
Grade 3	19	15
Outer third myoinvasion	17	4.3
Vascular space involvement	7	2.5
Microinvasion of cervix	15	1.5
Extrauterine (n=220=25%)		
Periaortic node	5	12
Pelvic node	5	12
Adnexal metastasis	4	12
Gross disease	5	12
Positive cytologic washings	6	2.4
Age ⩾75 years	16	1.8

Table 11.2. Survival rates (Gynecologic Oncology Group #33): endometrial cancer (n=895) (from Morrow *et al.*, 1991).

	No. of patients	*Survival (%)*
Uterine only (n=675)		
Grade 3	146	66
Deep myoinvasion	132	64
Positive vascular space involvement	56	64
Microinvasion of the cervix	109	84
Age ⩾71 years	121	64
Age ⩽51 years	100	95
Extrauterine (n=220)		
Positive periaortic nodes	48	42
Positive pelvic nodes	43	65
Positive adnexa	34	59
Gross disease	42	50
Positive peritoneal cytology	53	74

consisting of patients with zero or one, two, and three or four risk factors. These three risk groups were associated with five-year survival rates of 97%, 66%, and 17%.

Grade

In the FIGO revised grading system, the architectural growth pattern still serves as the basic parameter, but nuclear atypia incorporated with the architectural grade can raise the grade by one (Nielsen *et al.*, 1991). There is an acceptable interobserver reproducibility of 0.625 for grading. The reproducibility of the nuclear grade can be poor (0.55), while that of architectural grade is higher (0.70). Review of the literature shows a great variability in the definition of nuclear grading, indicating that the revised 1988 FIGO grading system is not applicable as a standard reference for studies of endometrial cancer before the definition of nuclear grading is standardized.

Histology

Squamous differentiation is identified in about 25% of endometrial carcinomas. Its significance has been the subject for debate for many decades. It is now advised that the terms adenoacanthoma and adenosquamous carcinoma be replaced by the descriptive term adenocarcinoma with squamous cell differentiation (Zaino *et al.*, 1991). The biologic behavior of endometrial carcinoma with squamous elements is similar to that of typical adenocarcinoma. The division of adenocarcinoma with squamous differentiation by depth of myometrial invasion and by architectural grade of the glandular component provides prognostic information that is superior to simple division into adenocarcinoma versus adenosquamous carcinoma.

Detection of endocervical involvement by endometrial carcinoma on fractional curettage is generally unreliable and often less than 50% of patients have histologic confirmation of endocervical tissue invasion (Carone *et al.*, 1991). Clear cell or serous adenocarcinoma has a tendency to contaminate the endocervical curettage.

Peritoneal Cytology

Conclusions regarding effective adjuvant therapy for positive washings are difficult to draw due to the small number of patients with positive cytology and the variety of treatments used. In an effort to resolve the current controversy about the importance of pelvic washings for cytologic analysis in endometrial cancer, 270 consecutive patients with neoplasms histologically limited to the uterus were studied (Kennedy *et al.*, 1993); 5% were positive for cytologic washings. Cytologic washings correlated with tumor grade and depth of myometrial invasion. Multivariate analysis indicated outer third invasion of the myometrium and positive washings predicted survival. The probability of a five-year survival in the total group was 85%, which decreased to 67% in patients with positive washings. Despite statistical significance as a prognostic variable, the overall clinical use of peritoneal cytology in planning postoperative adjuvant therapy is limited by its correlation with other prognostic factors and overall low rate of positivity.

DNA Analysis

There are conflicting reports related to the usefulness of the prognostic significance of DNA analysis (Stendahl *et al.*, 1991). Because of the multitude of independent clinical factors such as stage, age, histopathologic grade and myometrial invasion, it is difficult to determine if ploidy level and S-phase fraction are independently prognostically significant. Even when comparing S-phase fraction and DNA content, there are indications that S-phase fraction may be an independent factor within stage and grade.

In a multivariate analysis of all independent prognostic factors, DNA ploidy was an independent prognostic factor of uterine corpus cancer (Ikeda *et al.*, 1993). Not only in more advanced disease has DNA content analysis been reported to be significant, but in patients with Stage I the biologic characteristics of DNA content relate to tumor aggressiveness (Melchiorri *et al.*, 1993). It has been projected that DNA analysis could offer early objective evidence of an intrinsic, highly malignant phenotype.

DNA ploidy and proliferative activity in pretreatment curettage specimens did distinguish the majority of patients at high risk for extrauterine metastasis and relapse. Multivariate analysis identified proliferative index as the most cogent independent prognostic factor. Using pretreatment curettage specimens, cytometrically determined ribonucleic acid (RNA) may identify patients at high risk for extrauterine disease or pretreatment relapse (Podratz *et al.*, 1993). Flow cytometrically-determined RNA, S-phase fraction, DNA index, and proliferative index was measured in 140 paraffin-embedded curettage specimens containing endometrial cancer. Although clinical staging identified only 19% of patients with advanced disease, 40% with surgical Stage III and IV were aneuploid, 69% had an S-phase fraction of at least 9% and 69% had a proliferative index of at least 14%. Documented recurrences in cancer-related deaths correlated with non-diploid patterns with 50% recurrences and 54% deaths. S-phase fraction greater than 90% was associated with 67% recurrences and 75% deaths, while proliferative index equal to or greater than 14% was associated with 73% recurrences and 79% of deaths. DNA index (<1.5 versus >1.5) provides additional stratification of aneuploid tumors.

However, in a larger series of 400 Stage I and II patients considering multiple prognostic factors, DNA content did not maintain independent prognosis whereas S-phase fraction did correlate with time of recurrence (Wagenius *et al.*, 1992).

Surgical Staging and Treatment

Lymphadenectomy

The GOG has standardized the technique of selective node sampling for all GOG trials (*Table 11.3*). Morbidity and mortality of patients with endometrial carcinoma having total abdominal hysterectomy, bilateral salpingo–oophorectomy (TAH–BSO) alone or with selective pelvic and paraaortic lymphadenectomy is similar for each group. 'Selective node dissection' and 'no node dissection' patient groups have similar estimated blood loss and transfusion rates (Homesley *et al.*, 1992). The operative time is dependent upon the surgeon, the patient's weight and race, and estimated blood loss. The complications, such as wound infection, deep venous thrombosis or pulmonary embolus, are the same for both selective pelvic and paraaortic lymphadenectomy and total abdominal hysterectomy alone. The mortality is low and the same for each surgical group.

Pelvic and paraaortic lymphadenectomy can be added to the TAH–BSO in patients with endometrial cancer without a clinically significant increase in morbidity and mortality. Of 77 patients with endometrial cancer staged surgically without preoperative radiotherapy, 35 patients had TAH–BSO alone and 42 with lymphadenectomy (Larson *et al.*, 1992). The median number of lymph nodes removed was 18. Patients with lymphadenectomy had an increased operative time (129 minutes versus 87 minutes), increased blood loss (391–272) and a longer postoperative hospital stay. Notwithstanding, there was no difference in transfusion rate, febrile morbidity, postoperative ramifications or mortality.

Table 11.3. Selective pelvic and periaortic lymphadenectomy (Gynecologic Oncology Group definition, from Creasman *et al.*, 1987).

Pelvic nodal excision of tissue Nodal tissue excised from distal one-half of common iliac, anterior and medial aspects of external iliac and obturator fat anterior to obturator nerve
Aortic nodal excision of tissue Nodal tissue excised over the distal vena cava from the level of the inferior mesenteric artery to the mid common iliac arteries

Complete lymphadenectomy and thorough histologic processing with step serial sections for correct staging of patients with endometrial carcinoma is advocated (Girardi *et al.*, 1993). Of the patients with primary adenocarcinoma, 24% underwent pelvic lymphadenectomy with removal of a mean of 37 lymph nodes per patient. Of these patients 36% had lymph node metastasis and 37% of the lymph node metastases were 2 mm or less in diameter. The incidence of lymph node metastasis correlated with the depth of myometrial invasion, but not with histologic subtype and grade. Of the patients with positive nodes who had Stage I disease according to clinical classification (FIGO, 1971), 24 were upstaged to Stage III. Of the patients 37% (27 patients) of those patients (76 patients) who underwent lymphadenectomy were node positive. The entire series of patients reported was 322 and 24% of these (76 patients) underwent lymph node dissection. All patients with macroscopic metastasis to the paraaortic nodes developed recurrent cancer and only a small percentage of those with micrometastasis to the paraaortic nodes survived disease-free at five years.

Nevertheless, lymphadenectomy may not improve outcome for patients with endometrial carcinoma (Belinson *et al.*, 1992). Of 216 patients evaluated, 21 died. Analysis of these 21 patients by grade, depth of invasion, surgical stage, time of recurrence, site of recurrence, survival, protocol breaks and frozen section discrepancy did not indicate that lymphadenectomy would have prevented their recurrence. None of the patients had lymphadenectomies. All patients found to have positive paraaortic nodes died. No patient who received vaginal or pelvic radiation developed recurrence in the pelvis.

Omentum

Occult omental metastasis can be overlooked in patients with clinical Stage I carcinoma (Chen and Speigel, 1991). A routine histologic assessment of the omentum during primary surgery for 'Stage I' endometrial carcinoma revealed an 8% incidence of omental metastasis, the majority (5 of 8) of which were microscopic. Factors associated with omental metastasis are adnexal spread, cul-de-sac implantation, serous carcinoma, positive retroperitoneal lymph nodes and Grade 3 tumor.

Operative Endoscopy

Surgicopathologic staging can be performed laparoscopically with exploration of the abdomen and procurement of peritoneal cytology and pelvic and paraaortic lymph nodes. The combined laparoscopic and vaginal approach offers decreased morbidity to patients; this technique still captures the same pathologic information and surgical goal as the traditional transabdominal approach (Childers and Surwit, 1992). Postmenopausal patients with Stage I adenocarcinoma of the endometrium have been managed by this technique. The adnexa are ligated, mobilized laparoscopically and removed with the vaginal hysterectomy.

High-risk Groups and Surgical Treatment

The surgicopathologic findings can be used to divide surgical Stages I and II patients into low- and high-risk groups (*Table 11.4*). Surgery only, without lymphadenectomy, yields high survival rates with minimal complications for Stage IA and IB, Grade 1 (*Table 11.5*). Patients at high risk for pelvic node metastasis with Stages IB Grade 2, 3 and IC benefit from the discovery of positive pelvic nodes by full surgical staging with selective or complete pelvic lymphadenectomy followed by adjuvant whole pelvic radiation if indicated. Definitive prospective adjuvant radiation or chemotherapy clinical trials have not been completed. Postoperative progesterone is not effective.

Table 11.4. Endometrial carcinoma (from Creasman 1994 and Manëschi *et al.*, 1992).

Low risk
Myoinvasion <50%
Grade 1
Cervical gland involvement only
Confined to uterus
Negative pelvic and periaortic nodes
Negative peritoneal cytology
High risk
Myoinvasion ⩾50%
Grade 2, 3
Cervical stromal invasion
Extracorporeal
Positive pelvic/periaortic nodes
Positive peritoneal cytology

Adjuvant Therapy

Low-risk patients with Grade 1 tumors limited to the uterine body with myometrial invasion of no more than need 50% no adjuvant therapy and have a high survival. Survival is greater than 95% for FIGO surgical Stage IA and IB Grade 1. Tumor grade, myoinvasion, extent of spread, and lymph node status are the most common risk factors for recurrence.

Radiation

The earliest intracavitary radium treatment for uterine cancer was in 1908 (Rotman *et al.*, 1993). Refinements instituted preoperative irradiation of uterine and parauterine tissues. Preoperative intracavitary irradiation was entrenched as therapy for all endometrial cancers for four decades. In the 1950s and 1960s, the ability of external irradiation to eradicate cancer in regional lymphatic vessels facilitated the application of pelvic field radiation for Stage II and III, as well as recurrent disease. Surgical studies in the 1970s refined criteria for preoperative or postoperative external pelvic therapy for high-grade infiltrating Stage I cancers. In the 1980s a subset of patients was identified with high-grade lymph vascular invasion, clear cell or serous

Table 11.5. Surgical therapy of endometrial cancer (from Creasman, 1994).

Risk group (incidence)	*Pelvic nodes positive (%)*	*Surgery*	*Comment*
Low risk Stage IA and IB, Grade 1 (30%)	3	TAH–BSO	Grade 1 with deep invasion has a 10% positive pelvic node rate
High risk Stage IB, Grade 2, 3 (50%)	9	TAH–BSO + SLND	SLND for Grades 2 and 3
Moderate risk Stage IC Grades 1, 2, 3 (20%)	18	TAH–BSO + SLND	SLND is indicated in all patients with deep invasion

TAH–BSO, total abdominal hysterectomy, bilateral salpingo–oophorectomy; SLND, selective lymph node dissection.

histologic types or with positive peritoneal cytologic findings who were at high risk of developing metastatic disease in the paraaortic nodes and/or the upper abdomen for whom an extended field with whole abdominal radiation was advocated.

Paraaortic radiation

Periaortic nodal involvement diagnosed pathologically or lymphographically can be treated with preoperative, postoperative, and primary radiotherapy (Corn *et al.*, 1992). When pathologically diagnosed grossly involved nodes are debulked and all patients receive external beam to pelvic and periaortic portals, the actuarial survival is 46% for all patients. Relapse-free survival and pelvic control tends to improve among patients receiving surgery plus radiation in comparison to those treated with radiation alone. Distant metastases are more common among patients with high-grade lesions.

Yet, paraaortic field radiation has a significant complication rate and should be reserved for patients with histologic evidence of paraaortic metastases (Rose *et al.*, 1992). Of 26 patients, 17 received postoperative radiation therapy as part of their primary therapy, and 16 of the 17 (94%) received adjunctive hormonal therapy. Nine of the 17 patients (53%) are alive without evidence of disease with a median survival time of 27 months. Two of the 17 or 12% died of intestinal obstruction felt to be secondary to radiation enteritis, one of whom was disease free. There appeared to be no difference between microscopic and macroscopic nodal involvement. Of nine patients who did not receive radiation, seven have died. The survival difference remained significant in patients with microscopic, but not macroscopic, nodal disease.

Postoperative radiation

An assessment of the outcomes and patterns of recurrence in Stage III patients helps to guide adjuvant therapy (Greven *et al.*, 1991). Of 105 patients who underwent abdominal hysterectomy, 60 had node assessment and 45 had cytologic washings. All patients received postoperative external beam radiation to the pelvis or pelvis and paraaortic regions for pathologically positive paraaortic nodes. The five-year pelvic recurrence rate was 21% with multivariate analysis revealing the grade to be the strongest prognostic factor. Pathologic findings and the number of involved extrauterine sites were the most important prognostic factors for abdominal recurrence and other sites of distant relapse. The low-grade tumor with superficial myometrial penetration had a low distant relapse rate. Patients with high-grade tumors, deep myometrial penetration, clear cell or serous histologic types, or two or more involved extrauterine sites are at high risk for distant recurrence, which may include the abdomen.

The high dose-rate intracavitary rate of therapy with the Buchler afterloading system for vaginal vault radiation for carcinoma of the endometrium is convenient, safe and quick, and does not necessitate admission or sedation of the patient. In addition, it provides complete radiation protection for the staff (Thomas *et al.*, 1991). Retrospective analysis of high activity iridium-192 and the Buchler machine to treat the vaginal vault in patients with adenocarcinoma, most of whom received external beam radiotherapy to the pelvis, was compared to controls treated with low dose-rate intracavitary cesium ovoids. Complication rates, including vaginal stenosis, were no different and survival was similar.

Vaginal recurrence

Long-term survival can be obtained for patients with an isolated vaginal recurrence of endometrial cancer treated with aggressive local–regional radiation therapy (Morgan *et al.*, 1993). Of 34 patients with isolated vaginal recurrence treated with radiation, the five-year survival was 68%. The five-year survival for patients with local or regional recurrence was 44%. The tumor volume is an important prognostic factor. One of 17 patients with a tumor no larger than 4 cm relapsed while three out of nine with tumor sizes of at least 4 cm relapsed. None of the 16 patients treated with the combination of external beam therapy and brachytherapy failed locoregionally, while four of ten treated with either external beam therapy or brachytherapy relapsed.

Recurrent endometrial carcinoma when clinically confined to the vagina or pelvis can be associated with a poor survival. Local salvage therapy fails because a significant number of patients have occult distant metastasis at the time of relapse. In order to accurately assess disease status at the time of recurrence, a 'staging' procedure, which included laparotomy, selective pelvic and paraaortic lymphadenectomy, peritoneal biopsies and washings was performed (Hoekstra *et al.*, 1993). Three of eight patients had upper abdominal disease found at laparotomy. The presence of subclinical metastasis was associated with larger tumor size and elevated CA-125 antigen levels. Seven of eight patients are alive 21–61 months following salvage therapy. Since 38% of the patients with recurrent endometrial carcinoma clinically confined to the pelvis had occult upper abdominal disease, CT and/or surgical assessment is warranted, especially in those with elevated serum CA-125 levels or large tumors.

Serous carcinoma

Whole abdominal pelvic radiation may be considered as adjunctive therapy in serous carcinoma. The optimum management of this clinically aggressive histologic variant of endometrial adenocarcinoma is controversial. Additional adjuvant therapy such as chemotherapy needs to be considered for patients that present with metastasis. Stage I and II serous tumors may respond similarly to anaplastic carcinomas because the proclivity to early metastasis may account for poor survival.

Patients with Stage I serous carcinoma have been treated with radical hysterectomy, bilateral salpingo–oophorectomy with pelvic node sampling, adjuvant external pelvic radiation and four courses of cisplatin/epirubicin, and the outcome was better than for historical controls with none of the serous carcinoma patients relapsing during 32 months of follow-up (Rosenberg *et al.*, 1993).

Hormonal Therapy

Adjuvant hormone therapy did not improve cure rate because survival is influenced by the initial extent of disease (De Palo *et al.*, 1993). Patients with Stage IB, Grade 1 or 2 were randomized to no further treatment versus medroxyprogesterone acetate (MPA) 100 mg orally twice a day for 12 months. Patients with Stage IC and positive pelvic or paraaortic nodes were randomized to radiation therapy with or without MPA. There was a high relapse-free survival in 856 patients for both hormone and non-hormone groups.

There was no significant difference between the survival in the treatment group and in the control group in a prospective study devised to assess the effect of neoadjuvant MPA as part of the primary treatment of endometrial carcinoma in conjunction with surgery and radiotherapy (Vishnevsky *et al.*, 1993). The survival of 218 patients with Stage I adenocarcinoma of the corpus who received either neoadjuvant treatment with 300 mg daily MPA from diagnosis for 90 days or no adjuvant therapy was 84% and 69% at five and ten years, respectively, in the treatment group, and 79% and 71% in the control group.

Of 45 patients with endometrial carcinoma confined to the uterus except for malignant peritoneal cytology who were treated with one year of progesterone therapy (Piver *et al.*,1992), 36 underwent a second-look laparoscopy; 34 (95%) were negative and had negative repeat peritoneal cytology. After an additional year of progesterone therapy, two positive patients had negative peritoneal cytology at third-look laparoscopy. Of the 45 patients enrolled in the study, no patient has developed recurrent endometrial cancer.

Tamoxifen

Adjuvant hormone therapy may have to be administered for more than three years to endometrial carcinoma patients who have an unfavorable prognosis in order to obtain a prolonged remission of the disease. In a prospective randomized study of 540 primary endometrial carcinoma patients, the combination of oxyprogesterone caproate and tamoxifen increased the corrected survival after five years by 19% (Vishnevsky *et al.*, 1993).

Down-regulation of endometrial tumor progesterone receptors resulting from continuous progestin administration presumably leads to desensitization to progestin after initial growth inhibition (Satyaswaroop *et al.*, 1992). After an initial response, the tumors become resistant to continuous progestin administration. The characteristic progesterone receptor proteins were observed by Western blot analysis in tamoxifen-treated tumors while tumors treated with both tamoxifen and progestin are devoid of receptors. Combined treatment with tamoxifen and progestin effectively controlled human endometrial tumor growth in the nude mouse model.

Gonadotropin releasing hormones

Gonadotropin releasing hormone may be an ideal drug for new therapeutic hormonal approaches in endometrial cancer. Gonadotropin releasing hormone may have synergistic effects as an adjuvant treatment in the primary stages, relapsing endometrial cancer or refractory endometrial carcinoma (Kullander, 1992). The hypoestrogenic state induced theoretically leads to tumor regression. Gonadotropin releasing hormone agonists may have a role in complex endometrial hyperplasia and endometrial cancer where surgery is contraindicated.

Follow-up

Since recurrences are most common in the pelvis and lung, patients usually have follow-up pelvic examinations every 3–4 months for the first two years and at six-month intervals until five years. If the patient is considered to have a low risk, no other examinations are performed, but if the patient is at high risk a chest radiograph is obtained at six-month intervals for the first 2–3 years. At the time of any suspicious symptoms, more intensive imaging studies are obtained.

Tumor Markers

The combined value of four tumor markers in the follow-up of endometrial cancer has been analyzed using cancer antigen-125, squamous cell carcinoma antigen (SCC), cancer antigen CA-19.9 and CA-15.3 (Matorras *et al.*, 1992). The tumor markers were of limited value for the prediction of recurrences.

Advanced/Recurrent

Hormonal therapy may still have a role as a minimally toxic treatment and response rates are in the 20–25% range, but not of long duration.

Paclitaxel has activity (35% response rate in GOG Protocol # 86O) in advanced endometrial cancer and hopefully more new active agents will be identified along with doxorubicin and cisplatin.

Summary of Management Options

- The surgicopathologic findings can be used to divide surgical Stages I and II patients into low- and high-risk groups.
- Surgery alone without lymphadenectomy yields high survival rates with minimal complications for Stages IA and IB, Grade 1.
- Patients at high risk for pelvic node metastasis with Stages IB, Grade 2, 3 and IC benefit from the discovery of positive pelvic nodes by full surgical staging with selective or complete pelvic lymphadenectomy followed by adjuvant whole pelvic radiation, if indicated.
- Definitive prospective adjuvant radiation or chemotherapy clinical trials have not been completed. Postoperative progesterone is not effective.
- Whole abdominal radiation following surgical therapy may be beneficial for patients with disease confined to the abdomen and no one site of residual disease larger than 2 cm in its greatest diameter. Yet, adjuvant chemotherapy with doxorubicin and cisplatin may be as effective.
- The GOG is conducting a randomized trial of adjuvant whole abdominal radiation versus doxorubicin and cisplatin for the group of patients with less than 2 cm diameter residual disease.
- Hormonal therapy may still have a role as a minimally toxic treatment and response rates are in the 20–25% range, but not of long duration.
- Paclitaxel has activity (35% response rate in GOG protocol #860) in advanced endometrial cancer and hopefully more new active agents will be identified along with doxorubicin and cisplatin.

References

Aziz H, Rotman M, Hussain F *et al.* (1993) Poor survival of black patients in carcinoma of the endometrium. *Inter. J. Rad. Oncol. Biol. Phys.* **27:** 293–301.

Belinson JL, Lee KR, Badger GJ, Pretorius RG & Jarrell MA (1992) Clinical stage I adenocarcinoma of the endometrium—analysis of recurrence and the potential benefit of staging lymphadenectomy. *Gynecol. Oncol.* **44:** 17–23.

Brolmann HA, Van der Linden PJ, Bongers MY, Moret E & Meuwissen JH (1993) Ultrasonographic diagnosis of endometrial disorders: correlation with the histological results in 112 patients. *Nederlands Tildschrift voor Geneeskunde* **137(36):** 1823–1827.

Carone C, Tetu B, Laberge P, Bellemare G & Raymond PE (1991) Endocervical involvement by endometrial carcinoma on fractional curettage: a clinicopathological study of 37 cases. *Mod. Pathol.* **4(5):** 644–647.

Chen SS & Speigel G (1991) Stage I endometrial carcinoma. Role of omental biopsy and omentectomy. *J. Reprod. Med.* 36 **(9):** 627–629.

Childers JM & Surwit EA (1992) Combined laparoscopic and vaginal surgery for the management of two cases of stage I endometrial cancer. *Gynecol. Oncol.* **45(1):** 46–51.

Copperman AB, DeCherney AH & Olive DL (1993) A case of endometrial cancer following endometrial ablation for dysfunctional uterine bleeding. *Obstet. Gynecol.* **82:** 640–642.

Corn BW, Lanciano RM, Green KM *et al.* (1992) Endometrial cancer with para-aortic adenopathy: patterns of failure and opportunities for cure. *Int. J. Radiation Oncol. Biol. Phys.* **24(2):** 223–227.

Creasman W, Morrow C, Bundy B, Homesley H, Graham JE & Heller PB (1987) Surgicopathological spread patterns of endometrial cancer. *Cancer* **60:** 2034–2041.

■ Creasman WT (1994) Limited disease: Role of surgery. *Sem. Oncol.* **21:** 79–83.

De Palo G, Mangioni C, Periti P, Del Vecchio M & Marubini E (1993) Treatment of FIGO (1971) stage I endometrial carcinoma with intensive surgery, radiotherapy and hormonotherapy according to pathological prognostic groups. Long-term results of randomized multicentre study. *Eur. J. Cancer* **29A:** 1133–1140.

Del Maschio A, Vanzulli A, Sironi S, Spagnolo D, Belloni C *et al.* (1993) Estimating the depth of myometrial involvement by endometrial carcinoma. Efficacy of transvaginal sonography versus MR imaging. *Am. J. Roentgenology* **160:** 533–538.

Ferry J, Farnsworth A, Webster M & Wren B (1993) The efficacy of the pipelle endometrial biopsy in detecting endometrial carcinoma. *Aust. NZ. J. Obstet. Gynaecol.* **33(1):** 76–78.

Girardi F, Petru E, Heydarfadai M, Haas J & Winter R (1993) Pelvic lymphadenectomy in the surgical treatment of endometrial cancer. *Gynecol. Oncol.* **49(2):** 177–180.

Greven KM, Lanciano RM, Corn B, Case D & Randall ME (1991) Pathologic stage III endometrial carcinoma.

Prognostic factors and patterns of recurrence. *Cancer* **71(11):** 3697–3702.

Hoekstra CJ, Koper PC & Van Putten WL (1993) Recurrent endometrial adenocarcinoma after surgery alone: prognostic factors and treatment. *Radiother. Oncol.* **27(2):** 164–166.

Homesley HD (1992) Revised 1988 International Federation of Gynecology and Obstetrics staging systems for endometrial and vulvar cancer: An assessment. *Clin. Obstet. Gynecol.* **35:** 89–94.

Homesley HD, Kadar N, Barrett RJ & Lentz SS (1992) Selective pelvic and periaortic lymphadenectomy does not increase morbidity in surgical staging of endometrial carcinoma. *Amer. J. Obstet. Gynec.* **167:** 1225–1230.

■ Homesley HD & Zaino R (1994) Endometrial cancer: prognostic factors. *Sem. Oncol.* **21:** 71–78.

Ikeda M, Watanabe Y, Nanjoh T & Noda K (1993) Evaluation of DNA ploidy in endometrial cancer. *Gynecol. Oncol.* **50(1):** 25–29.

Indraccolo SR, Cecchi A, Thodos A, Brandi S & Carta G (1991) Possibility of the combined use of tumor markers in endometrial carcinoma. *Minerva Ginecol.* **43(10):** 461–463.

Kadar N, Malfetano J & Homesley H (1992) Determinants of survival of surgically staged patients with endometrial carcinoma histologically confined to the uterus: Implications for therapy. *Obstet. Gynecol.* **80:** 655–659.

Kennedy AW, Webster KD, Nunez C & Bauer LJ (1993) Pelvic washings for cytologic analysis in endometrial adenocarcinoma. *J. Reprod. Med.* **38(8):** 637–642.

Kubesik-Urek S, Shalan H & Kuraik A (1993) Early detection of endometrial cancer with transvaginal color Doppler. *Eur. J. Obstet. Gynecol. Reprod. Biol.* **49:** 46–49.

Kullander S (1992) Treatment of endometrial cancer with GnRH analogs. *Recent Results Cancer Res.* **124:** 69–73

Larson DM, Johnson K & Olson KA (1992) Pelvic and para-aortic lymphadenectomy for surgical staging of endometrial cancer: morbidity and mortality. *Obstet. Gynec.* **79:** 998–1001.

Macia M, Novo A, Ces J *et al.* (1993) Progesterone challenge test for the assessment of endometrial pathology in asymptomatic menopausal women. *Int. J. Gynaecol. Obstet.* **40(2):** 145–149

Magriples U, Naftolin F, Schwartz PE & Carcangiu ML (1993) High-grade endometrial carcinoma in tamoxifen-treated breast cancer patients. *J. Clin. Oncol.* **11:** 485–490.

Mangioni C, De Palo G, Marubini E & Del Vecchio M (1993) Surgical pathologic staging in apparent stage I endometrial carcinoma. *Int J. Gynecol. Cancer* **3:** 273–384.

Maly Z, Dorr A & Pilka L (1992) Results of transvaginal ultrasound screening for endometrial carcinoma in women at risk after menopause. *Cesk. Gynek.* **57:** 108–112.

Maneschi M, Maneschi F, Geraci P *et al.* (1992) Surgical pathological staging of endometrial carcinoma and results of treatment. *Eur. J. Gynaecol. Oncol.* **13:** 30–35.

Matorras R, Rodriguez–Escuderoi FJ, Diez J, Genolla J, Fombellida J & Ruibal A (1992) Monitoring endometrial adenocarcinoma with a four tumor marker combination. CA 125, squamous cell carcinoma antigen, CA 19.9 and CA 15.3. *Acta Obstet. Gynec. Scand.* **71:** 458–464.

Melchiorri C, Chieco P, Lisignoli G, Marabini A & Orlandi C (1993) Ploidy disturbances as an early indicator of intrinsic malignancy in endometrial carcinoma. *Cancer* **72(1):** 165–172.

Morgan JD 3rd, Reddy S, Sarin P, Yordan E, DeGeest K & Hendrickson FR (1993) Isolated vaginal recurrences of endometrial carcinoma. *Radiology* **189:** 609–613.

■ Morrow CP, Bundy BN, Durman RJ *et al.* (1991) Relationship between surgical–pathological risk factors and outcome in clinical stage I and II carcinoma of the endometrium: a Gynecologic Oncology Group study. *Gynecol. Oncol.* **40:** 55–65

Nielsen AL, Thomsen HK & Nyholm HC (1991) Evaluation of the reproducibility of the revised 1988 International Federation of Gynecology and Obstetrics grading system of endometrial cancers with special emphasis on nuclear grading. *Cancer* **68(10):** 2303–2309.

Parsons AK & Lense JJ (1993) Sonohysterography for endometrial abnormalities: preliminary results. *J. Clin. Ultrasound* **21(2):** 87–95.

Piver MS, Recio FO, Baker TR & Hempling RE (1992) A prospective trial of progesterone therapy for malignant peritoneal cytology in patients with endometrial carcinoma. *Gynecol. Oncol.* **47(3):** 373–376.

■ Podratz K, Wilson T & Gaffey T (1993) Deoxyribonucleic acid analysis facilitates the pretreatment identification of high-risk endometrial cancer patients. *Am. J. Obstet. Gynecol.* **168:** 1206–1215.

Rose PG, Cha SD, Tak WK, Fitzgerald T, Reale F & Hunter RE (1992) Radiation therapy for surgically proven para-aortic node metastasis in endometrial carcinoma. *Int. J. Rad. Oncol. Biol. Phys.* **24:** 229–233.

Rosenberg P, Boeryd B & Simonsen E (1993) A new aggressive treatment approach to high-grade endometrial cancer of possible benefit to patients with stage I uterine papillary cancer. *Gynecol. Oncol.* **48:** 32–37.

Rotman M, Aziz H, Halpern J, Schwartz D, Sohn C & Choi K (1993) Endometrial carcinoma. Influence of prognostic factors on radiation management. (Review) *Cancer* **71:** 1471–1479.

Sahakian V, Syrop C & Turner D (1991) Endometrial carcinoma: Transvaginal ultrasonography prediction of depth of myometrial invasion. *Gynecol. Oncol.* **43:** 270–279.

Satyaswaroop PG, Clarke CL, Zaino RJ & Mortel R (1992) Apparent resistance in human endometrial carcinoma during combination treatment with tamoxifen and progestin may result from desensitization following downregulation of tumor progesterone receptor. *Cancer Letters* **62(2):** 107–114.

Shipley CF 3rd & Nelson GH (1993) Seeking early medical attention after vaginal bleeding will not assure mild disease in postmenopausal endometrial carcinoma. *Am. J. Obstet. Gynecol.* **168(2):** 555–556.

Sironi S, Colombo E, Villa G *et al.* (1992) Myometrial invasion by endometrial carcinoma: assessment with plan and gadolinium-enhanced MR imaging. *Radiology* **185(1):** 207–212.

Stendahl U, Strano P, Wagenius G, Bergstrom R & Tribukait B (1991) Prognostic significance of proliferation in endometrial adenocarcinomas: a multivariate analysis of clinical and flow cytometric variables. *Int. J. Gynecol. Pathol.* **10(3):** 271–284.

Thomas H, Pickering DG, Dunn P, Kam KC, Stewart JS & Lambert HE (1991) Treating the vaginal vault in carcinoma of the endometrium using the Buchler afterloading system. *Brit. J. Radiol.* **64:** 1044–1048.

Varpula MJ & Klemi PJ (1993) Staging of uterine endometrial carcinoma with ultra-low field (0.02 T) MRI: a comparative study with CT. *J. Computer Assisted Tomography* **17(4):** 641–647.

Vishnevsky AS, Tsyrlina EV, Sofroniy DF *et al.* (1993) Criteria of endometrial carcinoma sensitivity to hormone therapy: pathogenetic type of the disease and the tumor reaction to tamoxifen. *Eur. J. Gynaecol. Oncol.* **14**(2): 139–143.

Vishnevsky AS, Bokhman YV & Loutfi G (1993) Favorable influence of adjuvant hormone therapy by oxyprogesterone caproate (OPC) and by its combination with tamoxifen on 5-year survival rate of surgical and combined treatment of primary endometrial carcinoma patients. *Eur. J. Gynaecol. Oncol.* **14**(2): 150–153.

Wagenius G, Bergstrom R, Strang P *et al.* (1992) Prognostic significance of flow cytometric and clinical variables in endometrial adenocarcinoma stages I and II. *Anticancer Res.* **12**(3): 725–732.

Zaino RJ, Kurman R, Herbold D *et al.* (1991) The significance of squamous differentiation in endometrial carcinoma. Data from a Gynecologic Oncology Group study. *Cancer* **68**(10): 2293–2302.

12 Mesenchymal Uterine Tumors

M Morris

Introduction

Mesenchymal tumors of the uterus present a particularly challenging problem for the oncologist. Since these tumors are uncommon, most practising clinicians do not have extensive experience in their treatment. The literature is similarly limited due not only to small numbers of patients to study, but to the confusion in terminology and the lack of efficacious therapies for advanced disease. Most studies are retrospective reviews over long time periods.

The most common mesenchymal tumors encountered are the malignant mixed mesodermal tumors (MMMT), leiomyosarcoma (LMS) and endometrial stromal sarcoma (ESS). The terminology is further defined in Chapter 10. For the purposes of this chapter on clinical management, adenosarcoma is considered in the category of MMMT. In this section, we will attempt to unravel the data regarding mesenchymal tumors and develop plans for therapeutic management.

Presentation

Mesenchymal tumors tend to occur in postmenopausal women. Olah *et al.* (1992) noted that women with MMMT tended to be older than those with LMS; for women with MMMT, 91% were postmenopausal while only 58% of women diagnosed with LMS were postmenopausal. This observation has been confirmed by others, with the average age of diagnosis of LMS ranging from 43–51 years (Hannigan and Gomez, 1979; Vardi and Tovell, 1980; Dinh and Woodruff, 1982) versus a mean age of 60 years for women with MMMT (Peters *et al.*, 1984). The onset and progression of symptoms may be quite rapid, especially in the more aggressive variants. The most common presenting symptom is abnormal vaginal bleeding, which occurs in 80–90% of affected women (Hannigan and Gomez, 1979; Vardi and Tovell, 1980; Dinh and Woodruff, 1982; De Fusco *et al.*, 1989; Larson *et al.*, 1990b). Other symptoms such as abdominal pain, vaginal discharge and increasing abdominal girth may also be seen in uterine sarcoma. Women with ESS have been noted to present with tumor protruding through the cervical os associated with bleeding (De Fusco *et al.*, 1989).

Occasionally, a LMS is detected in a leiomyoma that is rapidly increasing in size (Dinh and Woodruff, 1982). However, the incidence of LMS in leiomyomata is only in the range of 0.13–0.29% (Leibsohn *et al.*, 1990).

Uterine sarcomas are not known to be associated with the same risk factors as endometrial cancer. Peters *et al.* (1984) noted that of women diagnosed with uterine sarcoma, 9% had been on estrogen replacement therapy, 33% had hypertension and 17% were diabetic. It has been observed that 10–14% of women with MMMT had a history of previous pelvic radiation therapy, usually for cervical cancer (Peters *et al.*, 1984; Larson *et al.*, 1990a). Previous radiation may impact the selection of therapy for these women.

Diagnosis

There is no effective screening method for these tumors. For MMMT or ESS, a Pap smear may show abnormal cells. Nearly all patients experience abnormal vaginal bleeding, which is an indicator for an endometrial biopsy. A biopsy or curettage will identify MMMT or ESS in most cases. In the case of MMMT, it is not uncommon for the biopsy to be read as adenocarcinoma with the sarcomatous component only being recognized at the time of definitive surgery.

LMS may be difficult to detect preoperatively. In a woman with a rapidly enlarging pelvic mass, especially when associated with pain or abnormal bleeding, LMS should be considered. Ultrasound is an effective means of evaluating the uterus. LMS may appear as a 'fibroid,' but when there is sonographic evidence of necrosis or internal hemorrhage, a malignant diagnosis must be considered. Computed tomograph (CT) and magnetic resonance imaging (MRI) scanning are alternatives to ultrasound examination, but rarely add additional useful information. Occasionally, performing a curettage will confirm a diagnosis of LMS. A suspicious lesion may be biopsied under ultrasound guidance. Most often, however, the diagnosis is made intra- or postoperatively.

These lesions have no specific tumor markers associated with them. Peters *et al.* (1986) have reported an elevated CA-125 in five of six women with MMMT who had metastatic or recurrent disease. They also found CA-125 to be a useful indicator of response during therapy. As might be predicted, immunohistochemical analysis of MMMT has shown the CA-125 to be present in the glandular sections of the tumor, but absent in the sarcomatous areas (Podczaski *et al.*, 1993). It is probably worth screening patients with MMMT for CA-125 as a potential marker of the extent of disease.

It has been reported that patients with LMS may have an elevated lactate dehydrogenase (Seki *et al.*, 1992). The clinical usefulness of this observation is not known.

Staging

There is no internationally accepted standard for the staging of mesenchymal tumors of the uterus. By convention, the staging methodology from the International Federation of Gynecology and Obstetrics (FIGO) for endometrial cancer has been adopted for use for uterine sarcomas (*Table 12.1*). Therefore, most of the literature refers to clinical staging for reports including patients before the late 1980s. There is little information on surgical staging which is the currently accepted FIGO method. Some authors have tried to further subdivide the staging based on the depth of myometrial invasion and the site and extent of extrauterine disease, but the value of these observations is unclear. In the case of LMS, the degree of myometrial invasion is not relevant.

The distribution of stage of uterine sarcomas is similar to that observed for women with endometrial cancer. In a study of all uterine sarcomas, 60% were Stage I, 6% were Stage II, 18% were Stage III, 16% were Stage IV and 3% were unknown (Olah *et al.*, 1992). There is a tendency for patients with MMMT to present with a higher stage than those with LMS (Vardi and Tovell, 1980; Larson *et al.*, 1990a).

Preoperative evaluation of patients with uterine sarcoma is used to define the extent of disease before surgery. This evaluation must take into account the potential routes of metastasis: direct extension, lymphatic and hematogenous. MMMT and ESS have a similar spread pattern compared with endometrial carcinoma. There may be invasion of the myometrium, extension to the cervix, and in more advanced cases, spread to other pelvic tissues and peritoneal dissemination. It is not unusual to have pelvic or paraortic node metastases. Hematogenous spread is not common at initial presentation, but some women may present with lung or liver metastases. LMS may spread in a similar manner, although hematogenous spread, especially to the lung, is more common (Omura *et al.*, 1985).

Table 12.1. Staging of uterine sarcomas.

Stage I	Disease confined to the corpus
Stage II	Disease confined to the corpus and cervix
Stage III	Involvement of other pelvic tissues
Stage IV	Extrapelvic disease

Information about nodal metastases is more limited. In an autopsy study, Rose *et al.* (1989) noted a 41% incidence of pelvic node disease and a 38% incidence of paraortic metastases in MMMT. Goff *et al.* (1993) studied LMS and found nodal spread in 26.7% of patients, but all of these also had disseminated intraabdominal disease. None of seven patients with ESS had disease detected in the lymph nodes. Based on this, it is difficult to make any recommendations about node sampling in women with uterine sarcomas.

Patients with uterine sarcoma should have a careful physical examination with particular attention to the pelvic evaluation. The cervix should be visually inspected and palpated to determine if there is involvement with tumor. Assessment of uterine size, the adnexae and cul-de-sac will give additional information. Palpation of the abdomen, auscultation of the chest and a survey of node-bearing areas are also elements of the overall examination

A chest radiograph is an adequate screen for metastatic disease in the lungs. I do not routinely obtain other radiologic studies since the liver, abdominal cavity and pelvic and paraortic nodes will be evaluated at the time of surgery. For patients with MMMT, a preoperative CA-125 may indicate the presence of extrauterine disease. Additional studies should be obtained for patients who have symptoms of extrauterine disease.

Surgery and Surgical Staging

The most effective therapy for mesenchymal tumors of the uterus is surgery. Nearly all patients with gross or microscopic residual tumor will succumb to their disease, making early diagnosis and complete surgical extirpation of the tumor critical. There are very occasional patients who present too high a risk for surgery due to serious medical problems. Primary radiotherapy has been used as sole therapy for MMMT in the past. Using a combination of external beam therapy and brachytherapy, the Radiumhemmet has reported a worse survival when compared to patients who also received surgery, either with or without radiation therapy (Larson *et al.*, 1990b). Based on this, every attempt should be made to treat patients surgically.

The surgical approach to women with mesenchymal tumors is very similar to that for endometrial carcinoma. The abdomen should be opened with a vertical midline incision to gain access to the pelvis and upper abdominal structures. Cytologic washings should be obtained followed by a careful inspection of the pelvic–abdominal contents. Any suspicious areas should be biopsied or removed.

For patients with no evidence of extrauterine disease, a total abdominal hysterectomy should be performed. In most cases, a bilateral salpingo–oophorectomy should be performed concurrently. In the case of LMS or low-grade ESS that occurs in a woman under the age of 45 years who wishes to maintain ovarian function, consideration can be given to ovarian conservation. For women with MMMT or ESS, the ovaries may harbor metastatic disease and should be routinely removed.

There are no set criteria for surgical staging. Because of the potential for lymphatic spread, I recommend sampling of the pelvic and paraaortic nodes, the results of which may impact any adjuvant therapy. An omental biopsy is also routinely obtained, but an omentectomy has no benefit. Biopsies should be obtained from any suspicious areas in the abdomen or pelvis. Random sampling of normal-appearing peritoneal structures probably has little benefit.

For patients with advanced disease, surgical therapy should be tailored to the sites and volume of tumor based on the histology. If the cervix is grossly involved with tumor, especially if it is significantly enlarged, preoperative pelvic radiation followed by brachytherapy and an extrafascial hysterectomy is suggested. This will ensure that the gross disease is cleared and improves the potential for cure provided that extrauterine disease is not present.

The role of cytoreductive surgery for patients with extrauterine disease has not been clearly defined. When advanced disease is encountered, most gynecologic oncologists will attempt to remove tumor when feasible although this is a palliative maneuver. In the case of MMMT, since the metastases are usually carcinoma, there may be some improvement in progression-free survival when there is minimal residual tumor before the use of chemotherapy. There are no data to support this opinion, however, and radical procedures to debulk a uterine sarcoma are not warranted in most cases. There are instances where a patient will present with advanced disease and, perhaps, even distant metastasis. Hysterectomy is still a consideration in the patient who is experiencing vaginal bleeding, the purpose of surgery being to palliate this symptom. The use of pelvic radiation may also slow or stop uterine bleeding and should be considered, especially when the patient is medically unstable. There is no role for aggressive cytoreductive surgery when there are distant metastases or parenchymal liver metastases.

Following surgery, the operative findings and the report from the pathologist will guide further therapy, if any. Based on prognostic factors outlined below, patients receive either no further therapy, adjuvant therapy, or additional treatment for known residual disease.

Leiomyosarcoma

The most important prognostic factors in LMS are stage, mitotic count and tumor size. It is recognized that patients with any degree of extrauterine disease are not likely to survive. Vardi and Tovell (1980) noted that five-year survival was 36.8% for patients with Stage I LMS, but no patients survived five years who had Stages II–IV. The mitotic index is also a powerful predictor of survival with the critical point defined as greater than or equal to ten mitoses per ten high power fields (Hannigan and Gomez, 1979; Vardi and Tovell, 1980). Patients with larger lesions are less likely to survive, although this may or may not be independent of surgical stage.

Malignant Mixed Mesodermal Tumors

For women with MMMT, stage, depth of myometrial invasion, and histology are predictors of survival. There are some survivors of MMMT with advanced disease, although the five-year survival rate for Stage III disease is under 10% (Peters *et al.*, 1984; Larson *et al.*, 1990a; Silverberg *et al.*, 1990). For women with Stage I disease, the five-year survival rate is in the area of 35–45%. Note that this is a far worse prognosis when compared to the expected 80–90% five-year survival observed for women with Stage I adenocarcinoma of the endometrium. With MMMT, the depth of myometrial invasion usually can be measured, with deeper invasion correlating with poor survival (Peters *et al.*, 1984; Silverberg *et al.*, 1990).

For patients with MMMT, a study by the Gynecologic Oncology Group (GOG) revealed that the depth of myometrial invasion also correlated with the incidence of extrauterine disease (Silverberg *et al.*, 1990). The GOG study also noted that MMMT with a clear cell or serous component was also more likely to have extrauterine spread. As noted by others, the histologic nature of the metastatic deposits was most frequently carcinoma, with only 10% having pure sarcoma. Patients with involvement of the cervix or lymph vascular invasion also had a worse prognosis.

Endometrial Stromal Sarcoma

ESS has a wide range of clinical behavior based for the most part on the mitotic count. Stromal nodules or low-grade ESS usually behave in a benign fashion. After surgical extirpation there is little chance of recurrence. Low-grade ESS will sometimes recur, sometimes after a disease-free interval of many years (De Fusco *et al.*, 1989). Some ESS will have positive estrogen or progesterone receptors and these should be assayed at the time of primary surgery since hormonal therapy may play a role for such a patient. Surgical stage is also an important predictor of survival from ESS (De Fusco *et al.*, 1989; Chang *et al.*, 1990). In a study of 117 women with ESS, Chang *et al.* (1990) noted a 98% five-year survival for Stage I lesions compared to 38% for Stage III.

Adjuvant Therapy

Despite the fact that good information regarding prognostic factors for mesenchymal tumors can indicate which patients have a high risk for recurrent disease, the decision to use adjuvant therapy is a difficult one, primarily because there is little evidence that adjuvant therapy is helpful. The data on adjuvant therapy will be reviewed to give the practitioner some guidelines on which to base decisions.

Adjuvant Radiotherapy

Many women with uterine sarcoma have traditionally been treated with postoperative pelvic radiation therapy. In a review of 64 patients with Stage I mesenchymal tumors, Rose *et al.* (1987) found no improvement in the survival of women treated with radiation following surgery versus those treated with surgery alone. Echt *et al.* (1990) performed a similar retrospective study with 66 cases and found no improvement in survival, but did note a decrease in the rate of pelvic recurrence in women who received adjuvant radiotherapy compared to those treated with surgery alone. This finding is echoed in two other studies, which found only decreased rates of pelvic recurrence in those women treated with adjuvant radiotherapy (Sorbe, 1985; Covens *et al.*, 1987). In a review of 225 women treated by the GOG with mesenchymal tumors, there was no survival advantage following adjuvant radiotherapy for women with Stage I or II tumors, but radiation did appear to decrease the incidence of pelvic recurrence for both LMS and MMMT (Hornback *et al.*, 1986). The GOG study was a re-analysis of data gathered from a randomized trial that compared the use of adjuvant chemotherapy versus no further therapy. A problem in this study was that many women also received adjuvant radiotherapy in a non-randomized fashion, a fact that confounds the results of both analyses.

Proponents of adjuvant radiotherapy correctly point out that selection bias may influence the findings of retrospective studies. Women who were treated with adjuvant radiotherapy may have had worse prognostic factors compared to those who did not receive adjuvant therapy. There is no question that radiotherapy at least alters the natural history of mesenchymal tumors since the finding of a decreased rate of pelvic recurrence is a consistent theme in the literature.

In an often quoted literature review, Salazar and Dunne (1980) do recommend the use of adjuvant pelvic radiotherapy to decrease pelvic recurrence. They suggest treating patients with 50 Gy whole pelvic radiation followed by a vaginal cylinder to boost the vaginal cuff. While this regimen can be expected to have little serious toxicity, in the absence of an improvement in survival, the use of adjuvant radiotherapy must be questioned based on the additional cost and morbidity associated with that added treatment. A well-designed randomized trial should be conducted to provide a definitive answer to this question.

Adjuvant Chemotherapy

The use of adjuvant chemotherapy for women with Stage I mesenchymal tumors of the uterus has never been shown to have significant benefit. Some investigators have claimed potential benefit from adjuvant chemotherapy based on small single-arm trials. Peters *et al.* (1989) treated 17 women with Stage I MMMT and ESS with cisplatin and doxorubicin following primary surgery. With a median follow-up of 34 months, the calculated five-year survival rate was 75% which, they noted, was an improvement over historical controls. In another trial, seven women were treated with vincristine, dactinomycin and cyclophosphamide (VAC) following surgery for MMMT (Van Nagell *et al.*, 1986). Of the seven women, five remained disease free with a follow-up ranging from 48–73 months.

Piver *et al.* compared the results with surgery alone against surgery and adjuvant treatment with adriamycin for a small group of women with mixed histologies (MMMT and LMS) (Piver *et al.*, 1979) and another trial where the adjuvant therapy was cyclophosphamide, vincristine, adriamycin, and dimethyl-triazeno imidazole carboxamide (CYVADIC) (Piver *et al.*, 1982). Calculated five-year survival rates were 36% for surgery alone, 63% for surgery plus adriamycin, and 89% for surgery plus CYVADIC. While these results were encouraging, the small number of treated patients (total 30) and mixed histologies give these studies poor statistical validity.

In a study from M.D. Anderson Cancer Center, 34 patients received adjuvant chemotherapy with either doxorubicin or VAC following primary surgery for mesenchymal tumors of the uterus (Hannigan *et al.*, 1983b). This group was compared to 67 women who did not receive adjuvant chemotherapy. The use of chemotherapy had no apparent effect on survival or progression-free survival.

There has been only one randomized trial of adjuvant chemotherapy in uterine sarcoma. Because of slow accrual, this study took over ten years to complete. In this GOG trial, patients were randomized to receive doxorubicin versus no chemotherapy after primary surgery (Omura *et al.*, 1985). As mentioned above, this study was flawed by the non-random use of adjuvant radiotherapy. The study also mixed LMS, MMMT and ESS in the study design. However, the investigators found no difference in survival or progression-free survival between the two groups.

The use of adjuvant therapy remains controversial. There is little evidence that either chemotherapy or radiotherapy provides a significant protective benefit for women with Stage I disease. Because the prognosis for even early uterine sarcomas is so poor, many women receive some form of adjuvant therapy because the clinician feels the need to 'do something.'

Therapy for Advanced or Recurrent Disease

For women with documented extrauterine disease or recurrent disease, additional therapy is usually warranted. The usual treatment modality is systemic chemotherapy although there are clinical situations where either surgery or radiotherapy may play a role. The choice of therapy will depend on the timing and location of the recurrence, the type of symptoms the patient has, and the histologic type. For patients with MMMT, recurrence is most often in the peritoneum or in retroperitoneal nodes. About half will recur in the pelvis (Larson *et al.*, 1990a). Patients will often present with increasing abdominal girth, pain, or a mass on pelvic examination. The pattern of recurrence is very similar to that of endometrial cancer. For LMS, the presenting symptoms reflect the propensity for lung metastases followed by locoregional recurrence: 41% present with shortness of breath, 34% with pain and 31% with a pelvic mass or increasing abdominal girth (Vardi and Tovell, 1980). Hannigan and Gomez (1979) noted that the most common sites of extrapelvic disease were lung, bone and liver. Patients with high-grade ESS recur in the pelvis (50%) and at distant sites (50%) (De Fusco *et al.*, 1989). The most common site of distant recurrence of ESS is the lung (Chang *et al.*, 1990).

Surgery

As discussed above, cytoreductive surgery has a very limited role in the treatment of advanced disease. Debulking of intraperitoneal deposits in MMMT may provide some benefit as an adjunct to chemotherapy. This is probably not the case in advanced LMS or ESS. In the case of recurrent disease, secondary cytoreductive surgery for any of these tumor types cannot be justified except to palliate symptoms such as bowel obstruction. Patients with truly advanced disease have a short median survival whether additional surgery is performed or not. The expense and hospitalization time should be taken into account when considering surgical procedures in these women.

Some women with low-grade LMS or ESS have very indolent tumors which may repeatedly recur over long disease-free intervals. Some of these patients may benefit from repeated surgical resections to control symptoms. Surgical candidates must be carefully selected. The goal of the surgery is to provide relief from symptoms, and the feasibility of achieving this goal should be carefully assessed by physical examination and radiologic studies before starting. Very occasionally, a distant metastasis can be resected with good results (Levenback *et al.*, 1992).

Radiotherapy

Radiotherapy can also be used in a palliative manner for women with advanced or recurrent mesenchymal tumors of the uterus. For women who have not received adjuvant pelvic radiation, a small pelvic wall or vaginal recurrence can be treated with either external beam radiation, some type of implant, or both. Recurrent disease in other locations (e.g. supraclavicular nodes, lung, bone) can also be treated with palliative radiation. It is unlikely that radiation will be able to cure gross or palpable tumor, but it can relieve symptoms in selected cases.

Hormonal Therapy

High-grade mesenchymal tumors of the uterus are usually unresponsive to any form of hormonal manipulation. Low-grade ESS may be responsive to progestational therapy. The most commonly used regimen is megestrol, 40 mg four times daily. This has also been suggested as a treatment for low-grade LMS, although it has been difficult to find a well-documented response in the literature. Hormonal therapy for MMMT is strictly a placebo maneuver.

Chemotherapy

In distinction to the literature on adjuvant therapy for mesenchymal tumors of the uterus, there have been a number of well-designed phase II and III trials using chemotherapy to treat advanced or recurrent disease, most of which were conducted by the GOG. Some of these trials are summarized in *Table 12.2.*

Uterine sarcomas are often treated with the regimens used for other types of soft tissue sarcomas. The observation that these regimens often have less efficacy when treating uterine sarcomas confirms the differing biologic behavior compared to extrauterine sarcomas. Doxorubicin has been considered the 'standard' therapy, although the results with this agent are poor. In a randomized trial by the GOG, single-agent doxorubicin was compared to doxorubicin plus cyclophosphamide for women with MMMT, LMS or ESS. Both arms of this trial had an overall response rate of 19% (Muss *et al.*, 1985). Another 'standard' sarcoma drug is dimethyl-triazeno imidazole carboxamide (DTIC). In another randomized GOG trial with similar eligibility criteria, DTIC plus doxorubicin had an overall response rate of 24.2% versus a response rate of 16.3% for doxorubicin alone (Omura *et al.*, 1983). The difference between these two arms was not significant and no survival advantage was noted in the DTIC arm. Doxorubicin has been particularly disappointing in patients with MMMT. Gershenson *et al.* (1987) treated 15 patients for MMMT with single agent doxorubicin. There were no responders.

It has been observed that MMMT and LMS have very different response profiles to chemotherapy. Early reports tended to lump these tumors together, primarily to gather greater numbers of patients. More recent investigators have established separate clinical trials for patients with MMMT and LMS. The differences between these tumor types are illustrated in the trials with cisplatin, the drug that is most commonly used for gynecologic cancers.

Thigpen *et al.* (1986a) evaluated cisplatin at a dose of 50 mg m^{-2} repeated at three-week intervals for women with LMS. Of 33 patients evaluated, there was only one partial response (3%). The same regimen was used by the GOG for 63 women with MMMT (Thigpen *et al.*, 1986b). A complete response was noted in 8% and partial response in 11% (overall response rate 19%). Using a higher dose of cisplatin (75–100 mg m^{-2}), Gershenson *et al.* (1987) noted an overall response rate of 42%.

The drug that has recently attracted the most interest for mesenchymal tumors of the uterus has been ifosfamide: when given at a dose of 1.5 g m^{-2} daily for five days repeated every four weeks, a response rate of 32.2% was noted for MMMT and 17.2% for LMS (Sutton *et al.*, 1989, 1992). Ifosfamide is currently being evaluated in combination with other drugs for the treatment of mesenchymal tumors of the uterus.

Paclitaxel (Taxol) is currently undergoing evaluation as a single agent for the treatment of uterine sarcomas. There have been anecdotal reports of a response with this agent, but the overall activity is difficult to assess at this time.

Based on the literature, the use of ifosfamide should be considered, possibly with the addition of cisplatin, for the treatment of MMMT. For LMS, ifosfamide seems to have the most activity. There is less information about ESS. Peters *et al.* (1989) reported a 73% response rate to cisplatin and doxorubicin. The number of patients was small, however.

Even when patients with mesenchymal tumors of the uterus respond to chemotherapy, the progression-free interval tends to be short, with little, if any, impact on survival. There is no true 'standard' therapy, therefore, and most patients should be

Table 12.2. Chemotherapy trials for mesenchymal tumors of the uterus.

Authors	*Histology*	*n*	*Regimen*	*CR (%)*	*PR (%)*	*CR+PR (%)*
Piver *et al.*, 1982	Mixed	10	CYVADIC	11.5	11.5	23.0
Hannigan *et al.*, 1983	Mixed	74	VAC	13.3	15.6	28.9
Thigpen *et al.*, 1986	MMMT	63	CDDP 50 mg m^{-2} q3 wks	8.0	11.0	19.0
Muss *et al.*, 1990	MMMT	17	Mitoxantrone 12 mg m^{-2} q3 wks	0	0	0
Sutton *et al.*, 1989	MMMT	28	Ifos 1.5 g $m^{-2}\times 5$ days q3 wks	17.9	14.3	32.2
Gershenson *et al.*, 1987a	MMMT	15	Doxorubicin 90 mg m^{-2} q4 wks	0	0	0
Gershenson *et al.*, 1987b	MMMT	18	CDDP 75–100 mg m^{-2} q4 wks	8.0	33.0	42.0
Omura *et al.*, 1983	LMS	28	Doxorubicin 60 mg m^{-2} q3 wks			25.0
Thigpen *et al.*, 1986	LMS	33	CDDP 50 mg m^{-2} q3 wks	0	3.0	3.0
Muss *et al.*, 1990	LMS	12	Mitoxantrone 12 mg m^{-2} q3 wks	0	0	0
Slayton, 1987	LMS	28	VP–16 100 mg $m^{-2}\times 3$ days q4 wks	3.6	7.2	10.7
Sutton *et al.*, 1992	LMS	35	Ifos 1.5 g $m^{-2}\times 5$ days q3 wks	0	17.2	17.2
Peters *et al.*, 1989	ESS, MMMT	11	CDDP/doxorubicin	73	0	73

CYVADIC, cyclophosphamide, vincristine, adriamycin, and dimethyl-triazeno imidazole carboxamide; VAC, vincristine, dactinomycin and cyclophosphamide; CDDP, cisplatin; Ifos, ifosfamide; CR, complete response; PR, partial response.

considered for investigational therapy where available so that additional progress can be made in the treatment of uterine sarcomas.

Surveillance

Surveillance of asymptomatic patients following primary therapy is primarily aimed at detecting an early disease recurrence. This presumes that treatment of an early recurrence either prolongs the length or quality of life. Since nearly all women with recurrent disease are not curable and because very few asymptomatic patients will derive benefit from early therapy, it is difficult to be dogmatic about a surveillance scheme. There is a value to the support a patient is given upon being given a clean bill of health. I do, however, temper my enthusiasm for aggressive or frequent surveillance of the patient without symptoms.

During the first two years following therapy, it is suggested that patients are seen every 3–4 months and have a complete physical examination. The use of CA-125 should be considered in women with MMMT since a rise in this marker is predictive of recurrence. A chest radiograph may detect an early pulmonary metastasis, and I obtain one at every other visit. A Pap smear has little value since nearly all recurrent disease on the vaginal mucosa will be grossly visible. I do not routinely obtain CT or MRI scans as part of surveillance unless there was extrauterine disease that was eradicated by therapy. Again, the expense and discomforts associated with these tests must be weighed against the little (or no) value of early detection.

After the first two years, the surveillance interval may be lengthened to every six months until the five-year point is reached. After five years, the chance of recurrent disease is small.

Summary of Management Options

- Leiomyosarcoma (LMS) patients should initially be treated with total abdominal hysterectomy, bilateral salpingo-oophorectomy and staging biopsies. There is no evidence that adjuvant radiation therapy or chemotherapy is of benefit.
- For patients with advanced or recurrent LMS, the most active chemotherapeutic agents are ifosfamide and doxorubicin. Low-grade indolent lesions may benefit from repeat resection.
- Malignant mixed mesodermal tumor (MMMT) should be treated with total abdominal hysterectomy, bilateral salpingo-oophorectomy and staging biopsies. Cytoreductive surgery for advanced disease is probably not beneficial.
- Adjuvant therapy with radiation in MMMT may decrease the rate of pelvic failure, but has little or no impact on survival.
- Adjuvant chemotherapy for MMMT has no clear benefit. Recurrent or advanced disease is best treated with cisplatin or ifosfamide, possibly in combination.
- Women with endometrial stromal sarcoma (ESS) should undergo total abdominal hysterectomy, bilateral salpingo-oophorectomy and staging biopsies. Adjuvant therapy has no proven benefit.
- Recurrent high-grade lesions may be treated with ifosfamide, doxorubicin or cisplatin. When low-grade ESS lesions recur, consideration should be given to resection when possible, or hormonal therapy.

References

■ Chang KL, Crabtree GS, Lim-Tan SK, Kempson RL & Hendrickson MR (1990) Primary uterine endometrial stromal neoplasms. A clinicopathologic study of 117 cases. *Am. J. Surg. Pathol.* **14(5):** 415–438.

Covens AL, Nisker JA, Chapman WB & Allen HH (1987) Uterine sarcoma: an analysis of 74 cases. *Am. J. Obstet. Gynecol.* **156(2):** 370–374.

De Fusco PA, Gaffey TA, Malkasian G Jr, Long HJ & Cha SS (1989) Endometrial stromal sarcoma: review of Mayo Clinic experience, 1945–1980. *Gynecol. Oncol.* **35(1):** 8–14.

Dinh TV & Woodruff JD (1982) Leiomyosarcoma of the uterus. *Am. J. Obstet. Gynecol.* **144:** 817–823.

Echt G, Jepson J, Steel J *et al.* (1990) Treatment of uterine sarcomas. *Cancer* **66(1):** 35–39.

Gershenson DM, Kavanagh JJ, Copeland LJ, Edwards CL, Freedman RS & Wharton JT (1987a) High-dose doxorubicin infusion therapy for disseminated mixed mesodermal sarcoma of the uterus. *Cancer* **59(7):** 1264–1267.

Gershenson DM, Kavanagh JJ, Copeland LJ, Edwards CL, Stringer CA & Wharton JT (1987b) Cisplatin therapy for disseminated mixed mesodermal sarcoma of the uterus. *J. Clin. Oncol.* **5(4):** 618–621.

Goff B, Rice LW, Fleischhacker D, Muntz HG, Falkenberry SS, Nikrui N & Fuller AJ (1993) Uterine leiomyosarcoma and endometrial stromal sarcoma: lymph node metastases and sites of recurrence. *Gynecol. Oncol.* **50(1):** 105–109.

Hannigan EV, Freedman RS & Rutledge FN (1983a) Adjuvant chemotherapy in early uterine sarcoma. *Gynecol. Oncol.* **15(1)**: 56–64.

Hannigan EV, Freedman RS, Elder KW & Rutledge FN (1983b) Treatment of advanced uterine sarcoma with vincristine, actinomycin D and cyclophosphamide. *Gynecol. Oncol.* **15(2)**: 224–229.

Hannigan EV & Gomez LG (1979) Uterine leiomyosarcoma. *Am. J. Obstet. Gynecol.* **134(5)**: 557–564.

Hornback NB, Omura G & Major FJ (1986) Observations on the use of adjuvant radiation therapy in patients with stage I and II uterine sarcoma. *Int. J. Radiat. Oncol. Biol. Phys.* **12(12)**: 2127–2130.

■ Larson B, Silfversward C, Nilsson B & Pettersson F (1990a) Mixed Müllerian tumours of the uterus—prognostic factors: a clinical and histopathologic study of 147 cases. *Radiother. Oncol.* **17**: 123–132.

Larson B, Silfversward C, Nilsson B & Pettersson F (1990b) Endometrial stromal sarcoma of the uterus. A clinical and histopathological study. The Radiumhemmet series 1936–1981. *Eur. J. Obstet. Gynecol. Reprod. Biol.* **35(2-3)**: 239–249.

Leibsohn S, D'Ablaing G, Mishell D Jr & Schlaerth JB (1990) Leiomyosarcoma in a series of hysterectomies performed for presumed uterine leiomyomas. *Am. J. Obstet. Gynecol.* **162(4)**: 968–974.

Atkinson EN & Lewis J, Jr (1992) Resection of pulmonary metastases from uterine sarcomas. *Gynecol. Oncol.* **45(2)**: 202–205.

Muss HB, Bundy B, Di Saia PJ *et al.* (1985) Treatment of recurrent or advanced uterine sarcoma. A randomized trial of doxorubicin versus doxorubicin and cyclophosphamide (a phase III trial of the Gynecologic Oncology Group). *Cancer* **55(8)**: 1648–1653.

Muss, HB, Bundy BN, Adcock L & Beecham J (1990) Mitoxantrone in the treatment of advanced uterine sarcoma: A phase II trial of the Gynecologic Oncology Group. *Am. J. Clin. Oncol.* **13(1)**: 32–34.

■ Olah KS, Dunn JA & Gee H (1992) Leiomyosarcomas have a poorer prognosis than mixed mesodermal tumours when adjusting for known prognostic factors: the result of a retrospective study of 423 cases of uterine sarcoma. *Br. J. Obstet. Gynaecol.* **99(7)**: 590–594.

Omura GA, Blessing JA, Major F *et al.* (1985) A randomized clinical trial of adjuvant adriamycin in uterine sarcomas: a Gynecologic Oncology Group Study. *J. Clin. Oncol.* **3(9)**: 1240–1245.

Omura GA, Major FJ, Blessing JA *et al.* (1983) A randomized study of adriamycin with and without dimethyl triazenoimidazole carboxamide in advanced uterine sarcomas. *Cancer* **52(4)**: 626–632.

Peters WA, Bagley CM & Smith MR (1986) CA–125. Use as a tumor marker with mixed mesodermal tumors of the female genital tract. *Cancer* **58(12)**: 2625–2627.

Peters WA, Kumar NB, Fleming WP & Morley GW (1984) Prognostic features of sarcomas and mixed tumors of the endometrium. *Obstet. Gynecol.* **63(4)**: 550–556.

Peters WA, Rivkin SE, Smith MR & Tesh DE (1989) Cisplatin and adriamycin combination chemotherapy for uterine stromal sarcomas and mixed mesodermal tumors. *Gynecol. Oncol.* **34(3)**: 323–327.

Piver MS, Barlow JJ, Lele SB & Yazigi R (1979) Adriamycin in localized and metastatic uterine sarcomas. *J. Surg. Oncol.* **12(3)**: 263–265.

Piver MS, De Eulis TG, Lele SB & Barlow JJ (1982) Cyclophosphamide, vincristine, adriamycin, and dimethyltriazeno imidazole carboxamide (CYVADIC) for sarcomas of the female genital tract. *Gynecol. Oncol.* **14(3)**: 319–323.

Podczaski E, Kaminski P, Hackett TE, Olt GJ & Zaino R (1993) Tissue CA 125 and CA 19–9 in malignant, mixed mesodermal tumors of the uterus. *Gynecol. Oncol.* **49(1)**: 56–60.

Rose PG, Boutselis JG & Sachs L (1987) Adjuvant therapy for stage I uterine sarcoma. *Am. J. Obstet. Gynecol.* **156(3)**: 660–662.

Rose PG, Piver MS, Tsukada Y & Lau T (1989) Patterns of metastasis in uterine sarcoma. An autopsy study. *Cancer* **63(5)**: 935–938.

Salazar OM & Dunne ME (1980) The role of radiation therapy in the management of uterine sarcomas. *Int. J. Radiat. Oncol. Biol. Phys.* **6(7)**: 899–902.

Seki K, Hoshihara T & Nagata I (1992) Leiomyosarcoma of the uterus: ultrasonography and serum lactate dehydrogenase level. *Obstet. Invest.* **33(2)**: 114–118.

■ Silverberg SG, Major FJ, Blessing JA *et al.* (1990) Carcinosarcoma (malignant mixed mesodermal tumor) of the uterus. A Gynecologic Oncology Group pathologic study of 203 cases. *Int. J. Gynecol. Pathol.* **9(1)**: 1–19.

Slayton RE, Blessing JA, Angel C & Berman M (1987) Phase II trial of etoposide in the management of advanced and recurrent leiomyosarcoma of the uterus: a Gynecologic Oncology Group Study. *Cancer Treat. Rep.* **71(12)**: 1303–1304.

Sorbe B (1985) Radiotherapy and/or chemotherapy as adjuvant treatment of uterine sarcomas. *Gynecol. Oncol.* **20(3)**: 281–289.

Sutton GP, Blessing JA, Barrett, RJ & McGehee R (1992) Phase II trial of ifosfamide and mesna in leiomyosarcoma of the uterus: a Gynecologic Oncology Group study. *Am. J. Obstet. Gynecol.* **166(2)**: 556–559.

■ Sutton GP, Blessing JA, Rosenshein N, Photopulos G & Di Saia PJ (1989) Phase II trial of ifosfamide and mesna in mixed mesodermal tumors of the uterus (a Gynecologic Oncology Group study). *Am. J. Obstet. Gynecol.* **161(2)**: 309–312.

Thigpen JT, Blessing JA & Wilbanks GD (1986a). Cisplatin as second-line chemotherapy in the treatment of advanced or recurrent leiomyosarcoma of the uterus. A phase II trial of the Gynecologic Oncology Group. *Am. J. Clin. Oncol.* **9(1)** 18–20.

Thigpen JT, Blessing JA, Orr J Jr & Di Saia PJ (1986b) Phase II trial of cisplatin in the treatment of patients with advanced or recurrent mixed mesodermal sarcomas of the uterus: a Gynecologic Oncology Group Study. *Cancer Treat. Rep.* **70(2)**: 271–274.

Van Nagell J Jr, Hanson MB, Donaldson ES & Gallion HH (1986) Adjuvant vincristine, dactinomycin, and cyclophosphamide therapy in stage I uterine sarcomas. A pilot study. *Cancer* **57(8)**: 1451–1454.

Vardi JR & Tovell HM (1980) Leiomyosarcoma of the uterus: clinicopathologic study. *Obstet. Gynecol.* **56(4)**: 428–434.

13 Pathogenesis and Epidemiology of Ovarian Cancer

P Doyle
I dos Santos Silva

National and International Variations

Cancer of the ovary is one of the most common malignancies in women in industrialized countries: about 4200 new cases of ovarian cancer in England and Wales (Swerdlow and dos Santos Silva, 1993) and 21,000 in the USA (Yancik, 1993) are diagnosed each year. Mortality rates are only slightly lower than incidence rates and are a reflection of the poor prognosis. In England and Wales only 25% of women with the malignancy survive as long as five years after diagnosis although younger women do survive longer: 40% of those who are 35–44 years of age at diagnosis survive for five years compared to 17% of those aged 65–74 (Office of Population Censuses and Surveys, 1982). Because of its high incidence and poor prognosis, ovarian cancer represents the fifth most common cause of death from cancer among British and US white women.

It has long been recognized that ovarian cancer is more common in the industrialized than in the non-industrialized world, Japan being an exception. World statistics show that this international variation is considerable, the incidence in the highest-risk countries being five times greater than that in the lowest-risk countries (Muir *et al.*, 1987). The highest reported incidence rates are from Sweden, Norway and other affluent countries, whereas the lowest are from Japan and other Asian countries (Muir *et al.*, 1987). It seems unlikely, however, that this variation between countries is due to racial or genetic differences as migrants from low- to high-risk areas shift their risk to that of the host country. For example, first generation Chinese and Japanese women in the US have lower rates of ovarian cancer than US white women, but those in the second generation have rates similar to those of US women (King and Haenszel, 1973). Further evidence of environmental determinants of the disease is provided by the differences between women in different social classes in England and Wales: women in the upper (professional) social classes have a higher risk of developing ovarian cancer than women in the lower (manual worker) social classes (Beral *et al.*, 1978).

Ovarian cancer comprises a wide variety of histologic types, but relatively little is known about ethnic and international variations in the occurrence of the different cell types because diagnostic, histologic and coding criteria of these tumours have varied over time and from place to place. Data from the US Third National Cancer Survey showed that Japanese, Chinese, Hispano and black women living in the USA have similar incidences of non-epithelial tumours to white women, but have lower rates for all major epithelial tumour types (Weiss *et al.*, 1977; Weiss and Peterson, 1978). International data on histology published in Volume II of Cancer Incidence in Five Continents (Doll *et al.*, 1970) showed that the international gradient in risk was present for all histologic types except dysgerminomas (Berg and Baylor, 1973). It is, however, impossible to determine how much these findings were affected by diagnostic and coding artefacts.

The incidence and mortality rates from ovarian cancer increase rapidly with age until the sixth decade of life, after which they begin to plateau. Similar age curves have been described for all the main histologic types of epithelial ovarian tumours and also for sex-cord and mesenchymal tumours (Weiss *et al.*, 1977). Germ cell malignancies, however, have a distinct age pattern with an early sharp peak at 15–19 years of age, to which dysgerminomas and teratomas contribute equally, and a later broader peak at ages 65–69, mainly due to teratomas (Berg and Baylor, 1973; dos Santos Silva and Swerdlow, 1991).

Time Trends

Incidence of ovarian cancer (all ages combined) in England and Wales increased markedly from 1959–1987, but the trends differed by age: at ages 45 years and over, there was a marked increase in rates, whereas at ages 0–44 years there was a small decrease. The decline is now starting to reach older women. Mortality data for the years 1960–1991 showed similar patterns (dos Santos Silva and Swerdlow, 1995).

Analyses by year of birth show that the risk of ovarian cancer increased steeply for successive generations of women born before the turn of the

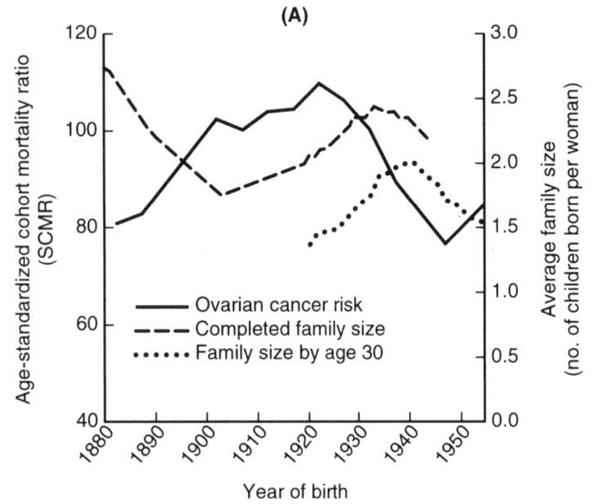

Average completed family size cannot be calculated for the most recent cohorts because they are still at childbearing ages. Therefore, data on the family size achieved by age 30 are also shown for cohorts born since 1920.

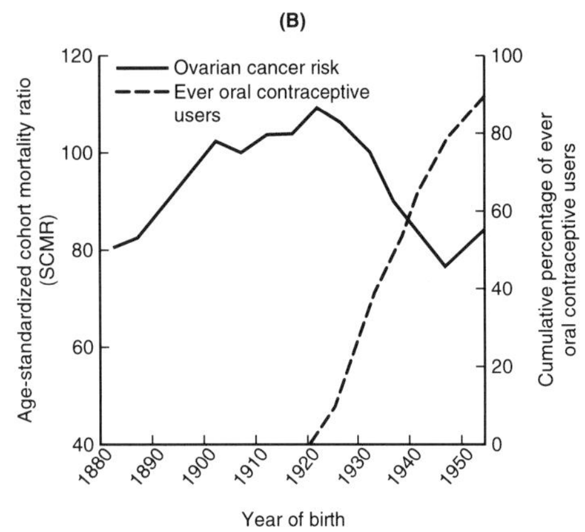

Data from Registrar General (1962–75), OPCS (1977–93), and dos Santos Silva & Swerdlow (1995). An SCMR of 110 indicates that the mortality for that particular cohort was 10% above the average for all women in this analysis, whereas an SCMR of 90 indicates it was 10% lower.

Figure 13.1. Mortality trends of ovarian cancer, family size (A) and cumulative percentage use of oral contraceptives (B) in women born 1880–1959, England and Wales, 1960–1991.

century, increased more slowly for cohorts thereafter (reaching a maximum for those born in the 1920s), and decreased for those born subsequently (*Figure 13.1*). The increase in risk for women born before the turn of the century paralleled marked declines in their fertility (*Figure 13.1A*). A similar negative relationship between ovarian cancer risk and family size was also seen in England and Wales and in the USA for an earlier period (Beral *et al.*, 1978). The fall in risk for women born after the 1920s was not accompanied by significant increases in fertility, but coincided with the introduction and increase in use of combined oral contraceptives (*Figure 13.1B*) (dos Santos Silva and Swerdlow, 1995).

Recent international trends in ovarian cancer incidence and mortality are also compatible with a protective effect of combined oral contraceptives (Coleman *et al.*, 1993; Mant and Vessey, 1994). In countries with a high prevalence of oral contraceptive use (e.g. Finland, Denmark, New Zealand, USA, Canada) there have been declines in risk (although more marked for mortality than incidence) for women born since the 1920s. Similarly to England and Wales, these declines were accompanied by decreases, not increases, in fertility (Mant and Vessey, 1994). A decreasing trend in the incidence of ovarian cancer for women born since the 1920s paralleling increases in the use of oral contraceptives was also observed in Sweden (Adami *et al.*, 1990). In contrast, in countries such as Japan where the prevalence of oral contraceptive use is very low (fewer than 1% of women in Japan used oral contraceptives in 1991 (Ogawa and Retherford, 1991)), risks have increased markedly in the last decades and show no indication of levelling off (Coleman *et al.*, 1993). The association between reproductive factors, oral contraception and ovarian cancer risk is discussed further in the next section.

The time trends described above mainly reflect trends for epithelial tumors, which account for more than 85% of all ovarian tumors (Weiss *et al.*, 1977). Very few data are available on trends in risk of other histologic types. Analyses of cancer registration data for England and Wales 1971–1984 showed that time trends in ovarian germ cell cancers were different at young and older ages: incidence increased at ages 0–44 years, but decreased at ages over 44 years (dos Santos Silva and Swerdlow, 1991). These diverging trends by age were mainly due to teratomas; there were no significant changes in the incidence of dysgerminomas during 1971—1984. Walker *et al.* (1984) also reported an increasing secular trend in ovarian germ cell cancer in young women (although mainly in dysgerminomas) and no significant changes at older ages in Los Angeles County during the period 1972–1981. Data on trends for other non-epithelial ovarian tumors are not available.

Risk Factors for Ovarian Cancer

Risk Factors Associated with a Decrease in Risk

Parity

It has been known for some time that reproductive factors influence a woman's risk of developing ovarian cancer. Single women have considerably higher rates of ovarian cancer than those who are married (Beral *et al.*, 1978) and sociodemographic differentials in fertility rates are consistent with the distribution of ovarian cancer in the general population. Ovarian cancer tends to be less common in lower socioeconomic groups (Beral *et al.*, 1978), Mormons (Enstrom, 1980), and Seventh-Day

Table 13.1. Risk factors for ovarian cancer.

Factors associated with decreased risk	*Factors associated with increased risk*
Increasing parity	Family history
Increasing age at first birth	Use of fertility drugs
Use of oral contraception	Radiation
Lactation	Dietary fat/milk consumption[1]
Tubal ligation/hysterectomy	Talc[1]
	Early menarche/late menopause[1]

[1]Associations not confirmed.

Adventists (Phillips, 1975), all of which experience relatively high fertility rates. In contrast, incidence rates are higher among nuns (Fraumeni *et al.*, 1969). Both case–control studies and cohort studies have clearly demonstrated the protective effect of births. Recent large collaborative studies involving the re-analysis of data from several centers in the USA (Whittemore *et al.*, 1992a) and Europe (Negri *et al.*, 1991), and a large national Swedish study (Adami *et al.*, 1994), have confirmed a decreasing risk with increasing parity. *Figure 13.2A* presents results from studies with 500 cases or more, and shows that women with four or more births have approximately half the risk of nulliparous women for epithelial ovarian cancer. The study by Adami *et al.* (1994) found a similar trend for non-epithelial cancer. There remains some controversy over the protective effect of uncompleted pregnancy in nulliparous women: Negri *et al.* (1991) reported a decreasing trend in risk with number of abortions, whereas Whittemore *et al.* (1992a) found that gravidity did not affect risk.

Age at first birth

Although not as clear and uncontroversial as parity, evidence for an effect of decreasing risk of epithelial ovarian cancer with increasing age at first birth (after adjustment for parity itself) is now good (Whittemore *et al.*, 1992a; Adami *et al.*, 1994) (see *Figure 13.2B*). The data from Sweden (Adami *et al.*, 1994) demonstrate a 10% reduction in risk for each five-year increment in age at first birth (see *Figure 13.2*), and a similar effect was found for non-epithelial ovarian cancers (Adami *et al.*, 1994). The Swedish study also examined temporal relationships between pregnancy and risk: a reduced risk soon after birth was found with the protective effect diminishing over time (Adami *et al.*, 1994).

Combined oral contraceptives

Oral contraceptives mimic pregnancy by suppressing ovulation and by reducing secretion of pituitary gonadotropins. As a result, one would expect oral contraceptives to reduce the risk of ovarian cancer. This relationship has now been assessed in more than 20 case–control studies conducted worldwide. Risk in ever-users range from 40–60% of that in never-users and the degree of protection increases with duration of use among ever-users (see *Figure 13.2C*): women who use oral contraceptives for five or more years experience about a 60% reduction in risk. The large majority of the studies not included in *Figure 13.2C* showed similar results. The magnitude of the negative association between oral contraceptives and ovarian cancer seems to be similar in developed and developing countries (The WHO Collaborative Study of Neoplasia and Steroid Contraceptives, 1989), and in white and black women (John *et al.*, 1993).

The protective effect of oral contraceptive use seems to persist for 15 years or more after cessation of use (Cancer and Steroid Hormone Study, 1987; Franceschi *et al.*, 1991b; Whittemore *et al.*, 1992a). In one of these studies (Franceschi *et al.*, 1991b) the protective effect was more marked for women who reported their first use before 25 years of age, but this finding was not observed in the other two studies (Cancer and Steroid Hormone Study, 1987; Whittemore *et al.*, 1992a). However, the separate effects of age at first use, time since first and last use, and duration of use are not easy to disentangle.

Most of the studies have been on invasive epithelial cancer and relatively little is known about the effect of oral contraception on other types of ovarian cancer. The pooled analysis of USA case–control studies suggests that the protective effect of oral contraceptives might be less strong for tumors of low malignant potential than for invasive tumors (Harris *et al.*, 1992), but this difference might be due to selection bias (i.e. the ovaries of oral contraceptive users might be screened more aggressively than those of non-users, and such screening might uncover borderline tumors not otherwise detected). Alternatively, the difference could reflect differences in pill formulation (i.e. the more recent, lower potency formulations used by the relatively young women at risk of borderline tumors may be less protective than the earlier high-dose formulations used by the older women at risk of invasive tumors). In this USA pooled analysis, oral contraceptives were associated with an increased risk of germ cell cancers and a decreased risk of stromal cancers, but there were no clear trends with duration of use (Horn–Ross *et al.*, 1992).

Breast feeding

Risch *et al.* (1983) were the first to report a protective effect of lactation. Although there is currently no overall consensus in the literature, the majority of large analytic studies have reported a protective effect

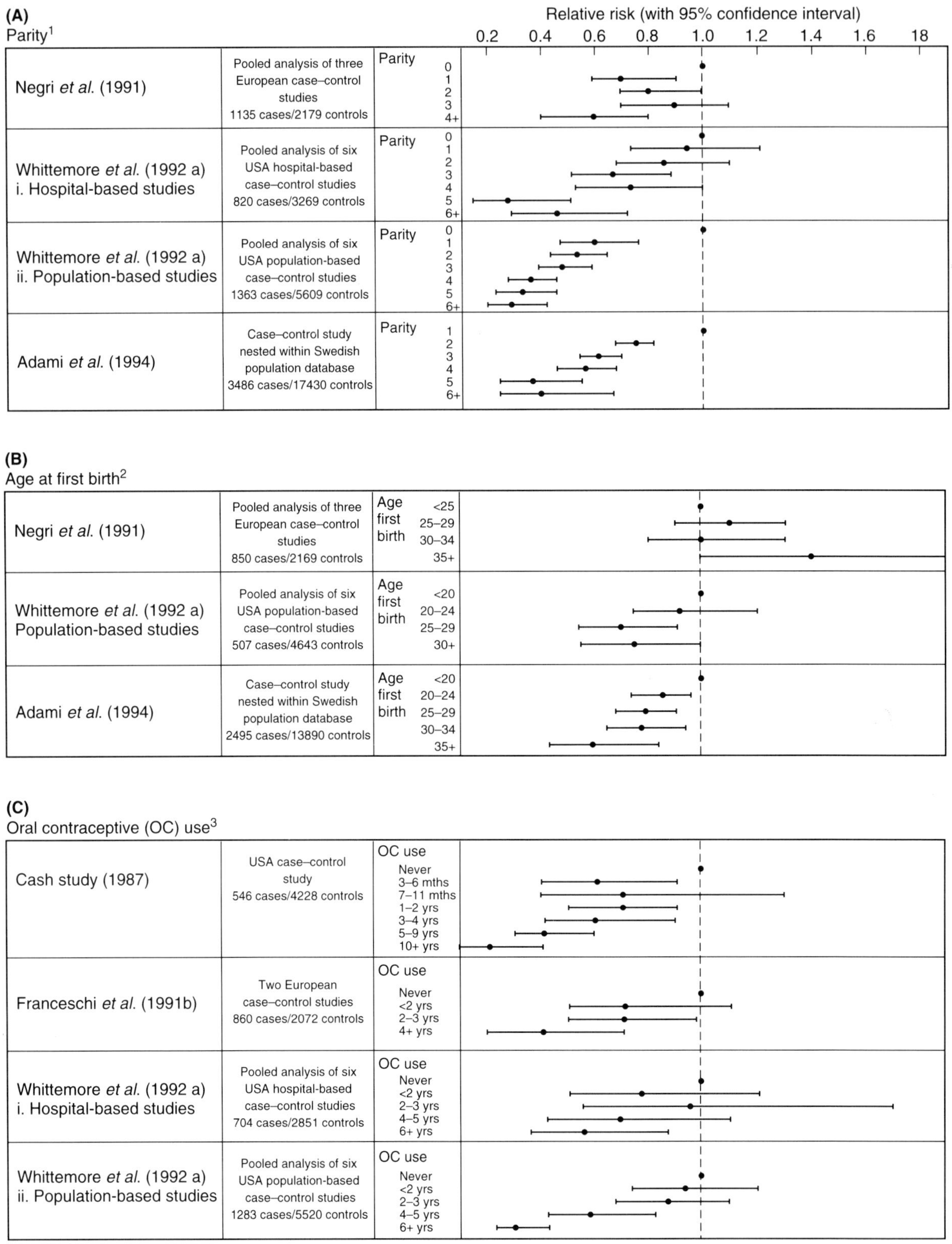

[1]Relative risk estimates adjusted for (at least) age and age at first birth. Risks presented relative to nulliparous women (but to parity 1 in Adami *et al.* data).
[2]Relative risk estimates adjusted for (at least) age and parity. Risks presented relative to that in younger group.
[3]Relative risk estimates adjusted for (at least) age and parity. Risks presented relative to that in never used oral contraceptive group.

Figure 13.2. Effect of parity (A), age at first birth (B) and use of oral contraceptives (C) on risk of epithelial ovarian cancer. Data extracted from studies reporting more than 500 cases.

of lactation (for review, see Shoham, 1994). From the pooled analysis of USA case–control studies, Whittemore *et al.* (1992a) reported an overall risk reduction of 1% for each month of breast feeding. In contrast, Rosenblatt *et al.* (1993) reported a reduction in risk with short-term lactation, but no further reduction in risk with additional months of lactation.

Tubal ligation and hysterectomy

Recent studies have suggested that tubal ligation or hysterectomy (with ovarian conservation) reduce the risk of subsequent ovarian cancer (Irwin *et al.*, 1991; Sightler *et al.*, 1991; Whittemore *et al.*, 1992a; Parazzini *et al.*, 1993). These observations may be a result of bias, in that early ovarian disease may be detected during surgery and the diseased ovary removed. However, not all surgery allows a view of the ovaries, and another explanation may be that surgery in some way impairs ovarian blood supply and so reduces ovulation (Whittemore *et al.*, 1992a; Whittemore *et al.*, 1992b; Parazzini *et al.*, 1993). Alternatively, tubal ligation and hysterectomy may prevent the access of carcinogens to the ovaries via the vagina, although there is only limited evidence that such carcinogens exist (see section on talc). Whatever the mechanism, the observed protective effects of pelvic surgery deserves further investigation since it offers a possible preventive strategy, especially for women at high risk of ovarian cancer.

Factors Associated with an Increase in Risk

Family history and genetic markers

There are many published reports of families with two or more ovarian cancer cases (for review see Amos and Struewing, 1993; Narod, 1994), and it has been recognized for some time that family history is a strong predictor of ovarian cancer risk. A recent combined analysis of case–control data from the USA, Canada, Greece and Japan found a 3.6-fold increased risk for women reporting a family member with the disease compared to those who did not (Amos and Struewing, 1993). Segregation analysis of families with a clustering of both ovarian and breast cancer cases has lead to the suggestion that a single dominant gene may be responsible for both (Lynch *et al.*, 1985), and genetic linkage studies have identified a marker gene on chromosome 17, called BRCA1, which predisposes those with the gene to both ovarian and breast cancer (Amos and Struewing, 1993; Narod, 1994). Although the presence of such a gene may confer a greatly increased risk, it must be pointed out that the proportion of all ovarian cancer cases which are of the familial ovarian carcinoma type may be as little as 1% (for review see Herbst, 1994).

Biochemical markers have been investigated and there is evidence that low levels of alpha-L-fucosidase, galactose-1-phosphate uridyl transferase and blood type A may confer increased risks for ovarian cancer (Amos and Struewing, 1993).

The use of fertility drugs

In the 1980s case reports of ovarian cancer in women undergoing assisted conception raised concern about the use of ovarian stimulants in infertility treatment (Fishel and Jackson, 1989). In 1992 Whittemore *et al.* (1992a) published some striking data from three USA case–control studies: infertile women who took fertility drugs were estimated to have a three-fold increase in risk (95% confidence interval 1.3–6.1) of epithelial cancer compared to women without a history of infertility. The risk for the smaller subgroup who never got pregnant was 27 times (95% confidence interval 2.3–315.6) that of nulliparous women who did not report infertility, whereas the risk for those who took drugs, but did achieve a pregnancy was not significantly different from the control group. These results generated a great deal of interest because of the potentially serious implications for the rapidly expanding assisted conception programs throughout the world (King, 1994; Shoham, 1994). However, as pointed out by Whittemore *et al.* (1992a), several possible explanations could account for the association between failed infertility treatment and ovarian cancer. The women may have taken drugs for longer periods and in greater doses because of the failure to become pregnant or they may have a certain type of infertility, such as ovulation problems, which may predispose them *a priori* to both infertility and ovarian cancer. A recent study of a group of infertile patients investigated these possibilities (Rossing *et al.*, 1994). In this infertile group, use of the drug clomiphene citrate for 12 months or more was associated with an increased risk of ovarian cancer (relative risk 11.1, 95% confidence interval 1.5–82.3), and this increased risk was present in women with and without ovulation problems. There were insufficient data to fully assess the role of other fertility drugs. The evidence to date is therefore suggestive of an independent role for clomiphene citrate as a risk factor for ovarian cancer, although larger studies are needed to test this hypothesis further.

Ionizing radiation

It is well-known that large radiation doses can cause cancer, but the impact of low-dose radiation is still debated. In a study of women who had radiotherapy for cervical cancer there was an overall deficit of subsequent ovarian cancers. Women who survived for 30 years or more, however, had a three-fold increase in risk (Day and Boice, 1983). Two follow-up studies of women given radiation treatment for benign gynecologic conditions showed an increased risk for pelvic cancer in general, but no increased risk for ovarian cancer in particular (Brinkley and Haybrittle, 1969; Smith and Doll, 1976).

Diet

International variations in risk, and the observation that incidence of ovarian cancer in second generation Japanese women born in the USA increased from the lower Japanese level to the higher USA level, highlight the possible role of dietary influences on ovarian cancer (King and Haenszel, 1973). Several studies have indicated that dietary fat may be a direct causal factor (Shoham, 1994; Risch *et al.*, 1994), although the evidence is not strong. Cramer *et al.* (1989) have highlighted the role of milk consumption in the etiology of ovarian cancer, and has proposed that increased dietary galactose consumption and low serum levels of galactose-1-phosphate uridyl-transferase (which prevents the degradation of galactose to glucose) is causal. Recent studies, however, have not confirmed these findings (Risch *et al.*, 1994; Herrington *et al.*, 1995).

Talc

The suggestion that talc may be involved in the etiology of ovarian cancer was made over 20 years ago when talc particles were detected in ovarian tumors (Wehner, 1994). It has been confirmed that talc particles can travel to the ovaries via the vagina, and Harlow *et al.* (1992) present data showing an association between talc and disease risk. Overall, however, the evidence in favour of a causal link between talc and ovarian cancer is not convincing (Wehner, 1994).

Pathogenesis

Two main hypotheses have been developed to explain the epidemiology of epithelial ovarian cancer. The first proposes a link between the number of ovulations and ovarian cancer, the so-called incessant ovulation hypothesis (Fathalla, 1971). The second suggests that exposure to high levels of gonadotropins increases the risk of ovarian cancer (Stadel, 1975). The observed decreasing risk with increasing parity, oral contraceptive use and breastfeeding, all of which suppress ovulation, fits with the incessant ovulation hypothesis. Perhaps surprisingly, published data on early menarche and late menopause do not show a consistent pattern of increasing risk (Franceschi *et al.*, 1991a; Whittemore *et al.* 1992a), as might be predicted by the incessant ovulation hypothesis. However, this may reflect the methodologic difficulties in recall of age at menarche and accurately determining a precise age at menopause. Also, starting or finishing menstruation may not accurately reflect ovulation patterns (Whittemore *et al.*, 1992b). The increased risk with the use of fertility drugs, which stimulate the ovary to produce multiple ovulations, and the protective effect of tubal ligation or hysterectomy, also support the incesant ovulation hypothesis. Parity, oral contraceptives and fertility drug use associations also fit the high gonadotropin hypothesis, but the breast feeding and pelvic surgery associations do not. The high gonadotropin hypothesis would predict a decreased risk for women taking hormone replacement therapy, but what little data there are do not show a protection effect (Whittemore *et al.*, 1992b). As suggested by Whittemore *et al.* (1992b) both hypotheses may be valid, with each explaining a fraction of all epithelial ovarian cancers. Recently, an additional hypothesis of a direct protective effect of pregnancy enabling clearance from the ovaries of cells that have undergone malignant transformation has been proposed (Adami *et al.*, 1994).

How far these hypotheses relate to non-epithelial ovarian cancer is difficult to assess because of the general lack of risk factor data on non-epithelial subtypes. The early age peak and the increase in incidence of ovarian germ cell cancers at young ages resembles testicular cancer epidemiology (Walker *et al.*, 1988; dos Santos Silva and Swerdlow, 1991) and it has been suggested that they may share at least some etiological factors. Early exposures in life, particularly oestrogen exposures *in utero*, have recently been investigated as potential risk factors for these cancers (Depue *et al.*, 1983; Walker *et al.*,1988).

Prevention

Of all the known risk factors for ovarian cancer, oral contraceptive use is the one that offers most scope for primary prevention. It has recently been estimated that five years of oral contraceptive use by nulliparous women can reduce their ovarian cancer risk to the level seen in parous women who have never used oral contraceptives, and that ten years of use by women with a positive family history can reduce the risk to a level less than that for women whose family history is negative and who have never use oral contraceptives (Gross and Schlesselman, 1994). Recent trends in the risk of ovarian cancer in countries with a high prevalence of oral contraceptive use seem to provide grounds for optimism. Also for women from families with the familial ovarian carcinoma syndrome, prophylactic oophrectomy once childbearing is completed has been suggested (Amos and Struewing, 1993).

Because of the lack of early symptoms, 65–75% of ovarian cancer cases present at an advanced stage of the disease, leading to a low survival rate (Austoker, 1994). During the past ten years studies of possible screening tools for secondary prevention in asymptomatic postmenopausal women have been investigated using the tumor marker called CA-125, abdominal ultrasound and bimanual pelvic examinations. Of the three, only CA–125 has proved useful (Austoker, 1994). In those with high risk, such as those with a family history of the disease or those with a positive CA-125 test, color Doppler ultrasound using a vaginal probe is currently being assessed as the second-line screening tool.

Summary of Core Information

- Ovarian cancer is one of the most common malignancies in women in most industrialized countries and represents the fifth most common cause of death from cancer among British and USA white women.
- Because of their rarity very little is known about the epidemiology of non-epithelial types of ovarian cancer.
- Factors associated with a decreased risk of ovarian cancer are parity, increased age at first birth, use of oral contraceptives, lactation, and previous tubal ligation and/or hysterectomy.
- Factors associated with an increased risk of ovarian cancer are family history, use of fertility drugs, ionizing radiation, and possibly fat and milk consumption, use of talc, early menarche and late menopause.
- The two main pathologic hypotheses propose that incessant ovulation and high gonadotropin levels are involved in the initiation of ovarian cancer.
- Of all the known risk factors for ovarian cancer, oral contraceptive use is the one that offers most scope for primary prevention, and in countries with a high prevalence of oral contraceptive use there have been recent declines in risk (although more marked for mortality than incidence).
- Secondary screening methods are currently being assessed and include tests for the tumor marker CA-125 and color Doppler ultrasound.

References

Adami H–O, Bergstrom R, Persson I & Sparen P (1990) The incidence of ovarian cancer in Sweden, 1960–1984. *Am. J. Epidemiol.* **132:** 446–452.

■ Adami H–O, Hsieh CC, Lambe M *et al.* (1994) Parity, age at first childbirth, and risk of ovarian cancer. *Lancet* **344:** 1250–1254.

Amos CI & Struewing JP (1993) Genetic epidemiology of epithelial ovarian cancer. *Cancer* **71:** 566–570.

Austoker J (1994) Screening for ovarian, prostatic, and testicular cancers. *Br. Med. J.* **309:** 315–320.

Beral V, Fraser P & Chilvers C (1978) Does pregnancy protect against ovarian cancer? *Lancet* **1:** 1083–1087.

Berg JW & Baylor SM (1973) The epidemiologic pathology of ovarian cancer. *Human Pathology* **4:** 537–547.

Brinkley D & Haybrittle JL (1969) The late effects of artificial menopause by radiation. *Br. J. Radiol.* **42:** 519–521.

Cancer and Steroid Hormone Study of the Centers for Disease Control and the National Institute of Child Health and Human Development (1987) The reduction in risk of ovarian cancer associated with oral-contraceptive use. *N. Engl. J. Med.* **316:** 650–655.

Coleman MP, Estève J, Damiecki P, Arslan A & Renard H (1993) *Trends in Cancer Incidence and Mortality.* IARC Scientific Publications no. 121. Lyon: International Agency for Research on Cancer.

Cramer DW, Harlow BL, Willett WC *et al.* (1989) Galactose consumption and metabolism in relation to the risk of ovarian cancer. *Lancet* **2:** 66–71.

Day NE & Boice JD (1983) *Second Cancer in Relation to Radiation Treatment for Cervical Cancer.* IARC Scientific Publications no. 52. p. 163. Lyon: IARC.

Depue RH, Pike MC & Henderson BE (1983) Estrogen exposure during gestation and risk of testicular cancer. *J. Natl Cancer Inst.* **71:** 1151–1155.

Doll R, Muir C & Waterhouse J (1970). *Cancer Incidence in Five Continents.* Vol. II. Geneva: International Union Against Cancer.

dos Santos Silva I & Swerdlow AJ (1991) Ovarian germ cell malignancies in England: epidemiological parallels with testicular cancer. *Br. J. Cancer* **63:** 814–818.

dos Santos Silva I & Swerdlow AJ (1995) Recent trends in incidence and mortality from breast, ovarian and endometrial cancers in England and Wales and their relation to changing fertility and oral contraceptive use. *Br. J. Cancer* **72:** 485–492.

Enstrom J (1980) Cancer mortality among Mormons in

California during 1968–75. *J. Natl Cancer Inst.* **65** 1073–1082.

Fathalla MF (1971) Incessant ovulation—a factor in ovarian nepolasia? *Lancet* **2:** 163.

Fishel S & Jackson P (1989) Follicular stimulation for high tech pregnancies: are we playing it safe? *Br. Med. J.* **299:** 309–311

Franceschi S, La Vecchia C, Booth M *et al.* (1991a) Pooled analyis of 3 European case-control studies of epithelial ovarian cancer: II. Age at menarche and at menopause. *Int. J. Cancer* **49:** 57–60.

Franceschi S, Parazzini F, Negri E *et al.* (1991b) Pooled analyis of 3 European case–control studies of epithelial ovarian cancer: III. Oral contraceptive use. *Int. J. Cancer* **49:** 61–65.

Fraumeni JF, Lloyd JW, Smith EM & Wagoner JK (1969) Cancer mortality among nuns: role of marital status in etiology of neoplastic disease in women. *J. Natl Cancer Inst.* **42:** 455–468.

Gross TP & Schlesselman JJ (1994) The estimated effect of oral contraceptive use on the cumulative risk of epithelial ovarian cancer. *Obstet. Gynecol.* **83:** 419–424.

Harlow BL, Cramer DW, Bell DA & Welch WR (1992) Perineal exposure to talc and ovarian cancer risk. *Obstetrics and Gynecology* **80:** 19.

Harris R, Whittemore AS, Itnyre J & Collaborative Ovarian Cancer Group (1992) Characteristics relating to ovarian cancer risk: collaborative analysis of twelve US case–control studies. III. Epithelial tumours of low malignant potential in white women. *Am. J. Epidemiol.* **136:** 1204–1211.

Herbst AL (1994) The epidemiology of ovarian carcinoma and the current status of tumor markers to detect disease. *Am. J. Obstet. Gynecol.* **170:** 1099–1107.

Herrington LJ, Weiss NS, Beresford SA *et al.* (1995) Lactose and galactose intake and metabolism in relation to the risk of epithelial ovarian cancer. *Am. J. Epidemiol.* **141:** 407–416.

Horn–Ross PL, Whittemore AS, Harris R, Itnyre J & Collaborative Ovarian Cancer Group (1992) Characteristics relating to ovarian cancer risk: collaborative analysis of twelve US case–control studies. VI. Non-epithelial cancers among adults. *Epidemiology* **3:** 490–495.

Irwin KL, Weiss NS, Lee NC & Peterson HB (1991) Tubal sterilization, hysterectomy, and the subsequent occurrence of epithelial ovarian cancer. *Am. J. Epidemiol.* **134:** 362–369.

John EM, Whittemore AS, Harris R, Itnyre J & Collaborative Ovarian Cancer Group (1993) Characteristics relating to ovarian cancer risk: collaborative analysis of seven U.S. case–control studies. Epithelial ovarian cancer in black women. *J. Natl Cancer Inst.* **85:** 142–147.

King TM (1994) Ovarian cancer and fertility drugs. *Cancer Bulletin* **64:** 181–184.

King H & Haenszel W (1973) Cancer mortality among foreign- and native-born Chinese in the United States. *J. Chron. Dis.* **26:** 623–646.

Lynch HT, Schuelke GS, Wells IC *et al.* (1985) Hereditary ovarian carcinoma: biomarker study. *Cancer* **55:** 410–415.

■ Mant JW & Vessey MP (1994) Ovarian and endometrial cancers. In: Doll R, Fraumeni Jr JF & Muir CS (eds) *Trends in Cancer Incidence and Mortality.* Cancer Surveys Vol. 19/20, pp. 287–307. New York: Cold Spring Harbor Laboratory Press.

Muir C, Waterhouse J, Mack T, Powell J & Whelan S (1987) *Cancer Incidence in Five Continents.* Vol V. IARC Scientific Publications no. 88. Lyon: International Agency for Research on Cancer.

Narod SA (1994) Genetics of breast and ovarian cancer. *British Medical Bulletin* **50:** 656–676.

Negri E, Francheschi S, Tzonou A *et al.* (1991) Pooled analysis of 3 European case–control studies: I. Reproductive factors and risk of epithelial ovarian cancer. *Int. J. Cancer* **49:** 50–56.

Office of Population Censuses and Surveys (1982) *Cancer Statistics Survival.* Series MB1 no. 9. London: HMSO.

Office of Population Censuses and Surveys (1977–1993) *Mortality Statistics for the years 1974–1991.* Series DH2 Nos 1–18. London: HMSO.

Ogawa N & Retherford RD (1991) Prospects for increased contraceptive pill use in Japan. *Studies in Family Planning* **22:** 378–383.

Parazzini F, Negri E, La Vecchia *et al.* (1993) Hysterectomy, oophrectomy, and subsequent ovarian cancer risk. *Obstetrics and Gynecology* **81:** 363–366.

Phillips RL (1975) Role of life-style and dietary habits in risk of cancer among Seventh-Day Adventists. *Cancer Research* **35:** 3513–3522.

Registrar General (1962–1975) *The Registrar General's Statistical Review of England and Wales 1960–1973.* London: HMSO.

Risch HA, Weiss NS, Lyon LJ, Daling JR & Liff JM (1983) Events of reproductive life and the incidence of epithelial ovarian cancer. *Am. J. Epidemiol* **117:** 128–139.

Risch HA, Jain M, Marrett LD & Howe GR (1994) Dietary lactose intake, lactose intolerance, and the risk of epithelial ovarian cancer in southern Ontario (Canada). *Cancer, Causes and Control* **5:** 540–548.

Rosenblatt KA, Thomas DB & Collaborative Study of Neoplasia and Steroid Contraceptives (1993) Lactation and the risk of epithelial ovarian cancer. *Int. J. Epidemiol.* **22:** 192–197.

■ Rossing MA, Daling JR, Weiss NS, Moore DE & Self SG (1994) Ovarian tumors in a cohort of infertile women. *New Eng. J. Med.* **331:** 771–776.

Shoham Z (1994) Epidemiology, etiology, and fertility drugs in ovarian epithelial carcinoma: Where are we today? *Fertility and Sterility* **62:** 433–448.

Sightler SE, Boike GM, Estape RE & Averette HE (1991) Ovarian cancer in women with prior hysterectomy: A 14-year experience at the University of Miami. *Obstetrics and Gynaecology* **78:** 681–684.

Smith PG & Doll R (1976) Late effects of X-irradiation in patients treated for metropathia haemorrhagica. *Br. J. Radiol.* **49:** 224–232.

Stadel BV (1975) The etiology and prevention of ovarian cancer. *Am. J. Obstet. Gynecol.* **123:** 772–774.

Swerdlow AJ & dos Santos Silva (1993) *Atlas of Cancer Incidence in England and Wales, 1968–85,* pp. 11. Oxford: Oxford University Press.

Walker AH, Ross RK, Pike MC & Henderson BE (1984) A possible rising incidence of malignant germ cell tumours in young women. *Br. J. Cancer* **49:** 669.

Walker AH, Ross RK, Haile RWC & Henderson BE (1988) Hormonal factors and risk of ovarian germ cell cancer in young women. *Br. J. Cancer* **57:** 418.

Wehner AP. (1994) Biologic effects of cosmetic talk *Fd. and Chem. Toxic.* **32:** 1173–1184.

Weiss NS & Peterson AS (1978) Racial variation in the incidence of ovarian cancer in the United States. *Am. J. Epidemiol.* **107:** 91–95.

Weiss NS, Homonchuk T & Young GL (1977) Incidence of the histologic types of ovarian cancer: The U.S. Third National Cancer Survey, 1969–1971. *Gynecologic Oncology* **5:** 161–167.

■ Whittemore AS, Harris R, Itnyre J & Collaborative Ovarian Cancer Group (1992a) Characteristics relating to ovarian cancer risk: collaborative analysis of 12 US case–control studies. II. Invasive epithelial ovarian cancers in white women. *Am. J. Epidemiol.* **136:** 1184–1203.

■ Whittemore AS, Harris R, Itnyre J & Collaborative Ovarian Cancer Group (1992b) Characteristics relating to ovarian cancer risk: collaborative analyis of 12 US case–control studies. IV. Pathogenesis of epithelial ovarian cancer. *Am. J. Epidemiol.* **136:** 1212–1220.

WHO Collaborative Study of Neoplasia and Steroid Contraceptives (1989) Epithelial ovarian cancer and combined oral contraceptives. *Int. J. Epidemiol.* **18:** 538–545.

Yancik R (1993) Ovarian cancer. Age contrasts in incidence, histology, disease stage at diagnosis, and mortality. *Cancer* **71:** 517–523.

14 Histopathology of Ovarian Neoplasia

W D Lawrence
P Papas

Surface Epithelial–Stromal Tumors

Surface epithelial tumors, formerly designated as common epithelial tumors, are so-named because of their derivation from the ovarian surface epithelium; the latter, despite its bland appearance by light microscopy, has tremendous metaplastic capabilities and can engender a bewildering array of histopathologic appearances that can mimic virtually any organ site in the female genital tract. The ovarian surface epithelium and the lining of the cervix, uterus, fallopian tubes and part of the vagina have a common histogenetic origin since the coelomic epithelium that covers the ovary gives rise to the müllerian lining of the aforementioned organs.

The seeming complexity of the classification of surface epithelial tumors is more readily understandable if the histopathologic criteria used for their classification are appreciated; such criteria include the cell type, the degree of cytologic atypia and the manner of growth. Surface epithelial tumors are largely comprised of five different cell types: serous, mucinous, endometrioid, clear cell and urothelial (transitional). The three degrees of cytologic atypia include benign, borderline (also referred to as low malignant potential) and malignant. The manner of growth alludes to the architectural configuration of tumor growth and indicates, for example, whether the neoplasm grows in a papillary exophytic fashion from the surface of the ovary or in an endophytic fashion into a cyst (*Table 14.1*). By evaluating the gross and microscopic characteristics of the neoplasm, these criteria are combined into a pathologic diagnosis. For example, an ovarian cyst lined by benign serous-type epithelium that is thrown into papillary excrescences would be classified as a serous papillary cystadenoma. Conversely, an ovarian carcinoma growing in an exophytic manner from the external surface of the ovary and composed of malignant serous epithelium would be categorized as a serous surface papillary carcinoma. Additionally, each category of surface epithelial tumor has a subgroup of biphasic tumors where (in addition to the epithelial contribution) a stromal, or mesenchymal, element comprises a neoplastic component of the tumor; the combination therefore gives rise to the 'surface epithelial–stromal' designation mentioned above. Consequently, a cystic ovarian tumor lined by serous epithelium and accompanied by a prominent fibrous neoplastic stroma would be subclassified as a serous cystadenofibroma.

The histologic typing of surface epithelial ovarian tumors is complex and difficult due to their diverse morphology and plethora of cell types; therefore, their classification has engendered considerable controversy over the past few decades (Lawrence, 1995). However, the World Health Organization (WHO) is presently the only body sanctioned by various clinical and pathology-oriented organizations to provide a uniform terminology using written criteria for each category. Regardless of the best attempts at uniform criteria, however, there exists considerable interobserver, as well as intraobserver, variation in their interpretation (Cramer, 1987). On the other hand, the WHO classification, despite its acknowledged deficiencies, has been widely accepted internationally and the use of the criteria set forth by the WHO, regardless of the previously mentioned inadequacies as well as those mentioned below, has resulted in an enhanced knowledge about the further classification and biologic behavior of ovarian tumors in general (Sobin and Scully, 1987). Consequently, the WHO classification, at times with slight modifications, will be used in this chapter.

Each of the clinicopathologically important histologic categories of surface epithelial tumors will be discussed separately. In addition to the various types of ovarian cancer, benign and borderline (low malignant potential) tumors are included in the discussion since the gynecologic oncologist frequently encounters them as pelvic masses.

Serous Tumors

Benign serous neoplasms are common, representing approximately one-fifth of all tumors of the ovary and occurring primarily in women of reproductive age. They tend to be bilateral more frequently than mucinous cystadenomas and involve both ovaries in approximately 20% of cases (Kliman *et al.*, 1986).

The so-called serous borderline tumors were separated from the clearly benign and clearly malignant serous tumors primarily because of their generally more indolent biologic behavior. The latter is true despite the finding in one-quarter to one-third

Table 14.1. Histologic classification of surface epithelial tumors of the ovary (modified from Scully, 1979).

A. Serous tumors
  1. Benign
    a. Cystadenoma and papillary cystadenoma
    b. Surface papilloma
    c. Adenofibroma and cystadenofibroma
  2. Borderline
    a. Cystadenoma and papillary cystadenoma
    b. Surface papilloma
    c. Adenofibroma and cystadenofibroma
  3. Malignant
    a. Adenocarcinoma, papillary adenocarcinoma and papillary cystadenocarcinoma
    b. Surface papillary carcinoma
    c. Malignant adenofibroma and cystadenofibroma

B. Mucinous tumors
  1. Benign
    a. Cystadenoma
    b. Adenofibroma and cystadenofibroma
  2. Borderline
    a. Cystadenoma
    b. Adenofibroma and cystadenofibroma
  3. Malignant
    a. Adenocarcinoma and cystadenocarcinoma
    b. Malignant adenofibroma and cystadenofibroma

C. Endometrioid tumors
  1. Benign
    a. Adenoma and cystadenoma
    b. Adenofibroma and cystadenofibroma
  2. Borderline
    a. Adenoma and cystadenoma
    b. Adenofibroma and cystadenofibroma
  3. Malignant
    a. Carcinoma
      i. Adenocarcinoma
      ii. Adenoacanthoma
      iii. Malignant adenofibroma and cystadenofibroma
    b. Endometrioid stromal sarcomas
    c. Mixed müllerian tumors

D. Clear cell tumors
  1. Benign
    a. Adenofibroma
  2. Borderline
  3. Malignant
    a. Carcinoma and adenocarcinoma

E. Brenner tumors
  1. Benign
  2. Borderline
  3. Malignant

F. Mixed epithelial tumors
  1. Benign
  2. Borderline
  3. Malignant

G. Undifferentiated carcinoma

H. Unclassified epithelial tumors

of women with borderline tumors of extraovarian disease of similar histology, placing the patient in a high stage category. Although the terminology of 'borderline malignancy' was accepted by the WHO and the International Federation of Gynecology and Obstetrics (FIGO) to designate these neoplasms, others prefer to use the term 'carcinoma of low malignant potential;' much discussion regarding the nature and nomenclature of such tumors has been elicited by both clinicians and pathologists since the two latter terms were accepted by both the WHO and FIGO in the early 1970s. In subsequent years, particularly in the past decade or so, several workers (Russell, 1984; Kurman and Trimble, 1993) have questioned the validity of the concept of 'borderline' tumors or 'carcinomas of low malignant potential.' Since any change in thinking regarding the biologic nature of a neoplasm is accompanied by a new nomenclature, these workers have proposed different designations to reflect the generally nonmalignant nature of the tumor that they favor. Accordingly, in one case, the term 'atypical proliferating tumor' has been suggested to replace the former borderline and low malignant potential categories. For example, the neoplasm formerly designated as 'serous papillary tumor of borderline malignancy' would be designated as 'atypical proliferating serous tumor' and the other cytologic varieties of surface epithelial–stromal tumors would be named in a similar manner. However, given the acknowledged, but as yet unresolved, controversy surrounding this important category of ovarian tumors, others have argued that the currently sanctioned WHO and FIGO classifications should occupy a prominent place in the pathology report to prevent misunderstanding among pathologists and clinicians and preclude the possibility of patient mismanagement, at least until resolution of the controversies has been achieved (Lawrence, 1995).

Despite the nosologic controversy surrounding borderline tumors, patients with such tumors tend to exhibit a much better prognosis than those with overtly invasive serous carcinomas; indeed, patients with serous borderline tumors have been shown by many workers to have markedly better five- and ten-year survival rates when compared with patients with serous cystadenocarcinomas. In fact, studies revealed five-year survival rates of 100% and 50% for borderline and invasive serous tumors (Fisher *et al.*, 1955), and 76% and 13% for the same tumor types, respectively, at ten years (Santesson and Kottmeier, 1968).

Patients with serous borderline tumors tend to be younger than patients with invasive serous carcinoma and they may live for many years, even with involvement of extraovarian pelvic tissues. The omentum and surfaces of the pelvic peritoneum, including the serosa of the uterus, fallopian tubes and cul-de-sac, may be seeded with so-called implants from the primary ovarian borderline tumor.

Patients with serous borderline neoplasms must be followed carefully because these tumors have been known to recur late, sometimes 10–20 years after removal of the primary tumor.

Serous carcinomas represent the most common ovarian malignancy, comprising almost half of such tumors. They occur in women mostly in the sixth and seventh decades, and both ovaries are involved in about half the cases. The relatively capacious nature of the pelvis and abdomen allows these neoplasms to reach large proportions before producing signs and symptoms. All too often, ascites and an increasing abdominal girth finally force the patient to seek medical attention at a time when the tumor is far advanced. Consequently, the five- and ten-year survival rates for serous carcinomas are dismal.

Grossly, serous cystadenomas are variably-sized neoplasms that have a smooth, glistening, pink-red external surface; they are usually unilocular, fluid-filled, and tense to palpation. On cut section, the cyst is filled with clear to straw yellow fluid that is usually thin, but may be mucoid in consistency. The inner lining of the collapsed cyst is smooth and gray–pink without surface papillations (*Figure 14.1*). Serous surface papillomas appear as small, soft and pink–red papillary excrescences arising from the ovarian surface.

On microscopic examination, the usually thin cyst wall of the serous cystadenoma is lined by an innocuous-appearing layer of tubal-type epithelium; the latter is characterized by columnar cells that may show slight stratification, as well as ciliated cells (*Figure 14.2*). The serous surface papilloma has an identical histologic picture except that it grows in an exophytic manner rather than into a cyst.

The serous borderline tumor likewise may be encountered as an exophytic or endophytic neoplasm. In the former case, the tumor is present as variably-sized papillary soft red–brown excrescences on the ovarian cortical surface (*Figure 14.3*); in the latter case, the tense cystic ovary may resemble the benign serous cystadenoma on external examination. Like the serous cystadenoma, the serous borderline tumor often contains a watery clear to straw-colored clear fluid; however, at times these tumors may produce a thick mucoid fluid that on gross examination may cause confusion with a mucinous tumor. On cut section variable amounts of the cyst wall are occupied by soft pink–tan to pink–red papillary excrescences (*Figure 14.4*); on section of the cyst wall or the ovarian cortex, the papillary character of the tumor is evident and it clearly does not invade the underlying tissues.

The microscopic appearance of serous borderline tumors is characteristic and similar regardless of whether the lesion is exophytic or endophytic. Although exhibiting a greater degree of proliferative

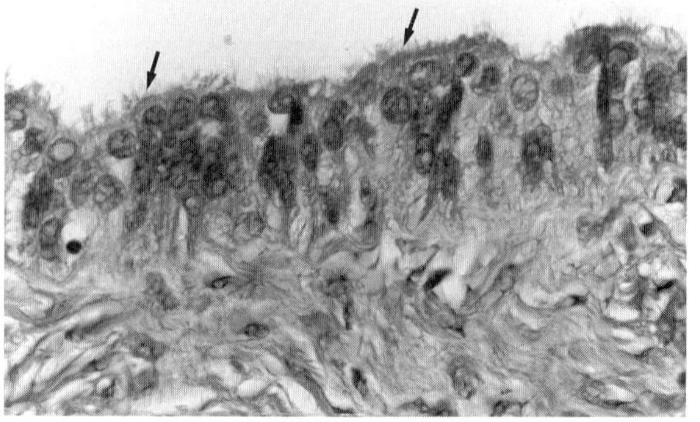

Figure 14.2. Serous cystadenoma. The cyst is lined by a pseudostratified epithelium that resembles that of the fallopian tube. Cilia (arrows) are present on the surfaces of the cells.

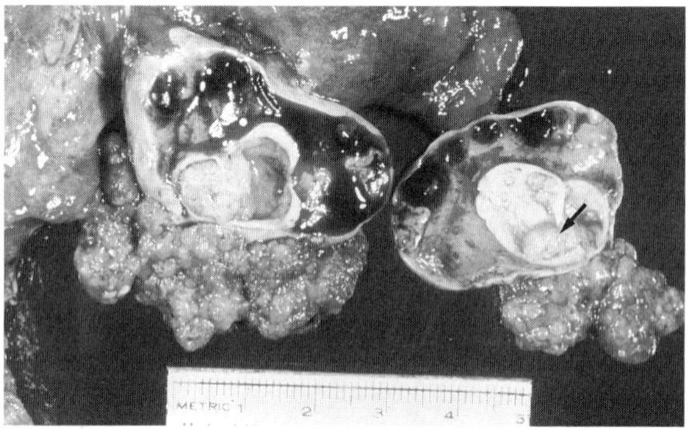

Figure 14.3. Serous papillary borderline tumor. The ovary has been bivalved to show both a small cystic component of serous borderline tumor (arrow) as well as the more prominent exophytic surface portion; the latter was soft, friable, and red–brown. Small blood-filled follicular cysts are present in a subcortical location on the opposite side of the ovary.

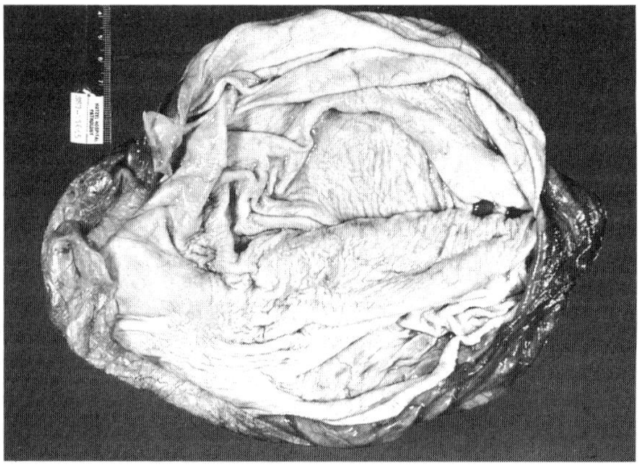

Figure 14.1. Serous cystadenoma. The entire cyst lining is smooth. The release of tension after evacuation of the clear fluid resulted in a wrinkled, convoluted surface, but no papillary excrescences are evident.

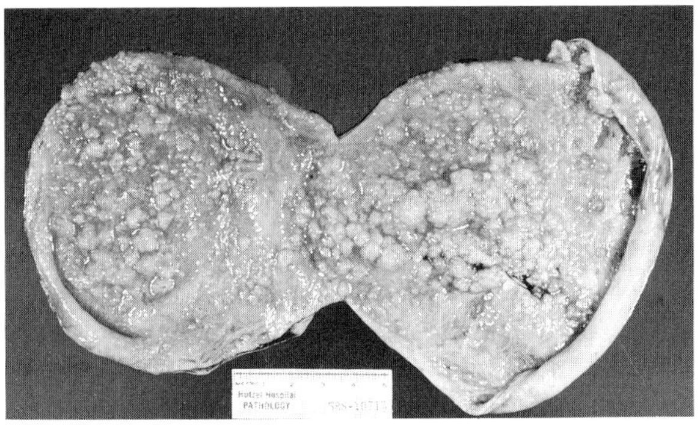

Figure 14.4. Serous borderline tumor. The cystic ovary has been opened and the inner surface is covered by variably-sized papillary excrescences that are pink–white and soft.

In surface papillary serous borderline tumors particularly, so-called 'implants' from the parent lesion are presumed, at least in many cases, to have 'seeded' the extraovarian tissues; the latter include the various peritoneal surfaces, including the omentum, the serosa of the tubes and the uterus, and even 'autoimplantation' on the surface of the ovary itself. Such 'implants' occur in approximately one-quarter to one-third of patients with a serous borderline tumor and microscopic examination reveals a histologic picture similar to the primary ovarian tumor. Importantly, however, the designation of borderline tumor is based on histopathologic examination of the primary ovarian tumor and not on the presence of implants or on their histology.

Work in the last decade has shown that implants of serous borderline tumors may be separated into

activity and atypia than the benign serous cystadenomas, serous borderline tumors generally show less atypia than the overtly serous carcinomas. Delicate papillary fronds of fibrovascular tissue, which arise from a cyst wall of fibrotic appearance, are lined by an atypical serous epithelium (*Figure 14.5*). Epithelial cells may exhibit considerable proliferative activity, resulting in their stratification and piling up; small, apparently 'pinched-off,' buds of tumor cells are generated by tangential cutting of such aggregates of tumor and appear to be free-lying. Although nuclear atypicality is generally not as severe as that of overt serous carcinomas, some borderline tumors exhibit significant nuclear pleomorphism and hyperchromatism. However, nuclear atypia alone does not appear to affect recrudescence of tumor or survival in low-stage tumors, in keeping with the currently held view that histopathologic criteria are of little value in predicting prognosis (Bostwick *et al.*, 1986). Mitotic activity is likewise less brisk than is generally seen in frankly invasive serous carcinoma. The use of special techniques such as DNA ploidy analysis using both flow and static image cytometry to predict the prognosis of serous borderline tumors has generated controversial results; some workers have claimed a good correlation between the presence of aneuploidy and prognosis (Kuhn *et al.*, 1989) whereas others (Harlow *et al.*, 1993) found little to none.

The cardinal histopathologic feature of serous borderline tumors is the absence of destructive invasion of the stroma. Although it is not unusual to see small single or aggregates of serous-type glands in the immediately subepithelial ovarian cortex, the typical desmoplastic response commonly seen around malignant glands, manifested by loosening of the stroma and a round cell infiltrate, is lacking. Such small single glands or aggregates of serous glands are frequently mistaken for invasive serous carcinoma, but should not be regarded as such.

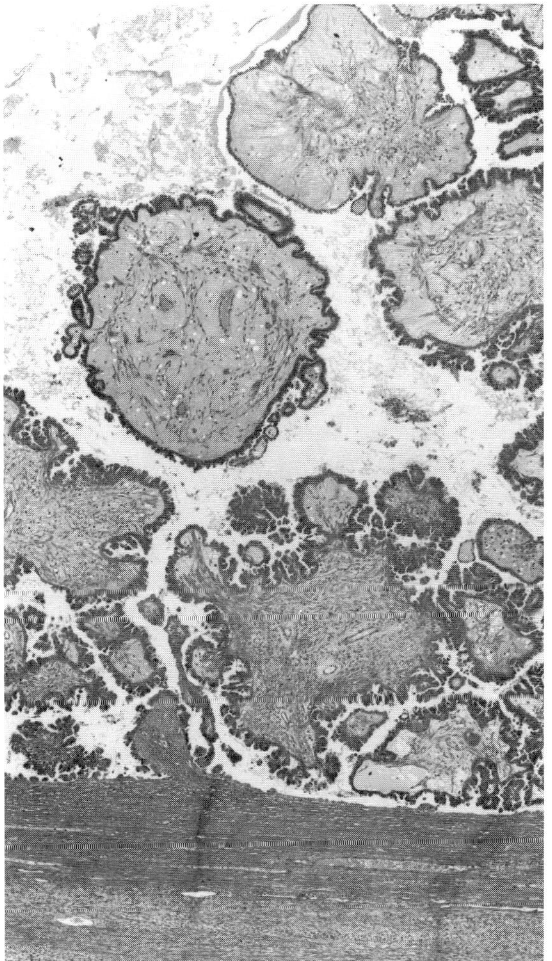

Figure 14.5. Serous borderline tumor. Numerous papillary excrescences arise from the inner surface of the cyst wall and project into the lumen. No invasion of the cyst wall is present.

two types: invasive and noninvasive, the latter being further divided into epithelial and desmoplastic subtypes. The desmoplastic implants are frequently surrounded by a prominent and exuberant desmoplastic reaction and a marked chronic inflammatory infiltrate. They often grow on the surface of the extraovarian tissues in a 'cake-like' fashion or involve the fibrous septae in between the lobules of the omental fat in an orderly manner. The epithelial subtype of implant frequently occurs either as single serous glands or small aggregates of such or as variably-sized, but usually minute, serous cysts containing atypical papillary serous epithelium, which are distributed over the peritoneal surfaces. Although surrounded by some degree of fibrosis, it is much less pronounced than that seen in the desmoplastic implant.

Psammoma bodies, concentrically laminated calcific concretions, are present in the majority of serous borderline tumors. In certain cases, only psammoma bodies remain in the implants and there are no residual borderline epithelial lesions. These may represent so-called 'burned out' foci of endosalpingiosis, a phenomenen that is the ectopic serous epithelial equivalent of endometriosis. Often both nonatypical and atypical endosalpingiosis may be demonstrated in the extraovarian peritoneal tissues of patients with serous borderline tumors. Such examples of endosalpingiosis also frequently accompany implants of serous borderline tumor. Consequently, some workers have suggested that at least a proportion of the so-called implants represent foci of atypical or borderline endosalpingiosis, implying a 'field effect' of coelomic metaplasia in the genesis of pelvic serous neoplasia (Russell, 1979; Genadry *et al.*, 1981; McCaughey, 1985). Subsequent investigators (Bell and Scully, 1990) have demonstrated the existence of extraovarian serous borderline tumors that may arise from the pelvic peritoneum with no involvement of the ovaries, supporting the previously mentioned susceptibility of the ovarian and extraovarian coelomic epithelium to the same carcinogenic influences.

About 30–40% of patients with extraovarian implants of serous borderline tumor die of their disease. Accordingly, Bell *et al.* (1988) have suggested that there may be a correlation between the more worrisome histopathologic features of peritoneal implants of serous borderline tumor (particularly with the 'invasive' implants) and prognosis. Indeed, an adverse prognosis was associated with implants exhibiting the following histologic features: invasion, severe cytologic atypia and mitotic activity. Bell *et al.* suggested that patients having serous borderline tumors with implants should be divided into high-risk and low-risk groups based on the previously mentioned criteria; furthermore they indicated that high-risk patients may benefit from adjuvant therapy if such adverse histopathologic features are present. Other investigators, however, have indicated that the clinical stage of the disease has greater prognostic importance than the histology of the implants and that, within a given stage, disease progression or recurrence does not appear to be influenced by invasive histologic characteristics (Michael and Roth, 1986).

Since borderline tumors generally tend to occur in younger patients than overt serous carcinomas, the preservation of reproductive capacity by conserving as much ovarian function as possible is often an issue in their treatment. A recent study investigated the frequency of persistence or recurrence of ovarian serous borderline tumors in 35 patients who underwent unilateral cystectomy, bilateral cystectomy, or unilateral cystectomy with contralateral oophorectomy or salpingo–oophorectomy. The frequency of ipsilateral persistence or recurrence in the cystectomized ovary was 8%; involvement of the resection margin of the cystectomy specimen or removal of multiple cysts was virtually always associated with persistence or recurrence of serous borderline tumor (Lim–Tan *et al.*, 1988).

In approximately two-thirds of the cases of frank serous carcinoma, the tumor involves both ovaries; the latter are likely to be large (more than half are greater than 15 cm in diameter) and either cystic, solid, or both. The ovaries are often irregularly shaped and show variable replacement by firm, friable, gray–tan to pink or yellow tissue (*Figure 14.6*). As with carcinomas arising in other body sites, hemorrhage and extensive necrosis are virtually constant gross features. The cystic portions of the tumor exhibit extensive soft papillary growths projecting into the lumens. A straw-colored to murky or hemorrhagic fluid may fill the cystic loculations. The tumor may involve contiguous organs such as the fallopian tubes, the uterus and the omentum, in the latter instance replacing the adipose tissue to form an 'omental cake.'

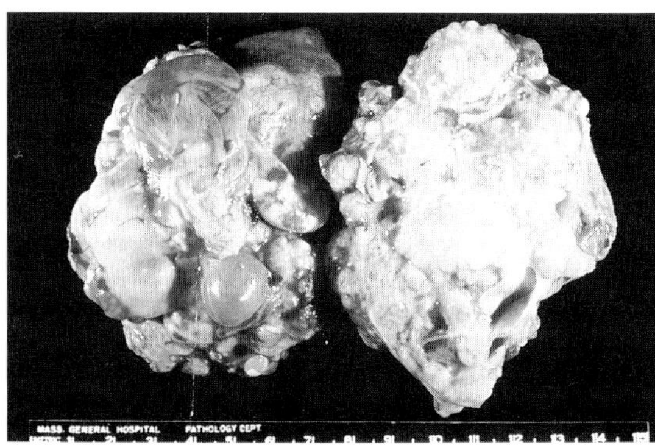

Figure 14.6. Serous papillary carcinoma. The enlarged ovary has been replaced by an irregularly-shaped, firm tumor, which was gritty and hard on cut section and showed extensive necrosis. Carcinoma had broached the cortex and was present on the surface of the ovary.

On microscopic examination, serous carcinoma may vary in its degree of differentiation. Low-grade tumors may be marked by extensive papillarity and nuclear atypia only slightly greater than that seen in serous borderline tumors. Even these low-grade tumors, however, are accompanied by the desmoplastic response of so-called 'destructive' invasion. Moderately- and poorly-differentiated serous carcinomas are characterized by decreasing degrees of papillarity so that in the latter the tumor grows in sheets, clusters and small nests of adenocarcinoma (*Figure 14.7*). Psammoma bodies in variable numbers are common, being present in approximately one-third of serous carcinomas (see inset *Figure 14.7*). In fact, on rare occasions, the entire tumor virtually is replaced by psammoma bodies, giving rise to the designation of psammocarcinoma for such a lesion (Scully, 1979). Psammocarcinoma is currently regarded as an extremely well-differentiated serous carcinoma, with a biologic behavior more akin to serous borderline tumor than to that of an overt serous carcinoma. The tumor is rare and specific pathologic criteria have been proposed for its diagnosis (Gilks *et al.*, 1990); therefore, among other findings, the designation of psammocarcinoma should be reserved for those very well-differentiated serous carcinomas in which at least three-quarters of the tumor is replaced with psammomatous calcification.

At the time of surgical exploration for an ovarian mass, additional samples for histopathologic examination should include contiguous adhesions of the ovarian tumor, since these may represent benign inflammation or malignant disease. Indeed, in patients with serous borderline tumors, adhesions from any site in the abdominopelvic cavity may be either of neoplastic or inflammatory origin. The pathologist's attention should be drawn to areas of adhesion or rupture to ensure their proper examination. The omentum should be inspected closely for metastases; however, tumor may not be grossly evident and as many as 20% of grossly negative omenta may show microscopic disease (Richardson, 1985).

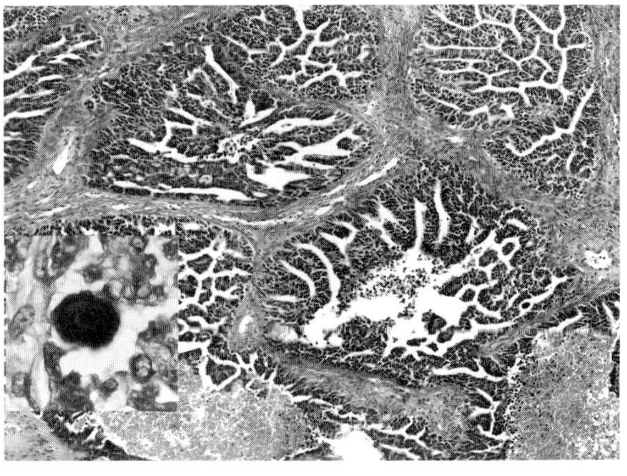

Figure 14.7. Serous papillary carcinoma. The tumor exhibits marked papillarity manifested by numerous delicate stalks that focally appear to 'pinch off' and lie within spaces. Extensive necrosis is present. Inset: A psammoma body composed of concentrically laminated calcifications sits among nests of serous papillary carcinoma.

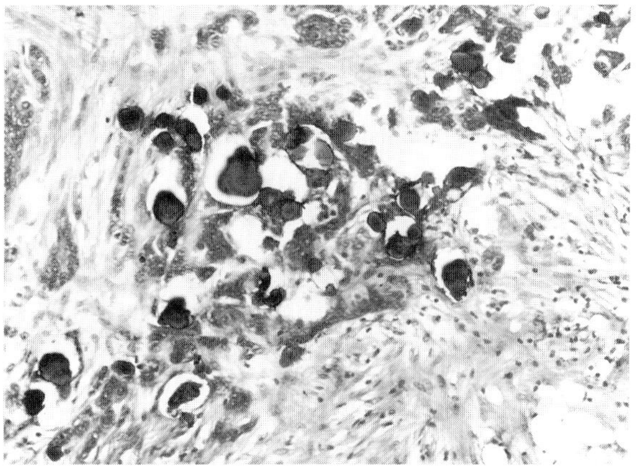

Figure 14.8. Pelvic serous carcinoma. The tumor has a histopathologic appearance similar to that of the usually primary ovarian serous carcinoma; numerous psammoma bodies are present and the carcinoma has elicited a marked desmoplastic and inflammatory response in the stroma. The ovaries in this case were small and were not involved by tumor.

In some patients, the pelvic organs are extensively involved by serous-type carcinoma with either minimal or no involvement of the ovaries; in the minimally involved ovary, the superficial cortex or the hilum is often invaded by small nests of serous carcinoma accompanied by a desmoplastic response (*Figure 14.8*). Current workers regard this lesion to be a primary serous carcinoma (pelvic serous carcinoma), arising by the previously mentioned mechanism of serous metaplasia of the coelomic epithelium. Regardless of its histogenesis, the tumor behaves in a manner similar to the ovarian lesion of the same nature (McCaughey, 1985; Lele *et al.*, 1988). Such lesions need not necessarily be invasive to spread over the coelomic surfaces (Richardson, 1985).

Some workers consider that the so-called serous surface papillary carcinoma is a distinct subtype of ovarian serous papillary carcinoma and pelvic serous carcinoma; such tumors are exophytic growths involving primarily the surface of the ovaries, which are often of normal size and shape, and exhibiting concomitant widespread peritoneal involvement. The clinical course appears to be more aggressive than the conventional type of ovarian serous papillary carcinoma with peritoneal implants (Gooneratne *et al.*, 1982; Mills *et al.*, 1988).

Mucinous Tumors

Mucinous tumors comprise approximately one-fifth of all ovarian tumors and like the serous tumors have benign, borderline and malignant categories of differentiation. The great majority are benign; borderline and malignant variants each make up less than 10% of all mucinous neoplasms. Patients with benign mucinous lesions are generally younger than those with borderline and malignant ones. Benign neoplasms are almost invariably unilateral, and the borderline and malignant tumors are bilateral in only 10% and 20% of cases, respectively.

A significant difference in prognosis between mucinous borderline tumors and overtly mucinous adenocarcinomas justifies their separation as distinct entities (similar to the situation between the serous borderline tumors and overtly invasive serous carcinomas). Indeed, the early series reported by Santesson and Kottmeier (1968) showed the ten-year survival of overt mucinous carcinomas to be half that of mucinous borderline tumors (68% versus 34%). Later investigators confirmed the generally excellent prognosis of mucinous borderline tumors (Hart and Norris, 1973), but noted that three patients with such lesions died after treatment. In addition to other reasons, the lethal nature of those tumors could be explained by sampling error and failure to document frank adenocarcinomatous elements. As will be discussed, mucinous tumors are notorious for their geographic variability and admixtures of benign, borderline and overtly malignant components.

Gross examination of mucinous tumors most frequently reveals them to be large (in fact they are generally the largest of the surface epithelial tumors) and multiloculated and to contain mucinous fluid that may vary considerably in its nature, from thick and viscid to watery (*Figure 14.9*).

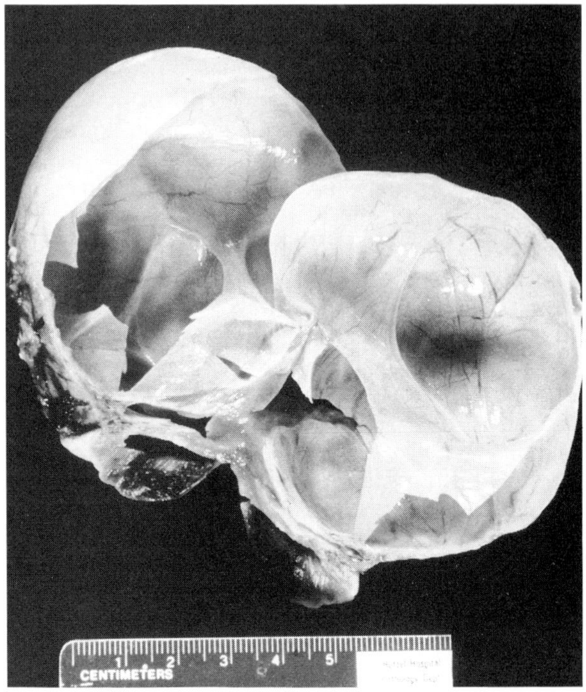

Figure 14.9. Mucinous cystadenoma. The tumor is multiloculated and contains a clear, slightly viscid, mucoid material. The inner lining of the cyst wall is smooth with a delicate vascular pattern, and no papillations or solid areas are evident.

The mucinous cystadenoma commonly exhibits a smooth external surface and is tense to palpation. On section, the inner cyst lining of the loculations is usually smooth without significant papillations. As indicated above, serous ovarian tumors can form significant amounts of intracystic mucin, so that microscopic examination may be necessary to establish the diagnosis. Microscopically, mucinous cystadenomas are lined by a single row of tall columnar cells in which the cytoplasm is filled with abundant mucin, depressing the nucleus to the basal aspect of the cell. Such an arrangement imparts a 'picket-fence' appearance to the epithelium.

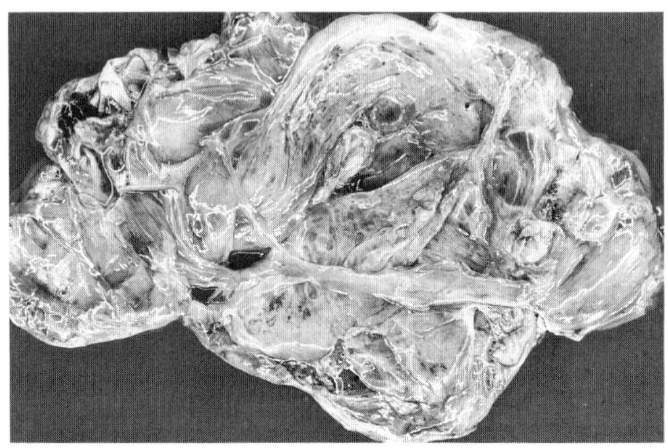

Figure 14.10. Mucinous borderline tumor. The ovary has been opened to reveal multiple cystic locules, all of which contained clear viscid mucoid material. All locules were opened and no solid areas were identified.

Mucinous tumors of borderline malignancy (tumors regarded in the formal WHO/FIGO classification as mucinous cystadenomas of borderline malignancy or mucinous carcinomas of low malignant potential) often have a gross appearance similar to the mucinous cystadenoma; however, the cyst lining of the locules has a greater tendency to exhibit papillary excrescences and thickening of the cyst walls than is seen in their benign counterparts (*Figure 14.10*). In general, the more complex appearance of the mucinous tumor on gross examination, the greater the chance that it harbors areas of borderline or overt malignancy on microscopic examination. Proper gross examination and adequate sampling of such lesions cannot be overemphasized; it is imperative that the tumor is sliced at sufficiently thin intervals to reveal areas of thickening or papillarity that may represent foci of borderline or frankly malignant change in an otherwise benign mucinous cystadenoma. Current recommendations are that at least one tissue section should be submitted for microscopic examination for each centimeter of the maximal diameter of the tumor; any area that looks different from the remainder of the tumor should be sampled.

On microscopic examination, the mucinous epithelium lining the cysts in a mucinous borderline tumor shows a greater degree of proliferative activity than that of benign forms. The lining is thrown into small papillae, exhibiting so-called tufting of the epithelium, and cellular stratification and atypicality are manifested by nuclear hyperchromatism, an increased nuclear-cytoplasmic ratio and enlarged nucleoli (*Figure 14.11*). In keeping with the proliferative nature of the borderline tumor, mitotic activity is often increased and despite the presence of cytologic atypia, the histopathologic criteria are generally insufficient to qualify as a bona fide carcinoma. As for the serous borderline tumors, the diagnosis of a mucinous borderline tumor is based on microscopic examination of the tumor. One of the requisites is that there is no evidence of stromal invasion; however, this is more difficult to assess in mucinous borderline tumors due to their tendency to grow as multiple variably-sized locules set in a fibrous stroma (*Figure 14.12*). Consequently, it is more difficult to judge whether such atypical cystic glandular aggregates represent areas of mucinous borderline tumor cut at an odd angle or whether they signify frank invasion of the stroma. Criteria that suggest overt carcinoma, either with or without true invasion, include the presence of a true cribriform glandular arrangement and a clearcut desmoplastic stromal response surrounding the often irregularly-shaped nests.

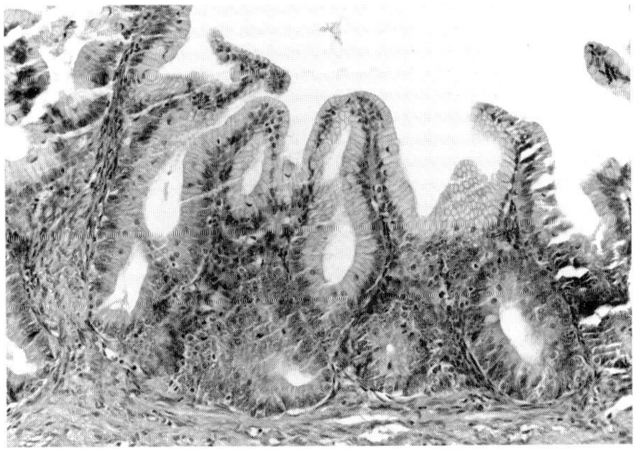

Figure 14.11. Mucinous borderline tumor. Higher magnification to illustrate the nuclear stratification, cellularity and mitotic activity in such tumors.

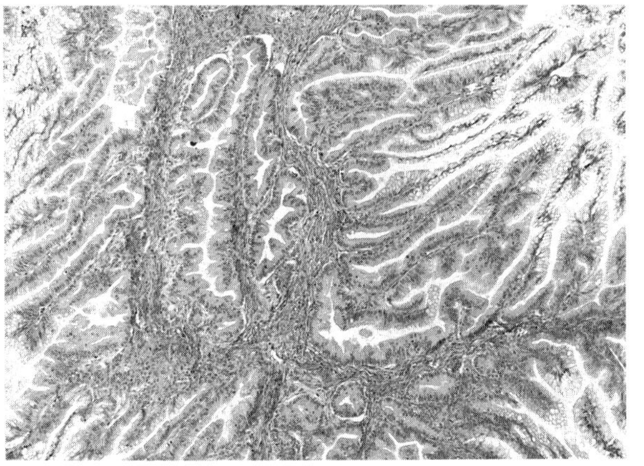

Figure 14.12. Mucinous borderline tumor. Although the tumor has a proliferative appearance with delicate papillary processes, no invasion with surrounding stromal response is evident and a cribriform arrangement of the glands is absent.

In an effort to establish more quantitative histologic criteria for the differentiation of mucinous borderline tumor from frank mucinous carcinoma, Hart and Norris studied 97 cases of the former and 39 cases of the latter; they concluded that a mucinous tumor with epithelial stratification exceeding three cell layers and, importantly, with associated significant nuclear atypia should be regarded as a mucinous adenocarcinoma (Hart and Norris, 1973). Additionally, recent investigators have attempted to grade mucinous borderline tumors based on the degree of cell layering, mitotic activity and, perhaps more importantly, nuclear characteristics; their results, in which three of 53 patients with mucinous borderline tumor died with recurrent tumor, indicate that grading of mucinous borderline tumors may have prognostic importance (Sumithran *et al.*, 1988). Others, however, have questioned the validity of histopathologic criteria (Russell, 1979; Govan *et al.*, 1983; Stahlsberg *et al.*, 1988), and some have suggested that only the histologic parameters of nuclear stratification and stromal invasion offer prognostic information, obviating the need for formal histologic grading (Chaitin *et al.*, 1985).

On gross examination, ovarian mucinous adenocarcinomas are frequently large and, in contrast to the benign and borderline variants, the external surface may contain areas where carcinoma has broached the cortical surface and is present there as irregular roughened foci (*Figure 14.13*). On cut section, necrosis and hemorrhage are frequently present, whereas these features are virtually never seen in mucinous borderline tumors. There may be great geographic variation in the cellular composition of mucinous tumors, with admixed mucinous cystadenoma and mucinous borderline tumor; similarly, these neoplasms may also harbor areas of mucinous carcinoma, further emphasizing the aforementioned importance of their proper

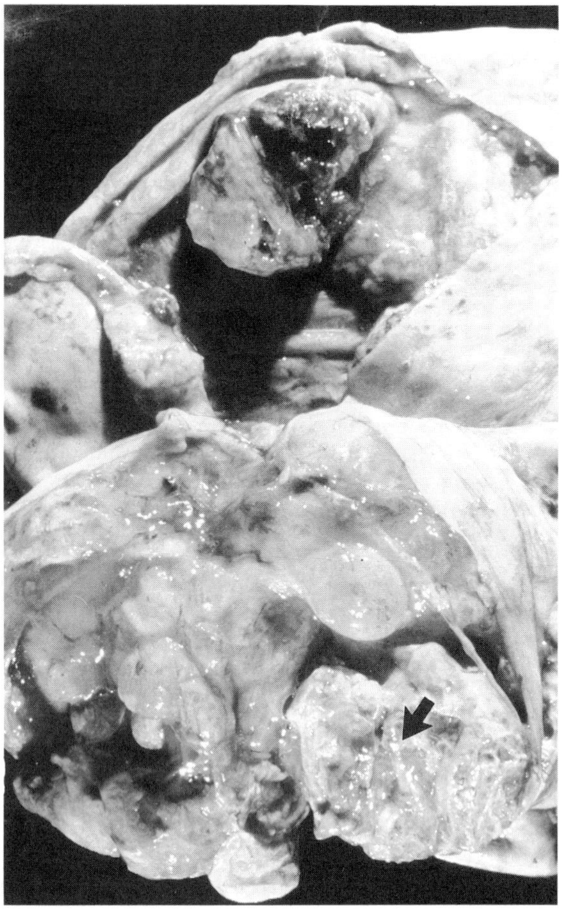

Figure 14.13. Mucinous cystadenocarcinoma. The ovary has been opened to reveal multiple, variably-sized locules that contained thick stringy mucin. Most of the cystic ovary consisted of mucinous borderline tumor; however, the nodule of solid tissue in the lower half of the specimen (arrow) represented an area of mucinous adenocarcinoma.

gross examination and adequate sampling. Some mucinous carcinomas, however, are predominantly solid and are composed almost entirely of pure carcinoma. Well-, moderately- and poorly-differentiated forms exist; the first of these is comprised of well-formed glands that show the cribriform arrangement of glands within glands and a lining of usually tall columnar cells containing abundant intracytoplasmic mucin, hyperchromatic nuclei, marked nuclear stratification and brisk mitotic activity. Those carcinomas exhibiting moderate and poor differentiation show progressive diminution in the ability to form glandular structures, as well as increasing nuclear atypia, often with numerous atypical mitotic figures.

In less than 5% of mucinous ovarian tumors, a concomitant neoplasm with distinctive gross and microscopic features occurs; the latter, referred to as pseudomyxoma peritonei, is characterized by often extensive involvement of the peritoneal cavity by gelatinous tumor that can be literally scooped out in some cases, but is difficult to evacuate in others because of its tendency to form locules surrounded by fibrous tissue (*Figure 14.14*).

In many of the cases of pseudomyxoma peritonei accompanied by ovarian tumors there are coincident mucinous neoplasms of the appendix. The ovarian tumor that is found in association with the appendiceal tumor and pseudomyxoma peritonei may be of any degree of malignancy; however, it frequently displays a borderline histologic pattern (*Figure 14.15*). Interestingly, the appendiceal lesion often has a borderline appearance, although some have classified such lesions as frank adenocarcinomas (Higa *et al.*, 1973). Since the histologic appearance of the invasive mucinous carcinoma cells within the pseudomyxoma peritonei is similar to that of both the appendiceal and ovarian lesions (see inset *Figure 14.15*) and since true borderline tumors of the ovary are by definition noninvasive, the carcinoma represented by pseudomyxoma peritonei may be a very well-differentiated mucinous carcinoma of gastrointestinal type arising in the appendix and/or the ovary. The well-known propensity of ovarian mucinous tumors to exhibit gastrointestinal differentiation lends some support to the argument (Scully, 1979) that some have designated as a 'field effect' phenomenon. However, current thinking (Young *et al.*, 1991; Prayson *et al.*, 1994) maintains that, in the great majority of cases of pseudomyxoma peritonei marked by concomitant ovarian and appendiceal neoplasms, the ovarian tumor represents metastases from the appendiceal tumor. Either tumor or both may rupture to produce the pseudomyxoma.

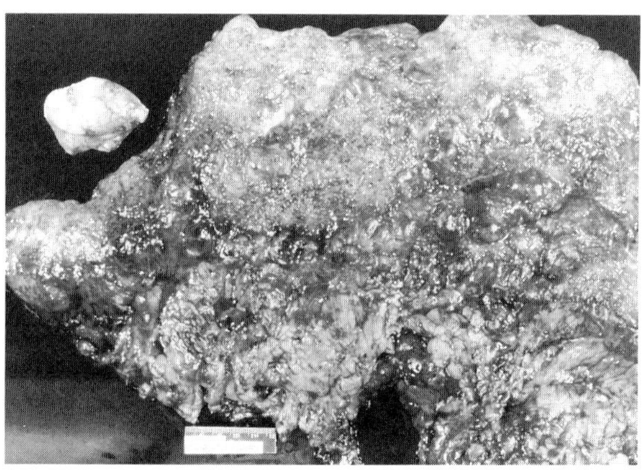

Figure 14.14. Pseudomyxoma peritonei and mucocele of the appendix. The omentum has been replaced by a gelatinous and fibrotic mass of firm tissue with a glistening surface. In the upper left hand corner of the photograph is the distended appendix that was filled with glairy mucus.

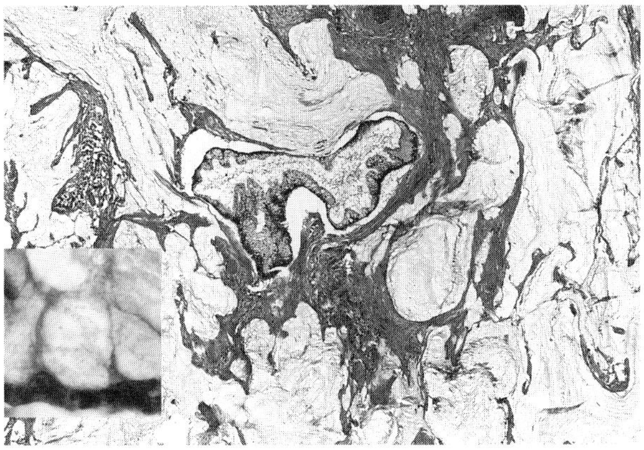

Figure 14.15. Pseudomyxoma peritonei. Scant aggregates of mucinous borderline-type tumor sit in lakes of mucin that are traversed by fibrous stroma. Inset: higher magnification of the tumor cells illustrating their mucin-distended cytoplasm depressing the nucleus to a basal position.

Rutgers and Scully (1988) separated ovarian mucinous borderline tumors by clinicopathologic criteria into those of müllerian and gastrointestinal types; in contrast to the intestinal type of ovarian mucinous borderline tumors, the müllerian variety occurred in younger patients, tended more often to be bilateral (40%), was smaller, and was more often associated with endometriosis; 20% were associated with implants and/or lymph node metastases and none was complicated by pseudomyxoma peritoneii. No deaths occurred in their series.

Endometroid Tumors

The designation endometrioid, meaning 'endometrium-like,' was chosen by the WHO (Serov *et al.*, 1973) to emphasize the similarity of such ovarian tumors to their counterparts in the endometrium, which they closely mimic and from which they may be histologically indistinguishable. Although one might postulate with a reasonable degree of confidence that endometrioid tumors arise from foci of ovarian endometriosis, they do not all exhibit concomitant endometriosis; indeed, most do not. In some cases, this may be due to overgrowth and destruction of benign endometriotic foci by the cancer, but is most probably related to the remarkable capacity of the ovarian surface epithelium for metaplastic differentiation toward other cell types. Benign endometrioid tumors are rare and are encountered most commonly as endometrioid adenofibromas (Bell and Scully, 1985).

There are no dependable gross characteristics that identify a tumor as being of endometrioid type; in fact, the finding of a carcinoma arising in a typical endometriotic 'chocolate cyst' of the ovary could just as likely represent a clear cell carcinoma as an endometrioid carcinoma, since the former is the surface epithelial tumor most frequently associated with endometriosis. The endometrioid tumors contain varying combinations of cystic and solid components, and papillarity may be evident. When endometrioid carcinomas are encountered within endometriotic cysts, one may be able to demonstrate that the tumor arises directly from areas of atypical endometriosis, a finding that supports the endometriotic origin of at least some endometrioid carcinomas (*Figure 14.16*) (Mostoufizadeh and Scully, 1980; Ballouk *et al.*, 1994). As for other ovarian carcinomas, endometrioid cancers commonly show necrosis and hemorrhage.

On microscopic examination, endometrioid carcinomas display the usual patterns encountered in their uterine counterparts; the tumors are composed of tubular-type glands in varying degrees of differentiation (*Figure 14.17*). Endometrioid carcinomas may exhibit squamous differentiation identical to that seen in the endometrioid adenocarcinoma with squamous differentiation (the former 'adenoacanthoma' and 'adenosquamous' carcinoma of the endometrium). In fact, when attempting to determine whether an ovarian tumor is of an endometrioid or another cell type, the finding of squamous elements is a useful histologic feature favoring the former. The ovary may in fact be the site of any of the endometrioid tumor types, including, for example, endometrioid adenofibromas and adenosarcomas, carcinosarcomas and endometrial stromal sarcomas.

Approximately 20–50% of endometrioid carcinoma of the ovary occur simultaneously with an endometrial adenocarcinoma, frequently of similar histologic appearance (Dockerty, 1954; Scully, 1979). These are regarded by most workers as synchronous

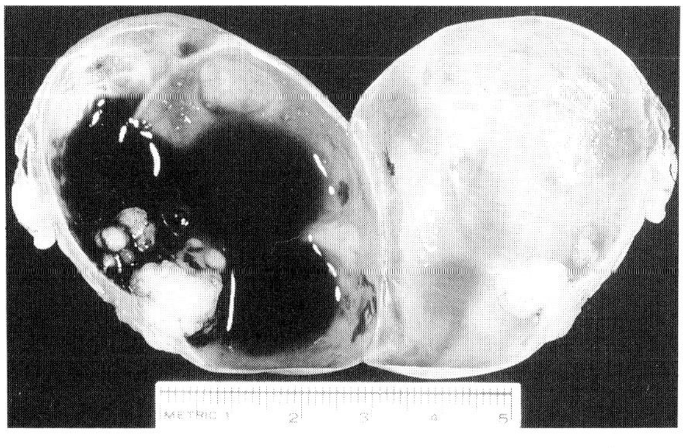

Figure 14.16. Endometrioid carcinoma. Most of the cystic ovary has a relatively smooth surface and represents an endometriotic cyst (note the dark appearance of the contained old blood); however, a papillary tumor, which shows gross invasion of the relatively thin cyst wall, represents an endometrioid carcinoma.

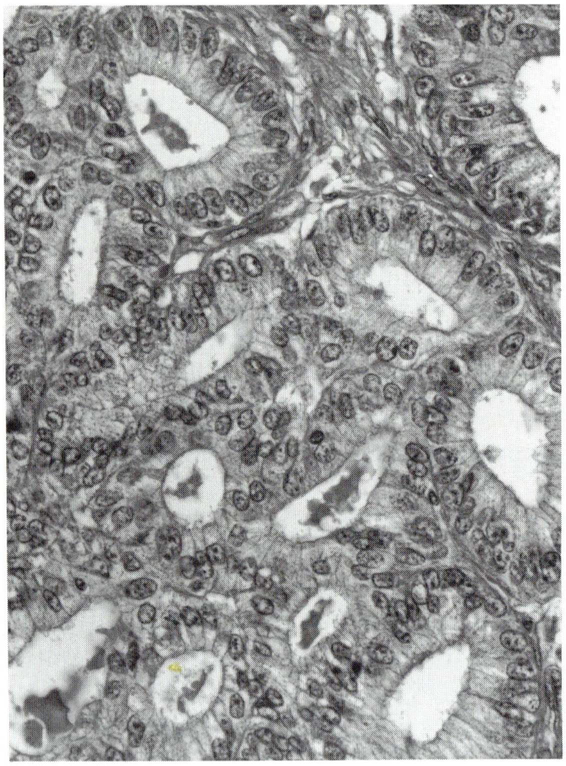

Figure 14.17. Endometrioid carcinoma. The well-differentiated tumor is composed of well-formed, tubular-type glands identical to those of an endometrial adenocarcinoma.

primaries since the endometrial adenocarcinoma is often well-differentiated, non-invasive and small. The frequent finding of surrounding precancerous glandular changes of atypical endometrial hyperplasia in particular, favor an endometrial origin. Furthermore, the long-term survival of patients having both an ovarian and an endometrial tumor is generally quite good, a finding that would be incongruous with metastatic dissemination from either site (Zaino *et al.*, 1984).

Clear Cell Tumors

Benign and borderline clear cell tumors of the ovary are very rare so that virtually all clear cell tumors encountered are malignant. Formerly classified as of mesonephric origin, the clear cell carcinoma is currently considered by most workers to be of müllerian origin. Some theorize that it is a variant of endometrioid carcinoma (Scully, 1979). Clear cell carcinoma is encountered most commonly in women in the fifth to eighth decades, with a mean age in the mid-fifties.

Like the endometrioid carcinoma, ovarian clear cell carcinoma lacks distinctive gross features; however, as previously mentioned, it is the surface epithelial tumor of the ovary that is encountered most frequently in association with ovarian endometriosis. Up to 40% have been reported as bilateral, but this may be related to the stage at the time of diagnosis since in one study only 3% of Stage I cases were bilateral (Aure *et al.*, 1971).

On microscopic examination, clear cell carcinoma has identical histologic features to those of other clear cell carcinomas of the upper and lower female genital tract. As its name implies, the tumor exhibits a clear cell component in most cases; however, the tumor may display a variety of histologic patterns. The clear cells *per se*, which contain abundant intracytoplasmic glycogen that is washed out during routine tissue processing, may be present in only relatively minor proportions. In its most easily recognizable form, clear cell carcinoma grows in solid sheets of round to polygonal cells. Other patterns include the characteristic hobnail cells, often lining hyalinized vascular papillae, as well as tubular and cystic forms (*Figure 14.18*). In support of the previously discussed theory concerning the endometrioid origin and kinship to clear cell carcinoma, admixed areas of endometrioid carcinoma may be encountered.

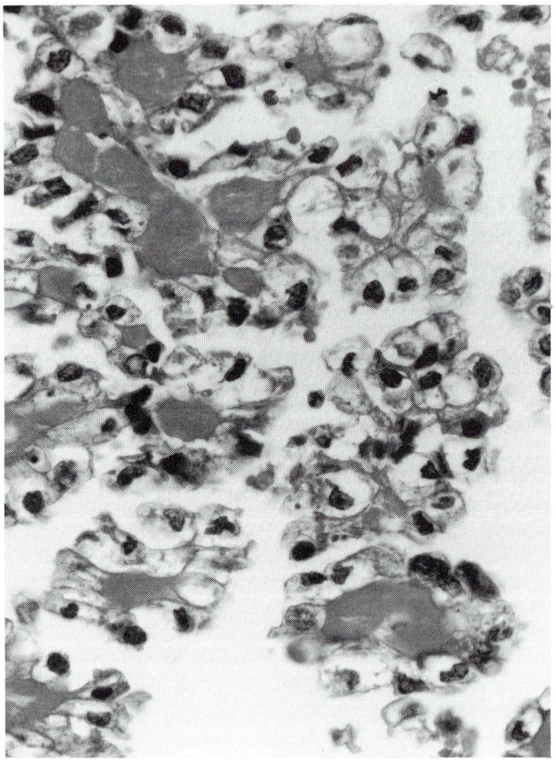

Figure 14.18. Clear cell carcinoma. The tumor is papillary with hyaline-appearing cores lined by clear cells, some of which have a hobnail appearance.

Urothelial Type Tumors

The Brenner tumor is yet another example of the exceedingly diverse metaplastic capacity of the ovary; differentiation in this case is toward an epithelium of urothelial type, but the tumors arising from such tissues have been retained in the surface epithelial category. Many workers believe that the Brenner tumor arises from the ovarian surface epithelium, the rationale provided by studies demonstrating continuity between it and parenchymal Brenner tumors (Arey, 1961). The epithelial element, however, represents only a very minor component of the tumor, which is comprised largely of ovarian stroma.

As with other surface epithelial ovarian tumors, the Brenner tumor exists in benign, borderline, and malignant forms; examples of the latter two categories are encountered only rarely. The benign Brenner tumor is relatively uncommon, is almost always unilateral, and usually occurs in patients in the fifth and sixth decades of life. The tumors vary widely in size, about half being only microscopic incidental findings, whereas others may attain sizes up to 8 cm; however, most of the larger Brenner tumors are around 2–3 cm in diameter. Grossly, they may be mistaken for fibromas on cut section since they are solid, tan–white to gray, and sometimes calcified (*Figure 14.19*); if the epithelial element is inconspicuous, the diagnosis may be missed on microscopic examination as well. That the Brenner tumor could be confused with an ovarian fibroma serves to emphasize the prominence of its fibrous-type stromal component. Scattered within the stroma in variable numbers are nests or islands of urothelial cells similar to those lining the urinary tract (*Figure 14.20*); coffee bean-shaped nuclei are a characteristic feature and resemble those observed in granulosa cell tumors.

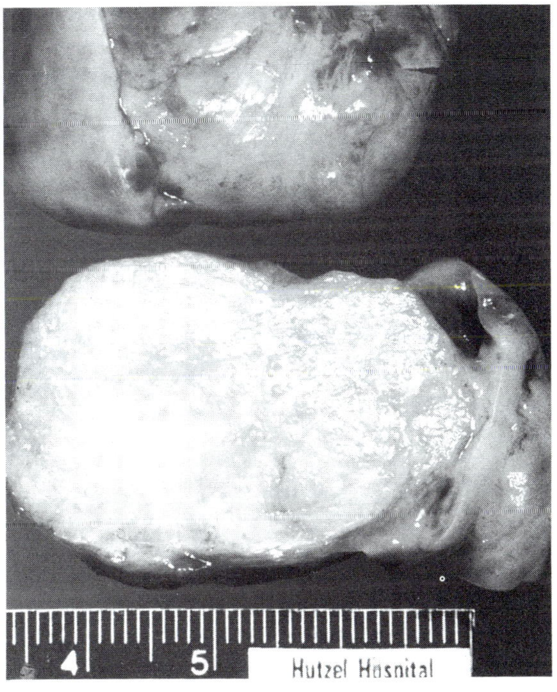

Figure 14.19. Brenner tumor. The uncut surface of the tumor was slightly lobulated (above), while the cut section was yellow–white and firm and occupied most of the ovarian parenchyma.

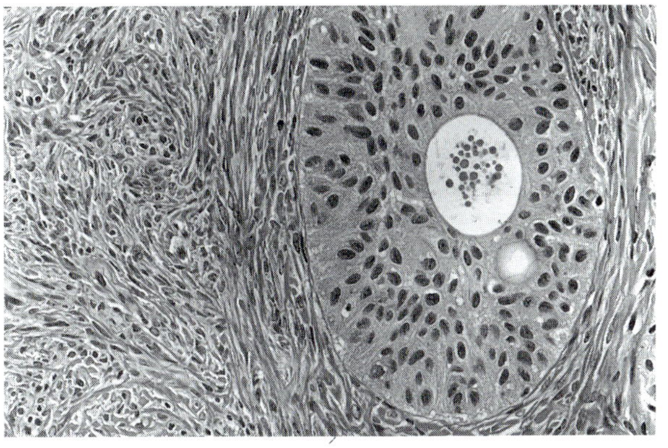

Figure 14.20. Brenner tumor. An island of urothelial-type cells is present in a dense fibrous stroma. Nuclear grooves imparting a 'coffee-bean'-like appearance can be appreciated in many of the cells.

Brenner tumors not uncommonly occur in association with cystic ovarian neoplasms; of the latter, the two most common are the mucinous cystadenoma and the benign cystic teratoma.

The classification of borderline and malignant variants of Brenner tumors is controversial; most, however, are accompanied by recognizable benign or atypical Brenner elements, which testify as to the origin of the tumor. The term borderline Brenner tumor denotes a (usually) cystic neoplasm that on microscopic examination resembles a Grade I papillary transitional cell carcinoma of the bladder. The use of the term borderline for such tumors has been criticized, since virtually none of them have exhibited any evidence of metastasis or recurrence. Consequently, the term proliferating Brenner tumor has been suggested as a replacement for the borderline category (Miles and Norris, 1972). In addition to the proliferating Brenner tumor, Roth *et al.* (1985) recognize a borderline variant of Brenner tumor that they categorize as of 'low malignant potential;' like the proliferating variant, the tumor is composed of papillary fronds, but these are lined by a high-grade noninvasive type of papillary transitional cell carcinoma or squamous cell carcinoma *in situ*. The number of such cases studied is small, so a larger series must be investigated before their separation as a distinct entity can be justified.

Austin and Norris (1987) identified a category of tumors that they designated as primary transitional cell carcinomas of the ovary; on histologic examination, the latter differed from malignant Brenner tumors only by the absence of coexistent recognizable Brenner components and were considered to arise by direct transformation of ovarian surface epithelium into urothelial carcinoma (transitional cell carcinoma). The ovarian transitional cell carcinoma appeared to be a more aggressive neoplasm than the malignant Brenner tumor since more than two-thirds presented in advanced stages compared with only one-fifth of the latter.

Sex Cord–Stromal Tumors

The term sex cord–stromal tumors was chosen by the WHO to include neoplasms composed of granulosa cells, Sertoli cells, Leydig cells, theca cells and ovarian stromal cells, the latter also being able to differentiate in a fibroblastic direction. Sex cord–stromal tumors can exist as pure forms of any of the aforementioned cell types, but frequently exhibit admixtures of the cellular elements in variable proportions and degrees of differentiation. Consequently, they can present a plethora of histologic patterns, a fact that has resulted in considerable and longstanding controversy over their classification (Fox, 1985). Although preferences in nosologic terminology exist among reputable investigators who have made enormous contributions to our understanding of sex cord–stromal tumors, we prefer to use the classification of the WHO (*Table 14.2*). As previously mentioned, the advantage of using standard and worldwide sanctioned terminology is that a better assessment of the natural history and biologic behavior of these neoplasms may be gained.

Sex cord–stromal tumors are rare, comprising approximately 5% or less of all ovarian tumors. Although functioning varieties afford the most dramatic examples, only a small minority generate hormonal symptoms.

Table 14.2. Histologic classification of sex cord–stromal tumors of the ovary (modified from Young & Scully, 1988).

Granulosa–stromal cell tumors
Granulosa cell tumor
Adult type
Juvenile type
Tumors in the thecoma–fibroma group
Thecoma
Typical
Luteinized
Fibroma–fibrosarcoma
Fibroma
Cellular fibroma
Fibrosarcoma
Sclerosing stromal tumor
Unclassified
Sertoli–stromal cell tumors
Leydig cell tumor
Sertoli–Leydig cell tumors
Well-differentiated
Intermediate differentiation
Poorly differentiated with heterologous elements
Gynandroblastoma
Sex cord tumor with annular tubules
Unclassified

Granulosa Cell Tumor

Granulosa cell tumors are often functioning tumors and represent the most common estrogenic ovarian neoplasm. They are considered to be low-grade malignant tumors, comprising 5–10% of cancers of the ovary.

Granulosa cell tumors exist in both adult and juvenile forms, the former occurring primarily in postmenopausal females and representing the most commonly encountered type. Such patients frequently exhibit clinical stigmata related to hyperestrinism, including postmenopausal bleeding associated with various grades of endometrial hyperplasia or adenocarcinoma. Premenopausal women with a granulosa cell tumor may complain of menometrorrhagia or even amenorrhea. In both groups of patients, the estrogen level may be elevated in the serum and in the urine.

On gross examination, granulosa cell tumors vary in size, representing incidental findings in some cases, but very large masses in others. They are virtually always unilateral. On section, the tumor may be solid, cystic or both (*Figure 14.21*). The cut surface is gray–tan to varying shades of yellow; the intensity of the yellow usually depends to a large degree on the lipid content of the tumor. At times, a higher grade tumor may be suspected on gross examination because of the rather common tendency for hemorrhage and necrosis. Some varieties exhibit extensive multiloculation; the cysts composing such locules frequently rupture so that on cut section the appearance is that of a blood-filled tumor. Additionally, the capsule may rupture in these types of granulosa cell tumor, resulting in hemoperitoneum.

On microscopic examination, a number of histopathologic patterns may be encountered in the adult granulosa cell tumor. The most well-known and common is the microfollicular pattern, in which islands of monotonous granulosa cells contain small round 'punched-out' spaces; these are not true

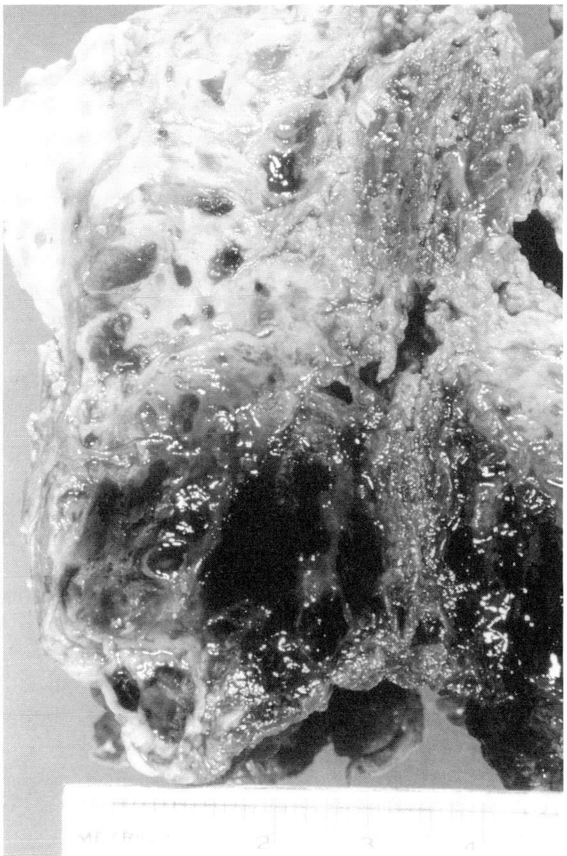

Figure 14.21. Granulosa cell tumor. The tumor is mostly solid; however, numerous cystic spaces are interspersed throughout. Foci of hemorrhage, a common finding in granulosa cell tumors, are seen in the lower portion of the specimen.

glandular lumens, but are spaces lined by granulosa cells with prominent 'coffee-bean' nuclei. Such structures are known as Call–Exner bodies and are almost pathognomonic of granulosa cell tumor (*Figure 14.22*). Nuclear grooves, although at least focally present in many adult granulosa cell tumors, are not a pathognomonic feature and may be seen in a variety of lesions, including the Brenner tumor. Other histopathologic patterns include the macrofollicular, trabecular and insular ones; however, the pattern that more often may be confused with other tumors, including undifferentiated carcinoma, is the diffuse, or sarcomatoid type. This particular neoplasm does not contain Call–Exner bodies or exhibit other more easily recognizable patterns, but rather grows as diffuse sheets of often spindle-shaped granulosa cells that show brisk mitotic activity.

The juvenile form of granulosa cell tumor has been described only relatively recently; as indicated by its name, the tumor occurs predominantly in young females during the first two decades of life (Young *et al.*, 1984). Juvenile granulosa cell tumors are virtually always unilateral and most are encountered as Stage I, which probably accounts for their generally good prognosis despite their sometimes alarming histologic appearance. Given their propensity to occur in younger patients, juvenile granulosa cell tumors may be confused with other ovarian tumors that primarily affect that age group, including germ cell tumors and small cell carcinoma of the ovary, the latter often being associated with hypercalcemia (Dickersin *et al.*, 1982). Distinction of the juvenile granulosa cell tumor from germ cell and small cell cancers, however, is important since there is a significant difference in its prognosis compared to that of the latter two neoplasms.

Grossly, the juvenile granulosa cell tumor may appear similar to its adult counterpart, but one of the most common appearances is that of a neoplasm with both solid and cystic components. The cysts not infrequently contain blood and the additional presence of necrosis may suggest a highly malignant neoplasm on gross examination.

On microscopic examination, the juvenile granulosa cell tumor usually exhibits one of two fairly distinctive histologic patterns, or combinations of either in variable proportions. One pattern is characterized by the presence of follicles that are usually large and irregular in configuration, often containing a mucinous secretion. The other is a solid pattern composed of granulosa cells arranged in a rather disorderly manner, not uncommonly showing

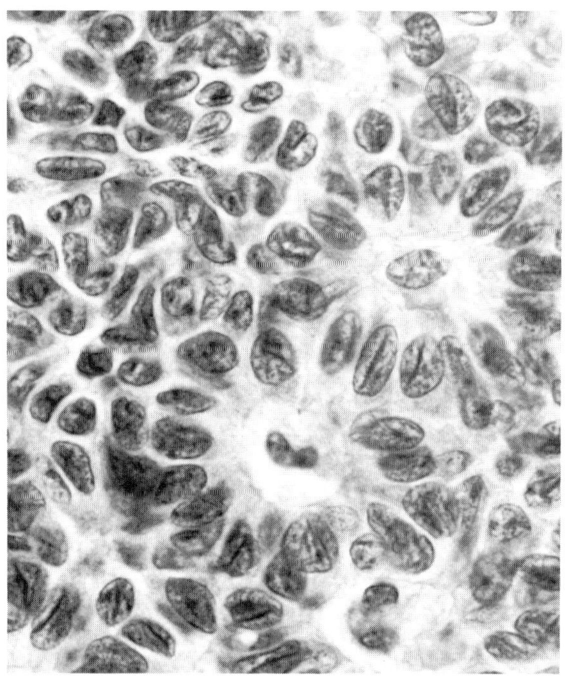

Figure 14.22. Granulosa cell tumor. Neoplastic granulosa cells with characteristic 'coffee-bean' nuclei are loosely arranged around spaces to form the pathognomonic Call–Exner bodies.

a marked degree of luteinization and containing nuclei that are more hyperchromatic and pleomorphic than those seen in the adult granulosa cell tumor; additionally, the nuclei are only rarely grooved (*Figure 14.23*). Mitotic figures may be quite numerous, adding further to the impression of a highly malignant tumor (Deppe and Lawrence, 1988).

Thecoma–Fibroma

This group of tumors is composed of ovarian stromal cells exhibiting differentiation toward either theca cells or fibroblastic-type cells. Like the granulosa cell tumor, the thecoma is usually estrogenic, but it is less common than the granulosa cell tumor and is generally seen in older women. Fibromas are usually non-functioning and are encountered most frequently in middle-aged females. Most of the tumors in the thecoma–fibroma group are unilateral and only rarely malignant. As with many sex cord–stromal tumors, thecomas vary in size, ranging from small incidental tumors to large, clinically palpable neoplasms. They are usually solid tumors that on cut section are firm and have variable shades of yellow to orange coloration, depending on their lipid content.

The microscopic appearance is dependent, as is the gross appearance, on the variable proportion of theca cells and fibroblasts. Theca cells have abundant cytoplasm that is either vacuolated or eosinophilic, the former appearance due to the loss of lipid from the cytoplasm during processing of the tissue.

The so-called luteinized thecoma is composed of islands of lutein cells (cells with abundant pink cytoplasm resembling the lutein cells of the corpus luteum) that are set in a background of otherwise unremarkable thecoma–fibroma (Zhang *et al.*, 1982).

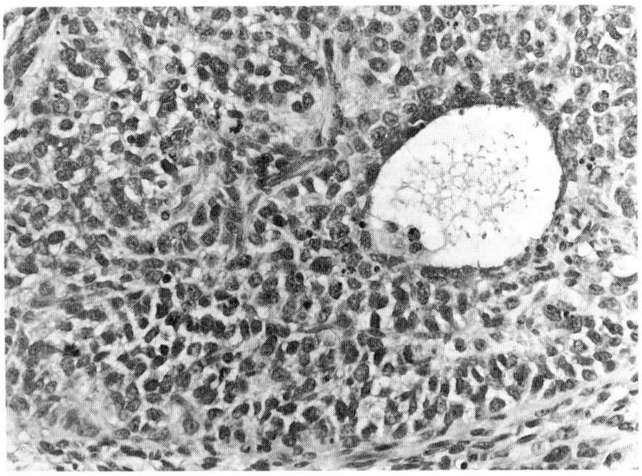

Figure 14.23. Juvenile granulosa cell tumor. The tumor grows as sheets of cells with hyperchromatic nuclei, only rarely exhibiting nuclear grooves. Small follicle-like spaces are sometimes present (upper right). Mitotic activity is brisk.

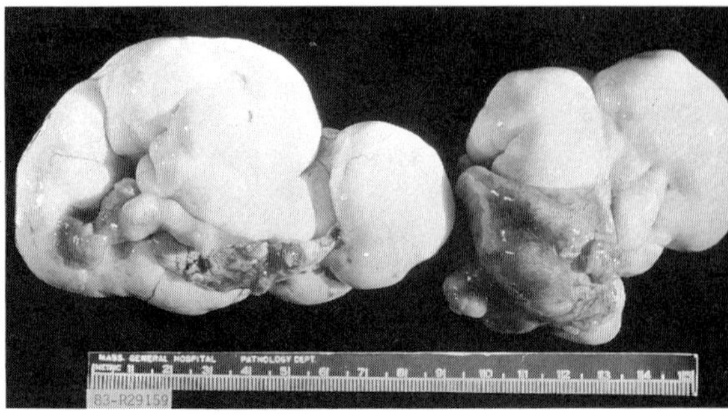

Figure 14.24. Bilateral fibromas. The ovaries are replaced by irregular, knobby tumors imparting a 'porcelain' appearance; the fibromas were heavy and difficult to section; however, they were not calcified.

These tumors are differentiated from the rare stromal Leydig cell tumor by the presence of intracellular crystalloids of Reinke in the latter. Almost half of the reported cases have been estrogenic, slightly more than one-third non-functioning, and a small minority have been androgenic.

Gross examination of a fibroma reveals a variably-sized firm, heavy, sometimes nodular tumor. The sectioned surface is usually whorled and pink–tan to white (*Figure 14.24*); however, variable amounts of calcification may either preclude or make sectioning difficult. The finding in a patient of bilateral fibromas should raise the question of the basal cell nevus syndrome; the latter occurs in young women and is more often associated with multiple fibromas.

Another syndrome that has rarely been associated with ovarian fibromas is Meigs' syndrome, defined as pleural effusions and ascites that occur simultaneously with an ovarian fibrous tumor, usually a fibroma, and that disappear after extirpation of the tumor. Weeping of serous fluid from the tumor apparently forms ascites and the fluid passes from the abdominal to the pleural cavity by either lymphatics or by a pathologic avenue between the two.

On microscopic examination, fibromas are comprised of ovarian stromal cells that resemble fibroblasts and produce collagen. A storiform or cartwheel pattern characterized by intersecting bundles of spindle-type cells may be observed and these may be accompanied by thick bands of fibrous tissue. Hyalinization and areas of edema may occur so that there may be confusion with so-called massive ovarian edema, a condition that may be related to ovarian fibromatosis (Young and Scully, 1984).

Although almost all fibromas have a bland histologic appearance and are relatively paucicellular, so-called cellular fibromas exist. As the name implies, such tumors exhibit increased cellularity accompanied by increased mitotic activity (Prat and Scully, 1981). Cellular fibromas usually show mild nuclear atypia and mitotic counts of 1–3 per ten high power fields. Their designation as a separate entity is justified by their potential for recurrence, especially when they are adherent to surrounding structures or have ruptured. Fibromas with greater degrees of mitotic activity (four or more per ten high power fields) and more severe nuclear atypia have been designated as fibrosarcomas and have overt malignant potential.

A tumor that has been described only relatively recently and has clinical and pathologic features that distinguish it from both thecomas and fibromas is the sclerosing stromal tumor (Chalvardjian and Scully, 1973). This neoplasm occurs in a younger age group, with a mean age in the late third decade, and are virtually always non-functioning.

Grossly, the sclerosing stromal tumor is almost always unilateral. Section of the mass reveals it to be well delimited from the surrounding ovarian parenchyma if the entire ovary has not been replaced. The sectioned surface is usually firm to rubbery, and reminiscent of both thecoma and fibroma (i.e. some foci are pink–tan and others have a yellowish coloration; *Figure 14.25*). Edema and areas of cystic degeneration may be prominent.

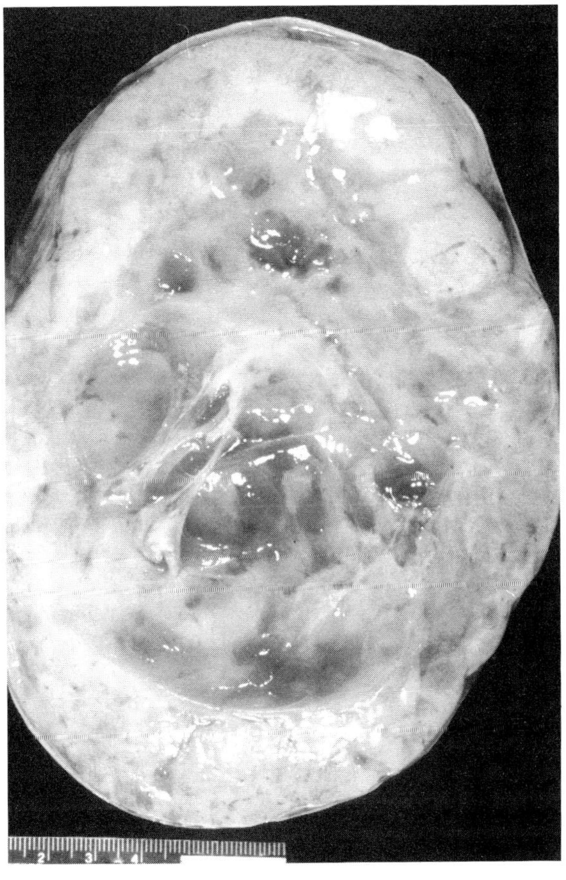

Figure 14.25. Sclerosing stromal tumor. Cut section of the neoplasm reveals central cystic degeneration and edema; the surface of the tumor was an admixture of yellow and tan–brown, reflecting the lipid-containing and fibrous components, respectively.

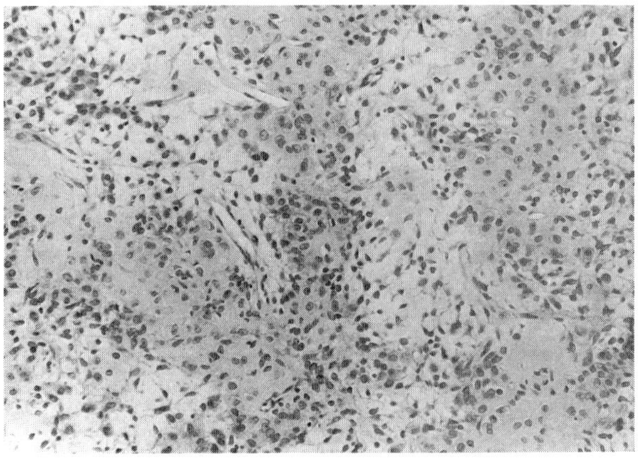

Figure 14.26. Sclerosing stromal tumor. Alternating more densely and sparsely cellular areas create a pseudolobular pattern to the tumor. A sclerotic background is evident.

Microscopic examination of the sclerosing stromal tumor shows a characteristic appearance composed of alternating areas of sparsely and densely cellular tissue; such an arrangement imparts a pseudolobular appearance to the neoplasm (*Figure 14.26*). In more densely cellular areas, the tumor is comprised of a mixture of larger vacuolated cells, probably representing weakly active lutein cells, and spindle cells.

No malignant example of sclerosing stromal tumor has been encountered.

Sertoli–Leydig Cell Tumors

Sertoli–Leydig tumors are among the rarest of ovarian tumors, representing far less than 1% of such neoplasms (Young and Scully, 1985). They occur predominantly in young females, with a mean age in the mid-twenties. Although commonly androgenic, many are non-functioning and a few are estrogenic.

According to the WHO, Sertoli–Leydig cell tumors are classified according to their cell type, degree of differentiation, and the presence or absence of heterologous elements (see *Table 14.2*). They are composed either exclusively of Sertoli cells or they contain admixtures of Leydig cells and stroma-derived fibroblasts. When present in any given tumor, the latter two cell types may vary in their numbers and degree of differentiation. Pure Leydig cell tumors also belong in this category.

On gross examination, Sertoli–Leydig cell tumors are almost invariably unilateral. They vary widely in size, but are frequently 10–20 cm in their greatest diameter. In general, the larger tumors tend to be more poorly differentiated. The external surface of the tumor is smooth and the contour of the ovary may be lobulated. On cut section, the Sertoli–Leydig cell tumor is most often solid, in contrast to the granulosa cell tumor, which more commonly exhibits cyst formation. The cut surface may be yellow to tan or brown, the former more evident in tumors with a higher lipid content. In those Sertoli–Leydig cell tumors with heterologous elements, the gross appearance reflects the nature of the individual elements; for example, those with mucinous elements may contain mucinous fluid, simulating a surface epithelial tumor of the mucinous variety. A variegated appearance of hemorrhage and necrosis, a hallmark of malignant tumors, is not a frequent feature except in the more poorly differentiated tumors (*Figure 14.27*).

Microscopic examination of Sertoli–Leydig cell tumors reveals a variety of histopathologic patterns. However, four types based on their degree of differentiation and the presence or absence of heterologous elements are currently recognized by the WHO (Serov *et al.*, 1973); these include well-differentiated types, those of intermediate differentiation, poorly-differentiated Sertoli–Leydig cell tumors, and those with heterologous elements. The latter are usually seen in association with tumors showing intermediate and poor differentiation.

Pure Sertoli cell tumors are most often well-differentiated and comprised of tubules that are either hollow or solid and lined by well-formed Sertoli cells (*Figure 14.28*). Some examples contain abundant intracytoplasmic lipid, the loss of which imparts a clear appearance to the cytoplasm after routine tissue processing. Leydig cells are either rare or absent. The histopathologic appearance of a well-differentiated Sertoli–Leydig cell tumor is similar to that of the pure Sertoli cell tumor except that Leydig cells are present in varying numbers.

The Sertoli–Leydig cell tumors of intermediate and poor differentiation represent a spectrum of both epithelial and stromal elements that may exhibit considerable intertumor as well as intratumor histopathologic variation. The Sertoli cell element

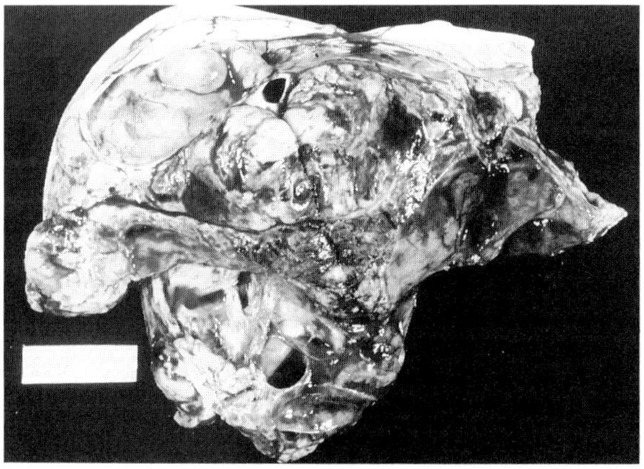

Figure 14.27. Sertoli–Leydig cell tumor – intermediate to poor differentiation. The ovary has been replaced by a large, irregularly lobulated tumor that on cut section shows extensive hemorrhage and necrosis.

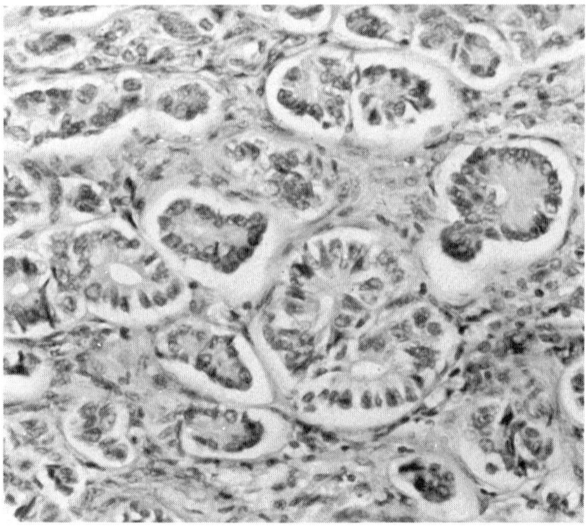

Figure 14.28. Well-differentiated Sertoli cell tumor. The neoplasm is composed of well-formed tubules that mimic the Sertoli cells of the testis.

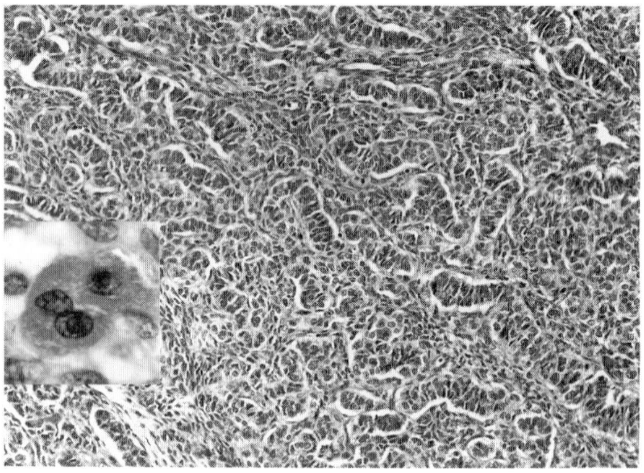

Figure 14.29. Sertoli–Leydig cell tumor – intermediate differentiation. Solid tubular configurations mimic the primitive sex cords of the embryonic testis. A cellular spindled stroma merges with the tubular component. Inset: Leydig cells exhibit abundant granular cytoplasm and are set in a loose spindled stroma.

may be present in the form of sheets, islands, and nests of immature Sertoli cells, without evidence of attempted tubule formation. Alternatively, the tumor may form thin cords without lumens that simulate the developing sex cords of the embryonic testis (*Figure 14.29*). Leydig cells may be present in variable numbers; indeed, they may be encountered in large numbers and such cells may contain abundant eosinophilic cytoplasm (see *Figure 14.29*). The Sertoli cell element may merge imperceptibly with the stromal component, which is generally comprised of spindled to round cells.

The heterologous elements found in the intermediate and poorly-differentiated forms of Sertoli–Leydig cell tumor are represented most frequently by glandular epithelium, usually of a mucinous type.

Contributing most commonly to the mesenchymal heterologous elements are cartilage and skeletal muscle. Despite the unusual appearance afforded by such foreign tissue derivatives in a Sertoli–Leydig cell tumor, the prognosis is usually determined by the grade of the sex cord elements.

Germ Cell Tumors

Germ cell tumors of the ovary form a heterogeneous array of neoplasms that comprise approximately 20–25% of all ovarian tumors (*Table 14.3*). Affecting mostly children and young women (Raney *et al.*, 1987), they represent the majority of ovarian tumors in the pediatric population; however, one-third are cancerous whereas only 4% of the germ cell tumors affecting all age groups are malignant. One reason for this observation is that the substantial majority of germ cell tumors is represented by the mature cystic teratoma (dermoid cyst), a common lesion that may comprise up to one-third of all benign ovarian neoplasms.

The progenitor cell of this group of neoplasms, the embryonic germ cell, is thought to arise in the yolk sac. These cells subsequently migrate to the ovary through the coelomic cavity and hindgut mesentery as well as via lymphatic channels to become incorporated into the sex cords of the developing ovary (Witschi, 1948). Migrating germ cells arrested on their journey to the ovary may give rise to midline benign or malignant germ cell tumors extrinsic to the gonads, thus explaining the presence of these tumors in extragonadal sites such as the mediastinum, retroperitoneum and sacrococcygeal region (Friedman, 1951).

Although most germ cell tumors are benign, metastases from malignant examples are often occult, requiring meticulous examination and histologic evaluation of the contralateral ovary, omentum, lymph nodes and adhesions. Additionally the liver, bowel and diaphragm should be inspected carefully during laparotomy, and if suspicious lesions are encountered, they should be biopsied for pathologic evaluation.

Table 14.3. Histologic classification of pure and mixed types of germ cell tumors of the ovary (modified from Talerman, 1994).

- I. Germ cell tumors
  - A. Dysgerminoma
  - B. Yolk sac tumor (endodermal sinus tumor)
  - C. Teratomas
    - 1. Immature (solid and/or cystic)
    - 2. Mature
      - a. solid
      - b. cystic (dermoid cyst)
      - c. cystic with malignant transformation
    - 3. Monodermal or highly specialized
      - a. Struma ovarii
      - b. Carcinoid
      - c. Others
  - D. Embryonal carcinoma
  - E. Choriocarcinoma
  - F. Polyembryoma
  - G. Combination germ cell tumor
- II. Mixed germ cell and sex cord–stromal tumors
  - A. Gonadoblastoma
  - B. Others
- III. Germ cell tumors arising in dysgenetic gonads
  - A. Pure gonadal dysgenesis
  - B. Mixed gonadal dysgenesis
  - C. Turner's syndrome
  - D. Testicular feminization

Dysgerminoma

Although dysgerminoma is a relatively uncommon ovarian cancer, representing only 3–5% of all ovarian malignancies, it is the most common malignant germ cell tumor and composes at least half of such malignant tumors of the ovary (Kurman and Petrilli, 1983). Dysgerminoma primarily affects younger women, exemplified by the following facts:

- 75% of them occur in the second and third decades;
- the median age of occurrence is 22 years (Asadourian and Taylor, 1969);
- it is the most frequently encountered ovarian malignancy during pregnancy (Scully, 1979).

While dysgerminoma is a very rare tumor in infancy, it is the ovarian malignancy most likely to be associated with gonadoblastoma and gonadal dysgenesis, Turner's syndrome, testicular feminization, hermaphroditism and ambiguous genitalia.

Although usually unilateral, dysgerminoma involves both ovaries with some frequency (Santesson, 1947; Mueller *et al.*, 1950); 10% of the bilateral cases are grossly evident, while an estimated 10–35% of cases show involvement of the contralateral ovary only on microscopic examination.

On gross examination, dysgerminomas usually have a smooth exterior surface, although on occasion foci of capsular rupture may be demonstrated in very large tumors. They tend to be large, with an average diameter of 15 cm, and are generally heavy and solid, with lobulated or bosselated contours (*Figure 14.30*). Cut section reveals the surface of the neoplasm to be fleshy, bulging and a homogeneous pink–tan color. Focal hemorrhage and necrosis may be seen, but large areas of hemorrhage or cystic change should suggest the possibility of admixed nondysgerminomatous germ cell components since

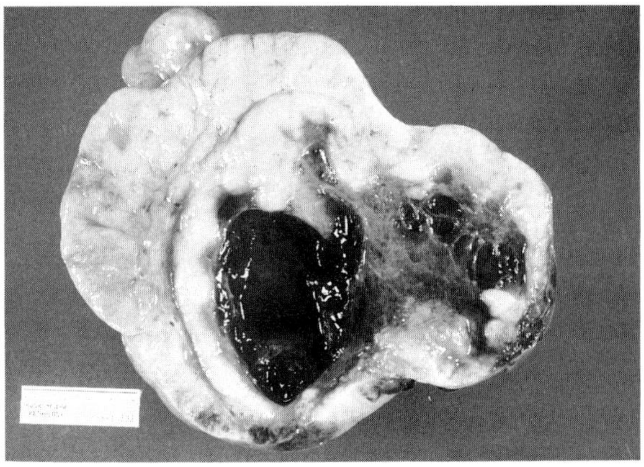

Figure 14.30. Dysgerminoma. A large, lobulated, firm tumor that was pink–tan on section shows central hemorrhage and cystic degeneration; although such foci should raise the question of nondysgerminomatous elements, none were found after extensive sampling.

approximately 20% of cases contain other germ cell components (Kurman and Petrilli, 1983).

On microscopic examination, dysgerminomas have a monotonous appearance, histologically identical to both extragonadal germinomas and testicular seminomas; the tumor grows as sheets of large polyhedral cells with abundant clear or lightly granular amphophilic cytoplasm that contains mostly glycogen, but some lipid (*Figure 14.31*). Cell borders are distinct. Nuclei are large and vesicular and contain one or more prominent nucleoli. Mitotic activity is variable. Delicate fibrous septae encompassing aggregates of tumor cells impart a lobulated appearance to the tumor, and the fibrous component is classically infiltrated by lymphocytes, which occasionally may organize themselves into lymphoid follicles. Less commonly, eosinophils, plasma cells, and even sarcoid-like non-caseating granulomas are noted (foreign body-type giant cells are seen in approximately 20% of the cases). The association of such lymphocytic or granulomatous infiltrates with an improved prognosis is controversial.

Some dysgerminomas harbor multinucleated syncytiotrophoblast-type giant cells that may produce clinically detectable levels of human chorionic gonadotropin (HCG) and/or contain immunohistochemically demonstrable HCG in tissue sections of the tumor. Such findings may cause confusion with a choriocarcinomatous component; however, both cytotrophoblast and syncytiotrophoblastic elements must be present to warrant that diagnosis. Although dysgerminomas associated with elevated serum levels of HCG should be thoroughly sampled to exclude an element of choriocarcinoma or embryonal carcinoma, in some instances the heightened serum levels may be explained by the presence of syncytiotrophoblastic giant cells. Consequently, a diligent search for them should be made since their presence without associated cytotrophoblastic elements does not appear to alter the prognosis unfavorably. Focal calcification may be present in areas of necrosis or hemorrhage; however, larger areas of calcification should raise the question of 'burnt out' gonadoblastoma.

In occasional cases, the differential diagnosis may include a poorly-differentiated adenocarcinoma, clear cell carcinoma and lymphoma; indeed, examples comprised of abundant thickened fibrotic stroma containing scattered germinoma cells have been confused with Hodgkin's disease or even a granulomatous inflammatory process, particularly in those examples containing foreign body giant cells. The presence of intracellular glycogen demonstrated by special stains in dysgerminoma, as well as placental alkaline phosphatase immunopositivity, aid in distinguishing dysgerminoma from these other entities.

Yolk Sac Tumor

The yolk sac tumor, or endodermal sinus tumor, represents the second most common malignant

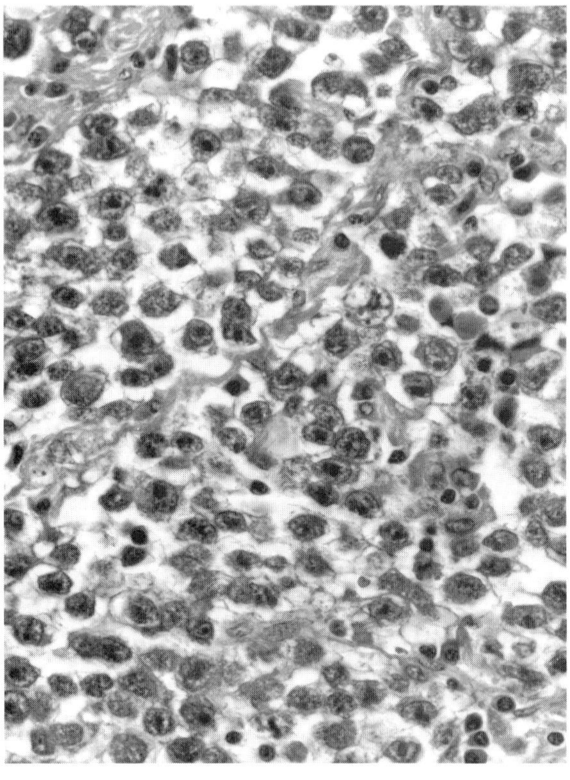

Figure 14.31. Dysgerminoma. The tumor grows as sheets of monotonous cells with pale to clear cytoplasm and round to oval nuclei with large prominent nucleoli. Small cells with dark nuclei represent the lymphocytic infiltrate characteristically found within such tumors.

ovarian germ cell tumor, although it accounts for only 1% of all malignant ovarian neoplasms (Kurman and Petrilli, 1983). It occurs over a relatively wide age range and may be encountered in infants and prepubertal females; however, the median age is 19 years. It rarely affects patients over the age of 40 years, the oldest reported case being 45 years of age (Kurman and Norris, 1976). Patients with a yolk sac tumor frequently present with the sudden onset of pelvic symptoms and a pelvic mass; elevated serum levels of alpha-fetoprotein (AFP) can be demonstrated serologically, while hCG levels are normal (Kurman *et al.*, 1979).

On gross examination, yolk sac tumors are typically unilateral and more often involve the right ovary; they range from 3–30 cm in their greatest dimension, with an average diameter of 15 cm. They frequently have a smooth external surface, although up to 25% of the tumors reveal evidence of having ruptured either preoperatively or during surgery. The cut surface is soft, usually pale yellow, and predominantly solid, with scattered variably-sized cysts imparting a honeycomb appearance. Large areas of necrosis, hemorrhage and cystic degeneration are common, while soft, friable and gelatinous tumor sometimes fills the pelvis. Of patients with a yolk sac tumor 14% have an ipsilateral teratoma and another 5% harbor a contralateral teratoma (Kurman and Petrilli, 1983).

On microscopic examination, the yolk sac tumor can exhibit a bewildering array of histologic appearances; in fact, as many as ten patterns have been reported, most of which have been described by Teilum (1959, 1965). In most examples, these patterns are admixed, although in some one pattern predominates, and a pure type is encountered very rarely. None of the histologic subtypes appears to have prognostic significance; however, recognition of the different patterns is important to prevent misdiagnosis and inappropriate treatment.

The microcystic or reticular pattern is characterized by a loose network of primitive, variably-sized spaces and channels lined by flattened or cuboidal cells with scanty cytoplasm and indistinct cellular borders. The nuclei may be large and mitotic activity is brisk. Intracellular and extracellular hyaline droplets are common. This pattern can occur in a pure form, but is dominant in only about 30% of the cases (Kurman and Norris, 1976).

The endodermal sinus, or festoon pattern, is the classic pattern associated with this neoplasm and is composed of abundant glomeruloid structures; the latter are composed of a fibrovascular core containing a single central vessel surrounded by a rim of primitive epithelioid cells with large vesicular nuclei. Such structures, which are thought to recapitulate the endodermal sinus of the rodent yolk sac, have been designated as Schiller–Duval bodies and are virtually pathognomonic of yolk sac tumor (*Figure 14.32*). However, it should be emphasized that approximately 25% of yolk sac tumors do not contain Schiller–Duval bodies. Mitotic activity in the endodermal sinus pattern is frequently brisk.

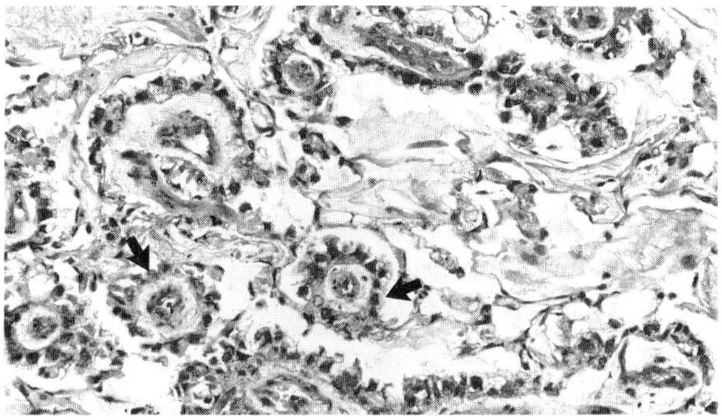

Figure 14.32. Yolk sac tumor (endodermal sinus tumor). Characteristic Schiller–Duval bodies (arrows) represented by fibrous cores with a central vessel and rimmed by anaplastic germ cells are present within a loose myxoid stroma.

Yolk sac tumors may be confused with clear cell carcinoma, which currently is regarded to be of müllerian origin (Scully and Barlow, 1967). Clear cell carcinomas, except those that arise in the vagina of younger women who have been exposed *in utero* to diethylstilbestrol, are generally seen in a much older age-group. A primary clear cell carcinoma occurring in the ovary of a prepubertal or adolescent female or even a young woman of reproductive age would be distinctly unusual.

Although mediastinal yolk sac tumors have been thought to occur only in males, recent workers have reported cases in females (Hawkins *et al.*, 1986).

Teratoma

Many workers feel that parthenogenetic development of a primordial germ cell best explains the histogenesis of a teratoma (Stevens, 1967), although some studies have challenged this concept (Sobis and Vandeputte, 1979). Teratomas characteristically contain elements arising from all three germ layers, although this is not an absolute requisite for making the diagnosis. A teratoma is generally classified as mature or immature depending on the degree of differentiation of its component tissues, the immature type being composed of more primitive embryonic-type tissues. Malignant behavior, manifested by recurrence and/or metastatic behavior, can be correlated with the amount of primitive tissue and its grade of immaturity; accordingly, these neoplasms must be sampled extensively and judiciously so that the histopathologic evaluation reflects the true proportions of mature and immature tissue.

Teratomas may be cystic or solid, and although such growth findings are typically associated with the mature and immature varieties, respectively, exceptions do occur. Mature teratomas may rarely undergo malignant transformation, an event that usually occurs in postmenopausal women. A small proportion of teratomas exhibit a very highly specialized monodermal differentiation, in which the teratomatous tissues originate from a single germ layer. Such tumors are thought to arise from a single germ cell following the first meiotic division.

Mature Teratoma

The mature teratoma is the most common ovarian tumor, constituting 20% of all ovarian neoplasms. Patients with a mature teratoma are most often in the third decade; however, 10% are postmenopausal (Kurman and Petrilli, 1983). In addition, mature teratomas account for approximately 50% of the ovarian neoplasms occurring in young females under 20 years of age (Scully, 1979).

Mature teratomas are generally asymptomatic unless they achieve sufficient size to cause abdominal pain or swelling. Complications are relatively frequent, with pain due to torsion the most common. Rupture into proximate hollow viscera, including the bladder, rectum and uterus, or the peritoneal cavity, may rarely occur, and other sequelae include infection (especially due to *Salmonella*), primary autoimmune hemolytic anemia, virilization, infertility problems and malignant transformation.

Mature teratomas may be either solid or cystic, with the latter comprising the vast majority. Bilaterality occurs in 10–15% of patients with mature cystic teratomas, but the mature solid teratomas are virtually always unilateral.

The mature cystic teratoma, or dermoid cyst, is usually less than 10 cm in diameter and has a smooth external surface and a thin wall. The cyst contents are typically composed of a thick, foul-smelling, greasy yellow–white mixture of sebum and hair. At one pole of the cyst, there is often an irregular nodule of solid tissue known as Rokitansky's protuberance, which usually contains bone, cartilage and/or fat. Roughly one-third of mature cystic teratomas contain a tooth, either protruding into the cyst lumen or embedded within the cyst wall (*Figure 14.33*). Mature solid teratoma, the less commonly encountered variant of benign teratoma, tends to be much larger, yet without hemorrhage and necrosis.

On microscopic examination, ectodermally-derived skin composed of keratinized stratified squamous epithelium and skin appendages is almost invariably the predominant constituent of the cyst wall, within which a foreign body reaction to extravasated keratin or cholesterol is often seen. Columnar epithelium lining either gastrointestinal-type and/or bronchial-type mucosa (endoderm) is present in approximately one-third of the cases.

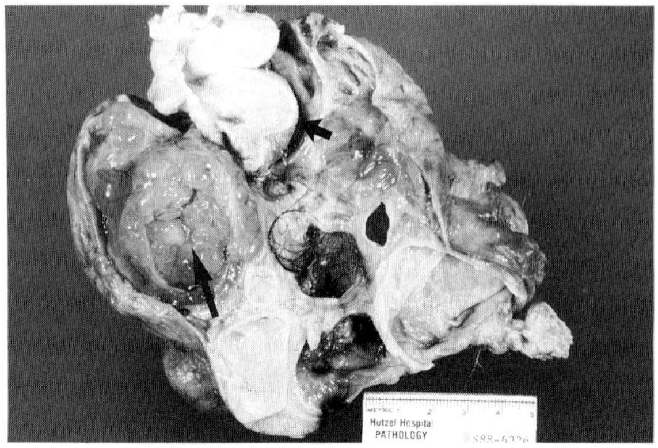

Figure 14.33. Mature cystic teratoma (dermoid cyst). The sectioned ovary contains the characteristic skin (small arrow), fat, hair and a tooth, as well as a multiloculated mucinous cystadenoma (large arrow).

Slightly more than two-thirds of mature cystic teratomas harbor fat and cartilage (mesoderm).

Malignant transformation occurs in only 1–2% of mature cystic teratomas and its occurrence is virtually confined to the postmenopausal age group. Ascites is an occasional clinical accompaniment, but in up to two-thirds of cases, invasion of contiguous structures and/or metastases have occurred by the time of diagnosis.

Macroscopically, teratomas with malignant transformation are often cystic, containing an intraluminal, partially necrotic mass that appears to invade the cyst wall. Although any histologic element of the teratoma may undergo malignant transformation, squamous cell carcinoma is by far the most frequently contained malignancy. Spread of the tumor typically occurs by direct extension into surrounding structures, a characteristic of squamous cell carcinomas occurring elsewhere.

Immature Teratoma

Immature teratoma is rare, but is the third most common ovarian germ cell cancer (Micha *et al.*, 1985), constituting approximately 25% of all such tumors (Kurman and Petrilli, 1983). Characteristically, it is observed in children under 15 years of age (Norris and Jensen, 1972), but sporadic cases have been reported in patients up to 40 years of age (Norris *et al.*, 1976).

At the time of diagnosis, three-quarters of patients complain of pelvic pain and have a clinically palpable mass. The latter can be explained by the fact that immature teratomas usually present as very large tumors; in fact, their median diameter is approximately 18 cm. Most have a smooth lobulated external surface and the cut surface is soft, varies from gray to pink, and exhibits extensive hemorrhage and necrosis (*Figure 14.34*). They are virtually always

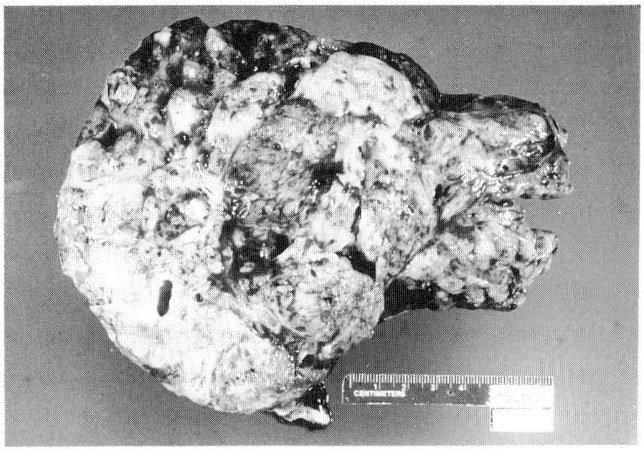

Figure 14.34. Immature teratoma. Cut section shows that the ovary has been replaced by a large solid mass with a variegated appearance. Darker areas represent hemorrhage and lighter ones, necrotic tumor.

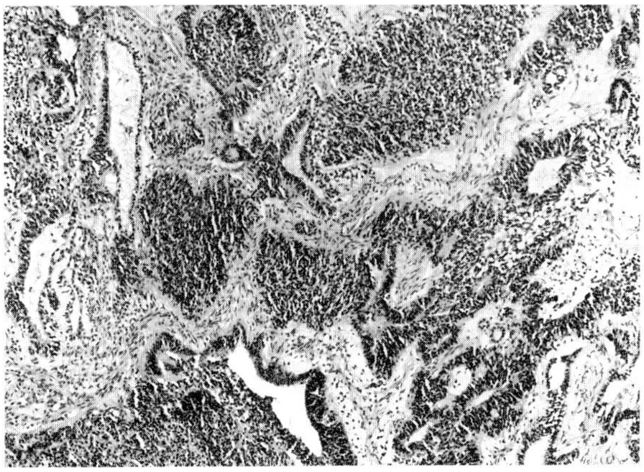

Figure 14.35. Immature teratoma – Grade III. The tumor was solid and largely composed of primitive neural tissue.

unilateral, a characteristic that allows conservation of the opposite gonad in most cases. Approximately 5% of ovaries contralateral to an immature teratoma harbor a mature cystic teratoma.

On microscopic examination, an immature teratoma is comprised of immature embryonic-type tissues derived from all three germ cell layers. Ectodermal derivatives are frequently observed, as are mesodermal representatives such as cartilage, bone and smooth muscle. Respiratory and gastrointestinal types of epithelium contribute to the endodermal components of these tumors. Histopathologic grading of the primitive cellular components of the tumor is based on their degree of immaturity and their relative proportions. The most commonly identified primitive component in immature teratomas is embryonic immature neural tissue; such tissue is often present in the form of neuroepithelium, neuroblastic tissue and atypical glia, and primarily determines the grade of the tumor (*Figure 14.35*). The histologic grade of immature teratomas may be correlated to some degree with biologic behavior, leading various workers to propose a grading system for them. The grading system given in *Table 14.4* has been adapted to include more quantitative information (Norris *et al.*, 1976).

Although immature teratomas may include several different tissue types that recapitulate various stages of primitive development, the least mature areas (i.e. the immature neural tissues) have the greatest tendency to metastasize; hence their relative proportions and degree of immaturity have an even greater impact on determining the grade of the tumor.

Direct extension and peritoneal implantation are the mechanisms of early spread, whereas lymphatic invasion and extraabdominal dissemination are manifestations of late spread. Once metastasis has occurred, the histologic grade of the metastasis appears to be the most reliable predictor of prognosis.

Teratomas with Specialized Tissue Derivatives

Three per cent of ovarian teratomas are comprised of a highly specialized tissue derivative of a single germ cell layer, as opposed to the usual three. When such monodermal derivatives are represented by thyroid tissue within an ovarian teratoma, the lesion is referred to as struma ovarii. To warrant this designation, however, the strumal (thyroid) component must comprise at least half of the tumor since some thyroid tissue occurs in 5–15% of teratomas (Caruso *et al.*, 1977). On microscopic examination, struma ovarii resembles mature thyroid tissue and is therefore composed of colloid-

Table 14.4. Histologic grading system for immature teratomas (modified from Norris *et al.*, 1976).

Grade 0	Wholly mature tissue
Grade 1	Most tissue is mature; immature neural tissue is limited to one low power field per slide (10 ×); rare mitoses; immature tissue usually comprised of glia embedded in primitive mesenchyme
Grade 2	Neural epithelium present in more than one low power field, but in less than or equal to three low power fields per slide
Grade 3	Abundant immature tissue present with neural epithelium in more than or equal to four low power fields per slide, often merging imperceptibly into sarcomatous stroma; mitoses common

containing follicles. Less than 20% of cases harbor contralateral ovarian teratomas.

Another rare monodermal variant of teratoma occurring in less than 1% of all such cases is the carcinoid tumor; the latter may occur as either the insular (midgut) or trabecular (foregut and hindgut) type (Robboy *et al.*, 1975, 1977). Histopathologic distinction between the two is clinically important. Approximately one-third of patients with the insular type manifest the carcinoid syndrome, whereas it does not apparently occur with the trabecular type of ovarian carcinoid (Robboy *et al.*, 1975). The carcinoid tumor exists as a grossly evident tan–yellow nodule or protuberance in the wall of a benign cystic or solid teratoma. On microscopic examination, the insular type is composed of small acini and clusters or islands of regular monotonous cells, whereas anastomosing rows and ribbons of uniform cells characterize the trabecular pattern. Primary carcinoids are not usually bilateral, although the contralateral ovary may harbor a benign cystic teratoma. Conversely, carcinoids are generally judged to be metastatic until proven otherwise.

Embryonal Carcinoma

Embryonal carcinoma accounts for only about 5% of ovarian malignant germ cell neoplasms (Kurman and Petrilli, 1983). It occurs in young females aged 4–28 years, with a median age of 15 years (Kurman and Petrilli, 1983). Such patients present with a relatively recent onset of abdominal and pelvic pain and most show clinical evidence of increased hormonal activity; in fact, precocious puberty is the most common clinical manifestation of the prepubertal age group which harbors this neoplasm.

On gross examination, embryonal carcinomas exhibit no distinguishing features but, like other germ cell cancers, tend to be large, bulky and soft. Unilateral tumors are the rule. The cut surface is variegated and gray to yellow–white, often with foci of hemorrhage and necrosis.

On microscopic examination, embryonal carcinoma is a morphologically heterogeneous tumor that has the potential to differentiate along somatic or extraembryonal pathways. Solid sheets of polyhedral large undifferentiated cells with vacuolated cytoplasm and indistinct cell borders make up the tumor. The nuclei are large and vesicular and contain 1–2 prominent nucleoli. Focally, gland-like formations and papillae may be seen. Mitotic figures are frequent and include bizarre forms. Scattered syncytiotrophoblastic giant cells are often present, but cytotrophoblast is lacking, obviating the diagnosis of concomitant choriocarcinoma. These tumors are often accompanied by a dysgerminoma, so careful inspection of the contralateral ovary should be performed routinely at the time of operation (Kurman and Norris, 1976).

Choriocarcinoma

Ovarian choriocarcinoma generally exists as a component of a mixed germ cell tumor, accompanied by one or all of the following: teratoma, yolk sac tumor, embryonal carcinoma and dysgerminoma. Ovarian choriocarcinoma in the pure form probably represents a metastatic gestational choriocarcinoma rather than a pure ovarian germ cell tumor or the exceedingly rare gestational choriocarcinoma arising from an ectopic ovarian pregnancy. Most cases of choriocarcinoma occur in young females with a median age of 13 years. Abdominal swelling and pain are present in approximately half the cases and precocious puberty is also evident in about half.

The hallmark gross feature of this tumor is its characteristic hemorrhage and necrosis, which are even present in metastases. Microscopically, two distinct cell populations are a requisite for the diagnosis of choriocarcinoma: multinucleated giant cells of the syncytiotrophoblastic type with abundant eosinophilic vacuolated cytoplasm and hyperchromatic nuclei tend to rim the aggregates of cytotrophoblastic cells. Syncytiotrophoblast elaborates hCG while cytotrophoblast does not. A third population of cells known as intermediate trophoblast may be seen in lesser amounts than the cytotrophoblastic and syncytiotrophoblastic elements; the former elaborate human placental lactogen.

Malignant Mixed Germ Cell Tumor

Mixed germ cell tumors comprise 8% of malignant ovarian germ cell tumors, a far smaller proportion than their counterparts in the testis, which account for about 40% of malignant germ cell tumors. Patients with ovarian mixed germ cell tumors tend to be young, with a median age of 16 years. Roughly 40% are found in prepubertal females, one-third of whom have signs and symptoms of precocious puberty (Kurman and Norris, 1976). The usual clinical manifestations are a relatively recent onset of abdominal pain and a growing abdominal mass.

On gross examination, the external surface is smooth and bosselated, and in a few examples the capsule is ruptured. Because they have an average diameter of 15 cm these tumors must be carefully sampled, especially since geographic variation in tissue types and degree of differentiation may exist from one area to another. Areas containing dysgerminoma are homogeneous, fleshy, soft, and lobulated, whereas foci of yolk sac tumor, choriocarcinoma and embryonal carcinoma tend to be hemorrhagic, necrotic and gelatinous. Teratomatous components are generally cystic and contain sebaceous or mucoid material.

Most mixed germ cell tumors contain only two components; the most common combination is dysgerminoma and yolk sac tumor (Kurman and Norris, 1976; Gershenson *et al.*, 1984). The various histologic types may either merge imperceptibly into one another or exist in different geographic loci, separated from each other by fibrous tissue. Quantitative estimates of component proportions as well as qualitative appraisals should be reported so that proper therapy may be instituted and the prognosis accurately determined. Poor prognostic indicators include:

- a size greater than 10 cm;
- greater than one-third of the neoplasm being comprised of yolk sac tumor, choriocarcinoma or Grade 3 immature teratoma (Kurman and Norris, 1976).

Most patients have Stage I disease and lack microscopic involvement of the contralateral ovary.

Mixed Germ Cell–Stromal Tumors

Mixed germ cell–stromal tumors are so designated because of the admixture of ample amounts of germinoma-type cells and stromal cells. The prototype tumor for this group is the gonadoblastoma, the neoplasm identified most frequently in patients with dysgenetic gonads; such patients usually have a Y chromosome (Scully, 1970) although gonadoblastomas do rarely occur in XX phenotypically-normal women (Bergher de Bacalao and Dominguez, 1969). Patients with gonadoblastoma range in age from 1–40 years. Often the streak gonads are bilateral and occasionally there is a streak gonad on one side and a normal testis on the other.

Grossly, gonadoblastomas may vary from a few millimeters to several centimeters in maximal dimension. They are bilateral in one-third of the cases; however, involvement of the contralateral ovary is often represented by microscopic disease. The cut surface varies from soft to firm to gritty, the texture depending on the absence or presence of calcification. A common and distinguishing feature is prominent dystrophic calcification, a finding that may be detected roentgenographically (*Figures 14.36 and 14.37*).

On microscopic examination, gonadoblastoma exhibits a biphasic pattern: nests and islands of germ cells resembling germinoma (seminoma or dysgerminoma) are admixed with immature sex cord derivatives; rounded hyaline bodies are interspersed within the nests and are composed of basement membrane material. Most cases are accompanied by cells within the stroma that resemble Leydig cells or lutein cells. About half of the cases of gonadoblastoma exhibit invasion of the ovarian parenchyma by the germinomatous element; the latter can vary in its extent from only microscopic to diffuse replacement of the gonad and obliteration of the gonadoblastoma that engendered it. Less commonly,

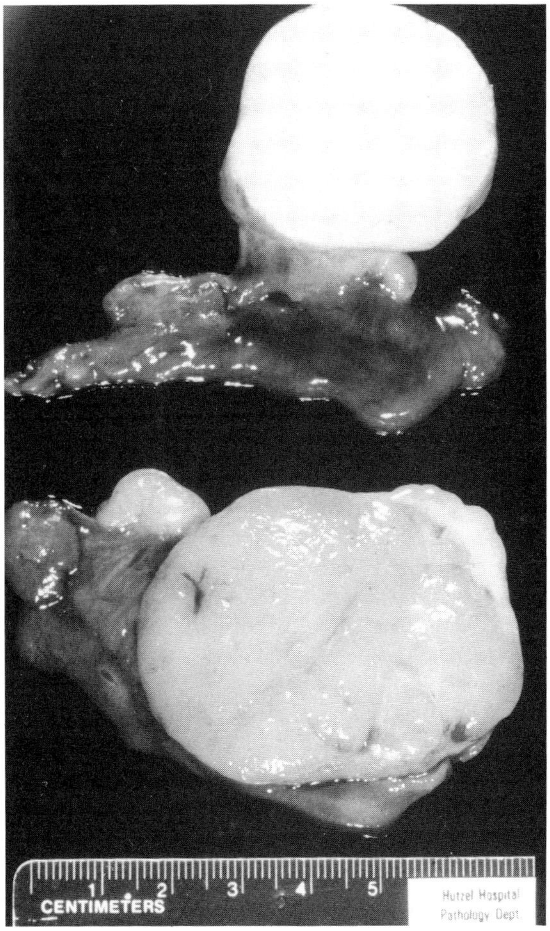

Figure 14.36. Gonadoblastoma and dysgerminoma. The patient had gonadal dysgenesis; the gonadoblastoma (above) was yellow–white, heavy and rock hard, requiring a band saw for sectioning. The dysgerminoma in the contralateral ovary (below) was lobulated, firm, and pink–tan. Both tumors replaced the ovary.

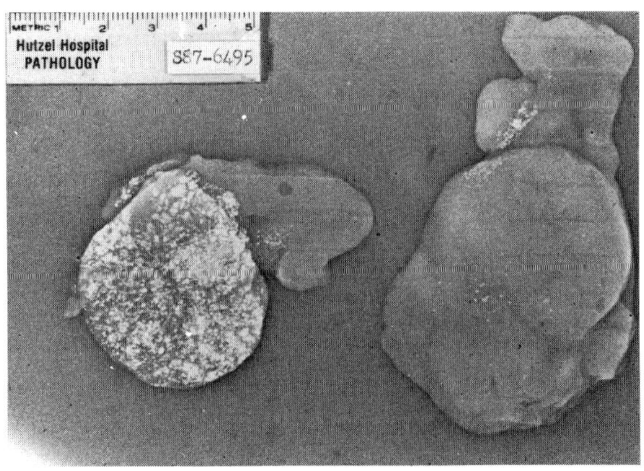

Figure 14.37. Gonadoblastoma and dysgerminoma. Xeroradiogram of the tumors in the previous figure. Note the extensive calcification evident in the gonadoblastoma; this may allow its identification in routine roentgenograms.

other more highly malignant germ cell elements such as yolk sac tumor, embryonal carcinoma or immature teratoma represent the invasive component.

Serologic and Immunohistochemical Markers

The presence of serologic markers determined by radioimmunoassay techniques enables the clinician to predict with a reasonable degree of assurance not only that the patient has a germ cell tumor, but at least some of its histopathologic elements; about two-thirds of germ cell tumors in the ovary can be expected to have an increase in hCG, aFP, or both markers (Kurman and Petrilli, 1983). Serologic markers are helpful, both in the early detection of germ cell tumors (since serologic markers often become elevated before clinically evident signs of disease), as well as in monitoring response to therapy. Lactic dehydrogenase (LDH) is another serum marker that is sometimes elevated in malignant germ cell tumors, and may also be used to follow the clinical status of patients (Schwartz and Morris, 1988). While patients are on therapy, serum levels of CA-125 have been found to parallel the pattern of hCG, aFP, and LDH; indeed, in one small series, elevated levels of CA-125 were found to be helpful not only in the detection of germ cell tumors, but also in their clinical follow-up (Altaras *et al.*, 1986).

More recently, germ cell tumors have been studied using immunohistochemical methods on paraffin-embedded tissue sections; these studies have shown that germinomas characteristically demonstrate focal vimentin positivity, whereas the tumor cells of embryonal carcinoma, choriocarcinoma and yolk sac tumor more typically show variable cytokeratin positivity, with vimentin staining only in the supporting stroma (Miettenen *et al.*, 1985a). Occasional examples of seminoma demonstrate focal keratin positivity (Miettenen *et al.*, 1985b). Choriocarcinoma, in particular, exhibits very strong keratin positivity, whereas keratin stains embryonal carcinoma and yolk sac tumor relatively weakly. Immature teratoma shows a variety of immunohistochemical staining reactions, the positivity depending on the component tissues. As might be expected, the areas with epithelial differentiation stain positively with cytokeratin while neuroglial areas are positive for neurofilaments and glial fibrillary acidic protein.

Metastatic Tumors of the Ovary

The ovaries are commonly the sites of metastatic spread from other primary tumors. Common extragenital sites include the breast and the gastrointestinal tract, particularly the stomach and colon; the most frequently encountered metastatic cancers, however, are those of the contiguous female genital tract. Carcinomas of the cervix very uncommonly metastasize to the ovaries, yet up to one-third or more of endometrial carcinomas have been found to involve the ovaries at autopsy (Scully, 1979). However, as previously noted, up to 25% of endometrial carcinomas have a synchronous ovarian primary of the endometrioid variety, identical in histology to the endometrial carcinoma. Although it may be difficult, if not impossible, to state with certainty whether the ovarian endometrioid carcinoma is primary or secondary, assessment of such should be attempted since the prognosis of the patient may be worse in the latter case. Certainly, if the endometrial carcinoma has already spread to one or both ovaries, there is a greater likelihood of its spread elsewhere. In those cases where the site of origin is controversial, some follow the FIGO criteria and classify the carcinomas as primary or secondary according to the manner of their clinical presentation (i.e. whether the patient presents with uterine bleeding or abdominal symptoms or signs).

Another type of endometrial carcinoma, designated as the uterine serous papillary carcinoma, has an identical histologic appearance to the ovarian carcinoma of the same name (Hendrickson *et al.*, 1982). The endometrial variant tends to invade the myometrium deeply, to show considerable myometrial vascular invasion, and to exhibit transtubal spread, seeding and growing over the peritoneal cavity in a manner similar to ovarian serous carcinoma. In some cases, the ovarian involvement is minimal and often restricted to the blood vessels of the hilum, factors that favor a metastasis from the endometrium.

Given the prevalence of breast carcinoma, the patient with either a single or with bilateral pelvic masses should be questioned carefully about a history of previous breast cancer in herself or relatives, and a breast examination should be performed to exclude that possibility. On the other hand, it is unusual for metastatic breast cancer to present as an ovarian tumor with concomitant signs and symptoms. Indeed, up to two-thirds of ovaries involved by metastatic breast cancer have been unremarkable on gross examination (Scully, 1979).

With regard to ovarian metastases from the gastrointestinal tract, the Krukenberg tumor is probably the best known. Most workers use this designation to denote a metastatic mucin-producing signet ring cell adenocarcinoma, usually of gastric origin. Recognition of this entity has assumed greater clinical significance because some investigators feel that this variety of gastric carcinoma has become more prevalent, particularly in young females (Antonioli and Goldman, 1982). The signet ring cells are so-named because their cytoplasm is distended

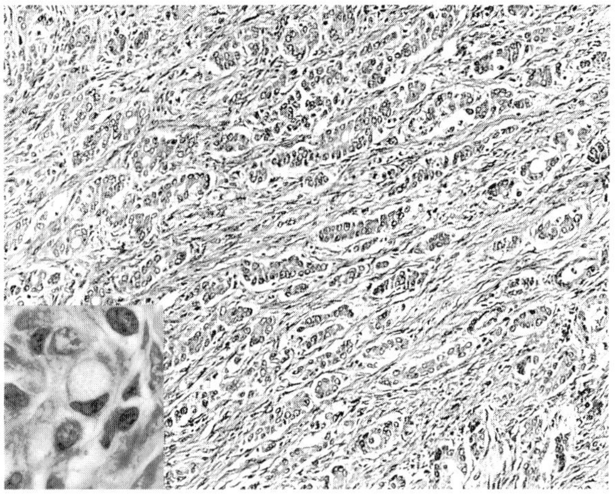

Figure 14.38. Krukenberg tumor – tubular type. Solid and hollow tubular-type configurations reminiscent of those that may be seen in Sertoli–Leydig cell tumors, endometrioid carcinomas or carcinoid tumors are present in a reactive fibrous stroma. Inset: close inspection reveals the presence of signet ring-type cells in which the cytoplasm is distended with mucin, pushing the nucleus to the periphery of the cell.

with mucin, compressing the nucleus to an eccentric position at the periphery of the cell and imparting an appearance similar to a signet ring (see inset *Figure 14.38*).

Additionally, Krukenberg tumors may elicit a prominent response from the ovarian stroma, which may be markedly luteinized and produce hormonal symptoms. In fact, virilization may be the presenting symptom and may raise the clinical question of virilizing Sertoli–Leydig cell tumor. A particular subtype, the so-called tubular Krukenberg tumor, which has been described relatively recently (Bullon *et al.*, 1981), has an even greater propensity for confusion with Sertoli Leydig cell tumors. Sex cord mimicry in the tubular Krukenberg tumor is made even more confusing by the concomitant luteinized stromal cells that may be misconstrued as Leydig cells.

Reactive, hormonally active, luteinized stromal cells are not just associated with gastric neoplasms, however, and metastatic colon carcinoma can produce a similar picture and cause confusion with sex cord–stromal tumors. A Sertoli–Leydig cell tumor, however, would be distinctly unusual in a perimenopausal or postmenopausal female, an age group in which metastatic tumors are more common.

A high index of suspicion is necessary to avoid misdiagnosis of a metastatic tumor as a sex cord–stromal tumor. The occurrence of bilateral tumors should make the diagnosis of Sertoli–Leydig cell tumor doubtful, since unilaterality is the rule for sex cord–stromal tumors. On the other hand, although many metastatic tumors are bilateral, unilateral involvement does occur and sometimes a normal-sized ovary may harbor microscopic metastases. The mucinous nature of metastatic gastrointestinal neoplasms hampers their gross and microscopic distinction from primary mucinous tumors (*Figure 14.39*), especially in light of the fact that primary ovarian mucinous tumors may show gastrointestinal differentiation. However, some features are useful in differentiating primary from metastatic cancer; the latter are commonly associated with significant amounts of necrosis and nuclear debris. As mentioned previously, gross or microscopic bilateral involvement is more frequent with metastatic gastrointestinal neoplasms. The presence within the same mucinous tumor of benign and borderline-appearing areas (the well-known geographic variation in mucinous ovarian neoplasms) is evidence supporting, but not unequivocally confirming, its primary nature. The tubular glands of a gastrointestinal metastasis may likewise be confused with endometrioid carcinoma; however, the aforementioned findings should serve to differentiate them (Young and Scully, 1988).

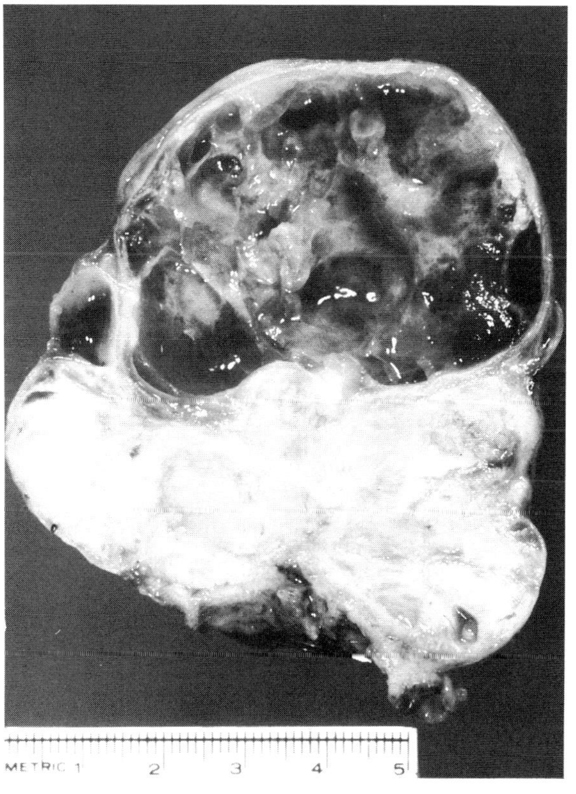

Figure 14.39. Metastatic colon carcinoma of the ovary. Cut section shows that the upper portion of the ovary contains a prominent mucinous component, mimicking a primary ovarian mucinous carcinoma. The lower portion exhibits a markedly firm cut surface, secondary to the reactive desmoplasia induced by the metastatic tumor.

Summary of Core Information

- Ovarian surface epithelial borderline tumors exhibit no destructive invasion and a degree of cytologic atypia and biologic behavior intermediate between overtly benign and malignant tumors.
- So-called 'implants' occur in one-quarter to one-third of serous ovarian borderline tumors and may represent seeding of extraovarian structures, *in situ* 'field effect' serous neoplasia, or both.
- Approximately one-quarter of endometrial adenocarcinomas are accompanied by a synchronous endometrioid carcinoma of the ovary similar to it in histologic appearance and grade.
- The mucinous ovarian tumors associated with pseudomyxoma peritoneii and a concomitant appendiceal mucinous neoplasm are probably metastatic in most cases, usually from the appendiceal tumor.
- The most common ovarian malignancies associated with endometriotic cysts are endometrioid carcinoma and clear cell carcinoma.
- The juvenile granulosa cell tumor most often occurs in younger patients, may have an ominous histologic appearance, and may be misdiagnosed as a more malignant ovarian neoplasm.
- Most Sertoli–Leydig cell tumors occur in younger women and are unilateral and androgenic.
- Dysgerminoma is the most common malignant germ cell tumor and is exquisitely radiosensitive and chemosensitive.
- Yolk sac tumors elaborate alpha-fetoprotein, which can be used to aid preoperative diagnosis and postoperative monitoring of clinical status for recurrence.
- The most common extragenital metastases to the ovary are from the breast and the gastrointestinal tract, particularly the stomach and the colon.

References

Altaros MM, Goldberg GL, Levin W *et al.* (1986) The value of cancer antigen-125 as a tumor marker in malignant germ cell tumors of the ovary. *Gynecol. Oncol.* **25:** 150–159.

Antonioli D & Goldman H (1982) Changes in the location and type of gastric adenocarcinoma. *Cancer* **50:** 775–781.

Arey LB (1961) The origin and formation of the Brenner tumor. *Am. J. Obstet. Gynecol.* **81:** 745–751.

Asadourian LA & Taylor HB (1969) Dysgerminoma. An analysis of 105 cases. *Obstet. Gynecol.* **33:** 370–378.

Aure JC, Hoeg K & Kolstad P (1971) Clinical and histologic studies of ovarian carcinoma. Long-term follow-up of 990 cases. *Obstet. Gynecol.* **37:** 1–9.

Austin RM & Norris HJ (1987) Malignant Brenner tumor and transitional cell carcinoma of the ovary: A comparison. *Int. J. Gynecol. Pathol.* **6:** 29–39.

Ballouk F, Ross JS & Wolf BC (1994) Ovarian endometriotic cysts. An analysis of cytologic atypia and DNA ploidy patterns. *Am. J. Clin. Pathol.* **102:** 415–419.

Bell DA & Scully RE (1985) Atypical and borderline endometrioid adenofibromas of the ovary. A report of 27 cases. *Am. J. Surg. Pathol.* **9:** 205–214.

■ Bell DA & Scully RE (1990) Serous borderline tumors of the peritoneum. *Am. J. Surg. Pathol.* **14:** 230–239.

Bell DA, Weinstock MA & Scully RE (1988) Peritoneal implants of ovarian serous borderline tumors. *Cancer* **62:** 2212–2222.

Bergher de Bacalao E and Dominguez I (1969) Unilateral gonadoblastoma in a pregnant woman. *Am. J. Obstet. Gynecol.* **105:** 1279–1281.

Bostwick DG, Tazelaar HD, Ballon SC *et al.* (1986) Ovarian epithelial tumors of borderline malignancy. A clinicopathologic study of 109 cases. *Cancer* **58:** 2052–2065.

Bullon A Jr, Arseaneau J, Prat J *et al.* (1981) Tubular Krukenberg tumors: a problem in histopathological diagnosis. *Am. J. Surg. Pathol.* **5:** 225–232.

Caruso PA, Marsh MR, Minkowitz S *et al.* (1971) An intense clinicopathologic study of 305 teratomas of the ovary. *Cancer* **27:** 343–348.

Chaitin BA, Gershenson DM & Evans HL (1985) Mucinous tumors of the ovary: a clinicopathologic study of 70 cases. *Cancer* **55:** 1958–1962.

Chalvardjian A & Scully RE (1973) Sclerosing stromal tumors of the ovary. *Cancer* **31:** 664–670.

Cramer SF (1987) Evaluation of reproducibility of the WHO classification of common ovarian cancers: emphasis on methodology. *Arch. Pathol. Lab. Med.* **111:** 819–829.

Deppe G & Lawrence WD (1988) Cancer of the ovary. In: Gusberg SB, Shingleton HM & Deppe G (eds) *Female Genital Cancer*, pp. 379–426. New York: Churchill Livingstone.

Dickersin GR, Kline IW & Scully RE (1982) Small cell carcinoma of the ovary with hypercalcemia. A report of eleven cases. *Cancer* **49:** 188–197.

Dockerty MB (1954) Primary and secondary ovarian adenoacanthoma. *Surg. Gynecol. Obstet.* **99:** 392–400.

Fisher ER, Krieger JD & Skirpan PJ (1955) Ovarian cystoma. Clinicopathologic observations. *Cancer* **8:** 437–445.

Fox H (1985) Sex cord–stromal tumors of the ovary. *J. Pathol.* **145:** 127–148.

Friedman NB (1951) The comparative morphogenesis of extragenital and gonadal teratoid tumors. *Cancer* **4:** 265–276.

Genadry R, Poliakoff S, Rotmensch J *et al.* (1981) Primary papillary peritoneal neoplasia. *Obstet. Gynecol.* **58:** 730–734.

Gershenson DM, Del Junco G, Copeland LJ *et al.* (1984) Mixed germ cell tumors of the ovary. *Obstet. Gynecol.* **64:** 200–206.

Gilks CB, Bell DA & Scully RE (1990) Serous psammocarcinoma of the ovary and peritoneum. *Int. J. Gynecol. Pathol.* **9:** 110–121.

Gooneratne S, Sassone M, Blaustein A *et al.* (1982) Serous surface papillary carcinoma of the ovary: a clinico-pathologic study of 16 cases. *Int. J. Gynecol. Pathol.* **1:** 258–269.

Govan DT, Anderson MC, Beilby JOW *et al.* (1983) Ovarian epithelial tumors of borderline malignancy: pathologic features and current status. The ovarian tumor panel of the Royal College of Obstetrics and Gynaecology. *Br. J. Obstet. Gynaecol.* **90:** 743–750.

Harlow BL, Fuhr JE, McDonald TW *et al.* (1993) Flow cytometry as a prognostic indicator in women with borderline epithelial ovarian tumors. *Gynecol. Oncol.* **50:** 305–309.

■ Hart WR & Norris HJ (1973) Borderline and malignant mucinous tumors of the ovary. Histologic criteria and clinical behaviour. *Cancer* **31:** 1031–1045.

Hawkins EP, Finegold MJ, Hawkins HJ *et al.* (1986) Nondysgerminomatous germ cell tumors in children; review of 89 cases from pediatric oncology group, 1971–1984. *Cancer* **58:** 2579–2584.

Hendrickson M, Ross J, Eifel P *et al.* (1982) Uterine papillary serous carcinoma. A highly malignant form of endometrial adenocarcinoma. *Am. J. Surg. Pathol.* **6:** 93–108.

Higa E, Rosai J, Pizzimbono RA *et al.* (1973) Mucosal hyperplasia, mucinous cystadenoma, and mucinous cystadenocarcinoma of the appendix. *Cancer* **32:** 1525–1541.

Kliman L, Rome RM & Fortune DW (1986) Low malignant potential tumors of the ovary: a study of 76 cases. *Obstet. Gynecol.* **68:** 338–344.

Kuhn W, Kaufmann M, Feichter GE *et al.* (1989) DNA flow cytometry, clinical and morphologic parameters as prognostic factors for advanced malignant and borderline ovarian tumors. *Gynecol. Oncol.* **33:** 360–367.

Kurman RJ & Norris HJ (1976) Endodermal sinus tumor of the ovary: a clinical and pathologic analysis of 71 cases. *Cancer* **38:** 2404–2419.

Kurman RJ & Norris HJ (1976) Embryonal carcinoma of the ovary: a clinicopathologic entity distinct from endodermal sinus tumor resembling embryonal carcinoma of the adult testis. *Cancer* **38:** 2420–2433.

Kurman RJ & Norris HJ (1976) Malignant mixed germ cell tumors of the ovary. A clinical and pathologic analysis of 30 cases. *Obstet. Gynecol.* **48:** 579–589.

Kurman RJ & Petrilli ES (1983) Germ cell tumors of the ovary: Pathology, biology, behavior and treatment. In: Griffiths CT & Fuller AF (eds) *Gynecologic Oncology*, pp. 103–153. Boston: Martinus Nijhoff.

Kurman RJ, Scardino PT, McIntire KR *et al.* (1979) Malignant germ cell tumors of the ovary and testis. An immunohistologic study of 69 cases. *Ann. Clin. Lab. Sci.* **9:** 462–466.

Kurman RJ & Trimble CL (1993) The behavior of serous tumors of low malignant potential: are they ever malignant? *Int. J. Gynecol. Pathol.* **12:** 120–127.

Lawrence WD (1995) The borderland between benign and malignant surface epithelial ovarian tumors: current controversy over the nature and nomenclature of "borderline" ovarian tumors. *Cancer*. **76(10):** 2138–2142

Lele SB, Piver MS, Matharu J *et al.* (1988) Peritoneal papillary carcinoma. *Gynecol. Oncol.* **31:** 315–320.

Lim-Tan S, Cajigas HE & Scully RE (1988) Ovarian cystectomy for serous borderline tumors: a follow-up study of 35 cases. *Obstet. Gynecol.* **72:** 775–781.

McCaughey WTE (1985) Papillary peritoneal neoplasia in females. *Pathol. Ann.* **20:** 387–404.

Micha JP, Kucera PR, Berman ML *et al.* (1985) Malignant ovarian germ cell tumors: a review of 36 cases. *Am. J. Obstet. Gynecol.* **152:** 842–846.

Michael H & Roth LM (1986) Invasive and noninvasive implants in ovarian serous tumors of low malignant potential. *Cancer* **57:** 1240–1247.

Miettinen M, Wahlstrom T, Virtanen I *et al.* (1985a) Cellular differentiation in ovarian sex cord–stromal and germ cell tumors studied with antibodies to intermediate filament proteins. *Am. J. Surg. Pathol.* **9:** 640–651.

Miettinen M, Virtanen I & Talerman A (1985b) Intermediate filament proteins in human testis and testicular germ cell tumors. *Am. J. Pathol.* **120:** 402–410.

Miles PA & Norris HJ (1972) Proliferative and malignant Brenner tumors of the ovary. *Cancer* **30:** 174–186.

Mills SE, Andersen WA, Fechner RE *et al.* (1988) Serous surface papillary carcinoma. A study of 10 cases and comparison with stage III–IV ovarian serous carcinoma. *Am. J. Surg. Pathol.* **12:** 827–834.

Mostoufizadeh M & Scully RE (1980) Malignant tumors arising in endometriosis. *Clin. Obstet. Gynecol.* **23:** 951–963.

Mueller CW, Topkins P & Lapp WA (1950) Dysgerminoma of the ovary – an analysis of 427 cases. *Am. J. Obstet. Gynecol.* **60:** 153–159.

Norris HJ & Jensen RD (1972) Relative frequency of ovarian neoplasms in children and adolescents. *Cancer* **30:** 713–719.

Norris HJ, Zirkin HJ & Benson WL (1976) Immature (malignant) teratoma of the ovary. A clinical and pathologic study of 58 cases. *Cancer* **37:** 2359–2372.

Prat J & Scully RE (1981) Cellular fibromas and fibrosarcomas of the ovary: A comparative clinico-pathologic analysis of seventeen cases. *Cancer*. **47:** 2663–2670.

■ Prayson RA, Hart WR & Petras RE (1994) Pseudomyxoma peritonei: a clinicopathologic study of 19 cases with emphasis on site of origin and nature of associated ovarian tumors. *Am. J. Surg. Pathol.* **18:** 591–601.

Raney RB Jr, Sinclair L, Uri A *et al.* (1987) Malignant ovarian tumors in children and adolescents. *Cancer* **59:** 1214–1220.

Richardson GS (1985) Common epithelial cancer of the ovary. Part I. *New. Engl. J. Med.* **312(7):** 415–424.

Robboy SJ, Norris HJ & Scully RE (1975) Insular carcinoid primary in the ovary. A clinicopathologic analysis of 48 cases. *Cancer* **36:** 404–418.

Robboy SJ, Scully RE & Norris HJ (1977) Primary trabecular carcinoid of the ovary. *Obstet. Gynecol.* **49:** 202–207.

Roth LM, Dallenbach-Hellweg G & Czernobilsky B (1985) Ovarian Brenner tumors. I. Metaplastic, proliferating and of low malignant potential. *Cancer* **56:** 582–591.

Russell P (1979) The pathological assessment of ovarian neoplasms. II. The proliferating "epithelial" tumors. *Pathology* **11:** 251–282.

Russell P (1984) Borderline epithelial tumors of the ovary: a conceptual dilemma. *Clin. Obstet. Gynecol.* **11:** 259–277.

Rutgers JL & Scully RE (1988) Ovarian müllerian mucinous papillary cystadenomas of borderline malignancy. A clinicopathologic analysis. *Cancer* **61:** 340–348.

Santesson L (1947) Clinical and pathological survey of ovarian tumors treated at the Radiumhemmet. I. Dysgerminomas. *Acta Radiol.* **28:** 643–668.

Santesson L & Kottmeier L (1968) General classification of ovarian tumors. In: Gentils F & Junqueiva AC (eds)

Ovarian Cancer, UICC Monograph Series, vol. 11, pp. 1–8. New York: Springer–Verlag.
Schwartz P & Morris JM (1988) Serum lactic dehydrogenase. A tumor marker for dysgerminoma. *Obstet. Gynecol.* **72:** 511–515.
Scully RE (1970) Gonadoblastoma. A review of 74 cases. *Cancer* **25:** 1340–1356.
■ Scully RE (1979) Atlas of Tumor Pathology. Second Series. Fascicle 16. *Tumors of the Ovary and Maldeveloped Gonads.* Washington, DC: Armed Forces Institute of Pathology.
Scully RE & Barlow JF (1967) "Mesonephroma" of ovary. Tumor of müllerian nature related to the endometrioid carcinoma. *Cancer* **20:** 1405–1417.
Serov SF, Scully RE & Sobin LH (1973) International Histological Classification of Tumors, No. 9. *Histologicacal Typing of Ovarian Tumors.* Geneva: World Health Organization.
Sobin L & Scully RE (1987) Histological typing of ovarian tumors. Editorial. *Arch. Pathol. Lab. Med.* **111:** 794–795.
Sobis H & Vandeputte M (1979) Teratoma induction in mice and rats in relation to the age of the visceral yolk sac. *Eur. J. Cancer.* **15:** 143–151.
Stahlsberg H, Susil BJ & Looi LM (1988) Observer variation in histological classification of malignant and borderline ovarian tumors. *Human Pathol.* **19:** 1030–1035.
Stevens LC (1967) The biology of teratomas. *Adv. Morphog.* **6:** 1–31.
Sumithran E, Susil BJ & Looi LM (1988) The prognostic significance of grade in borderline mucinous tumors of the ovary. *Human. Pathol.* **19:** 15–18.
Talerman A (1994) Germ cell tumors of the ovary. In: Kurman RJ (ed) *Blaustein's Pathology of the Female Genital Tract*, pp. 659–721. New York: Springer–Verlag.
Teilum G (1959) Endodermal sinus tumors of the ovary and testis. Comparative morphogenesis of the so-called mesonephroma ovarii (Schiller) and extra-embryonic (yolk sac–allantoic) structures of the rat's placenta. *Cancer* **12:** 1092–1105.
Teilum G (1965) Classification of endodermal sinus tumor (mesoblastoma vitellinum) and so-called "embryonal carcinoma" of the ovary. *Acta Pathol. Microbiol. Scand.* **64:** 407–429.
Witschi E (1948) Migration of the germ cells of human embryos from the yolk sac to the primitive gonadal folds. *Contrib. Embryol.* **32:** 67–80.
Young RH, Gilks CB & Scully RE (1991) Mucinous tumors of the appendix associated with mucinous tumors of the ovary and pseudomyxoma peritonei. A clinicopathological analysis of 22 cases supporting an origin in the appendix. *Am. J. Surg. Pathol.* **15:** 415–429.
Young RH & Scully RE (1984) Fibromatosis and massive edema of the ovary, possibly related entities: A report of 14 cases of fibromatosis and 11 cases of massive edema. *Int. J. Gynecol. Pathol.* **3:** 153–178.
Young RH & Scully RE (1985) Ovarian Sertoli–Leydig cell tumors: a clinicopathologic analysis of 207 cases. *Am. J. Surg. Pathol.* **9:** 543–569.
■ Young RH & Scully RE (1988) Ovarian sex cord–stromal tumors: problems in differential diagnosis. *Pathol. Annu. (part I)* **23:** 237–296.
Young RH, Dickersin GR & Scully RE (1984) Juvenile granulosa of cell tumor of the ovary. A clinicopathologic analysis of 125 cases. *Am. J. Surg. Pathol.* **8:** 575–596.
Zaino RJ, Unger ER & Whitney C (1984) Synchronous carcinomas of the uterine corpus and ovary. *Gynecol. Oncol.* **19:** 329–335.
Zhang J, Young RH, Arseneau J & Scully RE (1982) Ovarian stromal tumors containing lutein or Leydig cells (luteinized thecomas and stromal Leydig cell tumors). A clinicopathological analysis of fifty cases. *Int. J. Gynecol. Pathol.* **1:** 270–285.

15 Management of Epithelial Ovarian Cancer

R A F Crawford
J H Shepherd

Presentation

Ovarian cancer is the second most common gynecological malignancy after breast cancer and 1–2% of all women will develop it in their lifetime. Overall, ovarian cancer is the fifth commonest cancer occurring in women in the UK with nearly 6000 new cases a year (Austoker, 1994). In the USA, it was estimated that there would be 21,000 new cases of ovarian cancer in 1992 with 13,000 deaths (Boring *et al.*, 1992). Due to the position of the ovaries deep in the pelvis, the lack of specific symptoms and the insidious nature of the disease, the majority of these women (70%) present in an advanced stage with an overall prognosis of less than 30% five-year survival. Due to the late presentation there is a high mortality rate and ovarian cancer accounts for over half the deaths from gynecologic malignancy. In this chapter, the presentation and diagnosis of epithelial ovarian cancer (EOC) will be discussed followed by details relating to staging and the necessary surgery. The staging procedure as determined by the International Federation of Obstetrics and Gynecology (FIGO) will be discussed in relation to early stage disease. The use of advanced laparoscopic surgery in the management of women with benign and malignant ovarian disease will be reviewed. Primary, interval and secondary surgery will be defined and their specific value will be determined in advanced disease. The role of surgery in the palliative care of women with terminal ovarian cancer will be evaluated.

EOC increases in incidence with the woman's age and accounts for less than 30% of ovarian cancers in the teenage group and more than 80% in the postmenopausal age group (DiSaia and Creasman, 1993). Approximately 10% of women presenting with ovarian cancer are aged less than 40 years and 75% over the age of 50 years (Averette *et al.*, 1993). Gwinn *et al.* (1990) estimated a relative risk of EOC to be 0.6 (95% Cl 0.5–0.8) for women who had ever been pregnant. Despite the protective effect of pregnancy, the majority of patients (92%) in the American survey are multiparous (Averette *et al.*, 1993). The frequency of a second different malignancy in women with ovarian cancer is 14%.

There are few symptoms in early stage disease. In advanced cases, the woman often has only vague nonspecific complaints. The most common symptoms are related to extension of the disease outside the pelvis. Abdominal pain (53%) and swelling (46%) are the most frequent presenting symptoms (Averette *et al.*, 1993) with bloating (22%), pelvic pressure (18%), constipation (17%) and vaginal bleeding (13%) also recorded. In a series of 533 women with ovarian cancer registered in Scotland in 1987, only 48.2% of patients with ovarian cancer saw a gynecologist as their first contact with the hospital (Junor *et al.*, 1994) and the majority were seen by other specialists including general surgeons (34.9%) and physicians (13.6%). In this series, 33.8% of patients were admitted as an emergency. In view of the usual advanced nature of the disease, 50% of the women present with an abdominopelvic mass or ascites. There can be upper abdominal fullness due to omental involvement, the so-called 'omental cake.' Umbilical, inguinal and femoral herniae are more frequent due to the increased intraabdominal pressure. Occasionally, there is inguinal or axillary lymph node involvement and there may be a mass in the umbilicus—Sister Joseph's nodule. In advanced cases, pleural effusions and skin nodules may be present. Rarely, an ovarian cancer may present with signs of a distant metastasis such as in the brain (Izquierdo *et al.*, 1992). Although rare, ectopic hormone production can lead to Cushing's syndrome (cortisol—Marieb *et al.*, 1983) or Zollinger–Ellison syndrome (gastrin—Julkunen *et al.*, 1983). Paraneoplastic syndromes are associated with ovarian cancer such as humorally-mediated hypercalcemia associated with clear cell cancers (Allan *et al.*, 1984; Nussbaum *et al.*, 1990), cerebellar degeneration associated with Purkinje cell antibodies (Greenlee and Brashear, 1983), seborrheic keratosis (Holguin *et al.*, 1986), and arterial and venous thrombi due to chronic intravascular coagulation. Women with either adnexal masses that raise the suspicion of early stage disease or large abdominopelvic masses indicative of advanced disease should be managed by a suitably trained gynecologist. There is little place for the out-of-hours laparotomy performed by a doctor in training for the woman with advanced disease. In the unusual event of bowel obstruction as the primary presenting event, urgent advice should be sought from a specialized unit and the woman managed accordingly.

The preoperative assessment of the patient with known or suspected ovarian cancer is important. Clinical examination can give some idea of the extent of the peritoneal disease and the presence of ascites. The bidigital examination of the vagina and rectum can assess the involvement of the rectovaginal septum and Pouch of Douglas. At this examination, a cervical smear establishes that the cervix is normal, which is especially important if at surgery the cervix is left *in situ*. The cytologist should be warned that ovarian cancer is suspected because the smear may show adenocarcinoma cells of ovarian origin. Serum should be taken for tumor marker estimation. In a woman under 40 years of age, it is vital that alpha fetoprotein (AFP) and human β-chorionic gonadotrophin (HCG) are sent in addition to CA-125. If these specific markers for germ cell tumors are raised, the management is best transfered to a specialist center because these women can be cured even when they have advanced disease. If there is doubt as to the origin of the tumor other markers such as carcinoembryonic antigen, CA-19.9 and CA-15.3 can be helpful.

Various imaging modalities are used in the preoperative evaluation of women with ovarian cancer. The diagnosis is usually suspected when a pelvic ultrasound scan shows large multiloculated cysts with solid components. The ultrasound parameters that can be used to discriminate between benign and malignant lesions are the size, the number of loculi and thickness of their septations, the presence of inward papillary excresences, the overall echo density (how solid it appears) and the pulsatility index (using Doppler flow ultrasound). The transvaginal ultrasound brings the transducer closer to the pelvic organs allowing the use of higher frequency ultrasound, which gives greater resolution and is the preferred option in pelvic scanning (Steege, 1994). Obviously, in advanced disease, the trans-abdominal transducer can assess the liver and the retroperitoneum for metastatic involvement.

A chest radiograph, which is noninvasive and universally available, will detect Stage IV disease due to chest involvement. This use of chest radiography is in addition to the need from the anesthetic point of view. The presence of a malignant pleural effusion (confirmed cytologically) would alter our management because in our present protocols we would offer primary chemotherapy or only limited surgery.

A computerized tomographic (CT) scan is occasionally helpful as a preoperative investigation in advanced disease when there is doubt about the origin of the cancer. The preoperative CT and ultrasound scan do not correlate well with the operative findings regarding the size of tumor. The size of the intraabdominal mass measured at surgery was correctly predicted in 54% of cases by CT scan and 43% of cases by ultrasound scan (Guidozzi and Sonnendecker, 1991). The ultrasound scan of the liver is more sensitive than an isotope liver scan for detecting intraparenchymal metastases. We obtain a limited intravenous pyelogram (IVP) before surgery. This outlines the ureters in the pelvis, which can aid retroperitoneal dissection in the presence of a large pelvic mass and also excludes ureteric abnormalities. If the kidneys are not visualized on ultrasound scan or there is abnormal renal function, then an IVP is also justified. The routine use of a barium enema is not indicated because it does not predict in which cases bowel resection is required and there is often difficulty removing the residual contrast before surgery. The necessary preoperative investigations should be performed as an outpatient, sparing the patient a long and uncomfortable preoperative hospital stay.

All patients with advanced disease have a thorough bowel preparation (two sachets of sodium picosulphate with clear fluids over the two days before surgery) and are given antibiotic and thromboembolic prophylaxis covering the surgery. Four units of blood are available for the operation. In advanced disease, the surgery may take three or more hours and this should be taken into account when planning the operating list. In the infrequent situation when early stage disease is suspected, the woman should be counseled about the staging procedure. If she is young and wishes to preserve her fertility, then a limited procedure of unilateral salpingo–oophorectomy, staging and endometrial sampling can be considered. This will include some assessment of the contralateral ovary. In the older woman, consent should be obtained for a bilateral salpingo–oophorectomy, staging and probable hysterectomy. In advanced disease, the consent obtained should also include the possibility of a bowel resection and stoma formation.

The Lloyd–Davies position is used because this facilitates bowel resection if required. Mechanical foot and calf stimulation reduce the likelihood of venous thrombosis and are used throughout the operation and in the recovery room. Central venous pressure and arterial monitoring are often used. As a result of the bowel preparation, the patient is often slightly dehydrated and this coupled with the removal of large volumes of ascites and tumor can lead to hypotension. This can be avoided by starting an intravenous infusion before surgery. The length of the operation, the size of the wound and the exposure of the abdominal contents leads to considerable hypothermia, which can be circumvented by using patient warming devices. The use of an epidural or patient-controlled analgesic system for postoperative pain relief is of considerable benefit.

Staging

The incision of choice used for the staging and treatment of ovarian cancer is an extended midline.

This gives access to the whole abdomen and pelvis for a thorough laparotomy, which is the most important diagnostic objective. The staging of the woman with ovarian cancer is important because it will determine her prognosis and decide what treatment schedule she will receive. In the majority of patients, the stage will be obvious from the advanced nature of the disease. In early stage disease, surgery on its own can be curative and, therefore, this group of women who require no further treatment should be confidently defined.

The FIGO staging system (Crawford and Shepherd, 1994) reflects the pattern of spread of EOC (*Table 47.4*). EOC is thought to originate from the ovarian surface epithelium in inclusion cysts. Once invasion of the ovarian capsule has occurred, metastases spread: by direct extension and invasion of adjacent organs; by exfoliation of cells into the peritoneal fluid; via the lymphatics and bloodstream. The malignant cells in the peritoneal fluid circulate around the abdomen following colonic peristalsis in a clockwise fashion up the right paracolic gutter over the liver and down the left side of the abdomen. It is therefore apparent that all peritoneal surfaces are at risk of implantation. Spread via the lymphatic drainage of the ovarian primary along its vascular pedicle reaches the paraaortic and precaval region at the level of the renal vessels. Pelvic lymph drainage spreads to the external, internal iliac and obturator lymph nodes. Implants in the diaphragm may give rise to further metastases directly and via lymphatics into the pleural space. Rarely, lymphatic metastases may drain into the inguinal nodes via the round ligament. It is rare to have bloodborne spread in ovarian cancer until late in the disease when there is a large tumor volume. This demonstrates the contrast between the hostile environment of the serum and the relatively favorable milieu of the peritoneal fluid.

Staging of the woman with ovarian cancer starts with a careful laparotomy and documentation of the findings (*Table 15.1*). In advanced disease, care should be taken on opening the abdomen because there may be bowel adherent to the anterior abdominal wall. Ascites should be sent for cytologic assessment. In the absence of free fluid, a peritoneal lavage with 300 mls warm saline should be performed. Scrapings from the inferior surface of the diaphragm using a brush or spatula give a better cytologic yield than lavage alone (Luesley *et al.*, 1990). It should be noted that Stage IIIC is determined by the initial size of the abdominal implant. Stage IV relies on cytologic or histologic proof of the extraabdominal extension or the intraparenchymal hepatic involvement. There is interest in using laparoscopic techniques to complete the staging in early cancer (Querleu and LeBlanc, 1994), but it is too early to comment whether this technique is valid. After entering the abdomen through an appropriate incision and a suitable specimen has been taken for cytology, a bilateral salpingo–oophorectomy and total abdominal hysterectomy are performed. An infracolic omentectomy is performed and the tumor bulk is removed. In early stage disease, multiple peritoneal biopsies are performed, which include any nodularity or adhesions. A bilateral selective pelvic and paraaortic lymphadenectomy is also performed.

In early ovarian cancer, the staging is often suboptimal because the malignancy was not suspected. The significance of the accuracy of staging in Stage I disease can be seen in the improved survival seen over the last three decades by Venesmaa (1994) where there has been more accurate staging leading to less use of chemotherapy in true early stage disease. *Table 15.2* shows five-year survival rates per stage. Less than 25% of women with presumed early disease had an adequate staging because they did

Table 15.1. Staging procedure for ovarian cancer.

Appropriate surgeon
Gynecologic oncologist or suitably trained surgeon with knowledge of the natural history of ovarian cancer
Appropriate incision
Extended midline allowing access to upper abdomen and diaphragm
Cytology
Ascites, washings from paracolic gutters and pelvis with warmed saline
Diaphragmatic scrapes
Careful laparotomy with clear documentation
Biopsies from adhesions and any suspicious areas
Random biopsies from peritoneum on pelvic side wall, paracolic gutters and bowel
Bilateral salpingo–oophorectomy
Total abdominal hysterectomy
When conservative surgery is being performed see *Table 15.3*
When unable to remove the uterus, perform an endometrial sample (dilatation and curettage)
Bilateral selective pelvic and paraaortic lymphadenectomy

not have a suitable incision allowing acceptable visualization of the upper abdomen and diaphragm (Young *et al.*, 1983; Soper *et al.*, 1992). In early stage disease, ascites is not malignant in approximately half the women. In those cases without clinical ascites, about 20% have malignant cells in the peritoneal washings, hence the need to perform these washings. The infundibulopelvic ligament and broad ligament should be widely resected to ensure complete clearance of the tumour. If the preservation of fertility is required then a unilateral salpingo–oophorectomy is suitable when the disease is confined to one ovary and is well or moderately differentiated (*Table 15.3*).

The multiple random biopsies required by the staging procedure will detect occult or microscopic metastases in up to 10% of cases (Soper *et al.*, 1992). The macroscopic assessment of the omentum has poor sensitivity for the detection of small metastases (Buschbaum *et al.*, 1989). In early disease, we take only several portions of the omentum for evaluation rather than the whole infracolic omentum because it has a physiologic role other than as a site for metastases in this disease. In the presence of no gross extrapelvic disease, a selective pelvic and paraaortic lymphadenectomy should be performed. In apparent Stage I and II, 29% of patients will be upstaged to Stage IIIC by positive paraaortic lymph node biopsies (Young *et al.*, 1983). In the pelvis, the lymphatic tissue from the anterior and medial aspects of the external and internal iliac vessels and the obturator fossa is removed. The lymphatic chain anterior and lateral to the common iliac vessels, aorta and vena cava is removed up to the level of the renal arteries.

Table 15.2. Five-year survival rate of ovarian cancer per stage (from Venesmaa, 1994).

Stage	*Five-year survival (%)*
All stages	35–42
Stage I	70–100
Stage II	55–63
Stage III	10–27
Stage IV	3–15

Palpation of the nodal area is not sufficiently accurate for appropriate staging.

If at operation for benign indications, the adnexal mass appears to be malignant, it is important to confirm this histologically. This confirmation can be done by frozen section, though, occasionally a borderline tumour will be missed on this rapid processing. It is easier to complete the intended conservative operation, review the histology with the pathologist, and discuss the further management with the patient and also a specialist centre rather than perform radical surgery without consent. If the incision is inadequate, the surgeon has to decide whether to assess the abdomen correctly by performing a separate midline incision or extending the transverse incision laterally. It may be appropriate to decide on the management and future treatment including surgery based on limited staging and histology. The morbidity of a second laparotomy for staging is not inconsiderable (63%—Soper *et al.*, 1992) and a decision to reoperate may be taken if it appears that no adjuvant chemotherapy is required (i.e. to confirm early stage tumors).

Early Disease and Staging

The role of appropriate staging in early disease is still quite contentious. Less than 25% of cases will present with tumor confined to the pelvis. The Gynecologic Oncology Group/Ovarian Cancer Study Group in the USA have arbitrarily defined low-risk patients as having Stage IA/B, with well or moderate differentiation, and high-risk patients as having poorly-differentiated lesions, Stage IC and Stage II (Young *et al.*,1990). In the low-risk group of these women, surgery on its own can be curative and avoid any long-term effects of the chemotherapy, and in some of these patients, conservative surgery may be applicable (*Table 15.3*). Sevelda *et al.* (1990) reported a poorer prognosis for patients treated with unilateral salpingo–oophorectomy alone compared to patients who had a hysterectomy and bilateral salpingo–oophorectomy and this they attributed to less than adequate staging, although none of their patients underwent lymphadenectomy. Finn *et al.* (1992) commented in a series of 357 women with early stage EOC that only 30% had an appropriate

Table 15.3. Guidelines for conservative surgery of epithelial ovarian cancer.

- The patient must be of reproductive age and wishing to have further children
- The surgery must include a complete surgical staging. The abnormal adnexa is removed with a wide clearance of both the infundibulopelvic and broad ligaments. The contralateral ovary must be normal both in size and appearance. Biopsy may be indicated, but this may interfere with fertility due to adhesions.
- The FIGO stage should be Stage IA with well- or moderately-differentiated serious histology.
- Close follow-up is available with serum tumor marker estimation and pelvic ultrasound, preferably by the transvaginal route.
- When childbearing is completed, the contralateral ovary is removed.

lymphadenectomy in addition to other aspects of staging. This did not significantly improve the prognosis of the women concerned. In addition, they found that peritoneal washings as part of staging was an independent adverse factor. However, in the high-risk early stage group who would all receive adjuvant chemotherapy, it appears that adequate staging as defined by FIGO gives a significant survival advantage (Mayer *et al.*, 1992). The absolute five-year survival was 83% in those patients staged by a gynecological oncologist compared to 59% in those patients operated on by a non-oncological surgeon (either general obstetrician/gynecologist or general surgeon).

Laparoscopic Surgery and Ovarian Cancer

The initial management of a simple ovarian cyst in the premenopausal woman is usually expectant because a significant number are functional. The use of the oral contraceptive pill is useful to suppress ovulation. If it is larger than 10 cm in diameter or persistent then surgical removal is usually advised. Aspiration of these cysts either using ultrasound or at laparoscopy is not advisable because of the poor negative predictive value (i.e. the negative test excluding a malignant lesion) ranging from 58–98% (Nicklin *et al.*, 1994). Also, if the cyst is only aspirated, it will recur in two-thirds of cases regardless of histology. Laparoscopic adnexal surgery has developed considerably and spread widely since it was first described. The techniques for ovarian cystectomy, salpingo–oophorectomy and excision of endometriomas and dermoid cysts have been well described (Reich, 1987; Nezhat *et al.*, 1989; Daniell *et al.*, 1991 a&b; Nezhat *et al.*, 1991; Parker and Berek, 1993). Aware of the possible dangers of removing early ovarian cancers laparoscopically and therefore possibly compromising patient survival, gynecologists have relied heavily on preoperative ultrasound scanning and serum tumor marker estimation to select benign cases (*Table 15.4*). Most gynecologists would perform a laparotomy via a midline incision if there is a suspicion of malignancy. The incidence of malignant cysts occurring in patients where preoperative investigations wrongly suggest that the mass is benign ranges from 0.04–3.7% (Peterson *et al.*, 1990; Dreßler, 1991; Lehmann–Willenbrock *et al.*, 1991; Hulka *et al.*, 1992; Nezhat *et al.*, 1992; Canis *et al.*, 1994). At the Royal Marsden Hospital, London, 4.1% of new referrals with ovarian cancer in 1993/94 had laparoscopy involved in their initial management. If laparoscopy is used for the investigation and management of all adnexal masses in women regardless of the ultrasound and serum tumor marker findings, then the incidence of malignancy rises to 13% (Childers, personal communication). Although it is possible to carry out all the maneuvers required for the FIGO surgical staging of ovarian cancer including the pelvic and paraaortic lymph node dissection laparoscopically (Querleu and LeBlanc, 1994), we do not know if these minimal access techniques are as effective as accepted standard practice. As the long-term outcome for women whose ovarian cancer has been treated using minimal access techniques is not yet known, the use of laparoscopy in cases of ovarian cancer should be carefully audited.

Surgery in Advanced Disease

The majority of women present with advanced disease and the staging procedure is not complicated.

Table 15.4. Guidelines for selecting patients with adnexal masses suitable for laparoscopic surgery (from Crawford *et al.*, 1995).

Guidelines
American College of Obstetricians and Gynecologists (ACOG) guidelines for laparoscopic management of an adnexal mass
On USS* mass diameter <10 cm, cystic with a distinct border, no solid parts, no associated ascites or matted bowel
Normal CA-125 (<35 U/ml)
No family history of ovarian cancer
British Gynecological Cancer Society guidelines
On USS* mass diameter <8 cm, cystic with no solid elements, no multiloculation, not bilateral
Doppler scanning—no increased flow
Preoperative CA-125 should be known; if raised caution should be exercised before proceeding with minimal access surgery
No family history of ovarian cancer
Adnexal masses should be removed completely and if possible without rupture

*USS, ultrasound scan.

It is in these women that primary cytoreductive surgery is advocated. The objective of this surgery is to remove all macroscopic tumor or to reduce the bulk to smaller than a predetermined size or diameter (0.5–2 cm). Interval surgery applies to the situation where primary surgery has either not been attempted or has not been successful in reducing the tumor load to the desired size. The patient is then treated with a limited course of chemotherapy (3–4 courses) and the surgery, with radical intent, is repeated at a planned interval.

Secondary surgery includes a number of operation types. The second-look procedure refers to the surgery in women who have had a complete clinical response to primary surgery and adjuvant chemotherapy. Secondary cytoreduction refers to the clinical situation where there is either persistent disease despite surgery and chemotherapy or there is a recurrence. Palliative surgery is regarded as a surgical intervention when there are no curative therapeutic options remaining. At any time during the management of the woman with ovarian cancer, the surgeon may also need to obtain long-term intravenous or intraperitoneal access to administer chemotherapy or nutrition.

Primary Surgery

Successful removal of the tumor bulk in a woman with advanced ovarian cancer leads to a dramatic improvement in the patient's wellbeing and reduces the adverse effects of the cancer allowing the patient's recovery and ability to cope with adjuvant therapy. More than 25 years ago, it was suggested that women with advanced disease treated with irradiation had an improved survival if their initial tumor volume had been reduced using 'maximal surgical effort' (Munnell, 1968). In 1975, Griffiths reported a survival advantage for those women with Stage II and III disease who had no residual tumor following surgery and treatment with a single alkylating agent compared to those women who had less than 1.5 cm residual disease. Based on this work, the concept of maximal cytoreductive surgery was born. Many retrospective studies have been published that have shown impressive survival advantages for those women whose disease has been either macroscopically completely removed or reduced to a small size (39 months) compared to women whose disease has not been resected or not reduced to this size (17 months, Clarke–Pearson *et al.*, 1994). It is apparent from experience that in some cases the tumor volume at the beginning of surgery is small or that the tumor is easily removed favoring optimal cytoreduction. Complete cytoreduction, when all macroscopic disease is removed at surgery, is easy to document, although infrequently achieved. However, there is no clear consensus on the size and number of the tumor deposits remaining in a woman who has undergone optimal cytoreduction. Definitions of this optimal size to which tumor deposits should be reduced range from 0.5–2 cm (Hoskins and Rubin, 1991). This measurement refers to the largest diameter of the nodule remaining and obviously there is observer error in recording these measurements. As the measurement is a crude indication of the volume of disease remaining, it is apparent that there will be a significant difference in tumor volume between many small nodules, albeit optimally reduced in size, and a single nodule of larger diameter that is not below the arbitrary dimension. No account is taken of the confluent plaques that are often seen in the paracolic gutters and on the subdiaphragmatic surfaces. Unfortunately, no prospective randomized studies examining the role of cytoreduction in advanced ovarian cancer surgery have yet been published.

The surgery required in advanced ovarian cancer can be daunting for the surgeon as well as the patient. Often, the abdominal anatomy is distorted by large tumor plaques and the carcinomatosis has spread into the upper abdomen. The surgical objective is to remove as much of the macroscopic tumor as possible. The infracolic omentectomy often removes a considerable bulk of tumor. The space between the omental cake and the transverse colon is usually preserved allowing safe dissection. Ideally, a bilateral salpingo–oophorectomy and total abdominal hysterectomy are performed. The dissection is facilitated by the natural tendency of the ovarian cancer to remain intraperitoneal with little deep invasion. This allows the surgeon to debulk a 'frozen pelvis' safely by retroperitoneal dissection with a clear view of the major vessels and ureters. A retrograde hysterectomy allows removal of the tumor from the rectosigmoid and pouch of Douglas, avoiding a colonic resection (McCartney and Hudson, 1985). A decision has to be made as to whether further surgical endeavor to remove the remaining tumor is appropriate. Delgado *et al.* (1984) reported that only 17.3% of cases with Stage III disease had complete tumor excision and a further 10.7% had optimal debulking. Using a surgical approach involving bowel resection, twice this number can be optimally debulked (Soper *et al.*, 1991). In a report where the overall optimal cytoreduction was high (67% of cases), it appears that if the initial surgeon is a trained gynecologic oncologist, the proportion of patients undergoing optimal cytoreductive surgery can be increased to over 80% (Eisenkop *et al.*, 1992). The mean operative time, hospital stay, operative blood loss, blood transfusion and ileus were all significantly increased. However, it was not clear in this community-based study whether there was a selection bias for those patients referred for a specialist opinion. The perioperative mortality from the radical procedure in advanced ovarian cancer is 1% (Venesmaa and Ylikorkala, 1992) and the morbidity considerable. The surgical complications may delay the start of the adjuvant chemotherapy, which may be significant. In a review of published series, the surgical objective of optimal debulking was achieved in women with advanced disease in only one-third of cases (Hoskins, 1989).

In a meta-analysis, Hunter *et al.* (1992) reported that cytoreductive surgery had only a small effect on the overall survival of women with advanced ovarian cancer. They acknowledged that other benefits of the surgery such as relief of symptoms and improved quality of life were not addressed. This aspect was addressed by Blythe and Wahl (1982) in a small study comparing women who had undergone radical debulking surgery including bowel resection and stoma formation with those who had either no surgery or a limited procedure. They found that nearly 80% of women undergoing radical surgery 'enjoyed' life compared to 46% of the control group. However, the groups were not randomized before surgery and, therefore, the tumour biology could have been important in determining the surgeon's ability to perform optimal cytoreduction, which led to the improved wellbeing. Krag *et al.* (1989) reviewed a series of patients who had undergone radical debulking surgery as performed by Griffiths and they concluded that the biologic variables such as the histologic grade, the FIGO stage and initial tumor mass were independent prognostic factors and the extent of cytoreduction was not an independent predictor of survival. Potter *et al.* (1991) reported that patients who underwent extensive debulking procedures to achieve optimal cytoreduction including bowel resection and peritoneal stripping did not have an improved survival compared to those who had limited surgery with residual disease. Hoskins *et al.* (1992) reported that the survival in those women presenting with small volume disease was better than those women presenting with large volume disease, even when it was optimally debulked. This suggests that women with smaller volume disease (either earlier in its natural history or less aggressive) survive longer and that cytoreductive surgery cannot alter this. Hoskins *et al.* (1994) reported the results of an amalgamation of two trials addressing chemotherapy in women who had the degree of their surgery recorded. It was apparent that there was a difference in survival on the basis of residual disease. In their conclusion, the authors commented that in some patients the disease had inherent characteristics allowing complete surgical cytoreduction and at the same time affording their hosts longer survival.

To date, it appears that primary surgical cytoreduction in women with advanced disease should be attempted in a specialist center without necessarily recourse to bowel resection, peritoneal stripping or removal of other organs except when bowel obstruction is present or involvement has resulted in significant damage. In the rare situation where complete cytoreduction can be achieved, it may still be appropriate to perform radical surgery.

Interval Surgery

For the majority of women, the tumor cannot be macroscopically cleared at the primary surgery. Following chemotherapy, there is often a remarkable response and a number of investigators have reviewed their experience with interval surgery, where following either incomplete or inadequate primary surgery, a short course of chemotherapy (3–4 cycles) is given and then the woman undergoes radical reoperation. Wils *et al.* (1986) reported that patients who had responded to chemotherapy and then had interval cytoreduction had a survival rate close to those women who had primary surgical debulking followed by chemotherapy. Gershenson *et al.* (1989) reported that those women rendered operable by chemotherapy who then had complete debulking did not do as well as those who had the original complete debulking. Obviously, the questions of tumor biology and chemosensitivity were important. In women who have only had a biopsy at the primary operation, there may be some advantage to completing the primary surgery if there is a response to chemotherapy (Wiltshaw *et al.*, 1985; Ojeda–Gonzalez *et al.*, 1991). This group of patients is better assessed with the interval surgery procedure rather than in studies of secondary surgery. The benefit of this delayed primary surgery may otherwise bias the result from true secondary surgery. Lawton *et al.* (1989) presented a pilot project of interval debulking after chemotherapy cytoreduction where the operability as defined by achieving optimal debulking increased to 75% of cases. Unfortunately, the randomized study based on this initial report (Redman *et al.*, 1994) demonstrated no survival benefit for the women. An European Organization for Research and Treatment of Cancer (EORTC) collaborative study (Van der Berg *et al.*, 1995) has shown definite longer disease-free intervals and survival in those women with suboptimal primary surgery who then underwent interval debulking. The answer for this interesting group of patients remains to be clearly decided.

Secondary Surgery

There are several aspects of secondary surgery and these all need to be considered separately: the second-look operation, whether using laparoscopy or laparotomy, for the woman who has had adequate primary surgery, chemotherapy and appears to have a clinical complete response; the group of women who progress on primary treatment despite surgery and chemotherapy; and finally the group of women who appear to have a recurrence after a disease-free interval having had an initial good response.

Second-look procedure

Following initial surgery and platinum-based chemotherapy, 60–80% of women will have responded to treatment (Clarke–Pearson *et al.*, 1994) and a significant number will be clinically disease free. Traditionally, this group of patients then underwent an operative procedure to confirm the complete response. Rutledge and Burns (1966) adapted the second look procedure used in colorectal cancer to assess the response of women with ovarian cancer who had primary surgery and chemotherapy. This was then modified to include secondary cytoreduction for those women who had not had a complete pathologic response. It is undoubtedly the most sensitive method of determining the patient's status with respect to remaining disease (compared to CT scanning and tumor markers, Clarke–Pearson *et al.*, 1986), but there is no survival benefit for those women undergoing such a procedure (Cohen *et al.*, 1983; Wiltshaw *et al.*, 1985).

The reports on the role of second-look surgery are mixed as to their study design and initial objectives. A number of these reports were not randomized or prospective, included patients with preoperative measurable disease, disease progression on primary treatment or in bowel obstruction (therefore, not having second-look procedures by definition), had a range of entry criteria that changed during the duration of the study, had small numbers for evaluation, had limited primary or secondary surgery, or did not make the clinical management dependent on the results of the second-look surgery. Up to 40% of women with Stage III disease will have a negative second-look procedure (Potter *et al.*, 1992) and between 20–50% of these women will later have recurrence of their ovarian cancer (Podratz and Kinney, 1993). Increased age (over 70 years) appears to be a significant prognostic factor for finding residual tumor in those patients who are suitable for second-look surgery. There appears to be a survival advantage for those women who at the second-look procedure undergo secondary cytoreduction to no residual disease (Berek *et al.*, 1983; Hoskins *et al.*, 1989; Potter et *al.*, 1992), but as with primary cytoreduction, the ability to achieve this cytoreduction may be a result of the tumor biology rather than the chemotherapy or the surgical endeavor. It appears that the conversion of women with residual disease to a surgical complete response did not offer any survival benefit over those who had no cytoreductive surgery (Raju *et al.*, 1982). Even if there is a survival advantage for these women (Berek *et al.*, 1983; Hoskins *et al.*, 1989; Potter *et al.*, 1992), this group comprises some 5% of the total considered. Although there are no randomized studies evaluating the benefit of secondary debulking, Luesley *et al.* (1988) prospectively reviewed the role of secondary surgery following platinum chemotherapy. The only difference between the two arms receiving the second-line chlorambucil therapy was the second-look operation with secondary cytoreduction in one arm. There appeared to be no survival advantage for the group undergoing secondary surgery. Similarly, from the comparison of those women refusing second-look surgery with women who underwent the procedure (Omura *et al.*, 1989) and those women who underwent aggressive secondary cytoreduction (Miller *et al.*, 1992) there was no survival benefit from the surgery. The morbidity of the secondary procedures is probably less than primary radical surgery (Venesmaa and Ylikorkala, 1992), but is still notable at over 15% (Gallup *et al.*, 1987; Carson and Rubin, 1993). Traditionally, laparoscopy has not been favored in the second-look procedure because of the high incidence of adhesions limiting the view and increasing the complication rate. There is a high false negative-rate (up to 50%). With the advances in equipment and expertise, more extensive laparoscopic second-look procedures are possible (Querleu and LeBlanc, 1994), but it seems unlikely that they will alter the role for the second-look procedure. A possible role for the second-look procedure in women who have had a complete pathologic response may be to define a group who would benefit from consolidation therapy. This remains to be examined.

Second-effort debulking in patients with disease progression

The outlook for women who have progressive disease on first-line chemotherapy is poor and they do not respond well to other chemotherapy or surgical intervention. Usually they have been excluded from studies on secondary debulking. An interesting retrospective study (Morris *et al.*, 1989) showed that there was a longer median survival in those women who underwent second-effort debulking and had a residual less than 1 cm remaining than those who had greater residual disease. Also of note was that if the time interval between primary and secondary surgery was less than one year (i.e. progression of the disease through first-line surgery and chemotherapy) the patients had a survival of 7.3 months compared to 18.3 months in those whose surgical interval was greater than a year (i.e. true secondary debulking because the woman had a disease-free interval or had stable disease). This effect has been mirrored in the chemotherapy response as well. Essentially, in the absence of effective curative second-line chemotherapy, the morbidity of this second-effort debulking precludes its use.

Recurrence after a disease-free interval

If there has been a significant clinical remission, then it is important to re-evaluate the woman who has a supposed recurrence. After a significant disease-free interval of 3–4 years, we feel that repeat laparotomy and cytoreduction are important, especially to exclude a second malignancy. A number of studies have considered secondary cytoreduction in these cases, but have predominantly considered women who have relapsed within several years. Morris *et al.* (1989) found that there was no benefit, but Janicke *et al.* (1992) found a statistically significant survival advantage following this secondary cytoreduction. The criticism of these studies is that the group that relapses early is resistant to all types of therapy (surgery, first- and second-line chemotherapy); while the group that relapses later is relatively responsive to therapy (Markman *et al.*, 1991). In our unit, the early relapse group (less than one year from initial diagnosis) would be treated with second-line chemotherapy although the prognosis is poor. The moderate relapse group (1–3 years) would be rechallenged with first-line chemotherapy and a further good response would be expected. The late recurrence group (more than four years) would have a repeat laparotomy to confirm the diagnosis, radical surgery and first-line chemotherapy. It is in this group that there is a role for secondary surgery although it must be accepted that the tumor characteristics in these cases may be different to those of the majority of ovarian cancers.

Palliative Surgery

The nihilist may argue that all the discussion relating to secondary surgery should be included in this paragraph. We feel that women who have progressive disease and are no longer undergoing active treatment require palliative support. The predominant symptom in advanced incurable ovarian cancer is that of bowel obstruction. This obstruction may be in the small bowel, the large bowel, a combination of the two, or even a functional obstruction due to malignant infiltration and contraction of the mesentery. Other symptoms include abdominal distension and pressure, anorexia, nausea, vomiting and shortness of breath. The indication for surgery in these women needs to be carefully assessed in each case because the risks and morbidity of the proposed procedure may be more serious than the condition itself. Careful and sensitive management by a gynecologic oncologist familiar with the natural history of ovarian cancer and who has the capability of providing the full range of medical and surgical options for palliation is important. On the individual patient basis, therapeutic decisions can be made in conjunction with the woman and her family.

The decision to relieve bowel obstruction surgically is based on the clinical features that allow the gynecologic oncologist to determine whether the intervention will be successful and that the woman will recover from her surgery and survive long enough to benefit from the relief of her obstruction. The ability to predict a successful outcome to surgery is difficult. The initial reports suggested surgery was relatively useful. It appears that clinically detectable ascites, low serum albumin, a low lymphocyte count and clinical tumor status (the presence of palpable abdominal masses or distant metastases) are all important poor prognostic features with the serum albumin and tumor status as the most significant (Clarke–Pearson *et al.*, 1988). The tumor load cannot be changed before surgery. The nutritional status, as indicated by the low serum albumin, can be altered using total parenteral nutrition (TPN) and its use in the perioperative period is warranted. A review of home TPN in terminal ovarian cancer (August *et al.*, 1991) advised that there was no useful role for this technique because the patients died very rapidly compared to a group with advanced gastrointestinal malignancy. Due to the psychologic and emotional difficulties in stopping this treatment and also its high cost, we feel that TPN in terminal ovarian cancer is only indicated for the short term to allow a successful operative intervention. Consequently, there is a very limited use in our hospitals. Operative morbidity (up to 64%) and mortality (up to 32%) are significant and should be borne in mind before hasty surgery. The prognosis for women who are unable to have a definitive procedure (up to 24% of cases reported) is awful.

Rubin *et al.* (1989) tried unsuccessfully to determine preoperatively which patients would benefit from surgery. The gynecologic oncologist must be prepared to perform the entire range of surgery for obstruction from resection and re-anastomosis, through bypass to stoma formation or gastrostomy placement. Generally, most advise a bypass procedure over resection and anastomosis because it is quicker, there is less blood loss and less indication for a stoma. The use of a gastrostomy in those women where no surgery is possible avoids the use of a chronic nasogastric tube. We have found that few patients require continuous nasogastric drainage even when they have inoperable obstruction. Somatostatin analogs may reduce upper gastrointestinal secretion, reducing the volume of vomitus to an acceptable quantity and frequency. The use of a percutaneous endoscopically-placed gastrostomy may also be useful (Marks *et al.*, 1993).

In view of the difficulty in predicting which patient will benefit from surgery, the medical management of obstruction is more attractive. The survival following medical management of malignant obstruction is similar or longer than that of women managed surgically. A protocol, such as used at the

Royal Marsden Hospital, allows a simplified unit policy for the management of these women in acute or even subacute obstruction. The patient is hydrated via an intravenous infusion and the colic is relieved with opiate analgesia and antispasmodics. Constipation is relieved with laxatives taken orally and enemas rectally. Nausea and vomiting are actively managed with the range of anti-emetics available. The use of samastatin analogs and useful nasogastric drainage can be helpful. The analgesia and anti-emetic are usually given subcutaneously via a syringe driver. Corticosteroids can be helpful in relieving the obstruction. The team comprising the gynecologic oncologist, the medical oncologist and palliative care physician review the woman on a daily basis. Her symptoms and drug requirements are monitored and recorded on a flow chart. If it appears that surgery will benefit her, then she is scheduled for the most appropriate operation, performed by a suitable surgeon. Using a protocol of this nature, inappropriate surgery can usually be avoided. When the subacute or acute obstruction has resolved, a low residue diet is helpful. The long-term management of recurring subacute obstruction can then often be managed at home with conservative measures.

Summary of Management Options

- Preoperative preparation for surgery includes: consent for radical surgery; mechanical bowel preparation; prophylaxis against venous thrombosis and infection; and cross match for four units of blood.
- The primary operation should include: extended midline incision; cytology of ascites or peritoneal washings; bilateral salpingo–oophorectomy and total abdominal hysterectomy; multiple biopsies or cytoreduction of tumor; selective pelvic and paraaortic lymphadenectomy.
- The ideal surgical procedure is to remove all macroscopic disease without creating excessive morbidity and mortality.
- In the event of an unexpected cancer, perform staging at time of that operation as well as the other procedures outlined above.
- Use guidelines (*Table 15.3*) for laparoscopic surgery to avoid inadvertently encountering ovarian cancer.
- In advanced disease attempt cytoreduction to remove as much tumor as possible. The site and size of any remaining tumor should be carefully documented. Bowel resection is only indicated in cases of bowel obstruction.
- Consider an interval debulking procedure following several courses of chemotherapy.
- There is no survival advantage to second-look surgery following adequate primary surgery and chemotherapy in the presence of a complete clinical remission.
- It may be useful to identify a group of women suitable for consolidation therapy; however, there is no survival advantage to second-effort debulking.
- Palliative surgery can play a role in the management of ovarian cancer.

References

Allan SG, Lockhart SP, Leonard RC & Smyth JF (1984) Paraneoplastic hypercalcaemia in ovarian carcinoma. *Br. Med. J.* **288:** 1714–1715.

August DA, Thorn D, Fisher RL & Welchek CM (1991) Home parenteral nutrition for patients with inoperable malignant bowel obstruction. *J. Parent. Ent. Nut.* **15:** 323–327.

Austoker J (1994) Screening for ovarian, prostatic and testicular cancers. *Br. Med. J.* **309:** 315–320.

Averette HE, Hoskins W, Nguyen HN *et al.* (1993) National survey of ovarian carcinoma. I. A patient care evaluation study of the American College of Surgeons. *Cancer* **71:** 1629–1638.

Berek JS, Hacker NF, Lagasse LD, Nieberg RK & Elashoff RM (1983) Survival of patients following secondary cytoreductive surgery in ovarian cancer. *Obstet. Gynecol.* **61:** 189.

Boring CC, Squires TS & Tong T (1992) Cancer Statistics, 1992. *CA Cancer J. Clin.* **42:** 19–38.

Blythe JG & Wahl TP (1982) Debulking surgery: Does it increase the quality of survival? *Gynecol. Oncol.* **14:** 396–408.

Buschbaum HJ, Brady MF, Delgado G, Miller A, Hoskins WJ & Manetta A (1989) Surgical staging of carcinoma of the ovaries. *Surg. Gynecol. Obstet.* **169:** 226–232.

Canis M, Mage G, Pouly JL, Wattiez A, Manhes H & Bruhat MA (1994) Laparoscopic diagnosis of adnexal cystic masses: a 12-year experience with long term follow-up. *Obstet. Gynecol.* **83:** 707–712.

Carson LF & Rubin SC (1993) Secondary cytoreduction—Thoughts on the 'Pro' side. *Gynecol. Oncol.* **51:** 127–130.

Clarke–Pearson DL, Bandy L, Dudzinski M, Heaston D & Creasman WT (1986) Computed tomography in evaluation of patients with ovarian carcinoma in complete clinical remission: Correlation with surgical pathologic findings. *JAMA* **255:** 627–630.

Clarke–Pearson DL, DeLong ER, Chin NO, Rice R & Creasman WT (1988) Intestinal obstruction in patients with ovarian cancer: Variables associated with surgical complications and survival. *Arch. Surg.* **123:** 42–45.

■ Clarke–Pearson DL, Kohler MF, Hurteau JA & Elbendary A (1994) Surgery for advanced ovarian cancer. *Clin. Obstet. Gynecol.* **37:** 439–460.

Cohen CJ, Goldberg JD, Holland JF *et al.* (1983) Improved therapy with cis-platinum regimens for patients with ovarian carcinoma (FIGO stages III and IV) as measured by surgical end-staging (second look operation). *Am. J. Obstet. Gynecol.* **145:** 955–967.

Crawford RAF & Shepherd JH (1994) FIGO staging of gynaecological malignancies. *Contemp. Rev. Obstet. Gynaecol.* **6:** 137–141.

Crawford RAF, Gore ME & Shepherd JH (1995) Ovarian cancers related to minimal access surgery. *Br. J. Obstet. Gynaecol.* **102:** 726–730.

Daniell JF, Kurtz BR & Gurley LD (1991a) Laser laparoscopic removal of large endometriomas. *Fertil. Steril.* **55:** 692–695.

Daniell JF, Kurtz BR & Lee Ji–Yun (1991b) Laparoscopic oophorectomy: Comparative study of ligatures, bipolar coagulation and automatic stapling. *Obstet. Gynecol.* **80:** 325–328.

Delgado G, Oram DH & Petrilli ES (1984) Stage III epithelial ovarian cancer: the role of maximal surgical reduction. *Gynecol. Oncol.* **18:** 293–298.

DiSaia PJ & Creasman WT (1993) Chapter Epithelial Ovarian Cancer. *Clinical Gynecologic Oncology*, p. 336. St Louis: Mosby.

Dreßler F (1991) Zur endoskopischen Therapie von zystischen Ovarialtumouren und Paraovarialzysten. *Geburtsh. u. Frauenheilk.* **51:** 474–480.

Eisenkop SM, Spirtos NM, Montag TW, Nalick RH & Wang H–J (1992) The impact of subspeciality training on the management of advanced ovarian cancer. *Gynecol. Oncol.* **47:** 203–209.

Finn CB, Luesley DM, Buxton EJ *et al.* (1992) Is stage I epithelial ovarian cancer overtreated both surgically and systemically? results of a five year cancer registry review. *Br. J. Obstet. Gynaecol.* **99:** 54–58.

Gallup DG, Talledo OE, Dudzinski MR & Brown KW (1987) Another look at the second assessment procedure for ovarian epithelial carcinoma. *Am. J. Obstet. Gynecol.* **157:** 590–596.

Gershenson DM, Wharton JT & Copeland L (1989) Treatment of advanced epithelial ovarian cancer with cisplatin and cisplatin and cyclophosphamide. *Gynecol. Oncol.* **32:** 336–341.

Greenlee JE & Brashear HR (1983) Antibodies to cerebellar Purkinje cells in patients with paraneoplastic cerebellar degeneration and ovarian carcinoma. *Ann. Neurol.* **14:** 609–613.

Griffiths CT (1975) Surgical resection of tumour bulk in the primary treatment of ovarian cancer. *Monogr. Natl Cancer Inst.* **42:** 101–104.

Guidozzi F & Sonnendecker EWW (1991) Evaluation of preoperative investigations in patients admitted for ovarian primary cytoreductive surgery. *Gynecol. Oncol.* **40:** 244–247.

Gwinn ML, Lee NC, Rhodes PH, Layde PM & Rubin GL (1990) Pregnancy, breast feeding and oral contraceptives and the risk of ovarian cancer. *J. Clin. Epidemiol.* **43:** 559.

Holguin T, Padilla RS & Ampuero F (1986) Ovarian adenocarcinoma presenting with the sign of Leser–Trélat. *Gynecol. Oncol.* **25:** 128–132.

Hoskins WJ (1989) The influence of cytoreductive surgery on progression-free interval and survival in epithelial ovarian cancer. *Ballière's Clin. Obstet. Gynaecol.* **3:** 59–71.

Hoskins WJ, Bundy BN, Thigpen JT & Omura GA (1992) The influence of cytoreductive surgery on recurrence-free interval and survival in small-volume stage III epithelial ovarian cancer: A gynecologic oncology group study. *Gynecol. Oncol.* **47:** 159–166.

■ Hoskins WJ, McGuire WP, Brady MF *et al.* (1994) The effect of diameter of largest residual disease on survival after primary cytoreductive surgery in patients with suboptimal residual ovarian carcinoma. *Am. J. Obstet. Gynecol.* **170:** 974–980.

Hoskins WJ & Rubin SC (1991) Surgery in the treatment of patients with advanced ovarian cancer. *Semin. Oncology.* **18:** 213–221.

Hulka JF, Parker WH, Surrey MW & Phillips JM (1992) Management of ovarian masses: AAGL 1990 survey. *J. Reprod. Med.* **37:** 559–602.

Hunter RW, Alexander NDE & Soutter WP (1992) Meta-analysis of surgery in advanced ovarian carcinoma: Is maximum cytoreductive surgery an independent determinant of prognosis? *Am. J. Obstet. Gynecol.* **166:** 504–511.

Izquierdo MA, Ojeda B, Pallares C, Alonso MC & Matias–Guiu X (1992) Ovarian carcinoma preceded by cerebral metastasis: review of the literature. *Gynecol. Oncol.* **45:** 206–210.

Janicke F, Holscher M, Kuhn W *et al.* (1992) Radical surgery procedure improves survival time in patients with recurrent ovarian cancer. *Cancer* **70:** 2129–2136.

Julkunen R, Partanen S & Salaspuro M (1983) Gastrin-producing ovarian mucinous cystadenoma. *J. Clin. Gastroenterol.***5:** 67–70.

■ Junor EJ, Hole DJ & Gillis CR (1994) Management of ovarian cancer: referral to a multidisciplinary team matters. *Br. J. Cancer* **70:** 363–70.

Krag KJ, Canellos GP, Griffiths CT *et al.* (1989) Predictive factors for long-term survival in patients with advanced ovarian cancer. *Gynecol. Oncol.* **34:** 88–93.

Lawton FG, Redman CW, Luesley DM, Chan KK & Blackledge G (1989) Neoadjuvant (cytoreductive) chemotherapy combined with intervention debulking surgery in advanced unresected epithelial ovarian cancer *Obstet. Gynecol.* **73:** 61–65.

Lehmann–Willenbrock E, Mecke H & Semm K (1991) Pelviskopische Ovarialchirurgie—eine retrospektive Untersuchung von 1016 operierten Zysten. *Geburtsh. u. Frauenheilk.* **51:** 280–287.

Luesley DM, Blackledge G, Kelly K *et al.* (1988) Failure of second-look laparotomy to influence survival in epithelial ovarian cancer. *Lancet* **ii:** 599–603.

Luesley DM, Williams DR, Ward K & Lawton FG (1990) Peritoneal smears and lavage fluids in patients with epithelial ovarian cancer and benign gynaecological disease. *Acta Cytol.* **34:** 359–42.

Marieb NJ, Spangler S, Kashgarian M, Heimann A, Schwartz ML & Schwartz PE (1983) Cushing's syndrome secondary to ectopic cortisol production by an ovarian carcinoma. *J. Clin. Metab.* **57:** 737–740.

Markman M, Reichman B, Hakes T *et al.* (1991) Responses to second line cisplatin based intraperitoneal therapy in ovarian cancer: Influence of a prior response to intravenous cisplatin. *J. Clin. Oncol.* **9:** 1801–1805.

Marks WH, Perkal MF & Schwartz PE (1993) Percutaneous endoscopic gastrotomy for decompression in metastatic gynecologic malignancies. *Surgery, Gynecology & Obstetrics* **177:** 573–576.

Mayer AR, Chambers SK, Graves E *et al.* (1992) Ovarian cancer staging: Does it require a gynecologic oncologist? *Gynecol. Oncol.* **47:** 223–227.

McCartney AJ & Hudson CN (1985) Surgical treatment of localized disease: conservative and radical. In: Hudson CN (ed.) *Ovarian Cancer*, pp. 202–208. Oxford: Oxford University Press.

Miller DS, Spirtos NM, Ballon SC, Cox RS, Soriero OM & Teng NNH (1992) Critical reassessment of second-look exploratory laparotomy for epithelial ovarian carcinoma. *Cancer* **69:** 502–510.

Morris M, Gershenson D, Wharten T, Copeland L, Edwards C & Stringer A (1989) Secondary cytoreductive surgery for recurrent epithelial ovarian cancer. *Gynecol. Oncol.* **34:** 334–338.

Munnell EW (1968) The changing prognosis and treatment in cancer of the ovary: A report of 235 patients with primary ovarian cancer 1952–1961. *Am. J. Obstet. Gynecol.* **100:** 790–805.

Nezhat F, Nezhat C & Siefer SL (1991) Videolaseroscopy for oophorectomy. *Am. J. Obstet. Gynecol.* **165:** 1323–1330.

Nezhat F, Nezhat C, Welander CE & Benigno B (1992) Four ovarian cancers diagnosed during laparoscopic management of 1011 women with adnexal masses. *Am. J. Obstet. Gynecol.* **167:** 790–796.

Nezhat C, Winter W & Nezhat F (1989) Laparoscopic removal of dermoid cysts. *Obstet. Gynecol.* **73:** 278–280.

Nicklin JL, Van Eijkeren M, Athanasatos P, Wain GV & Hacker NF (1994) A comparison of ovarian cyst aspirate cytology and histology. The case against aspiration of cystic pelvic masses. *Aust. NZ J. Obstet. Gynaecol.* **34:** 546–549.

Nussbaum SR, Gaz RD & Arnold A (1990) Hypercalcaemia and ectopic secretion of parathyroid hormone by an ovarian carcinoma with rearrangement of the gene for parathyroid hormone. *New Eng. J. Med.* **323:** 1324–1328.

Ojeda-Gonzalez MB, Alvarez-Lopez I, Alonso-Munoz MC *et al.* (1991) Chemotherapy(CAP) for the treatment of advanced ovarian cancer and second-effort surgery in the second-look. *Gynecol. Oncol.* **48:** 7–12.

Omura GA, Bundy BN, Berek JS, Curry S, Delgado G & Mortel R (1989) Randomized trial of cyclophosphamide plus cisplatin with or without doxorubicin in ovarian cancer. A gynecologic oncology group study. *J. Clin. Oncol.* **7:** 457–465.

Parker WH & Berek JS (1993) Management of the adnexal mass by operative laparoscopy. *Clin. Obstet. Gynecol.* **36:** 413–422.

Peterson H, Hulka J & Phillips J (1990) American Association of Gynecologic Laparoscopists 1988 membership survey on operative laparoscopy. *J. Reprod. Med.* **35:** 587–589.

Podratz KC & Kinney WK (1993) Second-look operation in ovarian cancer. *Cancer* **71:** 1551–1558.

Potter ME, Hatch KD, Soong S-J, Partridge EE, Austin JM & Shingleton HM (1992) Second-look laparotomy and salvage therapy: A research modality only? *Gynecol. Oncol.* **44:** 3–9.

■ Potter ME, Partridge EE, Hatch KD, Soong S-J, Austin JM & Shingleton HM (1991) Primary surgical therapy of ovarian cancer: How much and when. *Gynecol. Oncol.* **40:** 195–200.

Querleu D & LeBlanc E (1994) Laparoscopic infrarenal paraaortic lymph node dissection for restaging of carcinoma of the ovary or fallopian tube. *Cancer* **73:** 1467–1471.

Raju KS, McKinna J, Barker GH, Wiltshaw E & Jones J (1982) Second-look operations in the planned management of advanced ovarian carcinoma. *Am. J. Obstet. Gynecol.* **144:** 650–654.

Redman CW, Warwick J, Luesley DM, Varma R, Lawton FG & Blackledge GRP (1994) Intervention debulking surgery in advanced epithelial ovarian cancer. *Br. J. Obstet. Gynaecol.* **101:** 142–146

Reich H (1987) Laparoscopic oophorectomy and salpingo-oophorectomy in the treatment of benign tubo-ovarian disease. *Int. J. Fertil.* **32:** 233.

Rubin SC, Hoskins WJ, Benjamin I, Lewis JL Jr (1989) Palliative surgery for intestinal obstruction in advanced ovarian cancer. *Gynecol. Oncol.* **34(1):** 16–19.

Rutledge F & Burns B (1966) Chemotherapy for advanced ovarian cancer. *Cancer* **96:** 761–770.

Sevelda P, Vavra N, Schemper M & Salzer H (1990) Prognostic factors for survival in stage I epithelial ovarian carcinoma. *Cancer* **65:** 2349–2352.

Soper JT, Couchman G, Berchuck A & Clark-Pearson D (1991) The role of partial sigmoid colectomy for debulking epithelial ovarian carcinoma. *Gynecol. Oncol.* **41:** 239–244.

Soper JT, Johnson P, Johnson V, Berchuck A & Clarke-Pearson DL (1992) Comprehensive restaging laparotomy in women with apparent early ovarian carcinoma. *Obstet. Gynecol.* **80:** 949–953.

Steege JF (1994) Laparoscopic approach to the adnexal mass. *Clin. Obstet. Gynecol.* **37:** 392–405.

Van der Berg MEL, van Lent M, Kobierska A *et al.* (1993) The effect of debulking surgery after induction chemotherapy on the prognosis in advanced ovarian cancer. *New Eng. J. Med.* **332:** 629–634.

■ Venesmaa P (1994) Epithelial ovarian cancer: Impact of surgery and chemotherapy on survival during 1977–1990. *Obstet. Gynecol.* **84:** 8–11.

Venesmaa P & Ylikorkala O (1992) Morbidity and mortality associated with primary and repeat operations for ovarian cancer. *Obstet. Gynecol.* **79:** 168–172.

Wils J, Blijham G, Naus A *et al.* (1986) Primary or delayed debulking surgery and chemotherapy of cisplatin, doxorubicin and cyclophosphamide in stage III–IV epithelial ovarian carcinoma. *J. Clin. Oncol.* **4:** 1068.

Wiltshaw E, Raju KS & Dawson I (1985) The role of cytoreductive surgery in advanced ovarian carcinoma of the ovary: An analysis of primary and second surgery. *Brit. J. Obstet. Gynaecol.* **92:** 522–527.

Young RC, Decker DG, Wharton JT *et al.* (1983) Staging laparotomy in early ovarian cancer. *JAMA* **250:** 3072–3076.

Young RC, Walton LA, Ellenberg SS *et al.* (1990) Adjuvant therapy in stage I and stage II epithelial ovarian cancer: Results of two randomized trials. *New. Eng. J. Med.* **322:** 1021–1027.

16 Epithelial Ovarian Cancer: Chemotherapy and Other Postoperative Therapy

G A Omura

Introduction

Only a minority of women with epithelial ovarian cancer present with early stage disease (Stage I or II), and a number of these recur following surgery. Nearly all of the recurrences are fatal. Because treatment of recurrence is unsatisfactory, high-risk early-stage patients are usually offered adjuvant chemotherapy after surgery. The majority of ovarian cancers present in advanced stages (III or IV) and are routinely treated with systemic chemotherapy; despite an initial 70–80% response rate in this subgroup, current therapy is inadequate, as demonstrated by the 5–20% long-term survivors.

This chapter reviews the primary chemotherapy of epithelial ovarian cancer, and addresses some controversial areas of patient management. The treatment of relapsed and refractory cases is briefly summarized. Unless otherwise noted, it is assumed that appropriate surgery has been completed.

Management of Early-stage Disease

Young *et al.* (1990) reported on two prospective randomized trials in which, following comprehensive surgical staging, patients with Stage I and II disease were divided into favorable and unfavorable prognostic groups. Borderline tumors were excluded. Women with Stage IA and IB carcinomas (Grades 1 and 2), were included in the favorable prognostic category. Eligibility criteria for the protocol studying unfavorable cases included Stage IA and B (Grade 3), IC, and Stage II. The favorable group ($n=81$) was randomized to no postoperative therapy versus oral melphalan (0.2 mg kg^{-1} d^{-1} for five days every 4–6 weeks for one year). The median follow-up was more than six years and there was no significant difference in the two treatment arms with regard to the five-year survival (91% versus 98%) or disease-free survival (94% versus 98%). Because of the similar excellent survival in both groups, it was concluded that postoperative therapy is not indicated for low-grade Stage I disease.

In the protocol for unfavorable cases ($n=141$), patients were randomized to a single intraperitoneal administration of 15 millicuries of colloidal radioactive phosphorus (^{32}P) or oral melphalan in the same dose schedule described above. No significant difference was observed between the two groups, with relapse rates of 19% in both treatment arms (five-year survival 78% and 81% respectively). ^{32}P was recommended as the control arm for a subsequent trial.

Bolis *et al.* (1992) gave an interim report of 83 eligible women with Stage IA and B (Grade 2 and 3) disease who were randomized to cisplatin 50 mg m^{-2} monthly for six courses or observation; disease-free survival favored the cisplatin (7/41 versus 14/42 relapses) ($p<0.028$), but there was no difference in overall survival. Of 176 patients with Stage IC disease randomized to cisplatin or intraperitoneal ^{32}P, disease-free survival was better in the cisplatin arm ($p=0.009$) (16/97 versus 27/79 relapses), but there was no statistically significant difference in overall survival. After recurrence, patients who had been on the observation or ^{32}P arm fared better with 'salvage' chemotherapy than those who had initially had cisplatin, presumably accounting for the lack of an overall difference.

Vergote *et al.* (1992) randomized 340 women with Stage I–IIIA disease (all grades) who were without residual tumor after staging laparotomy to receive either cisplatin (six courses) or irradiation (usually intraperitoneal ^{32}P, 7–10 millicuries) and demonstrated an equal survival rate in both groups. Grade was the only independent prognostic factor in Stage I cases. Disease-free survival rate in Stage I was 82% in the ^{32}P group and 79% after cisplatin. Late bowel complications after ^{32}P were relatively frequent, so the authors recommended against its continued use. At present, patients with unfavorable prognosis are randomized by the Gynecologic Oncology Group (GOG) to receive either ^{32}P or three cycles of cyclophosphamide (1000 mg m^{-2}) and cisplatin (100 mg m^{-2}); the results of this study should be of interest.

Currently, there are no trials that randomize the unfavorable prognostic group as defined above to a no further treatment arm after surgery. With only a limited number of women with early-stage and high-risk disease available for study, and the relatively high recurrence rate of 20% with adjuvant therapy, it has been difficult to gain acceptance of a study with an observation arm. However, the Medical Research Council (MRC) is attempting to deal with this problem in a current trial for early-stage cases by specifying that eligible patients are those the physician is uncertain should receive chemotherapy. Such cases are randomized to platinum-based chemotherapy or observation. Grade, cell type and stage are not prescribed. Whether that trial will accrue enough high-risk cases to answer the question remains to be determined.

It is not appropriate to compare current results to historic controls, because patients in past studies almost certainly were not as well staged as those in the more contemporary studies. Borderline tumors should be excluded since there is no evidence that they benefit from non-surgical treatment, and survival is more favorable.

Single Agent Therapy in Advanced Ovarian Carcinoma

The main agents with demonstrated activity in ovarian cancer include cisplatin (and carboplatin), paclitaxel, mustards, doxorubicin and hexamethylmelamine. Cisplatin has been regarded as the most active agent in the primary treatment of ovarian cancer, but its activity relative to paclitaxel is currently being studied by the GOG. In perhaps the largest experience, chemotherapy-naive Stage III and IV patients were treated with cisplatin 50 mg m^{-2} every four weeks; a 20% (35/173) surgical complete response rate and 19.4-month median survival were observed (Gruppo Interegionale, 1987).

Cisplatin versus Carboplatin

Carboplatin is another platinum coordination complex with a different toxicity profile compared to cisplatin. It has little or no nephrotoxicity or neurotoxicity, and can be administered more easily since it does not require intravenous hydration. The dose-limiting toxicity of carboplatin is myelosuppresion, primarily thrombocytopenia. Several prospective randomized trials comparing cisplatin to carboplatin (at about four times the dose) demonstrated equivalence in ovarian cancer; these results were supported by an MRC overview of 11 randomized clinical trials involving 2061 patients (Advanced Ovarian Cancer Trialists Group, 1991). For single agent therapy, carboplatin may be preferable, but in combination with marrow-toxic agents, cisplatin has some advantage because its marrow toxicity is limited.

Paclitaxel (Taxol)

Paclitaxel is a natural product that stabilizes cellular microtubules, thereby interfering with cell replication. In the first trial in ovarian cancer, 11 partial responses and one pathologic complete response were noted out of 40 patients, most of whom were heavily pretreated; in the subset considered platinum-resistant, 24% (6/25) responded (McGuire *et al.*, 1989). The results of this study were confirmed in other trials (Einzig *et al.*, 1992; Trimble *et al.*, 1993). In a subsequent European and Canadian study, the dosing of paclitaxel was evaluated, comparing 'high' dose (175 mg m^{-2}) versus low dose (135 mg m^{-2}) and short (three-hour) versus long infusions (24-hour) in patients with relapsed ovarian cancer (Swenerton *et al.*, 1993). The initial report indicated that paclitaxel may be given safely over three hours with premedication and that responses are more frequent in the 175 mg m^{-2} group compared to the 135 mg m^{-2} (24% versus 13% response). Neuropathy occurred more commonly in the 175 mg m^{-2} group (52% versus 33%). Another trial assessed a higher dose (250 mg m^{-2}) with growth factor support, yielding a 48% response rate (21/44) in platinum-resistant cases (Kohn *et al.*, 1994). Whether there is a survival benefit for higher dose paclitaxel is not established, but is being studied.

Alkylating Agents

The most commonly used mustards have included melphalan, cyclophosphamide, chlorambucil, and thiotepa. Recently, ifosfamide has been studied. The GOG experience with oral melphalan in Protocol #22 indicates an overall response rate of 37.5% (24/64) with a 20% clinical complete response rate in bulky Stage III and Stage IV disease (Omura *et al.*, 1983). Cyclophosphamide has been very popular in combination regimens, but there is only limited evidence that it has contributed to combinations.

Anthracyclines

Doxorubicin has an overall clinical response rate in the range of 30% (Young *et al.*, 1981) with one report of three clinical complete responses and three partial responses in 12 cases (DePalo *et al.*, 1977). Much higher doses (120 mg m^{-2} every three weeks for four doses) can be given, with considerably more toxicity, but high-dose doxorubicin has not been systematically studied in ovarian cancer (Wheeler *et al.*, 1982). The experience with single agent doxorubicin as primary treatment is not extensive since it was rapidly introduced into combination therapy.

Hexamethylmelamine

Hexamethylmelamine is a derivative of triethylene melamine that has been used in various schedules by mouth. The single agent experience has largely been with 8 mg kg^{-1} d^{-1} chronically or in 14-day courses. Using the former schedule in 22 previously untreated patients, there were seven clinical complete responses and three partial responses (Smith and Rutledge 1975).

Combination Chemotherapy

Despite a compelling rationale for combination chemotherapy, the evidence that drug combinations are superior to single agents in ovarian cancer has been seriously challenged. An MRC overview (meta-analysis) of 16 properly randomized trials using raw data from 3146 patients compared single non-platinum agents versus non-platinum combination chemotherapy (Advanced Ovarian Cancer Trialists Group, 1991) and showed no survival difference whatsoever (this overview included some additional analyses to be described below).

Several clinical trials have addressed the value of cisplatin-based therapy compared to regimens that have not included cisplatin. A randomized GOG study compared the combination of doxorubicin and cyclophosphamide with or without cisplatin in 440 patients with bulky Stage III and Stage IV disease and demonstrated a significant improvement in clinical complete response rate, response duration and overall survival with the addition of cisplatin (Omura *et al.*, 1986; Omura *et al.*, 1991). The median survival was 16.4 months for CA and 19.3 months for CAP; the estimated benefit was a 20% decrease ($p = 0.04$) in the relative death rate among those who received cyclophosphamide doxorubicin cisplatin (CAP). These findings were challenged by one aspect of the MRC overview in which, evaluating 1408 cases from eight randomized trials including the GOG study, no significant difference in overall survival between cisplatin and non-cisplatin treated groups was found. This discrepancy between the GOG trial and the overview might be explained by the fact that the other large trial (Gynecological Group, 1986) in the platinum/non-platinum overview routinely crossed patients over to cisplatin, a practice which was not part of the design of the GOG trial. At any rate, the clinical impact of cisplatin in advanced ovarian cancer is obviously more modest than originally thought.

Hexamethylmelamine Combinations

Since cyclophosphamide, hexamethylmelamine, doxorubicin and cisplatin all have activity in ovarian carcinoma, and since hexamethylmelamine and cisplatin are relatively nonmyelotoxic, it was reasonable to consider a combination of all four (variously known as CHAP, CHAD, or HEXA-CAP). However, most of the four drug combination trials did not have concurrent controls or large accruals and the results are not clearly better than what has been reported with CAP.

Neijt *et al.* (1991) conducted a randomized trial of CHAP versus cyclophosphamide and cisplatin in 191 advanced-stage ovarian cancer patients; they were unable to demonstrate any advantage for the CHAP regimen in either high- or low-volume disease groups.

It is disappointing, but should not be surprising, that the CHAP regimens have not given consistently improved results since the dose rate of each agent is compromised, and the compliance with prescribed doses of oral hexamethylmelamine is uncertain. The addition of hexamethylmelamine to 'full dose' melphalan gave a higher response rate than melphalan alone in bulky Stage III and Stage IV cases, but survival was identical (Omura *et al.*, 1983; Omura *et al.*, 1991).

CAP Versus CP

Four randomized clinical trials comparing cyclophosphamide and cisplatin (CP) versus cyclophosphamide, doxorubicin and cisplatin (CAP) individually failed to show a significant survival advantage with the addition of doxorubicin (Conte *et al.*, 1986; Gruppo Interegionale, 1987; Bertelsen *et al.*, 1987; Omura *et al.*, 1989). Because of these findings, the two-drug regimen of CP largely replaced the three-drug combination (CAP). However, a formal meta-analysis based on the raw data from the 1194 patients in these trials demonstrated a 7% difference in negative second-look rate ($p = 0.01$) and a 7% survival advantage at six years that are statistically significant in favor of the CAP regimen (Ovarian Cancer Meta-Analysis Project, 1991). There was a 15% reduction in the odds of death in favor of CAP ($p = 0.02$). Because the dose intensity of CAP was greater than CP in three of the trials, it is uncertain to what extent the benefit of CAP is from greater dose intensity and to what extent it is from the doxorubicin itself. Because the clinical impact of a 7% improvement in treatment outcome has been assumed to be very modest and because of its potential cardiac toxicity, doxorubicin has not been routinely reincorporated into the standard treatment regimen, but it warrants further study.

Cisplatin Alone or In Combination

A very revealing study already alluded to (Gruppo Interegionale, 1987), randomly compared cisplatin 50 mg m^{-2} every four weeks as a single agent to CP and to CAP. Despite greater dose intensity for the combinations, there was no significant difference in survival. The results did tend, however, to slightly favor the combinations, especially CAP. Although this was a large (P (cisplatin) = 173, CP = 181, CAP = 175 patients), well-done trial, it was not large enough to address the significance of small differences in outcome. By expanding the sample size to 838, the MRC overview was able to show a statistically significant advantage ($p = 0.03$) for cisplatin combinations over cisplatin alone, albeit a clinically small improvement. Since the results of the overview were, quite appropriately, not regarded as definitive, one outgrowth of that effort is an ongoing trial of moderately intensive carboplatin versus CAP being conducted by the MRC with a projected accrual of 2000.

Cisplatin plus Paclitaxel

A GOG trial in advanced ovarian cancer (suboptimal Stage III and IV cases) randomized cisplatin (75 mg m^{-2}) and cyclophosphamide (750 mg m^{-2}) versus cisplatin (75 mg m^{-2}) and paclitaxel (135 mg m^{-2}) given every three weeks for six courses. In an interim report, the clinical response rate in 290 evaluable patients with measurable disease was 63% for the cyclophosphamide/cisplatin and 79% for paclitaxel/cisplatin ($p < 0.01$); the rates of negative second-look were 19% and 26% respectively ($p = 0.07$). The median durations of progression-free survival (PFS) were 13.8 months (95% confidence interval 11.3–17.4) and 17.9 months respectively (95% confidence interval 14.6–undefined). The combination of cisplatin plus paclitaxel shows a significant survival advantage compared with cisplatin plus cyclophosphamide (McGuire *et al.*, 1995). At this point the question arises whether paclitaxel is more active than cisplatin. To further evaluate these two important agents, a GOG trial has been conducted comparing cisplatin (100 mg m^{-2}) versus paclitaxel (200 mg m^{-2}) versus paclitaxel (135 mg m^{-2}) plus cisplatin (75 mg m^{-2}) in bulky Stage III and Stage IV cases. The results should be available in the near future and will be of great interest.

Intraperitoneal Chemotherapy

It has been documented that intraperitoneal therapy produces objective responses in patients with persistent or recurrent ovarian cancer with small volume residual disease (Markman *et al.*, 1993). There is a potential 10- to 20-fold increase in drug exposure of the peritoneal surface by intraperitoneal administration of cisplatin compared to systemic exposure. Other drugs have been evaluated by the intraperitoneal route, such as carboplatin, doxorubicin, fluorouracil, melphalan, mitoxantrone, methotrexate and paclitaxel. However, the direct penetration of these agents into tumor tissue is limited to a few millimeters from the surface, so the common problem of relatively large tumor masses, even after debulking surgery, precludes the widespread application of this approach. Even in the most favorable cases, with microscopic to millimeter size residual disease, it is unclear whether the objective responses seen in as many as 30–50% of selected patients will translate into a survival benefit when this strategy is used as consolidation therapy or as second-line treatment for small-volume residual disease. Randomized trials are needed.

Recently, the use of intraperitoneal therapy as a component of initial management in ovarian cancer has been evaluated. In 1992 the Southwest Oncology Group and GOG completed a randomized trial comparing intraperitoneal cisplatin (100 mg m^{-2}) and intravenous cyclophosphamide (600 mg m^{-2}) versus intravenous cisplatin (100 mg m^{-2}) and intravenous cyclophosphamide (600 mg m^{-2}) each given every 21 days for six courses in small-volume Stage III disease. The results of that trial should be available soon. There is also a current GOG trial randomly comparing intensive carboplatin (every four weeks × 2) followed by intraperitoneal cisplatin (100 mg m^{-2}) and intravenous paclitaxel (135 mg m^{-2}) every 21 days × six courses versus cisplatin (75 mg m^{-2}) and paclitaxel (135 mg m^{-2}) every 21 days for six courses in small-volume Stage III disease ($\leqslant$1 cm). This study evaluates whether high-dose systemic chemotherapy (carboplatin) to 'debulk' the tumor initially, followed by the regional (intraperitoneal) treatment strategy, has an advantage over systemic therapy alone. Until the results of these trials are available the precise role for intraperitoneal chemotherapy as a component of primary treatment in ovarian cancer remains unsettled.

Dose Intensity

It has been assumed that higher drug doses and/or more drugs per unit of time would produce better results. However, the foregoing discussion has provided only limited support for the notion that more drugs are better. Only a few large scale trials have examined this issue with respect to cisplatin dose intensity in a prospective randomized fashion. Kaye *et al.* (1992) gave ovarian cancer patients cyclophosphamide 750 mg m^{-2} plus cisplatin 50 or 100 mg m^{-2}. Six courses were to be given. The randomization was stopped early after accruing 159 evaluable patients, because a significant survival advantage was observed for the double-dose cisplatin arm.

A larger trial (458 patients) compared 100 mg m^{-2} of cisplatin plus 1000 mg m^{-2} of cyclophosphamide for four courses versus 50 mg m^{-2} and 500 mg m^{-2} of the same drugs for eight courses in large-volume Stage III and Stage IV cases. There was much more toxicity, but no improvement in response rate or survival with the double-dose therapy (McGuire *et al.*, 1992). It is difficult to reconcile these results with those of Kaye *et al.*, except that the latter study probably had relatively more patients with small-volume disease (almost one third of those patients were Stage IC or II). The effect of dose might be easier to demonstrate in that setting. A potentially serious criticism of Kaye's study is the presence of an imbalance in performance status favoring the high-dose arm; moreover, no information was provided about the distribution of cell type, which some investigators regard as another important prognostic factor (Omura *et al.*, 1991). As a practical matter Kaye *et al.* concluded from their study that an intermediate dose of cisplatin (i.e. 75 mg m^{-2}), was more realistic in view of cumulative neurotoxicity with the double dose.

A third trial compared cisplatin at a dose intensity of 25 or 50 mg m^{-2} per week to the same total dose of 450 mg m^{-2} (75 mg m^{-2} every three weeks × six courses or 50 mg m^{-2} weekly × nine courses). With 296 eligible patients, an interim report did not indicate a significant improvement (Colombo *et al.*, 1993). A preliminary report on a fourth trial comparing 100 versus 50 mg m^{-2} of cisplatin, each in combination with epirubicin and cyclophosphamide has so far not shown a big difference, except in toxicity (Conte *et al.*, 1993). The weight of evidence does not suggest a consistent advantage for dose-intensive platinum therapy.

Duration of Therapy

Two trials have prospectively addressed the duration of cisplatin-based combination chemotherapy; randomized comparisons of five versus ten, and six versus 12 courses have shown no survival difference (Hakes *et al.*, 1992; Bertelsen *et al.*, 1993). Whether the lack of advantage for prolonged therapy can be generalized to paclitaxel-based regimens or to early stage ovarian cancer is unclear, but seems likely.

Post-remission Consolidation Therapy

After initial chemotherapy, even those with a negative second-look are at substantial risk of fatal recurrence. In one large chemotherapy trial (Omura *et al.*, 1989) of small-volume disease (≤1 cm residual lesions), 19/48 (40%) of women who began the study with residual disease and 16/39 (41%) of those who began without residual disease and then had a negative second-look had already progressed after only two years of follow-up! Clearly there is a need to consider further treatment in those with a negative second-look, but no standard recommendation can be made at this time. Studies are ongoing addressing this problem. For example, the GOG is comparing ^{32}P versus no further treatment and Southwest Oncology Group (SWOG) is randomizing alpha interferon versus no further treatment.

Curability with Drugs

The possible impact of chemotherapy on early-stage disease has already been discussed. To what extent does chemotherapy cure advanced cases? Prolonged follow-up is necessary to have confidence about the outcome, since recurrence and death may occasionally be observed even beyond seven years. With a minimum follow-up of ten years in a non-platinum trial, 9/319 (2.8%) of women who began with bulky Stage III or Stage IV cancer were alive and progression free at last contact; with at least seven years of follow-up in a CAP trial in a similar population, at least 178/198 (90%) had already progressed (Omura *et al.*, 1991). Another CAP trial which included small- as well as large-volume Stage III and Stage IV cases had 7.1% disease-free patients at ten years (Sutton *et al.*, 1989a). Similar results have been reported by others (Hoskins *et al.*, 1992) using cisplatin-based therapy. Thus, the likelihood of cure in advanced disease remains low. Whether cisplatin–paclitaxel regimens will improve the cure rate is to be hoped, but is not established.

Treatment of Relapsed or Refractory Ovarian Cancer

At present there is no convincing evidence that any approach will reproducibly cure relapsed or refractory ovarian carcinoma after failure of initial chemotherapy. A survival benefit from second-line treatment is also questionable. As a consequence, women desiring further treatment should be encouraged to participate in clinical trials of new agents. However, it is clear that (as with other types of cancer) patients who have shown an objective response to initial therapy and do not progress until at least 6–12 months have elapsed off treatment, have a good chance of responding again to the initial therapy. Those who have not responded at all or had only a brief response to initial therapy, should be entered in new drug trials and assessed as a separate group. Reports in the literature do not always distinguish between relapsed and refractory patients. A case in point is ifosfamide, an analog of cyclophosphamide, which has been reported to have a 20% response rate in women previously treated with CP or CAP (Sutton *et al.*, 1989b). It is not clear how many responding patients were truly refractory to cyclophosphamide. To the extent that ifosfamide is active after cyclophosphamide failure, it is interesting to wonder whether the typical five-day course of ifosfamide has an advantage over one day of cyclophosphamide; in other words, is the fractionation more important than the drug.

Although many drugs have some first-line activity in ovarian cancer, even a partial tabulation (*Table 16.1*) of second-line therapy indicates very few attractive options. Cisplatin and paclitaxel quickly stood out from the others, and were rapidly moved into first-line use. A few others worth some mention include hexamethylmelamine, etoposide and tamoxifen, the latter because of occasional responses and minimal toxicity (Ahlgren *et al.*, 1993). With a previous platinum response and a platinum-free interval of more than 12 months, the response rate to high-dose epirubicin was 9/20 (J. Vermorken, personal communication, April 1994), but most responses were partial despite a very select patient population. As patients increasingly receive both cisplatin and paclitaxel first-line, it is unclear whether any other current drugs will have utility as second line therapy; appropriate studies are needed.

Table 16.1. Some single agents for relapsed/refractory ovarian carcinoma.

	Response / Total (%)	*Reference*
Cisplatin	9/34 (27)	CRT **60:** 55 (1976)
Paclitaxel	12/45 (27)	AIM **111:** 273 (1989)
Epirubicin*	10/25 (40)	ASCO **10:** 190 (1991)
Esorubicin	2/26 (8)	IND **7:** 333 (1989)
Ifosfamide	8/41 (20)	JCO **7:** 1672 (1989)
Ifosfamide	7/57 (12)	JCO **10:** 243 (1992)
Etoposide	8/31 (26)	JCO **12:** 60 (1994)
Etoposide	2/24 (8)	CTR **63:** 2089 (1979)
Tamoxifen	18/105 (17)	*Cancer* **68:** 269 (1991)
Hexamethylmelamine	8/49 (16)	CTR **65:** 530 (1981)
Dianhydrogalactitol	6/39 (15)	*Gynecol. Oncol.* **15:** 381 (1983)
Gallium nitrate	3/26 (12)	AJCO **14:** 349 (1991)
Teniposide	3/26 (12)	CTR **70:** 1231 (1986)
Fluorouracil	3/29 (10)	*Gynecol. Oncol.* **46:** 326 (1992)
Fluorouracil	1/20 (5)	AJCO **15:** 494 (1992)
Echinomycin	2/22 (9)	AJCO **13:** 299 (1990)
Baker's antifol	2/26 (8)	IND **1:** 185 (1983)
Diaziquone	2/25 (8)	CTR **70:** 309 (1986)
N-methylformamide	3/41 (7)	IND **8:** 191 (1990)
Aminothiadiazole	2/32 (6)	AJCO **9:** 334 (1986)
Amonafide	1/21 (5)	AJCO **16:** 529 (1993)
Mitoxantrone	1/26 (4)	AJCO **7:** 737 (1984)
Amsacrine	1/23 (4)	AJCO **6:** 277 (1983)
Acivicin	1/24 (4)	IND **4:** 49 (1986)
Piperazinedione	1/31 (3)	AJCO **7:** 261 (1984)
PALA**	0/32	AJCO **7:** 257 (1984)
lomustine	0/31	CTR **61:** 1533 (1977)
Maytansine	0/29	AJCO **6:** 273 (1983)
Razoxane	0/21	CTR **68:** 439 (1984)
Vinblastine	0/19	IND **8:** 377 (1990)
Didemnin-B	0/16	AJCO **16:** 47 (1993)

*High dose; ** phosphonoacetyl-L-aspartate.

AJCO, *Amer. J. Clin. Oncol.*; AIM, *Ann. Intern. Med.*; ASCO, *Amer. Soc. Clin. Oncol. Proc.*; CTR, *Cancer Treat. Rep.*; IND, *Invest. New Drugs*; JCO, *J. Clin. Oncol.*

Biotherapy

Alpha interferon has modest activity in ovarian cancer, but interleukin-2 has been disappointing. Other approaches using monoclonal antibodies have recently been reviewed (Bookman and Berek, 1992) but cannot be recommended at present except on an experimental basis. Advanced bulky tumors are less likely to respond than relatively small tumor burdens, so appropriately designed trials will be especially important.

Autografting

There is increasing interest in megadose chemotherapy for cancer, including ovarian cancer, using agents with exclusively marrow toxicity (at more conventional doses), followed by hematopoietic reconstitution or 'rescue' with autologous marrow or with peripheral blood stem cells harvested with a cell separator. Cyclophosphamide doses can be increased seven-fold, melphalan six-fold, and thiotepa more than 30-fold before non-hematologic toxicities such as cardiac damage mucositis and/or central nervous system effects supervene. Carboplatin, etoposide and mitoxantrone can also be dramatically escalated using this approach. A combination of cyclophosphamide, mitoxantrone and carboplatin with doses as high as 120 mg kg^{-1}, 75 mg m^{-2} and 1500 mg m^{-2} respectively, followed by autografting, was used in a small group of ovarian cancer patients, resulting in clinical complete response in five and partial response in one (Stiff *et al.*, 1994). The responses lasted up to 30+ months. Similar studies are ongoing. Long-term follow-up is clearly needed as well as appropriate randomized trials.

Megadose chemotherapy and marrow rescue are potentially attractive in ovarian cancer because much higher doses of the drugs noted above can be given, but also because ovarian cancer does not commonly grow in the marrow. In addition, there is a relatively large group of patients who have small-volume residual after initial therapy, but have no really good standard treatment options subsequently. On the other hand, many potential candidates are in their 60s and 70s and may not survive such intensive therapy; it remains an unproven approach for ovarian cancer, and there is inconsistent financial support from insurance carriers for this costly treatment.

Radiation Therapy

There has been a longstanding interest in irradiation, either external or intraperitoneal, for ovarian cancer. Some very impressive long-term results have been reported in uncontrolled trials for small-volume disease; results that appear to readily surpass what is accomplished with chemotherapy (Thomas and Dembo, 1993). However, few randomized comparisons with chemotherapy in carefully staged patients have been reported, with conflicting results. Radiation oncologists point out that pelvic irradiation alone is inadequate treatment, even for Stage I since the entire peritoneal surface is at risk. Pelvic treatment plus intracavity ^{32}P is too toxic (Klaassen *et al.*, 1988). Whole abdominal irradiation must be limited in total dose because of toxicity to the spinal cord, liver, bowel and especially the kidneys. A tolerable dose to the upper abdomen is currently regarded as inadequate for gross residual disease. A large scale randomized trial of carefully staged Stage I Grade 3, Stage II and Stage III cases with microscopic residual, comparing cisplatin plus paclitaxel versus whole abdominal irradiation with analysis by intent to treat would be of great interest, but it has not been possible to carry out such a study in the USA. Studies of intraperitoneal ^{32}P in early-stage disease have already been discussed, and have shown no superiority for ^{32}P over chemotherapy.

In the study by Vergote *et al.* (1992) already mentioned, comparing ^{32}P versus cisplatin for Stage I–IIIA patients with no residual disease, there was a subset of 28 patients randomized to receive ^{32}P, but instead received whole abdominal irradiation (2200 Rad) with a pelvic boost because of intraperitoneal adhesions. The five-year disease-free survival rates for Stage I (all grades except borderline) were $94 \pm 6\%$ for whole abdominal irradiation and $79 \pm 4.4\%$ for cisplatin. This difference was not significant, presumably because of the small number irradiated. One wonders if the difference could be duplicated in a large scale trial. As a practical matter, however, there was a 21% incidence (6/28) of bowel obstruction without tumor recurrence after whole abdominal irradiation, limiting the appeal of this therapy.

Follow-up

It has already been indicated that the treatment of recurrent ovarian cancer is unsatisfactory; it follows that close monitoring for evidence of recurrence is therefore of limited value. Periodic general physical and pelvic examinations perhaps every 3–6 months, as well as an annual chest radiograph seem appropriate. In view of the possible late effects of chemotherapy such as myelodysplastic syndrome or acute leukemia, periodic blood counts should be obtained. The value of serial serum CA-125 determinations and abdominal CT scans is unclear, although many women expect them. When highly effective treatments for relapse become available, close follow-up may be important. In the meantime, the anxiety caused by suspicious findings or evidence of early recurrence should be balanced against the theoretical value of treating smaller volume recurrence.

Summary of Management Options

- Neither chemotherapy nor radioactive phosphorus is indicated for borderline tumors or Stage I well-differentiated ovarian carcinoma.
- Early-stage high-risk cases may benefit from adjuvant cisplatin, although a survival advantage has not been shown.
- Stage III and IV cases should be offered platinum-based therapy such as cisplatin plus paclitaxel for six courses, recognizing that the long-term benefit may be modest.
- Relapse after a negative second-look is common, but no specific recommendation can be made at present to prevent such relapses.
- Late recurrences after platinum-based chemotherapy may be retreated with carboplatin. Patients with an early recurrence can be offered paclitaxel (if not previously given) or investigational new drugs.
- The roles of intraperitoneal medication, megadose chemotherapy and whole abdominal irradiation remain unsettled.

References

■ Advanced Ovarian Cancer Trialists Group (1991) Chemotherapy in advanced ovarian cancer: an overview of randomized clinical trials. *Brit. Med. J.* **303:** 884–893.

Ahlgren JD, Ellison NM, Gottlieb RJ, Laluna F *et al.*, (1993) *J. Clin. Oncol.* **11:** 1957–1968.

Bertelsen K, Jakobsen A, Andersen JE *et al.* (1987) A randomized study of cyclophosphamide and cisplatinum with or without doxorubicin in advanced ovarian carcinoma. *Gynecol. Oncol.* **28:** 161–169.

Bertelsen K, Jakobsen A, Stroyler I *et al.* (1993) A prospective randomized comparison of 6 and 12 cycles of cyclophosphamide, adriamycin, and cisplatin in advanced epithelial ovarian cancer: a Danish Ovarian Study Group trial (DACOVA). *Gynecol. Oncol.* **49:** 30–36.

Bolis G, Colombo N, Favalli G *et al.* (1992) Randomized multicenter clinical trial in stage I epithelial ovarian cancer. *Proc. Am. Soc. Clin. Onc.* **11:** 225, abst. 714.

■ Bookman MA & Berek JS (1992) Biologic and immunologic therapy of ovarian cancer. *Hematol. Oncol. Clin. N. Am.* **6:** 941–965.

Colombo N, Pittelli MR, Parma G *et al.* (1993) Cisplatin (p) dose intensity in advanced ovarian cancer (AOC): a randomized study of conventional dose (DC) vs dose-intense (DI) cisplatin monochemotherapy. *Proc. Am. Soc. Clin. Oncol.* **12:** 255, abst. 806.

Conte PF, Bruzzone M, Chiara S *et al.* (1986) A randomized trial comparing cisplatin plus cyclophosphamide versus cisplatin, doxorubicin, and cyclophosphamide in advanced ovarian cancer. *J. Clin. Oncol.* **4:** 965–971.

Conte PF, Bruzzone M, Gadducci A *et al.* (1993) High doses versus standard doses of cisplatin (P) in combination with epidoxorubicin (E) and cyclophosphamide (C) in advanced ovarian cancer (AOC) patients (PTS) with bulky residual disease: a randomized trial. *Proc. Am. Soc. Clin. Oncol.* **12:** 273, abst. 880.

DePalo GM, DeLena M & Bonadonna G (1977) Adriamycin versus adriamycin plus melphalan in advanced ovarian carcinoma. *Cancer Treat. Rep.* **61:** 355–357.

Einzig AI, Wiernik PH, Sasloff J *et al.* (1992) Phase II study and long-term follow-up of patients treated with taxol for advanced ovarian adenocarcinoma. *J. Clin. Oncol.* **10:** 1748–1753.

Gruppo Interegionale Cooperativo Oncologico Ginecologia (1987) Randomised comparison of cisplatin with cyclophosphamide/cisplatin and with cyclophosphamide/doxorubicin/cisplatin in advanced ovarian cancer. *Lancet* **2:** 353–359.

Gynecological Group, Clinical Oncological Society of Australia and Sydney Branch, Ludwig Institute for Cancer Research. (1986) Chemotherapy of advanced ovarian adenocarcinoma: a randomized comparison of combination versus sequential therapy using chlorambucil and cisplatin. *Gynecol. Oncol.* **23:** 1–13.

Hakes TB, Chalas E, Hoskins WJ *et al.* (1992) Randomized prospective trial of 5 versus 10 cycles of cyclophosphamide, doxorubicin and cisplatin in advanced ovarian carcinoma. *Gynecol. Oncol.* **45:** 284–289.

Hoskins PJ, O'Reilly SE, Swenerton KD *et al.* (1992) Ten-year outcome of patients with advanced epithelial ovarian carcinoma treated with cisplatin-based multimodality therapy. *J. Clin. Oncol.* **10:** 1561–1568.

Kaye SB, Lewis CR, Paul J *et al.* (1992) Randomised study of two doses of cisplatin with cyclophosphamide in epithelial ovarian cancer. *Lancet* **340:** 329–333.

Klaassen D, Shelley W, Starreveld A *et al.* (1988) *J. Clin. Oncol.* **6:** 1254–1263.

Kohn EC, Sarosy G, Bicher A *et al.* (1994) Dose-intense taxol: high response rate in patients with platinum-resistant recurrent ovarian cancer. *J. Natl. Cancer Inst.* **86:** 18–24.

Markman M, Reichman B, Hakes T *et al.* (1993) Intraperitoneal chemotherapy in the management of ovarian cancer. *Cancer* **71:** 1565–1570.

McGuire WP, Rowinsky EK, Rosenshein NB *et al.* (1989) Taxol: a unique antineoplastic agent with significant activity in advanced ovarian epithelial neoplasms. *Ann. Int. Med.* **111:** 273–279.

McGuire WP, Hoskins WJ, Brady MF *et al.* (1992) A phase III trial of dose intense (DI) versus standard dose (DS) cisplatin (CDDP) and cytoxan (CTX) in advanced ovarian cancer (AOC). *Proc. Am. Soc. Clin. Oncol.* **11:** 226, abst. 718.

McGuire WP, Hoskins WJ, Brady MF *et al.* (1993) A phase III trial comparing cisplatin/cytoxan (PC) and cisplatin/taxol (PT) in advanced ovarian cancer (AOC). *Proc. Am. Soc. Clin. Oncol.* **12:** 255, abst. 808.

Neijt JP, Ten Bokkel Huinink WW, Van der Burg MEL *et al.* (1991) Long-term survival in ovarian cancer: mature data from the Netherlands Joint Study Group for Ovarian Cancer. *Eur. J. Cancer* **27:** 1367–1372.

Omura GA, Morrow CP, Blessing JA *et al.* (1983) A randomized comparison of melphalan versus melphalan plus hexamethylmelamine versus adriamycin plus cyclophosphamide in ovarian carcinoma. *Cancer* **51:** 783–789.

Omura G, Blessing JA, Ehrlich CE *et al.* (1986) A randomized trial of cyclophosphamide and doxorubicin with or without cisplatin in advanced ovarian carcinoma. *Cancer* **57:** 1725–1730.

Omura GA, Bundy BN, Berek JS *et al.* (1989) Randomized trial of cyclophosphamide plus cisplatin with or without doxorubicin in ovarian carcinoma: a Gynecologic Oncology Group study. *J. Clin. Oncol.* **7:** 457–465.

■ Omura GA, Brady MF, Homesley HD *et al.* (1991) Long-term follow-up and prognostic factor analysis in advanced ovarian carcinoma: the Gynecologic Oncology Group experience. *J. Clin. Oncol.* **9:** 1138–1150.

■ Ovarian Cancer Meta-Analysis Project (1991) Cyclophosphamide plus cisplatin versus cyclophosphamide, doxorubicin, and cisplatin chemotherapy of ovarian carcinoma: a meta-analysis. *J. Clin. Oncol.* **9:** 1668–1674.

Smith JP & Rutledge FN (1975) Random study of hexamethylmelamine, 5-fluorouracil, and melphalan in treatment of advanced carcinoma of the ovary. *Natl. Cancer Inst. Monogr.* **42:** 169–172.

Stiff PJ, McKenzie SR, Alberts DS *et al.* (1994) *J. Clin. Oncol.* **12:** 176–183.

Sutton GP, Stehman FB, Einhorn LH *et al.* (1989a) Ten-year follow-up of patients receiving cisplatin, doxorubicin, and cyclophosphamide chemotherapy for advanced epithelial ovarian carcinoma. *J. Clin. Oncol.* **7:** 223–229.

Sutton GP, Blessing JA, Homesley HD *et al.* (1989b) Phase II trial of ifosfamide and mesna in advanced ovarian carcinoma: a Gynecologic Oncology Group study. *J. Clin. Oncol.* **7:** 1672–1676.

Swenerton K, Eisenhauer E, Ten Bokkel Huinink W *et al.* (1993) Taxol in relapsed ovarian cancer: high *vs* low dose and short *vs* long infusion: a European–Canadian study coordinated by the NCI Canada Clinical Trials Group. *Proc. Am. Soc. Clin. Oncol.* **12:** 256, abst. 810.

Thomas GM & Dembo AJ (1993) Integrating radiation therapy into the management of ovarian cancer. *Cancer* **71:** 1710–1718.

■ Trimble EL, Adams JD, Vena D *et al.* (1993) Paclitaxel for platinum-refractory ovarian cancer: results from the first 1,000 patients registered to national cancer institute treatment referral center 9103. *J. Clin. Onc.* **11:** 2405–2410.

Vergote IB, Vergote–De Vos LN, Abeler VM *et al.* (1992) Randomized trial comparing cisplatin with radioactive phosphorus or whole-abdomen irradiation as adjuvant treatment of ovarian cancer. *Cancer* **69:** 741–749.

Wheeler RH, Ensminger WD, Thrall JH & Anderson JL (1982) High-dose doxorubicin: an exploration of the dose–response curve in human neoplasia. *Cancer Treat. Rep.* **66:** 493–498.

Young RC, Ozols RF & Myers CE (1981) The anchracycline antineoplastic drugs. *N. Engl. J. Med.* **305:** 139–153.

Young RC, Walton LA, Ellenberg SS *et al.* (1990) Adjuvant therapy in stage I and stage II epithelial ovarian cancer: results of two prospective randomized trials. *N. Engl. J. Med.* **322:** 1021–1027.

17 Non-epithelial Ovarian Cancer

S D Williams
G P Sutton

Ovarian Germ Cell Tumors

General Considerations

Ovarian germ cell tumors are a heterogeneous and complex group of diseases. Study of these fascinating neoplasms is hampered by their complexity and rarity. Much of the published literature tends to be anecdotal rather than prospective and there have been no randomized clinical trials. However, these neoplasms have importance beyond their numerical incidence because they typically occur in women of young age, and improvements in modern treatment have made these patients highly curable.

The neoplasms range from totally benign tumors to among the most rapidly progressive and malignant of any human tumors, and the usual onset is in the second or third decade. There are no clear-cut etiologic factors, although the incidence is substantially increased in women who have dysgenetic gonads. This observation is most notable in patients with gonadoblastoma, which as a frequent precursor of dysgerminoma can be considered to be a pre-malignant lesion.

The staging of ovarian germ cell tumors has been discussed in previous chapters. The same staging system used for epithelial tumors is used for this group. Of note, there is an appreciable incidence of retroperitoneal nodal metastases, particularly in dysgerminoma. The pathologic classification has also been described in an earlier chapter. Teratoma is graded according to the degree of immaturity present. At one end of the spectrum there is a benign solid or more usually cystic teratoma (the so-called dermoid cyst). At the other end are the immature teratomas, which are potentially malignant neoplasms with a prognosis for recurrence after local treatment related to grade. Recurrence after surgical treatment is somewhat unusual in well staged patients with Stage I Grade 1 disease, but the majority (approximately 85%) of patients with Stage I Grade 3 immature teratoma will have recurrence after local therapy only (Norris *et al.*, 1976). Finally, ovarian germ cell tumors frequently contain combinations of malignant elements and many patients are now classified as having mixed germ cell tumors.

Ovarian germ cell tumors occur principally in girls and young women, although they are occasionally seen in infants or older individuals. Median age at diagnosis is 16–20 years. These tumors, particularly dysgerminoma, are occasionally diagnosed during pregnancy or in the postpartum period.

Signs and symptoms are usually fairly typical. Abdominal pain associated with a palpable pelvic–abdominal mass is a common finding. Approximately 10% of patients will present with acute abdominal pain caused by rupture, hemorrhage or torsion of the tumor. This finding may be more common in patients with endodermal sinus tumor or mixed germ cell tumor and is frequently misdiagnosed as acute appendicitis, with the correct diagnosis made only at laparotomy. Other signs and symptoms that are occasionally seen include abdominal distension, fever and vaginal bleeding. A few patients show isosexual precocity, presumably due to human chorionic gonadotropin (HCG) production.

Many of these tumors produce the markers HCG and alphafetoprotein (AFP). Determination of marker levels is important in the initial diagnosis and subsequent follow-up. Patients with dysgerminoma will occasionally have an elevated HCG, but an AFP elevation is not consistent with this diagnosis and denotes the presence of other germ cell elements. Endodermal sinus tumor patients invariably have an elevated AFP, and choriocarcinoma patients, an elevated HCG. These markers should fall after surgery and during chemotherapy. A rising marker in a patient previously treated for an ovarian germ cell tumor is virtually diagnostic of recurrence, even if there is no other clinical or radiographic evidence of disease. The biologic half-life of HCG is 18–24 hours and that of AFP about five days. In other words, should marker production by the tumor immediately cease (e.g. due to total surgical excision), the serum level of HCG would decline by one-half every 18–24 hours and that of AFP every five days. During chemotherapy for advanced disease, HCG levels should decline by one log with each course. AFP decline, because of the much longer half-time, is less predictable.

Tumors Other Than Dysgerminoma

Tumors other than dysgerminoma have common characteristics that include rapid growth, the potential for intraperitoneal and nodal metastases, relative resistance to radiation and sensitivity to chemotherapy. Hematogenous metastases are also occasionally seen.

The majority of patients have Stage I disease at the time of diagnosis. Ideally, staging should be documented by thorough laparotomy as outlined for epithelial ovarian tumors. This initial surgical procedure establishes the pathologic diagnosis and initiates therapy. For patients with more advanced disease at the time of diagnosis, the role of 'debulking' surgery is controversial. The value of this has been taken as dogma by many gynecologic oncologists, but others have questioned its worth. For testicular germ cell tumors, a prospective clinical trial has shown that debulking surgery does not improve the prognosis in patients with bulky disease who receive chemotherapy, but there is no prospectively controlled information for ovarian germ cell tumors. However, in studies of the Gynecologic Oncology Group (GOG), there is a suggestion that patients with advanced disease who have surgical resection of as much tumor as possible have a higher chemotherapy complete remission rate than patients who, for whatever reason, are not debulked. Patients with bulky residual tumor after initial laparotomy fare considerably worse than patients with small-volume Stage III disease initially. Patients with bulky tumor debulked so that no residual tumor mass is larger than 1 cm have an intermediate prognosis (Williams *et al.*, 1989). The critical issue is whether the better prognosis of debulked patients is a function of the surgery or a biologic phenomenon related to the particular characteristics of that given tumor. In the absence of definitive information, it seems prudent, within the limits of good surgical practice, to attempt tumor debulking if there is a reasonable possibility of reducing maximum tumor diameter of all residual masses to less than 1 cm. This procedure should ordinarily not include bowel resection and must not preclude the prompt postoperative administration of chemotherapy, but it certainly should include omentectomy and excision of retroperitoneal nodal masses if feasible. As will be discussed, chemotherapy does not often result in amenorrhea or infertility and so reproductive organs should be preserved whenever possible, even if to do so would preclude successful debulking.

One of the great triumphs of cancer treatment in the 1970s and 1980s has been the development of effective chemotherapy for testicular germ cell tumors (Bosl *et al*,. 1986; Loehrer *et al.*, 1989). Most patients with these tumors will survive with the appropriate use of surgery and cisplatin-based combination chemotherapy. The lessons learned in prospective controlled clinical trials of testicular cancer have been applied to ovarian germ cell tumors, with many similarities and a few important differences.

Patients with established, incompletely resected, metastatic ovarian germ cell tumors should receive combination chemotherapy. These patients used to be treated with VAC (vincristine, dactinomycin and cyclophosphamide) or similar regimens (Creasman and Soper, 1985; Slayton *et al.*, 1985). This therapy had the ability to induce durable complete remission even in patients with advanced tumor. Unfortunately, many patients would either not respond initially or recur after an initial favorable response. In an early GOG trial, only 7/22 such patients were long-term survivors with VAC (Slayton *et al.*, 1985). Subsequent to the successes of cisplatin-based therapy for testicular germ cell tumors, similar regimens were evaluated in patients with ovarian germ cell tumors. In a subsequent GOG trial using the combination of cisplatin, vinblastine and bleomycin (PVB), 47/89 (53%) of patients are continuously disease-free with a median follow-up of 52 months (Williams *et al.*, 1989). The latest treatment failure occurred at 28 months. In addition, eight other patients had durable remissions with second-line therapy and a few other patients had non-progressive or slowly progressive immature teratoma. Four-year survival was about 70%. The administration of other chemotherapy before study entry and the presence of suboptimal residual Stage III or Stage IV disease adversely affected the outcome. Of note, however, 27% (8/30) who had no previous treatment and non-measurable (and presumably small-volume) tumor had persistent or progressive cancer. As noted above, patients who were debulked to optimal disease fared better than those who were not. Cell type and marker elevation were not obviously associated with outcome in this relatively small series.

Subsequent developments in testicular cancer defined the single agent activity of etoposide (VP-16) and later this agent was incorporated into combination regimens. A randomized trial then compared the 'standard' PVB regimen to one that substituted vinblastine for etoposide (BEP) (Williams *et al.*, 1987). The latter regimen had a similar level of efficacy overall; patients with a high tumor volume had an improved complete remission rate and survival. Also, BEP has less neurotoxicity and causes less abdominal pain and constipation than PVB. These adverse events are particularly important for ovarian germ cell tumor patients, many of whom have had recent surgery. Although not validated in a randomized clinical trial, these results seem, by available data, to also be applicable to the management of patients with ovarian germ cell cancer. The BEP regimen is shown in *Table 17.1*. Results of selected chemotherapy trials are shown

Table 17.1. The BEP regimen.

Cisplatin 20 mg m^{-2} days 1–5
Etoposide (VP-16) 100 mg m^{-2} days 1–5
Bleomycin 30 units intravenously weekly
3–4 courses given at 21-day intervals
Etoposide dose reduced 20% for patients with previous radiotherapy or episode of granulocytopenic fever

Table 17.2. Chemotherapy of advanced disease.

Institution	*Regimen*	*Prog free/total**	*Reference*
Gynecologic Oncology Group	PVB	47/89 (53)	(Williams *et al.*, 1989)
Stanford	PVB	4/4	(Carlson *et al*, 1983)
Cross Cancer Institute	PVB	8/10	(Taylor *et al.*, 1985)
M.D. Anderson	PVB	7/11	(Gershenson *et al.*, 1986b)
M.D. Anderson	BEP	5/6	(Gershenson *et al.*, 1990)

* Progression-free/total number of patients.

in *Table 17.2*. In general, these patients may fare slightly worse than their counterparts with testicular tumor of similar volume. This difference may be related to intrinsic biologic differences or, more likely, to underestimation of tumor volume because of intraperitoneal dissemination. Prognosis appears to be related to the amount of tumor present at the start of chemotherapy, but it does not appear to be related to the cell type, stage or marker elevation.

An area of controversy is the role of second-look laparotomy in the management of patients with ovarian germ cell tumors. Reassessment laparotomy is a surgical procedure commonly carried out in patients with epithelial ovarian cancer after completion of induction chemotherapy. The inherent inaccuracy of clinical staging, including newer tumor markers, in this situation is well known. It is less clear whether the findings of second-look laparotomy have a meaningful impact on patient management. Second-look laparotomy has also been recommended by many investigators for the routine management of ovarian germ cell tumors (Pippitt *et al.*, 1988; Curtin *et al.*, 1989), although others have questioned its use (Creasman and Soper, 1985; Gershenson *et al.*, 1986a).

The natural history and chemotherapeutic sensitivity of ovarian germ cell tumors are considerably different from their epithelial counterparts. Further, much of the literature devoted to the subject analyzed patients treated before the cisplatin era with a much longer duration of chemotherapy than is commonly given now. With relatively brief courses of cisplatin-based chemotherapy, nearly all patients with early stage disease and many patients with advanced tumor will be cured. In the male counterpart of this disease, testicular germ cell tumors, post-chemotherapy surgery is an important component of the overall management plan. In particular, some of these patients benefit from resection of persistent teratoma after chemotherapy.

To attempt to elucidate the role of reassessment laparotomy, the GOG experience with this procedure in ovarian germ cell tumors was recently reviewed (Williams *et al.*, 1994). All patients in this study were enrolled prospectively on one of three protocols that employed relatively brief cisplatin-based chemotherapy after initial surgical staging and cytoreduction. Of 45 surgical procedures carried out in patients who received three courses of cisplatin-based adjuvant therapy after complete tumor resection (see below), no tumor or mature teratoma was found in 43 and two patients had immature teratoma. One of the latter patients received further chemotherapy and one did not. Both of these patients and 44 of the total are disease free. Of 72 patients treated with similar chemotherapy for advanced incompletely resected tumor, 48 did not have teratoma elements in their primary tumor. At surgery, 45 of these 48 patients had no tumor and three had persistent endodermal sinus tumor or embryonal carcinoma. All three of the latter patients are dead despite further treatment. Teratoma elements were found in the primary tumor of 24 patients. Of these patients, 16 had mature teratoma at second-look, which in seven was bulky or progressive. Of the total 16, 14 remain disease free after surgical resection including six of the seven with bulky residual tumor. The conclusions from this relatively large series were that second-look laparotomy is not necessary in patients who are disease free after their initial surgical procedure or in those patients with advanced tumor that does not contain teratoma. However, enough patients with incompletely resected tumor initially that contains elements of teratoma benefit from the procedure to warrant its general use.

The growing favorable experience with chemotherapy for patients with advanced disease has profound potential ramifications for the management of patients with completely resected tumor. Patients with completely resected ovarian germ cell tumors have a risk of recurrence that ranges from 25% to nearly 100%, depending on cell type and stage (Norris *et al.*, 1976; Williams *et al.*, 1992). These patients routinely have been treated with postoperative adjuvant therapy, which in the era before the introduction of cisplatin was usually VAC or a similar regimen. While not studied in a randomized trial, it is likely that this regimen is effective, but some patients will still have a recurrence. In a trial of the GOG, 100 patients were treated with adjuvant VAC after complete resection of a Stage I, II or III ovarian germ cell tumor; 76 remain free of recurrence (Williams *et al.*, 1989). As cisplatin-based chemotherapy is clearly superior in the management of advanced disease, it seems logical to evaluate this regimen in patients with completely resected tumor.

There have been many anecdotal reports and smaller series that have suggested that cisplatin-based chemotherapy is potentially a more effective surgical adjuvant. The GOG elected to study this topic further in a large multi-institutional trial in early-stage ovarian germ cell tumor patients who were disease free after their initial surgical procedure. Of 93 patients eligible for this trial who received three courses of BEP after thorough surgical staging and complete resection of all known tumor, 89 patients are continuously free of germ cell cancer. Two other patients were found at second-look laparotomy to have small foci of immature teratoma; both remain clinically free of recurrence. One received subsequent alternate chemotherapy and one did not. Therefore, 91 of the 93 patients are currently free of germ cell cancer. Follow-up ranged from 4–90 months with 67 patients followed for more than two years. Acute toxicity was moderate and, notably, there were no serious pulmonary adverse events. It was concluded from this trial that three courses of BEP will nearly always prevent recurrence in well-staged patients with completely resected ovarian germ cell tumors and should be given to all such patients (Williams *et al.*, 1994). Selected 'adjuvant' series are summarized in *Table 17.3.*

Dysgerminoma

Dysgerminoma is the female equivalent of testicular seminoma. It differs from its nondysgerminomatous counterpart in several respects. First, it is probably somewhat more likely to be localized to the ovary at the time of diagnosis. Retroperitoneal nodal spread is more likely than for tumors other than dysgerminoma and intra-abdominal involvement less likely. Bilateral involvement is relatively common, occurring in 10–15% of patients and dysgerminoma is quite sensitive to radiotherapy.

Because of the rarity of dysgerminoma, the published series have tended to be retrospective reviews of patients treated over a many year time period. As such, most patients were not surgically staged as is now recommended. In most series, about 75% had Stage I tumors. However, it is likely that if they were carefully staged, only about two-thirds would have had Stage I disease. Many of these women were treated with postoperative radiotherapy. However, as pelvic radiotherapy is likely associated with a high incidence of sterility, the concept of observation after complete resection of Stage IA tumors was developed. Some investigators have thought that the size of the primary tumor is an important prognostic factor, with patients with tumors larger than 10 cm not being suitable for omission of radiotherapy (Krepart *et al.*, 1978). However, this approach has been challenged and most clinicians now believe that well staged patients with Stage IA involvement can be observed after unilateral salpingo–oophorectomy regardless of the size of the primary tumor if preservation of fertility is an issue and patients are compliant with follow-up (Thomas *et al.*, 1987). Careful follow-up is required because 15–25% will recur. Most recurrences will be noted in the first two years after primary surgery, but occasionally late recurrences are noted many years after initial treatment. Because of the sensitivity of this tumor to chemotherapy, virtually all patients can be successfully salvaged at the time of recurrence, assuming that the recurrence is diagnosed early when the tumor is of small volume.

In the past, many Stage I patients and all patients of higher stage have been treated with radiotherapy. Doses and fields used have varied according to stage and also investigator. In general, the hemi-pelvis or whole pelvis and paraaortic nodes are treated in patients with Stage IA or B disease. For patients with Stage III disease, the extent of radiation depends upon the area of involvement. Patients with retroperitoneal disease receive pelvic and retroperitoneal radiotherapy. Those with intraperitoneal tumor receive whole abdomen radiotherapy. Results of radiation therapy are reasonably good. For example, DePalo *et al.* (1987) report that all 13 stage I patients (12 Stage IA and one Stage IB) are alive and free of disease with a median follow-up of 77 months. Of 12 Stage III patients, the five-year relapse-free survival was 61.4%; overall survival was 89.5%. Median follow-up was 67 months. A number of other authors have reported similar results (Asadourian and Taylor, 1969; Thomas *et al.*, 1987; Bjorkholm *et al.*, 1990)

There is evolving chemotherapy experience in

Table 17.3. Adjuvant chemotherapy.

Institution	*Regimen*	*Prog free/total**	*Reference*
Gynecologic Oncology Group	BEP	89/93	(Williams *et al.*, 1994)
Stanford	PVB	5/5	(Carlson *et al.*, 1983)
Cross Cancer Institute	PVB	4/4	(Taylor *et al.*, 1985)
M.D. Anderson	PVB	4/4	(Gershenson *et al.*, 1986b)
M.D. Anderson	BEP	20/20	(Gershenson *et al.*, 1990)

*Progression-free/total number of patients.

ovarian dysgerminoma. A number of series comprised of small numbers of patients treated with PVB or BEP have reported high complete remission rates in patients with advanced dysgerminoma and excellent results in the adjuvant setting (Smales and Peckham, 1987; Newlands *et al.*, 1982; Gershenson *et al.*, 1990). In 1984, dysgerminoma patients became eligible for GOG chemotherapy protocols for the treatment of advanced ovarian germ cell tumors. Treatment was PVB in the first protocol. The second study is induction chemotherapy with BEP followed by consolidation with VAC. To date, 20 dysgerminoma patients are evaluable on these two protocols. All had Stage III or IV disease and most had suboptimal (more than 2 cm) residual tumor; 11 patients had clinically measurable tumor and ten responded completely. Of 14 patients who underwent second-look laparotomy, the results in all were negative, including the one patient who was only a clinical partial responder. Overall, 19 of the 20 are disease-free with a follow-up of 9–66 months (26 month median) (Williams *et al.*, 1991). It would seem that nearly all patients with advanced dysgerminoma who have not received previous radiation will be durable complete responders. Considering that patients with Stage III dysgerminoma would require extensive radiation and still have some risk of treatment failure and that such patients probably fare worse with subsequent chemotherapy, it is clear that these patients should be treated primarily with chemotherapy.

As discussed previously, second-look laparotomy is not required for patients with advanced disease whose tumors do not contain teratoma and for all patients who have had complete initial surgical resection. Patients with bulky dysgerminoma will frequently have clinically or radiographically detectable residual masses after chemotherapy. These residual masses are almost invariably fibrosis, and these patients do not require post-chemotherapy surgery or radiation.

As for other germ cell tumors, these results may have implications for the management of patients with resected early stage dysgerminoma deemed to require postoperative therapy. Late effects of chemotherapy will be discussed below. However, preliminary evidence is that chemotherapy-treated patients have a reasonably high likelihood of resuming menses and recovering fertility. Adjuvant chemotherapy will almost always prevent relapse in patients with tumors other than dysgerminoma; data are limited in dysgerminoma, but equally favorable. Therefore, patients who have an intact contralateral ovary, tube and uterus and who want to have a child and are deemed to require adjuvant therapy should be treated with chemotherapy and not radiation. It is also likely that similar therapy is also appropriate for patients in whom the fertility issue is moot because of the effectiveness and generally low toxicity of chemotherapy.

The role of tumor markers (HCG and AFP) should be discussed further. There are limited available data in dysgerminoma, but presumably the testicular seminoma experience will apply. In that situation, an HCG elevation is not inconsistent with pure dysgerminoma, but an AFP elevation connotes the presence of other germ cell elements and therapy should be as that given for tumors other than dysgerminoma. Therefore, a diagnosis of dysgerminoma, requires a normal AFP in addition to surgical pathology showing no other elements present.

Late Effects

The prognosis of patients with malignant ovarian germ cell tumors has dramatically improved with the evolution of modern combination chemotherapy. Nearly all these young patients will survive. Therefore, attention has increasingly been focused on the late effects of surgery, radiation, and chemotherapy.

Young patients with malignant ovarian germ cell tumors undergo at least one and sometimes multiple surgical procedures. Future infertility related to pelvic surgery with consequent peritoneal and tubal adhesions is well-described. The surgeon should practice a meticulous surgical technique and avoid unnecessary operative manipulation or maneuvers such as biopsy of a normal contralateral ovary. Another cause of infertility for these patients is unnecessary bilateral salpingo–oophorectomy and hysterectomy. This event will hopefully diminish in frequency as information about the current effectiveness of chemotherapy and the improved prognosis becomes more widely disseminated.

The data about the late effects of radiotherapy in dysgerminoma patients are fairly limited. However, radiotherapy in patients with lymphoma and Hodgkin's disease is associated with premature ovarian failure. The largest formal series of dysgerminoma patients is a retrospective review from M.D. Anderson Hospital (Mitchell *et al.*, 1991). In this study, 43 patients were evaluated by telephone interview and questionnaire. The results obtained were compared to an age-matched control group. The patients had been treated a median of 12.4 years before the study. Compared to controls, the patients had a higher frequency of passage of stools and were more likely to have dyspareunia. However, the general level of satisfaction with sexual function was high and comparable. A total of 19 patients had an intact uterus and at least one ovary. The majority of these patients have regular menses with hormonal support; of six who do not take hormonal support, three have resumed spontaneous menses. No patient had conceived.

The most serious potential late toxicity of chemotherapy is second malignancy, which is primarily acute non-lymphoblastic leukemia. This event is a known all-too-common complication of certain forms of chemotherapy for Hodgkin's disease and other situations characterized by relatively long-term alkylating agent therapy. Recent attention has been focused on the possible association between leukemia and treatment with epipodophylotoxins such as etoposide. The likely association of etoposide (and teneposide) therapy and the late development of leukemia has been noted in male germ cell tumors (Pedersen–Bjergaard *et al.*, 1991), lung cancer (Ratain *et al.*, 1987) and childhood lymphoblastic leukemia (Pui *et al.*, 1991). Many patients with epipodophylotoxin-related leukemia have a characteristic cytogenetic abnormality. The risk of leukemia appears to be related to dose and possibly schedule. In a series of 212 patients with male germ cell tumors, five of 82 patients with a total etoposide dose higher than 2000 mg m^{-2} developed leukemia. None of 130 patients with a total dose below this level were noted to have developed leukemia or myelodysplasia (Pedersen–Bjergaard *et al.*, 1991). In a group of 536 consecutive male germ cell tumor patients at Indiana University treated with etoposide-containing combination chemotherapy, five patients developed acute leukemia (Nichols *et al.*, 1993). Of these, three patients had primary mediastinal germ cell tumors, a situation in which leukemia is known to be part of the natural history. In the GOG adjuvant trial described above (Williams *et al.*, 1994), one of the 93 patients developed acute myelogenous leukemia (AML) that was clinically and morphologically consistent with etoposide-induced leukemia. Another patient developed a low-grade non-Hodgkin's lymphoma more that five years after chemotherapy. Lymphoma is not known to be associated with any of the agents of the BEP regimen nor is it known to be a part of the natural history of ovarian germ cell tumors. It is likely that this was a random event. The development of acute leukemia as a late event in patients treated with BEP is disturbing and mandates careful long-term follow-up, but is unusual, particularly in patients whose total etoposide dose is less than 1500–2000 mg m^{-2}. This rare event does not alter the risk–benefit ratio of treatment with BEP.

Another important consideration is, of course, the impact of chemotherapy on gonadal and reproductive function. There are sparse data about this issue in female germ cell tumor patients. However, anecdotally, many patients will resume menses after chemotherapy and a number of successful pregnancies have been reported. In the only study that has formally addressed this point (Gershenson, 1988), 33 of 40 patients who had an intact contralateral ovary, tube and uterus were having regular menses. Of 16 patients who had attempted pregnancy, 12 had become pregnant and had delivered 22 healthy infants. Many of these patients had received VAC and not cisplatin-based therapy. However, considering the numerous anecdotal reports and this study, it is likely that the likelihood of retaining fertility after treatment with chemotherapy is reasonably good. The impact of cisplatin-based chemotherapy on fertility is an important area for further study.

Other possible chemotherapy late effects include thromboembolic and coronary artery disease, hypertension, paresthesias and Raynaud's phenomenon. There are several case reports of coronary disease and stroke occurring in surprisingly young patients. A recent study has investigated these events in a prospectively-defined patient population. These patients were entered on an international study that investigated therapeutic alternatives in early-stage testicular cancer patients. The details of the treatment study have been published elsewhere (Williams *et al.*, 1987). In brief, there were three groups of patients that were defined prospectively. The first group received no chemotherapy. The second group received two courses of adjuvant cisplatin-containing treatment. The third group of patients received no chemotherapy initially, but later relapsed and were treated for metastatic disease with four courses of similar chemotherapy. Median follow-up was 5.1 years; information was collected by a patient-completed questionnaire. Treated patients had a significantly increased incidence of paresthesias. Cardiovascular disease was rare and of similar incidence in the chemotherapy-treated and untreated patients (Nichols *et al.*, 1992).

Stromal Tumors of the Ovary

Malignant stromal tumors of the ovary may be classified as either sex-cord or nonspecific in origin. Among the former are the lesions of the granulosa–stromal cell group, the Sertoli–stromal cell group and a few other rare lesions (*Table 17.4*). The nonspecific stromal tumors include mesenchymal tumors such as leiomyosarcoma and lymphoma, which arise from tissues that are not unique to the ovary.

Sex-cord–stromal tumors probably arise from the specialized mesenchyme of the embryonic genital ridge. Although many are benign, granulosa cell, Sertoli's cell and sex-cord tumors with annular tubules may be malignant.

Granulosa–Stromal Cell Tumors

The tumors are made up of granulosa cells and other components, such as theca cells of fibroblasts, and comprise approximately 2% of all ovarian neoplasms. The two most common lesions are the adult-type granulosa cell tumor (95%) and the juvenile granulosa cell tumor (5%).

Adult granulosa cell tumors occur in the perimenopausal years with a mean age of 50–53 years. Nonspecific symptoms such as abdominal

Table 17.4. Sex-cord–stromal tumors (adapted from Young and Scully, 1988).

Granulosa–stromal cell tumor
Granulosa cell tumor
Adult type
Juvenile type
Thecoma–fibroma group
Thecoma
Fibroma
Fibrosarcoma
Others
Sertoli–stromal tumors
Sertoli's cell tumor
Leydig's cell tumor
Sertoli–Leydig cell tumor
Gynandroblastoma
Sex-cord tumor with annular tubules
Unclassified

distension, pain or mass are common. Acute rupture with hemoperitoneum occurs in 10% of cases. Endocrine manifestations are observed in as many as 75% of patients. Most granulosa cell tumors produce estrogen and may cause symptoms such as amenorrhea, oligomenorrhea, menometrorrhagia, breast tenderness or postmenopausal bleeding. Occasionally, progesterone or androgens are secreted. The latter may result in virilization or hirsutism.

Endometrial changes ranging from atrophy to frank adenocarcinoma are observed. The incidence of hyperplasia may exceed 50% and endometrial adenocarcinoma may accompany adult granulosa cell tumors in up to 13% of cases (Evans *et al.*, 1980).

Grossly, these tumors vary greatly in size and may be discovered incidentally at the time of laparotomy for other indications or be large enough to visibly distend the abdoman. The average diameter is about 12 cm. Microscopically, granulosa cells are uniform in size and shape and possess a characteristic grooved nuclear membrane. Diverse numbers of theca cells and fibroblasts may accompany the granulosa cells.

Of adult granulosa cell tumors, 90% are Stage I at the time of diagnosis and less than 5% are bilateral (Bjorkholm and Silfversward, 1980). The spread pattern is similar to that of epithelial ovarian tumors and may include peritoneal surfaces or retroperitoneal lymph nodes. Conservative surgery is indicated in women who wish subsequent pregnancy, providing the tumor is adequately staged. Extirpation of the internal genitalia upon completion of childbearing is recommended. Isolated recurrences in the paraaortic lymph node chain suggest that appropriate staging is important at the primary operation. The propensity for late recurrences after primary therapy is a hallmark of adult granulosa cell tumors. Of 22 patients with a recurrence in the Mayo Clinic series (Evans *et al.*, 1980) five (23%) did so more than 13 years after the initial diagnosis.

Among Stage I tumors, size may be an important prognostic indicator. Fox *et al.* (1975) reported 100% ten-year survival for patients with tumors that were less than 5 cm in diameter, compared with 53% survival in patients with tumors exceeding 15 cm in diameter. Stenwig *et al.* (1978) observed similar survival rates (86.6% and 53.2%, respectively). Rupture of Stage I cancers was found to adversely affect survival (Bjorkholm and Silfversward, 1980). Although mitotic count was not a significant factor in Stage I tumors in this study, mitotic count and the degree of nuclear atypia were inversely correlated with survival in Stages II–IV. Poor survival (49% and 26% at ten years, respectively) was associated with higher stages in the series of Stenweg *et al.* (1979) and Bjorkholm and Silfversward (1980).

There is no evidence that adjunctive therapy for completely resected adult granulosa cell tumors is effective in reducing the risk of recurrence. Although the majority (122/180) of patients with Stage I disease in the study by Bjorkholm and Silfversward (1980) received postoperative radiotherapy, Stenwig *et al.* (1979) observed no difference in survival between 63 patients treated with surgery and radiotherapy and 51 treated with surgery alone. The value of adjunctive chemotherapy has never been assessed in patients with adult granulosa cell tumors. Since the risk of relapse in such patients with Stage I disease is low, most advocate no postoperative therapy.

Many drugs have been used in the treatment of patients with advanced or recurrent disease, although none has received a formal trial. Smith and Rutledge (1970) reported partial responses in six of 15 patients treated with alkylating agents. Two complete responses of 27 and 35 months' duration were described by Schwartz and Smith (1976) in patients receiving actinomycin D, 5-fluorouracil and cyclophosphamide. Three complete responses were observed among 13 patients treated with the same agents in a GOG trial (Slayton *et al.*, 1980). Colombo (1986) reported six complete and three partial responses in 11 patients with granulosa cell tumors treated with cisplatin, vinblastine and bleomycin. Response duration ranged from 6–36 months with a median of 13 months. The GOG is studying cisplatin, bleomycin and etoposide in attenuated doses in patients with advanced or recurrent disease.

Juvenile granulosa cell tumors are associated with sexual precocity in 80% of cases and account for 10% of cases of this syndrome in females (Young *et al.*, 1984). The lesions are confined to one ovary in approximately 98% of cases and are generally appreciable on abdominal or rectal examination. Although histologic findings may suggest an aggressive nature, tumors confined to the ovary generally have a favorable prognosis and may be treated by surgical excision alone.

Sertoli–Stromal Cell Tumors

These tumors are composed of Sertoli cells, Leydig cells and fibroblasts in varying proportions. They account for 0.5% of all ovarian cancers and have been termed androblastomas or arrhenoblastomas. Pure Leydig's cell tumors may cause virilization and are nearly always benign. Sertoli–Leydig tumors are subclassified according to the degree of histologic differentiation and cause virilization in about one-third of cases. The vast majority (98.5%) are unilateral and if well-differentiated rarely spread beyond the ovary of origin.

Prognosis is directly related to stage, with lesions of Stage II or greater associated with a grim prognosis despite therapy (Young, 1985); rupture of Stage I tumors of intermediate differentiation was associated with malignant behavior in 86% of cases compared with 45% of those remaining intact.

Surgery alone is adequate therapy for Stage I well-differentiated lesions. Radiotherapy and chemotherapy have been used with mixed results. Schwartz and Smith (1976) reported two complete responses of long duration in patients treated with vincristine, actinomycin D and cyclophosphamide.

Non-specific Stromal Tumors

Other non-epithelial tumors that rarely exhibit primarily ovarian involvement include carcinoid tumor, lymphoma and sarcoma. As opposed to their enteric counterparts, carcinoid tumors may produce carcinoid syndrome without hepatic involvement. They typically have only ovarian involvement only at the time of diagnosis and are treated by surgical excision.

Rarely, lymphoma patients will have ovarian involvement as the primary manifestation of disease. The diagnosis is ordinarily established at the time of surgery for an adnexal mass. Careful pathologic evaluation is of course indicated because the pathology of these tumors is sometimes quite difficult. Ordinarily a systemic disease process, malignant lymphomas are treated with the systemic chemotherapy used for lymphoma in general. The outcome of treatment is related to the specific type of lymphoma and the stage at diagnosis.

Ovarian sarcomas are rare and the most common histologic type is mixed müllerian tumor. Clinical presentation is very similar to that for epithelial ovarian cancer, but the mean age at diagnosis is about 65 years, which is about five years greater than that of patients with epithelial tumors. Surgical resection and appropriate staging are important and although the prognosis is poor, these patients benefit from systemic chemotherapy (Prendiville *et al.*, 1994).

Summary of Management Options

- Ideally, patients with ovarian germ cell tumors will have undergone initial thorough surgical staging as well as resection of the primary tumor and appropriate debulking. If at all possible, the contralateral ovary, tube and uterus should be preserved.
- Patients with tumors other than dysgerminoma and complete tumor resection should receive three courses of bleomycin, etoposide, platinol (BEP) with the exception of those with Stage I Grade I immature teratoma. Patients with incompletely resected tumor should probably receive four courses.
- Second-look laparotomy is not necessary except for those patients with incompletely resected immature teratoma.
- The majority of dysgerminoma patients have Stage IA disease at diagnosis. These patients can be treated with unilateral salpingo–oophorectomy and careful observation with regular pelvic examinations, abdominal computerized tomography and tumor markers.
- For dysgerminoma patients who have more advanced disease at diagnosis or for observed Stage I patients who develop a recurrence, systemic chemotherapy has replaced radiotherapy as the treatment of choice.
- Second-look laparotomy is not necessary, even for the dysgerminoma patient with a persistent radiographically-apparent mass that has not progressed.
- A special management problem is posed by patients who have dysgerminoma that has occurred in the setting of dysgenetic ovaries or gonadoblastoma. Fertility is not generally an issue in these patients and both ovaries should be removed with appropriate postoperative treatment depending on surgical stage.
- Of adult granulosa cell tumors 90% are Stage I at the time of diagnosis and less than 5% are bilateral. The spread pattern is similar to that of epithelial ovarian tumors and may include peritoneal surfaces and retroperitoneal lymph nodes. Conservative surgery is indicated in women who want a subsequent pregnancy, providing the tumor is adequately staged.

- The propensity for late recurrences after primary therapy is a hallmark of adult granulosa cell tumors.
- There is no evidence that adjunctive therapy for completely resected adult granulosa cell' tumors is effective in reducing the risk of recurrence.
- Juvenile granulosa cell tumors are associated with sexual precocity in 80% of cases and account for 10% of cases of this syndrome in females. The lesions are confined to one ovary in approximately 98% of cases.
- Although histologic findings may suggest an aggressive nature, juvenile granulosa tumors confined to the ovary generally have a favorable prognosis and may be treated by surgical excision alone.

References

Asadourian LA & Taylor HB (1969) Dysgerminoma: An analysis of 105 cases. *Obstet. Gynecol.* **33:** 370–376.

Bjorkholm E, Lundell M, Gyftodimos A & Silfversward C (1990) Dysgerminoma: the Radiumhemmet series 1927–1984. *Cancer* **65:** 38–44.

Bjorkjolm E & Silfversward C (1980) Prognostic factors in granulosa-cell tumors. *Gynecol. Oncol.* **11:** 261–274.

Bosl GJ, Gluckman R, Geller NL *et al.* (1986) VAB-6: An effective chemotherapy regimen for patients with germ-cell tumors. *J. Clin. Oncol.* **4(10):** 1493–1499.

Carlson RW, Sikic BI, Turbow MM & Ballon SC (1983) Combination cisplatin, vinblastine and bleomycin chemotherapy (PVB) for malignant germ-cell tumors of the ovary. *J. Clin. Oncol.* **1:** 645–651.

Colombo N, Sessa C, Landoni F *et al.* (1986) Cisplatin, vinblastrie, and bleomycin combination chemotherapy in metastatic granulosa cell tumor of the ovary. *Obstet. Gynecol.* **67:** 265–268.

Creasman, WT & Soper JT (1985) Assessment of the contemporary management of germ cell malignancies of the ovary. *Am. J. Obstet. Gynecol.* **153:** 828–834.

Curtin, JP, Rubin SC, Hoskins WJ *et al.* (1989) Second-look laparotomy in endodermal sinus tumor: A report of two patients with normal levels of alpha-fetoprotein and residual tumor at reexploration. *Obstet. Gynecol.* **73:** 893.

DePalo G, Lattuada A, Kenda R *et al.* (1987) Germ cell tumors of the ovary: The experience of the National Cancer Institute of Milan. I. Dysgerminoma. *Int. J. Radiat. Biol. Phy.* **13:** 853–860.

Evans AJ, Gaffey TA, Malkasian GD Jr & Annegers JF (1980) Clinicopathological review of 118 granulosa and 82 theca cell tumors. *Obstet. Gynecol.* **55:** 231–238.

Fox H, Agrawal K & Langley FA (1975) A clinicopathological study of 92 cases of granulosa cell tumor of the ovary with special reference to the factors infuencing prognosis. *Cancer* **35:** 231–241.

Gershenson DM (1988) Menstrual and reproductive function after treatment with combination chemotherapy for malignant ovarian germ cell tumors. *J. Clin. Oncol.* **6:** 270–275.

Gershenson DM, Copeland LJ & Del Junco G (1986a) Second-look laparotomy in the management of malignant germ cell tumors of the ovary. *Obstet. Gynecol.* **67:** 789–794.

Gershenson DM, Kavanaugh JJ, Copeland LJ *et al.* (1986b) Treatment of malignant nondysgerminomatous germ cell tumors of the ovary with vinblastine, bleomycin, and cisplatin. *Cancer* **57:** 1731–1737.

Gershenson DM, Morris M, Cangir A *et al.* (1990) Treatment of malignant germ cell tumors of the ovary with bleomycin, etoposide, and cisplatin. *J. Clin. Oncol.* **8:** 715–720.

Krepart G, Smith JP, Rutledge F & Declos L (1978) The treatment for dysgerminoma of the ovary. *Cancer* **41:** 986–990.

Loehrer PJ, Williams SD & Einhorn LH (1989) Testicular Cancer: The quest continues. *J. Nat. Cancer Inst.* **80:** 1373–1382.

■ Mitchell MF, Gershenson DM, Soeters RP *et al.* (1991) The long-term effects of radiotherapy on patients with ovarian dysgerminoma. *Cancer* **67:** 1084–1090.

Newlands ES, Begent RHJ, Rustin GJS & Bagshawe KD (1982) Potential for cure in metastatic ovarian teratomas and dysgerminomas. *Br. J. Obstet. Gynaecol.* **89:** 555–560.

Nichols CR, Breeden ES, Loehrer PJ *et al.* (1993) Secondary leukemia associated with a conventional dose of etoposide: review of serial germ cell tumor protocols. *J. Natl. Cancer Inst.* **85:** 36–40.

Nichols CR, Roth BJ, Williams SD *et al.* (1992) No evidence of acute cardiovascular complications of chemotherapy for testicular cancer: an analysis of the Testicular Cancer Intergroup Study. *J. Clin. Oncol.* **10:** 760–765.

Norris HJ, Zirkin HJ & Benson WL (1976) Immature (malignant) teratoma of the ovary. *Cancer* **37:** 2359–2372.

Pedersen–Bjergaard J, Hansen SW, Larsen SO *et al.* (1991) Increased risk of myelodysplasia and leukaemia after etoposide, cisplatin, and bleomycin for germ-cell tumours. *Lancet* **338:** 359–363.

Pippitt CH, Cain JM, Hakes TB *et al.* (1988) Primary chemotherapy and the role of second-look laparotomy in nondysgerminomatous germ cell malignancies of the ovary. *Gynecol. Oncol.* **31:** 268.

Prendiville J, Murphy D, Renninson J, Buckley H & Crowther D (1994) Carcinosarcoma of the ovary treated over a 10-year period at the Christie Hospital. *Int. J. Gynecol. Cancer* **4:** 200–205.

Pui C, Ribeiro RC, Hancock MI *et al.* (1991) Acute myeloid leukemia in children treated with epipodophyllotoxins for acute lymphoblastic leukemia. *N. Engl. J. Med.* **325:** 1682–1687.

Ratain MJ, Kaminer LS, Bitran JD *et al.* (1987) Acute nonlymphocytic leukemia following etoposide and cisplatin combination chemotherapy for advanced non-small-cell carcinoma of the lung. *Blood* **70:** 1412–1417.

Schwartz PE & Smith JP (1976) Treatment of ovarian stromal tumors. *Am. J. Obstet. Gynecol.* **125:** 402–409.

Slayton RE, Johnson G, Brady L & Blessing J (1980) Radiotherapy or chemotherapy in malignant stromal tumors of the ovary. *Proc. Am. Soc. Clin. Oncol.* 430.

Slayton RE, Park RC, Silverberg SG *et al.* (1985) Vincristine, dactinomycin, and cyclophosphamide in the treatment of malignant germ cell tumors of the ovary: a Gynecologic Oncology Group study (a final report). *Cancer* **56:** 243–248.

Smales E & Peckham MJ (1987) Chemotherapy of germ-cell ovarian tumors: first-line treatment of etoposide, bleomycin and cisplatin or carboplatin. *Eur. J. Can. Clin. Oncol.* **23:** 469–474.

Smith JP & Rutledge F (1970) Chemotherapy in the treatment of carcinoma of the ovary. *Am. J. Obstet. Gynecol.* **107:** 691–700.

Stenwig JT, Hazekamp JT & Beecham JB (1979) Granulosa cell tumors of the ovary. A clinopathological study of 118 cases with long-term follow-up. *Gynecol. Oncol.* **7:** 136–152.

Taylor MD, Depetrillo AD & Turner AR (1985) Vinblastine, bleomycin, and cisplatin in malignant germ cell tumors of the ovary. *Cancer* **56:** 1341–1349.

■ Thomas GM, Dembo AJ, Hacker NF & Depetrillo AD (1987) Current therapy for dysgerminoma of the ovary. *Obstet. Gynecol.* **70:** 268–275.

Williams SD, Birch R, Einhorn LH *et al.* (1987) Disseminated germ cell tumors: chemotherapy with cisplatin plus bleomycin plus either vinblastine or etoposide. *N. Engl. J. Med.* **316:** 1435–1440.

■ Williams S, Blessing JA, Liao S *et al.* (1994) Ajuvant therapy of ovarian germ cell tumors with cisplatin, etoposide, and bleomycin: a trial of the Gynecologic Oncology Group. *J. Clin. Oncol.* **12:** 701–706.

■ Williams SD, Blessing J, Slayton R *et al.* (1989) Ovarian germ cell tumors: adjuvant trials of the Gynecologic Oncology Group. *Proc. Amer. Soc. Clin. Oncol.* **8:** 150.

Williams SD, Blessing JA, DiSaia PJ *et al.* (1994) Second-look laparotomy in ovarian germ cell tumors: the Gynecologic Oncology Group experience. *Gynecol. Oncol.* **52:** 287–291.

Williams SD, Blessing JA, Hatch KD & Homesley HD (1991) Chemotherapy of advanced dysgerminoma: trials of the Gyncecologic Oncology Group. *J. Clin. Oncol.* **9:** 1950–1955.

Williams SD, Blessing JA, Moore DH *et al.* (1989) Cisplatin, vinblastine, and bleomycin in advanced and recurrent ovarian germ-cell tumors. *Ann. Int. Med.* **111:** 22–27.

■ Williams SD, Gershenson DM, Horowitz CJ & Scully RE (1992) Ovarian germ cell and stromal tumors. In: Hoskins W, Perez CA & Young RC (eds) *Principles and Practice of Gynecologic Oncology* pp. 715–730. Philadelpha: PA, JB Lippincott.

Williams SD, Stablein DM, Einhorn LH *et al.* (1987) Immediate adjuvant chemotherapy versus observation with treatment at relapse in pathological stage II testicular cancer. *New. Engl. J. Med.* **317:** 1433–1438.

Young RH, Dickersin GR & Scully RE (1984) Juvenile granulosa cell tumor of the ovary. A clinicopathological analysis of 125 cases. *Am. J. Surg. Pathol.* **8:** 575.

Young RH & Scully RE (1985) Ovarian Sertoli-Leydig cell tumors. *Am. J. Surg. Path.* **9:** 543–569.

Young RH & Scully RE (1987) Ovarian sertoli-leydig cell tumors. A clinicopathological analysis of 207 cases. *Am. J. Surg. Pathol.* **3:** 277.

Young RH & Scully RE (1988) Sex-cord-stromal, steroid cell, and other ovarian tumors with endocrine, para-endocrine, and paraneoplastic manifestations. In: Kurman RJ (ed.) *Blaustein's Pathology of the Female Genital Tract*, pp. 607–658. New York: Springer-Verlag.

18 Cancer of the Fallopian Tube

G Deppe

Introduction

Primary carcinoma of the fallopian tube is a rare malignancy accounting for 0.18–1.8% of all gynecologic malignancies (Hu *et al., 1950; McMurray et al.*, 1986). Approximately more than 1200 cases have been reported in the literature (Hurlbutt and Nelson, 1963; McMurray *et al.*, 1986; Tokunaga *et al.*, 1991). The experience of any one institution is limited. The average annual incidence of fallopian tube malignancy was found to be 3.6 per million women in an analysis of nine population-based cancer registries in the USA. Caucasian women had a 14% higher rate than Afro–American women (Rosenblatt *et al.*, 1989). Most fallopian tube cancers occur in women aged 52–64 years (Sedlis, 1978; Rosenblatt *et al.*, 1989).

The etiology of fallopian tube cancer is unknown. No risk factors have been identified. There is no causal relationship between tubal carcinoma and the commonly found chronic salpingitis.

Clinical Features

Most patients with fallopian tube carcinoma present with vaginal bleeding or discharge or abdominal pain or pressure (Yoonessi, 1979; Podratz *et al.*, 1986; Pfeiffer *et al.*, 1989; Pakisch *et al.*, 1990) (*Table 18.1*).

Hydrops tubae profluens refers to a syndrome characterized by a profuse, serous, watery, yellow intermittent discharge following colicky pelvic pain. This suggests a diagnosis of fallopian tube carcinoma (Sedlis, 1978) and is thought to be secondary to filling and emptying of a partially blocked tube. The pain is caused by tubal distension. Adenocarcinoma cells in cervical Pap smears, but negative findings at endometrial curettage, were found to be present in 10–20% of patients with tubal carcinomas (Fidler *et al.*, 1954; Yoonessi, 1979).

Frequent physical signs at presentation are a pelvic mass, abdominal mass and ascites (Yoonessi, 1979; Eddy *et al.*, 1984; Pakisch *et al.*, 1990). Correct preoperative diagnosis of fallopian tube carcinoma is uncommon (Eddy *et al.*, 1984; Podratz *et al.*, 1986). The diagnosis is usually established during laparotomy performed for a pelvic mass believed to be an ovarian or uterine neoplasm, fibroids or pelvic inflammatory disease. Computed tomography (CT) and magnetic resonance imaging (MRI) findings are usually not sensitive enough in the preoperative work-up to differentiate and locate the pelvic mass more accurately. However, higher resolution obtained by transvaginal ultrasound may be more helpful than CT in the diagnosis of suspected tubal carcinoma (Ajjimakorn and Bhamarapravati, 1991).

Pathology

The gross and microscopic features of fallopian tube carcinoma are similar to those of epithelial ovarian cancer. On gross examination the cancerous tube is usually diffusely swollen and sausage-shaped with fimbrial occlusion, often resembling hydrosalpinx, hematosalpinx or pyosalpinx (*Figure 18.1*). The lesion is present with equal frequency in the left or right tube. Most tumors arise in the ampullary region.

Differentiation between a primary tubal or primary ovarian malignancy can be extremely difficult. The vast majority are papillary serous adenocarcinoma. Histologically, the tumors were graded as papillary, alveolar or medullary adenocarcinoma (Hu *et al.*, 1950). This grading system is rarely used today. Most pathologists report the histologic grade as well-, moderate- or poorly-differentiated. The degree of histologic differentiation appears to be of less prognostic value than the stage of the tumor at presentation (Hanton *et al.*, 1966; Pfeiffer *et al.*, 1989) (*Figure 18.2*).

The ultrastructure of adenocarcinoma of the fallopian tube is similar to that of ovarian serous papillary carcinoma (Rorat and Fenoglio, 1976). No distinctive immunohistochemical parameters can differentiate fallopian tube malignancy from ovarian and other primary malignancies. Cancer antigen-125 (CA-125) can be detected immunohistochemically in benign and malignant lesions of ovary and fallopian tube (Neunteufel and Breitenecker, 1989). Principal diagnostic criteria suggested by Finn and Javert (1949), later modified by Hu *et al. (1950) and Sedlis (1978) may help in determining a tubal origin* (*Table 18.2*).

Spread

The pattern of spread of fallopian tube carcinoma is similar to that of epithelial ovarian cancer, occurring frequently by contiguous growth and intraperitoneal implantation. It may spread into the

Table 18.1. Most frequent presenting symptoms and signs of fallopian tube cancer.

- Vaginal bleeding or discharge
- Abdominopelvic pain or pressure
- Pelvic mass

Table 18.2. Pathologic criteria for diagnosis of primary fallopian tube malignancy.

- Main tumor is in the fallopian tube and arises from the endosalpinx
- Histologic pattern resembling the epithelium is identified
- Transition from benign to malignant epithelium should be present
- Ovaries and endometrium are either normal or contain a tumor that is smaller than the tumor in the tube

endometrial cavity or through the tubal ostium to the pelvic peritoneum, bowel or omentum. The fallopian tubes are supplied with a rich lymphatic network draining mainly through the mesosalpinx and infundibulopelvic ligaments into the paraaortic lymph nodes and occasionally via the lymphatics of the round ligaments to the inguinal nodes. Tamimi and Figge (1981) found paraaortic lymph node metastases in 33% of their patients.

Staging

The stage of disease is important in determining the prognosis of patients with fallopian tube cancer. It was only in 1991 that the International Federation of Gynecology and Obstetrics (FIGO) provided a standardized staging system for primary tubal carcinoma for the first time (see *Table 47.5*). It follows the ovarian cancer staging and is based on operative findings before tumor debulking.

Tumor Markers

As in ovarian cancer elevated serum CA-125 levels have been detected in patients with adenocarcinoma of the fallopian tube (Niloff *et al.*, 1984; Tokunaga *et al.*, 1989; Lootsma–Miklosova *et al.*, 1987; Kol *et al.*, 1990; Davies *et al.*, 1991). CA-125 titers (>35 u/ml) may predict the presence of tumor and can be used for monitoring the response to therapy or lack of it. Retroperitoneal lymph node metastases in patients with tubal cancer have been diagnosed through immunolymphoscintigraphy with the use of labeled fragments of monoclonal antibody OC-125 antibodies (Lehtovirta *et al.*, 1990).

Treatment

Due to the rarity of fallopian tube cancer no prospective controlled trials of treatment protocols have been carried out. Management has been individualized and has generally been similar to that of ovarian carcinoma.

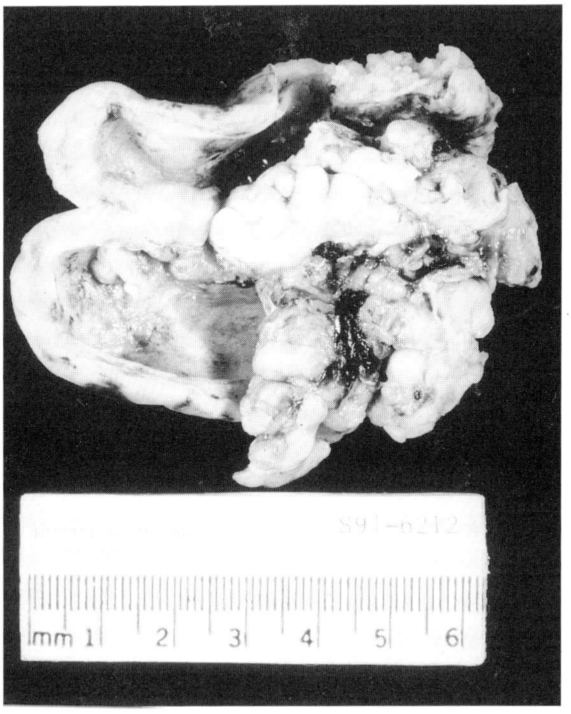

Figure 18.1. Papillary serous adenocarcinoma of the fallopian tube cut section reveals soft friable proliferating papillae.

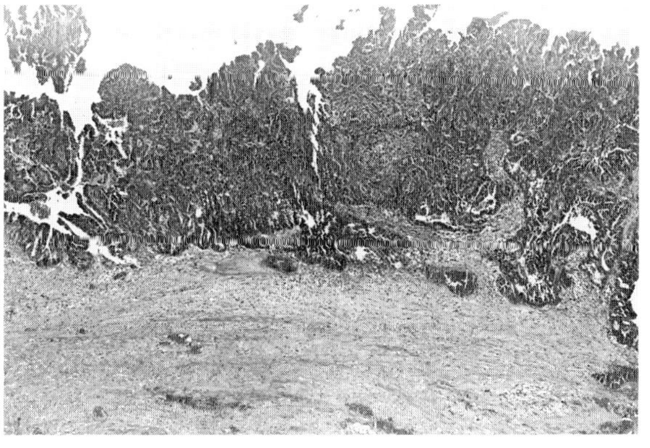

Figure 18.2. Papillary serous adenocarcinoma of the fallopian tube. Histologic appearance reveals prominent fibrous stalk and non-mucin producing neoplastic epithelial cells.

Table 18.3. Surgical management of fallopian tube cancer.

Peritoneal cytologic testing
Evaluation of extent of cancer
Pelvic/peritoneal surfaces
Diaphragm
Omentum
Aortic and pelvic lymph nodes
Total abdominal hysterectomy, bilateral salpingo–oophorectomy (unless there is desire for future childbearing in patients with Stage IA fallopian tube carcinoma), pelvic and aortic lymph node sampling, infracolic omentectomy and removal of all tumor possible

Surgery

Surgery is the cornerstone of initial treatment for primary fallopian tube carcinoma is surgery (*Table 18.3*). Patients should undergo a total abdominal hysterectomy and bilateral salpingo–oophorectomy. If there is no evidence of gross tumor spread, a selective pelvic and paraaortic lymphadenectomy and total omentectomy along with peritoneal washings should be performed. In patients with gross metastatic disease an effort should be made to remove as much tumor as possible. Unilateral salpingo–oophorectomy may be considered in patients with Stage IA well-differentiated fallopian tube cancer if complete surgical staging yields no other evidence of tumor and the patient wants to preserve her reproductive function.

Radiation Therapy

Radiation therapy has frequently been used in the treatment of patients with fallopian tube carcinoma (Henderson *et al.*, 1977; McMurray *et al.*, 1986; Podratz *et al.*, 1986; Peters *et al.*, 1988; Nordin, 1994). Definitive conclusions about its efficacy cannot be made because of difference in staging, type of surgical procedure and variability of technique of radiation used. A review of the literature failed to show a survival benefit from adjuvant pelvic radiotherapy (Roberts and Lifshitz, 1982).

Results from the Mayo Clinic suggested an improved survival with whole abdominal irradiation in patients with limited disease (Podratz *et al.*, 1986). The use of intraperitoneal radiocolloids or whole abdominal radiation with pelvic boost might be considered only for optimally debulked patients and for Stage I disease.

Chemotherapy

Systematic evaluation of chemotherapy has been restricted by the small numbers of patients available for treatment. Many reports in the literature were single case descriptions. These patients had previously been treated unsuccessfully with radiation therapy and surgery. Single alkylating agents such as thiotepa and melphalan alone or in combination with progestins have been reported to produce short-term responses. The rationale for the use of progestins was the histologic similarity of the tubal epithelium to the uterine endometrium and its similar cyclic response to the normal ovarian cycle (Boronow, 1973; Yoonessi, 1979; Deppe 1990).

Since 1980, cisplatin-containing combination chemotherapy regimens, mostly using cisplatin (50–100 mg m^{-2}) plus cyclophosphamide (500–600 mg m^{-2}) with or without doxorubicin (50 mg m^{-2}) have produced response rates ranging from 53–87%, with approximately 50% of patients with advanced stage surviving five years (Deppe *et al.*, 1980; Jacobs *et al.*, 1985; McMurray *et al.*, 1986; Peters *et al.*, 1989; Muntz *et al.*, 1989; Morris *et al.*, 1990; Rose *et al.*, 1990; Podratz *et al.*, 1986; Maxson *et al.*, 1987; Pakisch *et al.*, 1990; Nordin, 1994) (*Table 18.4*). Because of the clinical and histologic similarity between tubal and epithelial ovarian cancer patients response rates and survival are expected to be similar if treated with either the cisplatin (50–100 mg m^{-2}) or carboplatin (300–400 mg m^{-2}) combination chemotherapy (Pectasides *et al.*, 1994). Patients who are treated with carboplatin have a lower incidence of nausea, vomiting, peripheral neuropathy, renal toxicity and ototoxicity, but greater myelosuppression. There are no reports of taxol for tubal cancer, but one would anticipate that the platinum plus taxol combination will have a significant role in the treatment of this disease.

Second-look Surgery

Second-look laparotomy is defined as an exploratory laparotomy performed on a patient who is clinically free of disease and has a normal CA-125 following a prescribed course of chemotherapy. Its role in the management of fallopian tube carcinoma is debatable. It allows more accurate assessment of

Table 18.4. Suggested postsurgical treatment of adenocarcinoma of the fallopian tube.

Stage	*Therapy*
IA	None
IB and IC	Intraperitoneal ^{32}P or three courses of platinum-containing regimen
I–III (only if optimally debulked)	Six courses of platinum-containing regimen or whole abdominal radiation with pelvic boost
IV	Six courses of platinum-containing combination chemotherapeutic regimens

tumor status, permits secondary tumor debulking and provides important prognostic information. The influence of this procedure on survival appears to be limited. In the Memorial experience with 35 patients together with a collected series of 51 patients in the literature who underwent a second-look laparotomy for fallopian tube carcinoma following chemotherapy, approximately 80% of patients with a negative second-look procedure following platinum-based chemotherapy remained disease free. A second-look laparotomy was recommended for patients with Stage II–IV tubal cancer (Barakat *et al.*, 1993).

Sarcomas

Sarcomas of the fallopian tube are exceedingly rare (Imachi *et al.*, 1992; Jacoby *et al.*, 1993; Carlson *et al.*, 1993; Zorlu *et al.*, 1994), most constituting a malignant mixed müllerian tumor. Only 37 cases have been reported (Zorlu *et al.*, 1994) and of these only 16 contained heterologous components. Sarcomas have been found predominantly in postmenopausal women, and most patients present with advanced disease. Treatment should be surgery followed by postoperative chemotherapy with cisplatin combination chemotherapy.

Summary

Substantial progress has been made in understanding the biologic behavior of fallopian tube cancer and in assessing the disease status with transvaginal sonography and CA-125. However, most cases will only be diagnosed intraoperatively. A staging classification (FIGO) based on adequate surgical staging has been introduced. Because of the rarity of the disease, the currently used treatment strategies for epithelial ovarian cancer including the importance of surgical staging, the need for surgical debulking, the use of platinum-based combination chemotherapy, the role of second-look laparotomy and consolidation treatment are being employed. Five-year survival rates of 50% have been reported for patients with Stage III and IV fallopian tube cancer (Barakat *et al.*, 1991).

Summary of Management Options

- Total abdominal hysterectomy, bilateral salpingo–oophorectomy, peritoneal cytologic testing and selective pelvic and aortic lymphadenectomy is recommended for Stage I lesions.
- Unilateral salpingo–oophorectomy may be performed for a young women desirous of further childbearing found to have a Stage IA well-differentiated carcinoma of the fallopian tube.
- Total abdominal hysterectomy with bilateral salpingo–oophorectomy and removal of all gross tumor with an attempt to debulk all tumor deposits to 1 cm or smaller is recommended for patients with Stage II–IV disease.
- Whole abdominal radiation with pelvic boost or intraperitoneal colloids is effective for patients with negative nodes and minimal (<1 cm) residual disease.
- No postoperative therapy is needed for patients with unilateral well-differentiated tumors limited to tubal mucosa and negative peritoneal cytology.
- Combination chemotherapy consisting of cisplatin (50–100 mg m^{-2}) plus cyclophosphamide (500–600 mg m^{-2}) with or without doxorubicin (50 mg m^{-2}) every 3–4 weeks for 6–8 courses has produced complete responses and long-term survivals.
- A second look operation should be considered for patients with Stage II–IV tubal cancer.

References

Ajjimakorn S & Bhamarapravati Y (1991) Transvaginal ultrasound and the diagnosis of fallopian tubal carcinoma. *J. Clin. Ultrasound* **19:** 116–119.

Barakat RR, Rubin SC, Saigo PE *et al.* (1991) Cisplatin-based combination chemotherapy in carcinoma of the fallopian tube. *Gynecol. Oncol.* **42:** 156–166.

Barakat RR, Rubin SC, Saigo PE *et al.* (1993) Second-look laparotomy in carcinoma of the fallopian tube. *Obstet. Gynecol.* **82:** 748–751.

Boronow RC (1973) Chemotherapy for disseminated tubal cancer. *Obstet. Gynecol.* **42:** 62–66.

Carlson JA Jr, Ackerman BL & Wheeler JE (1993) Malignant mixed müllerian tumor of the fallopian tube. *Cancer* **71:** 187–192.

Davies AP, Fish A, Woodas R & Oram D (1991) Raised serum CA-125 preceding the diagnosis of carcinoma of the fallopian tube: Two case reports. *Br. J. Obstet. Gynecol.* **98:** 602–603.

Deppe G, Bruckner HW & Cohen CJ (1980) Combination chemotherapy for advanced carcinoma of the fallopian tube. *Obstet. Gynecol.* **56:** 530–532.

■ Deppe G (1990) Chemotherapy of fallopian tube neoplasm.

In: Deppe G (ed) *Chemotherapy of Gynecologic Cancer*, pp. 251–263. New York: Wiley–Liss.

■ Eddy GL, Copeland LJ & Gershenson DM (1984) Fallopian tube carcinoma. *Obstet. Gynecol.* **64:** 546–552.

Fidler HK, Loch DR & Van Couver BC (1954) Carcinoma of the fallopian tube detected by cervical smear. *Am. J. Obstet. Gynecol.* **67:** 1103–1111.

Finn WF & Javert CT (1949) Primary and metastatic cancer of the fallopian tube. *Cancer* **2:** 803–814.

Hanton EM, Malkasian GD JR, Dahlin DC *et al.* (1966) Primary carcinoma of the fallopian tube. *Am. J. Obstet. Gynecol.* **94:** 832–839.

Henderson SR, Harper RC, Salazar OM *et al.* (1977) Primary carcinoma of the fallopian tube. Difficulties of diagnosis and treatment. *Gynecol.* **5:** 168–179.

Hu CY, Taymor ML & Hertig AT (1950) Primary carcinoma of the fallopian tube. *Am. J. Obstet. Gynecol.* **59:** 58–67.

Hurlbutt FR & Nelson HB (1963) Primary carcinoma of the uterine tube. Report of 12 new cases. *Obstet. Gynecol.* **21:** 730–736.

Imachi M, Tsukamoto N, Shrigematsu T *et al.* (1992) Malignant mixed müllerian tumor of the fallopian tube: report of two cases and review of literature. *Gynecol. Oncol.* **47:** 114–124.

Jacobs AJ, McMurray EH, Parham J *et al.* (1985) Treatment of carcinoma of the fallopian tube using cisplatin, doxorubicin and cyclophosphamide. *Am. J. Clin. Oncol.* **9:** 436–439.

Jacoby AF, Fuller AF Jr, Thor AD *et al.* (1993) Primary leiomyosarcoma of the fallopian tube. *Gynecol. Oncol.* **51:** 404–407.

Kol S, Gal D, Friedman M & Paldi E (1990) Preoperative diagnosis of fallopian tube carcinoma by transvaginal sonography and CA-125. *Gynecol. Oncol.* **37:** 129–131.

Lehtovirta P, Kairemo KJ, Liewendahl K & Seppala M (1990) Immunolymphoscintigraphy and immunoscintigraphy of ovarian and fallopian tube cancer using F (ab[1]) 2 fragments of monoclonal OC 125. *Cancer Res.* **50(3 suppl):** 937s–940s.

Lootsma–Miklosova E, Aalders JG, Willemse PH & deBruijn HW (1987) Levels of CA-125 in patients with carcinoma of the fallopian tube: Two case histories. *Eur. J. Obstet. Gynecol. Reprod. Biol.* **24:** 231–235.

Maxson Wz, Stehman FB, Ulbright TM *et al.* (1987) Primary carcinoma of the fallopian tube: Evidence for activity of cisplatin combination therapy. *Gynecol. Oncol.* **26:** 305–313.

■ McMurray EH, Jacobs AJ, Perez CA *et al.* (1986) Carcinoma of the fallopian tube. Management and sites of failure. *Cancer* **58:** 2070–2075.

■ Morris M, Gershenson DM, Burke TW *et al.* (1990) Treatment of fallopian tube carcinoma with cisplatin, doxorubicin, and cyclophosphamide. *Obstet. Gynecol.* **76:** 1020–1024.

■ Muntz HG, Tarraza HM, Granai CO & Fuller AF Jr (1989) Primary adenocarcinoma of the fallopian tube. *Eur. J. Gynaecol. Oncol.* **10:** 239–249.

Neunteufel W & Breitenecker G (1989) Tissue expression of CA-125 in benign and malignant lesions of ovary and fallopian tube: A comparison with CA 19-9 and CEA. *Gynecol. Oncol.* **32:** 297–302.

Niloff JM, Klug TL, Schaetzl E *et al.* (1984) Evaluation of serum CA-125 in carcinoma of the fallopian tube, endometrium and endocervix. *Am. J. Obstet. Gynecol.* **148:** 1057–1058.

■ Nordin AJ (1994) Primary carcinoma of the fallopian tube. A 20-year literature review. *Obstet. Gynecol. Surv.* **49:** 349–361.

Pakisch B, Poschanko J, Stückschweiger G *et al.* (1990) Die Behandlung des primären Karzinoms der Tuba Fallopia. (Treatment of primary cancer of the fallopian tube.) *Geburtshilfe Frauenheilkunde* **50:** 593–596.

Pectasides D, Barbounis V, Sintilla A *et al.* (1994) Treatment of primary fallopian tube carcinoma with cisplatin-containing chemotherapy. *Am. J. Clin. Oncol.* **17:** 68–71.

Peters WA III, Anderson WA & Hopkins MP (1989) Results of chemotherapy in advanced carcinoma of the fallopian tube. *Cancer* **63:** 836–838.

■ Peters WA III, Anderson WA, Hopkins MP *et al.* (1988) Prognostic features of carcinoma of the fallopian tube. *Obstet. Gynecol.* **71:** 757–762.

Pfeiffer P, Mogensen H, Amtrup F & Honore E (1989) Primary carcinoma of the fallopian tube: A retrospective study of patients reported to the Danish Cancer Registry in a five year period. *Acta Oncol.* **28:** 7–11.

■ Podratz KC, Podczaski ES, Gaffey TA *et al.* (1986) Primary carcinoma of the fallopian tube. *Am. J. Obstet. Gynecol.* **154:** 1319–1326.

Roberts JA & Lifshitz S (1982) Primary adenocarcinoma of the fallopian tube. *Gynecol. Oncol.* **13:** 301–308.

Rorat E & Fenoglio C (1976) The ultrastructure of a poorly differentiated adenocarcinoma of the human tuba uterina. *Oncology* **33:** 167–169.

Rose PG, Piver MS & Tsukada Y (1990) Fallopian tube cancer. The Roswell Park Experience. *Cancer* **66:** 2661–2667.

Rosenblatt KA, Weiss NS & Schwartz SM (1989) Incidence of malignant fallopian tube tumours. *Gynecol. Oncol.* **35:** 236–239.

Sedlis A (1978) Carcinoma of the fallopian tube. *Surg. Clin. North Amer.* **58:** 121–129.

Tamimi HK & Figge DC (1981) Adenocarcinoma of the uterine tube: Potential for lymph node metastases. *Am. J. Obstet. Gynecol.* **141:** 132–137.

Tokunaga T, Miyazaki K & Okamura H (1991) Pathology of the fallopian tube. *Curr. Opin. Obstet. Gynecol.* **3:** 574–579.

Tokunaga T, Miyazaki K, Matsuyama S & Okamura H (1989) Serial measurement of CA-125 in patients with primary carcinoma of the fallopian tube. *Gynecol. Oncol.* **36:** 335–337.

Yoonessi M (1979) Carcinoma of the fallopian tube. *Obstet. Gynecol. Surv.* **34:** 257–270.

Zorlu OG, Cobanoglu O, Kuscu E *et al.* (1994) Malignant mixed müllerian tumor of the fallopian tube. *Acta Obstet. Gynecol. Scand.* **73:** 352–354.

19 Vulva: Pathogenesis and Epidemiology of Vulvar Cancer

V V Baker

Introduction

Neoplasms of the vulva are rare lesions, accounting for less than 5% of reported cases of gynecologic malignancies. The incidence of this disease is approximately 1.8 per 100,000 and has remained stable during the past two decades (Cramer and Cutler, 1974; Sturgeon *et al.*, 1992). Squamous cell carcinomas account for over 90% of primary vulvar neoplasms although a variety of histologic types arising from the stromal cells, skin appendages, and supporting structures may occur.

Squamous Cell Carcinoma of the Vulva

The search for risk factors associated with squamous cell carcinoma of the vulva has been the subject of numerous epidemiologic investigations. Consistent with observations made concerning other solid neoplasms, vulvar cancer is predominantly a disease of older women. Most diagnoses of vulvar cancer are made in the sixth decade or later (Franklin and Rutledge, 1972; Andreassin *et al.*, 1982; Menczer *et al.*, 1982). The association between advanced age and an increased incidence of cancer in general has been attributed to the accumulation of genetic mutations over a lifetime that may ultimately result in the appearance of a cancer.

A specific factor that appears to additionally increase this lifetime risk is cigarette smoking. Based upon a study of 22 women with invasive vulvar carcinoma, Newcomb *et al.* (1984) found that 60% of vulvar cancer patients were current smokers compared to only 33% of age-matched controls (observed risk=4.4). Brinton *et al.* (1990) reported a case–control study of 209 cases of squamous cell carcinoma of the vulva. Risk of disease was correlated with cigarette smoking. In addition, the number of lifetime sexual partners, a history of genital warts, and a history of previous abnormal Pap smears were also associated with risk of disease. Daling *et al.* (1992) conducted a population based case–control study and reported that the adjusted odds ratio for vulvar cancer was substantially elevated for women who smoked cigarettes. In addition, the risk increased in proportion to the number of cigarettes smoked.

The role of preinvasive and chronic vulvar lesions as risk factors has been postulated for decades. The coexistence of squamous dysplasia and invasive disease is well documented. This has been interpreted as indirect evidence that vulvar dysplasia may progress to invasive disease. Buscema *et al.* (1980) and Zaino *et al.* (1982) have reported that approximately 25% of invasive vulvar carcinomas have areas of vulvar intraepithelial neoplasia (VIN) III in adjacent epithelium. Leibowitch *et al.* (1990) found VIN III in 50% of 78 invasive squamous cell carcinomas of the vulva. The likelihood of finding VIN adjacent to invasive foci is related to the histologic pattern of the neoplasm. Both warty and basaloid carcinomas exhibit adjacent VIN in over two-thirds of cases (Kurman *et al.*, 1993). In contradistinction, keratinizing carcinoma of the vulva generally exhibits adjacent areas of hyperplastic dystrophy (Toki *et al.*, 1991). These observations indirectly support a model of vulvar cancer that may develop from dysplasia in a subset of patients. However, rigorous documentation of this progression is incomplete. A representative survey of reports published in the English language literature is presented in *Table 19.1* to illustrate the incidence of regression, persistence and progression of vulvar dysplasia.

Advanced age is also postulated to be an additive risk factor in the presence of vulvar dysplasia. A common clinical impression is that older patients are at greater risk of progression from dysplasia to invasive vulvar cancer compared to younger patients (Buscema *et al.*, 1980; Crum *et al.*, 1984; Leibowitch *et al.*, 1990). As an example, Barbero *et al.* (1990) reported a case of VIN I in a 69-year-old woman that progressed to invasive cancer during a 24-month period of time. In general, women younger than 40 years of age appear to be at minimal risk of progression to invasive disease. However, it is important to recognize that invasive cancer can and does occur in young women. Chafe *et al.* (1988) reported a series of 69 patients with presumed VIN who were treated by wide local excision of the vulva. Unexpected invasive cancer was found in 12 patients, the youngest of whom was 35.

In addition to advanced age, another factor that

Table 19.1. Published examples of regression, persistence and progression of vulvar intraepithelial neoplasia (VIN) lesions.

Authors	n	Duration of follow-up (yrs)	Recurrence or persistence	Progression	Regression
Treated patients					
Buscema *et al.*, 1980	102			3/102	
Caglar *et al.*, 1982	50		6/41	2/41	
Crum *et al.*, 1984	41	2–7		5/41	
DiPaola *et al.*, 1982	28		1/28		
Hording *et al.*, 1991	19	3–18		4/19	
Jones and McLean, 1986	32			1/32	
Ragnarrson *et al.*, 1987	74		21/74	3/74	
Ulbright *et al.*, 1982	18	1–5	3/18		2/18
Patients followed for VIN					
Bergeron *et al.*, 1987	2	6–40		2/2	
Buscema *et al.*, 1980	102	>5			2/102
Jones and McLean, 1986	4	2–8		4/4	

appears to influence the risk of progression of dysplastic lesions of the vulva to invasive ones is immunosuppression. Buscema *et al.* (1980) followed 106 patients with VIN III for 1–15 years and observed four cases of progression to invasive disease. Of these four cases, two occurred in postmenopausal women and two in immunosuppressed women. Depression of the immune system, particularly the cell-mediated arm, is associated with a generalized increase in cancer susceptibility. This increased susceptibility is best exemplified by the increased incidence of cancer in chronically immunosuppressed renal transplant patients. With respect to vulvar cancer, Sheil (1984) reported that vulvovaginal cancer was 39.6 times more frequent in renal transplant patients. Penn (1986) reported a 100-fold increase in the risk of vulvar and anal cancer in renal transplant patients. Preliminary observations suggest that the immunosuppression that accompanies human immunodeficiency virus (HIV) infection may also increase the risk of vulvar cancer and influence its biologic behavior (Levine *et al.*, 1994).

The metachronous occurrence of vulvar, vaginal and cervical cancers has been well documented in the English literature. Previous pelvic radiation therapy is a theoretical explanation for the development of vulvar cancer following treatment of cervical cancer although there are few reports to support this hypothesis. Although women with cervical cancer are at risk of a second neoplasm of the lower genital tract, there are very few reports of vulvar carcinomas in reports of post-radiation neoplasms (Palmer and Spratt, 1956; Novak and Woodruff, 1959; Czesnin and Wronkowski, 1978). The normal vulva does not appear to be particularly sensitive to radiation-induced transformation. If there is an increase in the relative risk, it appears to be very small.

As many as 30% of patients with invasive vulvar cancer will develop a second primary malignancy of the lower genital tract (Choo and Morley, 1980a, 1980b). In addition, as many as 30% of patients with carcinoma *in situ* of the vulva exhibit a second neoplasm of the lower genital tract (Bernstein *et al.*, 1983; Campion *et al.*, 1985). The occurrence of multicentric neoplasms of the lower genital tract led to the suggestion that a sexually-transmitted pathogen was acting upon susceptible tissues (Franklin and Rutledge, 1972).

There are several reports that indicate a relationship between syphilis and granulomatous diseases of the vulva and invasive vulvar cancer (Salzstein *et al.*, 1956; Green *et al.*, 1958; Franklin and Rutledge, 1972; Sengupta, 1981). However, associations do not equate with causation. It has not been determined whether these infectious diseases reflect causative factors or serve as markers of the passage of a sexually transmitted oncogenic agent.

The herpes simplex virus (HSV) has been evaluated as a potential oncogenic risk factor for neoplasms of the lower genital tract. However, HSV-specific DNA sequences are rarely detected in genital tumors. It has been postulated that HSV may damage host DNA through a 'hit and run' mechanism in which mutagenic changes, recombination and selective DNA amplification is followed by loss of HSV DNA from the host cell (Galloway and McDougal, 1983). In support of this hypothesis, Costa *et al.* (1990) reported the analysis of 12 vulvar neoplasms. Although HSV DNA was detected in only one neoplasm, eight of the 12 specimens were positive for HSV 2 ICP 11/12 protein and seven were positive for HSV 2 LA-1 protein.

There is considerable evidence that another sexually transmitted agent, the human papillomavirus (HPV), plays a central role in the pathogenesis of both premalignant and malignant squamous epithelial lesions of the lower genital tract. HPV-associated lesions, such as exophytic condyloma acuminata, are found in association with vulvar carcinomas in approximately 20–30% of cases (Josey *et al.*, 1976; Rhatigan and Saffos, 1977; Daling *et al.*, 1984). It has been suggested for decades that HPV-related lesions of the lower genital tract can undergo malignant change. Charlewood and Shippel (1953) first described spontaneous malignant transformation of a vulvar condyloma and there have been several additional reports since that time (Embrey, 1961; Shafeek *et al.*, 1979). However, there has been no documentation at the molecular level of spontaneous neoplastic transformation of benign exophytic condylomatous lesions of the vulva and the risk appears to be exceedingly small.

In contradistinction, neoplastic transformation of HPV-related lesions following exposure to genotoxic factors is well documented. Irradiation of verrucous carcinoma of the vulva, which is typically HPV 6-positive and demonstrates a somewhat indolent clinical course, is often followed by the emergence of a much more aggressive carcinoma (Rando *et al.*, 1986). In addition, ultraviolet irradiation of HPV DNA-positive lesions in patients diagnosed with epidermodysplasia verruciformis is followed by malignant transformation in a significant proportion of cases (Orth *et al.*, 1979).

The HPV is an 8 kilobase DNA virus that selectively infects squamous epithelial cells. HPV 16 and HPV 18 are or particular interest because they encode a protein, E6, which can bind to the gene product of the p53 tumor suppressor gene, resulting in abrogation of its normal anti-oncogene function. The p53 gene plays an important role in the regulation of the cell cycle. In the absence of normal p53 gene product activity, cells gain a proliferative advantage. Proliferating cells, which must replicate their DNA, are also at greater risk of DNA damage. Normally, when DNA damage occurs, levels of the p53 protein increase and transit through the cell cycle is delayed. During this delay, the DNA damage is repaired. When the E6 protein binds to the p53 gene product, transit through the cell cycle is not delayed and genetic mutations are propagated to subsequent generations. This permits the accumulation of genetic alterations that may ultimately contribute to cellular transformation. Undoubtedly, other mechanisms contribute to HPV-associated transformation. The presence of HPV 16 or HPV 18 DNA does not guarantee functional inactivation of the p53 protein activity by virtue of an E6 interaction. HPV-infected cells do not invariably synthesize a functional E6 protein. Bohm *et al.* (1993) studied four vulvar cancers and found that the HPV 16 mRNA transcripts initiated within the open reading frame of the E7 protein so that full length E7 protein was not encoded.

The significance of HPV in the pathogenesis of squamous cell carcinoma of the vulva is subject to question in view of the striking variation in the percentage of invasive squamous cell carcinomas of the vulva that contain HPV DNA (*Table 19.2*). Although some of this variation is undoubtedly due to sample size and the sensitivity of the detection technique used, it is unlikely that this is the only explanation for the observed disparities. Several authors have suggested that squamous cell carcinoma of the vulva may encompass at least two disease entities that can be differentiated by the age at diagnosis, histologic pattern, topographic distribution and presence or absence of HPV DNA (*Table 19.3*).

There is little information concerning specific genetic mutations in vulvar cancer. Walts *et al.* (1993) found immunohistochemical evidence of p53 expression in 86% of infiltrating squamous cell carcinomas of the vulva. Tervahauta *et al.* (1993) reported p53 expression in seven of eight vulvar carcinomas. The immunohistochemical detection of the p53 gene product implies that a mutation of the p53 gene is present. Data concerning specific point mutations of the p53 gene in vulvar carcinomas are not available.

Cytogenetic studies of vulvar neoplasms are also limited, but indicate that a variety of complex genetic alterations are present. Worsham *et al.* (1991) studied six squamous cell carcinomas of the vulva and found a number of complex chromosomal alterations. Abnormalities found in five of the six tumors included losses of 3p14-cen, 8pter-p11, 22qq13.1–p13.2, the short arm of inactive chromosome X, gains at 3q25-qter and 11q21 and rearrangement breakpoints at 5cen-q12.

Bartholin's Gland Carcinoma

Carcinoma of the Bartholin's gland accounts for 2–7% of vulvar cancers and 0.001% of female genital cancers (Barclay *et al.*, 1964). Chronic inflammation has historically been cited as a risk factor for this neoplasm although there is little supporting information. Boughton (1943) proposed that the increased percentage of squamous cell carcinomas reflected the progression of squamous metaplasia in response to chronic irritation. However, Leuchter *et al.* (1982) reviewed 90 cases reported through 1981 and noted that only 7.8% of patients had a history of inflammation of Bartholin's gland.

Approximately 50% of Bartholin's gland neoplasms are adenocarcinomas or squamous cell carcinomas. The remainder consist of adenoid cystic carcinoma, sarcoma and undifferentiated carcinoma. Copeland *et al.* (1986a) recorded the experience from the M.D. Anderson Hospital of 36 cases of primary Bartholin's gland carcinoma. Of the 36 cases, 27 were squamous cell carcinomas, six were adenocarcinomas, two were adenoid cystic carcinomas and one was an adenosquamous carcinoma. The medium age of diagnosis was 57 years with the age range extending from 23–86 years. The author noted that a delay in diagnosis was greater in women

Table 19.2. Survey of published reports of human papillomavirus (HPV) DNA-positive squamous cell vulvar cancers.

Authors	*n*	*No. positive for HPV DNA*	*Percentage positive for HPV DNA*	*Detection technique*
Pilotti *et al.*, 1984	21	9/14	64	I-HIST
Di Luca *et al.*, 1986	10	2/10	20	SBH
Macnab *et al.*, 1986	11	10/11	91	ISH
Gupta *et al.*, 1987a	12	11/12	92	ISH, I-HIST
Saito *et al.*, 1987	3	1/3	33	SBH
Sutton *et al.*, 1987	9	9/9	100	ISH
Bender *et al.*, 1988	27	16/27	59	ISH
Kasher and Roman, 1988	1	1/1	100	SBH
Kiyabu *et al.*, 1989	8	7/8	88	PCR
Venuti *et al.*, 1989	15	15/15	100	SBH, DBLOT
Costa *et al.*, 1990	12	4/8	50	ISH
Kulski *et al.*, 1990	2	1/2	50	ISH
Anderson *et al.*, 1991	42	12/42	28	ISH
Rusk *et al.*, 1991	31	7/31	23	DBLOT
Park *et al.*, 1991	6	4/6	67	ISH
Bloss *et al.*, 1991	21	10/21	48	SBH, PCR
Nuovo *et al.*, 1991	23	7/23	30	PCR
Leibowitch *et al.*, 1990				PCR
Hording *et al.*, 1993	62	19/62	31	PCR
Ansink *et al.*, 1994	60	19/60	32	PCR
Ogunbiyi *et al.*, 1994	33	25/33	76	PCR
Toki *et al.*, 1991	30	12/30	40	PCR
		13/30	43	ISH/PCR
Daling *et al.*, 1992	142	72/142	51	PCR
Mitchell *et al.*, 1993	169	14/88	16	ISH

I-HIST, immunohistochemistry; SBH, Southern blot hybridization; ISH, *in situ* hybridization (includes fluorescent *in situ* studies); PCR, polymerase chain reaction; DBLOT, dot blot.

Table 19.3. Relationship between human papillomavirus (HPV) DNA status, histological pattern, patient age and invasive vulvar cancer.

Characteristic	*Patient age <45 yrs*	*Patient age >50 yrs*
HPV DNA positive	Often	Less common
Histologic growth pattern of invasive carcinoma	Basaloid or warty	Keratinizing
Adjacent vulvar dysplasia	Common	Uncommon
Lesion distribution	Multifocal	Unifocal

younger than 45 years and cautioned that all vulvar masses be approached with a high index of suspicion for malignancy regardless of patient age.

Thirty-seven cases of adenoid cystic carcinoma of Bartholin's gland diagnosed and treated at the M.D. Anderson Hospital have also been reported (Copeland *et al.*, 1986b). The median age of diagnosis was 42 with a range of 25–76 years. Interestingly, seven of 14 patients who were less than 42 years of age were diagnosed during or soon after pregnancy. The significance of this observation is not known in the view of the small number of cases reported and the rarity of the lesion.

Paget's Disease of the Vulva

Extramammary Paget's disease most commonly involves the vulva and is primarily a disease of older women. Paget's disease of the vulva is a cutaneous adenocarcinoma of epidermal origin that is often associated with an underlying adenocarcinoma of the skin adnexa. It is believed to originate from eccrine or apocrine glands deep in the dermis (Nadji *et al.*, 1982; Mazoujian *et al.*, 1984). Strictly speaking, Paget's disease of the vulva is a dysplastic condition rather than an invasive neoplasm. It is notable because of its disputed association with second primary malignancies.

Chanda (1985) reviewed 197 cases of extramammary Paget's disease, 128 of which involved the vulva. Of 109 of the patients with vulva Paget's disease from whom follow-up information was available 31 were diagnosed with a second metachronous or synchronous malignancy. Of the 31 second primary neoplasms, 11 were cancers of the breast and 14 involved the genital tract.

Vulvar Melanoma

Although melanoma of the female genital tract is a rare diagnosis, it is the second most common primary neoplasm of the vulva. Approximately 3–4.8% of all melanomas arise on the vulva, which corresponds to the portion of skin covering this area of the body. However, only 0.1% of nevi occur on the vulva, suggesting that there may be some predilection to the development of melanoma in this area.

Hewett is credited with the first description of vulvar melanoma in 1861. Morrow and DiSaia (1976) analyzed 322 reported cases of vulvar melanoma in a detailed review, which was published in 1976. Since that time, over 150 additional cases have been reported in the English language literature.

In general, vulvar melanoma is a disease of postmenopausal Caucasian women and is most commonly diagnosed during the sixth decade. However, up to one-third of cases are diagnosed in premenopausal women, but it is only rarely diagnosed in prepubescent children.

Trauma and hormonal stimulation are often cited as two important etiologic factors in the pathogenesis of melanoma. A history of trauma has been reported in 20–40% of cases (Webster *et al.*, 1944; Pack *et al.*, 1947; Jorgsholm and Engdahl, 1955; Peterson *et al.*, 1962). However, this information is probably subject to bias and patient recall. In addition, the distribution of melanoma does not parallel those areas of the body subject to frequent trauma with the exception of the feet (Pack *et al.*, 1952).

Estrogen stimulation may result in enlargement and hyperpigmentation of nevi (Pack and Scharnagel, 1951; Allan and Spitz, 1953; Bischitz and Snell, 1958). However, conclusive evidence that estrogen-induced changes in nevi are precursors to malignant transformation is lacking. Based upon numerous case reports describing concomitant melanoma in pregnancy, many clinicians express the opinion that pregnancy adversely alters the course of melanoma. However, data from studies in which appropriate control groups have been chosen and matched with stage of disease fail to support this notion (George *et al.*, 1960; White *et al.*, 1961).

Summary of Core Information

- Vulvar cancer is a disease associated with multiple risk factors including advanced age, cigarette smoking, and immunosuppression.
- A role for the human papillomavirus (HPV) in the pathogenesis of vulvar cancer has not been established.
- Unlike cervical cancer, a model for the progression of vulvar dysplasia to invasive cancer has not been conclusively demonstrated.
- Although very rare, any mass of the Bartholin's gland must be evaluated to exclude a carcinoma.
- Paget's disease of the vulva is a dysplastic process and is uncommonly associated with invasive adenocarcinoma or a second primary.
- Melanoma of the vulva is the second most common vulvar cancer.

References

Allen AC & Spitz S (1953) Malignant melanoma. A clinico-pathological analysis of the criteria for diagnosis and prognosis. *Cancer* **6:** 1–45.

■ Anderson WA, Franquemont DW, Williams J, Taylor PT & Crum CP (1991) Vulvar squamous cell carcinoma and papillomaviruses: two separate entities? *Am. J. Obstet. Gynecol.* **165:** 329–336.

Andreassin B, Bock JE & Weberg E (1982) Invasive cancer in the vulvar region. *Acta Obstet. Gynecol. Scand.* **61:** 113–119.

Ansink AC, Krul MRL, DeWeger RA *et al.* (1994) Human papillomavirus, lichen sclerosus, and squamous cell carcinoma of the vulva: detection and prognostic significance. *Gynecol. Oncol.* **52:** 180–184.

■ Barbero M, Micheletti L, Preti M *et al.* (1990) Vulvar intraepithelial neoplasia: a clinocopathologic study of 60 cases. *J. Reprod. Med.* **35:** 1023–1028

Barclay DL, Collins CG & Macey HB (1964) Cancer of the Bartholin gland. A review and report of 8 cases. *Obstet. Gynecol.* **24:** 329–336.

Bender HG, Degen KW & Beck L (1988) Human papilloma virus findings in the perimeter of vulvo-vaginal malignancies. *Eur. J. Gynecol. Oncol.* **4:** 287–291.

Bernstein SG, Kovacs BR, Townsend DE & Morrow CP (1983) Vulvar carcinoma *in situ*. *Obstet. Gynecol.* **61:** 304–307.

Bergeron C, Naghashfar Z, Canaan C *et al.* (1987) Human papillomavirus type 16 in intraepithelial neoplasia (Bowenoid papulosis) and coexistent invasive carcinoma of the vulva. *Int. J. Gynecol. Pathol.* **6:** 1–11.

Bischitz PG & Snell RS (1958) Effect of ovariectomy, estrongens and progesterone on the activity of the melanocyte in the skin. *Nature* **181:** 1413.

■ Bloss JD, Liao SY, Wilczynski SP *et al.* (1991) Clinical and histologic features of vulvar carcinomas analyzed for human papillomavirus status: evidence that squamous cell carcinoma of the vulva has more than one etiology. *Hum. Pathol.* **22:** 711–718.

Bohm S, Wilczynski SP, Pfister H & Iftner T (1993) The predominant mRNA class in HPV16-infected genital neoplasias does not encode the E_6 or the E_7 protein. *Int. J. Cancer* **55:** 791–798.

Boughton TG (1943) Carcinoma of the Bartholin's gland. *Am. J. Surg.* **59:** 585–591.

Brinton A, Nasca PC, Mallin K *et al.* (1990) Care-control study of cancer of the vulva. *Obstet. Gynecol.* **75:** 859–866.

Buscema J, Woodruff D, Parmley TH & Genardry R (1980) Carcinoma *in situ* of the vulva. *Obstet. Gynecol.* **55:** 225–230.

Caglar H, Tamr S and Hreshchyshyn MM (1982) Vulvar intraepithelial neoplasia. *Obstet. Gynecol.* **60:** 346–349.

Campion MJ, Clarkson P & McCance DJ (1985) Squamous neoplasia of the cervix in relation to other genital tract neoplasia. *Clin. Obstet. Gynecol.* **12:** 265–280.

Chafe WC, Richards A, Morgan L & Wilkinson E (1988) Unrecognized invasive carcinoma in vulvar intraepithelial neoplasia (VIN). *Gynecol. Oncol.* **31:** 154–162.

Chanda JJ (1985) Extramammary Paget's disease: prognosis and relationship to internal malignancy. *J. Am. Acad. Dermatol.* **13:** 1009–1014.

Charlewood GP & Shippel S (1953) Vulvar condyloma acuminata as a premalignant lesion in the Bantee. *S. Afr. Med. J.* **27:** 149–151.

Choo YC & Morley GW (1980a) Double primary epidermoid carcinoma of the vulva and cervix. *Gynecol. Oncol.* **9:** 324–333.

Choo YC & Morley GW (1980b) Multiple primary neoplasms of the anogenital region. *Obstet. Gynecol.* **56:** 365–369.

Clarke EA, Morgan RW & Newman TM (1982) Smoking as a risk factor in cancer of the cervix: Additional evidence from case–control study. *Am. J. Epidemiol.* **115:** 59–66.

Copeland L, Sneige N, Gershenson DM *et al.* (1986a) Bartholin gland carcinoma. *Obstet. Gynecol.* **67:** 794–801.

Copeland LJ, Sniege N, Gershenson DM *et al.* (1986b) Adenoid cystic carcinoma of the Bartholin gland. *Obstet. Gynecol.* **67:** 115–120.

Costa S, Rotola A, Terzano P *et al.* (1990) Search for herpes simplex virus 2 and human papillomavirus genetic expression in vulvar neoplasia. *J. Reprod. Med.* **35:** 1108–1112.

Cramer DW & Cutler SJ (1974) Incidence and histopathology of malignancies of the female genital organs in the United States. *Am. J. Obstet. Gynecol.* **118:** 443–460.

Crum CP, Liskow A, Petras P, Keng WC & Frick HC (1984) Vulvar intraepithelial neoplasia/severe atypia and carcinoma *in situ*: a clinopathologic analysis of 41 cases. *Cancer* **54:** 1429–1434.

Czesnin K & Wronkowski Z (1978) Second malignancies of the irradiated area in patients treated for uterine cervix cancer. *Gynecol. Oncol.* **6:** 309–315.

Daling JR, Chu J, Weiss NS, Emel L & Tamini HK (1984) The association of condylomata acuminata and squamous carcinoma of the vulva. *Br. J. Cancer* **50:** 533–535.

Daling JR, Sherman KJ, Hislop TG *et al.* (1992) Cigarette smoking and the risk of anogenital cancer. *Am. J. Epidemiol.* **135:** 180–189.

Di Luca D, Pilotti S, Stefanon B *et al.* (1986) Human paillomavirus type 16 DNA in genital tumors: a pathological and molecular analysis. *J. Gen. Virol.* **67:** 583–589.

DiPaola GR, Rueda–Leverone G, Belardi MG and Vighi S (1982) Vulvar carcinoma in situ: a report of 28 cases. *Gynecol. Oncol.* **14:** 236–242.

Embrey MP (1961) Vulval carcinoma complicating condylomata acuminata. *J. Obstet. Gynecol. Br. Commonwth* **68:** 503–504.

Franklin WE & Rutledge FD (1972) Epidemiology and epidermoid carcinoma of the vulva. *Obstet. Gynecol.* **39:** 165–172.

Galloway DA & McDougall JK (1983) The oncogenic potential of herpes simplex viruses: evidence for a 'hit and run' mechanism. *Nature* **302:** 21–24.

George PA, Fortner JG & Pack GT (1960) Melanoma with pregnancy: a report of 115 cases. *Cancer* **13:** 854–859.

Green TM, Ulfender H & Meigs JV (1958) Epidermoid carcinoma of the vulva: An analysis of 238 cases. *Am. J. Obstet. Gynecol.* **75:** 834–847.

Gupta J, Pilotti S, Shah KV *et al.* (1987) Human papillomavirus associated early vulvar neoplasia investigated by in situ hybridization. *Am. J. Surg. Pathol.* **11:** 430–4.

Hewett P (1861) Melanosis of the labium and glands of the groin and pubes. *Lancet* **1:** 263.

Hording U, Kringsholm B, Andreasson B *et al.* (1991) Human papillomavirus in vulvar squamous cell carcinoma and in normal vulvar tissues: a search for a possible impact of HPV on vulvar cancer prognosis. *Int. J. Canc.* **55:** 394–396.

Jones RW and McLean MR (1986) Carcinoma in situ of the vulvar: A review of 31 treated and 5 untreated cases. *Obstet. Gynecol.* **68:** 499–504.

Jorgsholm V & Engdahl I (1955) Malignant melanoma. *Acta Radiol.* **44:** 417–433.

Josey WE, Nahmias AJ & Naib ZM (1976) Viruses and cancer of the lower genital tract. *Cancer* **38:** 552–533.

Kasher MS & Roman A (1988) Characterization of human papillomavirus type 6b DNA isolated from an invasive squamous carcinoma of the vulva. *Virology* **165:** 225–233.

Kiyabu MT, Shibata D, Arnheim N, Martin WJ & Fitzgibbons PL (1989) Detection of human papillomavirus in formalin-fixed, invasive squamous carcinomas using the polymerase chain reaction. *Am. J. Surg. Pathol.* **13:** 221–224.

Kulski JK, Demeter T, Mutavdzic S *et al.* (1990) Survey of histologic specimens of human cancer for human papillomavirus types 6/11/16/18 by filter *in situ* hybridization. *Am. J. Clin. Pathol.* **94:** 566–570.

■ Kurman RJ, Toki T & Schiffman H (1993) Basaloid and warty carcinoma of the vulva. Distinctive types of squamous cell carcinoma of the vulva frequently associated with human papillomavirus. *Am. J. Surg. Path.* **17:** 133–145.

Leibowitch M, Neill S, Pelisse M & Moyal–Barocco M (1990) The epithelial changes associated with squamous cell carcinoma of the vulva: A review of the clinical, histological and viral findings in 78 women. *Br. J. Obstet. Gynecol.* **97:** 1135–1139.

Leuchter RS, Hacker NF, Voet RL *et al.* (1982) Primary carcinoma of the Bartholin gland: A report of 14 cases and review of the literature. *Obstet. Gynecol.* **60:** 361–368.

Levine P, Maiman M, Zevalas E *et al.* (1994) *Invasive Vulvar Cancer and HIV Infection.* Orlando, Florida: The Society of Gynecologic Oncologists.

Macnab JCM, Walkinshaw SA, Cordiner JW & Clements JB (1986) Human papillomavirus in clinically and histologically normal tissues of patients with genital cancer. *N. Engl. J. Med.* **315:** 1052–1058.

Mazoujian G, Pinkus GS & Haageusen DE (1984) Extramammary Paget's disease, evidence for an apocrine origin. An immunoperoxidase study of gross cystic disease fluid protein 5, carcinoembryonic antigen and keratin proteins. *Am. J. Surg. Pathol.* **8:** 43–50.

Menczer J, Voliovitch Y, Modan B, Modan M & Steinitz R (1982) Some epidemiologic aspects of carcinoma of the vulva in Israel. *Am. J. Obstet. Gynecol.* **143:** 893–896.

Mitchell MR, Prasod CJ, Sihra EG *et al.* (1993) Second genital primary squamous neoplasms in vulvar carcinoma: viral and histopathologic correlates. *Obstet. Gynecol.* **81:** 13–18.

Morrow CP & DiSaia PJ (1976) Malignant melanoma of the female genitalia: A clinical analysis. *Obstet. Gynecol. Surv.* **31:** 233–271.

Nadji M, Morales AR, Girtanner RE *et al.* (1982) Paget's disease of the skin. An unifying concept of histogenesis. *Cancer* **50:** 2203–2207.

Newcomb PA, Weiss NS & Daling JR (1984) Incidence of vulvar carcinoma in relation to menstrual, reproductive and medical factors. *J. Natl. Cancer Inst.* **73:** 391–396.

Novak ER & Woodruff JD (1959) Postirradiation malignancies of the pelvic organs. *Am. J. Obstet. Gynecol.* **77:** 667–675.

Nouvo GJ, Delvenne P, MacConnell P *et al.* (1991) Correlation of histology and detection of human papillomavirus DNA in vulvar cancers. *Gynecol. Oncol.* **43:** 275–280.

Ogunbiyi OA, Scholefield JH, Robertson G *et al.* (1994) Anal human papillomavirus infection and squamous neoplasia in patients with invasive vulvar cancer. *Obstet. Gynecol.* **83:** 212–216.

Orth G, Jablonska S, Jarzabek–Chorzelska M *et al.* (1979) Characteristics of the lesions and risk of malignant conversion as related to the type of the human papillomavirus involved in epidermodysplasia verruciformis. *Cancer Res.* **39:** 1074–1082.

Pack GT, Pirzik SL & Scharnagel IM (1947) The treatment of malignant melanoma. *Calif. Med.* **66:** 283–287.

Pack GT & Scharnagel IM (1951) The prognosis for malignant melanoma in the pregnant woman. *Cancer* **4:** 324–334.

Pack GT, Lensen N & Gerber DM (1952) Regional distribution of moles and melanomas. *Arch. Surg.* **65:** 862–870.

Palmer JP & Spratt DW (1956) Pelvic carcinoma following irradiation for benign gynecologic diseases. *Am. J. Obstet. Gynecol.* **72:** 497–505.

Park JS, Jones RW, McLean MR *et al.* (1991) Possible etiologic heterogeneity of vulvar intraepithelial neoplasia. *Cancer* **67:** 1599–1607.

Penn I (1986) Cancers of the ano-genital region in renal transplant recipients. *Cancer* **58:** 611 616.

Petersen ND, Bodenham DC & Lloyd OO (1962) Malignant melanomas of the skin: a study of the origin, development, etiology, spread, treatment and prognosis. *Br. J. Plastic Surg.* **15:** 97–111.

Pilotti S, Rilke F, Shah KV, Delle Torre G & De Palo G (1984) Immunohistochemical and ultrastructural evidence of papilloma virus infection associated with *in situ* and microinvasive squamous cell carcinoma of the vulva. *Am. J. Surg. Pathol.* **8:** 751–761.

Ragnarsson B, Raabe N, Willems J, Pettersson F. (1987) Carcinoma in situ of the vulva: Long term prognosis. *Acta. Oncologica.* **26:** 277–280.

Rando RF, Sedlacek TV, Hunt J *et al.* (1986) Verrucous carcinoma of the vulva associated with an unusual type 6 human papillomavirus. *Obstet. Gynecol.* **67:** 70s–75s.

Rhatigan RM & Saffos RO (1977) Condyloma acuminatum and squamous carcinoma of the vulva. *South Med. J.* **70:** 591–594.

Rusk D, Sutton G, Look K & Roman A (1991) Analysis of invasive squamous cell carcinoma of the vulva and vulvar intraepithelial neoplasia for the presence of human papillomavirus DNA. *Obstet. Gynecol.* **77:** 918–922.

Saito J, Yutsudo M, Inoue M *et al.* (1987) New human papillomavirus tumors from Japanese patients. *Jpn. J. Cancer Res.* **78:** 1081–1087.

Salzstein SL, Woodruff JD & Novak ER (1956) Post-granulomatous carcinoma of the vulva. *Obstet. Gynecol.* **7:** 80–90.

Sengupta BS (1981) Carcinoma of the vulva in Jamaican women. *Acta Obstet. Gynecol. Scand.* **60:** 537–544.

Shafeek MA, Osman MI & Hussein MA (1979) Carcinoma of the vulva arising in condylomata acuminata. *Obstet. Gynecol.* **54:** 120–122.

Sheil AGR (1984) Cancer in organ transplant recipients: part of an induced immune deficiency syndrome. *Br. Med. J.* **288:** 659–661.

Sturgeon SR, Brinton LA, Devesa SS & Kurman RJ (1992) *In situ* and invasive vulvar cancer incidence trends (1973 to 1987). *Am. J. Obstet. Gynecol.* **166:** 1482–1485.

Sutton GP, Stehman FB, Ehrlich CE & Roman A (1987) Human papillomavirus DNA in lesions of the female genital tract: evidence for type 6/11 in squamous carcinoma of the vulva. *Obstet. Gynecol.* **70:** 564–568.

Tervahauta AI, Syrjanen SM, Vayrynen M *et al.* (1993) Expression of p53 protein related to the presence of human papillomavirus (HPV) DNA in genital carcinomas and precancer lesions. *Anticancer Res.* **13:** 1107–1111.

Toki T, Kurman RJ, Park JS *et al.* (1991) Probable nonpapillomavirus etiology of squamous cell carcinoma of the vulva in older women: a clinicopathologic study using *in situ* hybridization and polymerase chain reaction. *Int. J. Gynecol. Pathol.* **10:** 107–125.

Ulbright TM, Stehman FB, Roth LM *et al.* (1982) Bowenoid dysplasia of the vulva. *Cancer* **50:** 2910–2919.

Venuti A & Marcante ML (1989) Presence of human papilloma virus type 18 in vulvar carcinomas and its integration into the cell genome. *J. Gen. Virol.* **70:** 1587–1592.

Walts AE, Roeffler HP & Said JW (1993) Localization of p53 protein and human papillomavirus in anogenital squamous lesions and immunohistochemical and *in situ* hybridization studies in benign, dysplastic and malignant epithelia. *Hum. Pathol.* **24:** 1238–1242.

Webster JP, Stevenson TW & Stout AP (1944) The surgical treatment of malignant melanomas of the skin. *Surg. Clin. North Am.* **24:** 319–339.

White LP, Linden G, Berslow L & Harzfeld L (1961) Studies on melanoma: the effect of pregnancy on survival in human melanoma. *J. Am. Med. Assoc.* **177:** 235–238.

Worsham MJ, Van Dyke DL, Grenman SE *et al.* (1991) Consistent chromosome abnormalities in squamous cell carcinoma of the vulva. *Genes Chromosomes Cancer* **3:** 420–432.

Zaino RJ, Husseinzadeh N, Nahhas W *et al.* (1982) Epithelial alterations in proximity to invasive squamous carcinoma of the vulva. *Int. J. Gynecol. Path.* **1:** 143–147.

Zur Hausen H (1982) Human genital cancer: synergism between two virus infections or synergism between a virus infection and initiating events? *Lancet* **1:** 1370–1372.

20 Pathology of Malignant Vulvar Tumors

T P Rollason

Tumors of or Primarily Involving Surface Epithelium

Preinvasive Disease

Discussion and study of preinvasive disease of the vulva has been bedevilled by the profusion of terms used to define, on little clear histologic evidence, subgroups of intraepithelial neoplasia. All major international societies now recommend the use of the term vulvar intraepithelial neoplasia (VIN) to embrace all of these previous terms and subgroups, including the lesion that has been designated as 'Bowenoid papulosis.' VIN is divided into three grades dependent essentially on the level of epithelial involvement by undifferentiated neoplastic cells (*Figures 20.1 and 20.2*), but VIN III is considerably more common than the lower grades, which when identified are usually seen in association with VIN III. This terminology can equally be applied to intraepithelial neoplasia arising in association with vulvar 'dystrophies' *de novo* or in conjunction with human papillomavirus (HPV) effect.

Three variant patterns of VIN are described – warty, basaloid (the commonest type) and differentiated. The differentiated pattern differs from the others in that grading is really impossible as atypia is confined in almost all cases to the lower third of the epithelium and the rete pegs, where keratin pearls may form. This pattern is usually seen in pure form, whereas the others are commonly admixed (Kurman *et al.*, 1992), and tends to occur in older women, where it is commonly seen adjacent to foci of invasive carcinoma. VIN commonly extends into skin adnexal structures, often for more than 2 mm, and as the adnexae may be up to 5 mm deep, this must be borne in mind when local destructive techniques are employed.

The differentiation of warty changes (*Figure 20.3*) from lower grades of VIN histologically may be very difficult, but helpful features are the presence of abnormal mitoses, nuclear pleomorphism and loss of cellular maturation.

It should be stressed that it is unwise to extrapolate from histologic and terminologic similarity between VIN and CIN to biologic homology as there is evidence to indicate that VIN proceeds less frequently to invasive disease than CIN, particularly in the younger age group with coexistent HPV infection (Buscema *et al.*, 1980), though circumspection is necessary in view of the few cases observed long term without therapy. The very variable percentage of cases of invasive carcinoma of the vulva that show adjacent VIN in different series also casts doubt on VIN as the usual precursor of invasive squamous carcinoma of the vulva (Buscema *et al.*, 1980; Zaino *et al.*, 1982). Squamous hyperplasia is evident adjacent to invasive cancer more frequently than VIN in elderly women (Zaino, 1987) and when VIN is seen it is commonly of the differentiated type. In younger women, however, particularly those with early invasive lesions, 60% appear to have VIN of the common types (Kelley *et al.*, 1991).

Risk factors for progression of VIN to invasive carcinoma include age (above 60), immunosuppression and multifocal and midline disease (Buscema *et al.*, 1980; Jones and McLean, 1986; Sedlis *et al.*, 1987). A 'best guess' at risk of progression to invasion overall is probably 3–4% (Buscema *et al.*, 1980; Andreasson and Bock, 1985; Fiorica *et al.*, 1988). This compares to a risk of recurrence of VIN of perhaps 25% (Andreasson and Bock, 1985).

There is no clear evidence that the presence of HPV alters the outcome for VIN though older patients with 'warty' VIN may have an increased risk of progression compared to younger patients (Jones and McLean, 1986). Little data exist on the effects of aneuploidy, but there is a suggestion that low ploidy may equate with increased risk of invasion and high ploidy with persistence/recurrence of VIN (Fu *et al.*, 1981).

Superficially Invasive Squamous Carcinoma

No generally accepted definition of vulvar 'microinvasive' carcinoma exists. An excellent review of the problem has been presented by Wilkinson (1987).

The present International Federation of Gynecology and Obstetrics (FIGO) classification of Stage I disease confines itself to limiting the lateral extent of the tumor to 2 cm for inclusion in this category, but in early invasive tumors, depth rather than surface diameter has more importance. It is difficult to determine from published studies what criteria should be used to include early invasive vulvar carcinomas in any putative 'microinvasive' category. Some studies have shown no metastases to groin nodes with tumors up to a depth of 5 mm (Wharton *et al.*, 1974), whereas others suggest that a significant number (up to 30% in some series) will have metastasized at this depth (e.g. Buscema *et al.*, 1981;

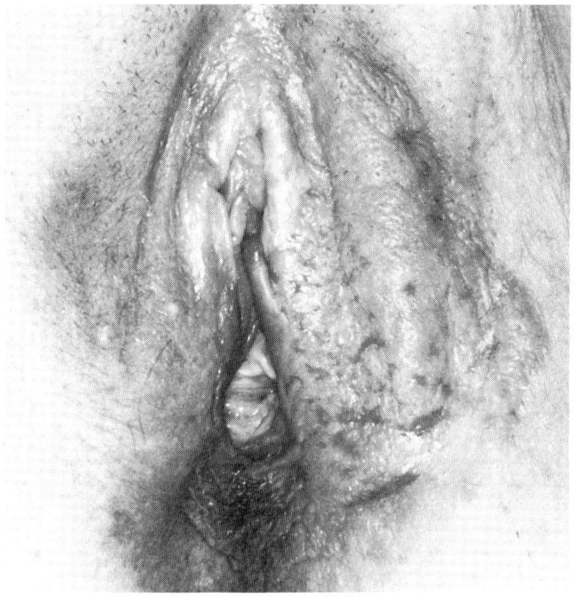

Figure 20.1. The left vulva shows diffuse epithelial thickening and focal excoriation. Histologically vulvar intraepithelial neoplasia (VIN) III was evident.

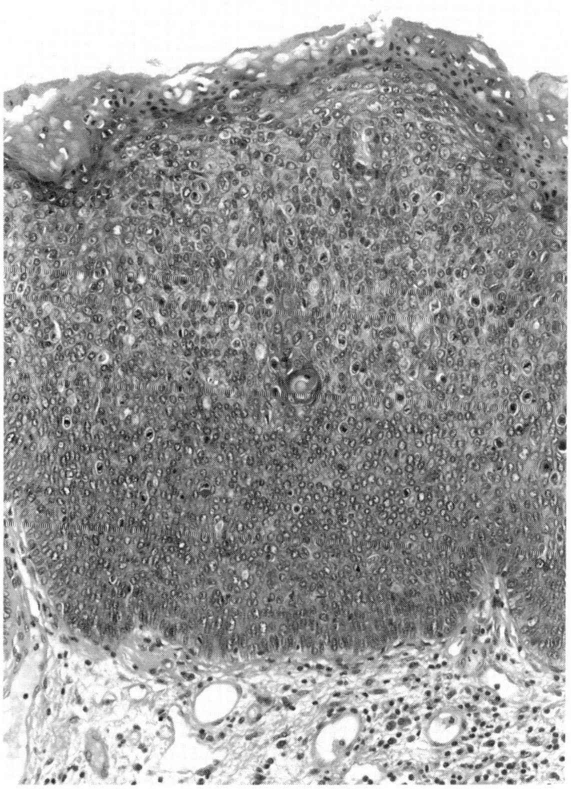

Figure 20.2. Vulvar biopsy showing intraepithelial neoplasia. Undifferentiated cells extend virtually to the surface, indicative of vulvar intraepithelial neoplasia (VIN) III.

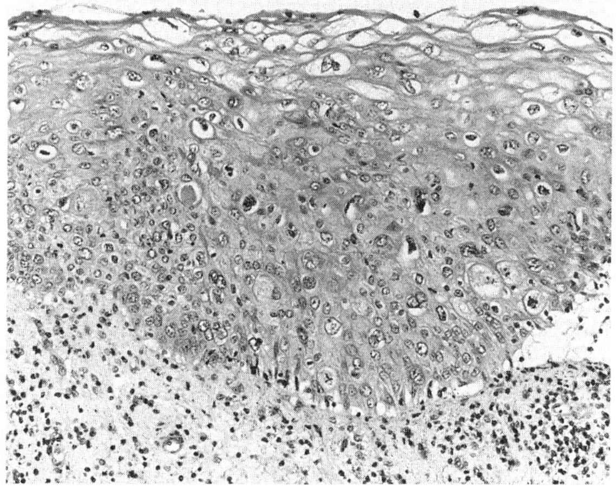

Figure 20.3. Vulvar biopsy showing florid human papillomavirus (HPV) effect (koilocytes and multinucleate cells). A probable abnormal mitosis is seen in the basal layers (center field). The occurrence of abnormal mitotic figures in the present state of knowledge must be taken to indicate coexistent vulvar intraepithelial neoplasia (VIN).

Donaldson *et al.*, 1981; Hacker *et al.*, 1984). Even at a maximum depth of invasion of 3 mm metastases have been reported in several series at varying rates (Donaldson *et al.*, 1981; Yoonessi *et al.*, 1983; Hacker *et al.*, 1984) and tumor volume studies have supported the tendency to spread at smaller size when compared to cervical carcinoma (Pickel and Haas, 1986). Comparison between studies is also hampered by the variable methods of measurement used. Dvoretsky *et al.* (1984) suggest total tumor thickness may be more useful and reproducible than depth of invasion, and Pickel and Haas have indicated that a tumor volume of 300 mm^3 or less may be best to define this group. In the light of the above problems it has been proposed that the term 'microinvasive' is avoided in vulvar carcinoma and a substage of FIGO Stage I disease be created consisting of tumors showing less than 1 mm depth of invasion, where risk of metastasis appears negligible, there being only two cases in the literature known to have metastasized (Van der Velden *et al.*, 1992). Depth of invasion should be measured from the epidermal–stromal junction of the most superficial adjacent dermal papilla to the deepest point of the tumor (Kurman *et al.*, 1992).

As with cervical disease it is clearly desirable that the presence or absence of vessel invasion be specifically noted in histologic reports (Donaldson *et al.*, 1981) and in view of the evidence that a diffuse or 'spray' pattern of invasive growth may indicate a poorer prognosis than a compact 'pushing' pattern (Barnes *et al.*, 1980; Wilkinson *et al.*, 1982) this should also be commented on. We suggest that the term 'confluent' (Barnes *et al.*, 1980; Hacker *et al.*,

1984) is best avoided because it is open to misinterpretation, and as Zaino (1987) points out, has been used in different senses by different authors. Tumor differentiation has not been convincingly demonstrated to correlate with prognosis (Dvoretsky *et al.*, 1984) though some dispute this (Sedlis *et al.*, 1987).

Invasive Squamous Carcinoma and Its Histologic Variants

Approximately 90–95% of all invasive tumors of the vulva are squamous (Andreasson *et al.*, 1982), but the tumor at this site makes up 8% or less of genital tract malignancy (Green, 1978; Andreasson *et al.*, 1982). Generally it is a disease of women over 50 years of age (Green, 1978), but the incidence in younger women does appear to be increasing (Andreasson *et al.*, 1982). Below the age of 40 years immunosuppressive medical conditions are common and most patients smoke (Carter *et al.*, 1993).

On gross examination these tumors are often ulcerated masses (*Figure 20.4*), but polypoid and diffuse plaque-like lesions are also not uncommon. No clear predilection for a particular site on the vulva is seen; most involve the labia (Japaze *et al.*, 1977). In one major series there was a tendency for the anterior half of the vulva to be more commonly involved than the posterior (Green *et al.*, 1958). Approximately 10% are multifocal. The tumors that follow granulomatous vulvar disease tend to be widespread and polypoid (Hay and Cole, 1969).

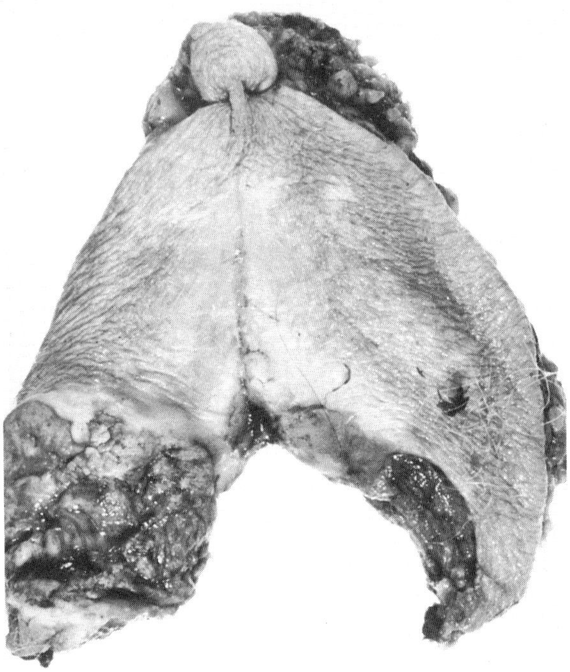

Figure 20.4. Total vulvectomy specimen. A large ulcerated nodular squamous carcinoma is present (lower left).

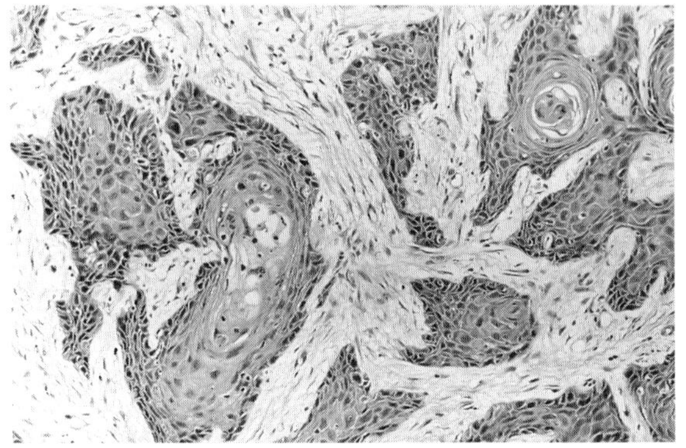

Figure 20.5. Vulvectomy specimen showing typical infiltrating well-differentiated keratinizing squamous cell carcinoma.

Most tumors are histologically well or moderately well differentiated, being composed of infiltrating tongues of eosinophilic cells showing keratinization, often with 'pearl' formation (*Figure 20.5*). Surgical staging by the FIGO method provides the most accurate prognostic information. Histologic grading of tumor differentiation has not been universally shown to be prognostically helpful (Hacker *et al.*, 1984) though some series have claimed good correlation (Boyce *et al.*, 1985; Rowley *et al.*, 1988; Hopkins *et al.*, 1991) and a grading method based on the percentage of undifferentiated cells has been recommended (Sedlis *et al.*, 1987). As with early invasive disease the 'spray' or diffuse pattern of invasion appears to confer a poorer prognosis, but no clear advantage is evident in grading nuclear cytoplasmic ratio, desmoplastic reaction, mitotic rate. One recent study showed considerable prognostic value in using a combination of tumor size, nuclear hyperchromasia and site (Bjerregaard *et al.*, 1993). The presence of vascular invasion (*Figures 20.6 and 20.7*) appears to be an important guide to the likelihood of lymph node metastasis (Iverson *et al.*, 1981; Hacker *et al.*, 1984; Boyce *et al.*, 1985; Rowley *et al.*, 1988; Hopkins *et al.*, 1991). Metastases are usually to groin nodes, which are almost invariably involved before more distant node groups.

To date there are few studies on ploidy and proliferation index in vulvar squamous carcinoma and no clear evidence of their prognostic use is available (Dolan *et al.*, 1993). Morphometry is not of proven value (Bjerregaard *et al.*, 1993).

Histologic variants of invasive squamous carcinoma

Verrucous carcinoma

When strict histologic criteria are applied these are relatively rare tumors with less than 50 vulvar

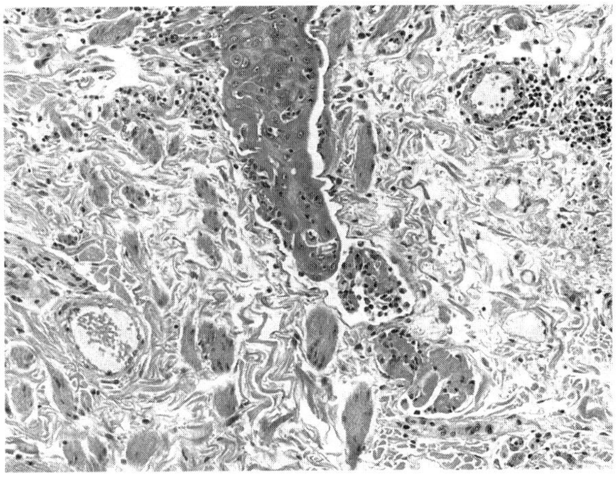

Figure 20.6. Vulvectomy specimen. Vessel invasion in invasive squamous carcinoma. The central thin-walled vein is filled by invasive squamous carcinoma and thrombus.

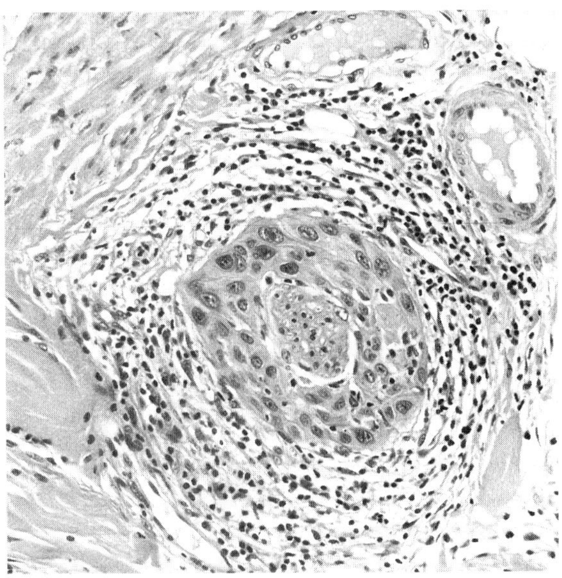

Figure 20.7. Vulvar biopsy – perineural lymphatic invasion. This is another type of vessel involvement in squamous carcinoma of the vulva. The small nerve seen centrally is cuffed by invasive squamous carcinoma in the lymphatics.

cases in the English literature (Isaacs, 1976; Brisigotti *et al.*, 1989). Macroscopically they are usually fungating, cauliflower-like masses, similar to large condylomata. It has been suggested that 50% are associated with 'classical' condylomata acuminata and HPV DNA has been demonstrated in these tumors, particularly type 6, but they are nonetheless predominantly tumors of postmenopausal women with a peak incidence in the sixth and seventh decades (Brisigotti *et al.*, 1989). The vulvar tumors are most often found on the labia majora and are typically malodorous.

Histologically verrucous carcinoma has a papillary pattern with virtually no cellular atypia. The epithelium is markedly thickened with florid hyper- and parakeratosis. Deep keratin-filled tunnels are seen, but clearly defined invasion is difficult to demonstrate (*Figures 20.8 and 20.9*). Groin lymph nodes are commonly enlarged due to infection, but metastases have not been described and extragenital tumors of this type also very rarely metastasize (Partridge *et al.*, 1980). Because of the bland histologic appearance it is imperative that any biopsy

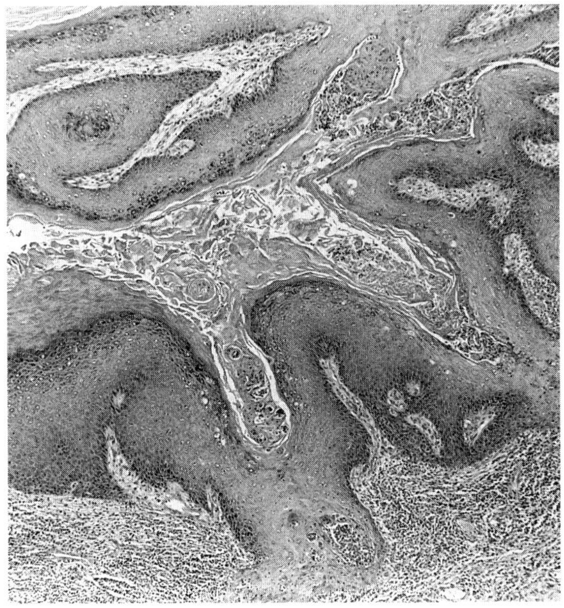

Figure 20.8. Simple vulvectomy specimen – verrucous carcinoma. The typical keratin-filled tunnels and coarsely papillary pattern of a verrucous carcinoma are evident.

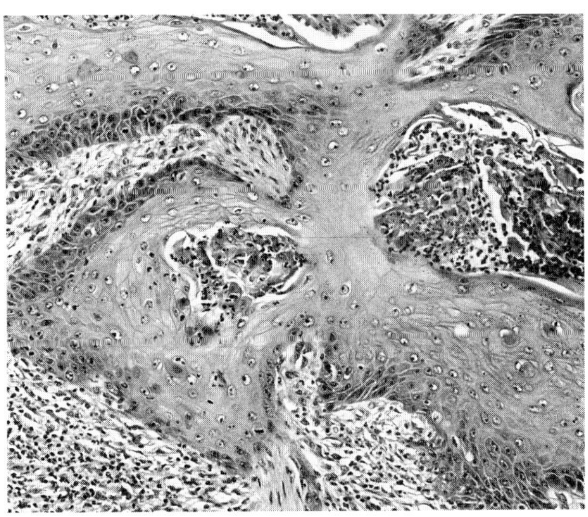

Figure 20.9. Vulvectomy specimen – verrucous carcinoma. There is a focus of stromal invasion (mid-lower edge of picture) arising from the squamous epithelium, which shows minimal nuclear atypia.

is of adequate size and depth. It was said in the past that irradiation of verrucous carcinomas led to alteration to a more aggressive tumor type with rapid progression and possibly metastasis, but for non-vulvar tumors this is probably not true and in the case of the vulva the position is unclear. Following wide and complete local excision prognosis is excellent.

It seems almost certain that this tumor is the same condition as the giant condyloma acuminatum of Bushke and Lowenstein, though some have disputed this (Partridge *et al.*, 1980); they are said to be inseparable on clinical appearance (Baird *et al.*, 1979). Verrucous carcinoma should not be confused with so-called 'warty' carcinoma, where the co-existence of very well-differentiated squamous cell carcinoma and HPV effect produces an exophytic tumor with coexistent koilocytosis, but with clear stromal invasion (Downey *et al.*, 1988; Kurman *et al.*, 1992). Such tumors have a prognosis possibly somewhat better than 'classical' keratinizing squamous cell carcinoma, but not as favorable as verrucous carcinoma.

When diagnosing very well-differentiated and verrucous carcinomas of the vulva the possibility of pseudoepitheliomatous hyperplasia should always be borne in mind because this mimics such tumors on occasion very closely. It is seen in association with many skin conditions, but in particular, may be seen on the vulva in association with benign granular cell tumors (Wolber *et al.*, 1991). An adequate deep biopsy is usually necessary for differential diagnosis.

Basaloid squamous cell carcinoma

These tend to occur in relatively young women (mean age in the mid 50s) and are usually associated with adjacent VIN. They also appear to be associated with a particularly high incidence of coexistent HPV infection, especially type 16, and synchronous or metachronous CIN and invasive squamous cell carcinoma of the cervix and vagina (i.e. they are a particular type of squamous cell carcinoma seen in association with 'lower female genital tract neoplasia syndrome', Kurman *et al.*, 1992). The prognosis is as yet unclear, but is probably similar to 'classical' keratinizing squamous cell carcinoma. Basaloid squamous carcinoma can be confused histologically with basal cell carcinoma and other small cell tumors.

Spindle cell squamous carcinoma

This tumor is composed histologically of pleomorphic spindle cells in a collagenous stroma. It may be very difficult to differentiate histologically from sarcoma, but immunocytochemistry may occasionally be helpful in this regard. It is a rare tumor with too few acceptable cases in the literature (Copas *et al.*, 1982) to assess relative prognosis.

Adenoid squamous carcinoma

This variant may be seen as an element in an otherwise typical squamous carcinoma or in 'pure' form and essentially consists of two elements – keratinizing squamous cells and acinar structures with dyskeratotic acantholytic cells in the center (Lasser *et al.*, 1974; Underwood *et al.*, 1978). Epithelial mucin is not present. Prognosis relative to squamous carcinoma generally is not known (Lasser *et al.*, 1974). This tumor should be differentiated from adenoid cystic carcinoma, which is a distinct entity (*vide infra*).

Basal Cell Carcinoma

Basal cell carcinomas usually occur on the light-exposed skin of the elderly, and although said to be rare on the vulva, are probably underreported. They usually present as a longstanding mass (Breen *et al.*, 1975), often on the anterior vulva, and possibly make up 4% of vulvar carcinomas (Cruz–Jimenez and Abell, 1975). Some authors suggest that they are rarely greater than 3 cm in diameter at presentation (Palladino *et al.*, 1969; Breen *et al.*, 1975), but others have found a wider size range with much larger tumors (Perrone *et al.*, 1987). Multicentricity is common and there is said to be a strong association with malignancy at other sites (Palladino *et al.*, 1969). Irradiation appears to be a predisposing cause. As at other sites, local invasion without metastasis is characteristic, though exceptions (six cases) are recorded (Perrone *et al.*, 1987; Gleeson *et al.*, 1994).

The vulvar tumor is histologically identical to tumors elsewhere, being composed of small dark 'undifferentiated' basal-type cells with a variable architectural pattern (*Figures 20.10 and 20.11*). An

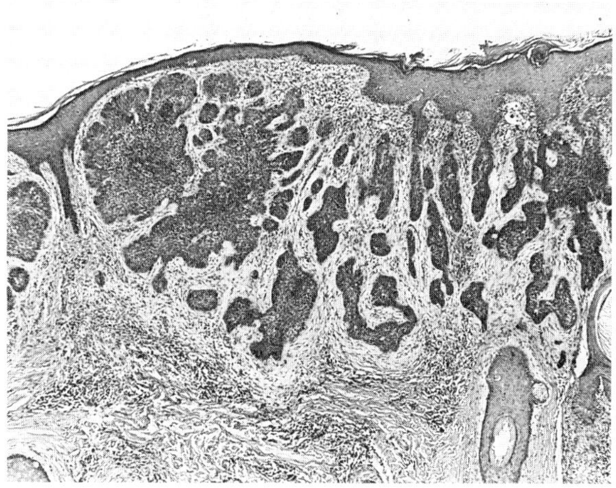

Figure 20.10. Vulvar biopsy – basal cell carcinoma. Low power photomicrograph showing a common pattern of basal cell carcinoma with irregular cords of dark cells infiltrating the dermis.

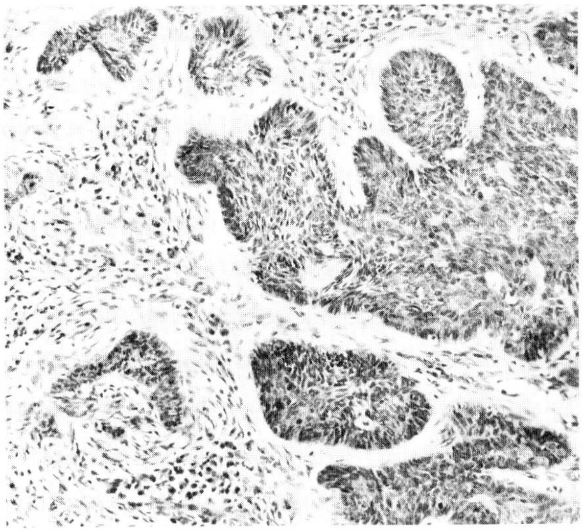

Figure 20.11. Vulvar biopsy – higher power view of the undifferentiated small dark cells of a basal cell carcinoma.

adenoid variant, which shows trabecular or gland-like structures in a dense stoma, has been described (Merino *et al.*, 1982). Basisquamous variants are also well described, but opinions vary on whether they represent true basal cell, squamous cell or intermediate neoplasms. The great majority probably behave as basal cell carcinomas. In cases where this apparent variant has metastasized only the squamous component has usually been seen at the metastatic site, suggesting that such cases were in reality squamous cell carcinomas.

Paget's Disease of the Vulva

Paget's disease of the vulva has generally been considered rare, making up approximately 2% of all vulvar malignancy (Taylor *et al.*, 1975) and differs from that of the breast in that only approximately one-fifth of cases have a demonstrable underlying carcinoma of adnexal structures (Baehrendtz *et al.*, 1994). Some cases, up to 40% in some series (Baehrendtz *et al.*, 1994), are associated with extragenital cancer (especially of the breast), other genitourinary tumors or basal cell carcinomas. In those cases without an underlying adenocarcinoma it is still unclear whether the primary site of origin is in ducts, surface epithelium or (most likely) at different sites in different cases. All three views have their proponents.

Macroscopically the disease appears as a scaly red area anywhere on the vulvar or perianal surface, usually in middle-aged or elderly women. Histologically, characteristic large pale Paget's cells, showing a distinct preference for the basal layers, are seen in the epithelium (*Figure 20.12*). These cells are often vacuolate and contain epithelial mucin. Melanin may be present due to transfer from melanocytes, and as the major differential diagnosis is intraepithelial superficial spreading malignant melanoma, immunocytochemistry may be very helpful in those cases where mucin histochemistry is equivocal. Immunohistochemistry has to date not been helpful in determining from superficial biopsies the presence of an underlying invasive tumor (Olson *et al.*, 1991).

Prognosis of Paget's disease is excellent if the disease is confined to the epithelium, though recurrences are common. With dermal invasion or an underlying adnexal carcinoma the prognosis worsens considerably (Jones *et al.*, 1979; Baehrendtz *et al.*, 1994) and metastases to regional nodes and elsewhere occur.

Malignant Melanoma

Malignant melanoma is an uncommon disease. Approximately 5% in white females are said to occur on the vulva (Ariel, 1981) making up 2–10% of vulvar malignancies (Chung *et al.*, 1975; Edington and Monaghan, 1980). These figures do not appear to have altered with the recent considerable increase generally in the incidence of malignant melanoma (Ragnarssonolding *et al.*, 1993). In a recent survey of the West Midlands of England, Bradgate *et al.* (1990) found only 60 cases over a 25-year period in an area with a population of 5 million. In this survey the tumor accounted for 2.2% of all melanomas in women and 3.6% of all vulvar malignant tumors.

Malignant melanoma at this site is said to be a disease of postmenopausal women. The mean age in our own series (Bradgate *et al.*, 1990) was 63 years (range 22–93 years). Impingement on or localization to 'mucosal' surfaces is seen in more than 60% of cases, manifest in some series as a preference for involvement of the clitoral area and labia minora (Morrow and Rutledge, 1972; Chung *et al.*, 1975).

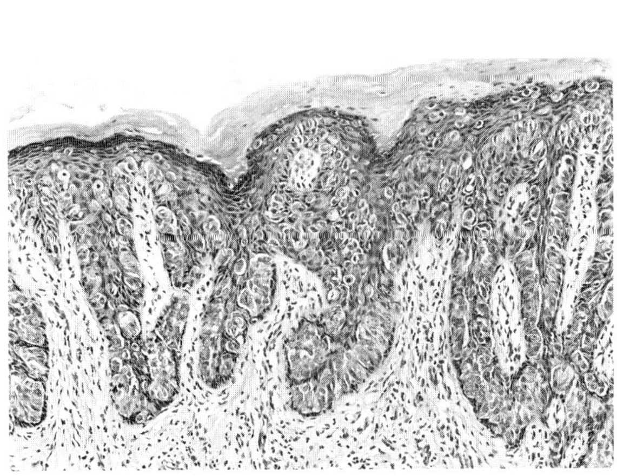

Figure 20.12. Vulvar biopsy showing large pale Paget's cells aggregating in the basal layers of the epithelium.

Macroscopically it may be pigmented or non-pigmented, nodular, flat or ulcerated (*Figure 20.13*). On the skin generally melanoma may be divided into four types: superficial spreading (pagetoid), nodular, acral lentiginous (including mucosal lentiginous) and lentigo maligna. In the great majority of cases lentigo maligna melanoma occurs on light-exposed skin. The relative proportions of the other types vary greatly in different series (Kendall Pierson, 1987) probably due to differences in definition of type. In our own series more than 50% were of invasive superficial spreading type.

Histologically, superficial spreading melanoma shows a 'radial' or *in situ* growth phase with nests of atypical melanocytes at all levels of the epidermis before the development of invasive foci (*Figure 20.14*). Acral lentiginous and lentigo maligna types also show a well-developed radial phase of different morphology. Nodular malignant melanoma manifests a 'vertical' (invasive) growth pattern from very early in the disease with an absent or slight intraepithelial component (extending no more than three rete ridges from the invasive zone). There is disagreement in the literature as to the prognostic usefulness of melanoma typing for malignant melanomas of the vulva (Podratz *et al.*, 1983; Johnson *et al.*, 1986; Bradgate *et al.*, 1990).

As with other skin sites the prognosis is likely to be closely determined by tumor depth. Depth is best assessed by direct measurement as described by Breslow rather than by Clark's levels. By inference from other sites the likely relevant depths will be up to 0.76 mm (prognosis excellent), 1.5 mm (intermediate group), and greater than 1.5 mm (prognosis poor). This hypothesis gains support from recent studies using depth measurement (Johnson *et al.*, 1986) and older studies using Clark's levels (Chung *et al.*, 1975; Jaramillo *et al.*, 1985). A considerable practical problem with the use of such depths for prognosis and treatment in vulvar tumors is that they tend to present late and prognostic bands of greater overall thickness may have more value at this site (Bradgate *et al.*, 1990).

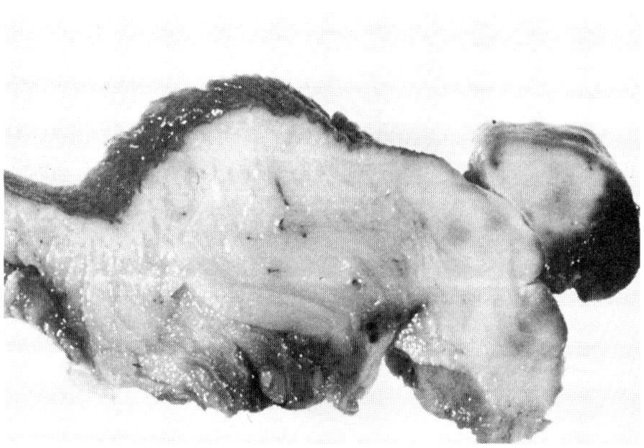

Figure 20.13. Vulvar excision biopsy sliced across to show a raised pigmented nodule and deep infiltrating zone of malignant melanoma.

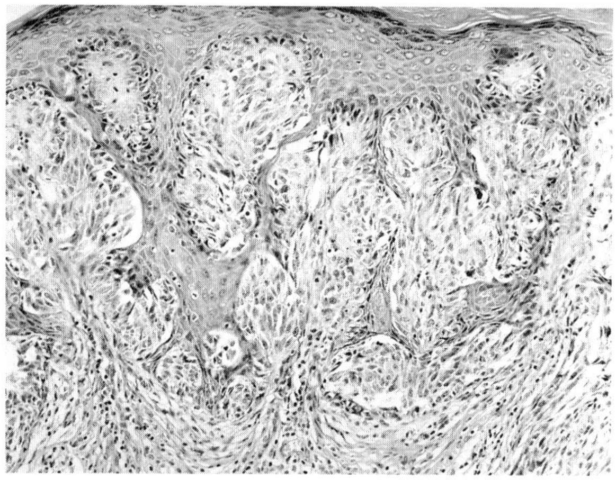

Figure 20.14. Vulvar biopsy showing the classical appearances of the superficial spreading variant of invasive malignant melanoma.

The FIGO staging system used for squamous carcinoma has been suggested not to correlate well with survival in malignant melanoma of the vulva (Podratz *et al.*, 1983), but others disagree (Johnson *et al.*, 1986; Bragdate *et al.*, 1990). Mitotic rate has been said by some to have prognostic importance (Johnson *et al.*, 1986; Bradgate *et al.*, 1990) as have the presence or absence of ulceration and the cell type (Bradgate *et al.*, 1990; Tasseron *et al.*, 1992). Morphometry has not been shown to be clearly useful (Tasseron *et al.*, 1992).

Epithelial Tumors of Glands and Adnexal Structures

Carcinoma of Bartholin's Glands

More than 200 cases of carcinoma of Bartholin's gland have been reported (Leuchter *et al.*, 1982; Wheelock *et al.*, 1984). The mean age at diagnosis is mid-fifties, but the age range is very wide. Presentation is usually with a mass, pain or discharge. Three criteria have been demanded in order to accept that a tumor is of Bartholin's gland origin: the tumor must arise in the usual area of Bartholin's gland, a transition from non-neoplastic to neoplastic tissue must be seen, and no primary tumor of similar type must be present at another site.

Adeno- and squamous carcinoma occur with almost equal frequency at this site making up 80% of malignant tumors. Variants of adenocarcinoma (e.g. papillary) are well described. Adenoid cystic carcinoma makes up a further 8–15% of carcinomas and shows the characteristic histologic pattern of cords and nests of cells, with a prominent myoepithelial cell layer, arranged around a dense hyaline core. The remaining tumors are transitional, adenosquamous and undifferentiated carcinomas, and malignant melanomas.

Tumors of Bartholin's gland typically spread locally and to regional nodes. Adenoid cystic tumors are slow growing with only 15% metastatic at the time of diagnosis, compared to 50% for adeno- and squamous carcinomas, but local recurrence is common.

Adnexal Tumors and Tumors of Breast-like Tissue

The great majority of sweat gland and other tumors are benign and the commonest at this site is the simple papillary hidradenoma. Clear cell hidradenomas are also described (Nielson, 1973) as are trichoepitheliomas, trichilemmomas and syringomas. Syringomas may be multiple and associated with pruritus. Proliferating trichilemmal tumors at this site may be mistaken histologically and clinically for squamous carcinomas (Avinoach *et al.*, 1989). Rare malignant examples of sweat gland tumors unassociated with Paget's disease have been described (Wick *et al.*, 1985) though the histologic appearance of the cases illustrated is not always convincing. Sebaceous carcinoma is also described (Jacobs *et al.*, 1986). Benign and malignant mixed tumors occur and it is suggested that they arise from sweat glands or Bartholin's glands (Rorat and Wallach, 1984).

Ectopic mammary-type tissue may be seen in the vulvar connective tissues. A range of mammary-type tumors, benign and malignant, are also described (Van der Putte, 1994) and a proportion of cases of vulvar Paget's disease may arise in such structures. Adenocarcinomas in the breast-type tissue are very rare, but usually appear to be small; they are virtually impossible to separate histologically from sweat gland carcinomas.

Sarcomas and Related Conditions

Leiomyosarcoma

Leiomyosarcoma appears to be the commonest of the vulvar sarcomas, which are rare tumors accounting for only approximately 1% of all vulvar malignancies. Only 15 cases of vulvar leiomyosarcoma had been reported up to 1980 (Audet-Lapointe *et al.*, 1980). Most appear to represent *de novo* tumors rather than malignant change in a leiomyoma and have usually presented as rapidly growing masses, greater than 5 cm diameter, in women in their 20s and 30s. Those cases not cured by wide local excision appear to have a protracted course with local recurrences, but widespread metastases may occur.

Diagnosis of malignancy at this site is best based on the presence of mitotic counts above ten per ten high power fields, pleomorphism, infiltrative margins and abnormal mitoses. Tavassoli and Norris (1979) reviewed 32 smooth muscle tumors of the vulva and found large size and high mitotic rate were the best predictors of recurrence, but none of their series metastasized; this is in contrast to the outcome seen by others (DiSaia *et al.*, 1971; Davos and Abell, 1976).

Fibrosarcoma

Fibrosarcomas occur over a wide age range (DiSaia *et al.*, 1971; Davos and Abell, 1976) and appear to have a poor prognosis. The diagnosis should be confined to tumors showing the classical herringbone pattern of interweaving spindle cells. Immunocytochemistry is imperative to exclude alternative tumors such as schwannoma and monophasic synovial sarcoma. Some tumors previously reported as fibrosarcomas might by modern criteria be better put into other diagnostic groups; even allowing for this they have been rarely reported.

Malignant Fibrous Histiocytoma

Said to be the second commonest vulvar sarcoma (Davos and Abell, 1976), malignant fibrous histiocytoma occurs in various subtypes of highly variable histologic pattern, but generally containing a fibroblast-like component together with histiocytic cells and often large bizarre cells. It classically presents as a large mass in a middle-aged woman. Widespread metastases have been reported in a proportion of cases (Hensley and Friedrich, 1973; Davos and Abell, 1976). Recent opinion suggests, however, that this diagnosis may simply represent a common differentiation pattern of several different tumors.

Occasional cases of dermatofibrosarcoma protuberans, a low-grade malignant variant of malignant fibrous histiocytoma, have been described in the vulva (Davos and Abell, 1976; Soltan, 1981; Agress *et al.*, 1983; Bock *et al.*, 1985). It may recur locally, but very rarely metastasizes. It is composed of spindle cells in an interweaving 'cartwheel' or 'storiform' pattern with infiltrative margins.

Aggressive Angiomyxoma

Aggressive angiomyxoma was first described by Steeper and Rosai (1983) and shows a predeliction for the vulva and paravaginal tissues of young women. Up until 1992 26 cases had been reported in the vulva, vagina, pelvic floor and perineum of women (Elchalal *et al.*, 1992). It is characterized by slow growth and extensive local recurrences and is locally infiltrative with very poorly-defined margins. Most recurrences occur within 3–4 years of primary surgery. Metastases are not described and the condition does not appear to be a true sarcoma.

Macroscopically the tumors are usually large (up to 60 cm), gelatinous and sticky (*Figure 20.15*). Histologically they show an abundant myxoid stroma with scattered collagen bundles and numerous vessels, some of which are thick walled. Glandular elements have been described. Some workers have favored a myofibroblast origin and immunocytochemistry (*Figure 20.16*) tends to support this, with immunohistochemical positivity for vimentin, actin and S100 protein (Elchalal *et al.*, 1992), but other studies by electron microscopy favor a purely fibroblast origin (Begin *et al.*, 1985).

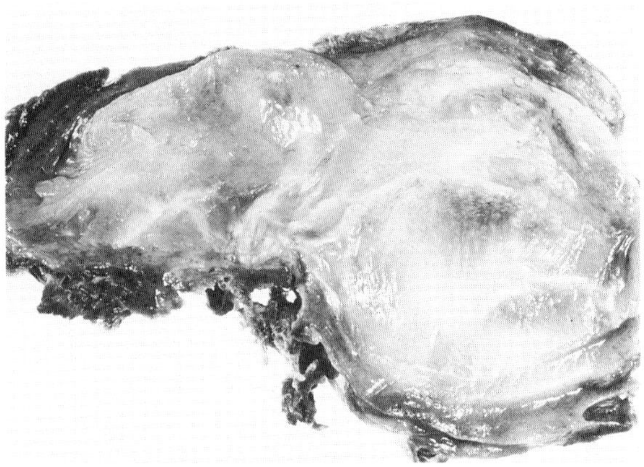

Figure 20.15. Pelvic mass from paravaginal and broad ligament area showing the typical myxoid appearance of aggressive angiomyxoma.

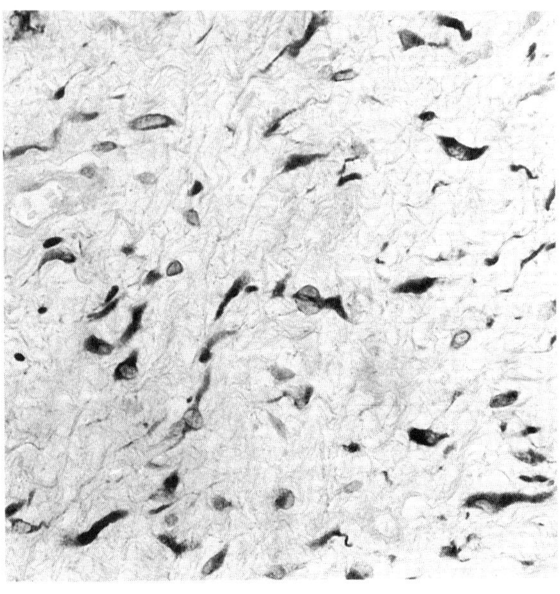

Figure 20.16. Paravaginal mass – aggressive angiomyxoma. Immunocytochemical stain demonstrating desmin (indicative of myocyte differentiation) in the stellate stromal cells.

Rhabdomyosarcoma

The embryonal variant typically seen in the vagina has been described on only three occasions in the vulva (Talerman, 1973; Hildebrand *et al.*, 1980; Copeland *et al.*, 1985a); in two cases the disease was fatal. It should be remembered that benign vulvar and vaginal fibroepithelial (pseudosarcomatous) polyps may superficially resemble embryonal rhabdomyosarcoma histologically (Mucitelli *et al.*, 1990) and care should be taken not to confuse the two. Vaginal rhabdomyosarcoma is virtually confined to infants and young children. Two cases of the alveolar variant of rhabdomyosarcoma (Copeland *et al.*, 1985b) have been described at this site. Other rhabdomyosarcomas have been reported, but their type was not stated (DiSaia *et al.*, 1971). Prognosis is generally poor.

Other Sarcomas

Malignant granular cell tumor (Robertson *et al.*, 1981), alveolar soft part sarcoma (Shen *et al.*, 1982), malignant schwannoma (DiSaia *et al.*, 1971; Davos and Abell, 1976), Kaposi's sarcoma (Hall, 1979; LiVolsi and Brookes, 1987), liposarcoma (LiVolsi and Brookes, 1987), malignant rhabdoid tumor (Perrone *et al.*, 1989) and epithelioid sarcoma (Hall *et al.*, 1980; Ulbright *et al.*, 1983) have all been described on the vulva and essentially behave similar to those at the more common sites of occurrence. Occasional cases are reported of vascular tumors including hemangiopericytomas (Davos and Abell, 1976).

Miscellanous Primary Tumors

Yolk sac (endodermal sinus) tumors occur rarely as primary vulvar tumors (Dudley *et al.*, 1983) as do mesotheliomas (Davos and Abell, 1976). Davos and Abell (1976) also reported an 'embryonal stromal sarcoma.' A suggested case of adenosarcoma arising in endometriosis has been described (Brookes and Wheeler, 1977).

Primary lymphomas are very rare, but this site has been stated to be the second commonest female genital tract site after the cervix (Young *et al.*, 1985;

Kurman *et al.*, 1992). Most appear to be of the diffuse large-cell type. They tend to occur in women of reproductive age and present as an erythematous mass.

Merkel cell tumors have occasionally been described and may be associated with VIN or invasive squamous carcinoma. They usually present as solitary or multiple intradermal nodules in elderly women and have a high risk of early metastasis to regional nodes (Copeland *et al.*, 1985c; Husseinzadeh *et al.*, 1988). Histologically they typically show the small cell pattern of neuroectodermal tumors, but may show trabecular, intermediate or small cell differentiation. They are reactive with neuroendocrine markers such as anti-chromogranin, but may be misdiagnosed as basal cell carcinomas, lymphomas or metastatic small cell bronchial or cervical carcinomas.

Metastatic Tumors

In a series of more than 260 cases of vulvar malignancy, Dehner found that 8% of tumors were metastatic (Dehner, 1973). Of 22 cases, ten were metastatic cervical squamous carcinomas. Metastatic endometrial carcinoma was next in frequency. Other metastases described are transitional cell carcinomas of the urethra and bladder (Dehner, 1973; Powell and Jones, 1983), carcinoma of the breast (Dehner, 1973; Mader and Friedrich, 1982), vagina, stomach, lung, ovary and kidney, and lymphoma. Metastatic choriocarcinomas, sarcomas and malignant melanomas have also been seen. Most metastases are within the labia majora. Bartholin's gland may be involved. The metastasis usually presents within 18 months of diagnosis of the primary tumor and few patients survive for more than 12 months.

Summary of Core Information

- Vulvar intraepithelial neoplasia (VIN Grades I, II, and III rather than mild, moderate, and severe squamous cell dysplasia/carcinoma *in situ*, respectively) is the recommended terminology for squamous intraepithelial neoplasia of the vulva.
- The progression rate of VIN to invasive cancer is variable but in general less frequent (3–4%) than that for cervical intraepithelial neoplasia (CIN).
- The term 'microinvasion', in squamous carcinoma, of the vulva should be avoided since there is no generally accepted definition; however, tumors in FIGO Stage I showing less than 1 mm of invasion have an almost negligible risk of lymph node metastasis.
- Moderately well- or well-differentiated squamous carcinoma is by far the commonest vulvar primary tumor.
- Basal cell carcinoma of the vulva is said to be rare, but is in reality probably an underreported tumor.
- An adequately-sized deep biopsy of verrucous carcinoma is necessary to examine the epithelial–stromal junction for invasion and prevent the misdiagnosis of a condylomatous lesion.
- Vulvar Paget's disease, in the majority of cases, does not have an underlying adenocarcinoma (as opposed to mammary Paget's disease).
- Anogenital Paget's disease is associated with an increased incidence of extragenital cancer, particularly from the breast or gastrointestinal tract.
- Prognosis in vulvar malignant melanoma is closely determined by tumor depth of invasion, a figure best derived by direct measurement.
- Although the vulva is an uncommon site for metastases, most come from other female genital tract tumors, particularly cervical squamous cell carcinoma, and involve the labia majora.

References

Agress R, Figge DC, Tamimi H & Greer B (1983) Dermatofibrosarcoma protuberans of the vulva. *Gynecol. Oncol.* **16**: 288–291.

Andreasson B, Bock JE & Weberg E (1982) Invasive cancer in the vulvar region. *Acta Obstet. Gynecol. Scand.* **6**: 113–119.

Andreasson B & Bock JE (1985) Intraepithelial neoplasia in the vulvar region. *Gynecol. Oncol.* **21**: 300–305.

Ariel IM (1981) Malignant melanoma of the female genital system: A report of 48 patients and review of the literature. *J. Surg. Oncol.* **16**: 371–383.

Audet-Lapointe P, Paquin F, Guerard MJ *et al.* (1980) Leiomyosarcoma of the vulva. *Gynecol. Oncol.* **10**: 350–355.

Avinoach I, Zirkin HJ & Glezerman M (1989) Proliferating trichilemmal tumor of the vulva. Case report and review of the literature. *Int. J. Gynecol. Pathol.* **8**: 163–168.

Baehrendtz H, Einhorn N, Pettersson F & Silfverswärd C (1994) Paget's disease of the vulva, the Radiumhemmet series 1975–1990. *Int. J. Gynecol. Cancer* **4**: 1–6.

Baird PJ, Elliot P, Stening M & Korda A (1979) Giant condyloma acuminatum of the vulva and anal canal. *Aust. NZ J. Obstet. Gynecol.* **19**: 119–122.

Barnes AE, Crissman JD, Schellhas HF & Azoury RS (1980)

Microinvasive carcinoma of the vulva: a clinicopathological evaluation. *Obstet. Gynecol.* **56:** 234–238.

Begin LR, Clement PB, Kirk ME *et al.* (1985) Aggressive angiomyxoma of pelvic soft parts: a clinicopathologic study of nine cases. *Hum. Pathol.* **16:** 621–628.

Bjerregaard B, Andreasson B, Visfeldt J & Bock JE (1993) The significance of histology and morphometry in predicting lymph node metastases in patients with squamous cell carcinoma of the vulva. *Gynecol. Oncol.* **50:** 323–329.

Bock JE, Andreasson B, Thorn A & Holck S (1985) Dermatofibrosarcoma protuberans of the vulva. *Gynecol. Oncol.* **20:** 129–135.

Boyce J, Fruchter RG, Kasambilides E *et al.* (1985) Prognostic factors in carcinoma of the vulva. *Gynecol. Oncol.* **20:** 364–377.

Bradgate M, Rollason RP, McConkey CC & Powell J (1990) Malignant melanoma of the vulva: A clinicopathological study of 50 cases. *Br. J. Obstet. Gynaecol.* **97:** 124–133.

Breen JL, Neubecker RD, Greenwald E & Gregori CA (1975) Basal cell carcinoma of the vulva. *Obstet. Gynecol.* **46:** 122–129.

Brookes JJ & Wheeler JE (1977) Malignancy arising in extragonadal endometriosis. A case report and summary of the world literature. *Cancer* **40:** 3065–3073.

Brisigotti M, Moreno A, Murcia C, Matias–Guia X & Prat J (1989) Verrucous carcinoma of the vulva. A clinicopathologic and immunohistochemical study of five cases. *Int. J. Gynecol. Pathol.* **8:** 1–7.

Buscema J, Stern J & Woodruff JD (1980) The significance of the histologic alterations adjacent to invasive vulval carcinoma. *Am. J. Obstet. Gynecol.* **137:** 902–909.

Buscema J, Stern JL & Woodruff JD (1981) Early invasive carcinoma of the vulva. *Am. J. Obstet. Gynecol.* **140:** 563–569.

Carter J, Carlson J, Fowler J *et al.* (1993) Invasive vulvar tumors in young women – A disease of the immunosuppressed? *Gynecol. Oncol.* **51:** 307–310.

Chung AF, Woodruff JM & Lewis JL (1975) Malignant melanoma of the vulva: a report of 44 cases. *Obstet. Gynecol.* **45:** 638–646.

Copas P, Dyer M, Comas FV & Hall DJ (1982) Spindle cell carcinoma of the vulva. *Diag. Gynecol. Obstet.* **4:** 235–241.

Copeland LJ, Gershenson DM, Saul PB *et al.* (1985a) Sarcoma botryoides of the female genital tract. *Obstet. Gynecol.* **66:** 262–266.

Copeland LJ, Sneige N, Stringer A *et al.* (1985b) Alveolar rhabdomyosarcoma of the female genitalia. *Cancer* **56:** 849–855.

Copeland LJ, Cleary K, Sneige N & Edwards CL (1985c) Neuroendocrine (Merkel cell) carcinoma of the vulva: a case report and review of the literature. *Gynecol. Oncol.* **22:** 367–378.

Cruz–Jimenez PR & Abell MR (1975) Cutaneous basal cell carcinoma of the vulva. *Obstet. Gynecol.* **36:** 1860–1868.

Davos I & Abell M (1976) Soft tissue sarcomas of the vulva. *Gynecol. Oncol.* **4:** 70–86.

■ Dehner LP (1973) Metastatic and secondary tumours of the vulva. *Obstet. Gynecol.* **42:** 47–57.

DiSaia PJ, Rutledge F & Smith JP (1971) Sarcoma of the vulva: report of 12 patients. *Obstet. Gynecol.* **38:** 180–184.

Dolan JR, McCall AR, Gooneratne S, Walter S & Lansky DM (1993) DNA ploidy, proliferation index, grade and stage as prognostic factors for vulvar squamous carcinomas. *Gynecol. Oncol.* **48:** 232–235.

Donaldson ES, Powell DE, Hanson MB & Van Nagell JR (1981) Prognostic parameters in invasive vulvar cancer. *Cancer* **11:** 184–190.

Downey GO, Okagaki T, Ostrow RS *et al.* (1988) Condylomatous carcinoma of the vulva with special reference to human papillomavirus DNA. *Obstet. Gynecol.* **72:** 68–73.

Dudley AG, Young RH, Lawrence WD & Scully RE (1983) Endodermal sinus tumour of the vulva in an infant. *Obstet. Gynecol.* **61:** 76s–79s.

Dvoretsky PM, Bonfiglio TA, Helmkamp BF *et al.* (1984) The pathology of superficially invasive thin vulvar squamous carcinoma. *Int. J. Gynecol. Pathol.* **3:** 331–342.

Edington PT & Monaghan JM (1980) Malignant melanoma of the vulva and vagina. *Br. J. Obstet. Gynaecol.* **87:** 422–424.

Elchalal U, Lifschitz–Mercer B, Dgani R & Zalel Y (1992) Case report. Aggressive angiomyxoma of the vulva. *Gynecol. Oncol.* **47:** 260–262.

Fiorica JV, Cavanagh D, Marsden DE, Shepherd JH, Ruffolo EH & Songster CL (1988) Carcinoma *in situ* of the vulva: 24 years experience in southwest Florida. *South Med. J.* **81:** 589–593.

Fu YS, Reagan JW, Townsend DE, Kaufman RH, Richart RM & Wentz WB (1981) Nuclear DNA study of vulvar intraepithelial and invasive squamous neoplasms. *Obstet. Gynecol.* **57:** 643–652.

Gleeson NC, Ruffolo EH, Hoffman MS & Cavanagh D (1994) Basal cell carcinoma of the vulva with groin node metastases. *Gynecol. Oncol.* **53:** 366–368.

Green TH (1978) Carcinoma of the vulva – a reassessment. *Obstet. Gynecol.* **52:** 462–469.

Green TH, Ulfelder H & Meigs JV (1958) Epidermoid carcinoma of the vulva: an analysis of 238 cases. I. Etiology and diagnosis. *Am. J. Obstet. Gynecol.* **75:** 834–847.

Hacker NF, Berek JS, Lagasse LD *et al.* (1984) Individualization of treatment for Stage I squamous cell vulvar carcinoma. *Obstet. Gynecol.* **63:** 155–162.

Hall DJ (1979) Kaposi's carcoma of the vulva: a case report and brief review. *Obstet. Gynecol.* **54:** 478–483.

Hall DJ, Grimes MM & Goplerud DR (1980) Epithelioid sarcoma of the vulva. *Gynecol. Oncol.* **9:** 237–246.

Hay DM & Cole FM (1969) Primary invasive carcinoma of the vulva in Jamaica. *J. Obstet. Gynaecol. Br. Commonwealth* **76:** 821–830.

Hensley GT & Friedrich EG (1973) Malignant fibroxanthoma: a sarcoma of the vulva. *Am. J. Obstet. Gynecol.* **116:** 289–291.

Hildebrand HF, Krivosic I, Grandier–Vazeille X *et al.* (1980) Perineal rhabdomyosarcoma in a newborn child: pathological and biochemical studies with emphasis on contractile proteins. *J. Clin. Pathol.* **33:** 823–829.

Hopkins MP, Reid GC, Vettrano IP, Morley GW (1991) Squamous cell carcinoma of the vulva: prognostic factors influencing survival. *Gynecol. Oncol.* **43:** 113–117.

Husseinzadeh N, Whesseler T, Newman N, Shbaro I & Ho P (1988) Neuroendocrine (Merkel cell) carcinoma of the vulva. *Gynecol. Oncol.* **29:** 105–112.

Isaacs JH (1976) Verrucous carcinoma of the female genital tract. *Gynecol. Oncol.* **4:** 259–269.

Iversen T, Abeler V & Aälders J (1981) Individualized treatment of Stage I carcinoma of the vulva. *Obstet. Gynecol.* **57:** 85–89.

Jacobs DM, Sandles LG & Leboit PE (1986) Sebaceous carcinoma arising from Bowen's disease of the vulva. *Arch. Dermatol.* **122:** 1191–1193.

Japaze H, Garcia Bunuel R & Woodruff JD (1977) Primary vulvar neoplasia. A review of *in situ* and invasive carcinoma 1935–1972. *Obstet. Gynecol.* **49:** 404–411.

Jaramillo BA, Ganjei P, Averette HE *et al.* (1985) Malignant melanoma of the vulva. *Obstet. Gynecol.* **66:** 398–401.

Johnson TL, Kumar NB, White CD & Morley GW (1986) Prognostic features of vulvar melanoma: a clinicopathological analysis. *Int. J. Gynecol. Pathol.* **5:** 110–118.

■ Jones RE, Austin C & Ackerman AB (1979) Extramammary Paget's Disease: a critical reexamination. *Am. J. Dermatopathol.* **1:** 101–132.

Jones RW & McLean MR (1986) Carcinoma *in situ* of the vulva: a review of 31 treated and five untreated cases. *Obstet. Gynecol.* **68:** 499–503.

Kelley JL III, Burke TW, Tornos C *et al.* (1992) Minimally invasive vulvar carcinoma: an indication for conservative surgical therapy. *Gynecol. Oncol.* **44:** 240–244.

Kendall Pierson K (1987) Malignant melanomas and pigmented lesions of the vulva. In: Wilkinson EJ (ed) *Pathology of the Vulva and Vagina,* pp. 155–179. New York: Churchill Livingstone.

■ Kurman RJ, Norris HJ & Wilkinson E (1992) Tumors of the vulva: In: *Tumours of the Cervix, Vagina, and Vulva,* pp. 179–255. Washington: Armed Forces Institute of Pathology.

Lasser A, Cornorg JL & Morris JM (1974) Adenoid squamous cell carcinoma of the vulva. *Cancer* **33:** 224–227.

Leuchter RS, Hacker NF, Voet RL *et al.* (1982) Primary carcinoma of the Bartholin gland: a report of 14 cases and review of the literature. *Obstet. Gynecol.* **60:** 361–367.

■ LiVolsi VA & Brookes JJ (1987) Soft tissue tumours of the vulva. In: Wilkinson EJ (ed) *Pathology of the Vulva and Vagina,* pp. 209–238. New York: Churchill Livingstone.

Mader MH & Friedrich EG Jr (1982) Vulvar metastasis of breast carcinoma. A case report. *J. Reprod. Med.* **27:** 169–171.

Merino MJ, Livolsi VA, Shwartz PE & Rudnicki J (1982) Adenoid basal cell carcinoma of the vulva. *Int. J. Gynecol. Pathol.* **1:** 299–306.

Morrow CP & Rutledge FN (1972) Melanoma of the vulva. *Obstet. Gynecol.* **39:** 745–752.

Mucitelli DR, Charles EZ & Kraus FT (1990) Vulvovaginal polyps. Histologic appearances, ultrastructure, immunohistochemical characteristics and clinicopathologic correlations. *Int. J. Gynecol. Pathol.* **9:** 20–40.

Nielsen NC (1973) Hidradenoma of the vulva. *Acta Obstet. Gynecol. Scand.* **52:** 387–389.

Olson DJ, Fujimura M, Swanson P & Okagaki Y (1991) Immunohistochemical features of Paget's disease of the vulva with and without adenocarcinoma. *Int. J. Gynecol. Pathol.* **10:** 285–295.

Palladino VS, Duffy JL & Bures GJ (1969) Basal cell carcinoma of the vulva. *Cancer* **24:** 460–476.

Partridge EE, Murad T, Shingleton HM *et al.* (1980) Verrucous lesions of the female genitalia. 2. Verrucous carcinoma. *Am. J. Obstet. Gynecol.* **137:** 412–418.

Perrone T, Twiggs LB, Adcock LL & Dehner LP (1987) Vulvar basal cell carcinoma: an infrequently metastasizing neoplasm. *Int. J. Gynecol. Pathol.* **6:** 152–165.

Perrone T, Swanson PE, Twiggs L, Ulbright TM & Dehner LP (1989) Malignant rhabdoid tumor of the vulva: is distinction from epithelioid sarcoma possible? A pathologic and immunohistochemical study. *Am. J. Surg. Pathol.* **13:** 848–858.

Pickel N & Haas J (1986) Microcarcinoma of the vulva. *J. Reprod. Med.* **31:** 831–835.

Podratz KC, Gaffey TA, Symmonds RE, Johansen KL & O'Brien PC (1983) Melanoma of the vulva: an update. *Gynecol. Oncol.* **16:** 153–168.

Powell CS & Jones PA (1983) Carcinoma of the bladder with metastasis in the clitoris. *Br. J. Obstet. Gynaecol.* **90:** 380–381.

Ragnarssonolding B, Johanson H, Rutgvist LE & Ringborg U (1993) Malignant melanoma of the vulva and vagina: trends in incidence, age distribution and long term survival among 245 consecutive cases in Sweden 1960–1984. *Cancer* **71:** 1893–1897.

Robertson AJ, McIntosh W, Lamont P & Guthrie W (1981) Malignant granular cell tumour (myoblastoma) of the vulva: report of a case and review of the literature. *Histopathology* **5:** 69–79.

Rorat E & Wallach RC (1984) Mixed tumours of the vulva: clinical outcome and pathology. *Int. J. Gynecol. Pathol.* **3:** 323–328.

Rowley KC, Gallion HH, Donaldson ES *et al.* (1988) Prognostic factors in early vulvar cancer. *Gynecol. Oncol.* **31:** 43–49.

Sedlis A, Homesley H, Bundy BN *et al.* (1987) Positive groin lymph nodes in superficial squamous cell vulvar cancer. A Gynecologic Oncology Group study. *Am. J. Obstet. Gynecol.* **156:** 1159–1164.

Shen JT, D'Ablang G & Morrow CP (1982) Alveolar soft part sarcoma of the vulva: report of first case and review of the literature. *Gynecol. Oncol.* **13:** 120–128.

Soltan MH (1981) Dermatofibrosarcoma protuberans of the vulva. Case report. *Br. J. Obstet. Gynaecol.* **88:** 203–205.

Steeper T & Rosai J (1983) Aggressive angiomyxoma of the female pelvis and perineum. *Am. J. Surg. Pathol.* **7:** 463–476.

Talerman A (1973) Sarcoma botryoides presenting as a polyp on the labium majus. *Cancer* **32:** 994–999.

Tasseron EWK, Van der Esch EP, Hart AAM, Brutel de la Riviere G & Aartson EJ (1992) A clincopathological study of 30 melanomas of the vulva. *Gynecol. Oncol.* **46:** 170–175.

Tavassoli FA & Norris FJ (1979) Smooth muscle tumours of the vulva. *Obstet. Gynecol.* **53:** 213–224.

Taylor PR, Stenwig JT & Klausen H (1975) Paget's disease of the vulva. *Gynecol. Oncol.* **3:** 46–60.

Ulbright TM, Brokaw SA, Stehman FB & Roth LM (1983) Epithelioid sarcoma of the vulva: evidence suggesting a more aggressive behaviour than extra-genital epithelioid sarcoma. *Cancer* **52:** 1462–1469.

Underwood JW, Adcock LL & Okagaki T (1978) Adenosquamous carcinoma of skin appendages (adenoid squamous cell carcinoma, pseudoglandular squamous carcinoma, adenoacanthoma of sweat gland of Lever) of the vulva. A clinical and ultrastructural study. *Cancer* **42:** 1851–1858.

Van der Putte SCJ (1994) Mammary-like glands of the vulva and their disorders. *Int. J. Gynecol. Pathol.* **13:** 150–160.

Van der Velden J, Kooyman CD, Van Lindert ACM & Heintz APM (1992) A Stage Ia vulvar carcinoma with an inguinal node recurrence after local excision. A case report and literature review. *Int. J. Gynecol. Cancer* **2:** 157–159.

Wharton J, Gallagher S & Rutledge FN (1974) Microinvasive carcinoma of the vulva. *Am. J. Obstet. Gynecol.* **118:** 159–162.

Wheelock JB, Goplerud DR, Dunn LJ & Oates JF (1984) Primary carcinoma of the Bartholin gland: a report of 10 cases. *Obstet. Gynecol.* **63:** 820–824.

Wick MR, Goellner JR, Wolfe JT & Su WPD (1985) Vulvar sweat gland carcinomas. *Arch. Pathol. Lab. Med.* **109:** 43–47.

■ Wilkinson EJ (1987) Superficially invasive carcinoma of the vulva. In: *Pathology of the Vulva and Vagina*, pp. 103–117. New York: Churchill Livingstone.

Wilkinson EJ, Rico MJ & Pierson KK (1982) Microinvasive carcinoma of the vulva. *Int. J. Gynecol. Pathol.* **1:** 29–39.

Wolber RA, Talerman A, Wilkinson EJ & Clement PB (1991) Vulvar granular cell tumors with pseudocarcinomatous hyperplasia: a comparative analysis with well differentiated squamous carcinoma. *Int. J. Gynecol. Pathol.* **10:** 59–66.

Yoonessi M, Goodell T, Satchidanand S *et al.* (1983) Microinvasive squamous carcinoma of the vulva. *J. Surg. Oncol.* **24:** 315–321.

Young RH, Harris NL & Scully RE (1985) Lymphoma-like lesions of the lower female genital tract: a report of 16 cases. *Int. J. Gynecol. Pathol.* **4:** 289–299.

Zaino RJ (1987) Carcinoma of the vulva, urethra and Bartholin's glands. In: Wilkinson EJ (ed) *Pathology of the Vulva and Vagina*, pp. 119–153. New York: Churchill Livingstone.

Zaino RJ, Husseinzadeh N, Nahas W & Mortel R (1982) Epithelial alterations in proximity to invasive squamous carcinoma of the vulva. *Int. J. Gynecol. Pathol.* **1:** 173–184.

21 Vulvar Intraepithelial Lesions

A Warwick
DM Luesley

In situ squamous cell carcinoma of the vulva was first described in 1922, but until recently the nomenclature, natural history and management of vulvar epithelial dysplasia has remained in a state of confusion. The increasing prevalence of vulvar intraepithelial neoplasia (VIN) (Shafi *et al.*, 1989), particularly in younger women (Buscema *et al.*, 1980), over recent years has brought to the fore the need to develop less radical treatment protocols. The increasing frequency of VIN appears to be a phenomenon of the last 25 years during which the incidence in the USA has doubled to 2.1/100,000 women; a similar trend is also apparent in the UK (Campion and Singer, 1987). The increasing incidence of VIN has not been mirrored by a similar increase in vulvar carcinoma (Sturgeon *et al.*, 1992), although any effect on the frequency of vulvar cancer secondary to rising incidence of VIN may not yet be apparent. A greater understanding of the natural history of VIN and the factors associated with high risk of progression to invasion have lead to the adoption of more conservative treatment regimens over recent years.

Definition

Before 1987 a plethora of descriptive histologic terms existed to describe squamous dysplasia of the vulva. In 1987 the term squamous intraepithelial neoplasia of the vulva or VIN was adopted by the International Society for the Study of Vulvar Disease (ISSVD) as the unifying term for those conditions where dysplastic keratinocytes are confined to the vulvar epithelium (Ridley *et al.*, 1989). These lesions are graded as VIN I, II or III according to the morphologic appearance with respect to the depth of epithelium occupied by neoplastic cells, together with their degree of differentiation and mutation. The VIN classification is therefore analogous to that used in the grading of cervical premalignant lesions.

Non-squamous VIN is also recognized and comprises Paget's disease, a derivation from skin appendages, and melanoma *in situ*. Paget's disease was first described in the breast (Paget, 1874) and has been recognized in the vulva since the turn of the century (Dubreuilh, 1901), but is less common than VIN. As with extragenital Paget's disease there is a strong association, as high as 25%, of current or subsequent malignancy of the lower genital tract, bladder and lower gastrointestinal tract (Ridley *et al.*, 1992; Baehrendtz *et al.*, 1994). Melanoma *in situ* is the least common of the VIN group, with the last reported series (Blickstein *et al.*, 1991) comprising three cases, all detected during pregnancy. Due to its rarity little is known of the natural history of melanoma *in situ* and the risk of malignant transformation.

Etiology

As with preinvasive disease at other sites in the female lower genital tract the human papillomavirus (HPV) is believed to have a strong association and the increasing frequency of HPV infection has seemingly paralleled the rise in VIN. Indeed there is a strong association between sexually transmitted diseases, including condylomata, and the development of VIN (Buckley *et al.*, 1984). The introduction of polymerase chain reaction (PCR) technology has increased the reported proportion of VIN lesions associated with HPV infection, although the risk of contamination during the use of PCR may lead to an overestimation of rates of HPV infection. The association of VIN with HPV appears to be a feature of VIN lesions in younger rather than older women (Crum *et al.*, 1982). The subtype most frequently detected in VIN lesions is HPV 16 (Hording *et al.*, 1991), with HPV 18 the next most prevalent (Buscema *et al.*, 1988). The precise role of HPV infection in the development of VIN and vulvar cancer remains to be elucidated, but incorporation of HPV DNA into the host genome appears to be an important event associated with the loss of normal cell control mechanisms. Aneuploidy is commonly found in VIN lesions of all severity and does not seem to be a marker for those lesions more likely to progress to invasion, in contrast to the association of aneuploidy with high-grade squamous intraepithelial lesions (SIL) of the cervix and progression to cervical cancer (Crum *et al.*, 1982).

Natural History

The risk of progression to vulvar carcinoma is ill understood, particularly in the case of VIN I and II. Reported estimates of the risk of progression for VIN III are generally less than 5% (Buscema *et al.*,

1980; Friedrich *et al.*, 1980). Factors associated with an increased risk of vulvar cancer include older age groups (Leibowitch *et al.*, 1990), unifocal disease and compromised immunity associated with immunosuppressive therapy in organ transplantation and connective tissue disease (Buscema *et al.*, 1980; Buckley *et al.*, 1984). Short-term immunosuppression such as that related to pregnancy, is associated with the development of VIN, but the majority of such lesions regress spontaneously after confinement, particularly when the disease is multifocal. The presence of VIN as a component of multifocal lower genital tract intraepithelial neoplasia is also associated with an increased risk of malignant progression (Jones and McLean, 1986). Progression of VIN to overt vulvar cancer has not been observed; however circumstantial evidence of progression arises from the reported presence of VIN III adjacent to vulvar carcinoma in 25–50% of cases (Buscema *et al.*, 1980; Leibowitch *et al.*, 1990).

Presentation

Age

Before the 1960s VIN was predominantly a disease of postmenopausal women (Woodruff *et al.*, 1973). However VIN has been described in women from the teenage years to old age, with a dramatic increase in the number of younger women affected in recent years (Crum *et al.*, 1984; Campion and Singer, 1987). The mean age for presentation with VIN has fallen from over 50 to under 38 years in the last 25 years (Bernstein *et al.*, 1983). The clinical form of the disease is related to age, with multifocal disease being commoner in younger women and unifocal disease more frequent in older women (Bornstein *et al.*, 1988). Furthermore multifocal VIN is commoner in those women who have undergone treatment for cervical intraepithelial neoplasia (CIN) (Andreasson and Bock, 1985).

Paget's disease is most commonly seen in the postmenopausal age group, mean age at presentation being 65 years; its occurrence in premenopausal women is uncommon (Baehrendtz *et al.*, 1994).

Symptoms

The most common presenting symptom of VIN and Paget's disease is that of pruritus vulvae, vulvar pain or a burning sensation (described in 38–72% of cases). Pruritus is of varying severity and often of a longstanding nature. In addition there may be an associated abnormal macroscopic appearance of the vulva in 14–40% of cases. VIN may be asymptomatic in as many as 50% of affected women and discovered as an incidental finding during examination of the lower genital tract such as colposcopic assessment of abnormal cervical cytology.

Site

VIN can affect any or all of the anatomical structures of the vulva and perineum. Disease affecting the posterior vulva, and the perineum in particular is more likely to exhibit features of early invasion (Schlaerth *et al.*, 1984).

Appearance

The macroscopic appearance of VIN is extremely variable; lesions may be white, lichenified, hyperkeratotic or ulcerated, reddened or pigmented, raised or flat. Therefore histopathologic assessment is required to differentiate VIN from other vulvar dermatoses. In addition both squamous and non-squamous VIN can mimic, and indeed, coexist, with non-neoplastic disease of the vulva. The pigmented form of VIN is more common in the premenopausal age group.

Associations

VIN is associated with other preinvasive disease of the lower genital tract, particularly CIL (Campion and Singer, 1987), with reported incidences as high as 80% (Bornstein *et al.*, 1988). This association is believed to reflect the association of premalignant disease with HPV infection of the lower female genital tract. Therefore assessment of the woman with VIN should include colposcopic examination of the cervix and vagina, because 25–71% of women will also have coexistent CIL and/or VAIN (Ferenczy, 1992). Preinvasive disease of the anal canal is reported in 14–35% of women diagnosed as having VIN (Schlaerth *et al.*, 1984).

As described above Paget's disease of the vulva is associated with underlying, often occult, malignancy and such women should undergo thorough investigation to exclude this possibility. The risk of future genital tract malignancy is also increased (Mitchell *et al.*, 1993), so these women should receive close long-term follow-up.

In addition to neoplastic conditions VIN often coexists with non-neoplastic epidermal dysplasia of the vulva such as lichen sclerosis and squamous cell hyperplasia.

Diagnosis

Symptomatology and Vulvar Appearance

The nonspecific symptoms and heterogeneous appearance of VIN lesions mean that they are unreliable in confirming the diagnosis, particularly as VIN can mimic the appearance of other vulvar dermatoses (Barbero *et al.*, 1990).

Exfoliative Cytology

Experience in the interpretation of vulvar cytology smears is limited, but the nuclear/cytoplasmic abnormalities described are similar to the classification used in cervical cytology. However the ability to differentiate between VIN III lesions and overt invasion cannot be reliably made from vulvar smears. The need for tissue biopsy to confirm the presence of VIN would seem to limit the potential use of exfoliative cytology as a diagnostic tool in the diagnosis of vulvar disease.

Colposcopy of the Vulva

Vulvar colposcopy has been advocated as a diagnostic tool in the identification of VIN and its differentiation from non-neoplastic vulvar disease (Forney *et al.*, 1977). The procedure can be time consuming due to the large surface area of epithelium to be examined and the identification of abnormal vascular patterns is hampered by the depth of the cutaneous keratin layer except in the skin of the labia minora and vestibule. The identification of abnormal vascular patterns is the main diagnostic criterion for invasive disease in common with cervical neoplasia. The principal benefit of vulvar colposcopy appears to be the identification of areas of early invasive disease within fields of VIN and the mapping of lesions before treatment. The application of lubricant jelly to the vulva may help to improve colposcopic examination and the use of acetic acid is useful in identifying VIN lesions in those areas with thin keratin layers. The application of toluidine blue has been advocated to identify areas of VIN, but there is a high false positive rate due to staining of areas of nonspecific inflammatory change and its use has therefore been abandoned in many centers.

Biopsy

Histologic assessment of a representative tissue sample is the only means presently available to obtain a precise diagnosis of VIN and exclude the presence of invasion. Such biopsies can be colposcopically directed and performed in the outpatient setting or obtained under general anesthesia.

The dermatologic Keyes punch is a useful tool and is suited to use in outpatient clinics under local anesthesia. The specimen obtained is of good histologic quality and multiple sites can be biopsied if appropriate. Large lesions or those in which invasion is suspected are best managed by excision biopsy under general anesthesia, with primary closure of the resulting skin defect.

Treatment

The documented low propensity for progression to invasion has led to the adoption of less radical therapy in recent years. This is particularly important in the management of the increasing numbers of younger women with VIN in whom the avoidance of mutilating genital tract surgery is of utmost importance. Furthermore the recognition that VIN can undergo spontaneous regression, particularly following pregnancy, brings into question the necessity to undertake treatment in all cases of VIN when close supervision following diagnosis may be appropriate in some cases.

In general terms the treatment modalities applied to VIN can be divided into excisional and ablative.

Excisional Treatment

The initial therapeutic strategy for preinvasive disease of the vulva was wide local excision, but the apparent high risk of developing vulvar cancer, especially in those women with multifocal disease led to the recommendation of total (simple) vulvectomy in the 1960s. The realization that treatment success and risk of recurrent disease was similar for vulvectomy and wide local excision (Forney *et al.*, 1977), has led to the abandonment of total vulvectomy in the management of VIN, therefore avoiding the adverse physical and psychologic effects of such mutilating surgery.

Recent reports have confirmed the effectiveness of wide local excision in eradicating VIN (Wolcott and Gallup, 1984). In addition the sexual and reproductive functions of the vulva are retained and recurrent disease can be managed by repeat excision. The success of treatment varies from 83–91%, but is markedly reduced if the excision margins are involved (Wolcott and Gallup, 1984; Andreasson and Bock, 1985); thus recurrence occurred in 46% of women with involved margins in one report (Campion and Singer, 1987). The apparent increased risk of invasive disease with lesions sited on the posterior vulva and perineum would suggest that local excision was particularly suited to these lesions, allowing histologic assessment of the complete lesion. VIN can involve the skin appendages: in 21% of cases the vulvar sebaceous glands are involved and in 32% hair follicles are affected. The mean thickness of the vulvar epithelium is 0.52 mm, with the average depth of VIN lesions being 0.1–1.9 mm (Benedet *et al.*, 1991). There is some variation in lesion thickness between hairbearing and non-hairbearing vulvar skin, the average being 0.77 mm and 0.69 mm, respectively (Schatz *et al.*, 1989). Therefore excision depth must take into account the likely involvement of pilosebaceous units and be of the order of 1 mm to confidently assume excision of affected skin appendages.

Skinning vulvectomy (Rettenmaier *et al.*, 1987) has been used as an alternative to standard total vulvectomy to decrease the morbitity associated with the latter. The success of treatment appears similar to other modalities with a recurrence rate of the order of 27%; the involvement of excision margins did not appear to play a significant role in determining the risk of recurrence following skinning vulvectomy and skin grafting. This technique may be of use in the management of women with widespread multifocal disease and allows better preservation of vulvar function than simple vulvectomy.

Ablative Treatment

The destruction of VIN can be achieved using physical modalities such as laser or by chemical means. The use of laser vaporization in the treatment of VIN followed its use in the management of CIL. The perceived advantages were the precision of use and the fact that large areas of vulvar skin could be treated without recourse to skin grafting because the depth of ablation can be arrested at the level of the reticular dermis from which epithelial regeneration will occur (Reid, 1985). Comparative studies of excisional and laser ablation demonstrate that both are equally effective, although some evidence exists to suggest that relapse occurs more quickly after ablation (Shafi *et al.*, 1989). This could be associated with VIN involving the skin appendages at a depth beyond the reticular dermis. Furthermore the ablation of large areas of vulvar epithelium that may contain foci of invasion not demonstrated in pretreatment biopsies is analogous to the argument used in preferring loop diathermy excision of the transformation zone over punch biopsy and ablation. Postoperative pain is considerable with healing taking several weeks, therefore excision may be preferred for the treatment of larger VIN lesions as well as when invasion is suspected from the vulvoscopic examination.

Cryotherapy has been used in the treatment of VIN, but is not generally recommended because of postoperative pain, sloughing and protracted healing, in addition to higher recurrence rates when compared to other treatment modalities. More recently the use of ultrasound described in a small series appears as successful as other ablative techniques (Rader *et al.*, 1991).

A number of chemotherapeutic agents have been used in the treatment of VIN and several have been shown to be effective, but the number of women included in each study is small so results are difficult to interpret. 5-Fluorouracil (5-FU) shows activity against several epithelial tumors and has been used as a topical application in VIN (Woodruff *et al.*, 1973). Response rates are variable, ranging from 75% (Krupp and Bohm, 1978), to complete failure (Forney *et al.*, 1977). The ability of 5-FU to eradicate VIN involving skin appendages is doubtful and may explain some of the treatment failures. Treatment is continued for a six-week period and repeated courses can be given; however therapy is complicated by painful tissue sloughing and prolonged healing. Dinitrochlorobenzene can be used in a similar manner to 5-FU with similar effects and results. Bleomycin has been used both as a topical application and as intradermal injections, but causes severe ulceration and has a poor response rate. The use of photosensitizing agents followed by laser therapy has proved initially disappointing, but further refinement may improve future results with this technique.

Follow-up

The uncertain malignant potential of VIN and its propensity to recur whichever treatment modality is used, makes long-term follow-up mandatory. Reported recurrence rates vary from 10% (Buckley *et al.*, 1985) to 22% (Crum *et al.*, 1984), and it seems likely that the longer the review period the higher the recurrence rate. The role of vulvoscopy has yet to be established, but it may be useful for detecting early invasion. A dedicated vulva clinic allows the assessment of treatment and the further scientific evaluation of the etiology and treatment of VIN.

Summary of Management Options

- Biopsy is essential to differentiate vulvar intraepithelial neoplasia (VIN) from non-neoplastic epithelial disorders of the vulva.
- Local excision appears the most appropriate management for localized disease, particularly if the perineum or perinal area is involved.
- Total (simple) vulvectomy probably has no role in the management of VIN, with skinning vulvectomy preferred when VIN is multifocal because vulvar function is better preserved.
- Long-term follow-up is required because of the high rate of recurrence and the unknown invasive potential of VIN.

References

Anderson M, Jordan J, Morse A & Sharp F (1992) *A Text and Atlas of Integrated Colposcopy*, pp. 179. London: Chapman and Hall.

Andreasson B & Bock JE (1985) Intraepithelial neoplasia in the vulvar region. *Gynecol. Oncol.* **21:** 300–305.

Baehrendtz H, Einhorn N, Pettersson F & Silfversward C (1994) Paget's disease of the vulva: the Radiumhemmet series 1975–1990. *Int. J. Gynecol. Cancer* **4:** 1–6.

Barbero M, Micheletti L, Preti M *et al.* (1990) Vulvar intraepithelial neoplasia: a clinocopathologic study of 60 cases. *J. Reprod. Med.* **35:** 1023–1028.

Benedet JL, Wilson PS & Matisic J (1991) Epidermal thickness and skin appendage involvement in vulvar intraepithelial neoplasia. *J. Reprod. Med.* **36:** 608–612.

Bernstein SG, Kovacs BR, Townsend DE & Morrow CP (1983) Vulvar carcinoma *in situ*. *Obstet. Gynecol.* **61:** 304–307.

Blickstein I, Feldberg E, Dgani R, Ben-Hur H & Czernobilsky B (1991) Dysplastic vulvar nevi. *Obstet. Gynecol.* **78:** 968–970.

Bornstein J, Kaufman RH, Adam E & Adler-Storthz K (1988) Multicentric intraepithelial neoplasia involving the vulva. *Cancer* **62:** 1601–1604.

■ Buckley CH, Butler EB & Fox H (1984) Vulvar intraepithelial neoplasia and microinvasive carcinoma of the vulva. *J. Clin. Pathol.* **37:** 1201–1211.

Buscema J, Woodruff D, Pharmley TH & Genadry R (1980) Carcinoma *in situ* of the vulva. *Obstet. Gynecol.* **55:** 225–230.

Buscema J, Naghashfar Z, Sawada E *et al.* (1988) The predominance of human papillomavirus type 16 in vulvar neoplasia. *Obstet. Gynecol.* **71:** 601–606.

Campion MJ & Singer A (1987) Vulval intraepithelial neoplasia: clinical review. *Genitourin. Med.* **63:** 147–152.

Crum CP, Fu YS, Levine RU *et al.* (1982) Intraepithelial lesions of the vulva: biologic and histologic criteria for the distinction of condyloma from vulvar intraepithelial neoplasia. *Am. J. Obstet. Gynecol.* **144:** 77–83.

Crum CP, Liskow A, Petras P, Keng WC & Frick HC (1984) Vulvar intraepithelial neoplasia (severe atypia and carcinoma *in situ*) A clinicopathologic analysis of 41 cases. *Cancer* **54:** 1429–1434.

Dubreuilh W (1901) Paget's disease of the vulva. *Br. J. Dermatol.* **13:** 407.

Ferenczy A (1992) Intraepithelial neoplasia of the vulva. In: Coppleson M (ed) *Gynecologic Oncology*, pp. 443–463. London: Churchill Livingstone.

Forney JP, Morrom CP, Townsend DE & DiSaia PJ (1977) Management of carcinoma *in situ* of the vulva. *Am. J. Obstet. Gynecol.* **127:** 801–805.

Friedrich EG, Wilkinson EJ & Fu YS (1980) Carcinoma *in situ* of the vulva: a continuing challenge. *Am. J. Obstet. Gynecol.* **136:** 830–838.

Hording U, Daugaard S, Iverson AK *et al.* (1991) Human papillomavirus type 16 in vulvar carcinoma, vulvar intraepithelial neoplasia, and associated cervical neoplasia. *Gynecol. Oncol.* **42:** 22–26.

Jones RW & McLean MR (1986) Carcinoma *in situ* of the vulva: a review of 31 treated and 5 untreated cases. *Obstet. Gynecol.* **68:** 499–503.

Krupp PJ & Bohm JW (1978) 5-fluorouracil topical treatment of *in situ* vulvar cancer. *Obstet. Gynecol.* **51:** 702–706.

■ Leibowitch M, Neill S, Pelisse M & Moyal-Baracco M (1990) The epithelial changes associated with squamous cell carcinoma of the vulva: a review of the clinical, histological and viral findings in 78 women. *Br. J. Obstet. Gynaecol.* **97:** 1135–1139.

Mitchell MF, Prasad CJ, Silva EG *et al.* (1993) Second genital primary squamous neoplasms in vulvar carcinoma: viral and histopathologic correlates. *Obstet. Gynecol.* **81:** 13–18.

Paget J (1874) On disease of the mammary areola preceding cancer of the mammary gland. *St Barth. Hospital Reports* **10:** 87.

Radar JS, Leake JF, Dillon MB & Rosenshein NB (1991) Ultrasonic surgical aspiration in the treatment of vulvar disease. *Obstet. Gynecol.* **77:** 573–376.

Reid R (1985) Superficial laser vulvectomy. *Am. J. Obstet. Gynecol.* **152:** 504–509.

Rettenmaier MA, Berman ML & DiSaia PJ (1987) Skinning vulvectomy for the treatment of multifocal vulvar intraepithelial neoplasia. *Obstet. Gynecol.* **69:** 247–250.

■ Ridley CM, Frankman O, Jones ISC *et al.* (1989) New nomenclature for vulvar disease: International Society for the Study of Vulvar Disease. *Hum. Path.* **20:** 495–496.

Ridley CM, Oriel JD & Robinson AJ (1992) *A Colour Atlas of Diseases of the Vulva*, pp. 68. London: Chapman and Hall.

Schatz P, Bergeron C, Wilkinson EJ, Arseneau J & Ferenczy A (1989) Vulvar intraepithelial neoplasia and skin appendage involvement. *Obstet. Gynecol.* **74:** 769–775.

Schlaerth JB, Morrow CP, Nalick RH & Gaddis O (1984) Anal involvement by carcinoma *in situ* of the perineum in women. *Obstet. Gynecol.* **64:** 406–411.

Shafi MI, Luesley DM, Byrne P *et al.* (1989) Vulval intraepithelial neoplasia – management and outcome. *Br. J. Obstet. Gynaecol.* **96:** 1339–1344.

Sturgeon SR, Brinton LA, Devesa SS & Kurman RJ (1992) *In situ* and invasive vulvar cancer incidence trends (1973 to 1987). *Am. J. Obstet. Gynecol.* **166:** 1482–1485.

■ Wolcott HD & Gallup DG (1984) Wide local excision in the treatment of vulvar carcinoma *in situ*: a reappraisal. *Am. J. Obstet. Gynecol.* **150:** 695–698.

Woodruff JD, Julian C, Puray T, Mermut S & Katayama P (1973) The contemporary challenge of carcinoma *in situ* of the vulva. *Am. J. Obstet. Gynecol.* **115:** 677–686.

22 Invasive Vulvar Cancer

K K Chan
C W Helm

Introduction

Although vulvar cancers account for only 3–4% of all gynecologic malignancies they are a cause of significant morbidity among those affected due to the site of the disease and the effects of treatment. At one time survival was extremely poor (Folsome, 1940), but the outcome was dramatically improved with the use of radical surgical excision. In recent years emphasis has focused on less radical surgery with reduced morbidity and better preservation of body image.

Due to the relative rarity of the condition and the special nature of the surgery, advances in the understanding and management of this condition have occurred mainly through the concentration of cases in specialized centers. If treatment for the individual patient is to be optimized and further advances made, vulvar cancer should continue to be treated in referral centers.

The histologic types of cancer of the vulva based on a report of 2877 cases (Sturgeon *et al.*, 1992) are squamous cell carcinoma (SCC) 82%, basal cell carcinoma 7%, malignant melanoma 7%, adenocarcinoma 2%, sarcoma 1%, other types 1%. This chapter will concentrate on the management of SCC.

Squamous Cell Carcinoma

Etiology and Epidemiology

The incidence of SCC increases steadily with age with the majority of cases occurring between the fifth and eighth decades (Sturgeon *et al.*, 1992). However, more cases are occurring in younger women.

Many risk factors are associated with the development of invasive SCC. Vulvar intraepithelial neoplasia (VIN) is analogous to intraepithelial neoplasia of the cervix (CIN). VIN has been reported adjacent to invasive SCC in 20–30% of cases (Buscema *et al.*, 1980), but the exact malignant potential of VIN is unknown and is thought to be less than for CIN. Since almost half the patients diagnosed with VIN are 20–40 years of age and with the annual incidence of *in situ* vulvar carcinoma nearly doubling from 1973–1987 and nearly tripling in white women less than 35 years of age the association is causing concern (Shafi *et al.*, 1989; Sturgeon *et al.*, 1992).

The role of human papillomavirus (HPV) remains unclear. Between 30–50% of vulvar carcinomas are associated with HPV infection (Bloss *et al.*, 1991; Ansink *et al.*, 1994), with both types 6/11 and 16 reported as being predominant (Sutton *et al.*, 1987; Neill *et al.*, 1990; Toki *et al.*, 1991). HPV has been reported to be more common or no more common in SCC in young patients (Andersen *et al.*, 1991; Husseinzadeh *et al.*, 1991; Ansink *et al.*, 1994).

The association of lichen sclerosus in resection specimens containing invasive SCC has been reported in from 4% (Buscema *et al.*, 1980) to up to 60% of cases (Neill *et al.*, 1990). However, only about 5% of patients with lichen sclerosus will develop a carcinoma (Kaufman *et al.*, 1974). Squamous cell hyperplasia with atypia is more commonly associated with invasive SCC in over 50% of cases (Kaufman *et al.*, 1974; Buscema *et al.*, 1980).

Lowered immunity due to disease or drugs used to treat connective diseases or prevent rejection of organ transplants is a risk factor, especially in young patients (Buscema and Woodruff, 1980; Friedrich *et al.*, 1980; Lindeque *et al.*, 1987; Carter *et al.*, 1993). Other factors include multiple sexual partners, current cigarette smoking, previous abnormal Pap smear (Brinton *et al.*, 1990) and warts (Woodruff and Novak, 1962; Daling *et al.*, 1984).

Presentation

Presenting symptoms include pruritus (71%), a vulvar lesion (58%), ulceration (28%), bleeding (26%), pain (23%) urinary tract symptoms (14%) and vulvar and vaginal discharge (13%) (Podratz *et al.*, 1983). There is often a delay in presentation, sometimes because of a reluctance of older women to present to their doctor. There may be a delay in diagnosis due to failure of the doctor to adequately assess a patient reporting symptoms of vulvar irritation.

Diagnosis

The diagnosis of cancer of the vulva can only be made histologically. Benign conditions such as lymphogranuloma inguinale and tuberculosis may mimic carcinoma and therefore all suspicious lesions on the vulva should be biopsied. If an incisional biopsy is made it should be full-thickness and include a segment of normal-appearing adjacent skin.

Spread

Carcinoma of the vulva spreads by direct invasion of surrounding tissues, by the lymphatics and rarely by the blood stream. Local spread may be to the urethra, vagina, anus, rectum and pubic bones.

Lymphatic spread principally passes through the superficial inguinal lymph nodes to the deep inguinal/femoral nodes and thence the pelvic nodes. The occurrence of metastatic disease in the deep inguinal nodes without involvement of the superficial nodes has been reported (Chu *et al.*, 1981). Direct lymphatic channels between the clitoris and both the pelvic and deep femoral nodes have been identified (Plentl and Friedman, 1971) and this potential route of spread must be borne in mind with clitoral area cancers.

Factors influencing involvement of the lymphatics are clinical node status (Homesley *et al.*, 1991), tumor thickness (Homesley *et al.*, 1991), lesion larger than 2 cm (Franklin and Rutledge, 1971; Monaghan and Hammond, 1984), histologic spray pattern (Crissman and Azoury, 1981), lymph–vascular space involvement and tumor grade (Parker *et al.*, 1975; Sedlis *et al.*, 1987; Homesley *et al.*, 1991).

Whereas tumors involving the midline can metastasize to the groin nodes on both sides, tumors no larger than 2 cm in dimension situated laterally on the vulva and away from the midline rarely metastasize to contralateral groin nodes (Hacker, 1990).

Staging

As in the case of other cancers the FIGO staging system for carcinoma of the vulva (see *Table 47.6*) attempts to allocate patients to stages that reflect prognosis in an accurate yet practical manner and are applicable to all patients. The reader is referred to Chapter 47 for an indepth discussion of stage of tumor as it relates to treatment planning.

Pre-treatment Assessment

Many patients with vulvar SCC require assessment Many patients with vulvar SCC require assessment under regional or general anesthesia. This allows a thorough examination of the lesion and assessment of spread. Other areas of the lower genital tract may be examined colposcopically for preinvasive and invasive disease. A cytologic smear of the vagina/cervix should be sent. Cystoscopy and proctosigmoidoscopy may also be necessary.

All patients require a chest radiograph. Computed tomography (CT) and magnetic resonance imaging (MRI) are both good for examining the abdomen and pelvis for pelvic and paraaortic lymph nodes and liver, but MRI is the best technique for assessing the degree of local spread in the case of large tumors with evidence of spread.

Before definitive surgery all patients need to undergo a medical assessment of fitness for surgery. If necessary, non-exenterative surgery may be performed under regional anesthesia. In addition, all patients who are to undergo vulvectomy require counselling with regard to postoperative changes in body image and sexual dysfunction.

Prognostic Factors

A large Gynecologic Oncology Group (GOG) study (Homesley *et al.*, 1991) showed by multivariate analysis that the most important factors affecting survival in carcinoma of the vulva are the extent of metastases in the groins (both laterality and number of nodes positive) and the size of the lesion. The number of positive groin nodes had previously been shown to be important (Curry *et al.*, 1980; Hacker *et al.*, 1983; Hoffman *et al.*, 1985) and more recently the degree of involvement of the node (Origoni *et al.*, 1992; Paladini *et al.*, 1994). Other investigators have reported that other surgicopathologic characteristics including lesion location, histologic differentiation, tumor thickness, status of microscopic resection margins and lymph–vascular space involvement are also of significance, depending on the stage of disease (Heaps *et al.*, 1990; Hopkins *et al.*, 1991; Rutledge *et al.*, 1991).

In early stage disease the depth of invasion is significant (Wilkinson, 1985). It has been reported that tumors showing evidence of HPV infection have a better prognosis (Husseinzadeh *et al.*, 1991; Ansink *et al.*, 1994).

Treatment

Surgery is the principal mode of treatment of vulvar carcinoma. Alternative modalities involving chemotherapy and radiation are being investigated for use in mainly advanced disease, but their role remains controversial.

The prognosis for patients with SCC of the vulva was transformed once radical resection of the primary carcinoma together with resection of the principal sites of lymphatic drainage to the groins and pelvis was accepted (Taussig, 1940; Way, 1948). The technique of Way, which became a widely used method involved resection of the primary tumor with an *en bloc* resection of the inguinal lymph nodes as well as removal of large areas of uninvolved skin in the groins, lower abdomen and perineum. Even with modifications, this procedure was associated with significant major complications including breakdown of the wounds in 50% of patients (Helm and Shingleton, 1992). Since the 1970s the trend has been for treatment to become less radical and more individualized. This more conservative approach has developed with regard to both excision of the primary tumor and excision of the lymph nodes.

Pelvic lymph node dissection was initially performed on all patients with carcinoma of the vulva and later only in selected patients (Monaghan and Hammond, 1984). However, a GOG study (Homesley *et al.*, 1986), which randomized patients who had undergone radical vulvectomy and bilateral groin node dissection and were found to have positive groin nodes to receive either surgical resection of the pelvic nodes on the side or sides of involved groin nodes or external beam radiotherapy to the pelvis and groins, reported that the patients receiving radiotherapy had a significantly improved survival rate at two years (68% versus 54%) with the major survival advantage being in the patients with suspicions or fixed ulcerated groin nodes or two or more positive nodes. Pelvic node dissection is now rarely performed for vulvar carcinoma.

The situation with regard to tumors involving the clitoris is still of concern for whereas large series of patients treated for such tumors do not report positive pelvic nodes in the absence of positive groin nodes (Piver and Xynos, 1977; Curry *et al.*, 1980), there are lymphatic channels passing from the clitoris directly to pelvic nodes without passing through the groins (Plentl and Friedman, 1971).

Wharton *et al.* (1974) suggested that lesions of less than 2 cm in size and with less than 5 mm depth of invasion could be treated with radical vulvectomy alone without lymph node dissection. Reports appeared documenting recurrence in the groin nodes of such patients who did not receive initial groin dissection (Nakao *et al.*, 1974; Jafari and Cartnick, 1976; Yazigi *et al.*, 1978; Crissman and Azoury, 1981), and data accumulated to show that only lesions with less than 1 mm depth of invasion were not at significant risk of nodal metastasis (Helm and Shingleton, 1992). Patients with a depth of invasion of more than 1 mm do require nodal dissection because there is a significant risk of nodal metastasis and if recurrence does develop in a groin that was not dissected at primary surgery the outcome is often fatal (Hacker, 1990). There are scattered reports of nodal recurrence in patients who did not undergo node dissection with tumors invading less than 1 mm (Buscema *et al.*, 1981; Atamdede and Hoogerland, 1989). The method used to measure depth of invasion should be stated clearly on all pathology reports. It has been suggested that the measurement be taken from the dermo–epidermal junction of the most superficial dermal papilla to the deepest point of invasion (Wilkinson, 1985). This method is of importance when tumors invade less than 5 mm; however, with larger tumors tumor thickness is often used.

Not all patients require bilateral node dissection since the incidence of positive contralateral nodes with negative ipsilateral groin nodes when the lesion size is no larger than 2 cm and not involving the midline is only 0.4% (two of 488 cases) (Hacker, 1990). Bilateral node dissection is advised for tumors close to or involving midline structures and lesions larger than 2 cm.

The question of whether the deep as well as the superficial inguinal nodes need to be removed has still not been resolved. DiSaia *et al.* (1979) stated that the superficial inguinal nodes act as sentinel nodes and provided these are removed and shown to be negative a deep dissection is unnecessary. However, there have been isolated reports of deep femoral node involvement in the absence of superficial inguinal node involvement (Chu *et al.*, 1981). It used to be thought that to excise all the deep femoral nodes it was necessary to strip the fascia lata from the entire femoral triangle. In fact, the deep femoral nodes lie close to the femoral vein and the sapheno–femoral junction medial to the femoral artery. None of these deep nodes lies distal to the lower edge of the cribriform fascia and so can they be removed through the cribriform fascia itself (Borgno *et al.*, 1990a; Borgno *et al.*, 1990b). Since they can be removed relatively easily without great morbidity, the deep femoral nodes should probably be removed in all patients undergoing groin node dissection.

For those patients who do need a groin node dissection, how much adjacent and overlying skin needs to be removed? Hacker *et al.* (1981) reported the results of a technique modifying the *en bloc* radical vulvectomy by using three separate incisions to perform radical vulvectomy together with complete inguino–femoral node dissection. The inguinal incisions ran parallel to the inguinal ligament. The idea of using triple incisions was similar to that of Taussig (1940), but the direction of Hacker's groin incisions was similar to that proposed by Basset (1912). Hacker reported good survival figures for 98 patients with SCC Stages I–III using this approach. Morbidity was much less than would be expected with the more radical approach, with only 14% of his patients having a major breakdown of the groin wounds.

It is difficult to prove conclusively that one technique is superior to another without a randomized controlled trial. No such study has been carried out, but a study was performed by Helm *et al.* (1992) in which patients undergoing triple incision surgery for SCC of the vulva and patients undergoing the traditional radical vulvectomy and *en bloc* inguino–femoral node dissection were matched for stage, lesion size, lesion site and lymph node status. There was no significant difference in survival, or disease-free survival between the two groups. As would be expected, the triple incision procedure took significantly less time, was associated with a lower mean blood loss and shorter hospital stay. When compared with 96 patients undergoing the traditional *en bloc* radical vulvectomy together with bilateral inguino–femoral (and in some cases pelvic) node dissection, wound complications were greatly reduced (Helm and Shingleton, 1992).

Isolated skin bridge recurrence in those undergoing triple incision procedures is rare (Hacker *et al.*, 1981; Christopherson *et al.*, 1985; Monaghan, 1987; Hoffman *et al.*, 1989). The available evidence supports the view that if a radical vulvectomy and bilateral groin node dissection is indicated, a triple incision technique should be recommended.

Vulvar excision

Way (1948) had established that a very wide resection of the vulvar lesion was vital to the chances of cure of cancer of the vulva and therefore radical excision was performed on even small tumors. The stimulus to a more conservative management of the vulvar primary was microinvasive disease of small dimensions occurring in young women in whom the mutilation of radical vulvectomy and *en bloc* groin node dissection was so devastating (Hughes, 1971; DiSaia *et al.*, 1979).

DiSaia suggested 'an alternative approach to carcinoma of the vulva.' He suggested wide local excision of a primary tumor no larger than 1 cm in diameter and with no more than 5 mm of stromal invasion, with a 3 cm margin together with bilateral dissection of the superficial inguinal lymph nodes. Patients found to have positive superficial nodes at surgery would undergo radical vulvectomy and bilateral inguino–femoral node dissection. All patients treated according to this protocol 18 were alive and free of disease at 7–74 months. Others followed using approaches using less radical surgery and selective sometimes unilateral lymphadenectomy (Iversen *et al.*, 1981; Hacker *et al.*, 1984b; Berman *et al.*, 1989; Burke *et al.*, 1990).

These approaches appear to result in survival compatible with that of more radical surgery and fears of an increased local recurrence rate as a result of less radical surgery proved to be unwarranted. Hacker *et al.* (1984b) found that the local recurrence rate was identical for lesions excised by radical vulvectomy or radical local excision.

Others have reported good results with the use of radical wide excision and selective lymphadenectomy (Berman *et al.*, 1989; Burke *et al.*, 1990). Although it has been customary to aim for a 2–3 cm margin around a carcinoma, one report suggests that a minimum of 1 cm may be all that is necessary (Heaps *et al.*, 1990). Whatever the extent of the excision, the dissection should be taken down to the superficial aponeurosis of the urogenital diaphragm and/or pubic periosteum in the line of the incisions. The possible types of excision for lesions confined to the vulva include a radical hemivulvectomy for a lateral lesion, an anterior or posterior vulvectomy for lesions placed anteriorly or posteriorly, or a radical total vulvectomy.

Locally advanced disease

SCC of the vulva may remain confined to the vulva for long periods of time. Such tumors can reach a considerable size (*Figure 22.1*) and cause considerable distress to patients. Even large tumors may be cured by radical surgery, the extent of which depends entirely on the extent of disease. The fundamental requirement for cure is complete excision of the tumor.

Removal of extensive areas of skin in the mons, groin, thigh or perineum may require the use of skin flaps to close the defect. These may vary from small simple transposition flaps to myocutaneous flaps using rectus abdominis, gracilis or tensor fascia lata. If vaginal reconstruction is necessary, rectus abdominis or gracilis myocutaneous flaps are widely used.

If the tumor involves the lower urethra, the distal 1 cm can be excised and continence may be maintained, although not guaranteed. The extent and site of vaginal involvement will dictate the amount of surgery. Involvement of the lower lateral walls can be dealt with by simple resection. If the tumor involves the anterior or posterior walls care

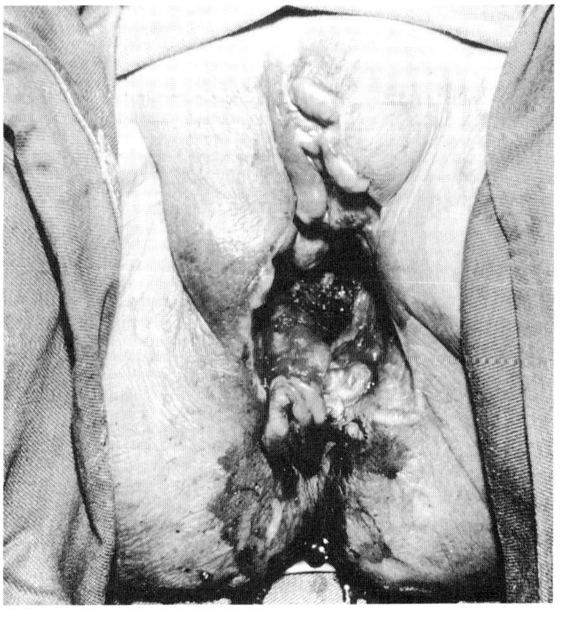

Figure 22.1. A relatively large carcinoma of the vulva.

must be taken not to damage the bladder or rectum while at the same time achieving clear margins around the tumor. Involvement of extensive amounts of the vagina will require removal of the bladder or anorectum depending on the site of involvement. The vagina may be replaced with gracilis or rectus abdominis myocutaneous flaps or the wound may be left open and allowed to granulate.

Where the lesion encroaches on the anus or there is a suspicion of this then the anterior one-third of the anus and sphincter can be excised without major impact on continence (Hoffman *et al.*, 1990). In many cases partial resection of the anus would be insufficient and anovulvectomy (Grimshaw *et al.*, 1991), anoproctectomy (Adams and Daly, 1979) or posterior exenteration can be used.

Anovulvectomy is a useful procedure in older women because it avoids the need for an extensive laparotomy in addition to the perineal procedure. It is extremely well tolerated. The operation is performed in two stages. In the first stage, a sigmoid end-colostomy is raised in the left iliac fossa by a trephine approach, if possible. Two weeks later in the perineal phase the tumor is excised widely, including the anus and lower rectum. The rectum is transected and left as a mucus fistula to the perineal wound. It is usually secured to the posterior edge of the residual vagina and to the skin margins.

Postoperatively, the patient will intermittently discharge a small amount of mucus from the rectum into the perineum. This is not usually a problem. Occasionally the mucus may be retained in the residual rectum and require release either digitally or by dilatation of the perineal opening.

Partial or total exenteration is performed when there is extensive involvement of either the bladder, upper urethra or anorectum, or where clear margins would be unobtainable with preservation of these structures (Cavanagh and Shepherd, 1982). Reconstruction of the vagina should be considered. In very elderly patients, this is not usually an issue. However, in younger patients, creation of a neovagina using either rectus abdominis or gracilis myocutaneous flaps creates a vagina and helps to fill the dead space in the pelvis.

Involvement of the pubic bones is a bad feature. Early involvement of the symphysis or pubic rami may be managed by removal of the involved bones. Preoperative chemoradiation should be considered in such cases.

Complications of surgery

Both the groin node dissection and vulvar wounds may break down, although much less when separate incisions are used. With separate incisions the incidence of major groin or vulvar wound breakdown is 3% versus 27% for the single incision technique (Helm and Shingleton, 1992). Other complications include acute infection, recurrent infection in the leg and chronic leg edema. The last is exacerabated in those patients who undergo postoperative radiotherapy. Other complications of the vulvar excision include introital stenosis and psychosexual problems.

Role of radiotherapy

Radiotherapy has not been widely accepted for the primary management of vulvar carcinoma because of the success of surgery and the complications of radiation. There is a definite role for radiotherapy as adjuvant therapy following surgical excision of the tumor in those patients with adverse prognostic features. These include close or positive surgical margins, residual unresectable disease and when more than one groin node is microscopically positive, there is replacement of a lymph node by tumor, or there is capsular breakthrough. Pelvic radiation should be considered when there are groin nodes metastases, particularly when the deep femoral nodes are involved or when the tumor involves the clitoral region. Despite its success in an adjuvant setting, radiotherapy cannot be used as a replacement for groin node dissection. The GOG set up a study (GOG Protocol 88) to test whether radiation therapy could substitute for bilateral inguinal lymphadenectomy in patients with vulvar cancer; 58 patients were recruited, and among the first 49 evaluable patients, there were five groin recurrences in the irradiated patients versus none in the operated group. The study was therefore terminated (Keys, 1993).

In advanced local disease, radiation has been used before surgery either alone or in combination with chemotherapy to reduce the size of the tumor and theoretically allow surgical excision without removal of either the bladder or anorectum. Boronow *et al.* (1987) gave preoperative radiation therapy to 37 patients with Stage III or Stage IV disease and achieved local control in 86% and spared most of them an exenteration. He reported a five-year survival of 75% with a single patient requiring total exenteration for recurrent disease. This concept has been supported by others (Hacker *et al.*, 1984a). However, the approach has not been widely accepted at the present time because the results of surgery are established in this situation and there is a major problem of where the surgical margin is taken at subsequent surgery. Even when surgical resection margins are clear of tumor, local recurrence can occur early suggesting occult residual disease.

Chemotherapy alone has been reported to be effective in eliciting a response in vulvar carcinoma (Kalra *et al.*, 1981). 5-Fluorouracil (5-FU) in combination with cisplatin or mitomycin C are used in combination with radiotherapy. Thomas *et al.* (1989) reporting the use of 5-FU and mitomycin C concomitant with radiotherapy advises keeping the daily fraction to 175 cGy to minimize the risk of late vulvar fibrosis, necrosis and atrophy. Most patients develop moist desquamation in the vulva and groins, and although this usually heals in 10–14 days, many patients require treatment interruption in the middle of the course. Side-effects of the radiation therapy include fistula formation and avascular necrosis of the femoral head.

Recurrent Carcinoma of the Vulva

The incidence of recurrence in the vulvar area varies from 3.6–70% depending on stage (Iversen *et al.*, 1981; Podratz *et al.*, 1982; Hacker *et al.*, 1984b; Boyce *et al.*, 1985). Patients who recur either distantly or in the groins do badly, with five-year survivals being 50% for vulvar recurrence and 10% for regional or distant recurrence (Podratz *et al.*, 1982). Radiotherapy allows salvage in a few patients (Miyazawa *et al.*, 1983; Prempree and Amornmarn, 1984; Simonsen, 1984), but overall results are poor (Buchler *et al.*, 1979; Thomas *et al.*, 1989).

Survival

Analysis of the results of treatment of 588 patients with SCC of the vulva revealed that for new FIGO Stages I, II, III and IV five-year survival was 98%, 85%, 74% and 31% (Homesley *et al.*, 1991).

Summary

The management of cancer of the vulva has changed from the universal application of radical surgery to all patients to individualized surgery for each patient in order to minimize the sequelae of treatment.

Summary of Management Options

- Tumors which are ⩽2 cm in their greatest dimension and are well- or moderately-differentiated with <1 mm depth of invasion and no lymph–vascular space involvement may be treated by radical local excision.
- Patients with tumors >2 cm in their greatest dimension or ⩽2 cm, but with a depth of invasion ⩾1 mm or lymph–vascular space invasion or of a poor grade, should undergo radical excision and inguino–femoral node dissection. This should be unilateral if the lesion lies lateral on the vulva and does not encroach the midline and bilateral if the lesion is >4 cm or lies close to or involves the midline. The site and size of the tumor defines the amount of resection necessary.
- When the lesion is locally advanced and therefore not excisable by a standard radical vulvectomy then more radical surgery is necessary. Chemoradiation may be considered, particularly when surgical cure would necessitate removal of either the bladder or anal sphincters.
- Radiotherapy should be used postoperatively for poor prognostic factors. Groin radiotherapy should be considered if groin node metastases are present (>1–2 microscopically positive nodes, extracapsular extension, large nodal metastases). Pelvic radiotherapy should be considered for patients with positive groin nodes, particularly if the deep femorals are positive. Therapy to the vulva should be considered for positive resection margins.

References

Adams J & Daly JW (1979) Proctectomy combined with vulvectomy for carcinoma of the vulva. *Obstet. Gynecol.* **54:** 643–646.

Andersen WA, Franquemont DW, Williams J *et al.* (1991) Vulvar squamous cell carcinoma and papillomaviruses: Two separate entities. *Am. J. Obstet. Gynecol.* **165:** 329–336.

Ansink AC, Krul MRL, DeWeger RA *et al.* (1994) Human papillomavirus, lichen sclerosus and squamous cell carcinoma of the vulva: detection and prognostic significance. *Gynecol. Oncol.* **52:** 180–184.

Atamdede F & Hoogerland D (1989) Regional lymph node recurrence following local excision for microinvasive vulvar carcinoma. *Gynecol. Oncol.* **34:** 125–128.

Basset A (1912) Traitement chirurgical operatoire de l'epithelioma primitif du clitoris. *Rev. Chir.* **46:** 546–570.

Berman ML, Soper JT, Creasman WT *et al.* (1989) Conservative surgical management of superficially invasive Stage 1 vulvar carcinoma. *Gynecol. Oncol.* **35:** 352–357.

Bloss JD, Liao S-Y, Wilczynzki SP *et al.* (1991) Clinical and histologic features of vulvar carcinomas analyzed for human papillomavirus status. *Hum. Pathol.* **22:** 711–718.

Borgno G, Micheletti L, Barbero M *et al.* (1990a) Topographic distribution of groin lymph nodes. *J. Repro. Med.* **35:** 1127–1129.

Borgno G, Micheletti L, Barbero M *et al.* (1990b) Deep femoral lymphadenectomy with preservation of the fascia lata. *J. Repro. Med.* **35:** 1130–1133.

Boronow RC, Hickman BT, Reagan MT *et al.* (1987) Combined therapy as an alternative to exenteration for locally advanced vulvovaginal cancer. *Am. J. Clin. Oncol.* **10:** 171–181.

Boyce J, Fruchter RG, Kasambilides E *et al.* (1985) Prognostic factors in carcinoma of the vulva. *Gynecol. Oncol.* **20:** 364–377.

Brinton LA, Nasca PC, Mallin K *et al.* (1990) Case–control study of cancer of the vulva. *Obstet. Gynecol.* **75:** 859–866.

Buchler DA, Kline JC, Tunca JC & Carr WF (1979) Treatment of recurrent carcinoma of the vulva. *Gynecol. Oncol.* **8:** 180–184.

Burke TW, Stringer CA, Gershenson DM *et al.* (1990) Radical wide excision and selective inguinal node dissection for squamous cell carcinoma of the vulva. *Gynecol. Oncol.* **38:** 328–332.

Buscema J, Stern J & Woodruff JD (1980) The significance of the histologic alterations adjacent to invasive vulvar carcinoma. *Am. J. Obstet. Gynecol.* **137:** 902–909.

Buscema J, Stern JL & Woodruff JD (1981) Early invasive carcinoma of the vulva. *Am. J. Obstet. Gynecol.* **140:** 563–569.

Buscema J & Woodruff JD (1980) Progressive histological alterations in the development of vulva cancer. A report of 5 cases. *Am. J. Obstet. Gynecol.* **138:** 146–150.

Carter J, Carlson J, Fowler J *et al.* (1993) Invasive vulvar tumors in young women – a disease of the immunosuppressed? *Gynecol. Oncol.* **51:** 307–310.

Cavanagh D & Shepherd JH (1982) The place of exenteration in the primary management of advanced carcinoma of the vulva. *Gynecol. Oncol.* **13:** 318–312.

Christopherson W, Buchsbaum HJ, Voet R & Lifschitz S (1985) Radical vulvectomy and bilateral groin lymphadenectomy utilizing separate groin incisions: report of a case with recurrence in the intervening skin bridge. *Gynecol. Oncol.* **21:** 247–251.

Chu J, Tamimi HK & Figge DC (1981) Femoral node metastases with negative superficial inguinal nodes in early vulval cancer. *Am. J. Obstet. Gynecol.* **140:** 337–339.

FIGO Committee on Gynecological Oncology (1989) Annual report on the results of treatment in gynecological cancer. *Int. J. Gynecol. Oncol.* **28:** 189–190.

Crissman JD & Azoury RS (1981) Microinvasive carcinoma of the vulva. *Diagn. Gynecol. Obstet.* **3:** 75–80.

Curry SL, Wharton JT & Rutledge F (1980) Positive lymph nodes in vulvar squamous carcinoma. *Gynecol. Oncol.* **9:** 63–67.

Daling JR, Chu J, Weiss NS *et al.* (1984) The association of condylomata acuminata and squamous carcinoma of the vulva. *Brit. J. Cancer* **50:** 533–537.

DiSaia PJ, Creasman WT & Rich WM (1979) An alternative approach to early cancer of the vulva. *Am. J. Obstet. Gynecol.* **133:** 825–832.

Folsome CE (1940) Benign and malignant tumors of the vulva. *JAMA* **114:** 1499–1503.

Franklin EW & Rutledge FD (1971) Prognostic factors in epidermoid carcinoma of the vulva. *Obstet. Gynecol.* **37:** 892–901.

Friedrich EG, Wilkinson EJ & Fu YS (1980) Carcinoma *in situ* of the vulva. A continuing challenge. *Am. J. Obstet. Gynecol.* **136:** 830–843.

Grimshaw RN, Ghazal Aswad S & Monaghan JM (1991) The role of anovulvectomy in locally advanced carcinoma of the vulva. *Int. J. Gynecol. Cancer* **1:** 15–18.

Hacker NF (1990) Current treatment of small vulvar cancers. *Oncology* **4:** 21–25.

Hacker NF, Berek JS, Juillard GJF & Lagasse LD (1984a) Preoperative radiation therapy for locally advanced vulvar cancer. *Cancer* **54:** 2056–2061.

Hacker NF, Berek JS, Lagasse LD *et al.* (1983) Management of regional lymph nodes and their prognostic influence in vulvar cancer. *Obstet. Gynecol.* **61:** 408–412.

Hacker NF, Berek JS, Lagasse LD *et al.* (1984b) Individualization of treatment for Stage 1 squamous cell vulvar carcinoma. *Obstet. Gynecol.* **63:** 155–162.

■ Hacker NF, Leuchter RS, Berek JS *et al.* (1981) Radical vulvectomy and bilateral inguinal lymphadenectomy through separate groin incisions. *Obstet. Gynecol.* **58:** 574–479.

Heaps JM, Fu YS, Montz FJ *et al.* (1990) Surgical-pathologic variables predictive of local recurrence in squamous cell carcinoma of the vulva. *Gynecol. Oncol.* **38:** 309–314.

Helm CW, Hatch K, Austin JM *et al.* (1992) A matched comparison of single and triple incision techniques for the surgical treatment of carcinoma of the vulva. *Gynecol. Oncol.* **46:** 150–156.

Helm CW & Shingleton HM (1992) The management of squamous cell carcinoma of the vulva. *Current Obstet. Gynecol.* **2:** 31–37.

Hoffman JS, Kumar NB & Morley GW (1985) Prognostic significance of groin lymph node metastases in squamous carcinoma of the vulva. *Obstet. Gynecol.* **66:** 402–405.

Hoffman MS, LaPolla JP, Roberts WS *et al.* (1990) Use of local flaps for primary anal reconstruction following perianal resection for neoplasia. *Gynecol. Oncol.* **36:** 348–352.

Hoffman MS, Roberts WS, Lapolla JP & Cavanagh D (1989) Recent modifications in the treatment of invasive squamous cell carcinoma of the vulva. *Obstet. Gynecol. Surv.* **44:** 227–233.

■ Homesley HD, Bundy BN, Sedlis A & Adcock L (1986) Radiation therapy versus pelvic node resection for carcinoma of the vulva with positive groin nodes. *Obstet. Gynecol.* **68:** 733–740.

■ Homesley HD, Bundy BN, Sedlis A *et al.* (1991) Assessment of current International Federation of Gynecology and Obstetrics staging of vulvar carcinoma relative to prognostic factors for survival. *Am. J. Obstet. Gynecol.* **164:** 997–1004.

Hopkins MP, Reid GC, Johnston CM & Morley GW (1992) A comparison of staging systems for squamous cell carcinoma of the vulva. *Gynecol. Oncol.* **47:** 34–37.

Hopkins MP, Reid GC, Vettrano I & Morley GW (1991) Squamous cell carcinoma of the vulva: prognostic factors influencing survival. *Gynecol. Oncol.* **43:** 113–117.

Hughes RR (1971) Early diagnosis and management of premalignant lesions and early invasive cancers of the vulva. *South Med. J.* **64:** 1490–1492.

Husseinzadeh N, DeEulis T, Newman N & Wesseler T (1991) HPV changes and their significance in patients with invasive squamous cell carcinoma of the vulva: A clinocopathologic study. *Gynecol. Oncol.* **43:** 237–241.

Iversen T, Abeler V & Aalders J (1981) Individualized treatment of Stage I carcinoma of the vulva. *Obstet. Gynecol.* **57:** 85–89.

Jafari K & Cartnick EN (1976) Microinvasive squamous cell carcinoma of the vulva. *Gynecol. Oncol.* **4:** 158–166.

■ Keys H (1993) Gynecologic Oncology Group randomised trials of combined technique therapy for vulvar cancer. *Cancer* **71:** 1691–1696.

Kalra JK, Grossman AM, Krumholz BA *et al.* (1981) Preoperative chemoradiotherapy for carcinoma of the vulva. *Gynecol. Oncol.* **12:** 256–260.

Kaufman RH, Gardner HL, Brown D & Beyth Y (1974) Vulvar dystrophies: an evaluation. *Am. J. Obstet. Gynecol.* **120:** 363–367.

Lindeque BG, Nel AE & DuToit JP (1987) Immune deficiency and invasive carcinoma of the vulva in a young woman: A case report. *Gynecol. Oncol.* **26:** 112–118.

Miyazawa K, Nori D, Hilaris BS & Lewis JT (1983) Role of radiation therapy in the treatment of advanced vulvar carcinoma. *J. Repro. Med.* **28:** 539–541.

Monaghan JM & Hammond IG (1984) Pelvic node dissection in the treatment of vulval carcinoma – is it necessary? *Brit. J. Obstet. Gynaecol.* **91:** 270–274.

Monaghan JM (1987) Vulvar carcinoma: the case for individualization of treatment. *Clin. Obstet. Gynecol.* **1:** 263–276.

Nakao CY, Nolan JF, DiSaia PJ & Futoran R (1974) "Microinvasive" epidermoid carcinoma of the vulva with an unexpected natural history. *Am. J. Obstet. Gynecol.* **120:** 1122–1123.

Neill SM, Lessana-Liebowitch M, Pelisse M & Moyal-Barrocco M (1990) Lichen sclerosis, invasive squamous cell carcinoma and human papillomavirus. *Am. J. Obstet. Gynecol.* **162:** 1633–1634.

Origoni M, Sideri M, Garsia S *et al.* (1992) Prognostic value of pathological patterns of lymph node positivity in squamous cell carcinoma of the vulva stage III and IVA FIGO. *Gynecol. Oncol.* **45:** 313–316.

Paladini D, Cross P, Lopes A & Monaghan JM (1994) Prognostic significance of lymph node variables in squamous cell carcinoma of the vulva. *Cancer* **74:** 2491–2496.

Parker RT, Duncan I, Rampone J & Creasman W (1975) Operative management of early invasive epidermoid carcinoma of the vulva. *Am. J. Obstet. Gynecol.* **123:** 349–355.

Piver MS & Xynos FP (1977) Pelvic lymphadenectomy in women with carcinoma of the clitoris. *Obstet. Gynecol.* **49:** 592–595.

Plentl AA & Friedman EA (1971) *Lymphatic System of the Female Genitalia.* Philadelphia: WB Saunders.

Podratz KC, Symmonds RE & Taylor WF (1982) Carcinoma of the vulva: analysis of treatment failures. *Am. J. Obstet. Gynecol.* **143:** 340–351.

Podratz KC, Symmonds RE, Taylor WF & Williams TJ (1983) Carcinoma of the vulva: analysis of treatment and survival. *Obstet. Gynecol.* **61:** 63.

Prempree T & Amornmarn R (1984) Radiation treatment of recurrent carcinoma of the vulva. *Cancer* **54:** 1943–1949.

Rutledge FN, Mitchell MF, Munsell MF *et al.* (1991) Prognosis indicators for invasive carcinoma of the vulva. *Gynecol. Oncol.* **42:** 239–244.

Sedlis A, Homesley H, Bundy BN *et al.* (1987) Positive groin lymph nodes in superficial squamous cell vulvar cancer. *Am. J. Obstet. Gynecol.* **156:** 1159–1164.

Shafi MI, Luesley DM, Byrne P *et al.* (1989) Vulval intraepithelial neoplasia – management and outcome. *Br. J. Obstet. Gynaecol.* **96:** 1339–1344.

Shanbour KA, Mannel RS, Morris PC *et al.* (1992) Comparison of clinical versus surgical staging systems in vulvar cancer. *Obstet. Gynecol.* **80:** 927–930.

Simonsen E (1984) Treatment of recurrent squamous cell carcinoma of the vulva. *Acta Radiol. Oncol.* **23:** 345–348.

■ Sturgeon SR, Brinton LA, Devesa SS & Kurman RJ (1982) *In situ* and invasive vulvar carcinoma incidence trends (1973–1987). *Am. J. Obstet. Gynecol.* **166:** 1482–1485.

Sutton GP, Stehman FB, Ehrlich CE & Roman A (1987) Human papilloma virus deoxyribonucleic acid in lesions of the female genital tract: evidence for type 6/11 in squamous carcinoma of the vulva. *Obstet. Gynecol.* **70:** 564–568.

Taussig FJ (1940) Cancer of the vulva. *Am. J. Obstet. Gynecol.* **40:** 764–779.

Thomas G, Dembo A, DePetrillo A *et al.* (1989) Concurrent radiation and chemotherapy in vulvar carcinoma. *Gynecol. Oncol.* **34:** 263–267.

Toki T, Kurman RJ, Park JS *et al.* (1991) Probable nonpapillomavirus etiology of squamous cell carcinoma of the vulva in older women: a clinicopathologic study using *in situ* hybridisation and polymerase chain reaction. *Int. J. Gynecol. Pathol.* **10:** 107–125.

Way S (1948) The anatomy of the lymphatic drainage of the vulva and its influence on the radical operation for carcinoma. *Ann. Royal Col. Surgeons Eng.* **3:** 187–209.

Wharton JT, Gallager S & Rutledge FN (1974) Microinvasive carcinoma of the vulva. *Am. J. Obstet. Gynecol.* **118:** 159–162.

Wilkinson EJ (1985) Superficial invasive carcinoma of the vulva. *Clin. Obstet. Gynecol.* **28:** 188–195.

Woodruff JD & Novak ER (1962) Premalignant lesions of the vulva. *Clin. Obstet. Gynecol.* **5:** 1102–1118.

Yazigi R, Piver MS & Tsukada Y (1978) Microinvasive carcinoma of the vulva. *Obstet. Gynecol.* **51:** 368–370.

23 Pathogenesis and Epidemiology of Breast Cancer

RA Smith
RM Giusti

Introduction

Breast cancer is the most frequently diagnosed malignancy among women in the USA (American Cancer Society, 1995). In 1995, the American Cancer Society estimates that 182,000 women will be diagnosed with breast cancer, and that 46,000 women will die from this disease (Wingo *et al.*, 1995). Among women in the USA, breast cancer accounts for one-third of all cancers detected, and nearly one-fifth of all cancer deaths. In the world, breast cancer is the most common cancer in women, accounting for more than half a million new cases annually (Stanley *et al.*, 1987). In developed countries it is the most common malignancy diagnosed among women. In developing regions, breast cancer is usually the second most frequently diagnosed cancer among women.

Pathogenesis and Etiologic Epidemiology

The basic etiology underlying the association between known risk factors and breast cancer is poorly understood, although it is generally accepted that higher levels of endogenous hormones, in particular estrogens, are an important factor in the etiology of the disease. Numerous factors have been associated with an increased risk of breast cancer, including early age at menarche, late age at menopause, nulliparity, late age at first live birth, obesity, exposure to high-dose radiation, not breast feeding, a history of some types of benign breast disease (e.g. proliferative disease with atypical hyperplasia, sclerosing adenosis), a history of lobular carcinoma *in situ,* a history of breast cancer and a family history of breast cancer in one or more first-degree relatives (Kelsey and Gammon, 1991; Kelsey, 1993). Lifestyle factors (i.e. a diet high in animal fats, alcohol consumption and a history of routine physical activity) have also been associated with breast cancer, although these data have not shown either a strong or consistent level of association, and as of this date offer little beyond the prudence of a healthy lifestyle as a potential preventive measure (Kelsey and Gammon, 1991; Kelsey, 1993; Bernstein *et al.,* 1994). The majority of risk factors for breast cancer are not particularly strong and are of little value for counseling women about individual risk. Among those risk factors that are relevant are a woman's age, her family history, and her personal history of breast cancer and biopsy-confirmed benign breast disease.

Family History and Increased Risk of Breast Cancer

Family background and its specific pattern are generally regarded as among the more important risk factors associated with breast cancer. In women with a first-degree relative with breast cancer, the risk of breast cancer is increased 2–3-fold compared with women without this risk factor Kelsey and Gammon, 1991). Having more than one affected first-degree relative likewise increases risk (Anderson, 1971 Schwartz *et al.*, 1985; Sattin *et al.*, 1985; Byrne *et al.*, 1991). An early age of onset or bilateral disease in the first-degree relative family member is also believed to increase risk of onset at an earlier age, although studies have not shown a consistent pattern (Sattin *et al.*, 1985; Ottman *et al.*, 1986; Claus *et al.*, 1990; Mettlin *et al.*, 1990). In a more recent study, Calle *et al.* (1993) found family history to be predictive of fatal breast cancer among young women, with the strongest association observed for women with a first-degree relative also diagnosed when younger than 50 years of age. In the presence of atypical hyperplasia in a benign breast lesion, the risk of breast cancer in a woman with a family history of breast cancer is five times the risk of a woman with atypical hyperplasia without a family history of breast cancer (Dupont and Page, 1985). There appears to be no measurable difference between the effect of breast cancer in a mother or sister; each has an adjusted relative risk of about 2.5. However, for women with a family history of breast cancer in both a mother and sister, the adjusted relative risk is 13.6, with a lifetime risk exceeding 50% (Schwartz *et al.*, 1985). Nearly as high a risk has been observed for women with a sister diagnosed with bilateral breast cancer before 40 years of age. However, these circumstances are rare. The proportion of women aged 40 years and older who report breast cancer in two first-degree relatives (mother and sister) is estimated to be less than 1% (Dawson and Thompson, 1990).

Two large studies have recently estimated the prevalence of a family history of breast cancer among women with breast cancer. Colditz *et al.* (1993) reported a family history in 6% of 2389 prospectively identified breast cancer cases in the Nurses' Health Study. In contrast, estimates from the Utah Population Database were as high as 19% (Slattery and Kerby, 1993). While the estimate from the Nurses' Health Study is likely to be low, based on the small family groups studied and the lack of information on paternal history, the estimate from the Utah study is likely be high based on the inclusion of more distant family members. Other studies suggest that the prevalence of family history among breast cancer patients lies somewhere between these two estimates. Most breast cancer patients will therefore not have had a family history to suggest an increased breast cancer risk, and clinicians are cautioned not to underestimate the risk among patients without a family history. With respect to the general population, data from the 1987 National Health Interview Survey of Cancer Epidemiology and Control (Dawson and Thompson, 1990) indicate that approximately 8% of women aged 40 years and older reported breast cancer in at least one primary relative (mother, sister, or daughter).

Assessing an individual's risk of breast cancer includes taking a detailed history of cancer occurrence in both the maternal and paternal lineage. As a guide to clinical management and counseling of women with a family history of breast cancer, Hoskins *et al.* (1995) stratified women with a family history of breast cancer into two groups, those at moderate-risk and those at high-risk. Moderate-risk families typically report breast cancer, often postmenopausal, in one or two family members in the absence of ovarian cancer or other defined familial syndromes. These families are a heterogeneous group, and probably include families that carry a mutation in a dominantly transmitted susceptibility factor with low penetrance, families with breast cancer related to multiple susceptibility factors or environmental exposures including lifestyle factors, and families with several sporadic rather than hereditary breast cancer cases. Several models for individual risk assessment have been developed and may be useful in counseling moderate-risk families (Claus *et al.*, 1991; Claus *et al.*, 1994; Benichou, 1993).

High-risk families have a high probability of having a mutation in a dominantly-inherited breast cancer susceptibility gene with high penetrance. These families are likely to be characterized by an early age of onset of breast cancer, bilateral or multifocal disease, and two or more first-degree relatives with breast and/or ovarian cancer. Some families are too small for the high risk to be apparent and may be mistakenly classified as at moderate-risk. Women with a high-risk family history account for an estimated 5% of all breast cancer cases and 25% of women diagnosed before 30 years of age (Claus *et al.*, 1991). The majority of the relatively small number of high-risk breast cancer families studied to date have demonstrated mutations in the recently sequenced breast cancer susceptibility gene BRCA-1, or linkage to a second gene locus associated with breast cancer susceptibility, BRCA-2. However, in 30% of high-risk families studied to date neither BRCA-1 mutations nor linkage to BRCA-2 have been documented. These families are assumed to carry yet unidentified genetic susceptibility factor(s).

A small number of high-risk families are affected by inherited syndromes associated with an increased breast cancer risk. These families can usually be identified on the basis of associated clinical findings. Where molecular markers of risk have been identified, the lifetime breast cancer risk for individual family members can be defined with a high degree of precision to be either close to 100% or comparable to the level of risk in the general population. High-risk families should be referred to multidisciplinary centers providing genetic counseling and access to genetic testing. Such families would be candidates for studies of intervention or prevention strategies and for registries.

Genetic Susceptibility to Breast Cancer

BRCA-1/BRCA-2

Identification of a gene locus on chromosome 17q (Hall *et al.*, 1990; Narod *et al.*, 1991) associated with hereditary breast cancer launched an intensive effort to identify and sequence gene(s) associated with breast cancer susceptibility. Miki *et al.* (1994), using positional cloning, identified a large gene spanning 17q12–q21 composed of 22 coding exons over an estimated 100 kb of genomic DNA. This gene encodes a protein of 1863 amino acids of yet unknown function. An increasing number of BRCA-1 mutations have been reported, and the risk associated with these mutations is currently being described. While developing a screen to detect individual mutations would be a daunting task, it appears that 86% of mutations result in a truncated protein suggesting the possibility that a simplified functional assay for BRCA-1 mutations could be developed (Shattuck–Eidens *et al.*, 1995).

A recent review from the Breast Cancer Linkage Consortium suggests an elevated risk of both breast and ovarian cancer (Easton *et al.*, 1995). Of note, significant excesses of both colon cancer and prostate cancer were also found among these families (Ford *et al.*, 1994). Refining the definition of the breast–ovarian cancer family syndrome to include those families with two or more cases of early-onset breast cancer (before 60 years of age), two or more cases of ovarian cancer, and no cases of male breast cancer, Narod *et al.* (1995) found most families (92%; 95% CI 0.76–1.00) to be linked to BRCA-1. Among breast–ovarian families defined in this way, Easton *et al.* (1995) have postulated two BRCA-1 alleles with heterogeneity of cancer risk, the first conferring a breast cancer risk of 62% and an ovarian cancer risk of 11%, and the second conferring a breast cancer risk of 39% and an ovarian cancer risk of 42%, by 60 years of age. The first allele appears to represent about 70% of BRCA-1 mutations. While little is currently known about the prognostic significance of a BRCA-1 mutation, one report suggests two factors associated with a poor prognosis (aneuploidy and higher S-phase fractions) to be more common among breast cancer patients from families linked to BRCA-1 or with a family history most consistent with BRCA-1 than among breast cancer patients from other hereditary breast cancer families (Lynch *et al.*, 1994). Paradoxically, patients likely to be from BRCA-1 families showed a longer disease-free survival. BRCA-1 mutations do not appear to be a common mechanism in the development of sporadic cancers (Futreal *et al.*, 1994).

A second breast cancer susceptibility gene, BRCA-2, has been localized to chromosome 13q12–13. Families linked to this locus appear to have a high risk of breast cancer, but a lower risk of ovarian cancer, and a higher risk of male breast cancer than has been observed with linkage to BRCA-1 (Wooster *et al.*, 1994).

Other genetic syndromes associated with breast cancer risk

A number of familial syndromes have been associated with an increased breast cancer risk. These account for a small number of breast cancer patients and are usually identifiable by other clinical manifestations. Perhaps the best known is the Li–Fraumeni syndrome, which is characterized by the development of a range of both childhood and adult cancers including breast cancer, soft tissue sarcoma, brain tumors, osteosarcoma, leukemia, adrenocortical carcinoma and possibly other tumor types. Family members typically develop cancers at an early age and frequently develop multiple primary cancer. The probability of family members developing any invasive cancer is high: 50% by 30 years of age and over 90% by 70 years of age (Young *et al.*, 1981). This syndrome has been associated with germline p53 mutations (Malkin *et al.*, 1990). Recommendations on testing for germline mutations among family members have been developed (Li *et al.*, 1992).

Cowden's disease, a rare autosomal dominant disorder, is characterized by multiple mucocutaneous lesions (facial trichilemmomas, acral keratoses and oral papillomas) and other hamartomas and tumors (thyroid tumors, fibrocystic breast disease, carcinoma of the breast, gastrointestinal polyps and lipomas) (Brownstein *et al.*, 1978; Starink, 1984).

Peutz–Jeghers syndrome, an autosomal dominant condition characterized by mucocutaneous pigmentation and gastrointestinal hamartomas, which are not considered to be premalignant, is associated with an increased risk of both gastrointestinal and non-gastrointestinal tumors (Spigelman *et al.*, 1989; Hizawa *et al.*, 1993), including bilateral breast cancer (Trau *et al.*, 1982).

Unlike the disorders described above, ataxia–telangiectasia (A–T) is an autosomal recessive syndrome. Homozygotes are characterized by distinctive neurologic findings and occulocutaneous telangiectasia. The A–T gene is associated with an unusual sensitivity to ionizing radiation and homozygotes have a 100-fold increased risk of cancer. Patients typically die before their mid-twenties from lymphoma or leukemia (Morrell *et al.*, 1986). Heterozygotes constitute approximately 1% of the population in the USA (Swift *et al.*, 1986). These individuals appear to have an elevated risk of cancer at all sites (Swift *et al.*, 1991). Female carriers have a five-fold increased risk of breast cancer. Diagnostic or occupational exposure to ionizing radiation has been associated with an increased risk of breast cancer among A–T carriers (Swift *et al.*, 1991).

Assessing Individual Risk of Breast Cancer

Genetic testing for breast cancer susceptibility

Recent progress in locating and sequencing genes that impart susceptibility to breast cancer (BRCA-1, BRCA-2) as well as the molecular definition of inherited disorders associated with increased breast cancer risk have led to the threshold of predictive testing for breast cancer susceptibility. Using molecular-based testing, the risk of a given individual within a high-risk family can be defined with a high degree of precision, separating those family members who carry the susceptibility factor and have a near 100% chance of developing breast cancer over their lifetime from other family members who have a breast cancer risk comparable to the general population. Indeed, predictive testing has been offered to a small number of families through linkage analysis and more recently through direct testing for mutations at several research centers. While such testing has proven to be a complex and laborious task due to the rapid development of advances in this area, the public's interest in predictive testing, and pressures for commercialization, it is likely that tests for breast cancer susceptibility genes will be available in the near future. Concerns about the potential misuse of predictive testing have led the American Society of Human Genetics (1994) and the National Advisory Council for Human Genome Research (1994) to issue position papers. These have argued against population-based genetic screening and stated that predictive testing should be done in the research setting with appropriate attention given to informing participants of the potential benefits as well as the potential risks of predictive testing, and to providing appropriate counseling and follow-up care. Several recent reviews have been published to assist clinicians in counseling patients concerning breast cancer risk (King *et al.*, 1993; Offit and Brown, 1994; Rowell *et al.*, 1994).

Assessing risk in moderate-risk families

For the majority of women with a family history of breast cancer who fall into the moderate-risk category, genetic testing for breast cancer susceptibility will not be appropriate. Nonetheless, clinicians should be prepared to assist patients in understanding how a family history of breast cancer impacts on their individual risk. This is critical in enabling patients to make informed decisions concerning additional risks and potential benefits they may incur from the use of exogenous estrogens (oral contraceptives, ovulatory agents, postmenopausal replacement estrogens), and through participation in breast cancer screening programs and chemopreventive trials.

Two models have been developed to quantitate an individual's risk of breast cancer. Gail and Benichou (1994) developed a risk assessment model based on the experience of women who volunteered for annual breast cancer screening in the Breast Cancer Detection Demonstration Project (BCDDP). This model incorporates five risk factors: age at menarche, age at first live birth, family history of breast cancer, number of previous breast biopsies, and the presence of atypical hyperplasia in a breast biopsy specimen to derive an individualized absolute risk, indicating the chance that a woman with a given risk factor profile will develop breast cancer in a specified time frame (Benichou, 1993; Gail and Benichou, 1994). A validation study of this trial suggests that this model is a good predictor of risk among white women screened according to the American Cancer Society Guidelines, but may overestimate risk for women who are not routinely screened (Bondy *et al.*, 1994). An interactive computer program using this model is available (Benichou, 1993).

A second model has been developed by Claus *et al.* using data from the Cancer and Steroid Hormone Study, a large, multicenter, population-based, case–control study conducted by the Centers for Disease Control and Prevention (Claus *et al.*, 1991; Claus *et al.*, 1994). Tables of cumulative risk that can be applied to most clinical setting are provided. This model is perhaps more applicable to the population not undergoing routine screening and also takes into account the age of onset of cancer among the affected family member(s). These and two other models, which are less frequently used, are described by Offit and Brown (1994).

These tools are useful because too often risk approximations are done on the basis of relative risks identified in the literature. However, the use of relative risk as a basis of estimating individual risk can be misleading for the simple reason that it is a comparative measure (i.e. it is a measure of risk for individuals with a known risk factor compared with the risk in individuals without the risk factor). The relative risk does not directly approximate the underlying probability of the event over time (i.e. a diagnosis of breast cancer). While relative odds may be greater by a factor of 2–3 times for a woman with a particular risk factor, the more important estimate is her risk during particular intervals (i.e. within one year, during one or more decades, or during a lifetime). For example, Gail and Benichou (1992) estimated the relative risk of breast cancer for a nulliparous woman aged 40 years whose mother developed breast cancer and who had no other risk factors to be 2.76 compared with women without that risk profile. Her absolute risk of developing breast cancer between 40 and 70 years of age was estimated to be 11.6%. Over that 30-year period, the risk of developing breast cancer as estimated in the lifetime risk calculations (which are based on a hypothetical cohort of women representing all risk profiles) is 7.47% (Feuer *et al.*, 1992). While these two estimates are not directly comparable, they are useful for illustrating that relative risk estimates alone may inflate the perception of risk for women with a certain risk profile. On the other hand, the risk between 40 and 70 years of age for a woman with a family history of breast cancer in two first-degree relatives can be estimated to be 21%, and will be higher if either or both had their disease diagnosed premenopausally. In this instance, the use of this kind of counseling may serve to heighten both the woman's and her provider's attention to the importance of a program of routine screening at regular intervals.

Several points are worth mentioning. With the exception of a family history and age, none of the identified risk factors is particularly strong, either alone or in combination. Genetic susceptibility results in a highly elevated risk, but is rare. While a majority of women have at least one confirmed risk factor, the majority of women diagnosed with breast cancer do not have a risk profile that suggests any practical potential for narrowing the targets for screening (Seidman *et al.*, 1982). Therefore, to date, efforts to design screening programs based on risk factor profiles have not proved productive since estimates of the effectiveness of targeting women on the basis of a handful of key risk factors such as family history, age at menarche and parity have shown that such a program would miss the majority of cases. From a public health standpoint, all women in appropriate age categories should therefore be screened according to recommended guidelines.

Strategies for Reducing the Risk of Breast Cancer

The majority of factors that influence a woman's risk of breast cancer such as hereditary, age, onset of menarche and menopause, are beyond her control. Others, such as the choice to have a full-term pregnancy before 20 years of age or increasing her parity are not easily modifiable for obvious reasons. Lifestyle modifications (a prudent diet, exercise, and reducing alcohol intake) have not been convincingly associated with a decreased breast cancer risk, but might be advised as measures consistent with good general health. For women with an average risk of breast cancer, routine screening according to recommended guidelines is the most important strategy to assure early detection. For women with a greater than average risk of breast cancer, intensified screening and chemoprevention have been proposed as protective methods. For women with an exceptionally higher risk, heightened surveillance, chemoprevention, and prophylactic mastectomy have all been considered. However, little is currently known about the efficacy of chemoprevention, screening, and prophylactic mastectomy for women with an increased risk of breast cancer, especially those with hereditary cancer syndromes.

Chemoprevention of breast cancer

Tamoxifen has been most widely used as a preventive agent (Nayfield *et al.*, 1991). The mechanism of action of tamoxifen is complex and not completely understood (Buckley and Goa, 1989; Jordan and Murphy, 1990; Nayfield *et al.*, 1991). It exerts both antiestrogenic and partial estrogenic effects. The partial estrogenic effects affect certain tissues including the endometrium. The antiestrogenic effects appear to be mediated through at least two mechanisms. Tamoxifen binds directly to the estrogen receptor resulting in a conformational change of the receptor, altered RNA transcription and decreased cell proliferation. It also appears to modulate the production of several polypeptide growth factors, inhibiting the estrogen-dependent secretion of transforming growth factor-alpha and epidermal growth factor and stimulating production of transforming growth factor-beta. Both transforming growth factor-alpha and epidermal growth factor bind to cell membrane receptors and promote breast cancer cell proliferation. Transforming growth factor-beta inhibits the growth of many epithelial cell lines, including estrogen receptor-negative breast cancer cells.

A large body of literature exists on the use of tamoxifen in the treatment of advanced disease and in the adjuvant treatment of early stage disease (Fisher *et al.*, 1989; Jordan, 1991; Early Breast Cancer Trialists' Collaborative Group, 1992). Overall survival and disease-free survival are increased in women over 50 years of age with adjuvant tamoxifen. Additionally, the pooled data from a number of adjuvant trials show a significant reduction in the rate of second primary breast cancers in the contralateral breast in the tamoxifen group versus the placebo control group and suggest an advantage to a longer use of tamoxifen. While the benefit for postmenopausal women has been clearly documented, the benefit to premenopausal women is less clear. The drug has been well tolerated in large trials and the effects of tamoxifen on lipid metabolism (Love *et al.*, 1990) and bone mineral density, which have been reported in several studies' suggest a potential benefit in protective effects from cardiovascular disease and osteoporosis. However, concerns about its long-term toxicity, primarily uterine cancer, but also liver disease, ocular toxicity, thrombosis and thrombophlebitis have been raised.

The apparent prevention of second primary breast cancers in the adjuvant setting has led to the use of tamoxifen as a chemopreventive agent in women with an increased risk of breast cancer. A large-scale, randomized, placebo-controlled study of the efficacy of tamoxifen for the chemoprevention of breast cancer has been initiated by the National Surgical Adjuvant Breast Project (NSABP). This trial will recruit an estimated 16,000 women aged 35–78 years. The Gail model mentioned previously has been used to assess the individual risk of breast cancer among participants. Women who are 60 years of age or older or women with a risk factor profile that makes their risk equivalent to that of a 60-year-old woman are eligible for randomization in this trial (Gail and Benichou, 1994). This trial remains controversial (Bush *et al.*, 1993; Love, 1993), primarily for the inclusion of premenopausal women, but provides a unique opportunity to establish the potential benefits and risks of this preventive therapy.

A large-scale, placebo-controlled Italian trial of the synthetic retinoid fenretinide is underway to assess the efficacy of this compound for the prevention of second breast malignancies in the contralateral breast of women with early stage ($T_{1,2}N_0$) disease (Decensi *et al.*, 1993). While there is less clinical experience with this agent, the trial was launched on the basis of strong preclinical data suggesting a chemopreventive effect in breast cancer models (Costa *et al.*, 1994). The drug appears to be well tolerated and side-effects include reduced ability to see in the dark and skin erythema. A Phase I chemoprevention study aimed at defining biomarkers and intermediate endpoints is now being carried out.

A number of other agents have been suggested for the chemoprevention of breast cancer (Kelloff *et al.*, 1993), but their potential use remains to be established. Hormonal manipulation of young women to effect a breast cancer risk reduction has also been suggested (Pike and Spicer, 1993; Henderson *et al.*, 1993; Russo and Russo, 1994). Again, the risks and benefits of such a potentially complex intervention remain to be assessed.

Intensified screening for early detection

There are currently no data to confirm that intensified screening of women with a genetic susceptibility to breast cancer results in a mortality reduction. One inherent problem is the fact that genetic susceptibility is associated with early onset of disease, a time at which a greater presence of breast densities poses a challenge to conventional imaging technology. It is possible that advances in breast imaging technology (digital imaging, breast magnetic resonance imaging, positron emission tomography scan) may improve the ability to detect small breast lesions in young women with dense breasts. More worrisome is the theoretical concern regarding exposure to low doses of ionizing radiation at a younger age among women with a genetic susceptibility to cancer or women who are A–T gene carriers. While the dose received in the course of routine mammographic screening poses little risk to the majority of women, it may adversely affect a small subgroup of women. However, it must be emphasized that these concerns are a matter of conjecture.

Prophylactic mastectomy

The use of bilateral prophylactic mastectomy to reduce breast cancer risk remains controversial. Indications for this procedure have been reviewed by several authors (Snyderman, 1984; Pressman, 1988; Danforth, 1990) and are most commonly a family history of two or more first-degree relatives with breast cancer, proliferative breast disease demonstrated in multiple biopsies, and breast scarring due to repeated breast biopsies in women with other risk factors for breast cancer with subsequent inability to evaluate the breast. As yet, there is no consensus on criteria. Nor has there been consistent agreement on the type of surgical procedure that should be performed to reduce the risk of breast cancer and whether the nipple–areola complex can be safely retained. While simple and subcapsular mastectomies have been used in the past, it is clear that more radical approaches, including the classic Halsted radical mastectomy do not result in an extirpation of all breast tissue (Temple *et al.*, 1991). Animal studies have suggested that a reduction in breast cancer risk, if effected, may not be proportional to the amount of breast cancer excised (Wong *et al.*, 1986; Nelson *et al.*, 1989). In fact, Nelson *et al.* (1989) have postulated that a reduction of breast tissue may lead to a paradoxical increase in breast cancer risk mediated by an increase in the secretion of prolactin.

There are currently little data concerning the efficacy of prophylactic mastectomy. Several cases reports of breast cancer following subcutaneous or simple mastectomy have been reported (Eldar *et al.*, 1984; Goodnight *et al.*, 1984; Ziegler and Kroll, 1991). Larger studies carried out to date have suggested breast cancer rates ranging from less than 1% to 19% (Humphrey, 1983; Woods, 1983; Pennisi and Capozzi, 1989). These studies are difficult to interpret because they have included heterogeneous patient groups, have used differing surgical approaches, and have had limited follow-up time. While the risk of cancer recurrence clearly needs to be established for defined high-risk subgroups, it is clear that prophylactic mastectomy does not eliminate the risk of breast cancer.

Trends in Incidence, Mortality and Survival in the USA

Estimates of disease burden in the USA are routinely calculated by several government agencies and the American Cancer Society. Incidence is estimated through the National Cancer Institute (NCI) Surveillance, Epidemiology and End Results (SEER) program (Ries *et al.*, 1994). Nine cancer registries, including five statewide registries (Connecticut, Hawaii, Iowa, New Mexico and Utah), and four urban areas (Detroit, Atlanta, San Francisco–Oakland and Seattle–Puget Sound) presently contribute incidence and survival data to the program. These areas represent approximately 9.5% of the USA population, and their combination is regarded as approximately representative of the USA. Mortality data are available from the National Center for Health Statistics (NCHS), which collects information on all deaths occurring in the USA. Each year the American Cancer Society estimates the number of new cases and deaths in the USA (and each of 50 states, the District of Columbia, and Puerto Rico) for all cancers (excluding non-melanoma skin cancer and carcinoma *in situ*) based on trends in incidence and mortality derived from the SEER database, and on cancer-related mortality data from NCHS (Ries *et al.*, 1994; American Cancer Society, 1995; Wingo *et al.*, 1995).

Incidence[1]

Early data from Connecticut (available since 1935) and data from 1973–1980 from SEER show a gradual annual increase over this period in the age-adjusted incidence rate of invasive breast cancer of approximately 1% per year (Devesa *et al.*, 1987). However, since 1980, the age-adjusted incidence of breast cancer increased from 85.0/100,000 to 112.3/100,000 in 1987, a relative increase over the period of 32% or an average increase of approximately 3% per year (*Figure 23.1*). Between 1987 and 1991, the incidence rate declined from 112.4 to 105.7/100,000 women, and then rose again to 110.2, indicating that the incidence rate is no longer increasing at the rate observed during the period 1980–1987, and the more recent trend (1987–1991) suggests that breast cancer incidence in the USA is either stabilizing or declining (Hankey *et al.*, 1993).

This dramatic increase in the incidence rate has been the focus of considerable clinical and public attention, with some arguing that the recent increase in rates qualifies as an 'epidemic.' Certainly the magnitude of the increase meets any definition of epidemic proportions, but to be true to the definition for this recent period (setting aside the question of the long-term trend) the shift in the trend would need to be explained by a change in the underlying risk. Such an abrupt increase in incidence would be difficult to explain for any malignancy. Rather, it appears that the marked increase in incidence is primarily accounted for by an increase in breast cancer screening rates, and further evidence for this conclusion has come from examination of screening trends and age-specific rates of detection.

As noted above, the recent trend in incidence, specifically the significant increase in rates between 1980 and 1987, has received considerable attention because of the interest in understanding the degree to which it represents a true increase in disease, a screening effect, or some combination of these two factors. There is little question that the dramatic increase in incidence occurred concomitant with the dramatic increase in screening and greater availability of mammography (Kessler, 1992; Smith and Haynes, 1992). According to Howard (1987), an evaluation of national surveys conducted between 1978 and 1983 indicated that only about 15–20% of American women had ever had a mammogram. However, by 1987, estimates from the NCI-sponsored Cancer Control Supplement to the National Health Interview Survey indicated that 39% of women aged 40 years and older had had a mammogram (Dawson and Thompson, 1990), and by 1992, according to estimates from the Mammography Attitudes and Usage Survey (MAUS), that number had increased to 74% (Horton *et al.*, 1992). While the majority of women have had at least one mammogram, a smaller proportion is screened routinely. Data from the Centers for Disease Control's Behavioral Risk Factor Surveillance System (BRFSS) in 48 participating states and the District of Columbia indicate (median values) that in 1992 64% of women aged 40–49 reported a mammogram in the previous two years, and 51% of women aged 50 years and older reported a mammogram in the previous year (American Cancer Society, 1994). During this time period a number of factors contributed to the increased use of mammography, including the growth of scientific support for the value of the procedure (Shapiro *et al.*, 1988; Hurley and Kaldor, 1992), increasing acceptance by providers (American Cancer Society, 1990), increasing acceptance by women (Horton *et al.*, 1992) and increasing access as measured by the growth in the number of installed dedicated mammography units (Brown *et al.*, 1990). Also

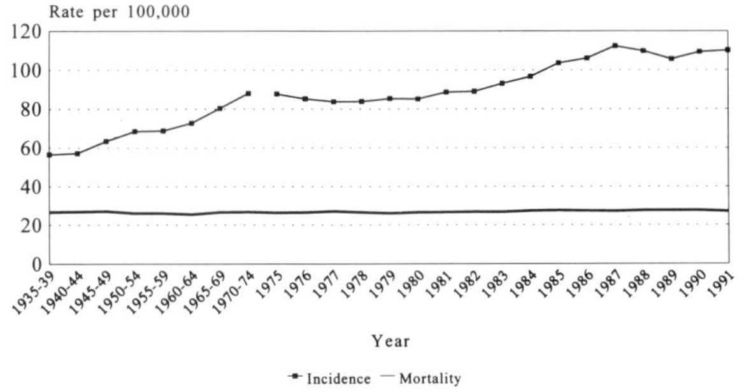

Figure 23.1. Breast cancer incidence and mortality rates of USA females, 1935–1991. (Incidence data are from the Connecticut Tumor Registry (1935–1974) and National Cancer Institute (NCI) Surveillance, Epidemiology and End Results (SEER) program (1975–1991). Mortality data are from the USA Vital Statistics. Rates are per 100,000 females, age-adjusted to the 1970 USA standard population.)

[1]Breast cancer statistics relating to different aspects of disease frequency are expressed in different ways. *Numbers* of new cases and deaths are usually expressed for a given year and have obvious intuitive value as a measure of disease burden. Incidence and mortality *rates* are more useful for comparisons between two different populations or for comparisons within a population over time. Because underlying population dynamics such as a change in mean age can influence both crude rates (number of cases per unit of population during a given time period) and numbers of cases and deaths. USA rates are typically standardized to the 1970 USA population. Because the incidence of breast cancer increases with increasing age, crude rates will increase over time in an ageing population on that basis alone. By removing the influence of age, trends in the age-standardized rates will be an expression of the trend in the underlying epidemiology of disease and/or the trend in detection. Age-specific rates, commonly calculated for five-year age groups, are usually regarded as directly comparable within and between populations. Unless otherwise specified, rates for all women in these discussions are expressed as the annual number of cases/100,000 women, age-adjusted to the 1970 USA population.

during this period, an increasing number of women reported that they were screened on a regular basis according to recommended guidelines or whenever their doctor recommended the test (Horton *et al.*, 1992).

However, recent analyses have also concluded that the entirety of the recent increase is not so easily explained. The analysis by White *et al.* (1990) points to screening as an explanation for the increase in women aged 55–64 years, but not entirely for women younger than 55 or older than 65 years. Likewise, Liff *et al.* (1991) suggest that the increase is accounted for by both an increase in the use of mammography and a true increase in the rate of disease. There is little question that a true increase of the disease is a factor in the recent increase in incidence. As noted earlier, there has been an observed average annual increase of slightly less than 1% per year measured by data from the Connecticut tumor registry before the widespread availability and use of mammography. In addition, Holford *et al.* (1991), using Connecticut Tumor Registry data, have shown higher age-specific incidence for successive cohorts of women born since 1870, providing indirect evidence that there is a true underlying increase in disease contributing in part to the recent increase in the incidence trend. However, recent analyses provide support for the hypothesis that the recent increase in the incidence trend has largely been a function of the influence of increased rates of case detection resulting from higher participation rates in screening (Feuer and Wun, 1992; Farwell *et al.*, 1993; Miller *et al.*, 1993).

Breast cancer is rare before 25 years of age (*Figure 23.2*), but the incidence increases measurably after that time. It is interesting to note the age-specific trends over the three time periods shown in *Figure 23.2*. Before the most recent period (shown here as average age-specific rates for 1987–1991), the breast cancer incidence rate was higher with each successive age group. However, the most recent data reveal a peak for the age group 75–79 years, followed by a decline in age-specific incidence. The specific reasons for this recent shift in the age–incidence trend are not conclusively established, but several hypotheses have been advanced. First, the shift in the age-specific pattern in recent years, specifically among older women, may be explained simply by different participation rates in screening and differences in lead time in older women compared to younger women (Kessler, 1992). Since the average lead time for breast cancer (i.e. the interval of time when breast cancer is detectable before the onset of clinical symptoms) increases with increasing age, a visible decline in incidence should be seen in subsequent cohorts of older women as a result of a previous increase in the participation rates of screening (Tabar *et al.*, 1987; Henderson, 1992). In contrast, a shorter lead time in younger women will contribute to a less striking increase in incidence, and hence a less apparent reduction in the incidence rate in subsequent age cohorts following an increase in screening. Another possible explanation to account for the changing age–incidence pattern relates to different levels of age-specific participation in screening. The proportions of women who have ever had and recently underwent mammography decrease substantially after 75 years of age (Dawson and Thompson, 1990). Inasmuch as age-specific incidence rates have not increased proportionally among older women at the same rate as those observed among women aged 60–79 years, the recent pattern may also be explained in part by a greater increase in breast cancer detection among women younger than 75 years resulting from higher rates of breast cancer screening. It is likely that some combination of these two explanations accounts for these age-specific patterns.

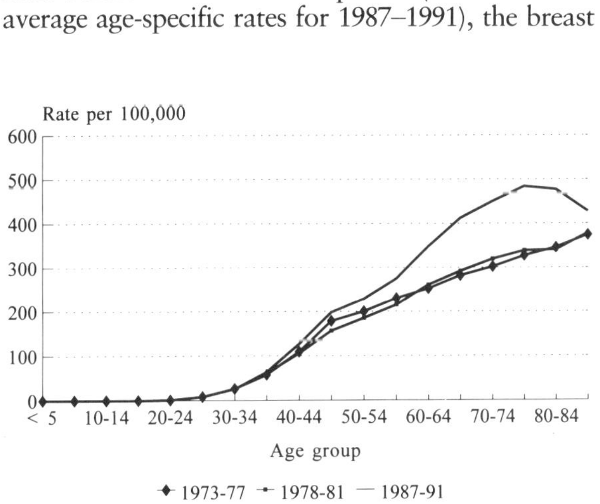

Figure 23.2. Average age-specific breast cancer incidence rates of USA females, 1973–1991. (Source: National Cancer Institute (NCI) Surveillance, Epidemiology and End Results (SEER) program. Rates are per 100,000 females within the specified age group.)

Overall, age-adjusted incidence rates are higher in white women (113.6/100,000) than in black women (95.1/100,000), although there are notable differences in age-specific rates and trends over time (*Tables 23.1 and 23.2*). In women aged 44 years and younger, age-specific incidence rates are higher in black women than in white women (see *Table 23.1*). In comparison, among women aged 45 years and older, age-specific incidence rates are between 18–36% higher in white women than in black women. Likewise, although the trend in increasing incidence between 1973 and 1991 has been similar in white and black women aged 50 years and older, in women under 50 years of age the increase in incidence over the same time period is nearly three times higher among black women than among white women (see *Table 23.2*)

Although there has been an overall increase in the age-adjusted incidence rate between 1973 and 1991, age-specific changes have differed markedly. Among women younger than 40 years of age, the incidence of breast cancer has declined slightly in some five-year age groups or remained essentially unchanged. Among women between 40–59 years of age an increase in incidence of 5–12.5% is apparent, while among women aged 60–79 years the increase in incidence has exceeded 40%. A much smaller increase in incidence is seen among women aged over 85 years, and this is probably a reflection of the comparatively lower rates of screening in this population. These trends, in particular those for younger women, may seem to contradict clinical experience (i.e. that the disease is increasing among all age groups). However, while the rate of disease may not have changed, the numbers of women from whom these rates are calculated has increased dramatically. For example, the impression that breast cancer incidence is increasing in women younger than 40 years of age is valid if measured by the presence of a growing number of newly diagnosed cases in this age group resulting from the growing numbers of women in this age category because increasingly larger numbers of women born since 1945 are over 30 years of age. In 1970 there were approximately 11,550,000 women aged 30–39 years, whereas in 1990 it is estimated there were 21,060,000 women in this age group, roughly a doubling of the number over the 20 years (Spencer, 1984). Even if age-specific incidence rates remain the same, the difference in the size of the population at risk means that the annual number of cases in this age group would nearly double, producing a reasonable impression of increasing incidence. Although age-specific breast cancer incidence rates are higher in the age group 50–59 years, the entry of post-war birth cohort women into the age group 40–49 years since 1985 means that in 1995 more women aged 40–49 are expected to be diagnosed with breast cancer in this age group compared with women aged 50–59 (33,800 versus 28,300). In 1985, approximately 57 million women were 35 years of age or older, and by the year 2025 it is estimated that 91 million women will be in this age group, an increase of 61%.

Table 23.1. Age-specific breast cancer incidence and mortality rates of USA females, by race, 1987–1991. (Source: National Cancer Institute (NCI) Surveillance, Epidemiology and End Results (SEER) program, and National Center for Health Statistics (NCHS) public use tape. Rates are new cases and deaths per 100,000 females in the specified age group.)

	Incidence		*Mortality*	
Age group	*Whites*	*Blacks*	*Whites*	*Blacks*
30–34	25.0	32.3	4.5	8.1
40–44	127.1	134.9	22.4	34.8
45–49	203.6	176.3	36.2	52.2
50–54	238.8	209.5	53.5	70.8
60–64	364.2	287.4	89.5	97.6
70–74	468.5	335.6	120.5	116.8
80–84	490.7	379.0	156.7	149.3

Mortality

The age-adjusted mortality rate from breast cancer has remained largely unchanged over the past 30 years (see *Figure 23.1*), ranging from an average of 26.0/100,000 for the period 1956–1958 to 27.4/100,000 for the period 1987–1991 (Hankey *et al.*, 1993; Ries *et al.*, 1994). The age-adjusted mortality rate among all females has increased 2.6% since 1973, from 26.9/100,000 to 27.0/100,000, averaging 0.2% per year (see *Table 23.2*). Although the overall rate has remained fairly stable, racial and age-specific differences, and differences in trends in mortality between 1973 and 1991 are noteworthy (Ries *et al.*, 1994). Overall, age-adjusted mortality rates for the period 1987–1991 are higher in black women (31.9/100,000) compared with white women (26.8/100,000). Black females aged 64 years and younger

Table 23.2. Trends in invasive breast cancer incidence and mortality in USA females by race and age, 1973–1991. (Source: National Cancer Institute (NCI) Surveillance, Epidemiology and End Results (SEER) program. Incidence data are from the SEER program; mortality data are from the National Center for Health Statistics (NCHS) public use tape.)

Trend 1973–1991	*All females*	*Whites <50 years*	*Whites >50 years*	*Blacks <50 years*	*Blacks >50 years*
Incidence					
Percentage change	23.9	8.5	31.8	26.1	32.0
Annual percentage change*	1.7	0.8	2.2	1.2	2.2
Mortality					
Percentage change	1.8	−14.0	4.0	2.0	26.3
Annual percentage change*	0.2	−0.8	0.3	0.8	1.5

*Estimated annual percentage change is significantly different from zero ($p < 0.05$).

have higher age-specific mortality rates than white women, whereas after 65 years of age white women have higher age-specific mortality rates, although the magnitude of the difference is much less than the differences observed in incidence rates (*Table 23.1*). Whereas the age-adjusted mortality rate has increased only slightly (1.8%) between 1973 and 1991 among white women, it has increased 17.4% among black women, from 26.3/100,000 in 1973 to 31.9/100,000 in 1991. As seen in *Table 23.2*, over this 18 year period (1973–1991), mortality rates decreased 14% in white women younger than 50 years (from 6.8/100,000 to 5.9/100,000), but increased by 2% in black women in this age group (from 8.9/100,000 to 9.2/100,000). Among women aged 50 years and older, mortality rates have increased among both white women (+4.0%) and black women (+26.3%). In fact, the mortality rate among black women aged 50 years and older, which was previously lower than the rate among white women, now is higher (1987–1991, 99.1 versus 93.1/100,000 women) (Ries *et al.*, 1994).

Stage at Diagnosis and Survival

The trend in stage of diagnosis is consistent with trends in early detection. As shown in *Figure 23.3*, the rate of cases diagnosed at Stage I has increased since 1980, and at a steeper rate since 1982, the period of time, as noted earlier, when mammography utilization rates were increasing. A similar pattern can be seen in the rate of cancer diagnosed *in situ* since 1982. Note that the rate of disease diagnosed at regional and distant stages has not changed appreciably during this time. More detailed information in stage shifts observed between 1983 and 1989 is shown in *Figures 23.4* and *23.5*. As can be seen, a significantly greater proportion of cases is being detected at more favorable stages among both black and white women, and among women younger than 50 years

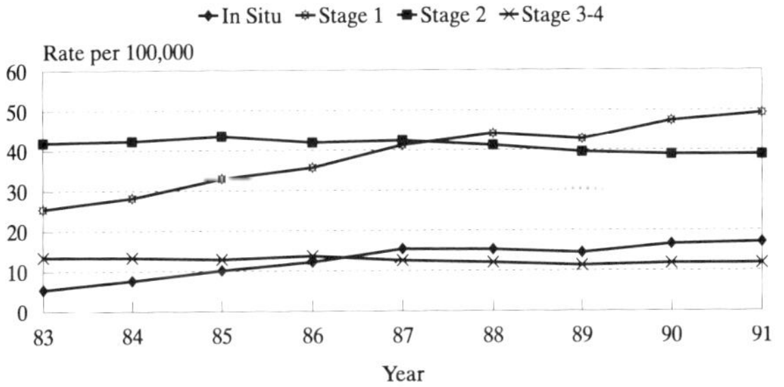

Figure 23.3. Breast cancer incidence rates by AJCC (American Joint Commission on Cancer) stage among USA females, 1983–1991. (Source: National Cancer Institute (NCI) Surveillance, Epidemiology and End Results (SEER) program. Rates are per 100,000 females, age-adjusted to the 1970 USA standard population.)

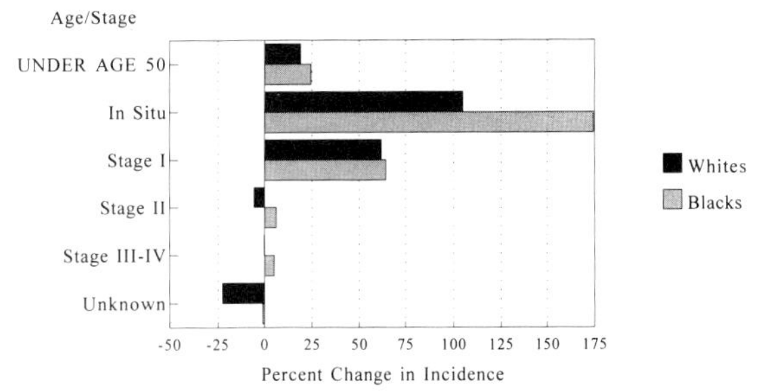

Figure 23.4. Female breast cancer by stage, percentage change in incidence, 1983–1991, for women less than 50 years of age. (Source: National Cancer Institute (NCI) Surveillance, Epidemiology and End Results (SEER) program, 1994.)

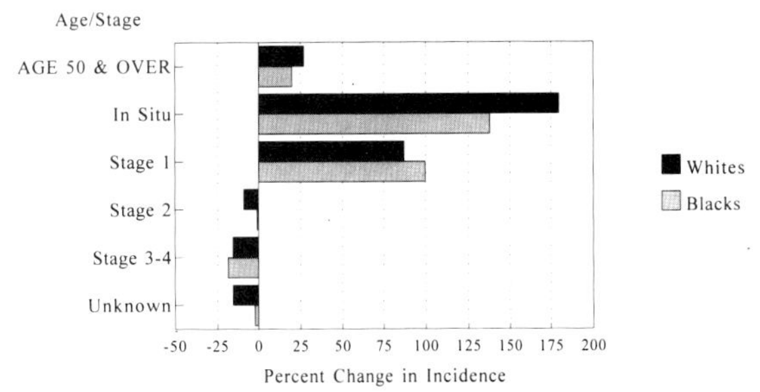

Figure 23.5. Female breast cancer by stage: percentage change in incidence, 1983–1991, for women over 50 years of age. (Source: National Cancer Institute (NCI) Surveillance, Epidemiology and End Results (SEER) program, 1994.)

Table 23.3. Breast cancer stage distribution by race, 1991. (Source: National Cancer Institute (NCI) Surveillance, Epidemiology and End Results (SEER) program, 1994.)

Stage	*White females*	*Black females*
In situ	12%	12%
Stage I	40%	26%
Stage II	32%	38%
Stage III	5%	9%
Stage IV	4%	6%
Unknown	7%	9%

of age, and aged 50 years and older. However, these improvements in stage at detection over time should not overshadow the fact that at present a significant percentage of all women, and especially black women, are diagnosed Stage II and above (*Table 23.3*).

Overall, breast cancer has a favorable survival rate. The current five-year survival rate for all stages of invasive disease is 81.3% (Ries *et al.*, 1994). Survival is also much improved if breast cancer is diagnosed early, with five-year survival rates

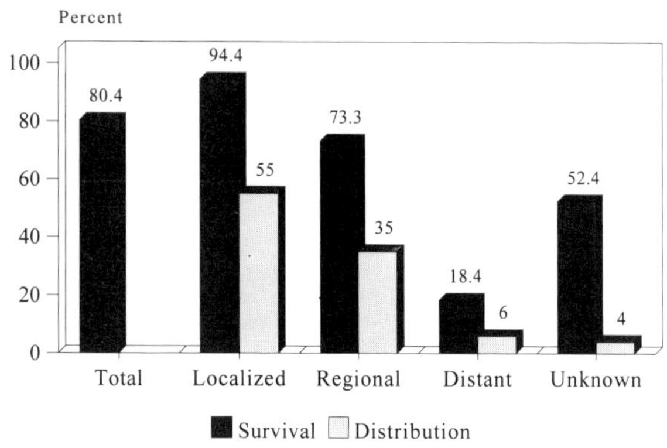

Figure 23.6. Historical stage distribution and five-year relative survival rates by stage among USA females, 1983–1990. (Source: National Cancer Institute (NCI) Surveillance, Epidemiology and End Results (SEER) program, 1994.)

exceeding 90% if invasive disease is diagnosed at a localized stage, as can be seen in *Figure 23.6* which shows five-year survival rates by stage and the comparative distribution of cases diagnosed at that stage for the period 1983–1990. As can be seen, breast cancers diagnosed at the regional or distant stage have a much poorer prognosis. Overall, five-year survival rates are lower in black women (65.8%) than in white women (81.6%), and poorer survival is seen at each stage of disease detection (Ries *et al.,* 1994). The overall poorer survival observed in black women compared to that of white women is largely attributable to later stage at diagnosis (Wells and Horm, 1992; Ries *et al.,* 1994). However, much of the difference attributable to race is a function of a higher poverty rate among black women than among white women. Of particular relevance is the influence of social class on both overall survival and disease-free survival. A recent analysis by Gordon *et al.* (1992) showed that taken alone, race significantly predicts shorter disease-free and overall survival, but after adjustment for the socioeconomic status of the patient, race ceases to be significant.

The most recent five-year survival data available for women diagnosed with breast cancer show a statistically significant improvement ($p<0.05$) in five-year survival for women with breast cancer diagnosed in 1983–1990 compared with average survival for women diagnosed between 1974–1976 (80.4% versus 74.3%) (Ries *et al.,* 1994). Comparisons of breast cancer incidence, survival, and mortality data, often lead to the questions about the associations between these different measurements, and how trends in one rate affect the others. As noted earlier, the incidence rate is a function of underlying true disease trends, as well as the social contribution of the availability of screening and diagnostic services and the motivation to use these services. The survival rate is a function of stage at detection, the availability of state-of-the-art treatment and host characteristics. The mortality rate in any given year is a function of incidence rates over time and the accompanying trend(s) in survival. For many, the absence of a visible and significant decline in the mortality rate has been viewed as paradoxical in the face of the recent increase in the use of mammography. However, this expectation must be tempered with the understanding that there is a certain measure of independence between these data that is a function of time. Presently, the most recent data from the NCI SEER program is from 1991, reflecting the normal lag between the calendar year of diagnosis, and a registry's ability to collect, process, and report summary statistics. The most recent five-year survival rate is for cases diagnosed in 1985, comparatively early during the recent period of increased availability and use of mammography. The mortality rate from breast cancer in any given year is a reflection of deaths from breast cancer among women diagnosed over many years previously. If the majority of deaths occur in women diagnosed with regional and distant disease, and it is cases diagnosed at this stage that have the poorest short-term survival, then significant near-term improvements in the mortality rate are unlikely to be seen without a significant shift in stage at detection from advanced disease to more favorable stages. While the recent trend in the greater use of mammography has been associated with a significant increase in the rate of disease detected at the *in situ* and localized stage, only since 1988 has there been a decline in the rate of breast cancer detected at the regional and distant stage. Therefore, the influence of greater participation in screening with mammography and the resulting improvements in lead time as measured by improvements in stage at detection and already visible in five-year survival rates, will take longer to be observed in mortality rates. However, as has been clearly demonstrated in clinical trials to date, a more favorable stage at detection does result in a reduction in mortality and this improvement in disease outcome should eventually be evident in summary statistics in the foreseeable future.

Lifetime Risk of Breast Cancer

The American Cancer Society estimates that one in nine women will be diagnosed with breast cancer in her lifetime. The lifetime risk of breast cancer has changed during the last five decades, largely as a function of increasing incidence and increasing longevity. In 1940 the risk to 85 years of age was estimated to be 1 in 20 (or 5%). By 1980, the risk was estimated to be 1 in 11 (or 9.1%) and by 1987, 1 in 9 (or 11.1%). The risk of being diagnosed with breast cancer or dying of breast cancer can be estimated

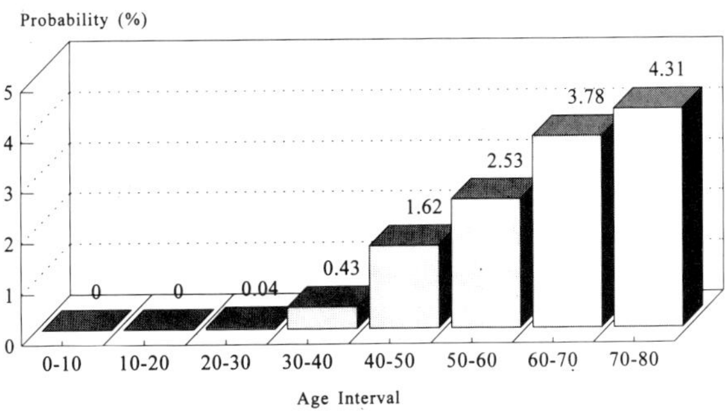

Figure 23.7. Probability of developing invasive breast cancer during specific age intervals, for white females in Surveillance, Epidemiology and End Results (SEER) areas, 1987–1988. (Source: Feuer *et al.*, 1992.)

for an interval from birth to some endpoint, arbitrarily defined as a lifetime, or for different intervals beginning at different ages. This probability is a function of two factors, which vary at different ages (i.e. the underlying incidence rate of disease, and the rate of survival, or removal from the interval by competing risks of dying from other causes) (Seidman *et al.*, 1985; Feuer *et al.*, 1992). The lifetime rate is a cumulative probability, and it can be expressed as a percentage.

The steadily increasing trend in lifetime risk is best explained by the interaction of increasing longevity and the increasing incidence of breast cancer. For women alive in 1940, 1970 and 1987, there has been a marked increase in the age-specific survival throughout a hypothetical lifetime. In 1987 compared with 1940, overall longevity is much improved and is apparent at every age interval. Although these gains in longevity are comparatively modest before 35 years of age over these three time periods, they are much more apparent as the population ages. During these same time periods, the age-specific incidence rate has increased in all age groups, but most notably among women aged 40 years and older. The combination of increasing incidence and increasing longevity has meant a steadily increasing risk of developing breast cancer.

The most recent rate (one in nine) is calculated to 85 years of age, although earlier rates were calculated to 110 years of age (Seidman *et al.*, 1985) and recent calculations have also estimated the risk beyond 85 years of age, which increases the estimate to one in eight (Feuer *et al.*, 1992). Any endpoint is arbitrary, since this exercise is designed to quantify risk over an interval of interest. For example, as seen in *Figure 23.7*, the average risk for a white female aged 30 years for the ten-year interval between the ages of 30 and 40 years is estimated to be 0.43%, or one in 232, compared with a lifetime risk from 0–85 years of 11.1%, or one in nine. However, between the ages of 60 and 70 years, a 60-year-old woman's risk is estimated to be 3.78%, or one in 26. Because lifetime risk is cumulative, the course of accumulated risk can be estimated by the summation of the decade risk shown in *Figure 23.7*. A woman's cumulative probability to 50 years of age is only approximately 2% (or one in 50), and the risk to age 60 years is less than half the potential risk as measured to age 80 years. For women who are concerned about breast cancer risk, these data may provide a measure of reassurance that average risk over periods of ten and 20 years is considerably less than the frequently expressed one in nine estimate. These estimates presume average risk, and as noted above will vary with more specific risk profiles.

Conclusion

Today, and for the foreseeable future, the greatest potential for reducing breast cancer mortality lies in the availability of comprehensive programs for the early detection and treatment of breast cancer. To realize the fullest potential of the proven technology, screening programs must achieve high rates of routine participation and must achieve high standards of quality at each step of the process. Coordination among providers is essential to assure quality of outcomes, and new guidelines issued by the Agency of Health Care Policy and Research (Bassett *et al.*, 1994) provide useful guidance for the individual provider and for women.

Summary of Core Information

- According to American Cancer Society estimates, breast cancer is the most frequently diagnosed malignancy among women in the USA.
- The basic etiology underlying the association between known risk factors and breast cancer is poorly understood, although it is generally accepted that higher levels of endogenous hormones, in particular estrogens, are an important factor in the etiology of the disease.
- The majority of risk factors for breast cancer are not particularly strong and are of little value for counseling women about individual risk. Among those risk factors that are relevant are a woman's age, her family history, and her personal history of

breast cancer and biopsy-confirmed benign breast disease.

- Assessing an individual's risk of breast cancer includes taking a detailed history of cancer occurrence in both the maternal and paternal lineage.
- Since 1980, the age-adjusted incidence of breast cancer increased from 85.0/100,000 to 112.3/100,000 in 1987, a relative increase over the period of 32%, or an average increase of approximately 3% per year.
- It appears that the marked increase in incidence is primarily accounted for by an increase in breast cancer screening rates, and further evidence for this conclusion has come from an examination of screening trends and age-specific rates of detection.
- The impression that breast cancer incidence is increasing in women younger than 40 years of age is valid if measured by the presence of a growing number of newly diagnosed cases in this age group resulting from the growing numbers of women in this age category as increasingly larger numbers of women born since 1945 exceed 30 years of age.
- The age-adjusted mortality rate from breast cancer has remained largely unchanged over the past 30 years, ranging from an average of 26.0/100,000 for the period 1956–1958 to 27.4/100,000 for the period 1987–1991.
- Survival is much improved if breast cancer is diagnosed early, with five-year survival rates exceeding 90% if invasive disease is diagnosed at a localized stage.

References

American Cancer Society (1994) *Cancer Risk Report: Prevention and Control, 1994.* Atlanta, Georgia: American Cancer Society.

American Cancer Society (1995) *Cancer Facts and Figures – 1995.* Atlanta, Georgia: American Cancer Society.

American Cancer Society (1990) Survey of physicians' attitudes and practices in early cancer detection. *CA* **40:** 77–101.

American Cancer Society (1993) *Mammography: Two Statements of the American Cancer Society.* Atlanta, Georgia: American Cancer Society Professional Education Publication.

American Society of Human Genetics (1994) Statement of the American Society of Human Genetics on genetic testing for breast and ovarian cancer predispoistion. *Am. J. Hum. Genet.* **55:** I–IV.

Anderson DE (1971) Some characteristics of familial breast cancer *Cancer,* **28:** 1500–1504.

■ Bassett LW, Hendrick RE & Bassford TL (1994) *Quality Determinants of Mammography. Clinical Practice Guideline No. 13.* AHCPR Publication No. 95–0632. Rockville, MD: Agency for Health Care Policy and Research, Public Health Service, US Department of Health and Human Services.

■ Benichou J (1993) A computer program for estimating individualized probabilities of breast cancer. *Comput. Biomed Res.* **26:** 373–382.

Bernstein L, Henderson BE, Hanisch R, Sullivan–Halley J & Ross RK (1994) Physical exercise and reduced risk of breast cancer in young women. *J. Natl. Cancer Inst.* **86:** 1403–1408.

Bondy ML, Lustbadder ED, Halabi S *et al.* (1994) Validation of a breast cancer risk-assessment model in women with a positive family history. *J. Natl. Cancer Inst.* **86:** 620–625.

Brown ML, Kessler LG & Rueter FG (1990) Is the supply of mammography machines outstripping need and demand? *Ann. Intern. Med.* **113:** 547-552.

Brownstein MH, Wolf M & Bikowski JB (1978) Cowden's disease: A cutaneous marker of breast cancer. *Cancer* **41:** 2393–2398.

Buckley MM & Goa KL (1989) Tamoxifen. A reappraisal of its pharmacodynamic and pharmacokinetic properties and therapeutic use. *Drugs.* **37:** 451–490.

Bush T & Helzlsouer K (1993) Tamoxifen for the primary prevention of breast cancer: A review and critique of the concept and trial. *Epidemiol. Rev.* **15:** 233–243.

Byrne C, Brinton LA, Haile RW *et al.* (1991) Heterogeneity of the effect of family history on breast cancer risk. *Epidemiology* **2:** 276–284.

Calle EE, Martin LM, Thun MJ *et al.* (1993) Family history, age, and risk of fatal breast cancer. *Am. J. Epidemiol.* **138:** 675–681.

Claus EB, Risch N & Thompson WD (1994) Autosomal dominant inheritance of early-onset breast cancer: Implications for risk prediction. *Cancer* **73:** 643–651.

Claus EB, Risch N & Thompson WD (1991) Genetic analysis of breast cancer in the cancer and steroid hormone study. *Am. J. Hum. Genet.* **48:** 232.

Claus EB, Risch NJ & Thompson WD (1990) Age at onset as an indicator of familial risk of breast cancer. *Am. J. Epidemiol.* **111:** 301–308.

■ Colditz GA, Willett WC, Hunter DJ *et al.* (1993) Family history, age, and risk of breast cancer. *JAMA* **270:** 338–343.

Costa A, Formelli F, Chiesa F *et al.* (1994) Prospects of chemoprevention of human cancers with the synthetic retinoid fenretinide. *Cancer Res.* **54:** 2032s– 2037s.

Danforth DN (1990) Prophylactic mastectomy to prevent cancer of the breast in high-risk patients. In DeVita VT Jr, Hellman S, Rosenberg SA (eds): *Cancer Prevention,* pp. 1–12 (December. Philadelphia, JB Lippincott Co.

Dawson DA & Thompson GB (1990) Breast cancer risk factors and screening; United States, 1987. National Center for Health Statistics. *Vital Health Statistics* 172 (10).

Decensi A, Formelli F, Torrisi R & Costa A (1993) Breast cancer chemoprevention: Studies with 4-HPR alone and in combination with tamoxifen using circulating growth factors as potential surrogate endpoints. *J. Cell Biochem.* **17G:** 226–233.

Devesa SS, Silverman DT, Young JL *et al.* (1987) Cancer incidence and mortality trends among whites in the United States, 1947–84. *J. Natl. Cancer Inst.* **79:** 701–770.

Dupont WD & Page DL (1985) Risk factors for breast cancer in women with proliferative breast disease. *N. Engl. J. Med.* **312:** 146–151.

■ Early Breast Cancer Trialists' Collaborative Group (1992) Systemic treatment of early breast cancer by hormonal, cytotoxic, or immune therapy. *Lancet* **339:** 1–15, 71–84.

Easton DF, Ford D, Bishop DT *et al.* (1995) Breast and ovarian cancer incidence in BRCA1-mutation carriers. *Am. J. Hum. Genet.* **56:** 265–271.

Eldar S, Mequid MM & Beatty JD (1984) Cancer of the breast after prophylactic subcutaneous mastectomy. *Am. J. Surg.* **148:** 692.

Farwell MF, Foster RS & Costanza MC (1993) Breast cancer and earlier detection efforts: realized and unrealized impact on stage. *Arch. Surg.* **128:** 510–514.

Feuer EJ & Wun LM (1992) How much of the recent rise in breast cancer incidence can be explained by increases in mammography utilization? *Am. J. Epidemiol.* **136:** 1423–1436.

Feuer EJ, Wun LM & Boring CC (1992) Probability of developing cancer. In: Miller BA, Gloeckler Ries LA, Hankey BF, Kosary CL & Edwards BK (eds) *Cancer Statistics Review 1973–89,* NIH Pub. No. 92–2789. National Cancer Institute.

■ Fisher B, Constantino J, Redmond C *et al.* (1989) A randomized clinical trial evaluating tamoxifen in the treatment of patients with node-negative breast cancer who have estrogen-receptor-positive tumors. *N. Engl. J. Med.* **320:** 479–484.

Ford D, Easton DF, Bishop DT *et al.* (1994) Risks of cancer in BRCA1-mutation carriers. *Lancet* **343:** 692–695.

Futreal PA, Liu Q, Shattuck–Eidens D *et al.* (1994) BRCA1 mutations in primary breast and ovarian carcinomas. *Science.* **266:** 120–122.

Gail MH & Benichou J (1994) Epidemiology and biostatistics program of the National Cancer Institute. *J. Natl. Cancer Inst.* **86:** 573–575.

Gail MH & Benichou J (1992) Assessing the risk of breast cancer in individuals. In DeVita VJ Jr, Hellman S, Rosenberg SA (eds): *Cancer Prev.* 1–15, Philidelphia, JB Lippincott Company, June.

Goodnight JE, Quagliana JM & Morton DL (1984) Failure of subcutaneous mastectomy to prevent the development of breast cancer. *J. Surg. Oncol.* **26:** 198–201.

Gordon NH, Crowe JP, Brumberg DJ & Berger NA (1992) Socioeconomic factors in race in breast cancer recurrence and survival. *Am. J. Epidemiol.* **135:** 609–618.

Hall JM, Lee MK, Morrow J *et al.* (1990) Linkage analysis of early onset familial breast cancer to chromosome 17q21. *Science* **250:** 1684–1689.

Hankey BF, Brinton LA, Kessler LG & Abrams J. (1993) Breast *1993 Cancer Statistics Review.* NIH Pub. No. 93–2789. Bethesda, Md: National Cancer Institute.

Henderson BE, Ross RK & Pike MC (1993) Hormonal chemoprevention of cancer in women. *Science* **259:** 633–638.

Henderson JC (1992) Biologic variations of tumors. *Cancer* **69** (Supplement): 1888–1895.

Hizawa K, Iida M, Matsumoto T, Kohrogi N *et al.* (1993) Cancer in Peutz–Jeghers syndrome. *Cancer* **72:** 2777–2781.

Holford TR, Roush GC & McKay LA (1991) Trends in female breast cancer in Connecticut and the United States. *J. Clin. Epidemiol.* **44:** 29–39.

Horton JA, Romans MC & Cruess DF (1992) Mammography attitudes and usage study, 1992. *Women's Health Issues* **2:** 180–188.

Hoskins KF, Stopfer JE, Calzone KA *et al.* (1995) Assessment and counseling for women with a family history of breast cancer. *JAMA* **273:** 577–585.

Howard J (1987) Using mammography for cancer control: An unrealized potential. *CA* **37:** 33–48.

Humphrey LJ (1983) Subcutaneous mastectomy is not a prophylaxis against carcinoma of the breast: opinion or knowledge? *Am. J. Surg.* **145:** 311–312.

■ Hurley SF & Kaldor JM (1992) The benefits and risks of mammographic screening for breast cancer. *Epidemiol. Rev.* **14:** 101–130.

Jordan VC & Murphy CS (1990) Endocrine pharmacology of antiestrogens as antitumor agents. *Endocr. Rev.* **11:** 578–610.

■ Jordan VC (1991) Overview from the international conference on long-term tamoxifen therapy for breast cancer. *J. Natl. Cancer Inst.* **84:** 231–234.

Kelloff GJ, Boone CW, Steele VE *et al.* (1993) Development of breast cancer chemopreventive drugs. *J. Cell Biochem.* **17G:** 2–13.

Kelsey JL & Gammon M (1991) The epidemiology of breast cancer. *CA* **41:** 146–165.

Kelsey JL (1993) Breast cancer epidemiology: summary and future directions. *Epidemiol. Rev.* **15:** 256–263.

Kessler LG (1992) The relationship between age and incidence of breast cancer: population and screening program data. *Cancer* (supplement) **69:** 1896—1903.

King MC, Rowell S & Love SM (1993) Inherited breast and ovarian cancer. What are the risks? What are the choices? *JAMA* **269:** 1975–1980.

Li FP, Garber JE, Friend SH *et al.* (1992) Recommendations on predictive testing for germ line p53 mutations among cancer prone individuals. *J. Natl. Cancer Inst.* **84:** 1156–1160.

Liff JM, Sung JFC, Chow WH *et al.* (1991) Does increased detection account for the rising incidence of breast cancer? *Am. J. Pub. Health* **81:** 462–465.

Love RR, Newcomb PA, Wiebe DA *et al.* (1990) Effects of tamoxifen therapy on lipid and lipoprotein levels in postmenopausal patients with node-negative breast cancer. *J. Natl. Cancer Inst.* **82:** 1327–1332.

Love RA (1993) The National Surgical Adjuvant Breast Project (NSABP) Breast Cancer Prevention Trial revisited. *Cancer Epidemiol. Biomarkers Prev.* **2:** 403–407.

Lynch HT, Marcus J, Watson, P & Page D (1994) Distinctive clinicopathologic features of BRCA1-linked hereditary breast cancer. *Proc. ASCO* **13:** 56.

Malkin D, Li FP, Strong LC *et al.* (1990) Germ line p53 mutations in a familial syndrome of breast cancer, sarcomas, and other neoplasms. *Science* **250:** 1233–1238.

Mettlin C, Croghan I, Natarajan N *et al.* (1990) The association of age and familial risk in a case–control study of breast cancer. *Am. J. Epidemiol.* **131:** 973–983.

■ Miki Y, Swensen J, Shattuck–Eidens D *et al.* (1994) A strong candidate for the breast and ovarian cancer susceptibility gene BRCA1. *Science* **266:** 66–71.

Miller BA, Feuer EJ & Hankey BF (1993) Recent incidence trends for breast cancer in women and the relevance of early detection: an update. *CA* **43:** 27—1.

Morrell D, Cromartie E & Swift M (1986) Mortality and cancer incidence in 263 patients with ataxia–telangiectasia. *J. Natl. Cancer Inst.* **77:** 89–92.

Narod SA, Feunteun J, Lynch HT *et al.* (1991) Familial

breast–ovarian cancer locus on chromosome 17q12-23. *Lancet* **338:** 82–83.

Narod SA, Ford D, Devilee P, Barkardottir RB *et al.* (1995) An evaluation of genetic heterogeneity in 145 breast–ovarian cancer families. *Am. J. Human Genet.* **56:** 254–264.

National Advisory Council for Human Genome Research (1994) Statement on use of DNA testing for presymoptomatic identification of cancer risk. *JAMA* **271:** 785.

Nayfield SG, Karp JE, Ford LG *et al.* (1991) Potential role of tamoxifen in prevention of breast cancer *J. Natl. Cancer Inst.* **83:** 1450–1459.

Nelson H, Miller SH, Buck D, Demuth RJ, Fletcher WS & Buehler P (1989) Effectiveness of prophylactic mastectomy in the prevention of breast tumors in C_3H mice. *Plast. Reconstruct. Surg.* **83:** 662–668.

Offit K & Brown K (1994) Quantitating familial cancer risk: A resource for clinical oncologists. *J. Clin. Oncol.* **12:** 1724–1736.

Ottman R, Pike MC, King MC *et al.* (1986) Familial breast cancer in a population-based series. *Am. J. Epidemiol.* **123:** 15–21.

Pennisi VR & Capozzi A (1989) Subcutaneous mastectomy data: a final statistical analysis of 1500 patients. *Aesthetic. Plast. Surg.* **13:** 15–21.

Pike MC & Spicer DV (1993) The chemoprevention of breast cancer by reducing sex steroid exposure: Perspectives from epidemiology. *J. Cell. Biochem.* **17G:** 26–36.

Pressman PI (1988) When we would recommend a prophylactic mastectomy. *Prim. Care Cancer,* **1:** 11.

■ Ries LAG, Miller BA, Hankey BF *et al. Cancer Statistics Review 1973-91: Tables and Graphs.* NIH Pub. No. 94–2789. National Cancer Institute.

Rowell S, Newman B, Boyd J & King MC (1994) Inherited predisposition of breast and ovarian cancer. *Am. J. Hum. Genet.* **55:** 861–865.

Russo J & Russo IH (1994) Toward a physiological approach to breast cancer prevention. *Cancer Epidemiol. Biomarkers Prev.* **3:** 353–364.

Sattin RW, Rubin Gl, Webster LA *et al.* (1985) Family history and the risk of breast cancer. *JAMA* **253:** 1908–1913.

Schwartz AG, King MC, Belle SH *et al.* (1985) Risk of breast cancer to relatives of young breast cancer patients. *J. Natl. Cancer Inst.* **75:** 665–668.

Seidman H, Mushinski MH, Gelb SK & Silverberg E. (1985) Probabilities of eventually developing or dying of cancer—United States, 1985. *CA* **35:** 36-56.

Seidman H, Stellman S & Mushinski MH (1982) A different perspective on breast cancer risk factors: Some implications of the nonattributable risk. *CA* **32:** 301–313.

Shapiro S, Venet W, Strax P & Venet L (1988) *Periodic Screening for Breast Cancer: The Health Insurance Plan Project and its Sequelae, 1963-1986.* Baltimore: Johns Hopkins Press.

Shattuck–Eidens D, McClure M, Simard J *et al.* (1995) A collaborative survey of 80 mutations in the BRCA1 breast and ovarian cancer susceptibility gene. *JAMA* **273:** 535–541.

Slattery ML & Kerby RA (1993) A comprehensive evaluation of family history and breast cancer risk. *JAMA* **270:** 1563–1568.

Smith RA & Haynes S (1992) Barriers to screening for breast cancer. *Cancer* **69** (supplement): 1968–1978.

Snyderman RK (1984) Prophylactic mastectomy: Pros and cons. *Cancer* **53:** 803.

Spencer G (1984) Projections of the population of the United States by age, sex, and race: 1983–2080. *Current Population Reports; Series P–25, no. 952.* Washington, DC: US Department of Commerce, Bureau of the Census, 1984.

Spigelman AD, Murday V & Phillips RKS (1989) Cancer and the Peutz–Jeghers syndrome. *Gut* **30:** 1588–1590.

Stanley K, Stjernsward J & Koroltchouk V (1987) Women and cancer. *World Health Statistics Quarterly* **40:** 267–278.

Starink TM (1984) Cowden's disease: Analysis of fourteen new cases. *J. Am. Acad. Dermatol.* **11:** 1127–1141.

Swift M, Morrell D, Cromartie E *et al.* (1986) The incidence and gene frequency of ataxia–telangiectasia in the United States. *Am. J. Hum. Genet.* **39:** 573–583.

Swift M, Morrell D, Massey RB & Chase CL (1991) Incidence of cancer in 161 families affected by ataxia–telangiectasia. *N. Engl. J. Med.* **325:** 1831–1836.

Tabar L, Fagerberg G, Day NE & Holmberg L (1987) What is the optimum interval between mammographic screening examinations?: An analysis based on the latest results of the Swedish two-county breast cancer screening trial. *Br. J. Cancer* **55:** 547–551.

Temple WJ, Lindsay RL, Magi E & Urbanski SJ (1991) Technical considerations for prophylactic mastectomy in patients at high risk for breast cancer. *Am. J. Surg.* **161:** 413–415.

Trau H, Schewach–Millet M, Fisher BK & Tsur H (1982) Peutz–Jeghers syndrome and bilateral breast carcinoma. *Cancer* **50:** 788–792.

Wells BL & Horm JW (1992) Stage at diagnosis in breast cancer: race and socioeconomic factors. *Am. J. Public Health* **82:** 1383–1385.

White E, Lee CY & Kristal AR (1990) An evaluation of the increase in breast cancer incidence in relation to mammography use. *J. Natl. Cancer Inst.* **82:** 462–465.

Wingo PA, Tong T & Bolden S (1995) Cancer statistics, 1995. *CA. Cancer J. Clin.* **4:** 8–30.

Wong JH, Jackson CF, Swanson JS *et al.* (1986) Analysis of the risk reduction of prophylactic partial mastectomy in Sprague–Dawley rats with 7,12-dimethylbenzanthracene-induced breast cancer. *Surgery* **99:** 67.

Woods JE (1983) Breast reconstruction: current state of the art. *Ann. Plast. Surg.* **145:** 541–550.

Wooster R, Neuhausen SL, Mangion J *et al.* (1994) Localization of a breast cancer susceptibility gene, BRCA2 to chromosome 13q12-13. *Science* **265:** 2088–2090.

Young JL, Perry CL & Asire AJ (1981) *National Cancer Institute Monograph 57, KY72* (NIH Publication No. 81–2330, Bethesda.

Zeigler LD & Kroll SS (1991) Primary breast cancer after prophylactic mastectomy. *Am. J. Clin. Oncol.* **14:** 451–454.

24 Pathology of Breast Cancer

D W Visscher
W D Lawrence

Introduction

The clinical and epidemiologic heterogeneity of breast neoplasia is reflected in a rich variety of histopathology. Until recently, though, homogeneous approaches to diagnosis and treatment of breast cancer limited the relevance of pathologic observations to clinical decision making. Widespread use of screening mammography, conservative surgery and adjuvant therapy have not only focused attention on pathologic features of malignant breast neoplasia, but have also materially altered the spectrum of disease submitted for pathologic examination. Moreover, recent developments in cytometric and molecular genetic technology have introduced novel concepts to the pathologic classification of breast neoplasms. At the present time, therefore, biological and clinical implications of classical histopathologic features in breast neoplasia are being revisited and, in some cases, re-formulated.

Preinvasive Neoplasia

There is near universal agreement that breast cancers evolve from preinvasive tumors (i.e. carcinomas *in situ*), defined histologically as a proliferation of malignant cells within the epithelial compartment or lumen of the duct–lobule system. Analogous processes characterize the adenoma–carcinoma and dysplasia–carcinoma sequences of colorectal and cervical neoplasia, respectively. Mammary carcinoma *in situ* is virtually always accompanied by lesser epithelial proliferations – hyperplasias which lack unequivocal histologic evidence of malignant transformation (Gallagher and Martin, 1969). This suggests that epithelial hyperplasias of the breast, which are currently regarded as a component of fibrocystic change, represent either an initial step or an accompanying process in breast tumorigenesis. The association between severe forms of hyperplasia and the subsequent development of clinical breast malignancy support this contention (London *et al.*, 1992).

Various hallmarks of fibrocystic change, including hyperplasia, are often diffuse and bilateral in patients with breast carcinoma (Gallager and Martin, 1969). This has been interpreted as evidence of a susceptibility to neoplastic transformation involving the mammary epithelium as a whole, or a 'field-effect' alteration. So called field-effect alteration is further implied by the significant frequency of occult preinvasive or invasive carcinomas (40–50%) in breasts contralateral to those with clinically recognized invasive malignancy (Ringberg *et al.*, 1991). Similarly, foci of disease in quadrants remote from incident lesions are observed in about one-third of *in situ* breast cancer cases (Rosen *et al.*, 1979). These findings imply that factors that provoke malignancy in breast epithelial populations are present throughout, or imposed diffusely on, the native tissue. It should be emphasized that, in contrast to hyperplasia, evidence of histologically malignant 'field-effect' alteration is extremely focal, requiring exhaustive sampling, and is generally inapparent on routinely sampled specimens (Smith *et al.*, 1992). Further, the frequency with which such abnormalities become clinically manifest as 'recurrences' or second primaries is considerably lower than their incidence as occult microscopic foci (*vide infra*).

The inherent problems with sequential sampling of breast tissue has done much to obscure the natural history of preinvasive neoplasia. Autopsy studies demonstrate that 6–25% of women in the population at large have microscopic, clinically inapparent, foci of carcinoma *in situ* (Wellings, *et al.*, 1975; Nielsen *et al.*, 1984; Alpers and Wellings, 1985). This high prevalence would suggest that not all preinvasive neoplasias of the breast are destined to become invasive lesions (i.e. within a limited time frame). Studies that report follow-up of patients with preinvasive breast neoplasia after biopsy only support this notion (Betsill *et al.*, 1978; Page *et al.*, 1982). Although such studies are biased by their inclusion of only a narrow histologic spectrum of lesions as well as by partial treatment, neither recurrence nor progression to invasion were inevitable. Those tumors that did recur, moreover, often became clinically evident after five years or more of follow-up.

In situ carcinoma of the breast accounted for only 1–3% of clinically diagnosed breast malignancies before 1988 (Rosner *et al.*, 1980; Simon *et al.*, 1992). Coincident with the widespread use of screening and diagnostic mammography, however, the incidence of preinvasive neoplasia has risen, and now represents up to 25% of breast malignancies diagnosed at some institutions (Graversen *et al.*, 1988; Lagios *et al.*, 1993). Given the considerations noted above, it is not entirely clear that the increasing rate of detection for *in situ* breast neoplasia reflects success exclusively in terms of diagnosing preinvasive breast cancer. It is possible that some of the screen-detected *in situ* carcinomas correspond to the biologically inert, focal lesions noted in the previously cited autopsy studies. Screen-detected invasive carcinomas are, in fact, more likely to be comprised of pathologically indolent subtypes as compared to symptomatic lesions (Anderson *et al.*, 1986). Presently, therefore, the biology of mammographically-detected breast lesions, particularly *in situ* carcinomas, is under close scrutiny.

Pathologic classification of *in situ* breast carcinoma is complex. The most important histologic stratification is based on the micro-anatomic distribution, or the apparent origin, of tumor cells (i.e. ductal carcinoma *in situ* (DCIS), or intraductal carcinoma, versus lobular carcinoma *in situ* (LCIS)). DCIS is then further subclassified by histopathologic features intrinsic to the neoplastic population, including the degree of nuclear anaplasia, architectural differentiation and presence of intraluminal necrosis. Recent authors, moreover, have advocated an additional subclassification of DCIS based on lesional size or histologic extent, which may vary considerably (Andersen *et al.*, 1987; Andersen *et al.*, 1988; Blichert–Toft *et al.*, 1990; Gump *et al.*, 1987). LCIS and DCIS are by no means mutually exclusive entities, and mixed cases are not uncommon. Similarly, invasive breast tumors, especially ductal carcinomas, often contain extensive areas of 'residual' carcinoma *in situ* (Silverberg and Chitale, 1973).

LCIS is a pathologically distinctive lesion characterized by filling and prominent distension of lobular acini by a monotonous population of cells with relatively small, uniform, cytologically-bland nuclei (*Figure 24.1A*). LCIS is non-palpable and mammographically undistinguished. Therefore, diagnosis virtually always represents an incidental histologic finding in breast tissue sampled to investigate a palpated lump or suspicious calcifications caused by an accompanying lesion, usually fibrocystic change (Van Dongen *et al.*, 1989). LCIS represents 20–30% of detected *in situ* neoplasias (Blichert–Toft *et al.*, 1988).

The epidemiologic features and biology of LCIS differ substantially from those of DCIS. First, the mean age at time of diagnosis for LCIS of approximately 50 years is significantly younger than that of DCIS, which is approximately 60 years. This is believed to reflect the differential responsiveness of lobule-based breast epithelium to endogenous hormones (i.e. estrogen). Second, breast carcinoma subsequently develops in only 15–25% of patients with LCIS treated with biopsy only, as opposed to 25–75% of patients with DCIS. Third, breast malignancies that occur in follow-up of LCIS are equally as likely to occur in either breast and may exhibit either ductal or lobular differentiation (*vide infra*) (Ketcham and Moffat, 1990; Rosen *et al.*, 1980). The former phenomenon reflects the near uniform multicentricity/bilaterality of LCIS. Indeed, some data suggest that when LCIS accompanies invasive breast neoplasia it may be a marker for family breast cancer history or for the clinical development of bilateral disease (Davis and Baird, 1984). Recurrences of DCIS, in contrast, usually occur close to the biopsy/excision site (i.e. in cases treated conservatively) and virtually always retain the ductal type of histology (Fisher *et al.*, 1986a). Finally, the interval between the diagnosis of LCIS and clinical recurrence/progression, which averages ten years, is lengthier than that of DCIS, which averages five years.

Pathologists may encounter considerable difficulty in distinguishing LCIS from a histologically similar lesion termed atypical lobular hyperplasia (ALH), which displays less prominent expansion and distortion of lobular acini. In the absence of a positive family history for breast cancer, patients with ALH have a risk of developing a subsequent breast malignancy that is approximately one-half that of LCIS (Page *et al.*, 1985). ALH and LCIS, therefore, may represent biologically similar processes that differ in degree, severity or level of development.

In contrast to the morphologic uniformity of LCIS, DCIS exhibits a more heterogeneous pathologic appearance (Schnitt *et al.*, 1988; Swain, 1992). Whereas LCIS is confined to the terminal duct lobular unit, DCIS may involve any segment of the duct–lobular system, including the nipple (i.e. Paget's disease). Nuclear cytologic features are highly variable, but abnormalities are generally more pronounced than in LCIS (*Figure 24.1B*). In some cases of DCIS, neoplastic cells form arborizing epithelial patterns (the so-called papillary and micropapillary types) or confluent glandular/bridging arrangements (the so-called cribriform type). Generally, these architecturally complicated variants of DCIS display relatively monotonous nuclei without dramatic enlargement. In other words, they are cytologically 'low grade' (*Figure 24.1C*). Micropapillary and cribriform types of DCIS may, on occasion, be difficult to distinguish from florid hyperplasias. One uncommon DCIS variant – clinging type – is difficult to recognize due to its cytologically low-grade features and its inconspicuous pattern of growth along the periphery of involved ducts. Cytologically low-grade forms of DCIS are generally accompanied by focal to numerous luminal microcalcifications, which are often apparent on mammographic images (Patchefsky *et al.*, 1989).

DCIS may also be characterized by intraluminal epithelial proliferation without papillary or gland-like arrangements (i.e. solid type). These cases typically exhibit conspicuously enlarged, pleomorphic nuclei, often with prominent nucleoli. In addition to microcalcifications, many of these

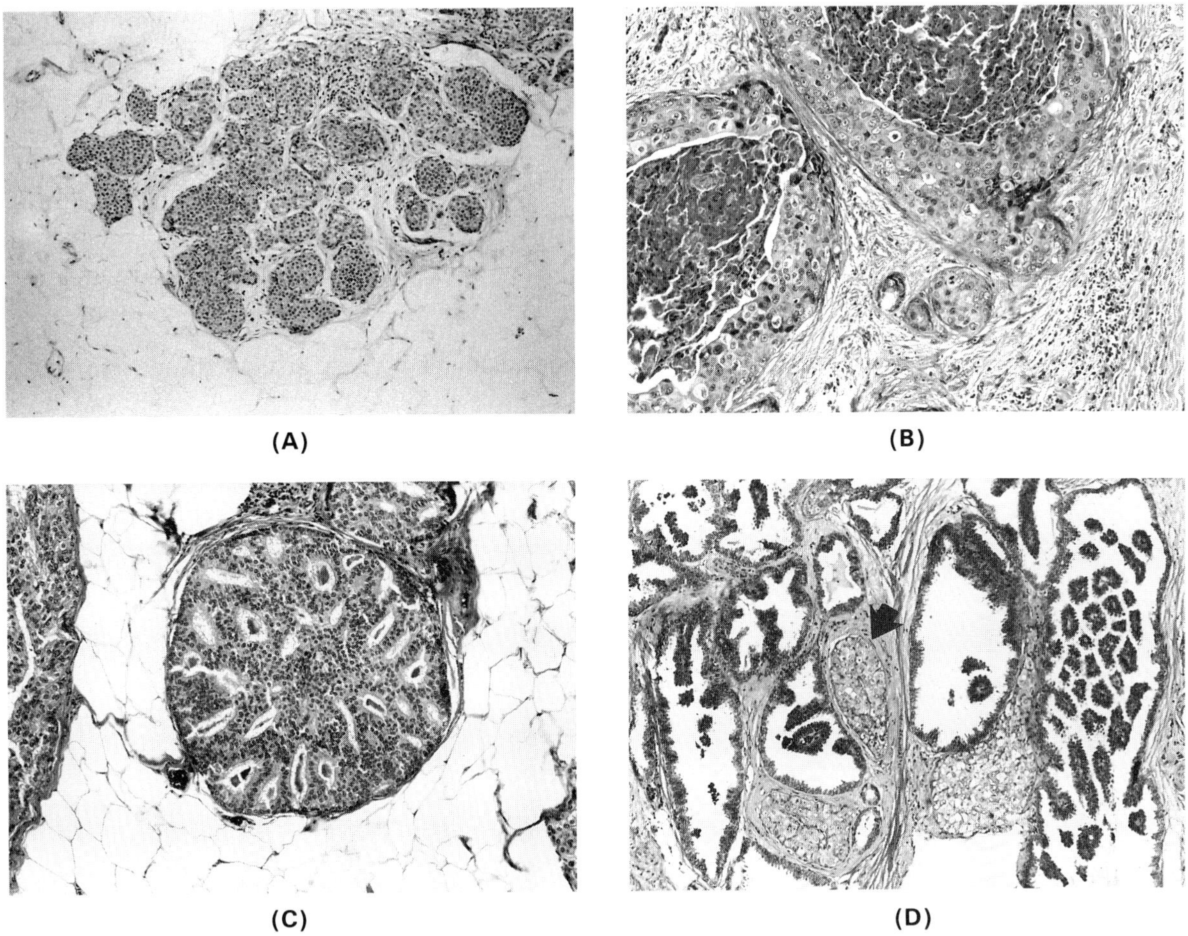

Figure 24.1. Carcinoma *in situ.* (**A**). Lobular carcinoma *in situ*, showing filling and expansion of acini by uniform cells with mild nuclear enlargement and pleomorphism. (**B**). Duct carcinoma *in situ*, high grade with solid growth, enlarged nuclei, prominent nucleoli and intraluminal necrosis. Note periductal fibrous and inflammatory host reaction. (**C**). Duct carcinoma *in situ*, low grade with smaller more monotonous nuclei and gland-like (cribriform) architectural differentiation. (**D**). Duct carcinoma *in situ* with mixed patterns. The predominant component is low grade (micropapillary). Focally, however, a solid high-grade pattern is apparent (arrow).

cytologically 'high-grade' preinvasive carcinomas display intraluminal necrosis, or so-called 'comedo' necrosis (see *Figure 24.1B*). Unlike most low-grade examples of DCIS, they are also accompanied by periductal fibrosis, edema and inflammation, which are components of a host stromal reaction. The host reaction, along with their generally greater extent, accounts for the greater likelihood for high-grade DCIS to present with a palpable mass.

There is a degree of morphologic overlap between pathologic subtypes of DCIS. Mixtures of various architectural patterns or cytologic grades are common (Fisher *et al.*, 1986b) (*Figure 24.1D*). At the present time there are no uniform, widely adopted criteria for the pathologic classification of these problematic examples and pathologists generally issue a descriptive report that catalog the various DCIS subtypes observed.

There are important clinical differences between low-grade and high-grade forms of DCIS. First, high-grade forms of DCIS (i.e. comedocarcinoma) display residual *in situ* and/or invasive neoplasm upon surgical re-excision significantly more often than low-grade cases (Fentiman *et al.*, 1986). At least one group of workers, moreover, has demonstrated that local recurrence of DCIS following partial mastectomy is significantly correlated with nuclear grade (Lagios *et al.*, 1989). Finally, although *in situ* neoplastic disease extent can be difficult to define objectively, it is generally believed that small (<25 mm) or microfocal lesions are less aggressive than larger diffuse or tumor-forming ones (Lagios, 1982; Andersen *et al.*, 1988).

In some examples of DCIS, pathologists are able to recognize microscopic invasion of host stroma by malignant cells. Such cases are often referred to as microinvasive carcinoma since the extent of invasion is superficial and minimal, and deemed insufficient to constitute a mass. Because host invasion implies a potential for metastasis there is at least a theoretical importance in distinguishing microinvasive from *in situ* carcinomas. Data that address the significance of microinvasive carcinoma as a diagnostic or clinical entity are limited. Axillary node metastasis in pathologically microinvasive DCIS is reported in 0–20% of cases, which is similar to the incidence of nodal metastasis in frankly invasive lesions less than 1 cm in diameter (Schuh *et al.*, 1986; Kinne *et al.*, 1989; Wong *et al.*, 1990).

Most experts agree that the term microinvasion is appropriate when applied to cases in which infiltrating neoplasm is unequivocally present in periodical or perilobular stroma yet the process is only discernible at a microscopic level. Such lesions should be accompanied by an approximate linear measurement (i.e. '0.5–1 mm in extent') in the diagnosis and are considered to have a low, yet measurable, potential for axillary metastasis. Cases in which there is blurring or irregularity of the duct-stroma interface or possible extension into stromal tissue have been called microinvasive by some pathologists; however, the clinical significance of this finding is unproven and probably insignificant. Therefore, the use of the term microinvasive in such cases is eschewed.

Invasive Carcinoma

The outcome of invasive breast neoplasia is exquisitely dependent on the extent of disease-spread or Stage. A survey of numerous population-based studies that employed multivariate statistical analysis revealed that the status of axillary lymph nodes is the most powerful prognostic factor, followed by tumor diameter (Visscher *et al.*, 1990). The relevance of regional lymph node involvement to poor outcome suggests that systemic colonization, presumably undetectable at the time of the initial clinical evaluation, is more likely when regional node metastasis is demonstrated. It should be noted, however, that regional lymphatic metastasis is neither a prescribed step, nor an obligate event, in the acquisition of the phenotypic traits that are necessary for hematogenous (systemic) metastasis (Koscielny *et al.*, 1988). Up to one-third of patients with 'node-negative' breast cancer, after all, will suffer distant relapse. The biology of regional lymph node metastasis is therefore not entirely analogous to that of osseous, cutaneous or visceral metastasis.

Although breast cancer patients are stratified clinically as 'node-positive' or 'node-negative' groups, there are several prognostically important pathologic subcategories of axillary involvement. First, prognosis worsens incrementally with increasing numbers of involved nodes. Outcome in patients with a single positive axillary node is, as a group, only marginally worse than otherwise similar node-negative patients. Workers have demonstrated that surgical 'levels' of the axillary lymph nodes become progressively involved in a more or less consecutive, or progressive, fashion. Therefore, although metastasis to 'high' axillary nodes is prognostically ominous, the poor outcome of such cases has been ascribed more to the overall number of involved nodes rather than to the location *per se* (Veronesi *et al.*, 1987).

The issue of whether a sufficient number of lymph nodes are examined to assure accurate staging is occasionally a problem in clinical settings. Kiricuta *et al.* (1994) have shown that in order to achieve a 90% certainty that the axillary nodes are negative, at least ten level I nodes must be examined. Several authors have reported that histologic serial sectioning (or special staining) of axillary nodes reveals occult micrometastases in 12–30% of node-negative patients (Rosen *et al.*, 1982; Elson *et al.*, 1993; Hainsworth *et al.*, 1993). Until recently, this finding was thought to have no clinical significance. Adverse prognostic relevance has now been suggested in larger series with longer follow-up intervals (Neville *et al.*, 1992; Hainsworth *et al.*, 1993). Occult deposits of neoplastic cells are not limited to regional lymph nodes. Bone marrow micrometastases have also been demonstrated in significant numbers (24%) of node-negative breast cancer patients (Redding *et al.*, 1983).

Neoplastic cells may also invade through the lymph node capsule into surrounding fatty connective tissue. This phenomenon has been shown to be associated with a higher frequency of disease recurrence (i.e. as compared to those cases having similar numbers of involved nodes without extracapsular spread) (Donegan *et al.*, 1993).

Taken together, these observations strongly suggest that there are clinically distinct subsets of node-positive breast carcinoma corresponding to nodal tumor burden. It is noteworthy, in this respect, that approximately one-third of node-positive breast cancer patients remain disease free indefinitely.

In contrast to nodal involvement, which is a reflection, albeit imperfect, of systematic colonization metastatic phenotype, tumor size is a more or less direct reflection of the number of cell doublings through which the neoplasm has passed. Stated another way, tumor volume is an indication of 'tumor age,' or the number of 'generations' that have evolved from the progenitor cell. It is enlightening to briefly analyze breast carcinoma in the context of tumor cell doublings. Empirical data indicate that in order to reach a size of 1 cm a neoplasm must undergo approximately 30 volume doublings and that 40 volume doublings would generate a 1 kg and therefore lethal tumor burden (Gullino, 1977). If it is assumed that the growth rate of a given neoplasm remains constant, these figures imply that at least one-half of the natural history of breast cancer (even screen-detected cases) is pre-clinical. Further, by comparing the sizes of primary and corresponding metastatic lesions, it has been extrapolated that the plenotypic factors responsible for the initiation of metastasis for most breast cancers probably emerge between the tenth and fifteenth volume doubling (i.e. during the pre-clinical phase). Accordingly, larger tumors are more likely to be associated with detectable metastases. Given these considerations it is hardly surprising that larger tumors are significantly more likely to be associated with axillary node metastases and that they usually recur after shorter intervals of follow-up than smaller tumors (Visscher *et al.*, 1990). It must be emphasized, however, that tumor size has prognostic relevance independent of its association with axillary node involvement, further demonstrating the biologic dichotomy between regional node and systemic metastasis noted earlier.

Although size is a good indication of tumor 'age' in terms of cell doublings it is not an accurate reflection of chronologic 'age' in terms of time, since there is considerable variation in growth rate among breast carcinomas. Empirically measured volume doubling times of breast malignancies range from 10–250 days. This explains the well-documented heterogeneous post-relapse course of breast neoplasia. In younger age groups (<50 years) volume doubling times are on average 2–3 times shorter than those of tumors in older patients (>70 years) (Peer *et al.*, 1993). Many recent investigators have developed technologically sophisticated means of assessing proliferation, and thereby, growth rate, in breast carcinoma. These include radiolabelled thymidine or bromodeoxyuridine uptake, flow cytometric DNA analysis, and immunohistologic detection of prolifcration-associated nuclear proteins. To a large extent, however, tumor cell proliferation is an inherent component of tumor differentiation, or morphologic 'grade.'

Numerous large studies have unequivocally demonstrated that tumor grade is a prognostic factor in breast carcinoma independent of tumor size and node status (Freedman *et al.*, 1979; Fisher *et al.*, 1984; Davis *et al.*, 1986; Contesso *et al.*, 1987). Depending on individual series, the difference in overall survival between well-differentiated and poorly-differentiated neoplasms within similarly staged patient cohorts ranges in the order of 30–60%. Further, poorly-differentiated tumors are not only more likely to have nodal metastases than well-differentiated tumors of similar size, but they typically recur earlier than well-differentiated tumors, compatible with a more rapid growth rate. Approximately two-thirds of recurrences in well-differentiated tumors occur after five years of follow-up. Most recurrences of poorly differentiated neoplasms, in contrast, become manifest within five years (Bloom and Richardson, 1957). Therefore, histologic differentiation reflects both metastatic phenotype and growth rate.

The biologically complex nature of tumor grade in breast carcinoma is apparent from the diversity of observations incorporated into its determination

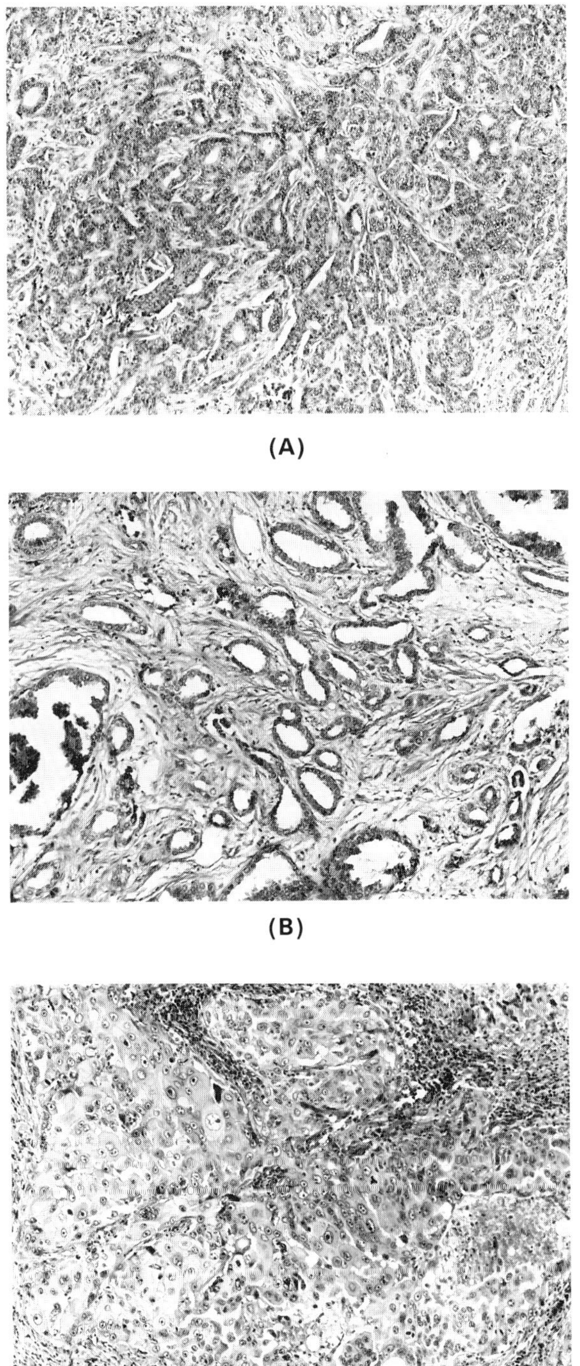

(A)

(B)

(C)

Figure 24.2. Differentiation in invasive breast carcinoma. (**A**). Moderately-differentiated ductal carcinoma with focal tubule formation and significant, but not marked, nuclear enlargement and pleomorphism. (**B**). Well-differentiated ductal carcinoma. All of the neoplastic elements form tubules and nuclei are uniformly small. This area is reminiscent of a favorable prognosis breast carcinoma subset (tubular carcinoma). (**C**). Poorly-differentiated ductal carcinoma with lack of appreciable glandular differentiation and bizarre pleomorphic nuclei.

(*Figure 24.2A–C*). Presently, most pathologists use the system of grading introduced by Scarff, and later systematically examined by Bloom and Richardson, in which nuclear enlargement/pleomorphism, mitotic activity and architectural features (i.e. formation of tubules) are each semiquantitated on a scale of 1 to 3 and then summated to provide a numerical score (Bloom and Richardson, 1957). A number of investigations have addressed the relative significance of each histologic component. In our opinion, the consensus of the published literature is that mitotic activity (i.e. proliferative fraction) is the most important variable (Baak *et al.*, 1985; Clayton, 1991). It should therefore come as no surprise that virtually any measure of tumor cell proliferative fraction is highly relevant to breast cancer outcome (Visscher *et al.*, 1990). Despite the biologically critical nature of proliferation, the other two components of the Scarff/Bloom/Richardson (SBR) score have also been shown to convey prognostically independent data (Fisher *et al.*, 1980). Clearly, however, the manner in which nuclear, architectural and proliferation-related features are combined into equally weighted parameters is somewhat artificial (Parl and Dupont, 1982; Rank *et al.*, 1987).

Despite its unquestionable prognostic relevance, histologic grading of breast carcinomas has not achieved the widespread clinical importance accorded to similar assessments in analogous tumor systems, such as prostatic or endometrial neoplasia. In part, this relates to the traditionally homogeneous nature of breast cancer management. Note, however, that one important parameter in determining therapy for breast cancer patients, viz. the presence of estrogen receptor protein, is exquisitely grade-related and in many ways represents a surrogate differentiation marker (Chabon *et al.*, 1982; Blanco *et al.*, 1990). A third factor that has limited the clinical value of morphologic differentiation is the inconsistency of breast tumor grading by pathologists, a problem which probably accounts, at least in part, for the poor reproducibility of breast cancer grading so frequently documented in the published literature (Stenkvist *et al.*, 1983; Theissig *et al.*, 1990).

Several conventional histopathologic parameters, in addition to grade/differentiation, have been reported to predict the clinical outcome of ordinary infiltrating carcinomas of the breast. Most frequently cited among these are: the presence/extent of tumor necrosis; the degree of peritumoral mononuclear inflammatory infiltrate; the character of the tumor–host interface (i.e. circumscribed versus infiltrative); and vascular invasion by tumor cells. With the possible exception of vascular invasion, reported correlations among these parameters and breast cancer survival have been less consistent than tumor differentiation. Furthermore, studies that systematically address their value with multivariate statistical analysis are limited in number; this is an important problem since these parameters are either strongly grade-associated or are present in relatively small subsets of breast carcinomas, thereby limiting their clinical use.

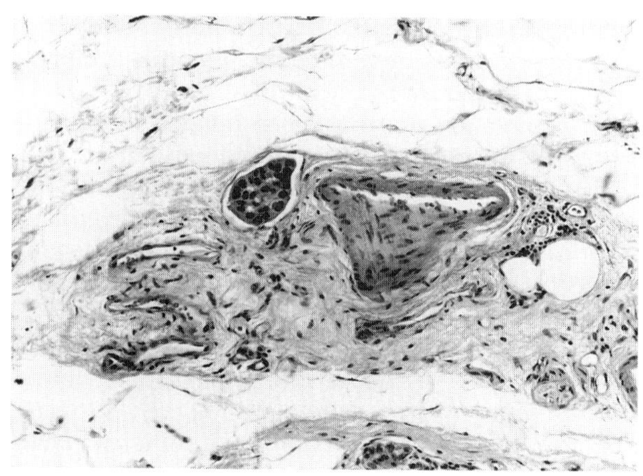

Figure 24.3. Angiolymphatic invasion. An embolus of malignant epithelial cells is present within the lumen of an endothelium-lined space.

Pathologists generally assess breast carcinomas for the presence of vascular (angiolymphatic) tumor cell emboli (*Figure 24.3*). Although this feature is correlated with both high grade and advanced stage, several authors have shown that tumors with vascular invasion recur 4–10 × more frequently than similarly staged cases without vascular invasion (Roses *et al.*, 1982; Bauer *et al.*, 1983). Particularly noteworthy is the adverse predictive significance of vascular emboli in node-negative patients with small (i.e. <2 cm) tumors (Rosen, 1983). Relatively stringent criteria were applied to the diagnosis of vascular permeation in the aforementioned studies, thereby avoiding confusion of intravascular tumor cell emboli with retraction artefacts associated with tissue processing. In our opinion, therefore, the finding of carefully assessed angiolymphatic space invasion is a reproducible marker of aggressive behavior in early stage breast cancer, a group in which prognostic biomarkers would be of considerable value. The problem with using vascular invasion as a prognostic factor is that only a limited number of node-negative tumors (10–20%) display clearcut angioinvasion in tissue sections.

Approximately one-quarter of invasive breast carcinomas belong to well-described, but uncommon or rare, histopathologic categories (Fisher *et al.*, 1975). Apart from their distinctive microscopic appearances, most of these breast cancer variants are characterized by epidemiologic, clinical, or prognostic features that differ from those of infiltrating ductal carcinoma, NOS (not otherwise specified). These characteristic features apply only to specialized breast carcinomas when present in pure form (in contrast to those admixed with ordinary infiltrating ductal carcinoma, as frequently occurs). Although we refer the reader to pathology texts for more detailed discussions of breast carcinoma subtypes, there are several categories which are worthy of specific mention.

Lobular Carcinoma

As its name implies, this subtype is usually accompanied by LCIS. In classic form, lobular carcinomas are comprised of small monotonous cells disposed individually or in single file without tubule formation (*Figure 24.4A & B*). Recently however, both large cell 'pleomorphic' and gland-like 'alveolar' variants have been described (Weidner and Semple, 1992). Lobular carcinoma is also characterized by a multifocal growth pattern in which areas of neoplasm are separated by residual benign tissue. For this reason, they often do not form discrete masses and their size may be underestimated by clinical or gross examination. Apart from their histologic appearance, lobular carcinomas differ from ductal carcinomas in their pattern of systemic metastasis, with significantly more frequent spread to meninges and abdominal viscera than ductal neoplasms (Harris *et al.*, 1984). They are also more frequently associated with a positive family history of breast cancer (Claus *et al.*, 1993). Although it is generally agreed that lobular carcinoma is more often multicentric and bilateral than ductal carcinoma (Simkouich, 1993), these features do not necessarily preclude conservative treatment of limited stage cases (Schnitt *et al.*, 1989; Poen *et al.*, 1992). The outcome of classic lobular carcinoma in terms of overall survival is similar to that of ductal carcinoma of equivalent stage. Disease-free interval, however, is typically lengthier, reflecting their generally lower proliferative fraction (Dicostanzo *et al.*, 1990; Ellis *et al.*, 1992). As implied by the recent description of higher grade variants, however, lobular carcinoma is not a homogeneous entity and its spectrum of clinical aggressiveness is considerable.

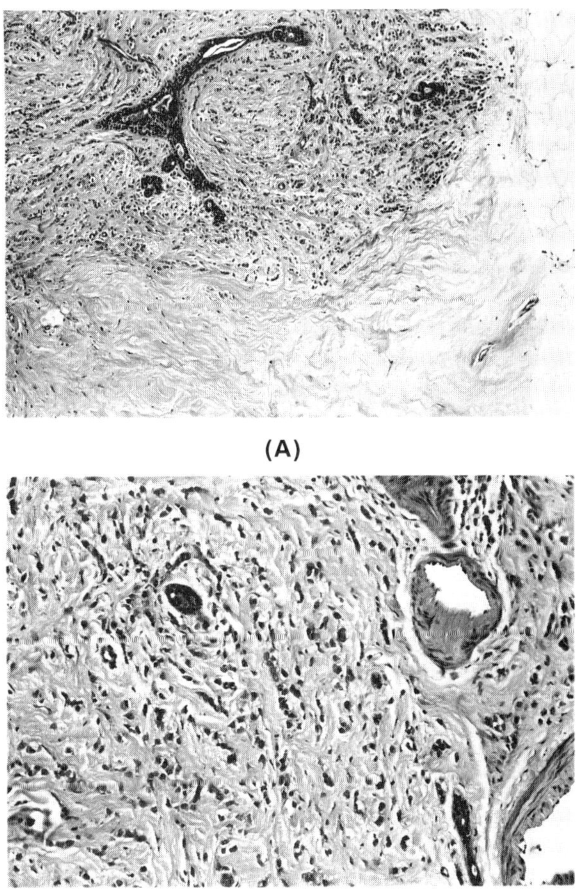

(A)

(B)

Figure 24.4. Lobular carcinoma. **A**. Neoplastic cells disposed individually and in single file permeate periductal/perilobular stroma. **B**. At higher magnification it can be appreciated that the neoplastic cells of this 'classical' lobular carcinoma are relatively small and monotonous. Note the absence of tubule formation.

Medullary Carcinoma

This uncommon, but not rare, neoplasm is characterized by the following constellation of histologic features:

- sheet-like or syncytial masses of cytologically high-grade cells without tubule formation;
- abundant, intimately-admixed mononuclear inflammatory infiltrates without stromal fibrosis;
- sharply demarcated, rounded interface with surrounding host tissue.

By virtue of their lack of stromal fibrosis, they typically have a fleshy nodular gross appearance, in contrast to the gritty stellate cut surface of most ordinary infiltrating ductal carcinomas.

Medullary breast carcinomas occur in a younger age group than other histologic types of breast carcinoma and they are usually estrogen receptor-negative (Stalsberg and Thomas, 1993). Despite their poorly differentiated histologic appearance, early studies suggested that these tumors had a more favorable prognosis than ordinary infiltrating ductal carcinoma (Ridolfi *et al.*, 1977). The early literature also emphasized the importance of distinguishing medullary carcinomas from histologically similar, but less well-circumscribed variants termed atypical medullary carcinomas, which were purported to behave in a manner similar to poorly-differentiated ductal carcinomas. Current authors dispute both the reproducibility of distinguishing 'typical' from 'atypical' medullary carcinoma as well as the putatively more favorable prognosis of the former (Neville *et al.*, 1992; Ellis *et al.*, 1992; Rigaud *et al.*, 1993). At the present time, therefore, the clinical relevance of tumors with 'medullary' histology is unclear.

Tubular and Mucinous Carcinoma

Both of these breast carcinoma variants are composed of slowly-proliferating cells with small uniform (i.e. low-grade) nuclear cytologic features, and when present in a pure form have a very favorable prognosis. They frequently occur as a component of ductal carcinoma NOS and under these circumstances the outcome reflects ductal phenotype (Parl and Richardson, 1983; Carstens *et al.*, 1985; Rasmussen *et al.*, 1987).

The term 'mucinous carcinoma' is applied to cases in which clumps of neoplastic cells appear to 'float' within pools of extracellular mucin. They are generally well-circumscribed, expansile lesions. Axillary metastasis of mucinous carcinoma occurs rarely; however, the prognosis has been shown to correlate with both maximal tumor diameter and the histologic degree of cellularity. Recurrences typically develop late. The median survival of fatal cases is over ten years (Clayton, 1986).

Tubular carcinomas are neoplasms in which more than 75% of the tumor cells form round gland-like structures with a single central lumen histologically. Most are less than 2 cm in diameter (McDivitt *et al.*, 1982). Their stroma is generally dense and fibrous. This neoplasm, like lobular carcinoma, is also associated with multicentricity and a family breast cancer history (Lagios *et al.*, 1980). Recurrences develop in approximately 10–20% of tubular carcinomas, generally after five years of follow-up.

There are two other favorable invasive breast carcinoma variants – papillary and cibriform. Each of these accounts for less than 2% of breast cancers.

Inflammatory Carcinoma

This term is applied to cases in which extensive angiolymphatic permeation by tumor cells results in an erythematous, diffusely indurated breast. As such, it is a clinical term. Generally, but not always, there is prominent tumor cell embolization within dermal angiolymphatic spaces, although the process may be limited to breast tissue *per se*. The underlying neoplasm is typically a poorly-differentiated infiltrating ductal carcinoma that is often larger than clinical examination suggests. Patients with inflammatory carcinoma are considered advanced stage and have a poor prognosis. It should be emphasized that the correlation between the 'inflammatory' clinical presentation and the extent of vascular tumor cell emboli is imperfect; the reason(s) for such a clinicopathologic discrepancy is unclear.

Pathologic Features in Relation to Conservative Therapy

A recurring theme in the recent breast cancer literature is the extent and pattern of disease spread, particularly as it relates to the adequacy of local surgical resection. In many cases of DCIS or invasive carcinoma, areas involved by neoplasm appear to be separated by variable amounts of benign tissue. This phenomenon is referred to as multifocality. It is to be distinguished from multicentricity, which is defined by most authors as non-contiguous involvement of multiple quadrants. The phenomena of multifocality and multicentricity imply that an independent origin of physically separated tumors along the lines of the 'field effect' alteration as previously discussed, is a feature of breast neoplasia subsets. Clearly, the significant incidence of occult contra-lateral neoplasia noted earlier would support the notion that breast neoplasis is in many ways a diffuse disease. On the other hand, authors who have performed careful three-dimensional reconstruction of apparently multicentric DCIS foci were able to demonstrate continuity between lesions in most cases (Holland *et al.*, 1985). In routine histologic sections these interconnections would have been obscured by the architectural tortuosity of the ductal system. It has been the authors' experience that virtually any neoplasm of the breast more extensive than a single microscopic focus is characterized by a degree of multifocal growth. The term multifocality, therefore, is seemingly relevant only in a descriptive sense.

'True' multicentricity, in contrast, has substantial theoretical and practical implications insofar as conservative surgical treatment of breast cancer is concerned. In essence, the presence of multicentric, or discontinuous, multiquadrant growth, implies that residual disease may remain in breast tissue following lumpectomy, even in cases with negative resection margins. To confound the issue, there is extreme variability in the reported frequency of multicentricity in breast neoplasia; in addition to confusion with multifocality, the latter reflects divergent pathologic criteria or methods used to define multicentricity. Most experts agree that 30–60% of DCIS cases (and virtually all cases of LCIS) are multicentric (Carter, 1986; Posner and Wolmark, 1992). A similar frequency is reported for invasive breast neoplasia.

An accumulating body of clinical data, however, would seem to downplay the actual clinical relevance of disease multicentricity in conservative therapy of breast cancer. First, Lagios *et al.* (1982) have reported that DCIS cases larger than 25 mm exhibited multicentricity in 54% and occult invasion in 46%, versus only 14% and 0% respectively for tumors less than 25 mm in extent. A similar association between size and multicentric growth has been observed with invasive carcinoma (Anastassiades *et al.*, 1993). These data seem to suggest geographic multicentricity is highly associated with, and perhaps reflects, heavy tumor burden (as opposed to an independent origin of separate tumors). Second, the pattern of parenchymal disease recurrence (for *in situ* or invasive disease) after conservative treatment, which is generally in the proximity of the surgical site, is additional evidence favoring the biologic and clinical importance of incident (versus occult multicentric) lesions (Fisher *et al.*, 1986). Evidence of 'field cancerization' appears unequivocal on the basis of observed bilaterality and multicentricity. However, it nevertheless appears that the clinically apparent neoplasm represents the biologically aggressive, and thereby most relevant, lesion. This conclusion is supported by the limited incidence (5–10%) of clinically bilateral breast neoplasia in the face of frequent, albeit focal, bilateral malignant alterations observed pathologically (Gallagher *et al.*, 1989; Webber *et al.*, 1981).

The issue of multicentric/multifocal growth is an important factor in pathologic assessment of biopsy or lumpectomy specimen margins. Although adequacy of excision materially impacts therapeutic decisions, pathologists differ in their approach and criteria for evaluation of resection margins. Indeed, it should be stated that fully documenting the histologic status of margins in breast specimens is not a trivial undertaking. In practice, a negative margin is largely defined by gross inspection. This factor, in addition to true multicentricity may help explain the frequent presence of residual disease (approximately 60%) in mastectomy specimens following biopsy of DCIS (Fentimen *et al.*, 1986). Even in biopsy/lumpectomy samples with pathologically negative margins, the frequency of residual disease approaches 30% (Frazier *et al.*, 1989). Studies have also correlated the extent of resection (or width of normal tissue) with the presence of residual disease in subsequent mastectomy specimens (Kinne, 1991). It is sobering to note that histologic examination is presently the only effective means of assessing the completeness of surgical resection, since mammographic images significantly underestimate disease extent in up to 35% of DCIS cases (Holland *et al.*, 1990).

The status of resection margins is often an issue in the clinical management of patients who are eligible for limited surgery. Virtually all of the accumulated outcome data on conservative treatment is based on gross excision of the mass with a variably-sized rim of 'normal' breast tissue. In most series the histologic status of surgical margins is either not considered or margins are not microscopically examined in a uniform standardized fashion. Despite this ambiguity, there is, nonetheless, evidence to suggest that adequacy of excision is a factor in breast cancer recurrence. As already noted, for example, most recurrences occur at or near the biopsy site. Indeed, two studies which addressed the issue (Schnitt *et al.*, 1985; Kurtz *et al.*, 1990) reported that tumors that were 'incompletely' excised recurred significantly more frequently than 'completely' excised tumors.

In general, pathologic features known to predict systemic relapse in patients treated with mastectomy – tumor size, grade, vascular invasion – are also useful in cases treated with less aggressive surgery (i.e. lumpectomy, wide excision, quadrantectomy) (Rosen *et al.*, 1986; Lash *et al.*, 1986). Unlike mastectomy patients, however, breast-conserving therapeutic interventions must address the subsequent detection and management of new lumps in the remaining parenchymal tissue. We employ the generic term 'lump' because not all suspicious masses that appear following conservative therapy are malignant. A significant number represent tissue induration attributable to fat necrosis (Chaudary *et al.*, 1988). This benign pathologic condition, which is presumably caused by therapy-related trauma, results in a mass due to prominent collections of fat-laden histiocytes with concomitant fibrosis.

Not all breast recurrences, moreover, present with a lump. Up to one-quarter are non-palpable and mammographically detected (Fowble *et al.*, 1990). It is also important not to confuse 'local' (i.e. parenchymal) recurrences in residual breast tissue with 'local' (i.e. skin/chest wall) recurrences in mastectomy patients. The latter are generally considered to be a harbinger of systemic dissemination. Parenchymal recurrence, in contrast, does not have the same implications and can generally be managed effectively without impairing overall survival (Calle *et al.*, 1986). Breast recurrences develop in approximately 10% of patients treated with conservative surgery and radiation therapy (Pierce and Harris, 1991). Interestingly, skin and chest wall recurrences occur earlier, within two years of mastectomy, than parenchymal recurrences, which usually develop after two years of follow-up (Kennedy and Abeloff, 1993).

One histologic feature that may predict parenchymal recurrence of breast carcinoma is the so-called extent of intraductal carcinoma. At least two independent groups have reported that breast recurrence is 2–4 times more likely if the estimated proportion of intraductal carcinoma exceeds 25% of the neoplasm (Harris *et al.*, 1984; Jacquemier *et al.*, 1990). The explanation for this association is not intuitively obvious. Schnitt *et al.* (1987) however, have shown that residual neoplasm in cases where mastectomy or re-excision was performed after gross excision of the tumor, was significantly more frequent and more widespread among tumors with extensive intraductal carcinoma. Of particular note in this study was the finding that the extent of intraductal carcinoma may be a better predictor of residual neoplasm near the biopsy site than histologically-negative resection margins.

Summary of Core Information

- Most breast biopsy specimens (60–80%) obtained to evaluate suspicious lumps or mammographic abnormalities represent fibrocystic changes or fibroadenoma.
- Fibrocystic lesions are a heterogeneous group of histologic abnormalities that are classified by degree of epithelial hyperplasia. Risk for breast malignancy in patients with proliferative fibrocystic changes is 2–10 times greater than the overall population, depending on the severity of hyperplasia.
- Invasive breast carcinomas arise from preinvasive neoplasms (carcinomas *in situ*), which are hypothesized to evolve from (preneoplastic) epithelial hyperplasias.
- Preinvasive breast neoplasia currently represents 10–25% of newly diagnosed breast malignancies, and is generally established through biopsy of calcifications detected in screening mammograms.
- The two major preinvasive lesions of the breast are ductal carcinoma *in situ* (DCIS, 70–85% of total) and lobular carcinoma *in situ* (LCIS, 15–30% of total).
- LCIS is usually nonpalpable, mammographically undistinguished, and often an incidental finding to a benign breast lesion. It is multicentric and bilateral.
- A subset (10–25%) of patients with LCIS develop breast malignancy; however, this often occurs after a protracted follow-up interval (mean of ten years) and frequently in the breast contralateral to the one with established LCIS (50%).
- High-grade DCIS (sometimes referred to as comedocarcinomas) and lesions larger than 25 mm in extent are more often associated with occult invasion and/or recurrences following conservative therapy.
- The clinical behavior of invasive breast carcinoma is deendent on both the extent (stage) and the intrinsic aggressiveness (grade) of the neoplasm.
- The status of axillary lymph nodes is the most useful prognostic parameter in invasive breast carcinoma.
- Up to one-third of axillary node-negative patients will experience distant metastases. Node-positive patients are a heterogeneous subset and up to one-quarter will remain disease free indefinitely.
- Intrinsic aggressiveness or grade of breast carcinomas is largely a reflection of the proliferative rate of neoplastic cells, although histologic evidence of angioinvasion is also significantly correlated with adverse outcome.
- There are a variety of histologic breast carcinoma subtypes, some of which (mucinous, tubular, cribriform) are characterized by indolent clinical behavior.
- Pathologic status of resection margins correlate with parenchymal recurrence in patients managed with breast conservation therapy. Parenchymal recurrences characteristically develop in or near the site of previous excision and do not necessarily portend an adverse outcome.
- A significant proportion of invasive breast carcinomas relapse in the ipsilateral skin and chest wall tissues. This is generally a harbinger of systemic disease dissemination.

Dedication

This chapter is dedicated to Lynda Lawrence Kemp (1950–1987), a victim of breast cancer.

References

Alpers CE & Wellings SR (1985) The prevalence of carcinoma *in situ* in normal and cancer-associated breasts. *Hum. Pathol.* **16:** 796–807.

Anastassiades O, Lakovou E, Stavridou N, Gogas J & Karameris A (1993) Multicentricity in breast cancer. A study of 366 cases. *Am. J. Clin. Pathol.* **99:** 238–243.

Andersen J, Blichert-Toft M & Dyreborg U (1987) *In situ* carcinoma of the breast. Types, growth pattern, diagnosis, and treatment. *Eur. J. Surg. Oncol.* **13:** 105–111.

■ Andersen JA, Nielsen M & Blichert-Toft M (1988) The growth pattern of *in situ* carcinoma in the female breast. *Acta Oncol.* **27:** 739–743.

Anderson TJ, Alexander F, Chetty U *et al.* (1986) Comparative pathology of prevalent and incident cancers detected by breast screening. *Lancet* **i:** 519–522.

Baak JPA, Van Dop H, Kurver PHJ & Hermans J (1985) The value of morphometry to classic prognosticators in breast cancer. *Cancer* **56:** 374–382.

Bauer TW, O'Ceallaign D, Eggleston JC, Moore GW & Baker RR (1983) Prognostic factors in patients with stage 1, estrogen receptor-negative carcinoma of the breast. A clinicopathologic study. *Cancer* **52:** 1423–1431.

Betsill WL, Rosen PR, Lieberman PH & Robbins GF (1978) Intraductal carcinoma. Long-term follow-up after treatment by biopsy alone. *JAMA* **239:** 1863–1867.

Blanco G, Holli K, Heikkinen M, Kallioniemi OP & Taskinen P (1990) Prognostic factors in recurrent breast cancer: relationships to site of recurrence, disease-free interval, female sex steroid receptors, ploidy and histological malignancy grading. *Br. J. Cancer* **62:** 142–146.

Blichert-Toft M, Andersen J & Dyreborg U (1990) *In situ* carcinomas of the female breast. Diagnostic and therapeutic aspects with special reference to histological growth patterns. Clinical Review. *Acta Chir. Scand.* **156:** 113–119.

Blichert-Toft M, Graversen HP, Andersen J, Dyreborg U & Green A (1988) *In situ* breast carcinomas: A population-based study on frequency, growth pattern, and clinical aspects. *World J. Surg.* **12:** 845–851.

Bloom HJG & Richardson WW (1957) Histological grading and prognosis in breast cancer. A study of 1409 cases of which 359 have been followed for 15 years. *Br. J. Cancer* **11(3):** 357–377.

Calle R, Vilcoq JR, Zafrani B, Vielh P & Fourquet A (1986) Local control and survival of breast cancer treated by limited surgery followed by irradiation. *Int. J. Rad. Oncol.* **12:** 873–878.

Carstens PHB, Greenberg RA, Francis D & Lyon H (1985) Tubular carcinoma of the breast. A long term follow-up. *Histopathology* **9:** 271–280.

Carter D (1986) Margins of "lumpectomy" for breast cancer. *Human Pathol.* **17:** 330–332.

Chabon AB, Goldberg JD & Venet L (1982) Carcinoma of the breast. Interrelationships among histopathologic features, estrogen receptor activity, and age of the patient. *Hum. Pathol.* **14:** 368–372.

Chaudary MM, Girling A, Girling S, Habib F, Millis RR & Hayward JL (1988) New Lumps in the breast following conservation treatment for early breast cancer. *Br. Can. Res. and Treat.* **11:** 51–58.

Claus EB, Risch N, Thompson WD & Carter D (1993) Relationship between breast histopathology and family history of breast cancer. *Cancer* **71:** 147–153.

Clayton F (1991) Pathologic correlates of survival in 378 lymph node-negative infiltrating ductal breast carcinomas. Mitotic count is the best single predictor. *Cancer* **68:** 1309–1317.

Clayton F (1986) Pure mucinous carcinomas of breast: Morphologic features and prognostic correlates. *Hum. Pathol.* **17:** 34–38.

Contesso G, Mouriesse H, Friedman S, Genin J, Sarrazin D & Rouesse J (1987) The importance of histologic grade in long-term prognosis of breast cancer: A study of 1,010 patients, uniformly treated at the Institut Gustave-Roussy. *J. Clin. Oncol.* **5:** 1378–1386.

Davis N & Baird RM (1984) Breast cancer in association with lobular carcinoma *in situ*. Clinicopathologic review and treatment recommendation. *Amer. J. Surg.* 1984 **147:** 641–645.

Davis BW, Gelber RD, Goldhirsch A *et al.* (1986) Prognostic significance of tumor grade in clinical trials of adjuvant therapy for breast cancer with axillary lymph node metastasis. *Cancer* **58:** 2662–2670.

DiCostanzo D, Rosen PP, Gareen I, Franklin S & Lesser M (1990) Prognosis in infiltrating lobular carcinoma – an analysis of "classical" and variant tumors. *Am. J. Surg. Path.* **14(1):** 12–23.

Donegan WL, Stine SB, Samter TG *et al.* (1993) Implications of extracapsular nodal metastases for treatment and prognosis of breast cancer. *Cancer* **72:** 778–782.

■ Ellis IO, Glaea M, Broughton N, Locker A, Blamey RW & Elston CW (1992) Pathological prognostic factors in breast cancer. II. Histological type. Relationship with survival in a large study with long-term follow-up. *Histopathology* **20:** 479–487.

Elson CE, Kufe D & Johnston WW (1993) Immunohistochemical detection and significance of axillary lymph node micrometastases in breast carcinoma. *Anal. and Qumt. Cytol. Histol.* **15:** 171–178.

Fentiman IS, Fagg N, Millis RR & Hayward JL (1986) *In situ* ductal carcinoma of the breast: implications of disease pattern and treatment. *Eur. J. Surg. Oncol.* **12:** 261–266.

■ Fisher B (1991) A biological perspective of breast cancer: contributions of the national surgical adjuvant breast and bowel project clinical trials. *Can. J. Clin.* **41:** 97–111.

Fisher ER, Sass R & Fisher B (1984) Pathologic findings from the National Surgical Adjuvant Project for Breast Cancers (Protocol No. 4) X. Discriminants for tenth year treatment failure. *Cancer* **53:** 712–723.

Fisher ER, Sass R, Fisher B *et al.* (1986a) Pathologic findings from the National Surgical Adjuvant Breast Project (Protocol 6) II. Relation of local breast recurrence to multicentricity. *Cancer* **57:** 1717–1724.

Fisher ER, Sass R, Fisher B, Wickerham L & Paik SM (1986b) Pathologic findings from the National Surgical Breast Project (Protocol 6) I. Intraductal carcinoma (DCIS). *Cancer* **57:** 197–208.

Fowble B, Solin LJ, Schultz DJ, Rubenstein J & Goodman RL (1990) Breast recurrence following conservative surgery and radiation: Patterns of failure, prognosis, and pathologic findings from mastectomy specimens with implications for treatment. *Int. J. Rad. Oncol.* **19:** 833–842.

Frazier TG, Wong RWY & Rose D (1989) Implications of accurate pathologic margins in the treatment of primary breast cancer. *Arch. Surg.* **124:** 37–38.

Freedman LS, Edwards DN, McConnell EM & Downham DY (1979) Histological grade and other prognostic factors in relation to survival of patients with breast cancer. *Br. J. Cancer* **40:** 4455.

Gallagher WJ, Koerner FC & Wood WC (1989) Treatment of intraductal carcinoma with limited surgery: Long-term follow-up. *J. Clin. Oncol.* **7:** 376–380.

Gallagher HS & Martin JE (1969) Early phases in the development of breast cancer. *Cancer* **25:** 1170–1178.

Graversen HP, Bilchert-Toft M, Dyreborg U & Andersen J (1988) *In situ* carcinomas of the female breast. Incidence, clinical findings and DBCG proposals for management. *Acta Oncol.* **27:** 679–682.

Gullino PM (1977) Natural history of breast cancer. Progression from hyperplasia to neoplasia as predicted by angiogenesis. *Cancer* **39:** 2697–2703.

Gump FE, Jicha DL & Ozello L (1987) Ductal carcinoma *in situ* (DCIS): A revised concept. *Surgery* **102:** 790–795.

Hainsworth PJ, Tjandra JJ, Stillwell RG *et al.* (1993) Detection and significance of occult metastases in node-negative breast cancer. *Br. J. Surg.* **80:** 459–463.

■ Harris JR, Connolly JL, Schnitt SJ *et al.* (1984) The use of pathologic features in selecting the extent of surgical resection necessary for breast cancer patients treated by primary radiation therapy. *Ann. Surg.* **201:** 164–169.

Harris M, Howell A, Chrissohou M, Swindell RIC, Hudson M & Sellwood RA (1984) A comparison of the metastatic pattern of infiltrating lobular carcinoma and infiltrating duct carcinoma of the breast. *Br. J. Cancer* **50:** 23–30.

Holland R, Hendriks JHCL, Verbeek ALM, Mravunac M & Schuurmans Stekhoven JH (1990) Extent, distribution and mammographic/histological correlations of breast ductal carcinoma *in situ*. *Lancet* **335:** 519–522.

Holland R, Veling SHJ, Mravunac M & Hendriks JHCL (1985) Histologic miltifocality of Tis, T1-2 breast carcinomas. Implications for clinical trials of breast-conserving surgery. *Cancer* **56:** 979–990.

Jacquemier J, Kurtz JM, Amalric R, Brandone H, Ayme Y & Spitalier JM (1990) An assessment of extensive intraductal component as a risk factor for local recurrence after breast-conserving therapy. *Br. J. Cancer* **61:** 873–876.

Kennedy MJ & Abeloff MD (1993) Management of locally recurrent breast cancer. *Cancer* **71:** 2395–2409.

Ketcham AS & Moffat FL (1990) Vexed surgeons, perplexed patients, and breast cancers which may not be cancer. *Cancer* **65:** 387–393.

Kinne DW (1991) The surgical management of primary breast cancer. *Can. J. Clin.* **41:** 71–84.

Kinne DW, Petrek JA, Osborne MP, Fracchia AA, DePalo AA & Rosen PR (1989) Breast carcinoma *in situ*. *Arch. Surg.* **124:** 33–36.

Kiricuta I–C, Warszawski N, Tausch J, Galimberti V & Zurrida S (1994) Incomplete axillary dissection in early breast cancer and the risk of erroneous staging. *Int. J. Oncol.* **4:** 661–666.

Koscielny S, Le MG & Tubiana M (1988) The natural history of human breast cancer. The relationship between involvement of axillary lymph nodes and the initiation of distant metastases. *Br. J. Cancer* **53:** 775–782.

Kurtz JM, Jocelyne J, Amalric R *et al.* (1990) Risk factors for breast recurrence in premenopausal and postmenopausal patients with ductal cancers treated by conservation therapy. *Cancer* **65:** 1867–1878.

Lagios MD (1992) Pathologic features related to local recurrence following lumpectomy and irradiation. *Sem. In Surg. Oncol.* **8:** 122–128.

Lagios MD, Margolin FR, Westdahl PR & Rose MR (1989) Mammographically detected duct carcinoma *in situ*. Frequency of local recurrence following tylectomy and prognostic effect of nuclear grade on local recurrence. *Cancer* **63:** 618–624.

Lagios MD, Rose MR & Margolin FR (1980) Tubular carcinoma of the breast. Association with multicentricity, bilaterality, and family history of mammary carcinoma. *Am. J. Clin. Pathol.* **73:** 25–30.

Lagios MD, Westdahl PR, Margolin FR & Roses MR (1982) Duct carcinoma *in situ*. Relationship of extent of noninvasive disease to the frequency of occult invasion, multicentricity, lymph node metastases, and short-term treatment failures. *Cancer* **50:** 1309–1314.

Lagios M, Wolmark N, Fowble B & Clark G (1993) Management of *in-situ* and minimally invasive carcinoma of breast cancer. *ASCO Educational Program* **Spring:** 59–82.

Lash RH, Bauer TW, Hermann RE & Esselstyn CB (1986) Partial mastectomy: pathologic findings and prognosis. *Hum. Pathol.* **17:** 813–822.

London SJ, Connolly JL, Schnitt SJ & Colditz GA (1992) A prospective study of benign breast disease and the risk of breast cancer. *JAMA* **267:** 941–944.

McDivitt RW, Boyce W & Gersell D (1982) Tubular carcinoma of the breast. Clinical and pathological observation concerning 135 cases. *Am. J. Surg. Pathol.* **6:** 401–411.

Neville AM, Bettelheim R, Gelber RD *et al.* (1992) Factors predicting treatment responsiveness and prognosis in node-negative breast cancer. *J. Clin. Oncol.* **10:** 696–705.

Nielsen M, Jensen J & Andersen J (1984) Precancerous and cancerous breast lesions during lifetime and at autopsy. A study of 83 women. *Cancer* **54:** 612–615.

Page DL, Dupont WD, Rogers LW & Landenberger M (1982) Intraductal carcinoma of the breast: Follow-up after biopsy only. *Cancer* **49:** 751–758.

■ Page DL, DuPont WD, Rogers LW & Rados MS (1985) Atypical hyerplastic lesions of the female breast. A long-term follow-up study. *Cancer* **55:** 2698–2708.

Parl FF & DuPont WD (1982) A retrospective cohort study of histologic risk factors in breast cancer patients. *Cancer* **50:** 2410–2416.

Parl FF & Richardson LD (1983) The histologic and biologic spectrum of tubular carcinoma of the breast. *Hum. Pathol.* **14:** 694–698.

Patchefsky AS, Schwartz GF, Finkelstein SD *et al.* (1989) Heterogeneity of intraductal carcinoma of the breast. *Cancer* **63:** 731–741.

Peer PG, Van Dijck JA, Hendriks JH, Holland R & Verbeek AL (1993) Age-dependent growth rate of primary breast cancer. *Cancer* **71:** 3547–3551.

Pierce SM & Harris JR (1991) The role of radiation therapy in the management of primary breast cancer. *Cancer J. Clinicians* **41:** 85–96.

Poen JC, Tran L, Juillard G *et al.* (1992) Conservation therapy for invasive lobular carcinoma of the breast. *Cancer* **69:** 2789–2795.

Posner MC & Wolmark N (1992) Non-invasive breast carcinoma. *Br. Can. Res. and Treat.* **21:** 155–164.

Rank F, Dombernowsky P, Jespersen NCB, Pedersen BV & Keiding N (1987) Histologic malignancy grading of invasive ductal breast carcinoma. A regression analysis of prognostic factors in low-risk carcinomas from a multicenter trial. *Cancer* **60:** 1299–1305.

Rasmussen BB, Rose C & Christensen IB (1987) Prognostic factors in primary mucinous breast carcinoma. *Am. J. Clin. Pathol.* **87:** 155–160.

Redding WH, Monaghan P, Imrie SF *et al.* (1983) Detection of micrometastases in patients with primary breast cancer. *Lancet* **ii:** 1271–1273.

Ridolfi RL, Rosen PR, Port A, Kinne D & Mike V (1977) Medullary carcinoma of the breast: A clinicopathologic study with 10 year follow-up. *Cancer* **40:** 1365–1385.

Rigaud C, Theobald S, Noel P *et al.* (1993) Medullary carcinoma of the breast. A multicenter study of its diagnostic consistency. *Arch. Pathol. Lab. Med.* **117:** 1005–1008.

Ringberg A, Palmer B, Linell F, Rychterova V & Ljungberg O (1991) Bilateral and multifocal breast carcinoma. A clinical and autopsy study with special emphasis on carcinoma *in situ*. *Eur. J. Surg. Oncol.* **17:** 20–29.

Rosen PP (1983) Tumor emboli in intramammary lymphatics. *Path. Ann.* **18(part 2):** 215–232.

Rosen PR, Braun DW & Kinne DE (1980) The clinical significance of pre-invasive breast carcinoma. *Cancer* **46:** 919–925.

Rosen PR, Kinne DW, Lesser M & Hellman S (1986) Are prognostic factors for local control of breast cancer treated by primary radiotherapy significant for patients treated by mastectomy? *Cancer* **57:** 1415–1420.

Rosen PR, Saigo PE, Braun DW, Beattie EJ & Kinne DW (1982) Occult axillary lymph node metastases from breast cancers with inflammatory lymphatic tumor emboli. *Amer. J. Surg. Pathol.* **6:** 639–641.

Rosen PR, Senie R, Schottenfeld D & Ashikari R (1979) Noninvasive breast carcinoma. Frequency of unsuspected invasion and implications for treatment. *Ann. Surg.* **3:** 377–382.

Roses DF, Bell DA, Flotte TJ, Taylor R, Ratech H & Dubin N (1982) Pathologic predictors of recurrence in Stage 1 (TINOMO) breast cancer. *Am. J. Clin. Pathol.* **78:** 817–820.

Rosner D, Bedwani RN, Vana J, Baker HW & Murphy GP (1980) Noninvasive breast carcinoma. Results of a national survey by the American College of Surgeons. *Ann. Surg.* **192:** 139–147.

Schnitt SJ, Connolly JL, Khettry U *et al.* (1987) Pathologic findings on re-excision of the primary site in breast cancer patients considered for treatment by primary radiation therapy. *Cancer* **59:** 675–681.

Schnitt SJ, Connolly JL, Recht A, Silver B & Harris JR (1985) Breast relapse following primary radiation therapy for early breast cancer. II. Detection, pathologic features and prognostic significance. *Int. J. Rad. Oncol.* **11:** 1277–1284.

Schnitt SJ, Connolly JL, Recht A, Silver B & Harris JR (1989) Influence of infiltrating lobular histology on local tumor control in breast cancer patients treated with conservative surgery and radiotherapy. *Cancer* **64:** 448–454.

Schnitt SJ, Silen W, Sadowsky NL, Connolly JL & Harris JR (1988) Ductal carcinoma *in situ* (intraductal carcinoma) of the breast. *New Eng. J. Med.* **318:** 898–902.

Schuh ME, Nemoto T, Penetrante RB, Rosner D & Dao TL (1986) Intraductal carcinoma. Analysis of presentation, pathologic findings, and outcome of disease. *Arch. Surg.* **121:** 1303–1307.

Silverberg SG & Chitale AR (1973) Assessment of significance of proportions of intraductal and infiltrating tumor growth in ductal carcinoma of the breast. *Cancer* **32:** 830–837.

Simkovich AH, Sclafani LM, Masri M & Kinne DW (1993) Role of contralateral breast biopsy in infiltrating lobular cancer. *Surgery* **114:** 555–557.

Simon MS, Schwartz AG, Martino S & Swanson GM (1992) Trends in the diagnosis of *in situ* breast cancer in the Detroit Metropolitan Area, 1973 to 1987. *Cancer* **69:** 466–469.

Smith BL, Bertagnolli M, Klein BB *et al.* (1992) Evaluation of the contralateral breast. The role of biopsy at the time of treatment of primary breast cancer. *Ann. Surg.* **216:** 17–21.

Solin LJ, Recht A, Fourquet A *et al.* (1991) Ten-year results of breast-conserving surgery and definitive irradiation for intraductal carcinoma (ductal carcinoma *in situ*) of the breast. *Cancer* **68:** 2337–2344.

Stalsberg H & Thomas DB (1993) Age distribution of histologic types of breast carcinoma. *Int. J. Cancer* **54:** 1–7.

Stenkvist B, Bengtsson E, Eiksson O *et al.* (1983) Histopathological systems of breast cancer classification: reproducibility and clinical significance. *J. Clin. Pathol.* **36:** 392–398.

Swain SM (1992) Ductal carcinoma *in situ*. *Cancer Invest.* **10(5):** 443–454.

Theissig F, Kunze KD, Haroske G & Meyer W (1990) Histological grading of breast cancer. Interobserver reproducibility and prognostic significance. *Path. Res. Pract.* **186:** 732–736.

Van Dongen JA, Harris JR, Pererse JL *et al.* (1989) *In-situ* breast cancer: The EORTC Consensus Meeting. *Lancet* **i:** 25–27.

Veronesi U, Rilke F, Luini A *et al.* (1987) Distribution of axillary node metastases by level of invasion. An analysis of 539 cases. *Cancer* **59:** 682–687.

■ Visscher DW, Zarbo RJ, Greenawald KA & Crissman JD (1990) Prognostic significance of morphological and flow cytometric DNA analysis in carcinoma of the breast. *Path. Ann.* **25:** 171–210.

Webber BL, Heise H, Neifeld JP & Costa J (1981) Risk of subsequent contralateral breast carcinoma in a population of patients with *in-situ* breast carcinoma. *Cancer* **47:** 2928–2932.

Weidner N & Semple JP (1992) Pleomorphic variant of invasive lobular carcinoma of the breast. *Hum. Pathol.* **23:** 1167–1171.

Wellings SR, Jensen HM & Marcum RG (1975) An atlas of subgross pathology of the human breast with special reference to possible precancerous lesions. *J. Natl. Cancer Inst.* **55:** 231–273.

Wong JH, Kopald KH & Morton DL (1990) The impact of microinvasion on axillary node metastases and survival in patients with intraductal breast cancer. *Arch. Surg.* **125:** 1298–1302.

25 Local Management of Breast Cancer

H R Chang
K I Bland

Surgery is the principal therapeutic modality for the comprehensive management of early and locally advanced breast cancer. Early breast cancer is defined as Stage I and II breast cancer. Locally advanced breast cancer (Stage IIIA, B) is defined as the presence of tumors greater than 5 cm, direct invasion of the skin or chest wall, or extensive nodal involvement. This chapter will detail the technical considerations of surgical treatment, use of irradiation, evaluation and selection of patients and the pathologic implications, as well as the results of treatment.

Evaluation of Breast Cancer

Presentation

Breast cancer primarily presents in middle-aged or elderly women; it is rare in young women and men. Typically two-thirds of the patients are peri- or postmenopausal women. Presenting indications include the appearance of a mass, nipple discharge, nipple and skin retraction, an eczematous nipple, pain, inflammation and abnormal mammography. The mammography may show a mass, microcalcifications, asymmetrical density or dermal thickening and distortion.

Diagnosis

Diagnosis of breast cancer is based on tissue and cytologic examinations of the mammary parenchymal abnormality. A palpable mass may be investigated by fine-needle aspiration (FNA). Cells of a solid mass or of bloody fluid from a cyst are forwarded for cytology evaluation. Bloody nipple discharge is also studied in a similar manner with cytology. When the results of the FNA are either negative or nondiagnostic (equivocal), open surgical biopsy is indicated. In the majority of patients, mammography is required before biopsy. The nonpalpable abnormality may be excised with a needle localization technique or evaluated by stereotactic biopsy. Patients with mammographic abnormalities may also be followed by interval mammography, depending on the level of suspicion as well as the experience of the clinician providing care to the patient.

Preoperative Evaluation

Once breast carcinoma is diagnosed, it is essential to clinically stage (TNM system, see below) the extent of the disease before planning its local management. Evaluation consists of the patient's history and physical examination, liver function tests, bilateral mammography, and chest radiography. A bone scan is not routinely employed in asymptomatic patients in the absence of an elevated alkaline phosphatase, palpable lymph nodes or a large primary tumor. It is required when any of these unfavorable parameters are present, especially advanced primary tumors or in patients with symptomatic bone or joint disease. A positive bone scan advances the stage of disease (Stage IV) and significantly impacts the treatment plan.

Staging

Pathologic staging after primary surgical treatment is crucially important in the management of breast cancer. Accurate pathologic staging defines the extent of the disease and the prognosis, and guides any additional regional or systemic treatment. Clinical staging alone is incorrect in more than 30% of patients in the assessment of metastatic lymph nodes, and frequently in the estimation of tumor size (diameter). When discrepancy exists between the clinical and histologic examinations, survival is estimated solely by the pathologic staging (Haagensen, 1986). The current staging for breast cancer published by the American Joint Committee on Cancer is based on the classification system of tumor (T), node (N), and metastasis (M) (Beahrs *et al.*, 1988) (see *Table 47.7*).

Surgical Treatment

Two principal surgical procedures have been used in treating primary operable breast cancer. Modified radical mastectomy has been the standard procedure, and breast conservation surgery has been the alternative. Both procedures are aimed at providing local–regional control of the breast cancer and proper staging.

Modified Radical Mastectomy

History

Development of the radical mastectomy is credited principally to William S. Halsted at the Johns Hopkins Hospital in 1882. He described extensive resection of the skin, breast and pectoralis major and minor muscles, as well as dissection of Levels I–III of the axillary nodes. Local recurrence associated with radical mastectomy was reported to be 6% at three years in 50 patients – an enormous technical achievement of the era in which local–regional recurrence exceeded 50% in operated patients. Radical mastectomy was the standard operation until the 1970s. A survey by the American College of Surgeons for carcinoma of the breast in the USA showed that between 1972 to 1981 the use of modified radical mastectomy increased from 27% to 78%; simultaneously, the use of radical mastectomy decreased from 50% to 3% (Wilson *et al.*, 1984). The shift to the alternative conservative approach resulted from data that confirmed that modified radical mastectomy achieved equivalent disease control while providing an enhanced appearance and improvement of anatomical function.

Operative technique

Modified radical mastectomy entails removal of the entire breast, including the nipple–areolar complex and axillary lymph nodes. This operation preserves the pectoralis major muscle. One version of the modified radical mastectomy, described in 1948 by David Patey of the Middlesex Hospital (London), is the Patey procedure, which requires removal of the pectoralis minor muscle and complete dissection of Level I–III axillary nodes (Patey and Dyson, 1948; Patey, 1967). A variant of the Patey modified radical mastectomy is the Auchincloss (Auchincloss, 1970) or Madden procedure (Madden, 1965), which preserves the pectoralis minor muscle. In Patey's procedure, the lateral pectoral nerve is generally sacrificed, which produces atrophy of the lower one-third of the pectoralis major muscle. In the procedure described by Auchincloss or Madden, both lateral and medial pectoral nerves are preserved, resulting in enhanced function of the pectoralis major muscle and improved breast reconstruction with prosthetic implants. For Stage I and II cancers, however, nodal dissection in the Auchincloss or Madden procedures is generally limited, and the interpectoral (Rotter's) and apical (Level III) axillary lymph nodes remain intact.

With the modified radical mastectomy, the entire ipsilateral breast and arm are draped free in the operative field (*Figure 25.1*). An elliptical incision encompassing the biopsy scar and nipple–areolar complex produces a scar of optimal cosmetic

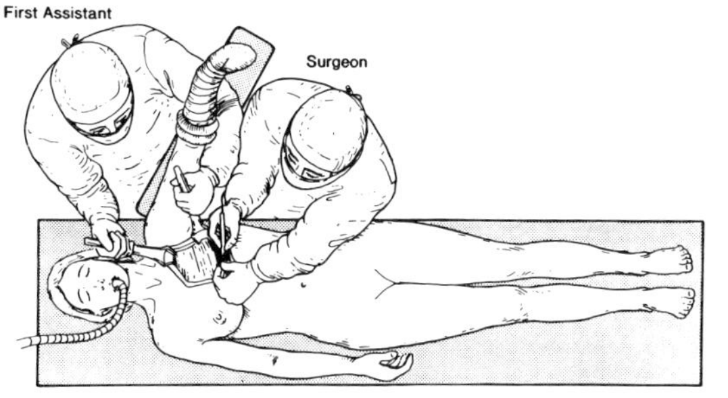

Figure 25.1. Position of the patient for left modified radical mastectomy at the margin of operative table. The first assistant is cephalad to the armboard and shoulder of the patient to allow access to the axillary contents without undue traction on major muscle groups. Depicted is the preferential isolation of the hand and forearm with an occlusive Stockinette cotton dressing secured distal to the elbow. This technique allows free mobility of the elbow, arm and shoulder to avoid undue stretch of the brachial plexus with muscle retraction. From Bland KI, Copeland EM III (eds) (1991) *The Breast: Comprehensive Management of Benign and Malignant Diseases*, p. 616. Philadelphia: WB Saunders.

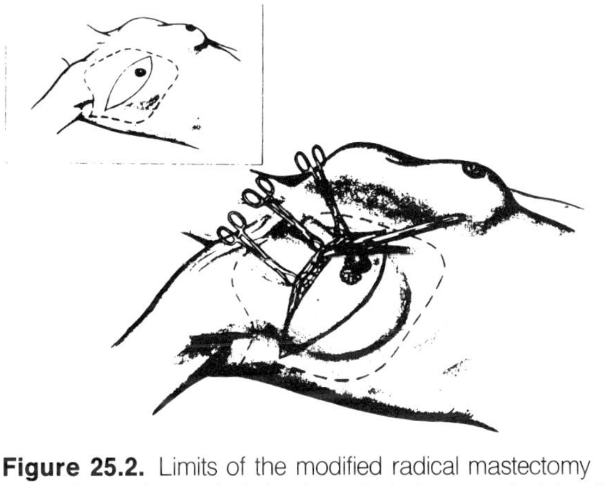

Figure 25.2. Limits of the modified radical mastectomy are delineated superiorly by the subclavius muscle, laterally by the anterior margin of the latissimus dorsi muscle, medially by the midline of the sternum, and inferiorly by the caudal extension of the breast approximately 3–4 cm inferior to the inframammary fold. Skin flaps for the modified radical technique are planned with relation to the quadrant in which the primary neoplasm is located. Adequate margins are ensured by developing skin edges 3–5 cm from the tumor margin. Incisions are planned so that they are developed perpendicular to the subcutaneous plane and are inclusive of skin and parenchymal tissue 3–5 cm around the neoplasm. Flap thickness is dependent on patient habitus and proportional lean body mass. Flaps should be 7–8 mm in thickness inclusive of the skin and tela subcutanea. Flap tension should be perpendicular to the chest wall with flap elevation deep to the cutaneous vasculature, which is accentuated by flap retraction. From Bland KI, Copeland EM III (eds) (1991) *The Breast: Comprehensive Management of Benign and Malignant Diseases*, p. 616. Philadelphia: WB Saunders.

appearance. The skin flaps developed at the avascular plane of the superficial mammary fascia are developed medially from the sternal border, laterally to the latissimus dorsi muscle, superiorly from the clavicle, and inferiorly to the level of the rectus sheath (*Figure 25.2*). The breast is then sharply detached from the chest wall and removed together with the pectoralis major fascia in a mediosuperior to lateroinferior direction (*Figure 25.3*). The pectoralis major muscle is preserved, but may be wedged if the tumor is located posteriorly or the biopsy cavity enters deeply into the muscle. Once the lateral border of the pectoralis major muscle is defined, the pectoralis fascia investing the axillary contents and the pectoralis minor muscle are incised (*Figures 25.4 and 25.5*). At this point, the patient's arm is flexed and elevated anterior to the chest to expose the axillary contents.

In the Patey procedure, the pectoralis minor tendon is divided at its origin from the coracoid process with digital protection of the neurovascular axillary structures (*Figure 25.6*). Once the tendon is divided, the length of the axillary vein is exposed and dissected medially from the costoclavicular ligament (also known as Halsted's ligament), to remove the lymphatic contents anterior and inferior to the axillary vein. Cephalad dissection (above) of the vein is technically dangerous and provides no therapeutic advantage and is to be strongly discouraged as neurovascular injury may result. The pectoralis minor muscle is then detached from its costal insertion and removed *en bloc* with the axillary contents. The medial pectoral nerve and the pectoral branch of the thoracoacromial artery and vein are preserved. The horizontally traversing intercostal brachial nerves will be encountered and may be divided to facilitate a thorough nodal dissection. Division of these nerves results in anesthesia of the posterior and medial aspect of the upper arm.

The long thoracic nerve lies deep to the intercostal brachial nerve and is invested by the serratus anterior fascia and can be identified near the medial aspect of the subscapular fossa. This nerve provides motor innervation to the serratus anterior muscle and should be preserved unless one finds grossly involved lymph nodes investing the nerve. Injury to this nerve results in the 'winged scapula' deformity and diminished shoulder strength. With clearing of the long thoracic nerve, the axillary dissection is extended laterally, and small branches of the axillary vessels are ligated and divided. The thoracodorsal nerve traverses the posterior axillary space beneath the axillary vessels, courses medially with the subscapular vessels, and crosses anteriorly to these vessels to provide motor innervation to the latissimus dorsi muscle. The thoracodorsal nerve is preserved,

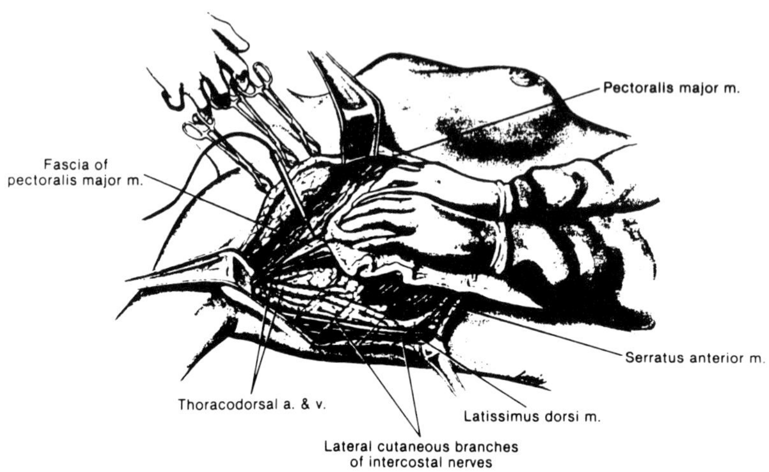

Figure 25.3. Elevation of the superior flap to the level of the subclavius muscle at the superiormost extent of the breast parenchyma. Skin flap thickness is constant at 7–8 mm from lateral to medial. Thereafter, dissection of the pectoralis major fascia from the pectoralis musculature may be completed with cold scalpel or electrocautery. Dissection commences lateral to medial in a plane that parallels the muscle bundles of the pectoralis major muscle from the origin of ribs 2–6 to insertion on the humerus. Counteraction in a caudal direction allows tension on the fascia to facilitate its removal from the pectoralis major. Perforator vessels from the lateral thoracic or anterior intercostal arteries are encountered as end-arteries that supply the pectoralis major and minor muscles. Thereafter, the inferior flap is elevated medially in similar fashion to the midline, inferiorly to the aponeurosis of the rectus abdominis tendon, and laterally to the anterior margin of the latissimus. The inferiormost portion of the breast is left intact following clearing of the superolateral margin of the pectoralis major. This maneuver ensures an *en bloc* resection of the axillary contents with the breast, leaving the axillary tail of Spence intact. From Bland KI, Copeland EM III (eds) (1991) *The Breast: Comprehensive Management of Benign and Malignant Diseases*, p. 617. Philadelphia: WB Saunders.

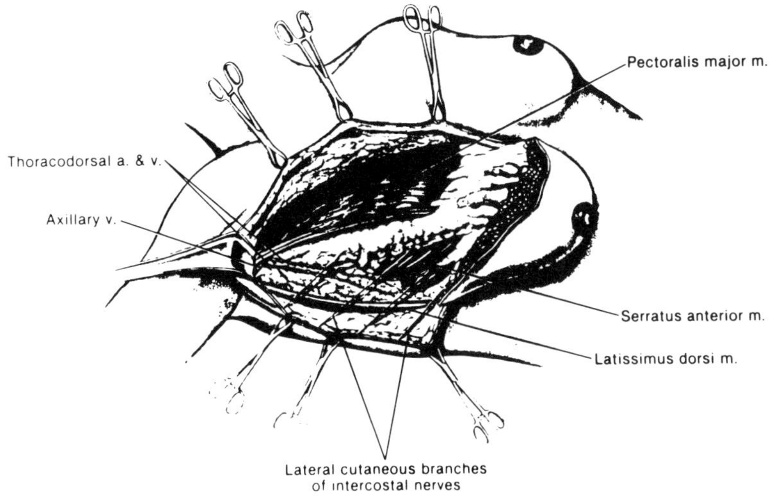

Figure 25.4. The completed superior and inferior flap with breast parenchyma intact with the axillary tail of Spence and the axillary contents. The pectoralis major is completely cleared of its fascia *en bloc* with the breast parenchyma. At this juncture, the pectoralis minor has not been exposed to allow access to the axilla (Level II and III nodes). The latissimus dorsi muscle has been dissected on its anterior surface to delineate the lateral boundary of dissection. Illustrated in this view is the cutaneous innervation of the skin of the lateral chest, axilla, and medial arm by intercostobrachial sensory nerves. These nerves are commonly divided in the course of dissection of the axilla and lateral skin flap following identification of the latissimus dorsi. From Bland KI, Copeland EM III (eds) (1991) *The Breast: Comprehensive Management of Benign and Malignant Diseases*, p. 618. Philadelphia: WB Saunders.

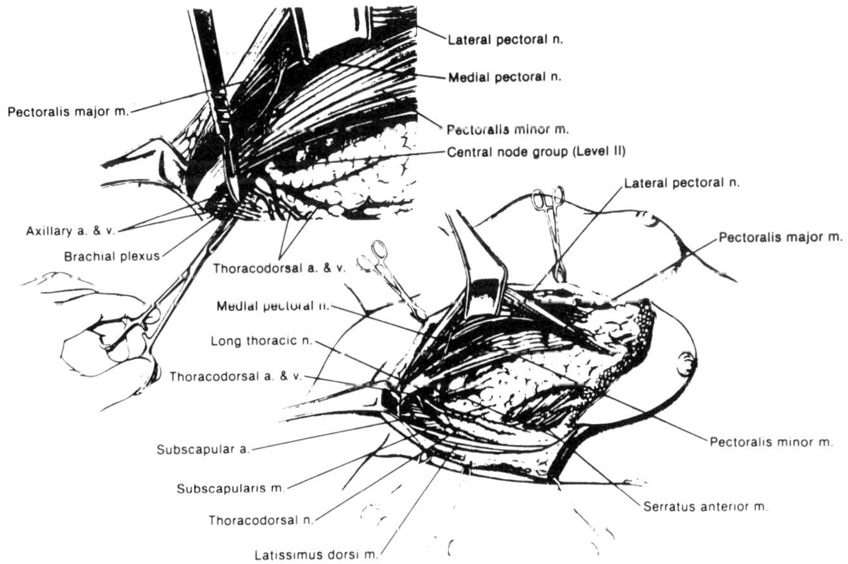

Figure 25.5. Juncture of the latissimus (unexposed) with the ventral surface of the axillary vein. Sharp division with a scalpel to incise the investing fascia of the axillary space. Following isolation of the tendinous portion of the pectoralis minor muscle with finger dissection, the insertion of this tendon on the coracoid process of the scapula can be readily identified. The surgeon must be cognizant of the anatomic location of the lateral neurovascular bundle and the laterally placed medial pectoral nerve, which takes origin from the medial cord. Every attempt should be made to preserve the medial pectoral nerve, as sacrifice of the main trunk may allow atrophy of the lateral head of the pectoralis major. Further, the lateral pectoral nerve, which takes origin from the lateral cord and is medially placed, should also be preserved. From Bland KI, Copeland EM III (eds) (1991) *The Breast: Comprehensive Management of Benign and Malignant Diseases*, p. 619. Philadelphia: WB Saunders.

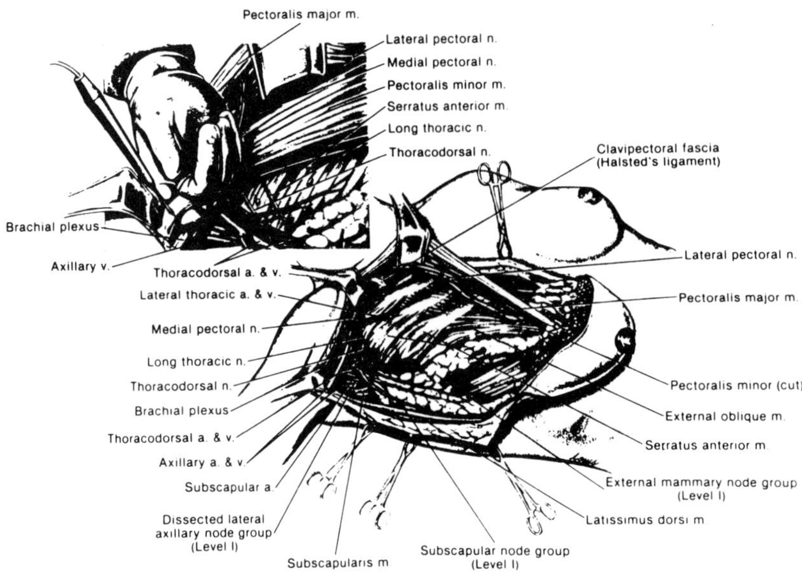

Figure 25.6. Digital protection of the brachial plexus for division of the insertion of the pectoralis minor muscle on the coracoid process. All loose areolar and lymphatic tissues are swept *en bloc* with the axillary contents to insure resection of the interpectoral (Rotter's) nodes. Dissection commences lateral to medial with complete visualization of the anterior and ventral aspects of the axillary vein. Dissection craniad to the axillary vein is inadvisable, for fear of damage to the brachial plexus and the infrequent observation of gross nodal tissue cephalic to the vein. Investing fascial dissection of the vein is best completed with the cold scalpel following exposure, ligation and division of all venous tributaries on the anterior and ventral surfaces. Caudal to the vein, loose areolar tissue at the junction of the vein with the anterior margin latissimus is swept inferomedially inclusive of the lateral (axillary) nodal group (Level I). Care is taken to preserve the neurovascular thoracodorsal artery, vein and nerve in the deep axillary space. The thoracodorsal nerve is traced to its innervation of the latissimus dorsi muscle laterally. Lateral axillary nodal groups are retracted inferomedially and anterior to this bundle for dissection *en bloc* with the subscapular (Level I) nodal group. Preferentially, dissection commences superomedially before completion of dissection of the external mammary (Level I) nodal group. Superomedial dissection over the axillary vein allows extirpation of the central nodal group (Level II) and apical (subclavicular) Level III group. The superomedialmost extent of the dissection is the clavipectoral fascia (Halsted's ligament). This level of dissection with the Patey technique allows the surgeon to mark, with metallic clip or suture, the superiormost extent of dissection. All loose areolar tissue just inferior to the apical nodal group is swept off the chest wall, leaving the fascia of the serratus anterior intact. With dissection parallel to the long thoracic nerve (respiratory nerve of Bell), the deep investing serratus fascia is incised. This nerve is closely applied to the investing fascial compartment of the chest wall and must be dissected in its entirety, cephalic to caudal to ensure innervation of the serratus anterior and avoidance of the 'winged scapula' disability. From Bland KI, Copeland EM III (eds) (1991) *The Breast: Comprehensive Management of Benign and Malignant Diseases*, p. 620. Philadelphia: WB Saunders.

but branches from it may be ligated without resultant functional or cosmetic deficit. Dissection is completed when the medial aspect of the latissimus muscle is cleared and when the lymphatic contents are divided from the serratus anterior muscle superficial to the long thoracic nerve (*Figure 25.7*). The specimen should be tagged to identify the nodes at Levels I through III, with the pectoralis minor muscle retained as a landmark.

In the Auchincloss and Madden modified radical mastectomy, the pectoralis minor muscle is cleared both medially and laterally and then retracted anteriorly and medially to expose Level II (central group) lymph nodes. Dissection is begun near the medial border of the pectoralis minor muscle. The lateral pectoral nerve is preserved. The remaining procedures are identical to those described for the Patey procedure.

Once the specimen is removed, hemostasis of the skin flaps, chest wall and axilla is achieved. Two soft Silastic closed-suction drains are inserted via separate stab wounds located inferiorly and laterally. A long drain is placed along the inferior flap curving medially then superiorly. A short drain is placed in the axilla below the level of the axillary vein. The drains are connected to continuous sealed bulb suction to facilitate seroma removal and allow adherence of the skin flap to the chest wall (see *Figure 25.7*).

Wound closure is performed in two layers: subcutaneous closure by interrupted absorbable sutures and skin closure by running subcuticular stitches of 3-0 nylon. Monofilament nylon

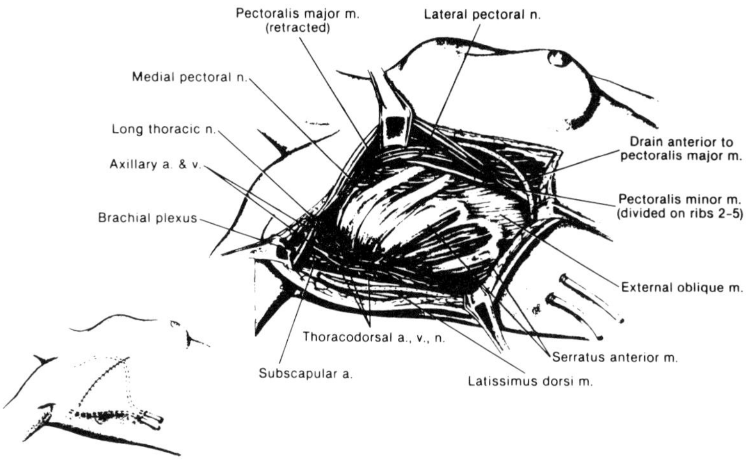

Figure 25.7. The completed Patey axillary dissection variant of the modified radical technique. The dissection is inclusive of the pectoralis minor muscle from origin to insertion of ribs 2–5. Both medial and lateral pectoral nerves are preserved to ensure innervation of the lateral and medial heads, respectively, of the pectoralis major. With completion of the procedure, remaining portions of this muscle are swept *en bloc* with the axillary contents to be inclusive of Rotter's interpectoral and the retropectoral groups.

Inset: Following copious irrigation with distilled water and saline, closed-suction Silastic catheters (18–20 French) are positioned via stab incisions placed in the inferior flap at the anterior axillary line. The lateral catheter is placed approximately 2 cm inferior to the axillary vein. The superior, longer catheter placed via the medial stab wound is positioned in the superomedial aspect of the defect anterior to the pectoralis major muscle beneath the skin flap. The wound is closed in two layers with 2–0 absorbable synthetic sutures placed in subcutaneous planes. Undue tension on the margins of the flap must be avoided; it may necessitate undermining of the tissues to reduce mechanical forces. The skin is optionally closed with subcuticular 4–0 synthetic absorbable sutures or stainless steel staples.

Following completion of wound closure, both catheters are irrigated copiously with saline to ensure patency and are connected and maintained on low to moderate continuous suction provided by reservoir portable vacuum bottles. Light bulky dressings of gauze are placed over the dissection site and taped securely in place with occlusive dressings. The surgeon may elect to place the ipsilateral arm in a sling to provide immobilization. From Bland KI, Copeland EM III (eds) (1991) *The Breast: Comprehensive Management of Benign and Malignant Diseases*, p. 621. Philadelphia: WB Saunders.

sutures slide easily and can be removed within one week of operation. Drains are removed usually 5–10 days postoperative when less than 30 ml over 24 hours is drained from each catheter. This technique obviates the need for wound binder or compression drawings.

Simple (Total) Mastectomy

Another version of modified radical mastectomy consists of complete removal of the breast without dissection of the axillary lymph nodes. The technique for simple (total) mastectomy is identical to the initial maneuvers of the modified radical mastectomy until that portion of the procedure when the breast is reflected along the lateral border of the pectoralis major and serratus anterior muscles (*Figure 25.8*). At this point, dissection is continued anterior to the intercostal brachial nerves to join the medioanterior border of the latissimus dorsi muscle. Two drains are placed inferiomedially and laterally. Patients with simple mastectomy do not sustain anesthesia of the inner arm, transient shoulder dysfunction or arm edema. In addition, they infrequently develop a seroma. Simple mastectomy has been the classical therapy for patients with ductal carcinoma *in situ* (DCIS). It has also provided effective disease control for patients who develop local recurrence following breast-conservation treatment.

Complications

Intraoperative complications

These include vascular and nerve damage, and rarely occur. They are easily identified and repaired. Immediate postoperative complications, such as pulmonary and myocardial events may occur, but are extremely infrequent due to the nature of the operation: short operating time, superficial procedure, and early ambulation.

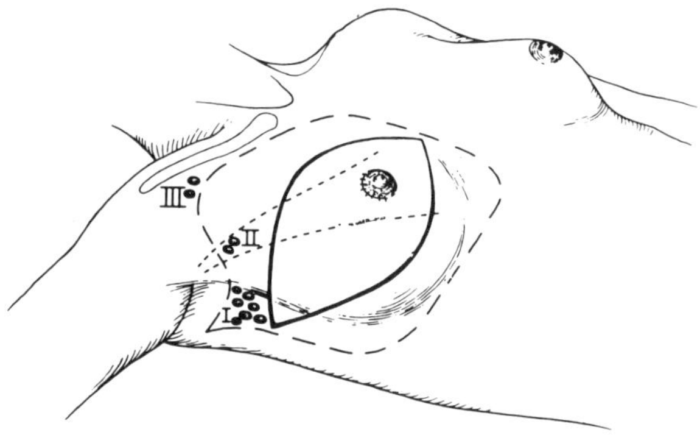

Figure 25.8. Limits of dissection for the extended simple mastectomy (dotted line). The dissection is inclusive of tumor and overlying skin, with an adequate skin margin to allow primary wound closure. Only Level I and lower Level II nodes are dissected *en bloc* with the breast. Modified from Bland KI, Copeland EM III (eds) (1991) *The Breast: Comprehensive Management of Benign and Malignant Diseases*, p. 654. Philadelphia: WB Saunders.

Early complications

These include infection, skin necrosis or seroma and are transient and easily treatable. Perioperative antibiotics are not used except in patients with a recent biopsy, personal history of diabetes mellitus, vasculitis, pre-existing infection or heart valve problem. The bacterium responsible for the wound infection is frequently *Staphylococcus aureus*. Antibiotics are effective in the therapy of post-operative cellulitis. Incision and drainage are rarely required to control the wound infection.

Flap necrosis occurs rarely. It results with tension of the skin closure, thin skin flaps or tight pressure dressings. Most skin necrosis is confined to small areas around the incision, which can be treated by local debridement and will heal with secondary intention (granulation). Wide excision and skin grafting are rarely necessary.

Seroma of the axilla and occasionally of the chest wall may occur following removal of the drains. Initially, seroma is best managed by frequent aspiration and by decreasing shoulder exercise via immobilization slings. However, repeated aspirations are inconvenient to the patient, increase the chance of infection and predispose the patient to long-term lymphedema of the arm. Recurrent prolonged seroma formation suggests open disruption of lymphatic channels as a consequence of nonadherence of skin flaps or proximal obstruction of residual lymphatics. Recurrent seromas often necessitate reinsertion of closed-suction systems.

Long-term complications

These include lymphedema of the arm or postmastectomy pain, which can be late manifestations of the operation. Lymphedema is prevalent and marked when complete (Levels I–III) axillary dissection and radiation to the axilla are combined. Lymphedema is also increased if there is wound infection or excessive exercise or injury of the arm. Any signs of swelling of the chest wound, axilla, or arm should be treated promptly and aggressively to minimize the extent of the swelling. Caution should be taken to avoid heavy lifting, venepuncture, or constrictive pressure of the arm and hand.

The other significant complaint is recurrent pain of the chest wall and axilla. This is usually associated with neuroma formation of sensory cutaneous nerves divided during axillary lymph node dissection. Excision is occasionally helpful for symptomatic relief; consistent, effective treatment is not available.

Lumpectomy and Axillary Dissection

Lumpectomy and axillary dissection are an alternative conservation therapeutic approach to modified radical mastectomy for patients with Stage I and II breast cancer. This breast-conservation surgery offers a superior cosmetic appearance and equivalent cancer control rates when compared to radical procedures. Radiation of the intact breast is an essential part of the treatment plan; this modality addresses the multicentric nature of the disease. Proper selection of patients for breast conservation is the key determinant of the treatment results, both tumor control and cosmetic appearance. Other critical considerations include appropriate design of the incision site and achieving tumor-free margins in the lumpectomy specimen. Important factors that influence the decision-making process and tumor control are summarized below:

- The size of the tumor and its anatomic location within the breast. If the diameter of the tumor is greater than 5 cm or its size is disproportionally large relative to the size of the breast or its particular location is unfavorable, modified radical mastectomy is advised over lumpectomy and axillary dissection.
- Multicentric cancers in different quadrants of the breast, as evidenced by palpable masses or mammography. This condition favors modified radical mastectomy.
- Persistent tumor involvement of the margins of the specimens with attempts at wide re-excision. This condition necessitates modified radical mastectomy because this presentation is indicative of multifocal disease within the index quadrant.
- Extensive DCIS implies that greater than 25% of the tumor involvement in the index quadrant of an invasive cancer has *in situ* features. Treatment of this condition by lumpectomy and

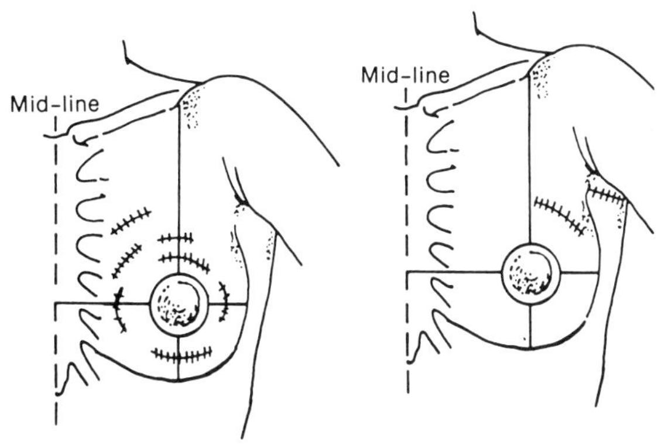

Figure 25.9. Recommended incisions. From Bland KI, Copeland EM III (eds) (1991) *The Breast: Comprehensive Management of Benign and Malignant Diseases*, p. 639. Philadelphia: WB Saunders.

axillary dissection has been reported to have a high incidence of locoregional failure, especially in younger women (<35 years) (Recht *et al.*, 1988).

- Lack of an adequate radiation facility or unfavorable patient factors such as non-compliance, fear of radiation, excessive obesity, or autoimmune collagen vascular disease. These factors suggest the necessity for modified radical mastectomy.
- Pregnancy and previous irradiation treatment to the breast. These conditions require modified radical mastectomy as the choice of therapeutic option.
- Patient preference in selecting the type of surgery.

Operative technique

Important technical issues in lumpectomy include placement of the incision, obtaining tumor-free margins and orientation of the tumor. Placement of the skin incision relies on four major points:

- A curvilinear skin incision following Langer's line is preferred in a majority of the cases (*Figure 25.9*). Radical incision at low mid-breast of mid-inner breast gives better cosmetic results and incorporates the biopsy scar.
- The incision should be placed relatively close to the tumor (*Figure 25.10*).
- The incision should be placed so that it can be incorporated into a mastectomy incision, if necessary.
- In the case of re-excision, a small elliptical section of skin surrounding the biopsy scar can be removed *en bloc* with the excised breast tissue.

The extent of the lumpectomy has also been debated (Olivotto *et al.*, 1989). It varies from quadrantectomy to wide excision to tumorectomy. In clinical practice, a margin of 1 cm is considered adequate. Removal of excessive breast tissue is cosmetically undesirable and therapeutically unnecessary (Chu *et al.*, 1984; Clarke *et al.*, 1985). A wider margin or mastectomy is preferred for patients with extensive invasive cancer (Recht and Harris, 1990; Vicini *et al.*, 1991). In the case of re-excision, the entire cavity is removed with 1 cm of normal tissue at the involved margin. Surface inking and/or suture/clip placement about the specimen is necessary for orientation of margins to be evaluated by the pathologist (*Figures 25.11 and 25.12*). A frozen section may not be needed when snap-frozen tissue (−70° Celsius) is being preserved to determine the estrogen receptor (ER) and progesterone receptor (PR) content. The tissue should be handled expeditiously to decrease the time of warm ischemia, which can artificially decrease the ER value (Clark *et al.*, 1976; Rosenthal, 1979; Bloom *et al.*, 1984; Ellis *et al.*, 1989a and b). Hemostasis is critical, as drainage of the lumpectomy site is discouraged. Subcutaneous closure and subcuticular skin closure result in a good cosmetic appearance.

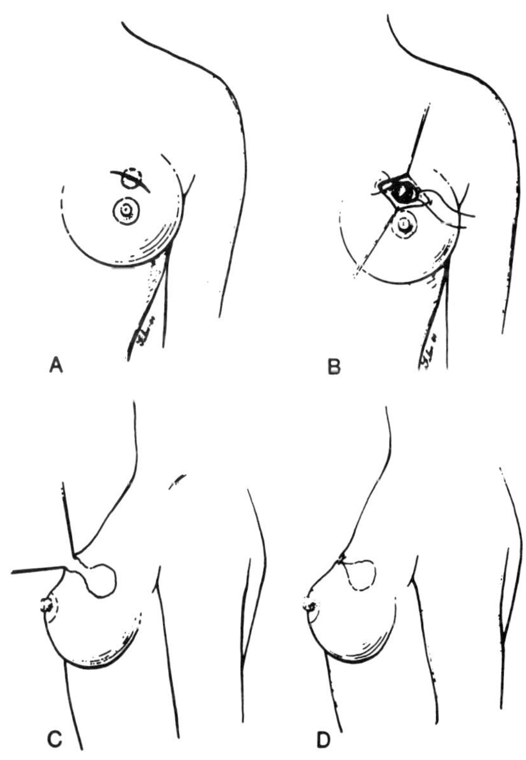

Figure 25.10. Techniques of lumpectomy. From Bland KI, Copeland EM III (eds) (1991) *The Breast: Comprehensive Management of Benign and Malignant Diseases*, p. 640. Philadelphia: WB Saunders. A, Skin incision; B, Excision biopsy; C, Biopsy cavity; D, Wound closure.

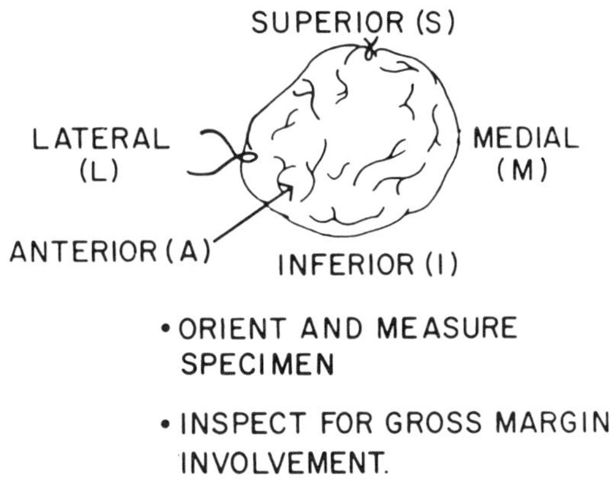

Figure 25.11. Orientation of the lumpectomy specimen. Modified from Bland KI, Copeland EM III (eds) (1991) *The Breast: Comprehensive Management of Benign and Malignant Diseases*, p. 641. Philadelphia: WB Saunders.

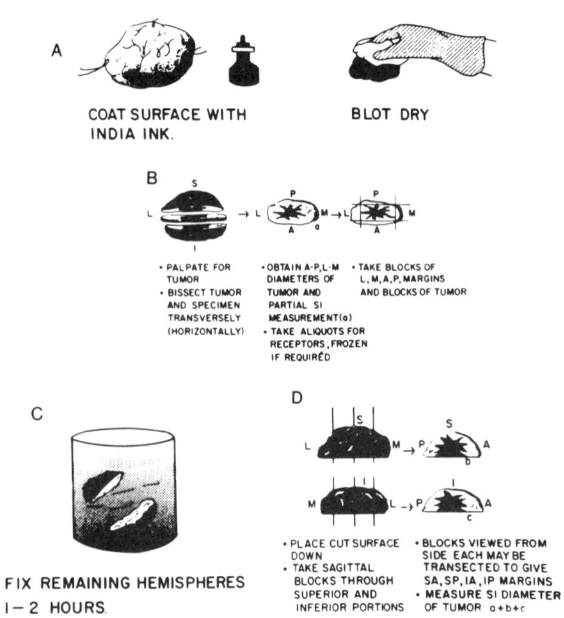

Figure 25.12. Preparation of specimen for determination of margin involvement. **A**. Application of India ink. **B**. Taking of blocks. **C**. Fixing tissue for additional blocks. **D**. Taking further blocks. From Bland KI, Copeland EM III (eds) (1991) *The Breast: Comprehensive Management of Benign and Malignant Diseases*, p. 641. Philadelphia: WB Saunders.

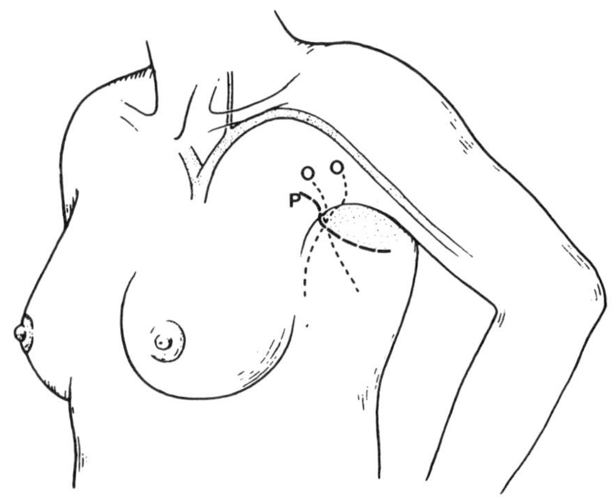

Figure 25.13. Illustration of preferred (P) and optional (O) incisions used in axillary dissection. Ideally, incisions are placed in skin folds that parallel Langer's lines. Incisions are preferably curvilinear with placement just caudal to the hairline of the axilla. Incisions depicted are oblique or vertically placed with the chest wall. As these O incisions cross the lines of tension (Langer's lines), delay in wound repair and inferior cosmetic results may be observed. From Bland KI, Copeland EM III (eds) (1991) *The Breast: Comprehensive Management of Benign and Malignant Diseases*, p. 582. Philadelphia: WB Saunders.

Axillary dissection is performed for staging purposes and to ensure control of regional disease. Two technical concerns include selection of the incision and the extent of the lymphadenectomy. In general, two separate incisions are made for the lumpectomy and axillary dissection. A variety of incisions have been used: the 'S'-shaped, vertical, and transverse. The transverse incision is used most frequently and is preferred by the authors (*Figure 25.13*). This incision is placed at the lower axilla inferior to the hair line extending from just posterior to the pectoralis major muscle to the anterior border of the latissimus dorsi muscle. Thick (6–8 mm) superior and inferior skin flaps are developed for a length of approximately 5 cm in each direction. The borders of the two muscles are delineated longitudinally throughout the wound. The remaining nodal dissection is essentially the same as described previously. Levels I and II lymph node dissections can be performed without sacrificing the pectoralis minor muscle. Drainage is required following a formal axillary dissection.

The major morbidities associated with axillary dissection are arm edema, nerve injury and shoulder dysfunction. Every effort should be made to diminish these untoward events. Minimal technical considerations that ensure postoperative neuromotor function include nerve identification and preservation, appropriate shoulder range of motion and the avoidance of infection, trauma and heavy lifting.

Several surgical issues in the local management of breast cancer deserve more detailed discussion. These are guidelines for re-excision of the lumpectomy site, contralateral biopsy and extent of the nodal dissection.

Re-excision

When biopsy is the initial procedure, three types of tumor biopsy margins exist: a negative margin (tumor greater than 2 mm from all inked margins);

a close margin (tumor less than or equal to 2 mm from the margin); and a positive margin (tumor at the margin). Surgeons are faced with deciding whether to remove more tissue. Frazier *et al.* (1989) reported that approximately 30% of the patients with negative or close margins had residual disease and 32.5% of the patients with involved margins had no residual tumor. They felt that pathologic margins were not the best guidelines for re-excision. In contrast, a subsequent study by Gwin *et al.* (1993) showed that 65% of the patients with positive margins had residual carcinoma and that 50% of these patients had invasive cancer. Although only 20% of the patients with close margins had residual tumor, all had either purely invasive cancer or invasive cancer associated with noninvasive components. These data suggest that patients with positive margins should, at the minimum, undergo re-excision to achieve an acceptable margin. Patients with close margins, particularly those with T2 tumors and those with poorly differentiated tumors, should also have additional local excision to minimize potential recurrence. An inadequate margin was reported to increase the local recurrence in patients receiving breast conservation surgery and radiation treatment (Ghossein *et al.*, 1992). With increasing volumes of tumor excised, recurrence was diminished.

Contralateral biopsy

Bilateral breast cancer occurs with a cumulative incidence of 5–20% (Fisher *et al.*, 1984; Fracchia *et al.*, 1985). It is important to recognize the risk and obtain an early diagnosis. Random biopsy of the contralateral breast is not indicated in most cases, including cases of infiltrating ductal cancer (IDC), DCIS, and lobular cancer *in situ* (LCIS). With IDC and DCIS, synchronous invasive lesions are poorly detected by nondirected biopsy (Moffat *et al.*, 1988; Carson *et al.*, 1994). LCIS is considered a marker for increased risk, but is clinically not to be considered a malignant or premalignant condition. Random biopsy of the contralateral breast in general, neither adds information nor alters the management plan. Patients with infiltrating lobular cancer (ILC), on the contrary, are at increased risk for synchronous bilateral breast cancer. Simkovich *et al.* (1993) reported that 10% of these patients were found by random biopsy of the contralateral breast to have invasive cancer, and an additional 6% were diagnosed with DCIS. Invasive cancer was observed in the contralateral breast at an increased frequency (24%) when the original lobular breast cancer harbored a multicentric component.

Extent of axillary dissection

Axillary lymph nodes are resected concomitant with definitive therapy of the primary breast cancer for the four following reasons:

- to allow proper staging;
- to provide useful prognostic information;
- to serve as a guide for subsequent treatment;
- for potential therapeutic benefit.

Axillary lymph node dissection (ALND) is recommended for all patients with invasive breast cancer. One may consider other alternatives for elderly patients with a guarded medical condition, or elderly with a dysfunctional shoulder, particularly if the tumor is small or the patient refuses node dissection.

In the absence of gross involvement of lymph nodes at Level III or of the highest node at Level II, axillary dissection including Levels I and II is considered optimal. Selective arguments to support Level I and II lymph node dissections are summarized as follows.

- Studies confirm that the total number of lymph nodes removed and the number of lymph nodes pathologically involved by cancer are critical for accurate staging, assessing prognosis, and establishment of the treatment plan (Fisher and Slack, 1970; Rosen *et al.*, 1983; Fisher *et al.*, 1993). Complete Level I and II dissections provide a sufficient number of lymph nodes for pathologic evaluation. Ideally, a minimum of ten nodes should be retrieved to ensure accurate pathologic staging of the axilla.
- 'Skip' metastasis was reported to be only 1% at Level III if the lower levels had no evidence of disease (Rosen *et al.*, 1983). Therefore, nodal staging achieved by Level I and II axillary dissections is highly accurate; nodal disease progression appears to be from echelon to echelon (e.g. Level I to Level II to Level III).
- In the absence of extracapsular tumor and numerous nodal metastases, Level I and II nodal dissections provide adequate regional control. When nodal disease is extensive, Level I and II nodal dissections are still appropriate unless the apical lymph nodes are grossly metastatic. Surgical resection provides superior regional control to chemotherapy and/or irradiation. Patients with extensive lymph node metastases should receive irradiation to the axilla and chest wall to reduce the high failure rates at these sites. The combination of radiation and full axillary dissection (Levels I–III) is most likely to result in marked edema of the chest and arm (Balch *et al.*, 1993) and should be avoided whenever possible.
- In addition to facilitating regional control, axillary dissection may improve survival rates of select subsets of patients (Pickren, 1961). Minimal microscopic nodal metastases discovered by serial sectioning when excised, were not shown to adversely affect survival in these patients compared to patients with truly negative

nodes (Wilkinson *et al.*, 1982). This implies that surgical removal of microscopically involved nodes provides therapeutic benefit.

Radiation Therapy

Radiation therapy is a crucial part of successful breast conservation treatment (Harris *et al.*, 1990; Wood *et al.*, 1991). Supervoltage radiation is directed to the whole breast in a dose of 45–50 Gy delivered in 4.5–5 weeks. The need for a radiation boost to the tumor bed is controversial. Patients with microscopic involvement of the margins may be treated with 'boost' irradiation both to the tumor bed and to several centimeters of margin. The radiation boost dose of 10–16 Gy is usually delivered in 5–8 fractions.

The axilla is not routinely irradiated if dissection of Levels I and II has been performed. An exception includes pathologic evidence of extracapsular extension of disease. Patients with numerous pathologically positive axillary lymph nodes or medial lesions have an increased risk for internal mammary and supraclavicular lymph nodes. Some radiotherapists favor radiation of these nodes to prevent subsequent regional site recurrence. Significant irradiation to the heart and lungs should be avoided.

Complications from radiation are infrequent when a proper conventional technique and adequate doses are used. Possible complications of this modality are carcinogenesis, decreased arm mobility, breast fibrosis, brachial plexopathy, radiation pneumonitis, late cardiac effect and arm edema.

Cosmetic Aspects of Breast Cancer Treatment

Cosmetic Results after Lumpectomy and Axillary Dissection

Approximately 90% of the patients treated with lumpectomy and axillary dissection have good-to-excellent cosmetic results over a long-term follow-up. Important surgical considerations include selection of the incision and avoiding removal of excessive uninvolved breast tissue to enhance cosmesis. The important radiation considerations are the accurate direction of radiation to the breast with a total dose limit of 50 Gy and the avoidance of axillary radiation in patients who have had extensive nodal dissection. This latter group includes patients treated with total ALND (Levels I–III). Concomitant chemotherapy combined with radiotherapy may increase breast fibrosis and should be avoided if possible.

Breast Reconstruction after Mastectomy

Breast reconstruction should be offered and explained to mastectomy patients. Unless patients do not desire reconstruction, consultation with a plastic surgeon is helpful in understanding the different methods of reconstruction and in timing the reconstructive surgery. Patients without advanced disease may have the reconstruction performed concomitant with mastectomy. The advantages of immediate reconstruction are those of skin preservation, one operation and hospitalization, as well as minimizing the emotional impact and suffering with the loss of a breast. The disadvantage of simultaneous reconstruction is a prolonged operative time. Most patients and surgeons prefer a staged approach, with the reconstruction procedure performed following completion of all therapeutic treatments. Certain patients, such as those with a high risk of local recurrence (e.g. advanced primary or extensive regional disease) may defer their reconstruction for two or more years.

The mastectomy site(s) may be reconstructed with either autologous tissues (myocutaneous flaps) or prostheses. Saline prosthesis has been gaining popularity over the silicone gel implant, which has the alleged risk of autoimmune disease and connective tissue disorders. To date, no conclusive objective evidence exists to support this claim. However, a systematic long-term follow-up of silicon gel prosthesis is warranted, to identify the types and frequency of any complications, as well as to understand the roles and mechanisms of prostheses to induce health hazards. The Food & Drug Administration (FDA) listed an additional six risk factors that are possibly associated with the use of silicone in inflatable breast prostheses. These risks include fibrous capsular contracture, leaks, infection, interference with early breast tumor detection, possible carcinogenicity and teratogenicity. Such allegations for the risk of prostheses are presently unfounded and are not supported by conclusive objective data. Therefore, these prosthetic materials are still being offered to patients who desire reconstruction following mastectomy.

An alternative method of breast reconstruction involves myocutaneous flaps transferred by a rotational or free-flap technique. The two muscles most commonly used are the transverse rectus abdominus myocutaneous (TRAM) flap and the latissimus dorsi myocutaneous flap. The advantages of flaps over prosthetic implants include the avoidance of any foreign materials in the body and the high probability of a durable and excellent cosmetic result. The disadvantages of using autologous flaps include the significantly longer operative period for reconstruction and the increased risk of complications at the donor or recipient tissue sites. Patients who cannot tolerate prolonged anesthesia or flap-related complications should be excluded from consideration of reconstruction.

Treatment Selection

Carcinoma in situ

The concept of *in situ* carcinoma of the breast was first introduced in the pathology literature by Broders in 1932. Subsequently, two types of *in situ* cancer have been identified, ductal (DCIS) and lobular (LCIS), depending on the cytologic features and patterns of growth. LCIS is a disease of small lobular ducts and lobules. DCIS is confined to the lactiferous or terminal ducts without invasion of the basement membrane or of the surrounding stroma.

Lobular cancer *in situ*

LCIS constitutes 30–50% of *in situ* breast cancers. This pathologic variant represents an increased risk (marker) for developing further breast cancer; the risk is estimated to be 20–30% in 15–20 years following diagnosis. Both breasts are at equal risk. Because of the bilaterality, multifocality, multicentricity, and nonmalignant nature of LCIS, close observation is recommended for life by most North American and European clinics. Obtaining a tumor-free margin for LCIS is not necessary, nor is axillary dissection. Irradiation is not advised. Ipsilateral mastectomy only reduces one-half of the risk. Contralateral biopsy is generally not helpful in changing the risk assessment and treatment plan, and is infrequently practiced today. Bilateral mastectomy may occasionally be performed in patients with an excessively high risk, especially a family history. Subcutaneous mastectomy is inadequate for eliminating the risk because this ill-conceived procedure leaves large volumes of residual breast tissue at risk for carcinogenesis.

Ductal cancer *in situ*

DCIS is a premalignant condition. Without treatment, invasive cancer will develop in the involved breast in approximately one-third of the patients within 5–10 years. DCIS accounts for 20% of all breast cancers. Its significant features include histologic heterogeneity, multifocality or diffuse presentation, and microinvasion. The conventional treatment for DCIS has been simple mastectomy. Axillary dissection is not part of the treatment because of a low incidence of nodal involvement (approximately 1.5%). The overall survival of DCIS patients following simple (total) mastectomy is estimated to be 99%.

Recently, breast conservation surgery for DCIS has been studied. For patients treated with lumpectomy and radiation treatment, the ten-year survival rate was 94%, and the local recurrence rate was 16% (Solin *et al.*, 1991). Bornstein *et al.* (1991) observed an eight-year local recurrence rate of 27%. In a prospective, randomized study, Fisher *et al.* (1993) reported a five-year local recurrence rate of 7% in patients who received radiation and lumpectomy. In patients with lumpectomy alone, the National Surgical Adjuvant Breast and Bowel Project (NSABP) reported a recurrence rate of 16.4%, suggesting that additional irradiation is an effective adjunct to conservative surgery for controlling DCIS. A follow-up well in excess of five years is necessary to document the true recurrence rate, because DCIS usually recurs after 5–10 years follow-up.

Schuh *et al.* (1986) found that patients with DCIS and microinvasion had much worse prognoses than patients with DCIS but without microinvasion. A high local recurrence rate of 20% and nodal metastasis of 20%, distant metastasis of 23%, and a death rate of 13% indicate that this condition should be optimally treated as invasive disease.

Invasive Breast Carcinoma

Early operable breast cancer

Public awareness of breast cancer and a wider application of mammography has resulted in frequent detection of Stage I and II breast cancers. Multiple prospective randomized trials have clearly demonstrated equivalent therapeutic results from modified radical mastectomy and breast conserving treatment in appropriately selected and staged patients (*Table 25.1*). Overall, survival and disease-free survival were statistically similar between the two treatments in all studies (*Table 25.2*). Among these trials, the local recurrences reported for breast conservation treatment were 4–19% and for mastectomy were 2–9%. More than one-half of the patients with breast recurrence were salvaged by total mastectomy. On the contrary, chest wall recurrence following mastectomy was an ominous sign of locoregional and systemic disease.

Among prospective randomized studies, the NSABP trial appears to be a landmark study. It had the largest sample size among similar studies. It set the surgical standards for removal of breast cancer; namely, the importance of tumor-free margins and conservative removal of normal breast tissue around the cancerous mass. This group demonstrated that radiation treatment to the whole breast is sufficient in most of the cases. Routine boost irradiation to the tumor bed and the lymph nodes are not necessary. Adjuvant systemic therapy in patients with positive lymph nodes concomitantly receiving irradiation was another important concept. Recently,

Table 25.1. Prospective randomized trials comparing mastectomy and breast-conservation treatment of primary operable breast cancer (from Winchester and Cox, 1992). (MRM, modified radical mastectomy; L, lumpectomy; Q, quadranectomy; RM, radical mastectomy; AD, axillary dissection; WE, wide excision.)

				Breast conservation		
Studies	*No. of patients*	*Maximum tumor size (cm)*	*Mastectomy*	*Surgery*	*Radiation therapy (Gy) (breast/boost)*	*References*
National Surgical Adjuvant Breast and Bowel Project (NSABP)	1219	4	MRM	L/AD	50/0	Fisher *et al.*, 1989
National Cancer Institute (NCI) (Milan)	701	2	RM	Q/AD	50/10	Veronesi *et al.*, 1986
Institute Gustave Roussy	179	2	MRM	L/AD	45/15	Sarrazin *et al.*, 1989
Danish Breast	905	None	MRM	WE/AD	50/10–25	Blichert–Toft, 1990 Blichert–Toft *et al.*, 1988
National Cancer Institute (NCI) (USA)	237	5	MRM	L/AD	45–50/15–20	Bader *et al.*, 1987 Glatstein *et al.*, 1990

Table 25.2. Survival and disease-free survivals of mastectomy and breast conservation treatment in prospective randomized trials.

		Overall survival % (rate)		*Disease-free survival % (rate)*	
Studies	*Endpoint (yrs)*	*Mastectomy*	*Breast Conservation*	*Mastectomy*	*Breast Conservation*
National Surgical Adjuvant Breast and Bowel Project (NSABP)	8	71	76	58	59
National Cancer Institute (NCI) (Milan)	10	78	79	76	77
Institute Gustave Roussy	10	79	78	56	65
Danish Breast Cancer Group	6	82	79	66	70
National Cancer Institute (NCI) (USA)	8	79	85	76	66

NSABP studies have been criticized for the inclusion of ineligible patients. Statistical re-analysis of the data after exclusion of these patients are available. The National Cancer Institute, on initial review, predicts no invalidation of the overall results of these studies. Outcome data with long term follow-up are essential.

Locally advanced breast cancer

Locally advanced breast cancers (T3 or T4 tumors) with or without N2 or N3 nodal metastases are associated with a very poor prognosis. In recent years a multimodal approach in which chemotherapy-induced tumor cytoreduction before surgery and/or radiation has proven to be an effective modality to enhance locoregional control of advanced local disease.

Multimodality therapy

Most studies report an objective response rate of 70% and a complete response rate that ranges from 15–30% for patients receiving multi-drug chemotherapy (Hortobagyi *et al.*, 1988). Non-inflammatory breast cancer of advanced stage (Stage III disease) responded better than inflammatory breast cancer (Hobar *et al.*, 1988). The five-year disease-free survival rates following multimodality treatment are approximately 80% and 45% in patients with Stage IIIA and inflammatory breast cancer, respectively (Swain and Lippman, 1989; Moore *et al.*, 1991). This remains the accepted regimen for treating patients with locally advanced breast cancer.

It may be argued that patients with inflammatory breast cancer have a short survival span and therefore surgery should not be advocated. Recent studies, however, confirm that survival is enhanced by the multimodality approach. Median survival has been increased from 20 months to approximately 60 months (Hagelberg *et al.*, 1984; Israel *et al.*, 1986; Kinne, 1993), and the five-year survival increased from 10 to 40% or better (Maloisel *et al.*, 1990). However, histologic disease usually remains despite a complete cytoreductive clinical response to the preoperative chemotherapy regimen (Israel *et al.*, 1986; Burton *et al.*, 1987). Radiation is not an effective substitute for surgery (Schafer *et al.*, 1987; Donegan and Padrta, 1990; Kinne, 1993). Radiation and surgery, however, are additive modalities – each enhances the cytoreductive effect of the other therapy.

Mastectomy in patients with locally advanced breast cancer

The procedure of choice in patients with locally advanced breast cancer is modified radical mastectomy. This technique ensures maximal local and regional control of the cancer while providing an assessment of prognosis following a comprehensive pathologic review of the specimen. Radical mastectomy is rarely used, unless a lesser procedure cannot encompass the disease (e.g. T4 tumor, fixation to chest wall). Simple mastectomy is not appropriate, since it affords the patient less regional disease control and prognostication.

Survival after the first recurrence of locally advanced breast cancer is poor; the mean time to death is five months (Kinne, 1993). Therefore, every effort should be made to secure primary control of the disease. In the majority of studies, the most significant predictor of survival is the number of metastatic lymph nodes existing after induction chemotherapy (McCready *et al.*, 1989). The five-year survival rates are 70% in patients with no positive lymph nodes and 3% in patients with numerous metastatic nodes ($p < 0.01$, Cox proportional hazards). This prognostic information is available only when the modified radical mastectomy is performed following induction chemotherapy.

Follow-up After Primary Treatment

The primary goal of follow-up care is to detect early recurrent disease and new primary breast cancer (Wickerham *et al.*, 1984; Cady, 1990; Kinne, 1990). Timely intervention may make recovery possible. Another follow-up goal is the monitoring of any potential sequelae resulting from the primary therapy. Follow-up programs are slightly different for patients treated with mastectomy than for those treated with breast conservation methods. After mastectomy, it is sufficient to examine the patient with laboratory studies every 3–6 months and with chest radiography and mammography once a year. A bone scan in asymptomatic patients is unnecessary and cost-ineffective. The NSABP reported positive bone scans in 0.6% of 7984 patients with breast cancer who were asymptomatic for bone involvement (Wickerham *et al.*, 1984).

For patients treated with lumpectomy and radiotherapy, follow-up requires an ipsilateral mammography every six months for the first two years and subsequently annually. Contralateral mammography is also performed once a year. Breast examinations are typically repeated every three months for the first three years and every six months for an additional two years. After five years without recurrent disease (NED status, no evidence of disease), patients can be followed on a yearly basis. Any interval changes in the radiated breast, such as increased thickening of tissues, lumps, nodularities and mammographic abnormalities require prompt investigation.

Local recurrences in patients postmastectomy and in those with breast-conservation surgery imply different prognoses. The majority of lumpectomy patients with local tumor recurrence may be salvaged by simple (total) mastectomy. More than one-half of these patients so treated are alive without disease at five years (Recht *et al.*, 1989). In contrast, most mastectomy patients presenting with chest wall recurrence are observed to have objectively demonstrable concurrent metastases. Very few of these patients are candidates for wide resection, with or without irradiation, performed with curative intent. Because almost all of these patients will eventually develop metastases, systemic therapy should be considered in patients with postmastectomy chest wall recurrence (Aberizk *et al.*, 1986).

Summary of the Management of Breast Cancer

The framework for the diagnosis and management and breast cancer is summarized in *Figure 25.14*. Major goals for care of patients with breast cancer include:

- establishment of early and accurate tissue diagnosis;
- proper clinical pathologic staging of disease;
- provision of suitable multimodal therapy;
- enhancement of disease-free and overall survival.

The follow-up program incorporates a lifelong commitment to detect any new or recurrent cancer and to provide psychosocial and functional support to these patients.

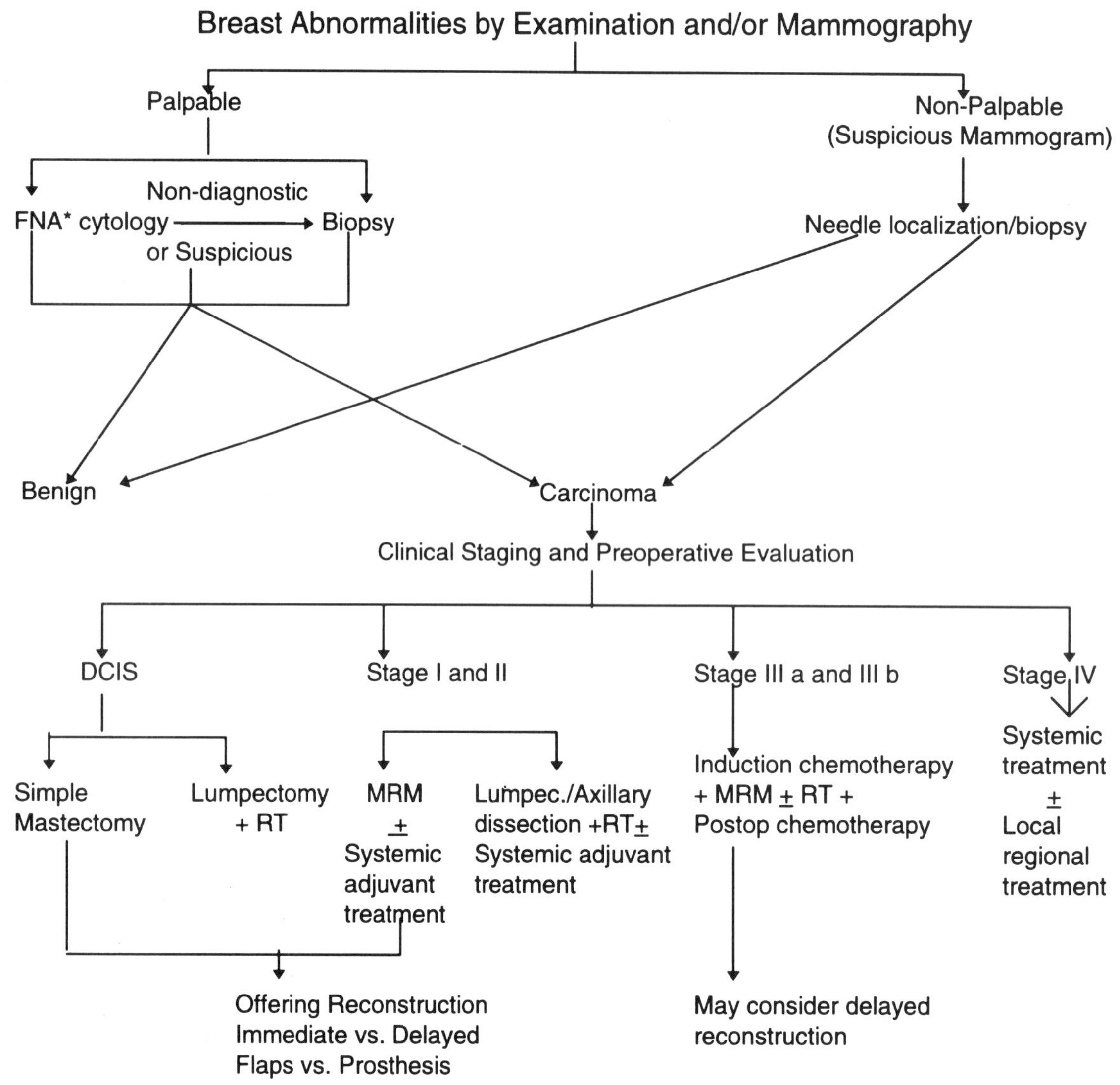

Figure 25.14. Algorithm for the management of breast carcinoma. (FNA, fine needle aspiration; DCIS, ductal carcinoma *in situ*, RT, radiation therapy; MRM, modified radical mastectomy.)

Summary of Core Information

- As a result of more frequent and rigorous mammographic screening, preinvasive breast neoplasia (carcinoma *in situ*) now accounts for up to 20% of breast malignancies. Approximately 30% of preinvasive breast carcinomas are lobular carcinoma *in situ*. The remaining preinvasive breast carcinomas (ductal carcinomas *in situ*) are pathologically heterogeneous.

- The clinical course and outcome of invasive breast carcinoma is extremely heterogeneous. The most powerful indices of prognosis (axillary lymph node status and tumor size) are determinants of disease extent or stage. Considerable clinical heterogeneity exists in node-positive breast cancer patients, roughly corresponding to axillary tumor burden (number of involved nodes).

- Although it is widely argued that gross involvement of resection margins correlates with local recurrence, considerably less is known about the significance of microscopic foci at or near the margins of resection. The current practice is to obtain microscopically tumor-free margins in breast-conservation surgery.

- Chest wall or cutaneous recurrences are not infrequent and are generally regarded as a manifestation of aggressive disease.

References

Aberizk WJ, Silver B, Henderson IC, Cady B & Harris JR (1986) The use of radiotherapy for treatment of isolated locoregional recurrence of breast carcinoma after mastectomy. *Cancer* **58:** 1214–1218.

Auchincloss H (1970) Modified mastectomy. *Am. J. Surg.* **119:** 506–509.

Bader J, Lippman ME, Swain SM *et al.* (1987) Preliminary report of the NCI early breast cancer (BC) study: A prospective randomized trial comparison of lumpectomy (L) and radiation (XRT) to mastectomy (M) for stage I and II BC. *Int. J. Radiat. Oncol. Biol. Phys.* **13(Suppl):** 160.

■ Balch C, Singletary E & Bland K (1993) Clinical decision-making in early breast cancer. *Ann. Surg.* **217:** 207–225.

Beahrs OH, Henson DE, Hutter RVP & Kennedy BJ (1988) *Manual for Staging of Cancer*, pp. 151–152. Philadelphia: JB Lippincott Company.

Blichert-Toft MA (1990) Danish randomized trial comparing breast conservation with mastectomy in mammary carcinoma. *Br. J. Cancer* **62(Suppl 12):** 15.

Blichert-Toft M, Brincker H, Andersen JA *et al.* (1988) A Danish randomized trial comparing breast-preserving therapy with mastectomy in mammary carcinoma. Preliminary results. *Acta Oncologica* **27:** 671–677.

Bloom ND, Johnson F, Pertshuck L & Fishman J (1984) Electrocautery: Effects on steroid receptors in human breast cancer. *J. Surg. Oncol.* **25:** 21–24.

■ Bornstein BA, Recht A, Connolly JL *et al.* (1991) Results of treating ductal carcinoma *in situ* of the breast with conservative surgery and radiation therapy. *Cancer* **67:** 7–13.

Broders AC (1932) Carcinoma *in situ* contrasted with benign penetrating epithelium. *JAMA* **99:** 1670–1674.

Burton GJ, Cox EB, Leight GS *et al.* (1987) Inflammatory breast cancer: effective multimodality approach. *Arch. Surg.* **122:** 1329–1332.

Cady B (1990) New diagnostic, staging, and therapeutic aspects of early breast cancer. *Cancer* **65:** 634–647.

Carson W, Sanchez-Forgach E, Stomper P *et al.* (1994) Lobular carcinoma *in situ*: observation without surgery as an appropriate therapy. *Ann. Surg. Oncol.* **1:** 141—146.

Chu AN, Cope O, Russo R & Lew R (1984) Patterns of local-regional recurrence and results in stages I and II breast cancer treated by irradiation following limited surgery. An update. *Am. J. Clin. Oncol. (CCT)* **7:** 221–229.

Clark JH, Erikson HA & Hardin JW (1976) Uterine receptor: Estradiol complexes and their interaction with nuclear binding sites. *J. Steroid Biochem.* **7:** 1039–1056.

Clarke DH, Le MG, Sarrazin D *et al.* (1985) Analysis of local-regional relapses in patients with early breast cancers treated by excision and radiotherapy: Experience of the Institut Gustave-Roussy. *Int. J. Radiat. Oncol. Biol. Phys.* **11:** 137–145.

Donegan WL & Padrta B (1990) Combined therapy for inflammatory breast cancer. *Arch. Surg.* **125:** 578–582.

Ellis LM, Wittliff JL, Bryant MS *et al.* (1989a) Lability of steroid hormone-receptors following devascularization of breast tumors. *Arch. Surg.* **124(1):** 39–42.

Ellis LM, Wittliff JL, Bryant MS *et al.* (1989b) Correlation of estrogen, progesterone and androgen receptor levels in breast cancer. *Am. J. Surg.* **157(6):** 577–581.

Fisher B & Slack NH (1970) Number of lymph nodes examined and the prognosis of breast carcinoma. *Surg. Gynecol. Obstet.* **131:** 79–88.

■ Fisher B, Costantino J, Redmond C *et al.* (1993) Lumpectomy compared with lumpectomy and radiation therapy for the treatment of intraductal breast cancer. *New Eng. J. Med.* **328:** 1581–1586.

■ Fisher B, Redmond C, Poisson R *et al.* (1989) Eight-year results of a randomized clinical trial comparing total mastectomy and lumpectomy with or without irradiation in the treatment of breast cancer. *New Eng. J. Med.* **320:** 822–828.

Fisher E, Fisher B, Sass R & Wickerham L (1984) Pathologic findings from the National Surgical Adjuvant Breast Project. (Protocol no. 4) XI: Bilateral breast cancer. *Cancer* **54:** 3002–3011.

Fracchia AA, Robinson D, Legaspi A *et al.* (1985) Survival in bilateral breast cancer. *Cancer* **55:** 1414–1421.

■ Frazier TG, Wong RWY & Rose D (1989) Implications of accurate pathologic margins in the treatment of primary breast cancer. *Arch. Surg.* **124:** 37–41.

■ Ghossein NA, Alpert S, Barba J *et al.* (1992) Breast cancer. Importance of adequate surgical excision prior to radiotherapy in the local control of breast cancer in patients treated conservatively. *Arch. Surg.* **127:** 411–415.

Glatstein E, Strauss K, Lichter A *et al.* (1990) Results of the NCI early breast cancer trial. *Proceedings of the NIH Consensus Development Conference*, June 18–21, pp. 32–33.

Gwin JL, Eisenberg BL, Hoffman JP *et al.* (1993) Incidence of gross and microscopic carcinoma in specimens from patients with breast cancer after re-excision lumpectomy. *Ann. Surg.* **218:** 729–734.

Hagelberg R, Jolly P & Anderson R (1984) Role of surgery in the treatment of inflammatory breast carcinoma. *Am. J. Surg.* **148:** 125–131.

Haagensen CD (1986) *Disease of the Breast.* Ed. 3. Philadelphia: WB Saunders.

Harris JR, Recht A, Connolly J *et al.* (1990) Conservative surgery and radiotherapy for early breast cancer. *Cancer* **66:** 1427–1438.

Hobar PC, Jones RC, Schouten J, Leitch AM & Hendler F (1988) Multimodality treatment of locally advanced breast carcinoma. *Arch. Surg.* **123:** 951–955.

Holleb AL (1992) Standards for breast-conservation treatment: A landmark report. *CA* **42:** 133–161.

■ Hortobagyi GN, Ames FC, Buzdar AU *et al.* (1988) Management of stage III primary breast cancer with primary chemotherapy, surgery, and radiation therapy. *Cancer* **62:** 2507–2516.

Israel L, Breau JL & Morere JF (1986) Two years of high dose cyclophosphamide and 5-fluorouracil followed by surgery after 3 months for acute inflammatory breast cancer. A phase II study of 25 cases with a median follow-up of 35 months. *Cancer* **57:** 24–28.

Kinne DW (1990) Staging and follow-up of breast cancer patients. *Cancer* **67(Suppl):** 1196–1198.

Kinne DW (1993) Controversies in primary breast cancer management. *Am. J. Surg.* **166:** 502–508.

Madden JL (1965) Modified radical mastectomy. *Surg. Gyn. Obst.* **121:** 1221–1230.

Maloisel F, Dufour P, Bergerat JP *et al.* (1990) Results of initial doxorubicin, 5-fluorouracil and cyclophosphamide combination chemotherapy for inflammatory carcinoma of the breast. *Cancer* **65:** 851–855.

McCready DR, Hortobagyi GN, Kau SW *et al.* (1989) The prognostic significance of lymph node metastases after preoperative chemotherapy for locally advanced breast cancer. *Arch. Surg.* **124:** 21–25.

Moffat FL, Ketcham AS, Robinson DS, Legaspi A & Irani H (1988) Breast cancer: management of the opposite breast. *Oncol.* **2:** 25–30.

Moore MP, Ihde JK, Crowe JP, Hakes TP & Kinne DW (1991) Inflammatory breast cancer. *Arch. Surg.* **126:** 304–306.

Olivotto IA, Rose MA, Osteen RI *et al.* (1989) Late cosmetic outcome after conservative surgery and radiotherapy: analysis of causes of cosmetic failure. *Int. J. Radiat. Oncol. Biol. Phys.* **17:** 747–753.

Patey DH (1967) A review of 146 cases of carcinoma of the breast operated on between 1930 and 1943. *Br. J. Cancer* **21:** 260–269.

Patey DH & Dyson WH (1948) The prognosis of carcinoma of the breast in relation to the type of operation performed. *Br. J. Cancer* **2:** 71–80.

Pickren JW (1961) Significance of occult metastases – a study of breast cancer. *Cancer* **14:** 1266–1271.

Recht A & Harris JA (1990) Selection of patients with early stage breast cancer for conservative surgery and radiation. *Oncol.* **4:** 23–30.

Recht A, Siddon RL, Kaplan WD, Andersen JW & Harris JR (1988) Three-dimensional internal mammary lymphoscintigraphy: implications for radiation therapy treatment planning for breast carcinoma. *Int. J. Radiat. Oncol. Biol. Phys.* **14(3):** 477–481.

Recht A, Schnitt SJ, Connolly JL *et al.* (1989) Prognosis following local or regional recurrence after conservative surgery and radiotherapy for early stage breast carcinoma. *Int. J. Radiat. Oncol. Biol. Phys.* **16:** 3–9.

Rosen PP, Lesser ML, Kinne DW & Beattie EJ (1983) Discontinuous or "skip" metastases in breast carcinoma. Analysis of 1228 axillary dissections. *Ann. Surg.* **197:** 276–283.

Rosenthal LJ (1979) Discrepant estrogen receptor protein levels according to surgical technique. *Am. J. Surg.* **138:** 681–689.

Sarrazin D, Le MG, Arriagada R *et al.* (1989) Ten-year results of a randomized trial comparing a conservative treatment to mastectomy in early breast cancer. *Radiother. Oncol.* **14:** 177–184.

Schafer P, Alberto P, Forni M *et al.* (1987) Surgery as part of a combined modality approach for inflammatory breast carcinoma. *Cancer* **59:** 1063–1067.

Schuh ME, Nemoto T, Penetrante RB, Rosner D & Dao TL (1986) Intraductal carcinoma. Analysis of presentation, pathologic findings, and outcome of disease. *Arch. Surg.* **121:** 1303–1307.

Simkovich AH, Sclafani LM, Masri M & Kinne DW (1993) Role of contralateral breast biopsy in infiltrating lobular cancer. *Surgery* **114:** 555–557.

Solin LJ, Recht A, Fourquet A *et al.* (1991) Ten-year results of breast-conserving surgery and definitive irradiation for intraductal carcinoma (ductal carcinoma *in situ*) of the breast. *Cancer* **68:** 2337–2344.

Swain SM & Lippman ME (1989) Systemic therapy of locally advanced breast cancer: review and guidelines. *Oncol.* **3:** 21–30.

Veronesi U, Banfi A, Del Vecchio M *et al.* (1986) Comparison of Halsted mastectomy with quadrantectomy, axillary dissection, and radiotherapy in early breast cancer: long-term results. *Eur. J. Cancer Clin. Oncol.* **22:** 1085–1089.

■ Vicini FA, Eberlein TJ, Connolly JL *et al.* (1991) The optimal extent of resection for patients with stages I or II breast cancer treated with conservative surgery and radiotherapy. *Ann. Surg.* **214:** 200–204.

Wickerham L, Fisher B & Cronin W (1984) The efficacy of bone scanning in the follow-up of patients with operable breast cancer. *Breast Cancer Res. Treat.* **4:** 303–307.

Wilkinson EJ, Hause LL, Hoffman RG *et al.* (1982) Occult axillary lymph node metastases in invasive breast carcinoma: Characteristics of the primary tumor and significance of the metastases. *Pathol. Ann.* **17:** 67–91.

Wilson RE, Donegan WL, Mettlin C *et al.* (1984) The 1982 national survey of carcinoma of the breast in the United States by the American College of Surgeons. *Surg. Gynecol. Obstet.* **159:** 309–318.

Winchester DD & Cox JD (1992) Standards for breast-conservation treatment. *CA – A Cancer Journal for Clinicians* **42(no 3):** 134–162.

Wood WC, Barringer TA, Daly JM *et al.* (1991) Treatment of early stage breast cancer. NIH Consensus Conference. *JAMA* **265:** 391–395.

26 Primary and Adjuvant Radiotherapy of Breast Cancer

M M Salter
R L S Jennelle

Breast Conservation

The traditional approach to breast cancer has been a surgical approach changing from radical mastectomy to modified radical mastectomy (MRM) in the 1970s. The 1980s brought conservation surgery and radiation as a definitive therapeutic option for many patients presenting with Stage I or II carcinoma of the breast. In June 1990, the National Institute of Health sponsored a consensus development conference on the treatment of early stage carcinoma of the breast. The panel concluded that "breast conservation treatment is an appropriate method of primary therapy for a majority of women with Stage I–II breast cancer and is preferable because it provides survival rates equivalent to those of total mastectomy and axillary dissection while preserving the breast" (NIH Consensus Conference, 1991). Despite this, a recent study revealed that a range of only 7–50% of women with early stage disease undergo breast preservation surgery.

Many retrospective European and North American trials using breast preservation and radiation therapy demonstrated that survival at 5–10 and 15 years was equal to that of mastectomy (Ray *et al.*, 1983; Harris *et al.*, 1981; Veronesi *et al.*, 1990; Pierquin *et al.*, 1991; Fowble *et al.*, 1991). Six prospective randomized trials have compared mastectomy and axillary dissection versus breast conserving surgery (Sarrazin *et al.*, 1989; Fisher *et al.*, 1992; Van Dongen *et al.*, 1992). These trials have shown no significant difference in the overall disease-free survival and distant disease-free survival.

Patient Selection

Who are candidates for breast preservation? Patients with clinical Stage I–II disease who will have an acceptable cosmetic result, a low risk of complications secondary to the radiotherapy and have a low risk for local recurrence are excellent candidates.

Tumor size and breast size

Primary tumor size includes any T1 or T2 tumor that can be adequately excised with clear margins. The related excision needs to be in proportion to the overall size of the breast. Initially, large pendulous breasts were felt to be a contraindication because of increased fibrosis and retraction. However, with proper treatment planning the result is often more pleasing than reconstruction and breast reduction mammoplasty.

Location

Tumors presenting in any quadrant and even centrally located tumors can be considered for breast conservation. The subareolar presentation requires excision of the nipple–areolar complex (Fowble *et al.*, 1992).

Contraindications to Breast Conservation

Underlying diseases

Collagen vascular disease (i.e. lupus, scleroderma) can lead to fibrosis, scarring and a painful breast when irradiated (Fleck *et al.*, 1989). Patients with these conditions are not candidates for breast conservation surgery. Uncontrolled severe diabetes, chronic obstructive pulmonary disease and myocardial disease with left breast cancer exclude breast conservation as a treatment choice. Uncooperative patients because of psychiatric disorders or dementia or for any reason are not candidates. Patients with a previous diagnosis of Hodgkin's disease or non-Hodgkin's lymphoma treated with irradiation to a supradiaphragmatic mantle and who develop breast cancer are not candidates for radiotherapy. Finally, pregnant patients whose radiation therapy cannot be delayed until after delivery are not candidates for breast conservation.

Age

Patient age has been a controversial issue with some retrospective data suggesting that there is an increased risk of local recurrence in women less than 35–40 years of age (Matthews *et al.*, 1988; Vicini *et al.*, 1990). Early information from the Joint Center for Radiation Therapy (JCRT) has suggested this greater risk is secondary to the increased presence of an extensive intraductal component in these young women and/or inadequate excision of the tumor (Recht, *et al.*, 1988). New data from this same institution (JCRT) and the University of Pennsylvania fail to reveal any significant difference in terms of survival, local control or regional control (Solin *et al.*, 1989). All of these patients had margins of resections known to be negative for tumor.

Multicentricity - possible contraindications

Patients who present with gross multicentric disease, clinically or mammographically, have an increased risk of local recurrence and are not candidates for breast conservation (Leopold *et al.*, 1989; Fowble *et al.*, 1993).

Histopathology

Patients with tumors that have an extensive intraductal component (EIC) have been thought to have a high local recurrence rate. What is EIC? It is simultaneous invasive carcinoma and an intraductal component of more than 25% of the primary tumor as well as intraductal carcinoma in the surrounding breast tissue away from the primary site. EIC may be related to age and is a pathologic predictor that the disease may be more extensive than clinically appreciated. Patients with EIC that has been completely excised with negative margins do not have an increased local recurrence rate and are candidates for breast conservation (Harris *et al.*, 1985). Other pathologic entities such as invasive lobular carcinoma and medullary or colloid carcinoma can be treated with breast conserving surgery and radiation (Weiss *et al.*, 1992). Nuclear grade, lymphatic or vascular invasion, and tumor necrosis have been implicated as bad pathologic predictors of local recurrence. At this time there is no consensus, and patients with any of the above components who have adequate local excision with negative margins should be considered as candidates for breast preservation.

Psychosocial

The psychosocial issues with regard to the patient's wishes and quality of life have been extensively reviewed. Making a decision when multiple treatment modalities are available with their accompanying risks and benefits is extremely difficult. The patient's active participation is required. There is no apparent proof for better psychologic adjustment in regard to changes of life patterns, fears, and concerns for mastectomy versus breast conservation. However, the women who have had breast conservation have better sexual functioning and preservation of body image (Kiebert *et al.*, 1991).

Surgical Factors

Surgical excision (i.e. wide local excision with a negative margin) is the optimal surgical intervention for removal of the primary tumor. Those patients who have had an incisional biopsy, unknown surgical margins, EIC with questionable margins or residual microcalcifications on mammograms (post-biopsy) should have re-excision for pathologic assessment and ultimate decision making. An axillary dissection separate from the primary site that includes Levels I–II appears not only to be adequate therapeutically and prognostically, but also produces less arm and breast edema than a complete axillary dissection (Solin *et al.*, 1988; Schmidt–Ullrich *et al.*, 1989; Vicini *et al.*, 1991; Solin *et al.*, 1991; Margolese, 1992).

Radiation Treatment

The radiation therapy delivery requires attention to detail and should be given only in facilities that understand the complexity of the total problem. Cooperation between the mammographer, pathologist, surgeon, radiation and medical oncologist is essential.

Equipment

Radiation therapy equipment including four or six MEV linear accelerators, simulator, and a treatment planning computer are necessary. Cobalt-60 (^{60}Co) is adequate in the absence of a linear accelerator. Excellent physics, dosimetry and a well-trained technical staff are essential.

Dose

Radiation treatment is delivered five days/week at a dose of 180–200 cGy/fraction for a total of 4500–5000 cGy in 4.5–5 weeks. The entire breast is treated with tangent or oblique fields, each field being treated daily.

Portals

A tissue compensator or wedges are used to ensure homogeneity of dose throughout the breast. The treatment field extends superiorly to the level of the sternoclavicular joint, inferiorly to 1.5 cm below the inframammary fold, medially to the midline and laterally to include the mid to posterior axillary line. The underlying chest wall, including muscles and ribs, is included. Careful treatment planning is essential to avoid excessive radiation to the underlying lung and to the heart if tumors are located within the left breast.

Boost dose

A boost dose of 1000–1500 cGy to the area of the primary tumor is common practice. This is usually given by means of external beam using appropriate energy electrons or interstitial iridium-192 (^{192}Ir) (Fowble *et al.*, 1989; Recht *et al.*, 1991). External beam boost is routinely done at the end of therapy, but the interstitial boost can be done at the time of the axillary dissection. The added dose is controversial in patients with negative margins and is currently being investigated in an EORTC trial.

Regional nodal irradiation

The irradiation of regional nodes in patients with a negative axillary dissection is not warranted. However, in patients with positive axillary nodes there is no consensus and this area remains controversial (Fowble *et al.*, 1989; Recht *et al.*, 1991).

Integration of Chemoradiotherapy

Adjuvant chemotherapy has become an essential part of the management of early stage breast cancer and has resulted in a decrease in the incidence of local breast recurrence when compared to that of surgery and radiation alone. The sequencing of chemoradiotherapy has been controversial and many schedules have been used (e.g. chemotherapy followed by radiotherapy, radiotherapy followed by chemotherapy, concomitant chemoradiotherapy or radiotherapy given in the middle of the chemotherapy regimen) (Recht *et al.*, 1992).

A small increase has been noted in complications (e.g. pneumonitis, rib fractures and poorer cosmesis) when concurrent chemotherapy is used (Danoff *et al.*, 1983; Abner *et al.*, 1991; Wazer *et al.*, 1992; Pierce *et al.*, 1992). There is no conclusive answer to the optimal sequence of therapy.

Local Recurrence

Local recurrence in the breast is a risk the patient must take if she chooses breast conservation. The 5–15 year local recurrence rates are now available from large studies and reveal a 5–10% recurrence rate at five years and a 10–20% recurrence rate at ten years with stabilization at 15 years. There are local regional recurrence rates post mastectomy and those studies available reveal no difference in the recurrence rate at ten years (10–20%) when compared to breast preservation studies (Clark *et al.*, 1982; Kurtz *et al.*, 1987; Pierquin *et al.*, 1991; Clark *et al.*, 1992). It is most important that patients who undergo breast-conserving therapy are followed-up with physical examinations and mammograms. Most often the recurrences will be found on physical examination with only one-third being detected solely by mammography (Stomper *et al.*, 1987; Kurtz *et al.*, 1989; Dershaw *et al.*, 1992; Vicini *et al.*, 1992). The median time to recurrence for a true or marginal recurrence is three years. The incidence of recurrence in a separate quadrant increases with time, and recurrences after ten years should be considered new tumors.

A palpable mass or induration during the immediate post-radiation time is usually resolving seroma or fat necrosis. Patients who recur have a 90% invasive histology and 85–90% of the patients are operable and present without distant metastases. The standard treatment is mastectomy with locoregional control in 90% of the patients (Fowble *et al.*, 1990).

The impact of local recurrence on ultimate survival is unclear. Most series demonstrate no statistical difference in survival between women who suffer a local recurrence after conservative therapy and those who do not (Calle *et al.*, 1986; Kurtz *et al.*, 1988; Haffty *et al.*, 1989; Haffty *et al.*, 1991; Van Dongen *et al.*, 1992). Other series have shown a decrease in survival when the recurrence occurred within the first five years (Kurtz *et al.*, 1990).

Ductal carcinoma *in situ*

Ductal carcinoma *in situ* (DCIS) comprises about 15% of all breast cancers and is defined as carcinoma confined to the pre-existing duct system of the breast without microscopic evidence of penetration of the basement membrane. Before the widespread use of screening mammography, DCIS was an infrequent diagnosis and was almost always associated with a palpable breast mass. The impact of screening has increased the frequency of this diagnosis and 20–30% of the lesions detected by this method are DCIS.

DCIS has traditionally been treated with mastectomy, either unilateral or bilateral. In a few instances local excision has been used. The concept of a lesser procedure for this disease has been reviewed and a randomized trial has been completed looking at wide excision plus radiation (National Surgical Adjuvant Breast Project (NSABP) B-17). In summary, the incidence of second ipsilateral tumors was significantly decreased by adding radiation therapy. Surgery followed by radiation is felt to be more appropriate than lumpectomy alone (Fisher *et al.*, 1993).

To further confuse the issue Lagios *et al.* have explored the use of excision alone in mammographically-detected lesions. Their results revealed a crude recurrence rate of 10.1% at four years and 14% actuarial at ten years. A majority of the recurrences were found mammographically with 50% being invasive cancer. The groups of patients met strict criteria – all lesions were mammographically detected, less than 2.5 cm, had negative margins of excision and there were no residual microcalcifications on post-biopsy mammography. Interestingly, the median tumor size was 5 mm. There was a 19% recurrence rate in lesions with high nuclear grade and comedo histologic subtype (Lagios *et al.*, 1989).

A collaborative analysis of cases of DCIS from nine institutions has a median follow-up of 18 months. Patients were treated with breast-conserving surgery and irradiation. The results revealed a cause-specific survival rate of 97% with a ten-year local failure rate of 16%, again with 50% of the recurrences being invasive cancer. This paper supports high overall survival, cause-specific survival, and freedom from distant metastasis (Solin *et al.*, 1991).

Because of the long natural history of DCIS, prolonged and careful follow-up is recommended. At this time breast-conserving surgery should be considered as an alternative to mastectomy for appropriately selected patients. With the many reports in the literature not comparable to one another the issue is indeed confusing and decisions still difficult.

Advanced Breast Cancer

Postmastectomy Adjuvant Radiotherapy

The routine use of postmastectomy radiotherapy is controversial. Papers both supporting and refuting its usefulness have appeared in the literature. Since the advent of multi-agent chemotherapy, routine adjuvant radiotherapy has been largely abandoned. The true value of postmastectomy radiotherapy is difficult to glean from the studies that have been done. Many of them have suffered from inadequate technique and study design. The American experience is most influenced by the results of the NSABP study B-04 (Fisher *et al.*, 1981). The results of this study failed to demonstrate any advantage for extended field radiotherapy especially for distant metastasis. Unfortunately, since it incorporated all patients with breast cancer whatever their prognostic category, its power in subset analysis is somewhat decreased. In any event, based upon these results adjuvant radiotherapy following radical surgery fell into a period of disfavor in the USA.

One analysis of the world literature incorporating radiotherapy without chemotherapy would suggest that there is no benefit and perhaps an increase in mortality (Cuzick *et al.*, 1987). Other authors suggest that there is a difference favoring radiotherapy (Strom *et al.*, 1991) or in certain subgroups of patients (Edland, 1988). M.D. Anderson Hospital has also published their results which, when compared retrospectively with an older NSABP surgery-only series may show a benefit (Tapley *et al.*, 1982).

It is interesting to note that there is a suggestion that extended field radiotherapy may potentially affect the rate of distant metastasis (Auquier *et al.*, 1992). This effect was observed only for node-positive patients, but was of statistical significance and seen in two studies. This would lead one to consider the possibility that increased local control of breast cancer may decrease the rate of distant metastasis.

The question of radiotherapy alone after mastectomy is largely moot. Patients with bad prognostic findings will almost uniformly receive chemotherapy. In the modern era, the question is whether local radiotherapy can contribute to the management of the postmastectomy patient who is to receive chemotherapy. The best support for adding radiotherapy is the ongoing results of the Danish Breast Cancer Co-operative Group (DBCG) (Overgaard *et al.*, 1990). This large study suggests that there is a small, but significant absolute survival advantage in the premenopausal group as well as a significant increase in disease-free survival and local control in all groups. The group with the most benefit appeared to be women under the age of 45 years with four or more positive lymph nodes. It is also interesting to note that chemotherapy was unable to prevent local recurrence adequately unless combined with radiotherapy.

Similar results are also seen for high-risk postmenopausal women. In a randomized study of radiotherapy, radiotherapy plus tamoxifen, chemotherapy (CMF) or chemotherapy plus tamoxifen, improved local control and recurrence-free survival was seen in the groups receiving radiotherapy. There was also a trend toward improved survival with radiotherapy, but this did not achieve statistical significance (Rutqvist *et al.*, 1990).

Analysis of the Eastern Cooperative Oncology Group studies of patients receiving adjuvant chemotherapy also suggest that there is a subgroup of patients who could benefit from adjuvant radiation (Fowble *et al.*, 1988). Overall, it is worthwhile to consider adding radiotherapy to mastectomy and chemotherapy when the tumor is larger than 5 cm or when four or more lymph nodes are involved.

Radiation Technique

The optimal fields of radiotherapy remain undefined as yet. The majority of the studies cited employ extended field radiotherapy including the supraclavicular, axillary and internal mammary nodal regions as well as the chest wall. *Figure 26.1* shows the regions that are typically included, but the radiotherapeutic technique is beyond the scope of

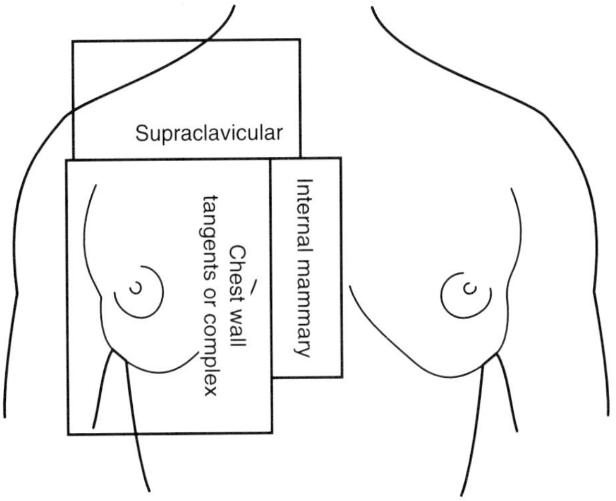

Figure 26.1. Regions typically included in extended field radiotherapy.

this chapter. Lesser radiotherapy (chest wall or chest wall plus supraclavicular nodal region) has not been adequately compared, but is commonplace when radiotherapy is used in the USA.

Radiotherapy in Unresectable Disease

Unresectable disease is a term that encompasses many different situations. Patients can be medically unresectable because of their inability to tolerate anesthesia or surgically unresectable because of tumor factors. Usually factors such as chest wall fixation, skin infiltration, axillary nodal fixation, satellite nodules, inflammatory carcinoma or supraclavicular nodal involvement imply disease that is classically outside the domain of surgery. This is an unusual presentation of breast cancer in developed countries, accounting for about 10–20% of all cases. Unfortunately it is more common in the developing countries.

The treatment used most often in the past has been primary radiotherapy. This technique can provide local management of the cancer with acceptable morbidity. Therapy of locally advanced disease requires doses in excess of those typically given for adjuvant treatment. Doses higher than 60 Gy are required to achieve local control, and there is a dose–response relationship. Dose increments of 15 Gy can decrease the chance of local failure by a factor of two (Arriagada *et al.*, 1985).

As expected, the risk of complications is related to total dose, the area treated and the technical aspects of administration. The patients who receive the highest doses to the most extensive area are often those treated with primary radiotherapy. An analysis of treatment-related complications in the above cited study have been analyzed with respect to treatment and tumor characteristics (Arriagada *et al.*, 1993). The improved local control achieved with high-dose radiotherapy must be carefully balanced with the increased incidence of complications, but the treatment is well tolerated and can prevent the complications associated with uncontrolled local disease.

Recently, combination chemotherapy, in addition to local treatment, has been advocated in the management of unresectable disease. Patients with locally advanced disease have a high rate of distant failure, which is theoretically addressed by chemotherapy. In addition, there is evidence from the studies cited in the previous section that chemotherapy may contribute to improving local control.

Two randomized and prospective trials have been conducted to address these theories. Both studies employ extended field therapy as described above. The first is a series reporting on 118 patients randomized between radiotherapy, radiotherapy plus twelve cycles of chemotherapy (CMF) and tamoxifen, and radiotherapy sandwiched between eight cycles of chemotherapy (CMF alternating with AV) (Schaake–Koning *et al.*, 1985). The results of this study failed to demonstrate any advantage over radiotherapy alone for survival, complete response, local control or relapse-free survival. The second study was conducted by the EORTC. 363 evaluable patients with locally-advanced disease received radiotherapy and were then randomized between observation, chemotherapy (CMF × 12), endocrine therapy, or chemotherapy combined with endocrine therapy (Rubens *et al.*, 1989). Combined therapy demonstrated an advantage in local control, but not in survival or metastatic rate. The local effects were seen in both pre- and postmenopausal women, but were most pronounced for the postmenopausal group. It was concluded that present cytotoxic and hormonal manipulation remained of only marginal value in this patient population, and that the benefits were limited to improved local control. It is felt that increasing the radiation dose may be able to increase local control in the radiotherapy alone arm without the need to add chemotherapy. It would seem reasonable to consider the use of up-front chemotherapy in this patient group. The large tumor mass can serve as an objective measure of response, and the decrease in tumor volume would theoretically improve the effectiveness of local therapy. These theoretical advantages should be weighed against the very real increase in morbidity from chemotherapy when deciding a course of therapy. Further evaluation is warranted before any final conclusion can be reached.

Complications of High-dose Radiotherapy

The complications of high-dose radiotherapy are similar to those of the lower doses employed in adjuvant radiation. Those have been covered elsewhere and will not be repeated here. In addition to an increased risk of fibrosis of the soft tissues and rib fractures, there is a very real danger of cardiac toxicity from the internal mammary field. The Oslo data demonstrate an increased morbidity from cardiac events, which may be due to the hormonal manipulation, the internal mammary nodal radiation, or some combination of the two (Host *et al.*, 1986).

Another area of concern is damage to the brachial plexus. As the total dose is increased, the often disabling complication of brachial plexopathy becomes more prominent. In a subset of patients from the DBCG study cited above an analysis of the rate of brachial plexopathy was performed (Olsen *et al.*, 1993). The findings indicated that the rate of disabling plexopathy was 5%, with a rate of 9% for mild symptoms. The addition of chemotherapy increased the risk of damage to the brachial plexus. The most common signs and symptoms were paresthesia (100%), hypesthesia (74%), weakness (58%), decreased muscle stretch reflexes (47%) and pain (47%). Unfortunately, no effective therapy exists to treat this complication.

Summary of Management Options

- Breast conservation is acceptable management for the majority of women with Stage I or II breast cancer.
- Cosmesis is the goal of breast conservation treatment, and as such, cosmetic concerns are the most important factors when selecting this mode of therapy.
- The presence of multicentricity or collagen vascular disease may sway the choice away from breast conservation and toward mastectomy.
- Radiation therapy should be given with appropriate equipment and by staff well trained in breast conservation techniques.
- The optimal timing of chemotherapy and radiotherapy has not yet been determined, but concurrent therapy can adversely affect cosmetic outcome.
- Local recurrence rates of 10–20% at ten years are to be expected, but this does not adversely affect survival.
- Breast conservation therapy is also appropriate in the management of ductal carcinoma *in situ* (DCIS).
- The addition of irradiation to mastectomy is indicated in certain situations for advanced tumors treated with mastectomy.
- The use of radiation alone or with chemotherapy in advanced and unresectable disease is appropriate and potentially curative.
- The role of neoadjuvant chemotherapy in advanced disease is attractive, but unproven when compared to standard therapy.
- Complications are a rare, but potentially debilitating, consequence of irradiation for breast cancer, and the patient must be carefully counselled before making a decision to proceed.

References

Abner AL, Recht A, Vicini FA *et al.* (1991) Cosmetic results after surgery, chemotherapy, and radiation therapy for early breast cancer. *Int. J. Radiat. Oncol. Biol. Phys.* **21:** 331–338.

Arriagada R, Mouriesse H, Rezvani A *et al.* (1993) Radiotherapy alone in breast cancer. Analysis of tumor and lymph node radiation doses and treatment-related complications. The experience of the Gustave–Roussy Institute and the Princess Margaret Hospital. *Radiother. Oncol.* **27:** 1–6.

Arriagada R, Mouriesse H, Sarrazin D, Clark RM & Deboer G (1985) Radiotherapy alone in breast cancer. I. Analysis of tumor parameters, tumor dose and local control: the experience of the Gustave–Roussy Institute and the Princess Margaret Hospital. *Int. J. Radiat. Oncol. Biol. Phys.* **11:** 1751–1757.

Auquier A, Rutqvist LE, Host H, Rotstein S & Arriagada R (1992) Post-mastectomy megavoltage radiotherapy: the Oslo and Stockholm trials. *Eur. J. Cancer* **28:** 433–437.

Calle R, Vilcoq RJ, Zafrani B *et al.* (1986) Local control and survival of breast cancer treated by limited surgery followed by irradiation. *Int. J. Radiat. Oncol. Biol. Phys.* **12:** 873–878.

Clark RM, McCulloch PB, Levine MN *et al.* (1992) Randomized clinical trial to assess the effectiveness of breast irradiation following lumpectomy and axillary dissection for node-negative breast cancer. *J. Natl. Cancer Inst.* **84:** 683–688.

Clark RM, Wilkinson RH, Mahoney LJ *et al.* (1982) Breast Cancer: A 21 year experience with conservative surgery and radiation. *Int. J. Radiat. Oncol. Biol. Phys.* **8:** 967–975.

Cuzick J, Stewart H, Peto R *et al.* (1987) Overview of randomized trials of postoperative adjuvant radiotherapy in breast cancer. *Cancer Treat. Rep.* **71:** 15–29.

Danoff BF, Goodman RL, Glick JH *et al.* (1983) The effect of adjuvant chemotherapy on cosmesis and complications in patients with breast cancer treated by definitive irradiation. *Int. J. Radiat. Oncol. Biol. Phys.* **9:** 1625–1630.

Dershaw DD, McCormick B, Osborne MP *et al.* (1992) Detection of local recurrence after conservative therapy for breast carcinoma. *Cancer* **70:** 493–496.

Edland RW (1988) Does adjuvant radiotherapy have a role in the postmastectomy management of patients with operable breast cancer – revisited. *Int. J. Radiat. Oncol. Biol. Phys.* **15:** 519–535.

■ Fisher B, Costantino J, Redmond C *et al.* (1993) Lumpectomy compared with lumpectomy and radiation therapy for the treatment of intraductal breast cancer. *N. Engl. J. Med.* **328:** 1581–1586.

Fisher B, Redmond C and others for the National Surgical Adjuvant Breast and Bowel Project (1992) Lumpectomy for breast cancer: an update of the NSABP experience. *J. Natl. Cancer Inst. Monographs* **11:** 7–13.

■ Fisher B, Redmond C, Poisson R *et al.* (1989) Eight-year results of a randomized clinical trial comparing total mastectomy and lumpectomy with or without irradiation in the treatment of breast cancer. *N. Engl. J. Med.* **320:** 822–828.

Fisher B, Wolmark N, Redmond C, Deutsch M & Fisher E (1981) Findings from NSABP Protocol No. B-04: Comparison of radical mastectomy with alternative treatments. II. The clinical and biological significance of medial-central breast cancers. *Cancer* **48:** 1863–1872.

Fleck R, McNeese MD, Ellerbroek NA *et al.* (1989) Consequences of breast irradiation in patients with pre-existing collagen vascular diseases. *Int. J. Radiat. Oncol. Biol. Phys.* **17:** 829–833.

Fowble BL, Solin LJ, Schultz DJ *et al.* (1991) Ten year results of conservative surgery and irradiation for Stage I and II breast cancer. *Int. J. Radiat. Oncol. Biol. Phys.* **21:** 269–277.

Fowble B, Solin LJ, Schultz DJ *et al.* (1992) Breast recurrence and survival related to primary tumor location in patients undergoing conservative surgery and radiation for early-stage breast cancer. *Int. J. Radiat. Oncol. Biol. Phys.* **23:** 933–939.

■ Fowble B, Solin LJ, Schultz DJ *et al.* (1990) Breast recurrence following conservative surgery and radiation: patterns of failure, prognosis, and pathologic findings from mastectomy specimens with implications for treatment. *Int. J. Radiat. Oncol. Biol. Phys.* **19:** 833–842.

Fowble B, Solin LJ, Schultz DJ *et al.* (1989) Frequency, sites of relapse, and outcome of regional node failures following conservative surgery and radiation for early breast cancer. *Int. J. Radiat. Oncol. Biol. Phys.* **17:** 703–710.

Fowble B, Yeh IT, Schultz DJ *et al.* (1993) The role of mastectomy in patients with Stage I–II breast cancer presenting with gross multifocal or multicentric disease or diffuse microcalcifications. *Int. J. Radiat. Oncol. Biol. Phys.* **27:** 567–573.

Fowble B, Gray R, Gilchrist K *et al.* (1988) Identification of a subgroup of patients with breast cancer and histologically positive axillary nodes receiving adjuvant chemotherapy who may benefit from postoperative radiotherapy. *J. Clin. Oncol.* **6:** 1107–1117.

Haffty BG, Fischer D, Beinfield M *et al.* (1991) Prognosis following local recurrence in the conservatively treated breast cancer patient. *Int. J. Radiat. Oncol. Biol. Phys.* **21:** 293–298.

Haffty BG, Goldberg NB, Fischer D *et al.* (1989) Conservative surgery and radiation therapy in breast carcinoma: local recurrence and prognostic implications. *Int. J. Radiat. Oncol. Biol. Phys.* **17:** 727–732.

Harris JR, Botnick L, Bloomer WD *et al.* (1981) Primary radiation therapy for early breast cancer: The experience at the joint center for radiation therapy. *Int. J. Radiat. Oncol. Biol. Phys.* **7:** 1549–1552.

Harris JR, Connolly JL, Schnitt SJ *et al.* (1985) The use of pathologic features in selecting the extent of surgical resection necessary for breast cancer patients treated by primary radiation therapy. *Ann. Surg.* **201:** 164–169.

Host H, Brennhovd IO & Loeb M (1986) Postoperative radiotherapy in breast cancer – long-term results from the Oslo study. *Int. J. Radiat. Oncol. Biol. Phys.* **12:** 727–732.

Kiebert GM, De Haes JCJM & Van de Velde CJH (1991) The impact of breast-conserving treatment and mastectomy on the quality of life of early-stage breast cancer patients: A review. *J. Clin. Oncol.* **9:** 1059–1070.

Kurtz JM, Amalric R, Brandone H *et al.* (1989) Local recurrence after breast-conserving surgery and radiotherapy. *Cancer* **63:** 1912–1917.

Kurtz JM, Amalric R, Brandone H *et al.* (1988) Results of salvage surgery for mammary recurrence following breast-conserving therapy. *Ann. Surg.* **207:** 347–351.

Kurtz JM, Amalric R, Delouche G *et al.* (1987) The second ten years: long-term risks of breast conservation in early breast cancer. *Int. J. Radiat. Oncol. Biol. Phys.* **13:** 1327–1332.

Kurtz JM, Spitalier JM, Amalric R *et al.* (1990) The prognostic significance of late local recurrence after breast-conserving therapy. *Int. J. Radiat. Oncol. Biol. Phys.* **18:** 87–93.

Lagios MD, Margolin FR, Westdahl PR *et al.* (1989) Mammographically detected duct carcinoma *in situ*. *Cancer* **63:** 618–624.

Leopold KA, Recht A, Schnitt SJ *et al.* (1989) Results of conservative surgery and radiation therapy for multiple synchronous cancers of one breast. *Int. J. Radiat. Oncol. Biol. Phys.* **16:** 11–16.

Margolese R (1992) Surgical considerations in selecting local therapy. *J. Nat. Cancer Inst. Monographs* **11:** 41–48.

Matthews RH, McNeese MD, Montague ED *et al.* (1988) Prognostic implications of age in breast cancer patients treated with tumorectomy and irradiation or with mastectomy. *Int. J. Radiat. Oncol. Biol. Phys.* **14:** 659–663.

■ NIH Consensus Conference (1991) Treatment of early-stage breast cancer. *JAMA* **265:** 391–395.

Olsen NK, Pfeiffer P, Johannsen L, Schroder H & Rose C (1993) Radiation-induced brachial plexopathy: neurological follow-up in 161 recurrence-free breast cancer patients. *Int. J. Radiat. Oncol. Biol. Phys.* **26:** 43–49.

■ Overgaard M, Christensen JJ, Johansen H *et al.* (1990) Evaluation of radiotherapy in high-risk breast cancer patients: report from the Danish Breast Cancer Cooperative Group (DBCG 82) Trial. *Int. J. Radiat. Oncol. Biol. Phys.* **19:** 1121–1124.

Pierce SM, Recht A, Lingos TI *et al.* (1992) Long term radiation complications following conservative surgery (CS) and radiation therapy (RT) in patients with early stage breast cancer. *Int. J. Radiat. Oncol. Biol. Phys.* **23:** 915–923.

Pierquin B, Huart J, Raynal M *et al.* (1991) Conservative treatment for breast cancer: long-rerm results (15 years). *Radiother. Oncol.* **20:** 16–23.

Ray GR, Fish VJ, Lee RH *et al.* (1983) Biopsy and definitive radiation therapy in Stages I and II carcinoma of the female breast. *Int. J. Radiat. Oncol. Biol. Phys.* **9:** 23–28.

Recht A, Come SE & Harris JR (1992) Integration of

conservative surgery, radiotherapy, and chemotherapy for patients with early-stage breast cancer. *Semin. Radiat. Oncol.* **2:** 107–115.

Recht A, Connolly JL, Schnitt SJ *et al.* (1988) The effect of young age on tumor recurrence in the treated breast after conservative surgery and radiotherapy. *Int. J. Radiat. Oncol. Biol. Phys.* **14:** 3–10.

Recht A, Pierce SM, Abner A *et al.* (1991) Regional nodal failure after conservative surgery and radiotherapy for early-stage breast carcinoma. *J. Clin. Oncol.* **9:** 988–996.

Rubens RD, Bartelink H, Engelsman E *et al.* (1989) Locally advanced breast cancer: the contribution of cytotoxic and endocrine treatment to radiotherapy. An EORTC breast cancer co-operative group trial (10792). *Eur. J. Cancer Clin. Oncol.* **25:** 667–678.

Rutqvist LE, Cedermark B, Glas U *et al.* (1990) Randomized trial of adjuvant tamoxifen combined with postoperative radiation therapy or adjuvant chemotherapy in postmenopausal breast cancer. *Cancer* **66:** 89–96.

Sarrazin D, Le MG, Arriagada R *et al.* (1989) Ten-year results of a randomized trial comparing a conservative treatment to mastectomy in early breast cancer. *Radiother. Oncol.* **14:** 177–184.

Schaake–Koning C, Hamersma van der Linden E, Hart G & Engelsman E (1986) Adjuvant chemo- and hormonal therapy in locally advanced breast cancer: a randomized clinical study. *Int. J. Radiat. Oncol. Biol. Phys.* **11:** 1759–1763.

Schmidt–Ullrich R, Wazer DE, Tercilla O *et al.* (1989) Tumor margin assessment as a guide to optimal conservation surgery and irradiation in early stage breast carcinoma. *Int. J. Radiat. Oncol. Biol. Phys.* **17:** 733–738.

Solin LJ, Fowble BL, Schultz DJ *et al.* (1991) The significance of the pathology margins of the tumor excision on the outcome of patients treated with definitive irradiation for early stage breast cancer. *Int. J. Radiat. Oncol. Biol. Phys.* **21:** 279–287.

Solin LJ, Fowble B, Martz KL *et al.* (1988) Definitive irradiation for early stage breast cancer: The University of Pennsylvania experience. *Int. J. Radiat. Oncol. Biol. Phys.* **14:** 235–242.

Solin LJ, Fowble B, Schultz DJ *et al.* (1989) Age as a prognostic factor for patients treated with definitive irradiation for early stage breast cancer. *Int. J. Radiat. Oncol. Biol. Phys.* **16:** 373–381.

Solin LJ, Recht A, Fourquet A *et al.* (1991) Ten-year results of breast-conserving surgery and definitive irradiation for intraductal carcinoma (cuctal carcinoma *in situ*) of the breast. *Cancer* **68:** 2337–2344.

Stomper PC, Recht A, Berenberg AL *et al.* (1987) Mammographic detection of recurrent cancer in the irradiated breast. *AJR* **148:** 39–43.

Stotter A, Atkinson EA, Fairston BA *et al.* (1990) Survival following locoregional recurrence after breast conservation therapy for cancer. *Ann. Surg.* 166–172.

Strom EA, McNeese MD, Fletcher GH *et al.* (1991) Results of mastectomy and postoperative irradiation in the management of locoregionally advanced carcinoma of the breast. *Int. J. Radiat. Oncol. Biol. Phys.* **21:** 319–323.

Tapley ND, Spanos WJJ, Fletcher GH *et al.* (1982) Results in patients with breast cancer treated by radical mastectomy and postoperative irradiation with no adjuvant chemotherapy. *Cancer* **49:** 1316–1319.

Van Dongen JA, Bartelink H, Fentiman IS *et al.* (1992) Randomized clinical trial to assess the value of breast-conserving therapy in Stage I and II breast cancer, EORTC 10801 trial. *J. Natl Cancer Inst. Monographs* **11:** 15–18.

Van Dongen JA, Bartelink H, Fentiman IS *et al.* (1992) Factors influencing local relapse and survival and results of salvage treatment after breast-conserving therapy in operable breast cancer: EORTC trial 10801, breast conservation compared with mastectomy in TNM Stage I and II breast cancer. *Eur. J. Cancer* **28A:** 801–805.

Veronesi U, Salvadori B, Luini A *et al.* (1990) Conservative treatment of early breast cancer. *Ann. Surg.* **211:** 250–259.

Vicini FA, Eberlein TJ, Connolly JL *et al.* (1991) The optimal extent of resection for patients with Stages I or II breast cancer treated with conservative surgery and radiotherapy. *Ann. Surg.* **214:** 200–205.

Vicini FA, Recht A, Abner A *et al.*(1992) Recurrence in the breast following conservative surgery and radiation therapy for early-stage breast cancer. *J. Natl Cancer Inst. Monographs* **11:** 33–39.

Vicini F, Recht A, Abner A *et al.* (1990) The association between very young age and recurrence in the breast in patients treated with conservative surgery (CS) and radiation therapy (RT). *Int. J. Radiat. Oncol. Biol. Phys.* **19:** 132.

■ Wazer DE, DiPetrillo T, Schmidt–Ullrich R *et al.* (1992) Factors influencing cosmetic outcome and complication risk after conservative surgery and radiotherapy for early-stage breast carcinoma. *J. Clin. Oncol.* **10:** 356–363.

Weiss MC, Fowble BL, Solin LJ *et al.* (1992) Outcome of conservative therapy for invasive breast cancer by histologic subtype. *Int. J. Radiat. Oncol. Biol. Phys.* **23:** 941–947.

27 Adjuvant Systemic Therapy of Breast Cancer

J J Perry
H B Muss

Introduction

Breast cancer remains the most common cancer of American women. The American Cancer Society has estimated that in 1994 there will be 183,000 new patients accounting for 32% of all newly diagnosed female malignancies. Breast cancer is also the second leading cause of cancer mortality in women and will result in an estimated 46,000 deaths (Boring *et al.*, 1994). Adjuvant systemic therapy is defined as the use of systemic treatment with endocrine therapy, chemotherapy or immunotherapy, alone or in combination, either before, during or after definitive treatment of the primary breast lesion. The objective of adjuvant therapy is to improve survival. This chapter will discuss the use of adjuvant systemic therapy in women with early stage breast cancer.

The effectiveness of adjuvant therapy in increasing overall survival in women with both node-negative and node-positive early stage breast cancer has made such treatment a viable option for the majority of women currently diagnosed with breast cancer (Early Breast Cancer Trialists' Collaborative Group, 1992; Olivotto *et al.*, 1994). Over the last decade and with the increased use of screening mammography, the majority of women now diagnosed with breast cancer have smaller node-negative lesions, while the number of patients presenting with advanced locoregional or metastatic disease has decreased. Detailed information concerning the staging of breast cancer has been presented earlier in this monograph. This chapter will discuss the rationale and current role of adjuvant systemic therapy in women with early-stage breast cancer.

The Biologic Rationale of Adjuvant Therapy

The goal of adjuvant therapy is to eliminate small, clinically occult micrometastases arising from the hematogenous spread of malignant cells from the primary lesion before diagnosis. Adjuvant treatment is therefore based on the probability that distant metastases have occurred; the probability of cancer spread is based on staging, histologic and biologic information (see below). The rationale of adjuvant therapy is based on the following.

- Currently, patients with clinically detectable, overt metastatic breast cancer are incurable.
- There are no effective means for diagnosing occult metastases (micrometastases).
- Small tumors have a higher percentage of cells in the cell cycle (higher growth fraction) than large tumors.
- Chemotherapy is most effective in tumors with high growth fractions.
- Smaller tumors are less likely to have developed drug resistance.
- Smaller tumors are less likely to be necrotic and drug delivery should be favorable.
- Patients without overt metastatic disease are generally healthier and more likely to tolerate toxicity due to chemotherapy than women with symptomatic or bulky metastatic disease.

An excellent review of these concepts is available (Bonadonna, 1992). Physicians and patients may have great difficulty in recommending and selecting adjuvant treatment. First, there are major differences in recurrence risks among patients with different stage lesions. Second, adjuvant treatment is an evolving discipline and there is considerable controversy concerning treatment selection among physicians, including those considered experts in this area. Third, long-term follow-up for many trials is not available. Last and most importantly, patient preferences based on the risk and benefits of such treatment may vary greatly.

The Overview Analysis of Adjuvant Therapy

A large number of adjuvant trials involving thousands of breast cancer patients have been performed over the past 20 years. The majority of these trials have involved relatively small numbers of patients and were not designed to detect small, but clinically significant, differences in efficacy between treatments. Through combined analysis (termed overview or meta-analysis) of the major trials, the relative benefits of adjuvant therapy for major subgroups of patients with breast cancer can be estimated.

In 1984, the Early Breast Cancer Trialists Collaborative Group was formed with the objective of conducting an international overview analysis of adjuvant systemic therapy. The first meta-analysis was performed in 1987 and evaluated the five-year results of adjuvant treatments (Early Breast Cancer Trialists' Collaborative Group, 1988). The updated meta-analysis was conducted in 1991, and provided ten-year follow-up data for a total of 75,000 women enrolled on 133 randomized trials, including tamoxifen, chemotherapy, ovarian ablation and immunotherapy trials (Early Breast Cancer Trialists Collaborative Group, 1992). These 75,000 women represented approximately 90% of patients entered on randomized trials before 1985, including published and unpublished trials.

In the meta-analysis, the results of the adjuvant therapies were expressed in terms of proportional benefit or percentage reduction in the annual odds of recurrence or death. The impact of the proportional benefit in clinical terms depends upon the underlying recurrence or death rate without treatment. To illustrate this, consider three clinical subsets of 100 patients each, and treatment estimated to produce a 30% proportional benefit (*Table 27.1*). These data illustrate the major differences in survival

Table 27.1.

	Ten-year recurrence rate (%)		
	Without treatment	*With treatment*	*Absolute benefit*
Low risk	10	7	3/100 patients
Moderate risk	50	35	15/100 patients
High risk	80	56	24/100 patients

benefit from treatment (lives saved) based on the risk of recurrence. Although the proportional benefit is the same for each group, clearly the absolute benefit is greatest in the high-risk subgroup. *Table 27.2* lists the major results of the ten-year International Overview. Combination chemotherapy reduces the odds of recurrence (28% ±3) and death (17% ±3) for all women, although the benefit was greater for younger women. Further subset analyses demonstrated that the proportional benefit reductions were similar for node-positive and node-negative patients, but the absolute improvement in ten-year survival was about twice as great for node-positive patients. Additional observations were that combination chemotherapy was superior to single agents, and shorter duration therapy (3–6 months) was as effective as longer duration therapy. An important finding was that the benefit of combination chemotherapy persisted beyond five years, with survival curves continuing to diverge at ten years.

Tamoxifen therapy reduced the odds of recurrence and mortality in all age groups (25% ±2 for recurrence; 16% ±2 for mortality) when compared to no treatment. The magnitude of the benefit on disease recurrence was greater for patients of at least 50 years of age, but women less than 50 years of age also had a statistically significant reduction when treated with tamoxifen.

Regarding the influence of nodal status, tamoxifen produced statistically significant benefits on recurrence-free and overall survival in node-positive and node-negative subgroups, although node-positive patients had a greater degree of absolute benefit. The benefit from tamoxifen was greater in patients with estrogen receptor (ER)-positive tumors who had a 36% reduction in annual odds of death; of note however patients with ER-negative tumors (<10 fmol mg^{-1}) also showed a smaller, but statistically significant, 16% reduction in mortality with tamoxifen use. Patients with tumors containing

Table 27.2. International overview of adjuvant therapy – overall effects of adjuvant combination chemotherapy and tamoxifen therapy versus no therapy. ([ ] denote statistically unstable results)

	Typical percent reduction (± SD) in annual odds of:					
	Recurrence			*Death*		
Category of trial	*Any age*	*<50 yrs*	*≥50 yrs*	*Any age*	*<50 yrs*	*≥50 yrs*
Chemotherapy versus no chemotherapy	28±3	36±5	24±3	17±3	24±5	13±4
Node-negative	26±7	[26±10]	[27±9]	18±8	[6±13]	[23±11]
Node-positive	30±3	41±5	23±4	18±3	30±6	11±4
Tamoxifen versus no tamoxifen	25±2	12±4	29±2	16±2	6±5	20±2
Node-negative	26±4	22±8	28±4	17±5	[19±12]	16±5
Node-positive	28±2	11±4	33±2	18±2	5±5	22±3
Estrogen receptor-negative	13±4	3±8	16±5	11±5	[−5±9]	16±6
Estrogen receptor-positive	32±3	19±6	36±3	21±3	13±8	23±4

high ER levels ($\geqslant$100 fmol mg^{-1}) derive the greatest benefit from tamoxifen (42% and 28% reductions in annual odds of recurrence and mortality respectively). As with combination chemotherapy, the benefit of tamoxifen therapy persisted between five and ten years of follow-up.

In the overview analysis it was also possible to estimate whether combinations of tamoxifen plus chemotherapy offer an advantage over either treatment alone. For patients of 50 years of age and over a significant effect was seen only in recurrence when comparing trials of chemotherapy plus tamoxifen versus tamoxifen alone. Significant reduction of the odds of both recurrence and mortality was seen in older patients receiving chemotherapy plus tamoxifen compared to chemotherapy alone. For patients less than 50 years of age, studies of chemotherapy plus tamoxifen compared to chemotherapy alone did not demonstrate significant improvements in either recurrence or survival with the addition of tamoxifen. The latter analysis was limited by the smaller number of patients accrued in such trials.

The overview analysis also provided information about the role of ovarian ablation (surgery, radiation or drugs). For women of 50 years and over there was no significant effect of ovarian ablation either on recurrence-free survival or overall survival. However, an unanticipated finding was that women less than 50 years of age had a highly significant improvement in recurrence-free survival (26% proportional benefit) and in overall survival (25% proportional benefit). There was the suggestion of an additive effect when combining chemotherapy and endocrine ablation in this age group, but the reliability of this determination was limited by the small number of patients analyzed. Regarding trials of adjuvant immunotherapy, the conclusion reached from the overview analysis was that this modality had no impact on recurrence-free or overall survival.

Adjuvant Systemic Therapies

Endocrine Therapy

The most commonly used endocrine agent in the adjuvant setting is tamoxifen. Tamoxifen, an antiestrogen with weak estrogen agonist properties, displays similar response rates as other endocrine regimens in women with advanced breast cancer, but with the least toxicity (Muss, 1992). In the overview, tamoxifen therapy significantly decreased the annual odds of recurrence and death in both node-negative and node-positive women; a reduction was seen in both ER-positive and ER-negative patients. Also, durations of tamoxifen therapy for longer than two years were associated with greater benefit (Fisher *et al.*, 1987; Early Breast Cancer Trialists' Collaborative Group, 1992), and current trials are evaluating the efficacy of tamoxifen given for periods of ten years and longer (Tormey and Jordan, 1984; Breast Cancer Trials Committee, 1987; Fisher *et al.*, 1989).

Major toxicities of tamoxifen include hot flashes (more common in premenopausal women), thromboembolic phenomena (occurring in about 1% of patients) and endometrial cancer (occurring in an estimated 2/1000 patients/year (Muss, 1992; Fisher *et al.*, 1994a). Asymptomatic patients on tamoxifen who have an intact uterus are advised to have pelvic examinations yearly. Further evaluation, including consideration of endometrial biopsy, should be considered for patients with symptoms. Other toxicities, including vaginal dryness or discharge and mood changes, are usually mild; retinopathy is rare. The cost of tamoxifen in the USA currently ranges from 60–100 dollars/month of treatment.

In addition to its beneficial effects on recurrence and survival, tamoxifen has other benefits in postmenopausal women due to its weak estrogen agonist activity. Tamoxifen significantly reduces serum cholesterol levels (about 15%), and decreases the concentration of low density lipoproteins, improving the lipid profile (Spicer *et al.*, 1990). In the overview, tamoxifen significantly decreased the annual odds of developing contralateral breast cancer by approximately 40%, and was associated with a reduction in non-cancer-related deaths (mostly cardiovascular) of 12% ($p=0.05$). The findings of the Scottish adjuvant tamoxifen trial showed a highly significant decrease in death from myocardial infarction in postmenopausal patients receiving tamoxifen (5% of deaths in the tamoxifen group versus 10% in the observation group) (McDonald and Stewart, 1991), and similar findings were recently reported in the Stockholm Breast Cancer Study (Rutqvist and Mattsson, 1993). Also, preliminary data indicate that vertebral bone density may be maintained in postmenopausal women taking tamoxifen (Love *et al.*, 1992).

The overview analysis indicated that ovarian ablation was similar to chemotherapy in improving breast cancer survival in premenopausal women. Many physicians and patients find ovarian ablation by surgical or radiotherapeutic means objectionable, and ablation has not been widely used in the USA. The introduction of gonadotropin releasing hormone (GnRH) agonists has provided a more acceptable and extremely effective method for 'chemical ablation' in premenopausal women (Harvey, 1988; Muss, 1992). Several weeks of treatment with GnRH analogues reduces follicle stimulating hormone, luteinizing hormone and estradiol concentrations to castrate levels. In one recent randomized trial a GnRH analogue displayed similar efficacy to the same GnRH analogue plus tamoxifen in pre- and perimenopausal women with advanced breast cancer (Nicholson *et al.*, 1990), and GnRH analogues are currently being evaluated in premenopausal women in the adjuvant setting.

Chemotherapy

The first generation of randomized clinical trials of adjuvant chemotherapy for breast cancer used single agent melphalan (Fisher *et al.*, 1975), and combination chemotherapy with cyclophosphamide, methotrexate and 5-fluorouracil (CMF) (Bonadonna *et al.*, 1976). These and other studies demonstrated the benefit of adjuvant chemotherapy in this setting, with ten-year results confirmed in the International Overview analysis previously discussed (Early Breast Cancer Trialists' Collaborative Group, 1992).

The anthracycline doxorubicin (Adriamycin®), is probably the single most effective drug in the treatment of metastatic breast cancer and was introduced into adjuvant therapy trials beginning in the early and mid-1980s. Most combination chemotherapy regimens in the overview trials used the CMF combination. To date, comparative trials of CMF versus doxorubicin-based therapy have not shown improvements in recurrence-free or overall survival benefit for the doxorubicin-containing regimen. Nevertheless, doxorubicin-based adjuvant regimens have been increasingly employed, particularly for patients with multiple positive lymph nodes.

Commonly used adjuvant chemotherapy agents and regimens are listed in *Table 27.3*, along with toxicities most frequently encountered. With the use of shorter treatment periods (usually six months or less) and improved supportive care (including newer, more effective antiemetics), contemporary adjuvant chemotherapy programs are generally well tolerated. While no specific adjuvant combination chemotherapy has proven to be superior, it is clear from several studies that dose reductions should generally be avoided. In the first CMF trial from the Milan group, the lack of a survival benefit for postmenopausal (node-positive) patients was retrospectively attributed to the use of lower initial doses of CMF and arbitrary dose reductions in older patients (Bonadonna and Valagussa, 1981). The Cancer and Leukemia Group B (CALGB) recently conducted a randomized study in node-positive patients using three dose schedules of cyclophosphamide, doxorubicin and fluorouracil (CAF): CAF 600/60/600 mg m^{-2} every four weeks for four cycles, 400/40/400 mg m^{-2} every four weeks for six cycles, and 300/30/300 mg m^{-2} every four weeks for four cycles. The low dose arm had (statistically significant) inferior three-year disease-free and overall survival results compared to the higher dose arms (Wood *et al.*, 1994).

The concept of dose-intensity in adjuvant therapy has been explored in a number of adjuvant trials. Results from several large Phase II studies appear to demonstrate a benefit in disease-free survival for patients at high risk for metastatic disease using this approach. In the subgroup of patients with ten or more positive axillary lymph nodes, five-year relapse-free survival results are poor, ranging from 22–45% using conventional CMF or CAF schedules (Jones *et al.*, 1987; Kau *et al.*, 1990). Abeloff (1992) treated 64 patients with operable breast cancer and at least ten positive nodes using a 16-week intensive regimen employing cyclophosphamide, doxorubicin, methotrexate with Leucovorin rescue, vincristine, and 5-fluorouracil. At a median follow-up of 40 months, the disease-free survival is 53% (95%

Table 27.3. Commonly used adjuvant chemotherapy regimens and toxicities.

Regimens

CMF = Cyclophosphamide, methotrexate, 5-fluorouracil

CAF = Cyclophosphamide, doxorubicin (Adriamycin), 5-fluorouracil

CMFP = CMF + Prednisone

CA = Cyclophosphamide and Adriamycin

Common toxicities	Agent
Nausea and vomiting	C, A
Alopecia	A
Fatigue	All
Weight gain	All regimens (etiology unclear)
Mouth sores	A, M, F
Premature menopause	C, A
Febrile neutropenia (uncommon)	All regimens
Hemorrhagic complications (uncommon)	All regimens
Thrombosis (uncommon)	All regimens
Cardiomyopathy from doxorubicin (less than 1%)	A
Secondary leukemia (rare, less than 0.05%)	Alkylating agents (C)

confidence interval 38–65%). Based on these promising results, an intergroup adjuvant study was conducted by the Eastern Cooperative Oncology Group (ECOG), the Southwest Oncology Group (SWOG) and the CALGB for patients with node-positive, hormone receptor-negative breast comparing the 16-week dose-intensive program to conventional CAF. This study has completed accrual and results are awaited. Peters *et al.* (1993) have investigated the role of high-dose cyclophosphamide, carmustine and cisplatin with autologous bone marrow transplantation as consolidation therapy following four cycles of conventional dose CAF in 85 patients with Stage II or III breast cancer involving ten or more axillary nodes. Early results at a median follow-up of 2.5 years show relapse-free survival of 72% (95% CI 56–82%), with a 12% transplant-related mortality. The CALGB and SWOG are presently conducting a randomized study comparing high-dose and low-dose consolidation with cyclophosphamide, carmustine and cisplatin following four cycles of CAF in this high-risk subset of breast cancer patients.

At least one major randomized study has failed to demonstrate a benefit for dose-intensity. National Surgical Adjuvant Breast Program (NSABP) B-22 treated cyclophosphamide dose-intensity in patients with positive axillary lymph nodes (Dimitrov *et al.*, 1994). The control group was treated with 'standard' cyclophosphamide 600 mg m^{-2} intravenously every three weeks for four cycles, versus two intensified cyclophosphamide schedules: 1200 mg m^{-2} intravenously every three weeks for two cycles versus 1200 mg m^{-2} intravenously every three weeks for four cycles. All patients received doxorubicin 60 mg m^{-2} intravenously every three weeks for four cycles. Disease-free survival at three years was similar for the three groups (73%, 70% and 74%, respectively).

Doxorubicin dose-intensity in the adjuvant setting is also being investigated. The CALGB has recently initiated an intergroup trial with ECOG and SWOG involving three dose levels of doxorubicin (60 mg m^{-2} versus 75 mg m^{-2} versus 90 mg m^{-2}) every three weeks for four cycles along with cyclophosphamide 600 mg m^{-2} for patients with three or more positive axillary lymph nodes. This protocol also involves a second randomization to Paclitaxel or no further therapy.

Follow-up After Initial Therapy

There is considerable debate concerning the role of follow-up evaluation after primary therapy (Schapira and Urban, 1991; Wertheimer, 1991; Schapira, 1993). Numerous investigators have demonstrated that a brief follow-up visit that includes an interim history and physical examination will detect recurrence in more than 75% of patients. Serum chemistry profiles and complete blood counts, routine chest radiographs, radionuclide bone scans and other expensive imaging studies add great cost, but only small additional yield in detecting early recurrence in asymptomatic patients (Muss *et al.*, 1988). Recently two large randomized trials have compared intensive (history and physical examination, chest radiograph and bone scan) and clinical (history and physical examination only) follow-up strategies (Del Turco *et al.*, 1994; GIVIO investigators, 1994). In both trials there was no evidence of a survival advantage for the intensively followed group. In one of these trials, relapses were more frequently detected in patients receiving intensive follow-up (Del Turco *et al.*, 1994). In the second trial, both relapse-free and overall survival were similar for the intensively followed and clinically followed groups (GIVIO investigators, 1994); moreover, quality of life perception, emotional well-being, social functioning, symptoms and satisfaction with care did not differ between the two groups. The investigators in both trials concluded that the routine use of laboratory and imaging tests should be discouraged. Our suggested guidelines for follow-up evaluation are presented in *Table 27.4*.

Table 27.4. Follow-up after primary therapy.

	Frequency of examination	
	Years 0–5	*After five years*
History and physical examination	Every 3–4 months	Every 6–12 months
Mammogram[1]	Yearly	Yearly
Complete blood count and biochemical profile[2]	Every 6–12 months	Yearly
Chest radiograph[2]	Yearly	Yearly
Other studies[3]	As indicated	As indicated

[1]In patients tested with lumpectomy and breast irradiation, more frequent mammograms (every 4–6 months) are generally recommended for the first three years.
[2]Of questionable value; may be omitted depending on the cost and local standards of care.
[3]Tumor marker studies, skeletal radiographs, radionuclide and computerized tomographic scans are not necessary in asymptomatic patients. Appropriate studies should be obtained for patients with signs or symptoms of recurrence.

Because standards of follow-up care vary greatly in the USA and are not well defined, we have continued to recommend yearly chest radiography and laboratory work for such patients pending development of more formal consensus guidelines. Mammography, however, should be continued on a yearly basis for all patients.

Treatment Recommendations

Because the impact of current adjuvant therapy on disease-free and overall survival is modest at best, prospective clinical trials are still necessary to test promising hypotheses, new agents, combinations of agents and new treatment modalities in order to make progressive advances in the treatment of early stage breast cancer.

For patients not on clinical trials, the consensus recommendations from the Fourth International Conference on Adjuvant Therapy of Primary Breast Cancer (St. Gallen, Switzerland, February 1992), can be used to guide therapy (see below) (Glick *et al.*, 1992). Decisions regarding adjuvant therapy should always take into account individual patient characteristics, including other medical illnesses, treatment preferences and psychosocial status.

Node-negative Patients

More than 50% of new patients with breast cancer in 1995 will be diagnosed with node-negative breast cancer. Overall, such women have a generally favorable prognosis with ten-year disease-free survival estimates of 70–75%. Great differences exist in recurrence risk. For women with ductal carcinoma *in situ* (DCIS), the risk of developing distant metastases is less than 2–3%. Patients with DCIS with only a small area of microinvasion also appear to have an excellent prognosis, but more data are needed (Matsukuma *et al.*, 1991; Rosner *et al.*, 1991). Adjuvant therapy is not recommended for such patients. The major controversy concerning treatment selection in node-negative patients involves the management of women with invasive lesions less than or equal to 1 cm in their largest diameter. Prognostic factors such as tumor size, histologic grade, and ER and PR expression can help predict patients with intermediate and high recurrence risk; tumor proliferative activity (S-phase), protease expression (e.g. cathepsin-D) and molecular markers (for example erbB-2 and p53) may prove to be of even greater value (McGuire and Clark, 1992; Clark *et al.*, 1993), but factors that would help to consistently define extremely low-risk patients (e.g. <5% recurrence risk) are needed. A list of currently available prognostic factors for node-negative patients are listed in *Table 27.5*. Although such factors help define high-risk node-negative patients, they add little if any information to tumor size measurements in defining risk for women with small (<1 cm) tumors. Therefore, an overall recurrence rate of about 10% over a 10–20 year period appears the best assessment of risk at this time (Rosen *et al.*, 1992). Also, there are no universally agreed models that are capable of defining the relative role of each factor in predicting recurrence; moreover, not all factors provide independent information. Current recommendations for the management of node-negative patients are presented in *Table 27.6*.

Node-positive Patients

Results from the updated International Overview indicate that all patients with node-positive tumors

Table 27.5. Prognostic factors for node-negative breast cancer.

Factor	Effect: Favorable	Effect: Unfavorable	Survival difference between groups
Tumor size	Small	Large	About 10% decrease for each 1 cm in size (1 cm=90% survival)
Hormone receptor status (estrogen and progesterone)	Positive	Negative	About 5–10%
Menopausal status	Post	Pre	<5%
Tumor grade	Low	High	About 10%
DNA content (ploidy status)	Normal	Abnormal	Little if any
S phase fraction	Low	High	About 10%
ErbB2 (HER2/neu) oncogene*	None	Expression	Little if any
p53 expression*	Low	High	Little if any
Cathepsin D*	Low	High	5–10%

*Still under research study and not generally available from commercial reference laboratories.

Table 27.6. Consensus treatment recommendations for node-negative patients: St. Gallen recommendations (modified from Glick *et al.*, 1992).

	*Minimal/low risk**	*Good risk***	*High risk****
Premenopausal			
Hormone receptor-positive	No treatment versus tamoxifen	Tamoxifen	Chemotherapy plus tamoxifen
Hormone receptor-negative	No treatment versus tamoxifen	Tamoxifen	Chemotherapy
Postmenopausal			
Hormone receptor-positive	No treatment versus tamoxifen	Tamoxifen	Tamoxifen plus chemotherapy
Hormone receptor-negative	No treatment versus tamoxifen	Tamoxifen	Chemotherapy plus tamoxifen
Elderly (>70 yrs)			
Hormone receptor-positive	No treatment****	Tamoxifen	Tamoxifen
Hormone receptor-negative	No treatment****	Tamoxifen	Tamoxifen

*Minimal low risk: includes patients with DCIS, patients with invasive cancers <1 cm in size detected by mammogram, and patients with tubular, colloid, or papillary tumors <2 cm in size.
**Good risk: includes patients with hormone receptor-positive tumors greater than 1 cm, but less than 2 cm, with favorable histologic type and low nuclear grade.
***High risk: includes patients with hormone receptor-negative tumors ≥1 cm, estrogen receptor-positive tumors >2 cm, and nuclear grade III tumors.
****In selected circumstances, given the patient's medical condition and treatment preference, tamoxifen could be administered.

Table 27.7. Consensus treatment recommendations for node-positive patients (modified from Glick *et al.*, 1992).

	Hormone-receptor-positive	*Hormone-receptor-negative*
Premenopausal	Chemotherapy ± tamoxifen	Chemotherapy
Postmenopausal	Tamoxifen ± chemotherapy	Chemotherapy ± tamoxifen
Elderly (>70 yrs)	Tamoxifen	Chemotherapy*

*In selected circumstances, given the patient's medical condition and treatment preferences, chemotherapy could be administered. We believe tamoxifen should be offered to these patients based on the overview analysis.

should receive adjuvant therapy (Early Breast Cancer Trialists' Collaborative Group, 1992). Treatment recommendations from the Fourth International Conference on Adjuvant Therapy (St Gallen) for the major subgroups of node-positive patients are outlined in *Table 27.7*. Combination chemotherapy regimens of proven benefit are listed in *Table 27.3*. Issues regarding the role of doxorubicin (patient subgroups, optimal dose, schedule, combinations) and dose-intensification may be further clarified following analyses of maturing and ongoing prospective randomized trials.

Clinical Trials

Important questions regarding how to best combine cytotoxic and endocrine treatments for particular subgroups (defined by axillary lymph node, hormone receptor and menopausal status) need to be addressed in large, well-designed, prospective randomized clinical trials. All newly diagnosed women should be evaluated for entry into current clinical trials (*Table 27.8*). Referral of the breast cancer patient to a medical oncologist is appropriate after primary diagnosis for discussion and decisions regarding adjuvant therapy. Information of interest to the medical oncologist is listed in *Table 27.9*.

Neoadjuvant Therapy and Treatment of Large Primary Lesions

The use of chemotherapy before definitive resection of the primary breast lesion has been gaining in popularity. Such treatment has the potential benefit of tumor reduction before surgical or irradiation-induced perturbation of the tumor bed. Moreover, the potential benefit of such treatment might be estimated from the clinical and pathologic evaluation of the primary lesion after several cycles of chemotherapy and before definitive surgery. A recent randomized trial of the NSABP (B-18) compared four cycles of chemotherapy with cyclophosphamide and doxorubicin (CA) given either before or after definitive surgery (lumpectomy or mastectomy) (Fisher *et al.*, 1994b). Preliminary data from this trial showed that preoperative chemotherapy resulted in complete or partial response of the primary lesion in 80% of patients. The correlation between tumor response to therapy and relapse-free and overall survival has not yet been analyzed. Further follow-up

Table 27.8. Current active phase III cooperative group protocols (compiled from Physicians Data Query, June 1994).

Group(s)	Stage	Treatment arms
Node-positive trials		
Group(s)	*Stage*	*Treatment arms*
CALGB ECOG SWOG NCCTG	PS I–IIIA ER+ or − Pre- or postmenopausal	S: C+A 60 mg $m^2 \times 4$ / C+A 75 mg $m^2 \times 4$ / C+A 90 mg $m^2 \times 4$ → Paclitaxel / No further therapy
SWOG ECOG CALGB NCCTG NCI-C	PS I–IIIA ER+ Postmenopausal	S: Tamoxifen / CAF+tamoxifen / CAF→tamoxifen
IBCSG	PS I–IIIA ER+ or − Peri or postmenopausal	S: AC × 4→16-week gap→CMF × 3 → Tamoxifen / Toremifene AC × 4→No gap →CMF × 3 → Tamoxifen / Toremifene
IBCSG	PS I–IIIA ER+ or − Premenopausal	S: AC × 4→16-week gap→CMF × 3 → Tamoxifen / No further therapy AC × 4→No gap →CMF × 3 → Tamoxifen / No further therapy
IBCSG	PS I–IIIA ER+ Peri- or postmenopausal	S: AC+toremifene / AC+tamoxifen / Tamoxifen / Toremifene
IBCSG	PS I–IIIA ER+ Premenopausal	S→Ovarian ablation → Tamoxifen / AC × 4→tamoxifen
NCI-C	PS I–II ER+ or − Pre- or perimenopausal	S→CMF, CEF, or AC → Tamoxifen / No further therapy
CALGB SWOG	PS I–IIIA ⩾10 involved nodes ER+ or − Pre- or postmenopausal	S→CAF × 4 → High-dose C/CDDP/BCNU+ABMT/ASCT / Low-dose C/CDDP/BCNU
ECOG	PS I–IIIA ⩾10 involved nodes ER+ or − Pre- or postmenopausal	S→CAF × 4 → High-dose C/thiotepa+ABMT / No further therapy
Node-positive trials		
Group(s)	*Stage*	*Treatment arms*
IBCSG	T1–3 psN0 M0 ER+ or − Pre- or postmenopausal	S: CMF / Goserelin / CMF→Goserelin
IBCSG	CS T1–3 N0 M0 ER+ or − Age >70 years	S: Axillary node clearance→Tamoxifen / Tamoxifen
NSABP B-21	Clinically occult invasive cancer	Lumpectomy+breast RT → Tamoxifen / Placebo
NSABP B-23	PS I–II ER− Pre- or postmenopausal	S: AC → Tamoxifen / No further therapy CMF → Tamoxifen / No further therapy

Table 27.8. *Continued*

Trials for both node-positive and node-negative patients

Group(s)	*Stage*	*Treatment arms*
SWOG	PS I-IIIA 0–3 involved lymph nodes ER+ or − Pre- or postmenopausal	S → CA S → A→C
CRC	CS I-II 0 or any number of involved nodes ER+ or − Age <50 years	S → Tamoxifen S → Endocrine ablation S → No further therapy
CRC	CS I-II 0 or any number of involved nodes ER+ or − Age ≥50 years	S → Tamoxifen × 2 years S → Tamoxifen × 5 years
Other trials		
NSABP B-24	DCIS Pre- or postmenopausal	Lumpectomy + breast RT → Tamoxifen Lumpectomy + breast RT → Placebo

Abbreviations

CALGB	Cancer and Leukemia Group B	CMF	Cyclophosphamide, methotrexate, 5-fluorouracil
SWOG	Southwest Oncology Group	CEF	Cyclophosphamide, epirubicin, 5-fluorouracil
ECOG	Eastern Cooperative Oncology Group	CDDP	Cisplatin
NCCTG	North Central Cancer Treatment Group	BCNU	Carmustine
PS	Pathologic stage	ABMT	Autologous bone marrow transplantation
S	Surgery (lumpectomy or mastectomy with axillary node dissection)	ASCT	Autologous stem cell transplantation
		NSABP	National Surgical Adjuvant Breast Program
C	Cyclophosphamide	RT	Radiation therapy
A	Doxorubicin (Adriamycin®)	CRC	Cancer Research Campaign Clinical Trials Centre (London)
ER	Estrogen receptor		
NCI-C	National Cancer Institute of Canada	CS	Clinical stqge
CAF	Cyclophosphamide, doxorubicin, 5-fluorouracil	DCIS	Ductal carcinoma *in situ*
IBCSG	International Breast Cancer Study Group		
AC	Doxorubicin, cyclophosphamide		

Table 27.9. Helpful information for medical oncology referral.

Patient characteristics	Pathology*
Significant co-morbid medical problems	Presence of necrosis, vascular or lymphatic involvement
Major abnormalities on physical examination	Percentage of invasive and intraductal cancer
Complete blood count	Tumor size (maximum diameter by pathologic examination)
Biochemical profile including liver and renal function	Number of axillary nodes removed
Chest radiograph	Number of axillary nodes positive for tumor
Mammographic report	Estrogen and progesterone receptor information
Clinical stage (TNM)	
Type of initial treatment	
Mastectomy or lumpectomy	Social environment
Radiation therapy – type, center, treating radiotherapist	Physical and mental function
Pathology*	Family and social support
Histologic type	Access to clinic (transportation)
Tumor grade	Financial resources (co-insurance)

*This information is generally available in the pathology report. All pathology reports, including needle aspiration cytology, excisional biopsy, lumpectomy or mastectomy surgical pathology reports should be provided. Estrogen and progesterone receptor results are often sent to reference laboratories and may be reported separately.

will be needed to determine if preoperative chemotherapy results in significant improvements in either relapse-free or overall survival.

For women with sizeable primary lesions, several courses of preoperative chemotherapy can be given to reduce the size of the primary lesion allowing for 'lumpectomy' and breast conservation. In one study, almost 80% of 161 patients with breast cancers larger than 3 cm had tumor shrinkage to less than 3 cm after three or four courses of preoperative chemotherapy and only four patients progressed (Bonadonna *et al.*, 1990). Preoperative chemotherapy for women with large primary lesions (>4 cm) makes breast conservation an option for almost all women.

Summary of Management Options

- Adjuvant treatment for early stage breast cancer is an evolving discipline. Current regimens have led to modest, but clinically important, improvements in both relapse-free and overall survival.
- Promising new regimens, especially those that are associated with major toxicity and high cost, should be tested in randomized trials. When available, patients should be offered the opportunity of clinical trial participation.
- Adjuvant therapy is recommended for most of the 50% of new patients with breast cancer who have negative nodes.
- With regards to neoadjuvant chemotherapy, complete or partial responses of the primary (large) lesion occurred in 80% of patients in a recent randomized trial.
- Tamoxifen therapy reduced the odds of recurrence and mortality in all age groups when compared to no treatment. The magnitude of the benefit on disease recurrence was greater for patients of 50 years of age and over, but women less than 50 years of age also had a statistically significant reduction.
- For women aged 50 years and over there was no significant effect of ovarian ablation either on recurrence-free survival or overall survival. However, women less than 50 years of age had a highly significant improvement in recurrence-free survival and in overall survival.
- Tamoxifen significantly decreased the annual odds of developing contralateral breast cancer by approximately 40%, and was associated with a reduction in non-cancer-related deaths (mostly cardiovascular) of 12%.
- The introduction of gonadotropin releasing hormone (GnRH) agonists has provided a more acceptable and extremely effective method for 'chemical ovarian ablation' in premenopausal women.

References

Abeloff MD (1992) High-dose adjuvant chemotherapy for high-risk breast cancer. *Rec. Res. Cancer Res.* **127:** 177–183.

Bonadonna G, Brusamolino E, Valagussa P *et al.* (1976) Combination chemotherapy as an adjuvant treatment in operable breast cancer. *N. Engl. J. Med.* **294:** 405–410.

Bonadonna G, Veronesi U, Brambilla C *et al.* (1990) Primary chemotherapy to avoid mastectomy in tumors with diameters of three centimeters or more. *J. Natl. Cancer Inst.* **82:** 1539–1545.

■ Bonadonna G (1992) Evolving concepts in the systemic adjuvant treatment of breast cancer. *Cancer Res.* **52:** 2127–2137.

Bonadonna G & Valagussa P (1981) Dose-response effect of adjuvant chemotherapy in breast cancer. *N. Engl. J. Med.* **304:** 10–15.

Boring CC, Squires TS, Tong T & Montgomery S (1994) Cancer statistics, 1994. *CA* **44:** 7–26.

Breast Cancer Trials Committee, Scottish Cancer Trials Office (MRC) (1987) Adjuvant tamoxifen in the management of operable breast cancer: the Scottish trial. *Lancet* **2:** 171–175.

Clark GM, Wenger CR, Beardslee S *et al.* (1993) How to integrate steroid hormone receptor, flow cytometric, and other prognostic information in regard to primary breast cancer. *Cancer* **71:** 2157–2162.

Del Turco MR, Palli D & Cariddi A (1994) Intensive diagnostic follow-up after treatment of primary breast cancer. *JAMA* **271:** 1593–1597.

Dimitrov N, Anderson S, Fisher B *et al.* (1994) Dose intensification and increased total dose of adjuvant chemotherapy for breast cancer: findings from NSABP B-22. *Proc. Am. Soc. Clin. Oncol.* **13:** 64 (abstract).

Early Breast Cancer Trialists' Collaborative Group (1988) Effects of adjuvant tamoxifen and of cytotoxic therapy on mortality in early breast cancer. An overview of 61 randomized trials among 28,896 women [see comments]. *N. Engl. J. Med.* **319:** 1681–1692.

■ Early Breast Cancer Trialists' Collaborative Group (1992) Systemic treatment of early breast cancer by hormonal, cytotoxic, or immune therapy. 133 randomised trials involving 31,000 recurrences and 24,000 deaths among 75,000 women. *Lancet* **339:** 1–15, 71–85.

Fisher B, Brown A, Wolmark N *et al.* (1987) Prolonging tamoxifen therapy for primary breast cancer. Findings from the National Surgical Adjuvant Breast and Bowel Project clinical trial. *Ann. Intern. Med.* **106:** 649–654.

Fisher B, Carbone P, Economou SG *et al.* (1975) L-phenylalanine mustard (L-PAM) in the management of primary breast cancer. *N. Engl. J. Med.* **292:** 117–123.

Fisher B, Costantino JP, Redmond CK *et al.* (1994a) Endometrial cancer in tamoxifen-treated breast cancer patients: findings from the National Surgical Adjuvant Breast and Bowel Project (NSABP) B-14 [see comments]. *J. Natl. Cancer Inst.* **86:** 527–537.

Fisher B, Redmond C, Dimitrov NV *et al.* (1989) A randomized clinical trial evaluating sequential methotrexate and fluorouracil in the treatment of patients with node-negative breast cancer who have estrogen-receptor-negative tumors. *N. Engl. J. Med.* **320:** 473–478.

Fisher B, Rockette H, Robidoux A *et al.* (1994b) Effect of preoperative therapy for breast cancer on local-regional disease: first report of NSABP B-18. *Proc. Am. Soc. Clin. Oncol.* **13:** 64 (abstract).

GIVIO investigators (1994) Impact of follow-up testing on survival and health-related quality of life in breast cancer patients. *JAMA* **271:** 1587–1592.

Glick JH, Gelber RD, Goldhirsch A & Senn H (1992) Meeting highlights: Adjuvant therapy for primary breast cancer. *J. Natl. Cancer Inst.* **84:** 1479–1485.

Harvey HA (1988) Luteinizing hormone-releasing hormone agonists in the treatment of breast cancer. [Review]. *Cancer Treat. Res.* **39:** 39–49.

Jones SE, Moon TE, Bonadonna G *et al.* (1987) Comparison of different trials of adjuvant chemotherapy in stage II breast cancer using a natural history data base. *Am. J. Clin. Oncol.* **10:** 387–395.

Kau SW, Buzdar A, Fraschini G, Hug V, Holmes F & Hortobagyi G (1990) Impact of adjuvant chemotherapy with FAC in patients with $\geqslant 10$ positive nodes operable breast cancer. *Proc. Amer. Soc. Clin. Oncol.* **9:** 24 (abstract).

Love RR, Mazess RB, Barden HS *et al.* (1992) Effects of tamoxifen on bone mineral density in postmenopausal women with breast cancer [see comments]. *N. Engl. J. Med.* **326:** 852–856.

Matsukuma A, Enjoli M & Toyoshima S (1991) Ductal carcinoma of the breast. An analysis of proportions of intraductal and invasive components. *Pathol. Res. & Practice* **187:** 62–67.

McDonald CC & Stewart HJ (1991) Fatal myocardial infarction in the Scottish adjuvant tamoxifen trial. *Br. Med. J.* **303:** 435–437.

McGuire WL & Clark GM (1992) Prognostic factors and treatment decisions in axillary-node-negative breast cancer [see comments]. *N. Engl. J. Med.* **326:** 1756–1761.

Muss HB (1992) Endocrine therapy for advanced breast cancer: a review. *Breast Cancer Res. Treat.* **21:** 15–26.

Muss HB, McNamara MJ & Connelly RA (1988) Follow-up after stage II breast cancer: a comparative study of relapsed versus nonrelapsed patients. *Am. J. Clin. Oncol.* **11:** 451–455.

Nicholson RI, Walker KJ, McClelland RA *et al.* (1990) Zoladex plus tamoxifen versus Zoladex alone in pre- and peri-menopausal metastatic breast cancer. *J. Steroid Biochem. Molec. Biol.* **37:** 989–995.

■ Olivotto IA, Bajdik CD, Plenderleith IH *et al.* (1994) Adjuvant systemic therapy and survival after breast cancer. *N. Engl. J. Med.* **330:** 805–810.

Peters WP, Ross M, Vredenburgh JJ *et al.* (1993) High-dose chemotherapy and autologous bone marrow support as consolidation after standard-dose adjuvant therapy for high-risk primary breast cancer. *J. Clin. Oncol.* **11:** 1132–1143.

Rosen PP, Groshen S & Kinne DW (1992) Survival and prognostic factors in node-negative breast cancer: results of long-term follow-up studies. *J. Natl. Cancer Inst. Monographs* **11:** 159–162.

Rosner D, Lane WW & Penetrante R (1991) Ductal carcinoma *in situ* with microinvasion. A curable entity using surgery alone without need for adjuvant therapy. *Cancer* **67:** 1498–1503.

Rutqvist LE & Mattsson A (1993) Cardiac and thromboembolic morbidity among postmenopausal women with early-stage breast cancer in a randomized trial of adjuvant tamoxifen. The Stockholm Breast Cancer Study Group [see comments]. *J. Natl. Cancer Inst.* **85:** 1398–1406.

Schapira DV (1993) Breast cancer surveillance – a cost-effective strategy. *Breast Cancer Res. Treat.* **25:** 107–111.

Schapira DV & Urban N (1991) A minimalist policy for breast cancer surveillance. *JAMA* **265:** 380–382.

Spicer D, Pike MC & Henderson BE (1990) The question of estrogen replacement therapy in patients with a prior diagnosis of breast cancer. *Oncology* **4:** 49–59.

Tormey DC & Jordan VC (1984) Long-term tamoxifen adjuvant therapy in node-positive breast cancer: a metabolic and pilot clinical study. *Breast Cancer Res. Treat.* **4:** 297–302.

■ Wertheimer MD (1991) Against minimalism in breast cancer follow-up. *JAMA* **265:** 396–397.

Wood WC, Budman DR, Korzun AH *et al.* (1994) Dose and dose intensity of adjuvant chemotherapy for stage II, node-positive breast carcinoma [see comments]. *N. Engl. J. Med.* **330:** 1253–1259.

28 Metastatic Breast Cancer

L N Harris
M E Lippman

Metastatic breast cancer is one of the greatest challenges facing the oncologist. Few other malignant diseases can recur anywhere from a few months to a few decades after the diagnosis and treatment of the primary disease. Metastatic disease may have a myriad of presentations. Breast cancer can be indolent or aggressive, widespread or localized, and this undoubtably reflects the heterogeneous nature of the disease itself. This 'jack of all trades' is, unfortunately, also a master. It is commonly sensitive to therapy at first recurrence, but then, with few exceptions, follows a course of relapse and death of the patient from chemoresistance. The challenge then, is not only to diagnose and treat this disease, but to keep foremost in mind the value of quality of life in a disease which is rarely curable.

Epidemiology

Breast cancer is a common malignancy in women in developed countries, occurring in 12% of women, with 3.5% of women dying of this disease in the USA during the last decade. (Harris *et al.*, 1992). In addition, its incidence has increased significantly since the 1930s with a 1.2% per year increase until the early 1980s and a 4% per year increase between 1982 and 1986 (Connecticut tumor registry). Although some argument exists as to the significance of this recent increase given potential biases (improved diagnosis, reporting), the numbers alone speak for the health problem at hand.

If left untreated, breast cancer is fatal. The most significant impact on survival from the disease is, indisputably, the advent of surgical removal of the primary tumor. Early studies from the Middlesex hospital (Bloom *et al.*, 1962) recounting the natural history of breast cancer indicate that untreated breast cancer patients have a median survival of 2.7 years. Surgical intervention has reduced the mortality to 50% at ten years. Adjuvant therapies, including endocrine manipulation and chemotherapy, have had a modest, but significant, impact on survival (Early Breast Cancer Trialists' Collaborative Group, 1992). Despite the 30% risk reduction, a significant minority of breast cancer patients (40%) will still relapse and die of metastatic disease. The overwhelming clinical challenge remains the skilful treatment of recurrent disease and the ongoing search for new therapies that may significantly impact on mortality.

Impact of Therapy on Survival

Metastatic disease is, essentially, incurable. The one possible exception to this is locoregional recurrence. In-breast recurrence, as seen following breast-conserving procedures, has a far less grave outcome. These entities should be clearly distinguished in one's mind and will therefore be discussed separately from the treatment of distant metastasis. While adjuvant therapy has allowed a modest improvement in overall survival, this has not been clearly demonstrated in the treatment of metastatic disease. The reason for this lies in the fact that direct comparisons of treatment versus observation have not been done due to an understandable reluctance on the part of both the physician and patient not to intervene once a recurrence is evident. The ideal study, in theory, would be a randomization of patients with known disease and individual characteristics to treatment versus none. As this study will never be done for ethical reasons, how then do we sort out the question of benefit from therapy? Attempts to address this have been made using three methods of data analysis:

- Retrospective studies. When treated cohorts are compared with untreated historical controls, several studies have shown improved survival. Todd *et al.* (1983) showed a median survival increase from 21 months in 1920 to 41 months in 1970 when looking at series of breast cancer patients from Yale. Although fraught with the inherent biases of comparison with historical controls such as lead-time bias, recent improvement in diagnostic techniques and ancillary care, it is unlikely that these account for all of the improvement in overall survival.
- Comparison of responders and non-responders. Clearly, patients who respond to systemic therapy have a longer survival than those that do not. Most studies in metastatic breast cancer support this contention, implying that effective therapy may improve survival. The potential error in this assumption is that the patients who respond do not otherwise harbor characteristics that themselves predict for longer survival. For example, patients with estrogen receptor (ER)-positive

disease and a long disease-free interval are likely to do better than the converse, regardless of treatment.

- Comparison of different treatment regimens. Doxorubicin-containing regimens have a higher response rate and longer median survival from time of treatment onset than other multiagent regimens (e.g. cyclophosphamide, methotrexate and 5-fluorouracil – CMF). A recent overview (A'Hern *et al.*, 1988) indicates that the higher response rate predicts for a longer overall survival. While there is no 'no treatment' arm in these studies, it seems reasonable to suggest that therapy has some impact, particularly when there is no evidence that chemotherapy has a negative impact on the natural history. However, the impact on overall survival, even when the response rate is projected to 90%, is modest at best (of the order of 4–6 months) (*Table 28.1*).

Although evidence for a modest improvement in survival is implied, it has been harder to show that patients with disseminated disease are cured. Dose-intensive chemotherapy is being evaluated in this regard, but due to insufficient length of follow-up, it is too early to determine if a tail exists on the survival curve. In the meantime, 'standard-dose' therapy is usual practice. How, then, do we justify this treatment with its attendant toxicities to our patients with metastatic breast cancer when little is gained in objective terms? The answer lies in unequivocal evidence of benefit in quality of life for patients on systemic therapy.

Table 28.1. Effect of chemotherapy on survival of patients with metastatic breast cancer: hypothetical examples derived from overview analysis of 50 randomized trials comparing two or more chemotherapy regimens with unequal response rates (modified from A'Hern RPA *et al.*, 1988).

Response rate (%)	*Median survival (months)*
50*	18*
60	20.6
70	22.9
80	24.4
90	23.7

*Baseline assumption that patients treated with a regimen inducing a 50% response rate would have a median survival of 18 months. The other values in the table have been calculated from a fitted regression equation derived from the relationship between the odds ratio of the response rate of the regimen with the higher response rate divided by that with the lower response rate and the hazard ratio of the median survival (the median survival of patients on the regimen with the higher response rate divided by that of patients on the regimen with the lower response rate).

Palliation and Quality of Life

If systemic therapy for metastatic disease does not have a major impact on survival, and does not cure metastatic breast cancer, other endpoints must be assessed. Palliation and quality of life therefore become of paramount importance. Do patients benefit from systemic therapy in these terms? Although counter-intuitive, studies seem to indicate that this is indeed the case. Measures of symptom control have been assessed in a number of trials. Of note is the consistent observation that the percentage of patients who achieve relief from pain considerably exceeds the percentage of responders (complete and partial) (Brunner *et al.*, 1975). In addition, quality of life measures have been recently incorporated into studies of metastatic breast cancer patients. Examples are the Nottingham Health Profile (NHP), Linear Analogue Self-Assessment (LASA) and Qualitator (QoL). A number of studies show improved scores in patients on continuous treatment versus intermittent therapy or standard versus low-dose treatment (Tannock *et al.*, 1988). Surprisingly, it appears in this setting that 'more is better.' The contribution of 'placebo effect' and the psychologic effect of treatment is impossible to determine.

Finally, certain treatments that are unlikely to affect survival are undeniably helpful in palliating symptoms. Examples include drainage of pleural/pericardial effusion, irradiation of painful bone lesions and other sites (e.g. choroidal, brain and spinal cord metastases), and surgical control of local disease. While it is unlikely that these modalities significantly prolong life, no one disputes their use because they undoubtly have palliative benefit.

Diagnosis of Metastatic Disease

The same questions may be put to the idea of 'early diagnosis' of metastatic disease. Does the patient stand to benefit by knowing about a recurrence early or in an asymptomatic stage? Similar quandaries are encountered when trying to address this question. It would be difficult to convince any patient with known metastatic disease, whether asymptomatic or not, to receive no treatment, therefore these studies are not available. Some retrospective studies do support a modest improvement in survival in patients diagnosed earlier. Whether this is due to the biology of disease (e.g. earlier treatment, less resistant clones as per the Goldie–Coldman hypothesis, 1979) or lead-time bias is undetermined, although evidence from the adjuvant treatment of breast cancer supports the concept that earlier diagnosis improves outcome. It seems reasonable then, where practical, to diagnose metastatic disease at the stage where therapy may be of most benefit.

Certain groups undoubtly achieve benefit from early detection and these include patients with in-breast recurrences and some patients with locoregional disease. In-breast recurrence after conservative treatment has a much better prognosis than distant recurrence, statistically comparable with the diagnosis of primary node-positive disease (Recht *et al.*, 1989). This fact supports breast screening in patients with physical examination and mammography on a regular basis. It is felt that six-monthly screening of the affected breast is likely only useful for the first three years (Hassell *et al.*, 1990), due to the higher rate of in-breast recurrence during this time period. In addition, patients who have been diagnosed with a breast cancer have an increased incidence of a second primary (estimated at about 0.8% per year). This reinforces the need for breast screening.

Locoregional recurrence has a much poorer prognosis than in-breast recurrence. Nonetheless, there appears to be a small subset of patients who enjoy long disease-free intervals after secondary local therapy and some may, in fact, be cured (Aberizk, *et al.*, 1986). Whether time of treatment intervention influences this survival is unclear; however, patients with these recurrences do benefit from early detection in order to optimize local control.

Certain patients with visceral disease may achieve benefit from early detection, in theory, as both liver and lung metastases are more easily treated when the tumor burden is lower before performance status is compromised. Whether routine screening for these entities using chest radiography and liver imaging is beneficial has been called into question. Two Italian randomized studies were recently published examining the efficacy of three-monthly follow-up with history and physical examination alone versus the same follow-up with the addition of regular blood tests, chest radiography, liver ultrasound and bone scan (GIVIO, 1994; Del Turco *et al.*, 1994). Neither study was able to demonstrate a difference between 'intensive' versus control follow-up with respect to overall survival. Quality of life measures were assessed in one of the two studies and, again, no difference was seen between the two groups. When questioned about their preference for follow-up, it is interesting to note that 70% of women in the GIVIO study indicated a preference for routine diagnostic testing, even in the absence of symptoms. The use of intensive screening for visceral disease requires re-evaluation, although follow-up with history, physical examination and simple blood tests is probably cost-effective. Both studies did incorporate symptom-directed testing, and it is clear that this is indicated. Symptoms such as anorexia, weight loss, malaise and right upper quadrant pain should be assessed with liver ultrasound or computerized tomography (CT) scan. Although routine chest radiography in addition to clinical examination may not be appropriate, it should be performed if there are pulmonary complaints.

Bone disease is a common first site of metastasis and should be screened for by routine history and physical examination. The benefit of plain films or

Table 28.2. Oncogenes in human breast cancer. (DFS, disease-free survival; OS, overall survival; CT, chemotherapy.)

Gene	*Synonyms*	*Mode of activation*	*Clinical correlation*
c-erbB-2 Van De Vijver *et al.* (1991) Slamon *et al.* (1987), Nicholson *et al.* (1990), Muss *et al.* (1994)	HER2/neu	Amplification in 20–30%	Grade, number of positive lymph nodes, DFS, OS, hormone and CT resistance
c-erbB-1 Lippman *et al.* (1989), Nicholson *et al.* (1990)	Epidermal growth factor receptor (EGFR)	Amplification in 4–14%	Hormone resistance
c-myc Mackay *et al.* (1990)	None	Amplification in 4–32%	Inconsistent association with number of positive lymph nodes, inflamatory cancer, poor prognosis
c-Ha-ras-1 Mackay *et al.* (1990)	H-ras Harvey ras p21 protein	Point mutation leading to RNA and protein overexpression	Increase in activated p21 (ras) protein in higher grade, T3 and 4 tumors, metastatic disease (progression)
Int-1 Van De Vijver *et al.* (1991)	Wnt-1 (*Drosophila* wingless gene)	Amplification (infrequent)	No correlation with prognosis
Int-2 Van De Vijver *et al.* (1991)	Fibroblast growth factor (FGF)	Amplification in 5–23%	Increased local recurrence, lymph node metastasis, poor prognosis
c-erbB-3 Rajlcumai *et al.* (1994)	HER3	Over expression	Positive lymph nodes
c-erbB-4	HER4	Not studied	Not studied

bone scans in the absence of symptoms is questionable. Central nervous system metastases are rare as a first site of metastasis and should be screened for by history and physical examination alone. Symptoms such as headache, nausea and vomiting, mental changes and sensorimotor changes should be investigated promptly. CT of the brain, lumbar puncture, plain films of the spine and CT magnetic resonance imaging (MRI) of the spinal cord may be useful for specific symptom complexes.

The use of biologic markers for screening is of unproven benefit. Certainly, tumor associated antigens such as carcinoembryonic antigen and CA-15.3 may be of use in following a patient with recurrent disease, particularly if disease is difficult to evaluate. Since there is currently no evidence that treatment of asymptomatic elevations in a tumor marker is useful it seems reasonable to perform these tests at the diagnosis of first recurrence.

Certain oncogenes are expressed in human breast cancer and are associated with clinical outcome (*Table 28.2*). The erbB-2 (HER-2/neu) oncogene product is the most extensively studied (Slamon *et al.*, 1987) and correlates with a worse prognosis in node-positive patients. Whether patients with erbB2 overexpression can be followed with recently described measures of circulating antigen is under study (Hayes *et al.*, 1989). If early detection is possible, these patients might be ideal for targetting new modalities of therapy (e.g. dose-intensive therapy) aimed at irradicating minimal disease or biologic therapies directed against the erbB2 protein, which are now entering clinical trials.

Treatment

Once the diagnosis of metastatic breast cancer is made, the treatment decision involves a number of variables. It is important to keep in mind that some of the variables, which denote prognosis and treatment in the adjuvant setting, are no longer useful in the metastatic setting (except in an academic sense). For example, nodal status, while of critical importance in predicting liklihood of relapse, has no further clinical use once the disease has recurred. Several factors do retain their prognostic and therapeutic significance, however. The most important of these factors are discussed below.

Factors with Prognostic and Therapeutic Significance

Estrogen and progesterone receptor status

These nuclear steroid receptors are known to have both prognostic and therapeutic significance and are therefore generally determined at the time of initial diagnosis. They can be measured by a number of techniques, the most commonly accepted method being enzyme immunoassay from a sample of the primary tumor (Chamness *et al.*, 1979). This method requires tissue which is snap-frozen at the time of biopsy and thus may be a limitation in small tumors. As a result, immunohistochemical assays using paraffin-embedded tissue have been developed, which allow the measurement of steroid receptors using a smaller tissue sample. Recent reports indicate that the latter method is useful in this setting and may be widely applicable (Allred, 1993).

Due to clonal heterogeneity, ER receptor status in the metastatic tumor may not concur with that determined at the time of primary diagnosis. It has been shown that the presence and amount of ER measured at time of recurrence predicts for response to endocrine therapy independently of site or extent of disease and previous therapy (Allegra *et al.*, 1980). Where practical, measurement of ER in the recurrence should be undertaken.

Although ER-positive/progesterone receptor (PR)-negative tumors have a lower response rate to anti-estrogens than ER-positive/PR-positive tumors (32% versus 71%) (McGuire *et al.*, 1978), the clinical use of measuring PR levels in metastatic patients has not been determined. Most patients with recurrent disease (even ER-negative) will receive a trial of hormonal therapy sometime during their course because these interventions are relatively non-toxic and options are limited. More recent studies have shown that certain mutations in the PR may make it constitutively active, even in the absence of ER (Fuqua *et al.*, 1991).

Menopausal status

Menopausal status is of unquestionable value in deciding on adjuvant therapy for primary breast cancer. This may not hold true for the metastatic setting, however. Although premenopausal women have a worse prognosis than postmenopausal women with respect to rate of relapse, particularly at 35 years of age and under, when all prognostic indicators are taken into account, age is not an independent predictor of response to treatment. The confusion lies in the fact that a higher proportion of premenopausal women have ER-negative tumors and visceral disease, which tend to behave more aggressively. This means that other factors should be taken into account when making treatment decisions for premenopausal women. For example, a young woman with ER-positive, locally recurrent breast cancer has a similar prognosis to an older woman with such a history. Knowledge of menopausal status is useful when endocrine therapy is being considered because certain hormonal maneuvers are effective in this subgroup and not in postmenopausal patients (e.g. oophrectomy, luteinizing hormone releasing hormone (LHRH) agonists). The opposite is also true (e.g. aminoglutethimide is not effective in ovulatory women).

Disease-free interval

The time between primary diagnosis and recurrence of breast cancer is important from both a prognostic and therapeutic point of view (Cutler, 1974). Long disease-free interval, over two years is associated with more indolent disease, which is more likely to respond to endocrine therapy. In addition, if the patient has received adjuvant treatment (which is becoming more common), the time to treatment failure predicts liklihood of second response to the same treatment. This applies mainly to chemotherapy because most women who relapse after adjuvant endocrine therapy are still on that treatment at the time of relapse. Patients who relapse less than two years after systemic chemotherapy are unlikely to respond to that same regimen and should be offered an alternative. Chemotherapy is usually indicated in this setting because the short disease-free interval implies aggressive disease. Patients who relapse after a long disease-free interval usually do so with more indolent bone or soft tissue disease and are therefore somewhat more likely to respond to endocrine manipulations.

Site of relapse

Information regarding the sites of relapse is important in both prognosis and treatment of metastatic breast cancer patients and underscores the need to do a full metastatic work-up at the time of first recurrence. Visceral disease (e.g. lung, liver, brain) carries a poor prognosis in comparison with soft tissue and bone disease. While overlap exists, for example some patients with liver or lung metastases can have excellent therapeutic responses and prolonged survival, most patients with visceral disease have aggressive disease with a dismal prognosis (median survival one year, Zinser *et al.*, 1987). Systemic chemotherapy is indicated in these patients due to the low response rate to endocrine treatment and the rapidity of disease progression. Soft tissue and bone disease, depending on the clinical setting, can usually be treated with hormonal maneuvers and other measures (surgery, radiation, local treatments).

Biologic markers

As we come to understand the biology of breast cancer through cellular and molecular biologic studies, several markers for disease behavior have been identified. These 'markers' are products of normal cellular genes, which when mutated or de-regulated in some fashion, can contribute to malignant behavior. Two members of the epidermal growth factor receptor family (EGF-R or c-erbB-1 and HER-2/neu or c-erbB-2) have been shown to have prognostic significance in the adjuvant setting (Nicholson *et al.*, 1990). While this may have little relevance once the patient has metastatic disease, recent studies have shown a negative correlation with response to endocrine therapy in metastatic patients whose tumors overexpress C-erbB-2 or EGF-R. In addition, erbB-2 may predict resistance to some chemotherapeutic regimens (CMF) and sensitivity to others (doxorubicin-containing) Muss *et al.*, 1994). The potential for biologically-directed therapeutics is an exciting possibility if these results are confirmed.

Metastatic breast cancer is a complex clinical problem that requires both the art and science of medicine. Effective palliation depends upon understanding the biology of the disease in all its manifestations and a sensitivity to the needs and preferences of the particular patient.

Endocrine Therapy

After surgical extirpation, manipulation of the hormonal milieu with varying forms of endocrine therapy is the oldest form of breast cancer treatment. Observations dating back nearly a century show that a proportion of breast cancers will regress following oophorectomy. In addition, many experimental studies have demonstrated that estrogens are critically responsible for the growth of ER-positive breast cancer (Lippman, 1989). In particular, estrogens appear to regulate critical growth factors and their receptors in ER-positive tumors (Lippman *et al.*, 1986). Although the mechanism of breast cancer control by estrogen withdrawal has been thought to be 'cytostatic' based on *in vitro* observations of breast cancer cell lines being shifted into G0 (resting phase of the cell cycle), there is some evidence that anti-estrogens may be cytocidal *in vivo*. When Michigan cancer foundation-7 (MCF-7) breast cancer cells are injected into nude mice and estrogens are subsequently withdrawn, apoptosis or programmed cell death can be seen in regressing tumors (Kyprianou *et al.*, 1986). Removal of sources of estrogens such as the ovary and adrenal or therapy with anti-estrogens results in tumor regression and relief of symptoms in many patients. The choice of endocrine therapy (in the first instance) and the specific modality relate to aforementioned factors (e.g. ER/PR status, menopausal status, disease-free interval).

Approximately 30% of unselected patients will respond to some form of endocrine manipulation (Henderson, 1989). If estrogen receptor status is taken into account, 50–75% of ER-positive tumors will show a response, while only 5–10% of ER-negative tumors respond. The degree of positivity is also important because tumors with an ER measurement higher than 50 fmol mg^{-1} protein are associated with a 77% response to endocrine therapy as opposed to 30% in tumors with an ER measure of 10–20 (Allegra *et al.*, 1980) (*Table 28.3*). Other clinical characteristics associated with a response to endocrine treatment include long disease-free interval (over two years), performance status, bone or soft tissue disease and a previous response to hormonal therapy.

With a few notable exceptions, most forms of endocrine treatment give similar response rates (*Table 28.4*). Median duration of response is 12–18 months although many patients will respond to a second (50%) and third-line (30%) hormonal maneuver, which can extend survival for 2–3 years or more. These subsequent responses depend heavily on the response to initial therapy with the minority of ER-positive patients responding to a second-line treatment if they do not respond initially (although the response rate is quoted as high as 30% in a review by Byar *et al.*, 1979). Given equivalent efficacy, the choice of endocrine therapy is usually based on the side-effect profile of a given treatment and ease of administration. The exceptions to this are as follows.

- Oophorectomy, which is only effective in patients who are actively menstruating or within one year from cessation of menses.
- High-dose estrogen therapy and aromatase inhibitors may be useful in the treatment of postmenopausal patients but appear to give lower response rates in premenopausal women, probably because of the specific mechanism-of-action (see later discussion).
- LHRH agonists are more effective in premenopausal women due to the modulation of ovarian function. Response rates in postmenopausal women appear to be quite low (i.e. 11%, Saphner *et al.*, 1993).
- Androgens and corticosteroids. Although the combination of these drugs with tamoxifen may increase response rates (Tormey *et al.*, 1983), their independent use gives a lower response rate (approximately 20% for androgens, 5–10% for corticosteroids) and therefore these agents should not be used as first-line (see *Table 28.4*).

Specific hormonal treatments

Adrenalectomy/hypophysectomy

These forms of surgical castration were the mainstay of treatment of metastatic breast cancer before the

Table 28.3. Objective response rate to endocrine therapy as a function of the amount of estrogen receptor. (Reprinted from *Eur. J. Cancer* **16**, Allegra J, Lippman M, Thompson E *et al.* Estrogen receptor status: An important variable in predicting response to endocrine therapy in metastatic breast cancer, 1980, with kind permission from Elsevier Science Ltd, The Boulevard, Langford Lane, Kidlington, OX5 1GB, UK.)

Estrogen receptor (fmol mg^{-1} cytoplasmic protein)	*Response rate*			
$0 \leq ER < 10$	3/33 (9%)	$p > 0.05$ (rows 1–2)	$p < 0.001$ (rows 1–3)	$p < 0.00001$ (rows 1–4)
$10 \leq ER \leq 20$	3/10 (30%)			
$20 < ER < 50$	7/11 (63%)			
$ER \geq 50$	24/31 (77%)			

Table 28.4. Response rates of unselected patients to endocrine therapies (reprinted with permission from Harris *et al*, 1993).

Therapy	*No. of patients*	*Response rate (%)*	*Range (%)*
Tamoxifen*	1269	32	16–52
Oophorectomy‡	3380	33	21–41
Progestins*	3479	31	9–67
Aminoglutethimide†	1153	32	16–43
Luteinizing hormone releasing hormone (LHRH) analogs	293	40	32–45
Estrogens*	1683	26	15–38
Androgens*	2250	21	10–38
Adrenalectomy*	3739	32	23–46
Hypophysectomy	1174	36	22–58

*Primarily postmenopausal patients.
†Exclusively postmenopausal patients.
‡Exclusively patients premenopausal or within one year of last menstrual period.

introduction of newer methods. Although the response rates are similar to those of other modalities, these methods have been supplanted by less morbid interventions.

Ovarian ablation

Response rates to ovarian ablation in premenopausal women are approximately 32%. Although never compared directly in controlled clinical trials, response rates to surgical oophorectomy versus radiation-induced menopause appear to be quite similar (Henderson, 1991). The latter may have a prolonged time to the onset of treatment effect, however, and this should be kept in mind when treating patients with metastatic disease. Surgical ablation involves an operative procedure with its attendant risks and in general should be used in situations where radiotherapy is contraindicated. In addition to low response rates in postmenopausal women, it has been documented that patients less than 35 years of age have a low response rate (less than 20%) to ovarian ablation and therefore this is not the optimal treatment of such patients (Dao, 1972)

Side-effects of ovarian ablation, apart from surgical or radiotherapy-associated morbidity, are those expected with a premature induction of menopause (e.g. hot flushes, mood changes, vaginal dryness). Although early induction of the menopause does carry with it the risk of accelerated osteoporosis and cardiovascular disease, these patients do not generally survive long enough to manifest such symptoms.

Medically-induced ovarian ablation by LHRH agonists will be discussed in a later section.

Tamoxifen

Tamoxifen is an anti-estrogenic compound that interacts with the ER in breast cancer cells and causes a number of effects on transcription of this and other genes (Lerner and Jordan, 1990). When studied in MCF-7 breast cancer cells, tamoxifen produces a reduction in thymidine incorporation, suppression of DNA polymerase and a reduction in cell growth rate. The drug may have other mechanisms of action against breast cancer including the release of the inhibitory growth factor, tumor-derived growth factor β (TGF-β). This may explain responses seen in ER-negative patients. While inhibiting breast cancer growth *in vitro*, tamoxifen also acts as a partial agonist of estrogenic activity in other cells. This may explain some of the positive effects seen in patients on tamoxifen treatment including reduction of low density lipoprotein cholesterol and maintenance of bone density. It may also account for the proliferative effects seen on the endometrium and increased risk of endometrial cancer in patients so treated as observed in the National Surgical Adjuvant Breast and Bowel Program (NSABP-B14) and other studies (Van Leeuwen *et al.*, 1994).

The standard dose of tamoxifen is 10 mg twice a day, although based on pharmacokinetics a dose of 20 mg once a day is also acceptable. Higher doses have been investigated with no clear improvement in response rate or time to treatment failure (Tormey *et al.*, 1983). In general, tamoxifen is standard treatment for postmenopausal patients at the time of first recurrence, provided the patient has not taken the drug in an adjuvant setting within the preceding year. Extensive or rapidly growing visceral disease is also a relative contraindication. The use of tamoxifen as a first-line agent in premenopausal patients with metastatic disease is controversial. Two randomized studies published simultaneously in the *Journal of Clinical Oncology*, 1986, have been conducted to answer this question. In the larger of the two, no difference in response rate between treatment with tamoxifen versus oophorectomy was seen. In addition, secondary response rate after crossover was higher in the tamoxifen followed by oophorectomy arm than the reverse (33% versus 11%) (Ingle *et al.*, 1986; Buchanan *et al.*, 1986). It has been suggested that oophorectomy is superior to tamoxifen in the treatment of visceral metastases (Sawka *et al.*, 1986). While it seems intuitively difficult to accept that tamoxifen could be as efficacious as oophorectomy in young women with relatively high circulating estrogen levels, particularly when adjuvant studies indicate less benefit in premenopausal versus postmenopausal women, the evidence suggests their equivalence in the metastatic setting. It seems reasonable then to recommend either treatment modality in the appropriate premenopausal patient.

Although tamoxifen has a long list of side-effects, few occur with any frequency and those that are common tend to be non-prohibitive. Hot flushes, which tend to subside over time, are observed in approximately 30% of patients. The contribution of the drug to these side-effects may be much lower due to the proportion of perimenopausal women who may be experiencing this symptom already. Mild nausea occurs in fewer than 10% and may be abrogated by taking the medication with meals or at bedtime. Occasional headache and dizziness may occur and a transient thrombocytopenia or leukopenia has been observed. None of these side-effects have had serious consequences or dictate withdrawal of the medication. Elevated liver function tests may necessitate discontinuation of the drug. Several toxicities have come to light in the recent past as women on adjuvant tamoxifen have longer survival rates. The most serious of these include retinal and corneal changes and an increased risk of endometrial cancer (aforementioned). Annual ophthamologic and gynecologic examinations are therefore prudent although the enthusiasm for these should be tempered by the clinical situation.

Thrombophlebitis occurs in 1–3% of patients, but the increased risk of this phenomenon in metastatic cancer patients in general makes etiology difficult to determine. Pulmonary embolus occurs rarely.

Newer anti-estrogens with less agonist activity and/or more potent anti-tumor effect are now being investigated. Examples are toremifene, droloxifene and ICI-164384. Preliminary studies show similar response rates and toxicities to those of tamoxifen with some patients responding to these agents after failing tamoxifen. Further randomized studies are underway.

Estrogens

Surprisingly, estrogens themselves in pharmacologic doses are quite effective in the treatment of metastatic breast cancer. It has been proposed that estrogens work via a direct toxic effect through the ER, although this has not been clearly proven. Due to their considerable toxicity (nausea and vomiting, fluid retention, thrombophlebitis) they have been supplanted by other agents and are now rarely used.

Progestins

Although the mechanism of action of progestins on breast cancer is not entirely understood, experimental evidence suggests a dose-dependent inhibition of the hypothalamic–pituitary axis and a decrease of autocrine growth factors (Lippman, 1989).

Both medroxyprogesterone acetate (MPA) and megestrol acetate are effective in breast cancer, the former more commonly used in Europe and the latter in the USA. Direct comparisons with tamoxifen have generally shown equivalency, although a recent randomized study has shown an increased response rate to MPA versus tamoxifen in untreated patients (50% versus 30%) and a slightly longer time to progression (8.8 months versus 5.4 months) (Castiglione Gertsch *et al.*, 1993). Toxicities were also higher in the MPA arm.

Standard dosing of MPA is 400 mg qd and of megestrol acetate is 40 mg, four times a day. It may be that higher doses are more effective, based on some preliminary studies which led to a current study by CALGB of megestrol acetate 160 mg versus 800 mg versus 1600 mg. Results are not yet available.

Toxicities from progestational agents are more undesirable than those of tamoxifen and include weight gain in 20–50%, fluid retention, hypertension, hyperglycemia and vaginal bleeding in 5–10% of patients. Less than 10% of women experience hot flushes. In general, the toxicity profile of these drugs has placed them second-line in the treatment of metastatic breast cancer with endocrine therapy.

Based on observations of antiproliferative effects in breast cancer cell lines (Schneider *et al.,* 1989), certain antiprogestational agents are currently under evaluation in this clinical setting. Mifepristone (RU-486) and onapristone are two such agents which have activity in breast cancer cell lines. A Phase II study is currently underway to evaluate responses in patients with advanced cancer.

Aromatase inhibitors

Aminoglutethimide is the main agent in this class and shows similar efficacy to other hormonal agents. It has two separate mechanisms of action which seem to be dose-related. At higher doses (250 mg twice a day to four times a day) the drug blocks adrenal conversion of cholesterol to pregnenolone, a precursor of estrogen synthesis. Due to the blockade of adrenal steroid production, patients on these doses require corticosteroid replacement therapy. The aromatization reaction, which occurs in peripheral tissues and involves conversion of androstenedione to estrone as well as testosterone to estradiol, is blocked at lower doses (125 mg four times a day). Although standard therapy has been 250 mg twice a day to four times a day with hydrocortisone replacement (40 mg daily in divided doses), lower doses may give similar response rates and reduce the need for steroid replacement (Harris *et al.*, 1986). If 125 mg twice a day is ineffective, escalating to a higher dose may produce responses. The adrenal gland is indirectly the main source of estrogens in the postmenopausal women (through peripheral conversion of androgens). Ovarian production of estrogen is not sufficiently abolished by these drugs due to hypothalamic–pituitary compensation; therefore, they are only indicated in women whose ovaries no longer function. This can be assessed by measuring levels of pituitary function in young patients whose menopausal status is uncertain.

Toxicities of aminoglutethimide include lethargy and other central nervous system side-effects (due to its similarity to the sedative glutethimide), a rash in 20%, which usually does not require discontinuation of the drug and may respond to an increase in hydrocortisone dosage, and steroid-related symptoms. The latter may manifest as addisonian or cushingoid symptoms, depending on the adequacy of the hydrocortisone dosage in a given patient, and should be closely monitored. Mild to moderate leukopenia and thrombocytopenia may occur from 2–7 weeks after administration and complete blood counts are indicated.

In general, aminoglutethimide with or without hydrocortisone replacement is indicated as third-line therapy, although there is evidence that bone metastases respond particularly well, which argues for its use as a second-line agent in the appropriate setting.

Newer aromatase inhibitors (e.g. 4-OH androstenedione) are currently under investigation and have progressed to clinical trial.

Androgens and corticosteroids

While these agents have some efficacy in the treatment of metastatic breast cancer, the response rates are lower than with other agents and therefore they are generally reserved for patients who have failed all other endocrine therapies. The most commonly used androgen is fluoxymestrone (Halotestin) at a dose of 10 mg twice a day. Side effects are those of virilization. Cholestatic jaundice has also been observed. Corticosteroids probably have minimal activity against breast cancer when used alone, but their positive effects on energy, appetite and sense of wellbeing may be useful in the pre-terminal stages of disease.

Danazol is a synthetic steroid with multiple endocrine effects, the main one being inhibition of pituitary function. Although it has been used alone and in combination with other endocrine treatments for metastatic breast cancer, it is not particularly active (17% response rate) and has several undesirable side-effects (lethargy, peripheral edema, hot flushes).

Luteinizing hormone-releasing hormone agonists

These agents have recently been implemented in the premenopausal setting as a form of 'medical oophrectomy.' Follicle stimulating hormone and luteinizing hormone are transiently increased and then fall to low levels. Response rates are much higher in premenopausal women (not unexpectedly) in the range of 32–50% (Harvey *et al.*, 1985). As aforementioned, postmenopausal women have an exceedingly low, 11%, response rate. Side-effects are minimal and include amenorrhea and postmenopausal symptoms. Ovarian function may resume on withdrawal of the drug and this should be kept in mind when choosing further therapy. Due to the low toxicity, reversibility and comparable efficacy to standard forms of oophorectomy, these agents are likely to supplant radiation and surgical methods of castration in the future.

Combinations of hormonal treatments

A number of combinations have been investigated in the past (tamoxifen +/− fluoxymestrone, MPA, aminoglutethimide, danazol). Although response rates are generally higher, no improvement in overall survival is seen and the combined toxicities probably do not warrant concurrent use (Henderson, 1991).

Chemotherapy

Chemotherapy is, in general, reserved for patients who have failed endocrine therapy or whose disease is less likely to respond to hormonal maneuvers. The latter includes those with rapidly progressive visceral disease, a disease-free interval less than 2 years and ER-negative primary tumors. The patient should, ideally, have measurable lesions and no co-morbid disease serious enough to preclude the use of cytotoxic agents.

Polychemotherapy in this setting gives objective responses in approximately two-thirds of patients with a median duration of response of less than 1 year. A complete response occurs in fewer than 20% (*Table 28.5*). Although the minority, a number of patients achieve long disease-free periods of quality life and prolonged survival after treatment with chemotherapy. The choice of chemotherapy for first-line treatment is between two well-studied drug regimens: alkylator-based (e.g. cyclophosphamide/ methotrexate/5-fluorouracil – CMF) and doxorubicin-containing combinations.

Alkylator-based regimens

Cyclophosphamide-containing regimens (or other alkylator-based combinations e.g. L-PAM (melphalan), chlorambucil) have been studied extensively in the metastatic setting. Combinations of CMF (with cyclophosphamide given in oral or intravenous form) are felt to give the highest response rates with the least toxcity. Vincristine and prednisone were included in the original 'Cooper regimen' and have been evaluated in randomized trials with and without these drugs. Vincristine is not felt to contribute substantially to the regimen and adds neurotoxicity. The addition of prednisone may lead to higher response rates, but the added toxicity of 40 mg of the drug daily for two weeks may not justify its added benefit, particularly as overall survival is not altered (Canellos *et al.*, 1976). The administration of cyclophosphamide by oral versus intravenous form was felt to be equivalent based on phase II studies; however, a recent article has cast some doubt on this assumption. The European Organization for the Research and Treatment of Cancer (EORTC) compared 'classical CMF' with

Table 28.5. Response to and survival after treatment with commonly used drug combinations for metastatic breast cancer (modified from Henderson, 1987).

Percentage of patients with a response	43–82
Percentage with a complete response	4–27
Time to response (wks)	
Median	7–14
Maximum	72
Duration of response (months)	
Median	5.3–13
Maximum	180+
Survival of responders (months)	
Median	14.8–33
Maximum	180+

the three-weekly intravenous schedule in postmenopausal patients with advanced breast cancer and found the former to be superior in both response rate (48% versus 29%) and overall survival (17 months versus 12 months) (Engelsman *et al.*, 1991).

Doxorubicin-based regimens

Doxorubicin, either alone or in combination with other drugs gives 10–20% higher response rates than alkylator-based regimens. Some randomized studies show a nonsignificant 3–6 month improvement in survival (Tormey *et al.*, 1984). Because of the added toxicity of increased alopecia and the potential risk of cardiac failure, and given a favorable second-line response to doxorubicin (30–40%) some groups advocate initial treatment with CMF. However the higher response rates do lead to an improved quality of life (measured by various scales) and the modest improvement in survival may justify the added toxicity.

Dosage and duration of treatment

A number of studies have clearly shown that suboptimal chemotherapy doses reduce response rates and overall survival (Tannock *et al.*, 1988; Blomqvist *et al.*, 1993). Quality of life has also been shown to be superior in patients on full-dose CMF compared to that of patients on low-dose epirubicin despite higher toxicity (Fraser *et al.*, 1993). Therefore it is not appropriate to reduce chemotherapy dosages unnecessarily in this setting with the hope of minimizing side-effects. The role of increasing dose intensity (mg/m^2 per week) in breast cancer is less well defined and the topic of considerable debate. While retrospective studies show a relationship between increased dose intensity and improved therapeutic outcome in metastatic patients (Hryniuk and Bush, 1984), whether this extrapolates to an increase over and above standard doses is an open question. Studies are currently underway investigating the use of bone marrow transplant and/or growth factor support in intensifying chemotherapy dose. Initial results do indicate improved response rates, but the duration of response and overall survival have not been significantly different between high-dose and standard-dose chemotherapy in the metastatic setting (*Table 28.6*).

The optimum duration of chemotherapy treatment in metastatic breast cancer has not been clearly established. While it has been shown that continuous chemotherapy (cyclophosphamide + doxorubicin (CA) or CMF) is superior to three months' induction with reinduction at disease progression (Coates *et al.*, 1987), another study has shown that patients treated with CMFVP (CMF plus vincristine and prednisone) for six months followed by observation and reinduction had a slightly improved survival compared with the same regimen given continuously (Smalley *et al.*, 1976). A more recent study from the Piedmont Oncology Group treated patients with six cycles of CAF (cyclophosphamide, doxorubicin, 5-fluorouracil) followed by randomization to either observation or maintenance therapy with CMF (Muss *et al.*, 1991). In this study, patients on the continuous chemotherapy arm had a longer median survival (21.1 months versus 14.8 months). Unfortunately, of 250 patients who entered this study, only 145 were randomized to the latter part of the study and when this population was considered, no difference in overall survival was seen. In addition, neither of the latter studies incorporated formal measures of quality of life, which are now felt to be imperative in this setting. In summary then, optimum dosage should be maintained for at least six months of induction chemotherapy. The decision to continue treatment should be based on symptoms and the patient's level of comfort with either continuing or discontinuing treatment.

Salvage chemotherapy

A number of agents are known to have activity in breast cancer and can be used once patients have failed CMF and doxorubicin-containing regimens.

Mitomycin C and vinblastine are effective for some tumors resistant to the above agents. Infusional 5-fluorouracil has been used extensively and may give response rates as high as 50% in heavily pretreated patients (Chang *et al.*, 1989). The addition of folinic acid to 5-fluorouracil in conjunction with mitoxantrone has shown considerable second-line activity (65%) in several Phase II studies (Hainsworth,

Table 28.6. High-dose chemotherapy (HDC) versus standard chemotherapy (SC) for metastatic breast cancer. (NS, not stated.)

Study	*Disease-free survival (months)*	*Overall survival (months) HDC versus SC*	*Complete remission rate (%) HDC versus SC*	*Overall response rate (%) HDC versus SC*	*Response duration (months) HDC versus SC*
Hillner *et al.*, 1992	NS	27.4 versus 21.4	40 versus 20	75 versus 50	NS
Antman and Souhami, 1993	NS	NS	74	NS	NS
Eddy, 1992	NS	16.0 versus 16.6	36 versus 8	NS	8 versus 9.6

1993). The efficacy of this combination as first-line therapy is currently being compared to CMF in a randomized trial.

Newer agents

Paclitaxel, and other members of the taxane family have recently been added to the armory of treatment for metastatic breast cancer. The compound contains a 16-carbon taxene ring, is derived from the Pacific yew, *Taxus brevifolia* and has a unique mechanism of action. It appears to promote microtubule assembly and inhibit depolymerization, thereby interfering with cytoskeletal integrity and mitosis, inducing G_2M arrest of cells. Although the compound was identified many years ago, only recently has technology allowed it to be purified in a form that can be administered to patients. Treatment regimens vary from 4–96 hour infusions, 125–250 mg/m^2. In patients who have failed one or more regimens, impressive response rates of 50–60% are seen (Hortobagyi and Holmes, 1994). Studies are currently underway to evaluate its efficacy as a first-line therapy. Vinorelbine, another inhibitor of microtubule structure, is also being investigated in breast cancer patients both in Europe and the USA. Response rates of 43–52% are observed in untreated patients (Vogel *et al.*, 1994).

Drug resistance

Overcoming resistance to currently used chemotherapeutic agents is an area of intense activity. Reversing the 'multidrug resistance' phenotype by inhibitors of p-glycoprotein and glutathione transferases are currently being studied.

Biologic therapies

A large number of growth factors and their receptors have been identified that play a role in breast cancer tumorigenesis. These include members of the EGFR family (EGFR, erbB-2) and their ligands (TGF-α, EGF, PDGF, ndf/heregulin), insulin-like growth factors and fibroblast growth factors (Lippman and Dickson, 1986). The latter group is probably involved in angiogenesis in breast tumors. A number of trials are currently underway using specific inhibitors of these factors including pentosan polysulfate, CAI (a novel calcium-channel blocker), medroxyprogesterone, vitamin D analogues and others.

Another, less obvious mechanism of action is being exploited in some biologic therapies. It is generally accepted that chemotherapeutic agents preferentially kill rapidly dividing cells through a number of cellular pathways. It follows then that agents that may increase the fraction of dividing cells in a tumor to a significant degree may allow synergistic effects when administered with chemotherapy. Various growth factor receptors are known to induce mitogenesis and increased growth fraction in both tumor cell lines and experimental tumors. In order to exploit this concept, a number of investigators are currently combining conventional chemotherapeutic agents and antibodies to, for example, EGFR and the erbB-2 receptor (Norton *et al.*, 1994; Shawver *et al.*, 1994). These antibodies have been shown to bind to their respective receptors and activate signalling without inducing growth stimulation, possibly explaining the synergistic effects seen with these combinations.

Radiotherapy

Radiotherapy plays an important adjunctive role in the treatment of metastatic breast cancer. Breast tumor cells are quite sensitive to radiotherapy and can be retreated in some circumstances. Bone lesions that produce pain, instability or impending fracture can usually be well-controlled with radiation with minimal side-effects. Other sites that are amenable to this treatment are skin and soft tissue, spinal cord, leptomeninges, choroid and brain disease. The latter will be discussed further in the next section.

Special Problems

Bone Metastases and Hypercalcemia

In most instances, bone metastases will be multiple in the metastatic setting and should therefore be treated with systemic therapy in addition to radiotherapy and surgery where appropriate. The best choice for systemic therapy will depend on the clinical situation, as previously discussed. Radiotherapy to all lesions is not feasible and should therefore be limited to isolated painful areas or lesions that invade bone cortex, involve over 50% of the bone diameter or are larger than 2.5 cm in their greatest dimension (Cornell and Lane, 1987). Surgical stabilization may be appropriate for lesions that have already fractured or do not respond to radiotherapy. In addition, worrisome lesions in the axial skeleton may require this intervention. The use of isotopes such as strontium-89 and others in treating extensive skeletal metastases has shown some interesting results with reduction of bone pain in 83% of breast cancer patients in one study (Robinson, 1990). The exact role still needs clarification.

Hypercalcemia is not uncommon, with approximately 5–10% of all patients developing this condition at some time in the course of metastatic disease. Hydration and stabilization of fluid and electrolyte status is mandatory in all patients. While standard measures have included the administration of corticosteroids, mithramycin or calcitonin in the past, these modalities have to a large extent been replaced by the use of bisphosphonates. These compounds (etidronate, pamidronate, clodronate) are highly effective, relatively non-toxic and can be used repeatedly. In fact, a recent study by Paterson *et al.* (1993) has reported the efficacy of clodronate in oral form in reducing the incidence of fractures in women with bone metastases. This is being further evaluated in randomized trials.

Lymphangitic Disease and Pleural Effusion

Spread of breast cancer through the lung lymphatics can be difficult to diagnose. A chest radiograph may appear normal initially, although CT scan of the chest can give further information. Reticulonodular infiltrates on the chest radiograph may have other causes as well in this population (e.g. infection, drug toxicity) and should be ruled out using clinical and laboratory means before embarking on treatment. Systemic chemotherapy is nearly always indicated in this setting because endocrine therapy is unlikely to produce a rapid response rate. Despite the serious nature of this site of recurrence, median survival at one year can be as high as 80% and two-year survival rate, 30% (Henner, 1987).

Pleural effusion, while tending to follow a more indolent course, is a very common problem in metastatic breast cancer with more than 50% of patients developing this condition (Henner, 1987). In many cases, intermittent thoracentesis or pleurodesis with sclerosing agents (bleomycin, tetracycline) can control symptoms, the choice between them depending on the patient's projected survival. Systemic therapy is generally indicated, although more non-toxic endocrine therapies may be considered in this situation.

Central Nervous System Metastases

Brain metastases

Parenchymal brain lesions are usually multifocal in breast cancer patients and may present with a number of symptom constellations. Nausea and vomiting, headache, ataxia, changes in mental status, focal neurologic deficit and seizure are the most common. Treatment involves the use of corticosteroids (usually dexamethasone) to reduce peritumoral edema in conjunction with whole brain radiotherapy. Carefully selected patients with a single focus should be considered for surgical extirpation, which may improve survival in this setting (Patchell *et al.*, 1990). Unfortunately, isolated brain metastases are rare in patients with metastatic breast cancer. Systemic chemotherapy may also help control disease, but should not be used in isolation.

Spinal cord compression

Spinal cord compression is a medical emergency and usually presents with lateralizing weakness and/or sensory deficit. A rapid diagnosis must be made, usually by plain film in conjunction with CT/myelography, although MRI may be a better diagnostic tool (Byrne, 1992). Prompt introduction of corticosteroids and radiotherapy can significantly reduce morbidity from permanent neurologic deficit.

Leptomeningeal disease

Carcinomatous meningitis can be a very difficult diagnosis in breast cancer patients as it often presents insidiously with headache, mental changes and fleeting sensorimotor deficits. Diagnosis, too, may be problematic because CT scans of the brain and bone radiographs may be normal. Repeated lumbar puncture for cytology and myelography are necessary to make the diagnosis. Once confirmed, the introduction of intrathecal chemotherapy is almost always indicated because this disease is too diffuse to be treated with radiotherapy alone. Methotrexate and cytosine arabinoside (Ara-C) and thiotepa are the most commonly used agents (Wasserstrom *et al.*, 1982). Median survival from leptomeningeal disease is quite poor (seven months) and most patients will die from systemic disease within a year.

Conclusions

Metastatic breast cancer is a complex disease which has and will continue to challenge us for decades. Although some in-roads have been made in the treatment of this devastating illness, we are far from satisfied with our ability to manage the continuing morbidity and mortality it inflicts. With careful patient evaluation and awareness of quality of life as an endpoint we can attempt to provide optimal treatment. Only through innovative thinking and further understanding of its biologic origins will we ever impact on the human suffering caused by metastatic breast cancer.

Summary of management options

- In-breast recurrence after conservative treatment carries a prognosis statistically comparable with the diagnosis of primary node-positive disease; therefore six-monthly screening of the affected breast is indicated for the first three years after primary diagnosis of breast cancer and yearly thereafter.
- Although patients with visceral disease may achieve benefit from early detection because both liver and lung metastases are more easily treated when the tumor burden is low, routine screening using chest radiography and liver imaging has been called into question. At the present time it seems reasonable to follow breast cancer patients with a history, physical examination and blood tests (complete blood count and liver function tests) with further investigations to be performed when dictated by symptoms.
- Bone disease is a common first site of metastasis and should be screened for by history and physical examination. Plain films or bone scans in the absence of symptoms are not indicated.
- Once the diagnosis of metastatic breast cancer is made, the treatment decision involves a number of variables including estrogen receptor level in the primary tumor, menopausal status, disease-free interval and site of recurrence. In general, all patients should receive a trial of endocrine therapy although certain conditions (rapidly progressive visceral disease, central nervous system metastases) preclude this.
- Most forms of endocrine treatment give similar response rates and therefore their use is dictated by the side-effect profile of a given treatment and the ease of administration. The exceptions to this are: oophorectomy, which is only effective in patients who are actively menstruating or within one year from cessation of menses; high-dose estrogen therapy and aromatase inhibitors, which may be useful in the treatment of postmenopausal patients, but give lower response rates in premenopausal women; luteinizing hormone releasing hormone (LHRH) agonists, which are more effective in premenopausal women due to the modulation of ovarian function; androgens and corticosteroids, the independent use of which is associated with a lower response rate (approximately 20% for androgens, 5–10% for corticosteroids) so therefore these agents should not be used first line.
- Chemotherapy is usually reserved for patients who have failed endocrine therapy or whose disease is less likely to respond to hormonal maneuvers. The choice of chemotherapy for first-line treatment is between alkylator-based (e.g. cyclophosphamide/methotrexate/5-fluorouracil – CMF) and doxorubicin-containing combinations. The added toxicity of increased alopecia and potential risk of cardiac failure and a favorable second-line response to doxorubicin (30–40%) lead some groups to advocate initial treatment with CMF. Higher response rates to doxorubicin-containing regimens lead to improved quality of life and the modest improvement in survival may justify the added toxicity.
- High-dose chemotherapy with growth factor support or bone marrow transplantation has led to improved response rates in the metastatic setting; however, little evidence for improved overall survival exists and this approach should still be considered as experimental.
- Newer endocrine and chemotherapeutic agents (e.g. LHRH agonists, paclitaxel) have shown considerable activity in metastatic breast cancer and show promise for the future.
- Bone metastases are usually multiple in the metastatic setting and should be treated with systemic therapy in addition to radiotherapy and surgery where indicated.
- Hypercalcemia occurs in 5–10% of metastatic breast cancer patients and should be treated with hydration and stabilization of fluid and electrolyte status followed by corticosteroids, mithramycin or calcitonin. The latter two agents have to a large extent been replaced by the use of bisphosphonates.
- Parenchymal brain lesions are usually multifocal in breast cancer patients and treatment involves the use of corticosteroids in conjunction with whole brain radiotherapy. Carefully selected patients with a single focus should be considered for surgical extirpation, which may improve survival in this setting.
- Spinal cord compression is a medical emergency and prompt introduction of corticosteroids and radiotherapy can significantly reduce morbidity from permanent neurologic deficit.

References

Aberizk WJ, Silver B, Henderson IC *et al.* (1986) The use of radiotherapy for treatment of isolated locoregional recurrence of breast carcinoma after mastectomy. *Cancer* **58:** 1214–1218.

A'Hern RP, Ebbs SR & Baum MB (1988) Does chemotherapy improve survival in advanced breast cancer? A statistical overiew. *Br. J. Cancer* **57:** 615–618.

Allegra J, Lippman M, Thompson E *et al.* (1980) Estrogen receptor status: An important variable in predicting response to endocrine therapy in metastatic breast cancer. *Eur. J. Cancer* **16:** 323–331.

Allred DC (1993) Should immunohistochemical examination replace biochemical hormone receptor assays in breast cancer? *Am. J. Clin. Pathol.* **99(1):** 1–3.

Antman KH & Souhami RL (1993) High-dose chemotherapy in solid tumors. *Ann. Oncol.* **4 (Suppl 1):** S29–S44.

Blomqvist C, Elomaa I, Pissanen R *et al.* (1993) Influence of treatment schedule on toxicity and efficacy of cyclophosphamide, epirubicin and fluorouracil in metastatic breast cancer: a randomized trial comparing weekly and every 4-week administration. *J. Clin. Oncol.* **11(3):** 467–473.

Bloom HJG, Richardson WW & Harrier EJ (1962) Natural history of untreated breast cancer (1805–1933). *Br. J. Med.* **2:** 213–221.

Brunner KW, Sonntag RW, Martz G *et al.* (1975) A controlled study in the use of combined drug therapy for metastatic breast cancer. *Cancer* **36:** 1208–1219.

Buchanan RB, Blamey RW, Durrant KR *et al.* (1986) A randomized comparison of tamoxifen with surgical oophorectomy in premenopausal patients with advanced breast cancer. *J. Clin. Oncol.* **4:** 1325–1330.

Byar D, Sears M & McGuire W (1979) Relationship between estrogen receptor values and clinical data in predicting the response to endocrine therapy for patients with advanced breast cancer. *Eur. J. Cancer* **15:** 299–310.

Byrne TN (1992) Spinal cord compression from epidural metastases. *N. Eng. J. Med.* **327(9):** 614–619.

Canellos GP, Pocock S, Taylor S *et al.* (1976) Combination chemotherapy for metastatic breast carcinoma. *Cancer* **38:** 1882–1886.

Castiglione-Gertsch, Pampallona S, Varini M, Cavalli F, Brunner K, Senn HJ, Goldhirsch A & Metzzer U (1993) Primary endocrine therapy for advanced breast cancer. To start with Tamoxifen or with medroxyprogesterone acetate? *Ann. Oncol.* **4:** 735–740.

Chamness GC & McGuire WL (1979) Methods for analyzing steroid receptors in human breast cancer. In: McGuire WL (ed) *Breast Cancer, Advances in Research and Treatment,* vol 3, p. 149. New York: Plenum.

Chang AYC, Most C & Pandya KJ (1989) Continuous intravenous infusion of 5-fluorouracil in the treatment of refractory breast cancer. *Am. J. Clin. Oncol.* **12(5):** 453–455.

Coates A, Gebski V, Stat M *et al.* (1987) Improving the quality of life during chemotherapy for advanced breast cancer. *N. Eng. J. Med.* **317(24):** 1490–1495.

Cornell CN & Lane JM (1987) Specific sites of metastatic disease and emergencies: Management of pathologic fractures. In: Harris JR, Hellman S, Henderson IC & Kinne DW (eds) *Breast Diseases,* pp. 525–532. Philadelphia: JB Lippincott.

Cutler S (1974) Classification of extent of disease in breast cancer. *Semin. Oncol.* **1:** 91–96.

Dao TL (1972) Ablation therapy for hormone-dependent tumors. *Annu. Rev. Med.* **23:** 1–18.

■ Del Turco MR, Palli D, Cariddi A *et al.* (1994) Intensive diagnostic follow-up after treatment of primary breast cancer. A randomized trial. *JAMA* **27(20):** 1593–1597.

Early Breast Cancer Trialists' Collaborative Group (1992) Systemic treatment of early breast cancer by hormonal, cytotoxic or immune therapy: 133 randomized trials involving 31,000 recurrences and 24,000 deaths among 75,000 women. *Lancet* **339:** 1–15, 71–85.

Eddy DM (1992) High-dose chemotherapy with autologous bone marrow transplantation for the treatment of metastatic breast cancer. *J. Clin. Oncol.* **10:** 657–670.

Engelsman E, Klign JCM, Rubens RD *et al.* (1991) 'Classical' CMF versus a 3-weekly intravenous CMF schedule in postmenopausal patients with advanced breast cancer. *Eur. J. Cancer* **27(8):** 966–970.

Fraser SCA, Dobbs HJ, Ebbs SR *et al.* (1993) Combination or mild single agent chemotherapy for advanced breast cancer? CMF vs epirubicin measuring quality of life. *Br. J. Cancer* **67(2):** 402–406.

Fuqua SAW, Charness GC, Benedix MG *et al.* (1991) Progesterone receptor gene restriction fragment length polymorphisms in human breast tumors. *J. Natl. Cancer Inst.* **83:** 1157–1160.

■ GIVIO Investigators (1994) Impact of follow-up testing on survival and health-related quality of life in breast cancer patients. A multicenter randomized controlled trial. *JAMA* **271(20):** 1587–1592.

Goldie JH & Coldman AJ (1979) A mathematical model for relating the drug sensitivity of tumors to their spontaneous mutation rate. *Cancer Treat. Rep.* **63:** 1727–1733.

Hainsworth JD (1993) The use of mitoxantrone, 5-fluorouracil and high-dose leucovorin in the treatment of advanced breast cancer. *Ann. Oncol.* **4 (Suppl 2):** S37–S40.

Harris AL, Cantwell BMJ, Sainsbury JR *et al.* (1986) Low dose aminoglutethimide (125 mg twice daily) with hydrocortisone for the treatment of advanced postmenopausal breast cancer. *Breast Cancer Res. Treat.* **7:** 1–44.

■ Harris JR, Lippman ME, Veronesi U & Willett W (1992) Breast cancer. *N. Eng. J. Med.* **327(5):** 319–478.

Harris JR, Morrow M & Bonnadonna G (1993) Cancer of the breast. In: Devita VT *et al.* (eds) *Cancer: Principles and Practice of Oncology,* 4th edition, p. 1250. Philadelphia, PA: JB Lippincott.

Harvey HA, Lipton A, Max DT *et al.* (1985) Medical castration produced by the HRH analogue leuprolide to treat metastatic breast cancer. *J. Clin. Oncol.* **3:** 1068–1072.

Hassell PR, Olivotto IA, Mueller HA *et al.* (1990) Detection of recurrence after conservative surgery and radiation therapy. *Radiology* **176:** 731–735.

Hayes DF, Carney W, Tondini C *et al.* (1989) Elevated circulating c-neu oncogene product in patients with breast cancer. *Br. Cancer Res. Treat.* **14:** 135.

Henderson IC (1987) Chemotherapy for advanced disease. In: Harris JR, Hellman S, Henderson IC & Kinne DW (eds) *Breast Diseases,* pp. 428–479. Philadelphia: JB Lippincott.

■ Henderson IC (1991) Endocrine therapy of metastatic breast cancer. In: Harris JR, Hellman S, Henderson IC & Kinne DW (eds) *Breast Diseases,* 2nd ed, pp. 559–587. Philadelphia: JB Lippincott.

■ Henner WD (1987) Specific sites of metastatic disease and emergencies: Lymphangitic spread of carcinoma of the breast. In: Harris JR, Hellman S, Henderson IC & Kinne DW (eds) *Breast Diseases,* pp. 538–540. Philadelphia: JB Lippincott.

Henner WD (1987) Specific sites of metastatic disease and emergencies: Malignant effusions in breast cancer. In: Harris JR, Hellman S, Henderson IC & Kinne DW (eds) *Breast Diseases,* pp. 540–558. Philadelphia: JB Lippincott.

Hillner BE, Smith TJ & Desch CE (1992) Efficacy and cost-effectiveness of autologous bone marrow transplantation in metastatic breast cancer. *JAMA* **267:** 2055–2061.

Hortobagyi GN & Holmes FA (1994) Paclitaxel (taxol) therapy in breast cancer management. *Cancer Invest.* **12 (Suppl 1):** 31–32.

Hryniuk W & Bush H (1984) The importance of dose intensity in chemotherapy of metastatic breast cancer. *J. Clin. Oncol.* **2:** 1281–1288.

■ Ingle JN, Krook JE, Green SJ *et al.* (1986) Randomized trial of bilateral oophorectomy versus tamoxifen in premenopausal patients with metastatic breast cancer. *J. Clin. Oncol.* **4:** 178–185.

Kyprianou N, English HF, Davidson NE & Issacs JT (1986) Programmed cell death during regression of the MCF-7 human breast cancer following estrogen ablation. *Cancer Res.* **51:** 162–166.

Lerner LJ & Jordan VC (1990) Development of antiestrogens and their use in breast cancer: eighth Cain memorial award lecture. *Cancer Res.* **50(14):** 4177–4189.

■ Lippman ME, Dickson RB, Bates S *et al.* (1986) Autocrine and paracrine growth regulation of human breast cancer. *Breast Cancer Res. Treat.* **7:** 59–70.

Lippman ME & Dickson RB (1989) Mechanisms of growth control in normal and malignant breast epithelium. *Rec. Prog. Horm. Res.* **45:** 383–593.

Mackay J. Thompson AM, Coles C & Steel CM (1990) Molecular lesions in breast cancer. *Int. J. Cancer* **5:** 47–50.

McGuire WL, Horwitz KB, Zava DT *et al.* (1978) Progress in endocrinology and metabolism: hormones in breast cancer: Update 1978. *Metabolism* **27:** 487–501.

Muss HB, Case LD, Richards II F *et al.* (1991) Interrupted versus continuous chemotherapy in patients with metastatic breast cancer. *N. Eng. J. Med.* **325(19):** 1342–1348.

■ Muss HB, Thor AD, Berry DA *et al.* (1994) c-erbB-2 expression and response to adjuvant therapy in women with node-positive early breast cancer. *N. Engl. J. Med.* **330:** 18, 1260–1266.

Nicholson S, Wright C, Sainsbury RC *et al.* (1990) Epidermal growth factor receptor (EGFr) as a marker for poor prognosis in node-negative breast cancer patients: neu and tamoxifen failure. *J. Steroid Biochem. Molec. Biol.* **37:** 811–814.

Norton L, Baselga J, Fan Z *et al.* (1994) Rationale for the use of chemotherapy plus growth factor receptor blockage in the treatment of breast cancer. *Cancer. Invest.* **12 (Suppl 1):** 43–44.

Patchell RA, Tibbs PA, Walsh JW *et al.* (1990) A randomized trial of surgery in the treatment of single metastases to the brain. *N. Eng. J. Med.* **322:** 494–500.

Paterson AHG, Powles TJ, Kanis JA *et al.* (1993) Double-blind controlled trial of oral clodronate in patients with bone metastases from breast cancer. *J. Clin. Oncol.* **11(1):** 59–65.

Rajlcumai T, Cullick WJ (1994) The typelgrowth factors in human breast cancer. *Breast Cancer Res. Treat* **29:** 3–9.

Recht A, Schnitt SJ, Connolly JL *et al.* (1989) Prognosis following local or regional recurrence after conservative surgery and radiotherapy for early stage breast carcinoma. *Int. J. Radiat. Oncol. Biol. Phys.* **16:** 3–9.

Robinson RG (1990) Systemic radioisotopic therapy of primary and metastatic bone cancer. *J. Nucl. Med.* **31:** 1326–1327.

Saphner T, Troxel AB, Tormey D *et al.* (1993) Phase II study of goserelin for patients with postmenopausal metastatic breast cancer. *J. Clin. Oncol.* **11(8):** 1529–1535.

Sawka CA, Pritchard KI, Paterson AHG *et al.* (1986) Role and mechanism of action of tamoxifen in premenopausal women with metastatic breast carcinoma. *Cancer Res.* **46:** 3152–3156.

Schneider M, Michna H, Nishino Y *et al.* (1989) Antitumor activity and mechanism of action of different anti-progestins in experimental breast cancer models. *J. Steroid Biochem.* **34:** 447–453.

Shawver LK, Mann E, Elliger SS, Dugger TC & Arteaga C (1994) Ligand-like effects induced by anti-erbB-2 antibodies do not correlate with and are not required for growth inhibition of human carcinoma cells. *Cancer Res.* **54:** 1367–1373.

Slamon DJ, Clark GM, Wong SG *et al.* (1987) Human breast cancer: Correlation of relapse and survival with amplification of the HER-2/neu oncogene. *Science* **235:** 177–182.

Smalley RV, Murphy S, Huguley CM *et al.* (1976) Combination versus sequential five-drug chemotherapy in metastatic carcinoma of the breast. *Cancer Res.* **36:** 3911–3916.

Tannock IF, Boyd NF, DeBoer G *et al.* (1988) A randomized trial of two dose levels of cyclophosphamide, methotrexate and fluorouracil chemotherapy for patients with metastatic breast cancer. *J. Clin. Oncol.* **6:** 1377–1387.

Todd M, Shoag M & Cadman E (1983) Survival of women with metastatic breast cancer at Yale from 1920 to 1980. *J. Clin. Oncol.* **1:** 406–408.

Tormey DC, Lippman ME, Edwards BK *et al.* (1983) Evaluation of tamoxifen doses with and without fluoxymesterone in advanced breast cancer. *Ann. Int. Med.* **98:** 139–144.

■ Tormey DC, Weinberg VE, Leone LA *et al.* (1984) A comparison of intermitten vs. continuous and of adriamycin vs. methotrexate 5-drug chemotherapy for advanced breast cancer. *Am. J. Clin. Oncol.* **7:** 231–239.

Van de Vijver MJ & Nusse R (1991) The molecular biology of breast cancer. *Biochim. Biophysic. Acta* **1072:** 33–50.

Van Leeuwen FE, Benraadt J, Ceobergh JWW *et al.* (1994) Risk of endometrial cancer after tamoxifen treatment of breast cancer. *Lancet* **343:** 448–452.

Vogel CL, Bertsch LA & Hohneker JA (1994) Navelbine: a promising new drug with a favorable toxicity profile for breast and non-small cell lung cancer. *Cancer Invest* **12 (Suppl 1):** 17–18.

Wasserstrom WR, Glass JP & Posner JB (1982) Diagnosis and treatment of leptomeningeal metastases from solid tumors: experience with 90 patients. *Cancer* **49:** 759–772.

Zinser JW, Hortobagyi GN, Buzdar AU *et al.* (1987) Clinical course of breast cancer patients with liver metastases. *J. Clin. Oncol.* **5(5):** 773–782.

29 Pathogenesis and Epidemiology of Gestational Trophoblastic Neoplasia

A Ilancheran

Introduction

The term trophoblastic neoplasia designates the clinical condition caused by a spectrum of chorionic tumors that may originate either from the placenta or from the germinal cells of the gonads of either sex. This chapter will deal with those that directly result from a pregnancy (i.e. gestational trophoblastic neoplasms, GTN).

Classification

Before the pathogenesis and epidemiology of GTN are discussed it is vital to be clear about the nomenclature used in GTN because this has been a major source of confusion both for the pathologist and the epidemiologist. GTN remains unique among tumors in that malignancy is often diagnosed and treated without a histologic basis. Histologic and clinical terms are used interchangeably and this has led to conflicting epidemiologic data.

The original classification was proposed by Ewing in 1910. He devised a morphologic classification under the broad term 'chorioma' with the subdivisions shown in *Table 29.1*.

The term 'chorioadenoma destruens' was used to denote a particular type of hydatidiform mole (HM) which was mainly locally invasive into the myometrium and maintained its villous structure. Hence Ewing considered it to be an intermediate stage between HM and choriocarcinoma (CC). However, this entity can rarely metastasize and result in fatality. This was recognized by Prawirohardjo *et al.* in 1957, who replaced the term with a new term, villous choriocarcinoma. Tow (1966) in Singapore adopted this classification and included a new term, 'clinical choriocarcinoma.' This entity included patients who showed a pulmonary shadow on chest radiography, who had persistently raised human chorionic gonadotropin (HCG) levels or a positive pelvic angiogram, but without any histologic diagnosis of CC. In clinical practice, all these patients were treated in identical fashion to true CC (i.e. with chemotherapy). More recently, the term 'chorioadenoma destruens' has been replaced by the straightforward descriptive term 'invasive mole' (IM) (Park, 1971).

Table 29.1. Ewing's morphologic classification of chorioma.

1. Hydatid mole
2. Chorioadenoma destruens
3. Choriocarcinoma

4a. Syncytial endometritis

4b. Syncytioma

The term 'syncytial endometritis' is considered a misnomer (Elston, 1987) for it is clear now that the appearance in this condition is simply that of normal physiologic permeation of the gestational implantation site by the interstitial trophoblast. It is non-neoplastic. Similarly, the term 'syncytioma' has now been replaced by the term 'placental site trophoblastic tumor' (PSTT).

In order to bring some uniformity and in an attempt to standardize reporting of data, the Scientific Group of the World Health Organization recommended in 1983 that the terms shown in *Table 29.2* be used in the histopathologic and clinical nomenclature.

Pathogenesis

Trophoblasts have an inherent property of invasiveness involving both chemical and physical mechanisms. They usually burrow as deeply as the stratum compactum of the endometrium. Around day 11–12, the blastocyst has penetrated into the endometrium and comes to lie beneath the surface epithelium. In the course of erosion into the maternal endometrium, some trophoblasts become detached and are carried in the systemic circulation to reach distant parts of the body, most frequently the lungs. Attwood and Park (1961), among others, have shown that trophoblastic deportation is an apparently innocuous and almost physiologic phenomenon. It is well tolerated in normal women. They found some clearly identifiable trophoblastic cells in the lungs of nearly half of 220 patients reviewed. There is an obscure defense mechanism whereby most of the emboli are presumably quietly and uneventfully held in check and removed. The normal trophoblast therefore shows some of the characteristics of malignancy,

Table 29.2. Histopathologic and clinical nomenclature recommended by the World Health Organization Scientific Group, 1983.

A. Histopathologic terms
1. Hydatidiform mole (HM)
   1a. Complete hydatidiform mole (CHM)
   1b. Partial hydatidiform mole (PHM)
2. Invasive mole (IM)
3. Choriocarcinoma (CC)
4. Placental site trophoblastic tumor (PSTT)

B. Clinical terms
A. Gestational trophoblastic disease (GTD) – a general term that covers HM, IM, CC and PSTT, when histology is available
B. Gestational trophoblastic tumor (GTT) – a disease state in which there is clinical evidence of invasive mole or choriocarcinoma, but no histology is available. This category is further subdivided according to antecedent pregnancy, as post-mole, post-abortion, post-delivery, or unknown pregnancy
C. Metastatic trophoblastic tumor (MTT) – a disease state in which there is GTT that has extended beyond the body of the uterus

such as invasiveness, rapid growth and embolization.

Despite the vast advances made in its diagnosis and treatment, the actual derivation of trophoblastic disease is still a matter of inference and conjecture. Many abortuses show cystic alterations in a proportion of their chorionic villi similar to that seen in a HM. This is referred to as 'hydropic degeneration.' However, the marked discrepancy between the great frequency of such minimal changes and the relatively low incidence of a recognizable HM, has led to the postulation that there must be a continuum, a spectrum from simple hydropic change in a spontaneous abortion through to a classical HM (Hertig and Edmonds, 1940). They hypothesized that the primary defect was in the ovum; blighting of the ovum, with the resultant failure of the fetal circulation in the presence of actively secreting trophoblasts resulted in hydropic changes. This theory does not explain the prominent trophoblastic hyperplasia seen in HM. Park (1971), on the other hand, suggested that the primary defect was in the trophoblast itself and that the hyperplasia of this layer results in hydropic changes by oversecretion into the stroma. This may lead to total hydropic changes resulting in a blighted ovum and HM or partial change allowing the embryo to develop. The nature of the triggering mechanism for these pathogenetic changes remains largely obscure.

The field of cytogenetics has shed some light towards the understanding of the pathogenesis of GTN. For many years it had been generally agreed that moles were predominantly female in genetic sex (i.e. 46XX) (Park, 1957; Tominaga and Page, 1966). These findings were derived from the crude technique of Barr body estimation. However, more refined cytogenetic techniques used in recent years have demonstrated convincingly that the majority of complete moles are of 46XX constitution (Kajii and Ohama, 1977; Vassilakos *et al.*, 1977; Szulman and Surti, 1978; Lawler *et al.*, 1982). A more astounding fact that came out of these studies was that unlike a normal conceptus in which a haploid set of 23 chromosomes is contributed by each parent, complete moles contained a diploid complement of exclusively paternally-derived chromosomes (Kajii and Ohama, 1977; Jacobs *et al.*, 1980; Lawler *et al.*, 1982).

Two mechanisms have been suggested for this androgenetic parthenogenesis. The majority of the classic CHM with a 46XX karyotype come about through the fertilization of an 'empty egg' by a haploid sperm (23X). This duplicates itself (endo-reduplication) to give rise to a 46XX complement (*Figure 29.1*). In other words, the majority of CHM are from a homozygous zygote. Rarely, heterozygous CHM may result from fertilization of an 'empty egg' by two sperms (dispermy), one containing a 23X and the other a 23Y chromosomal set (Surti *et al.*, 1982). Approximately, 3–13% of CHM are heterozygous, with a 46XY karyotype (Wake *et al.*, 1978; Surti *et al.*, 1979). Very rarely, heterozygous 46XX CHM have been described (Fisher and Lawler, 1984). Moles with 46YY complement are never seen because at least one X chromosome is required for survival (Szulman and Surti, 1978). Although the androgenetic origin of CHM is generally accepted, very recent data suggest that the pathogenesis of

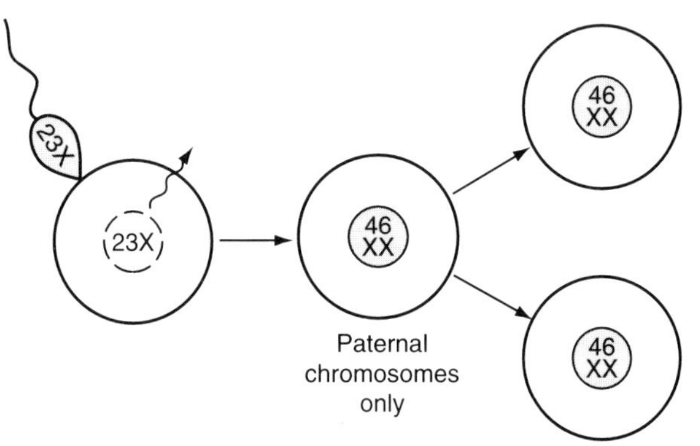

Figure 29.1. Paternal chromosomal origin of a complete classic mole (46XX). Left to right: an entry of a normal spermatozoon with a haploid set of 23X into an egg whose 23X haploid set is lost; the egg is 'taken over' by the paternal chromosomes, which duplicate (without the cell's division) to reach the requisite complement of 46. Observe that virtually the same result can be obtained through a fertilization by two spermatozoa gaining entry into an 'empty egg' (dispermy). (By courtesy of Szulman, 1984a.)

CHM may be more heterogeneous than previously suspected (Kovacs *et al.*, 1991). In a study of 22 consecutive CHM, it was demonstrated, using molecular genetic 'fingerprinting' methods, that 60% of these moles contained alleles consistent with a completely homozygous androgenetic origin. The remaining 40% were heterozygous for marker alleles; half of these were completely androgenic in origin and the other half contained alleles from the maternal genome. Therefore there was biparental contribution to the genesis of the moles. In a very recent study, Fisher and Newlands (1993), using the rapid polymerase chain reaction, showed that five of seven PHM studied had contributions from both parents to the molar genome.

The PHM, which is characterized by the presence of fetal parts, microscopic hydropic change and focal trophoblastic hyperplasia, is genetically abnormal and is usually triploid (Szulman and Surti, 1978), possessing 69 chromosomes instead of the normal 46 (*Figure 29.2*) with a maternal complement. Conversely, the majority of triploid conceptuses (86%) have histologic features of a partial mole (Szulman *et al.*, 1981). Some other cytogenetic abnormalities have also been described with PHM: various trisomies, 45X and 46XX karyotypes have been recorded (Jacobs *et al.*, 1982). When triploidy is present in PHM, the chromosome complement is XXY in 70%, XXX in 27% and XYY in 3% of the cases (Szulman and Surti, 1978). This extra haploid set of chromosomes may result from abnormal fertilization by dispermy (each with a haploid set of chromosomes), monospermy (with a diploid XY) or by digyny (maternally-derived 46XX, after failure of meiotic division, fertilized by haploid sperm).

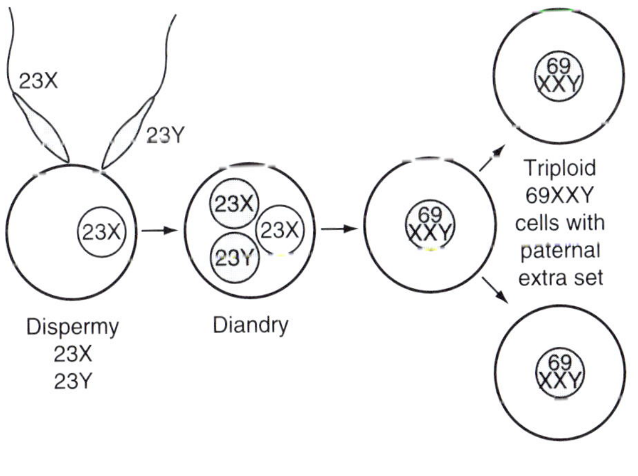

Figure 29.2. Triploid chromosomal origin of a partial mole (69XXY – dispermy). Fertilization of an egg equipped with a normal 23X complement by two independently produced spermatozoa (dispermy) to give a total of 69 chromosomes. Observe that triploidy can also result through the fertilization by a spermatozoon carrying the father's total complement of 46XY (paternal meiosis-I error). (By courtesy of Szulman, 1984b.)

These cytogenetic studies indicate that abnormal fertilization is probably the key factor in the development of CHM and PHM. Although the exact mechanism by which these chromosomal aberrations cause a molar change is unknown, it has been suggested that the ratio between the paternal and maternal haploid chromosomes may be important (Surti *et al.*, 1986). They hypothesized that the formation of a mole is associated with an excess of paternal contribution to the zygote. The higher the ratio of paternal to maternal chromosomes, the greater the molar change. CHM show a 2:0 ratio while PHM show a 2:1 ratio. This also implies that there can be a range of phenotypes of moles. Recent flow cytometric studies have shown a blurring of the apparently sharp division of mole into CHM and PHM (Hemmings *et al.*, 1987). These studies have shown that morphologic CHM may have triploidy, and histologically typical PHM may have a diploid karyotype. Surti *et al.* (1986) described tetraploid moles, some having the appearance of CHM and others PHM. It therefore appears that the morphologic appearance of a hydatidiform mole may not accurately predict its karyotype.

The chromosome complement of IM, CC and PSTT have not been well studied yet. The rarity of the occurrence of these conditions together with the fact that tissue diagnosis is not needed to diagnose or treat these conditions, has made it difficult to study these tumors. Makino *et al.* (1963) reported two cases of choriocarcinoma with aneuploidy. In a study of three post-molar CCs, Wake *et al.* (1981) found them to be heterozygous with a wide range of modal chromosomes. In another study of CCs and IMs, Davis *et al.* (1984) found that 14 of 19 (73%) CCs and two of four (50%) IMs showed positive Y chromatin. In a study of four established CC cell lines, no common karyotype or ploidy were noted (Shepard *et al.*, 1985).

The relationship between HM, IM and CC is still not clear. Persistent trophoblastic disease may follow both CHM and PHM, but the risk of subsequent CC is much greater for patients with CHM (Elston, 1987). Wake *et al.* (1984) have demonstrated that the heterozygous moles are associated with a much higher incidence of persistent trophoblastic disease than the homozygous moles, but Fisher and Lawler (1984) did not find a preponderance of heterozygosity in their cases of persistent trophoblastic disease. Frequent mutations were found at many loci of chromosomes in a study of CHM (Kovacs *et al.*, 1991). These authors suggest that these mutations may reflect the generalized genetic instability and that this may be related to subsequent malignant change. Further studies using these modern techniques will hopefully unravel the mysteries of this fascinating condition.

Epidemiology of Trophoblastic Neoplasia

The epidemiologic study of trophoblastic neoplasia is fraught with difficulties. There are many reasons for this, not least of which is the lack of uniform nomenclature. While histologic diagnosis may be the only objective, acceptable criterion, the nature of the disease is such that in many cases no histologic evidence of the disease may be available, and management is carried out on the basis of high levels of HCG, radiologic disease or clinical suspicion. Many other confounding factors affect the population at risk, which is exclusively women in the reproductive age group. The age of first marriage or first intercourse may affect the number of years of exposure to the risk of conception. Moreover, effective contraception and sterilization would have a great impact on the risk. For every conception that is prevented, a possible mole is averted. The incidence would be greatly affected by the abortion rate – both spontaneous and induced. Contraception, sterilization and abortion all constitute indirect prophylaxis against trophoblastic diseases and may be the reason why in countries like Singapore many fewer cases are seen now than 20 years ago.

A report of the World Health Organization Scientific Group (1983) identified three obstacles to the interpretation of most of the published studies on the epidemiology of trophoblastic disease. Firstly, as mentioned previously, many reports lack a clear,

Table 29.3. Incidence of hydatiform mole and choriocarcinoma by regions.

			Hydatiform mole per 1000			*Choriocarcinoma per 10,000*		
Country	*Authors*	*Period of study*	*Pregnancies*	*Deliveries*	*Live births*	*Pregnancies*	*Deliveries*	*Live births*
Hospital-based								
Africa								
Nigeria	Ayangade (1979)	1966–75	—	1.7	—	—	9.9	—
Nigeria	Junaid (1984)	—	—	3.04	—	—	—	—
Asia								
Singapore	Teoh *et al.* (1971)	1963–65	—	1.2	—	—	—	—
Philippines	Acosta-Sison (1959)	1955–57	1.1	—	—	—	—	—
	Baltazar (1976)	1970–74	—	—	—	—	—	1.7
Indonesia	Poen and Djojopranato (1965)	1962–63	10	11.6	—	15.3	17.7	—
Taiwan	Wei and Ouyang (1963)	1951–60	—	8	—	—	20.2	—
North America								
USA	Brewer and Gerbie (1967)	1959–64	—	—	—	0.5	0.6	—
Hawaii	Jacobs *et al.* (1982)	—	—	—	4.6	—	—	—
Latin America								
Mexico	Marquez-Monter *et al.* (1968)	1961–65	4.6	—	—	3.5	—	—
Population-based								
Asia								
Singapore	Shanmugaratnam *et al.* (1971)	1959–64	—	—	—	—	—	1.1
North America								
USA	Hayashi *et al.* (1982)	1970–77	1.1	—	—	—	—	—
USA	Yen and MacMahon (1968)	—	—	—	—	—	—	1.4
Latin America								
Paraguay	Rolon and De Lopez (1979) (1979)	1960–69	0.2	—	—	0.2	—	—

precise and reproducible case definition of the disease. Secondly, these reports are subject to errors in ascertaining the 'at risk' population. Hospital-based studies tend to overreport the number of gestational trophoblastic diseases because these 'problem pregnancies' are more likely to receive hospital care than uncomplicated pregnancies, many of whom may deliver at home, especially in developing countries. Again in many of these countries, cases of CC may die without receiving any medical attention or autopsy. Thirdly, reported cases of trophoblastic neoplasia are difficult to interpret because different denominators have been used (e.g. number of deliveries, number of live births, number of pregnancies). Ideally, the preferred denominator would be all the women who have conceived. The reported incidences of HM and CC are given in *Table 29.3*. The large geographic differences in the incidence of HM are probably due mainly to the methodologic difficulties mentioned above. Most reports of high incidence of HM come from developing countries with single hospital-based studies. However, if the population-based studies from North America, South Asia and Europe are compared, the differences are much less. Overall rates in these population studies range from 0.2–1.96 cases per 1000 pregnancies; whereas, incidence rates from hospital-based studies range from 0.7–11.6 (WHO Scientific Group, 1983). Similarly, for CC, the figures for population-based studies are 0.2–0.53 and for hospital-based studies, 0.2–19.1. However, two carefully controlled studies suggest that there might be a real geographic difference in the incidence of HM. In a study from Japan, Ishizuka (1976) reported an incidence of 1:522 pregnancies, while Womack and Elston (1985) reported that the incidence of HM in the UK was 1:1400 pregnancies. When the incidence per live births were compared in these two studies, it was 1:342 in Japan and 1:1364 for UK, a four times higher incidence in Japan. In an unpublished study conducted for the World Health Organization in 1983 in which 2000 consecutive first trimester abortions performed at the Kandang Kerbau Hospital, Singapore were sent for tissue analysis, this author found seven cases of PHM and one case of CHM, an incidence very similar to that of developed countries.

The geographic variation in the incidence may be a reflection of the racial distribution of the population. However, this aspect has not been well studied. In a study from Hawaii, a multiracial community, McCorriston (1968) found that the Japanese had a much higher incidence than the Caucasian population. In Singapore, which consists of three main racial groups, Teoh *et al.* (1971) found that the incidence was higher in Indians than in Chinese and Malays. In the USA, blacks have been reported to have a higher incidence in one study (Yen and MacMahon, 1968), but a lower rate in another (Hayashi *et al.*, 1982).

Several risk factors have been identified with the development of trophoblastic disease and these may indirectly affect the incidence. The most common of these is maternal age. Women at the extremes of reproductive age groups seem to be at a higher risk. Teenagers have been shown to have a moderately elevated risk of HM (Hayashi *et al.*, 1982; La Vecchia *et al.*, 1984; Bagshawe *et al.*, 1986). Studies in several countries have shown an increased risk of HM in women over 35 years of age (Teoh *et al.*, 1971; Nakano *et al.*, 1980; Hayashi *et al.*, 1982; La Vecchia *et al.*, 1984). The risk increases further with age to almost ten-fold beyond the age of 40 (Bagshawe *et al.*, 1986). Women in developing countries tend to conceive more at these age extremes and this may be partly responsible for the higher incidence in these countries. One study in Italy (La Vecchia *et al.*, 1984) indicated that even the paternal age may be important. In this study it was reported that there was an increased risk of GTN when fathers were over 45 years of age, after adjustment for maternal age. Another risk factor appears to be a previous HM pregnancy. The risk of a second HM is about 1.3% increasing to 15.4% (Bagshawe *et al.*, 1986) to 28% (Sand *et al.*, 1984) for the third HM. Other factors that do not consistently affect the incidence of HM include age of menarche, consanguinity, smoking, contraceptive use, infertility and nutritional status. The interested reader should refer to the excellent review on the epidemiology of moles by Bracken (1987).

CC or malignant GTN has the same epidemiological risk factors as HM. The single most important risk factor is an antecedent molar pregnancy. There is a 500–1000-fold increased risk of malignant sequelae after a CHM compared with a normal-term delivery (Ratnam and Ilancheran, 1982). The risk is much lower after a PHM (Berkowitz *et al.*, 1979). Malignant sequelae have also been found to be more common in women with blood group A (Dawood *et al.*, 1971). The risk is even higher if these women have an O spouse (Bagshawe, 1976).

Summary of Core Information

- Gestational trophoblastic neoplasia (GTN) encompasses a wide spectrum of disorders ranging from the benign hydatidiform mole to the malignant choriocarcinoma.
- Cytogenetically, two distinct forms of molar pregnancy have been identified, namely complete and partial hydatidiform moles.
- Recent advances in cytogenetics have shed some light on the pathogenesis of GTN. Abnormal fertilization seems to be the key factor in the development of moles from the conceptus.
- Epidemiologic studies of GTN suggest a much higher prevalence of the disease in the East and in Africa, but a closer look at the data indicates that this may be due to the type of population studied rather than a real difference in the incidence.

References

Acosta–Sison H (1959) Observations which may indicate the etiology of hydatidiform mole and explain its high incidence in Philippines and Asiatic countries. *Philippines J. Surg.* **14:** 290–293.

Attwood HD & Park WW (1961) Embolism to the lungs by trophoblast. *J. Obstet. Gynaecol. Br. Cwlth.* **68:** 611–617.

Ayangade O (1979) Gestational trophoblastic disease in Nigeria – a 10 year review. *E. Afr. Med. J.* **56:** 278–282.

Bagshawe KD (1976) Risk and prognostic factors in trophoblastic neoplasia. *Cancer* **38:** 1373–1385.

Bagshawe KD, Dent J & Webb J (1986) Hydatiform mole in England and Wales 1973–1978. *Lancet* **ii:** 673–677.

Baltazar JC (1976) Epidemiological features of choriocarcinoma. *Bull. WHO* **54:** 523–532.

Berkowitz RS, Goldstein DP, Mare AR & Bernstein MR (1979) Proliferative sequelae after evacuation of partial hydatidiform mole. *Lancet* **ii:** 804–805.

■ Bracken MB (1987) Incidence and aetiology of hydatidiform mole: an epidemiological review. *Br. J. Obstet. Gynaecol.* **94:** 1123–1135.

Brewer JI & Gerbie AB (1967) Early development of choriocarcinoma. In: Holland JF & Hreshchyshyn MM (eds) *Choriocarcinoma. Transactions of a Conference of the International Union against Cancer*, pp. 33–36. Berlin: Springer Verlag.

Davis JP & Foster KJ (1984) Sex assignment in gestational trophoblastic neoplasia. *Am. J. Obstet. Gynecol.* **148:** 722–725.

Dawood MY, Teoh ES & Ratnam SS (1971) ABO blood group in trophoblastic disease. *J. Obstet. Gynecol. Br. Cwlth.* **78:** 918–923.

Elston CW (1987) Gestational trophoblastic disease. In: Fox H (ed) *Haines & Taylor Obstetrical and Gynaecological Pathology*, 3rd Edition, pp. 1045–1078. London: Churchill Livingstone.

Ewing J (1910) Chorioma: a clinical and pathological study. *Surg. Gynecol. Obstet.* **10:** 366–392.

Fisher RA & Lawler SD (1984) Heterozygous complete hydatidiform mole: do they have a worse prognosis than homozygous complete moles? *Lancet* **ii:** 51.

Fisher RA & Newlands ES (1993) Rapid diagnosis and classification of hydatidiform moles with polymerase chain reaction. *Am. J. Obstet. Gynecol.* **48:** 563–569.

Hayashi K, Bracken MB, Freeman DH Jr & Hellenbrand K (1982) Hydatidiform mole in the United States (1970–1977): a statistical and theoretical analysis. *Am. J. Epidemiol.* **115:** 67–77.

Hemmings JD, Quirke P, Womack C *et al.* (1987) Diagnosis of molar pregnancy and persistent trophoblastic disease by flow cytometry. *J. Clin. Pathol.* **40:** 615–620.

Hertig AT & Edmonds HW (1940) Genesis of hydatidiform mole. *Arch. Path.* **30:** 260–291.

Ishizuka N (1976) Studies in trophoblastic neoplasia. *Gann* **18:** 203–216.

Jacobs PA, Wilson CM, Sprenkle JA, Rosenheim NB & Migeon BR (1980) Mechanism of origin of complete hydatidiform mole. *Nature* **286:** 714–716.

■ Jacobs PA, Hunt PA, Matsuura JS, Wilson CC & Szulman AE (1982) Complete and partial hydatidiform moles in Hawaii: cytogenetics, morphology and epidemiology. *Br. J. Obstet. Gynaecol.* **89:** 258–266.

Junaid TA (1984) Epidemiologic aspects of gestational trophoblastic disease in Ibadan, Nigeria. In: Patillo RA & Hussa RO (eds) *Human Trophoblast Neoplasms*, pp. 177–185. Plenum Press: New York.

Kajii T & Ohama K (1977) Androgenic origin of hydatidiform mole. *Nature* **268:** 633–634.

Kovacs BW, Shabarahrami B, Tast DE & Curtin JA (1991) Molecular genetic analysis of complete hydatidiform moles. *Cancer Genet. Cytogenet.* **54:** 143–152.

La Vecchia CL, Parazzini F, Decarli A *et al.* (1984) Age of parents and risk of gestational trophoblastic disease. *J. Natl. Cancer Inst.* **73:** 639–642.

Lawler SD, Povey S, Fisher RA & Pickthall VJ (1982) Genetic studies on hydatidiform moles. II. The origin of complete moles. *Ann. Hum. Genet.* **46:** 209–222.

Makino S, Sasaki MS & Fukushima T (1963) Preliminary notes on the chromosomes of human chorionic lesions. *Proc. Jap. Acad.* **39:** 54–58.

Marquez–Monter H, De la Vega GA, Ridaura C & Robles M (1968) Gestational choriocarcinoma in the general hospital of Mexico. Analysis of forty cases. *Cancer* **22:** 91–98.

McCorriston CC (1968) Racial incidence of hydatidiform mole. A study in a contained polyracial community. *Am. J. Obstet. Gynecol.* **101:** 377–381.

Nakano R, Sasaki Y, Yamoto M & Hata H (1980) Trophoblastic disease: analysis of 342 patients. *Gynecol. Obstet. Invest.* **11:** 237–242.

Park WW (1957) The occurrence of sex chromatin in chorionepithelioma and hydatidiform moles. *J. Path. Bact.* **74:** 197–206.

Park WW (1971) *Choriocarcinoma. A Study of its Pathology*, pp. 15–20. London: Heinemann.

Poen HT & Djojopranato M (1965) The possible etiologic factors of hydatidiform mole and choriocarcinoma. *Am. J. Obstet. Gynecol.* **92:** 510–513.

Prawirohardjo S, Martionao KS & Sutomo T (1957) *Hydatidiform Mole and Choriocarcinoma on Indonesia. First Asiatic Congress of Obstetrics and Gynecology*, pp. 112–129. Tokyo.

Ratnam SS & Ilancheran A (1982) Disease of the trophoblast. *Clin. Obstet. Gynecol.* **9:** 539–564.

Rolon PA & De Lopez BH (1979) Malignant trophoblastic disease in Paraguay. *J. Reprod. Med.* **23:** 94–96.

Sand PK, Lurain JR & Brewer JI (1984) Repeat gestational trophoblastic disease. *Obstet. Gynecol.* **63:** 140–144.

Shanmugaratnam K, Muir CS, Tow SH *et al.* (1971) Rates per 100,000 births and incidence of choriocarcinoma and malignant moles in Singapore. *Int. J. Cancer* **8:** 165–175.

Shepard DM, Fisher RA, Lawler SD (1985) Karyotypic analysis and chromosome polymorphism in four choriocarcinoma cell lines. *Cancer Genet. Cytogenet.* **16:** 251–258.

Surti U, Szulman AE & O'Brien S (1979) Complete (classic) hydatidiform mole with 46 XY karyotype of paternal origin. *Hum. Genet.* **51:** 153–155.

Surti U, Szulman AE & O'Brien S (1982) Dispermic origin and clinical outcome of three complete hydatidiform moles with 46 XY karyotype. *Am. J. Obstet. Gynecol.* **144:** 84–87.

Surti U, Szulman AE, Wagner K, Leppert M & O'Brien SJ (1986) Tetraploid partial hydatidiform moles: two cases with a triple paternal contribution and a 92, XXXY karyotype. *Hum. Genet.* **72:** 15–21.

Szulman AE (1984a) The syndromes of partial and complete molar gestation. *Clin. Obstet. Gynecol.* **27(1):** 177, Fig. 5.

Szulman AE (1984b) The syndromes of partial and complete molar gestation. *Clin. Obstet. Gynecol.* **27(1):** 178, Fig. 6.

■ Szulman AE & Surti U (1978) The syndromes of hydatidiform mole. I. Cytogenetic and morphologic correlations. *Am. J. Obstet. Gynecol.* **131:** 665–671.

Szulman AE, Philippe E, Boue JG & Boue A (1981) Human triploidy: association with partial hydatidiform moles and nonmolar conceptuses. *Hum. Pathol.* **12:** 1016–1021.

Teoh ES, Dawood MY & Ratnam SS (1971) Epidemiology of hydatidiform mole in Singapore. *Am. J. Obstet. Gynecol.* **110:** 415–420.

Tominaga T & Page EW (1968) Sex chromatin of trophoblastic tumours. *Am. J. Obstet. Gynecol.* **96:** 305–309.

Tow WSH (1966) The classification of malignant growths of the chorion. *J. Obstet. Gynaecol. Br. Cwlth.* **73:** 1000–1001.

Vassilakos P, Riotten G & Kajii T (1977) Hydatidiform mole: two entities. A morphologic and cytogenetic study with some clinical considerations. *Am. J. Obstet. Gynecol.* **127:** 167–170.

Wake N, Takagi N & Sasaki M (1978) Androgenesis as a cause of hydatidiform mole. *J. Natl. Cancer Inst.* **60:** 51–53.

Wake N, Chapman V, Matski S & Sandberg AA (1981) Chromosomes and cellular origin of choriocarcinoma. *Cancer Res.* **41:** 3137–3143.

Wake N, Seki T, Fujita H *et al.* (1984) Malignant potential of homozygous and heterozygous complete moles. *Cancer Res.* **44:** 1226–1230.

Wei PY & Ouyang PC (1963) Trophoblastic disease in Taiwan. *Am. J. Obstet. Gynecol.* **85:** 844–849.

Womack C & Elston CW (1985) Hydatidiform mole in Nottingham: a 12 year retrospective epidemiological and morphological study. *Placenta* **6:** 95–105.

■ World Health Organization Scientific Group (1983) *Gestational Trophoblastic Disease. WHO Technical Report Series* 692. Geneva: World Health Organization.

Yen S & MacMahon B (1968) Epidemiologic features of trophoblastic disease. *Am. J. Obstet. Gynecol.* **101:** 126–132.

30 Pathology of Gestational Trophoblastic Disease

H Fox

Introduction

The term 'gestational trophoblastic disease' is, by convention, restricted to hydatidiform moles, choriocarcinomas and placental site tumors, these all being defined in purely morphologic terms. By contrast, a diagnosis of 'persistent trophoblastic disease' implies a biochemical abnormality (i.e. a persistently elevated, or increasing, level of human chorionic gonadotropin (HCG) following a molar pregnancy) and lacks any specific morphologic connotation.

The term 'gestational trophoblastic neoplasia' is sometimes used as an alternative to gestational trophoblastic disease and indeed many seem to feel, often at a subliminal level, that these various conditions represent a neoplastic spectrum, with moles at the benign end, choriocarcinoma at the malignant extreme, and invasive hydatidiform mole being equivalent to a neoplasm of borderline malignancy. This is a misleading approach for there is nothing to suggest that a hydatidiform mole, of any type, is a form of neoplasia; it is, without question, a specific form of abortion. A choriocarcinoma is usually considered to be neoplastic, but as will be discussed later, even this may in some cases be no more than an unusual type of pregnancy and the only undoubtedly neoplastic entity within this group of conditions is the placental site trophoblastic tumor.

Hydatidiform Moles

During the last few decades molar disease has been divided into complete and partial hydatidiform moles, the distinction between these two entities being based on their differing morphologic and cytogenetic features (Vassilakos *et al.*, 1977; Szulman and Surti, 1978a, 1978b). The later application to moles of such techniques as flow cytometry and DNA fingerprinting, although largely confirming the existence of two differing types of molar pregnancy has, however, tended to blur the sharpness of the distinction between the two forms.

Morphology

A complete mole is characterized by diffuse vesicular change, which involves to a greater or lesser degree the entire villous population, thus producing the classical 'bunch of grapes' appearance; the mass of villous tissue is markedly increased, to an extent that an *in situ* mole can fill or even distend the uterus (*Figure 30.1*), no remnant of a normal placental shape is discernible and neither a fetus nor a gestational sac is present. Histologic examination confirms that all the villi are swollen and edematous, some very markedly, but others only minimally (*Figure 30.2*); central cistern formation is common. It is usually maintained that trophoblastic hyperplasia is a characteristic feature of a complete mole, but in reality the degree of trophoblastic proliferation in such lesions is often no greater, and sometimes less, than that seen in the normal first trimester placenta. It is the pattern, rather than the degree, of trophoblastic proliferation that is abnormal in a

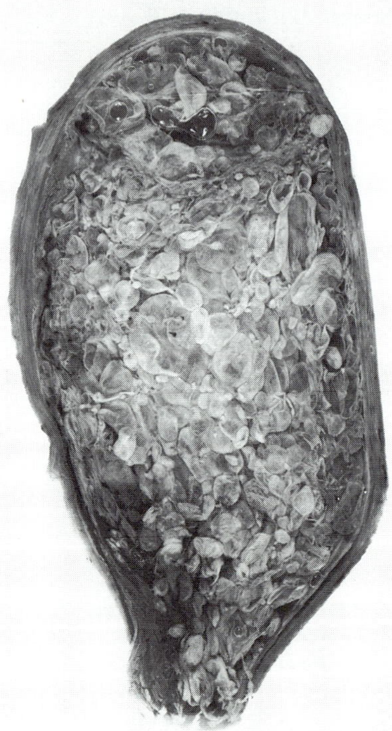

Figure 30.1. A uterus enlarged and distended by a complete hydatidiform mole; no normal placental tissue is present and all the villi show vesicular distension.

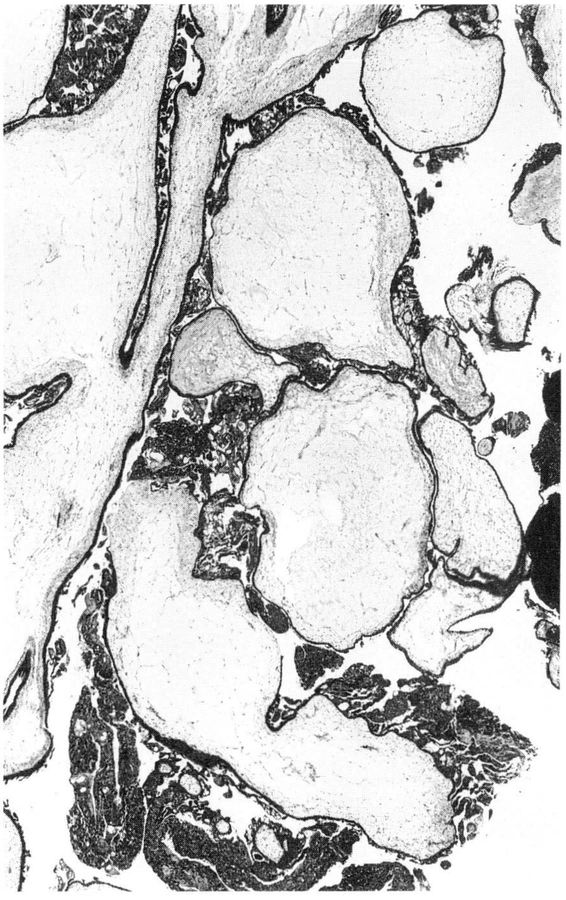

Figure 30.2. Complete hydatidiform mole. The villi are all of abnormal appearance, being distended and showing early central cistern formation; atypical trophoblastic proliferation is present.

complete mole; while in a normal pregnancy trophoblast proliferates along one side or at one pole of a villus, in a complete mole the villous trophoblastic proliferation is either circumferential or multifocal. A moderate degree of nuclear atypia is commonly present in molar trophoblast, though this is often no more marked than that seen in the trophoblast of placentas from normal first trimester pregnancies. Because of the use of ultrasound, anembryonic gestations and hence molar pregnancies are now being diagnosed at an earlier stage of gestation than in the past: in these early lesions the classical vesicular appearances of a complete mole may not be apparent (Paradinas, 1994), and in such cases the abnormal pattern of trophoblastic proliferation and the presence of polypoid villi become key factors in the recognition of a molar pregnancy.

A partial mole differs in numerous respects from a complete mole: it is commonly associated with a fetus, retains a placental shape and does not have an increased villous mass. Only a proportion of the villi show gross vesicular change, these being scattered within normal placental tissue. Histologically (*Figure 30.3*) the presence of both edematous swollen villi and villi of normal size, albeit often with an unusually fibrotic or cellular stroma, is confirmed. The vesicular villi commonly have a very irregular, scalloped outline, this resulting in the 'Norwegian fjord' appearance: cutting of some of these deep indentations in cross-section results in the presence of so-called 'trophoblastic inclusions' within the villous stroma. There is abnormal trophoblastic proliferation, which as, with complete moles, is usually either circumferential or multifocal; the degree of trophoblastic proliferation is usually not only less than that seen in complete moles, but is less than that encountered in normal first trimester placentas. The villous trophoblast frequently has a somewhat vacuolated or 'lacy' appearance. It should be noted that the use of the word 'partial' to describe a mole does not mean that one portion of the placenta is normal and another portion molar. This latter situation is encountered if a complete mole is part of a dizygotic twin pregnancy and associated

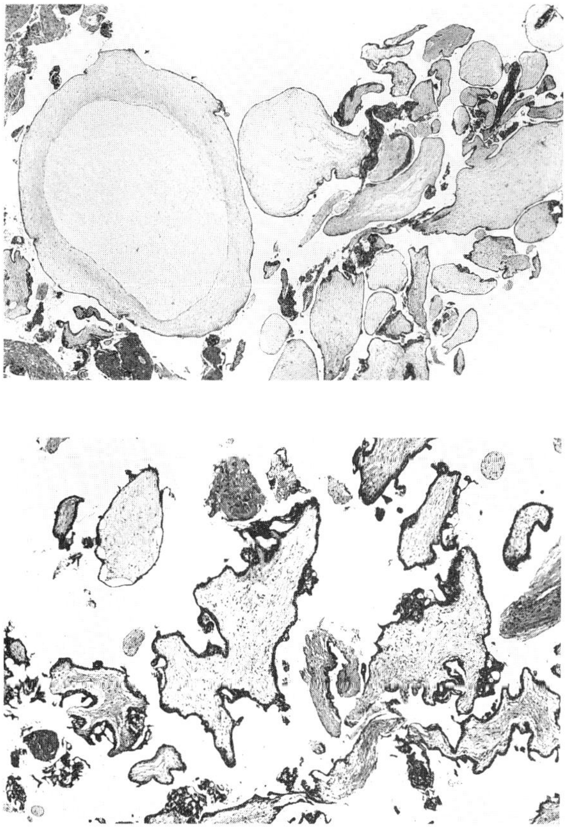

Figure 30.3. Upper: a partial hydatidiform mole. A mixture of large vesicular villi and small villi of normal configuration is present. Lower: partial hydatidiform mole. Villi of irregular outline, the so-called 'Norwegian fjord' appearance, are admixed with a small number of villi of normal configuration.

with a normal twin (Miller *et al.*, 1993; Stellar *et al.*, 1994; Popek, 1994); in such pregnancies one placenta is molar and the other non-molar, while in a true partial mole there is an intermingling of molar and non-molar villi with the molar villi distributed throughout the entire placenta.

Cytogenetics

It has been recognized for some time that complete moles are androgenetic (i.e. all their nuclear DNA is paternally derived) (Kajii and Ohama 1977); furthermore approximately 95% of complete moles have a 46XX chromosomal constitution, the remainder having a 46XY karyotype (Szulman and Surti, 1978a). Banding studies have shown that the vast majority of 46XX complete moles are derived from a single sperm (monospermic or homozygous moles) while all 46XY moles and a small minority of 46XX moles are derived from two sperms (dispermic or heterozygous moles). A hypothetical model has been proposed to explain these findings, namely that homozygous moles are due to fertilization of a 'dead' ovum (i.e. one containing no viable genomic material) by a single haploid sperm, which then undergoes endoreduplication of its genetic material without cell division (Jacobs *et al.*, 1980), and that heterozygous moles result from entry into a 'dead' ovum of two haploid sperms, which then fuse and replicate (Surti *et al.*, 1982). It has to be stressed that this concept is purely theoretical and that the true nature of a 'dead' ovum has never been determined.

Partial moles contain both paternal and maternal genomic material and the vast majority are chromosomally triploid, usually 69XXY, but sometimes 69XXX or 69XYY (Lawler *et al.*, 1982). It is of course known that not all triploid gestations are associated with molar change in the placenta and it is now clear that if the extra chromosomal load is of paternal origin a partial mole will result, while if the extra chromosomal content is contributed from the mother, a non-molar placenta will develop (Jacobs *et al.*, 1982).

This relatively simple subdivision into androgenetic diploid complete moles and biparentally-derived triploid partial moles is not, however, the whole story. Cytogenetic studies have yielded a few instances of triploid and tetraploid complete moles and of diploid and tetraploid partial moles (Teng and Ballon, 1984; Surti *et al.*, 1986; Vejerslev *et al.*, 1987; Lage *et al.*, 1989). Further, flow cytometric studies, although in general confirming that most complete moles are diploid and most partial moles triploid, have nevertheless rather consistently revealed small subpopulations of diploid partial moles and triploid complete moles (Hemming *et al.*, 1987; Lage *et al.*, 1992; Koenig *et al.*, 1993; Lage and Popek, 1993). To complicate the matter further there have been very occasional instances of androgenetic partial moles and biparently-derived complete moles (Vejerslev *et al.*, 1987), entities for which there is, at the moment, no plausible explanation.

Triploid complete moles may well be due to three haploid sperms entering a 'dead' ovum, but many of the reported diploid partial moles have in reality been examples of a complete mole with an accompanying concomitant non-molar twin pregnancy; nevertheless, a distinct entity of diploid partial mole does exist, which, it has been suggested, merits consideration as a separate third type of molar pregnancy (Vejerslev *et al.*, 1991), such cases possibly being a result of uniparental disomy.

The fact that not all molar gestations fit neatly into a rigid classification raises the currently unsolved question as to how the different varieties of mole should be defined; should the diagnosis rest on the morphologic findings, upon the cytogenetic data or upon DNA studies?

Postmolar Disease

In the UK about 8% of patients who have had a complete mole develop persistent trophoblastic disease (Womack and Elston, 1985; Bagshawe *et al.*, 1986): the figure in the USA is rather higher because of the use of different diagnostic criteria. The actual basis of persistent trophoblastic disease is generally unknown: there may have been incomplete removal of the mole, but it is equally possible that many of these cases are invasive hydatidiform moles with residual molar tissue within the myometrium or its vasculature; it is also possible that some are early choriocarcinomas. It is thought that the risk of development of a clinically overt choriocarcinoma following a complete mole is in the region of 5%.

The incidence of persistent trophoblastic disease following a partial mole has been much disputed, but there is now no doubt that it occurs, though the magnitude of the risk is very much lower than is that for complete moles (Bagshawe *et al.*, 1990; Rice *et al.*, 1990; Lage *et al.*, 1991; Goto *et al.*, 1993). The eventual risk of choriocarcinoma in patients with partial moles is also unknown: choriocarcinomas have been reported following partial moles (Looi and Sivanesaratnam, 1981; Bagshawe *et al.*, 1990; Gardner and Lage, 1992), but this in itself does not necessarily mean that this condition increases the risk of a choriocarcinoma because it can follow a normal pregnancy.

Prognostic Factors

As it is widely agreed that all women who have had a molar pregnancy should enter a follow-up surveillance program there is no practical point in attempting to define those cases at most risk of developing postmolar disease. Nevertheless, from a purely theoretic viewpoint it is of interest to consider if a high-risk group can be defined. It was at one time considered that the risk of eventual postmolar disease was directly related to the degree of trophoblastic proliferation in the mole, but this has proved not to be the case (Elston and Bagshawe, 1972; Genest *et al.*, 1991), and 'grading' of moles in terms of their degree of trophoblastic proliferation has now been abandoned. Attempts to forecast those cases at greatest risk for postmolar disease by the use of cell proliferation markers and flow cytometry (Hemming *et al.*, 1988; Fukunaga *et al.*, 1993; Cheung *et al.*, 1993) have failed, but it has been maintained that heterozygous (dispermic) moles have a much higher risk of subsequent postmolar complications that homozygous (monospermic) moles (Wake *et al.*, 1987). Doubts have, however, been cast upon this claim by the failure to find any association between the presence of a Y chromosome, detected by the polymerase chain reaction, in a mole and an excess incidence of postmolar disease (Mutter *et al.*, 1993).

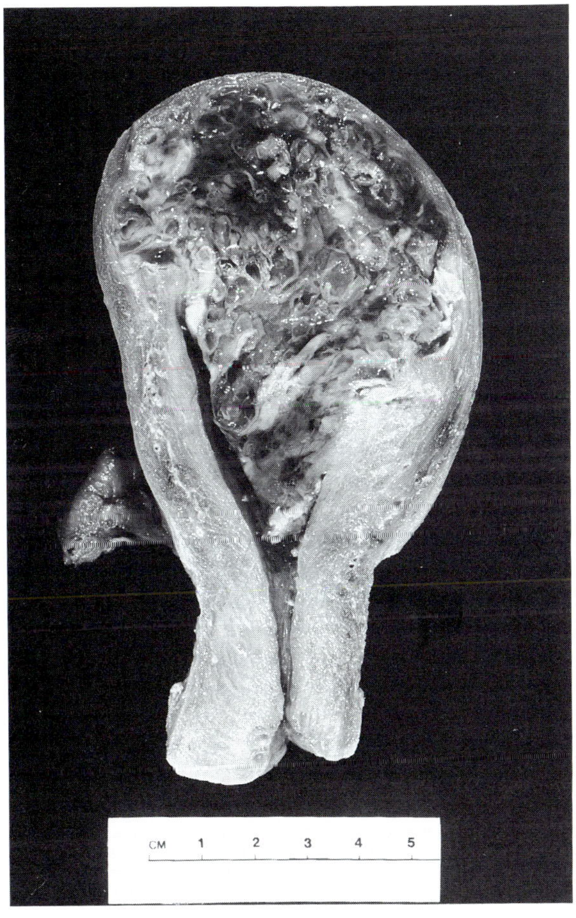

Figure 30.4. Invasive hydatidiform mole. The uterus is occupied by a hydatidiform mole, which is invading deeply into the myometrium. At one point the mole infiltrates almost to the serosa. (Courtesy of Professor DO'B Hourihane, Dublin.)

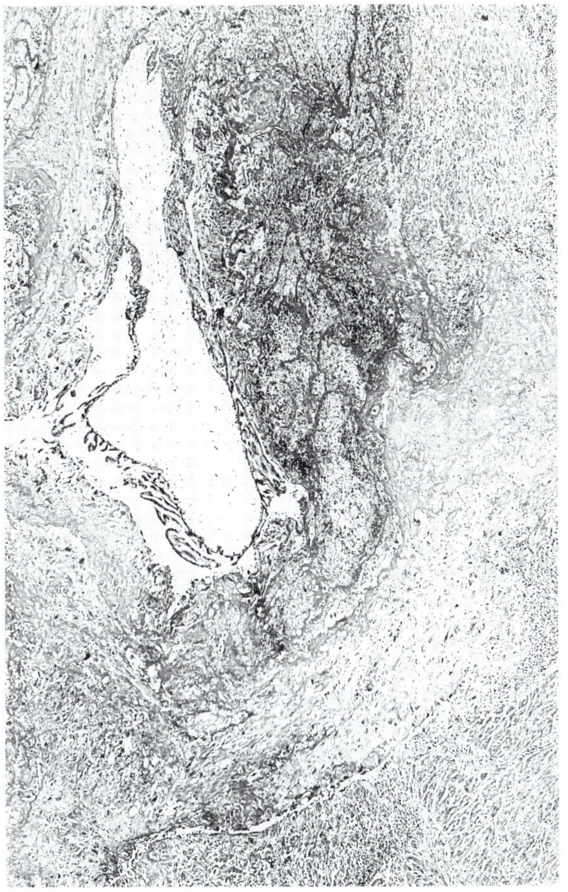

Figure 30.5. Invasive hydatidiform mole. The myometrium contains deeply penetrating molar villi six months after a diagnosis of hydatidiform mole had originally been made. Chemotherapy for persistent trophoblastic disease had failed to control bleeding and hysterectomy was carried out.

Invasive Hydatidiform Mole

An invasive hydatidiform mole is one that penetrates into the myometrium or invades the uterine vasculature. A deeply invasive mole usually becomes clinically evident several weeks after apparently complete evacuation of a mole, the patient usually presenting with hemorrhage. If a hysterectomy is performed at this stage the appearances range from a small hemorrhagic focus in the myometrium to a large deeply cavitating hemorrhagic lesion of the uterine wall (*Figure 30.4*): rarely, a mole penetrates the full thickness of the myometrium, leading either to uterine perforation or to extension of the mole into adjacent structures such as the broad ligament. The histologic distinction from a choriocarcinoma is dependent upon finding molar villi within the uterine wall (*Figure 30.5*), these more commonly being seen in the myometrial vascular channels than between the myometrial fibers.

Invasive moles have in the past caused death from uterine bleeding or perforation, but their mortality rate is now virtually zero because of the success achieved in their treatment by a limited course of chemotherapy. In fact the diagnosis of an invasive mole, which can only be made with certainty on a hysterectomy specimen, is now almost obsolete because nearly all invasive moles are subsumed into the category of persistent trophoblastic disease.

It has to be stressed that the invasive capacity of some moles is not an indication that they are neoplastic. Normal trophoblast has the ability to invade both the myometrium and the uterine vessels, while villi from a normal placenta can invade deeply into or even through the uterine wall to give rise to a placenta increta or a placenta percreta, both of which are the exact non-molar equivalents of an invasive mole.

Molar tissue can be transported via the bloodstream to extrauterine sites, particularly to the vagina and lungs: the transported molar trophoblast can then grow in these sites to form nodules that are either clinically or radiologically detectable. The development of 'metastatic' lesions implies that molar trophoblast has entered the uterine vessels and hence their presence is taken as *de facto* evidence of the presence of an invasive mole; the 'metastatic' nodules are not, however, usually associated with evidence of molar invasion of the myometrial tissues.

The 'metastatic' nodules usually appear several weeks after evacuation of a mole from the uterus, but may occur concurrently with a mole or can be the presenting symptom of such a lesion. Vaginal lesions form hemorrhagic submucous nodules, the true nature of which only becomes apparent when microscopy reveals the presence of villous structure (Elston, 1976), a finding that rules out a diagnosis of choriocarcinoma. Pulmonary lesions can cause hemoptysis, but are usually an asymptomatic radiologic finding: histologic examination of these will also reveal their content of villi (Ring, 1972; Johnson *et al.*, 1979). These extrauterine lesions may resolve spontaneously, but are commonly treated with limited chemotherapy, which achieves excellent results.

The fact that molar trophoblast is transported to extrauterine sites is not an indication of neoplastic behavior. Trophoblast enters the maternal blood stream in every normal pregnancy (Mueller *et al.*, 1990) and is transported to sites such as the lung (Attwood and Park, 1961), but this transported trophoblast only gives rise to detectable lesions if it is molar in nature.

Choriocarcinoma

Approximately 50% of choriocarcinomas follow a molar pregnancy, 30% occur after an abortion and 20% follow an apparently normal gestation. The time interval between the antecedent pregnancy and the clinical presentation of a choriocarcinoma is very variable, ranging from a few weeks or months to 15 years.

Morphology

Within the uterus (*Figure 30.6*) a choriocarcinoma forms single or multiple hemorrhagic nodules, which are often accompanied by local metastases to the cervix and vagina. The neoplastic masses consist of a central area of hemorrhagic necrosis and usually, though not invariably, a peripheral rim of viable tumor tissue. The central, sometimes complete, necrosis of the neoplastic tissue is a reflection of the fact that a choriocarcinoma has no intrinsic blood supply, relying for its oxygenation on its ability to invade the uterine blood vessels. Therefore only the growing edge of the tumor is adequately oxygenated, the remainder undergoing ischemic necrosis.

Histologically, a choriocarcinoma has a biphasic structure (*Figure 30.7*) that recapitulates, often to a striking degree, that of the trophoblast of the normal

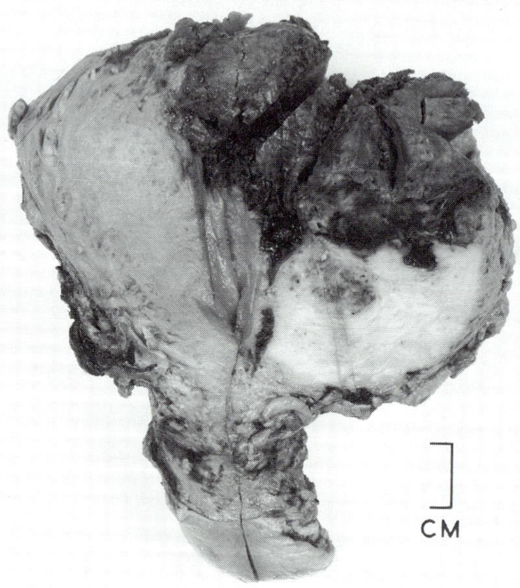

Figure 30.6. Choriocarcinoma. Section of a uterus showing a hemorrhagic mass of choriocarcinoma in the uterine body (from Elston, 1987, with permission).

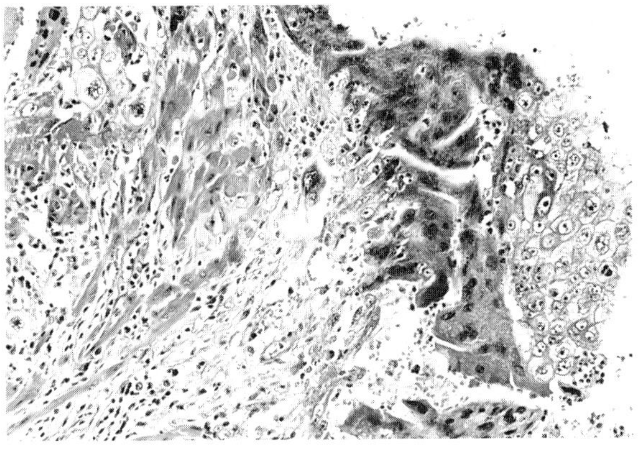

Figure 30.7. Choriocarcinoma. Myometrium to the bottom is infiltrated by tumor tissue in which two distinct components can be seen: the darkly staining syncytiotrophoblast and the pale staining cytotrophoblast with vesicular nuclei to the top; no villi are present.

implanting blastocyst, with central sheets or cores of cytotrophoblast being 'capped' by a peripheral rim of syncytiotrophoblast. The trophoblastic cells in a choriocarcinoma commonly show no greater degree of atypia and mitotic activity than is seen in an implanting blastocyst. Villi are never present in an extraplacental choriocarcinoma and the presence of villous structures negates a diagnosis of choriocarcinoma.

Because of the need to obtain an oxygen supply a choriocarcinoma is avariciously invasive of vascular channels in the myometrium. The tumor cells tend to form solid plugs within the myometrial vasculature (*Figure 30.8*) and although there is often extravascular extension, the malignant trophoblast tends to infiltrate between the muscle fibers with very little tissue destruction. The propensity for vascular invasion is the basis for the predominantly hematogenous dissemination of a choriocarcinoma to sites such as the lungs, brain, liver, kidney and gastrointestinal tract (*Figure 30.9*): large tumor emboli may impact within the pulmonary arteries. Lymph node deposits of a choriocarcinoma are usually tertiary metastases from a large extrauterine lesion.

Origin

Choriocarcinomas may follow either a normal or a molar pregnancy, more commonly the latter; there is a considerable gap in our knowledge as to the relationship between the previous pregnancy and the subsequent choriocarcinoma. Is the neoplasm actually derived from the trophoblast of the previous pegnancy and if so what has been happening to this trophoblast during the intervening months or years? The application of genetic techniques, such as the study of cytogenetic polymorphism (Chaganti *et al.*, 1990), DNA restriction fragment length polymorphism assays (Azuma *et al.*, 1990; Osada *et al.*, 1991; Fisher *et al.*, 1992) or the study of tandem repeat regions amplified by the polymerase chain reaction (Suzuki *et al.*, 1993), has shown that some, but by no means all, choriocarcinomas are androgenetic. It has been demonstrated that some of these androgenetic tumors were derived from a previous molar gestation despite the fact that in two such cases there had been a full-term normal delivery intervening between the molar pregnancy and the development of the choriocarcinoma (Fisher *et al.*, 1992; Suzuki *et al.*, 1993). In one of these cases the time interval between the mole and the choriocarcinoma was ten years and it is difficult to understand how tissue from the mole remained in the uterus for that length of time and throughout a later normal pregnancy to then subsequently undergo a neoplastic resurgence.

Some points are, however, becoming clearer. It is seeming increasingly probable that many, possibly most or even all, choriocarcinomas that follow an apparently normal pregnancy are in reality metastases from an undetected small intraplacental choriocarcinoma. Only a small number of intraplacental choriocarcinomas have been described (Brewer and Mazur, 1981; Tsukamoto *et al.*, 1981; Fox and Laurini, 1988; Christopherson *et al.*, 1992; Lage and Roberts, 1993) and in nearly all the choriocarcinoma was very small and easily overlooked unless the placenta was meticulously examined. One case (Hallam *et al.*, 1990) is of particular interest insofar as a patient developed an apparently primary choriocarcinoma soon after a normal pregnancy: re-examination of the placenta at that time revealed a tiny intraplacental choriocarcinoma. Intraplacental choriocarcinomas are histologically identical to extraplacental choriocarcinomas, but are often separated from the normal villous population by villi with a surrounding mantle of choriocarcinoma-like trophoblast, which has replaced the normal trophoblast.

If choriocarcinomas following a normal pregnancy are in reality metastases from an intraplacental choriocarcinoma, are those which follow a molar gestation similarly derived from an intramolar choriocarcinoma? This is certainly a possibility, for one such lesion has been described (Heifetz and Csaja, 1992), though it was not associated with subsequent disease. The prolonged time interval in some cases between a molar pregnancy and the development of an overt choriocarcinoma does, however, suggest that by no means all postmolar choriocarcinomas are derived from such lesions and it is certainly conceivable that some choriocarcinomas are new pregnancies that evolve directly into a choriocarcinoma, the choriocarcinoma *ab initio* that has long been considered as a possibility

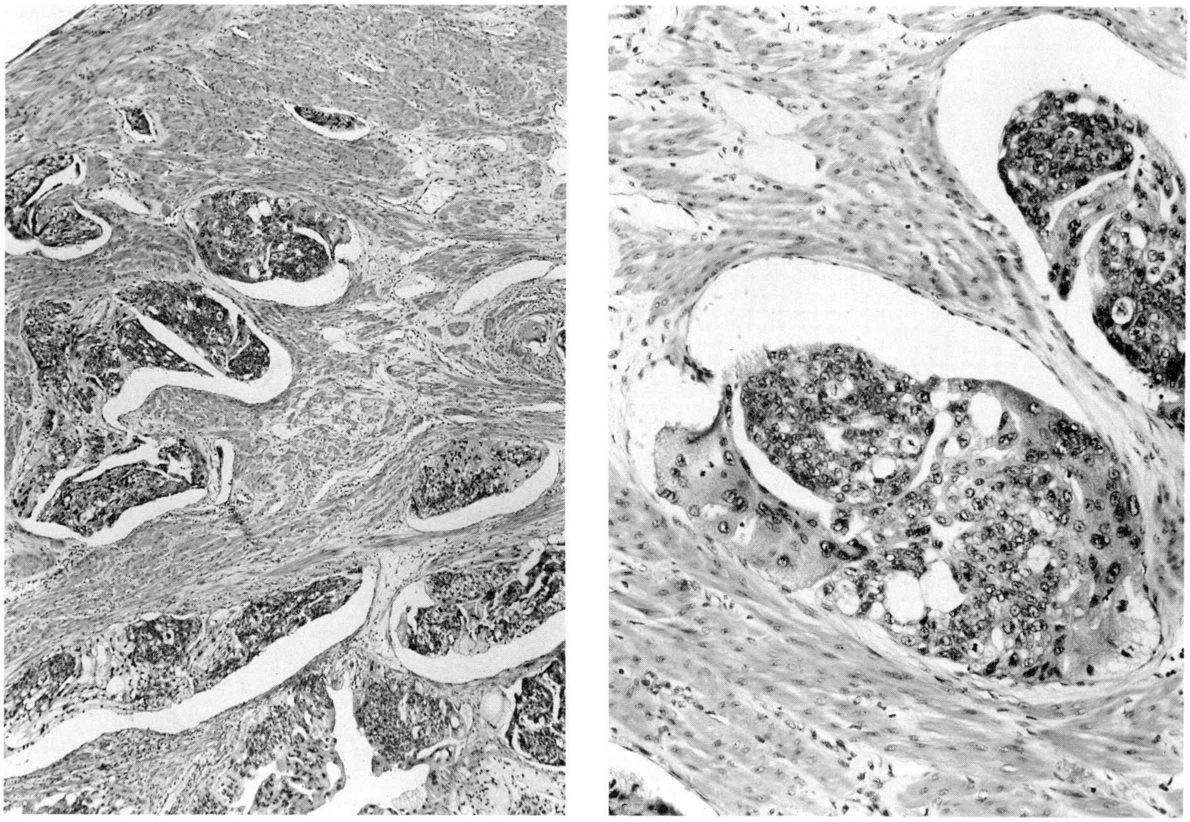

Figure 30.8. Choriocarcinoma. Permeation of the uterine vasculature by choriocarcinoma. The tumor is present in dilated vascular sinuses, but the intervening myometrium is intact. Right: tumor embolism has impacted in a venous sinus (from Elston, 1987, with permission).

(Acosta–Sison, 1955). This raises the question, however, as to whether such pregnancies should be considered as truly neoplastic or simply as aberrant gestations. It is true that they invade vessels and spread to distant sites, but so does normal trophoblast. They resemble acutely the trophoblast of the normal implanting blastocyst and their response to methotrexate, although quite different to that of virtually every other neoplasm, is not unlike that of a normal, but ectopic, early gestation. This is, of course, speculation, but nevertheless the possibility that some choriocarcinomas are simply abnormal pregnancies should not be dismissed too lightly.

Placental Site Trophoblastic Tumor

Placental site trophoblastic tumor is an uncommon tumor that is derived from the extravillous trophoblast of the placental bed (sometimes referred to as 'intermediate trophoblast'). In the vast majority of cases the neoplasm develops after a normal pregnancy, with only 5% occurring after a molar gestation (Lage and Young, 1993). Patients present at anything from a few weeks to 18 months after the antecedent pregnancy with a complaint of irregular vaginal bleeding or, perhaps more commonly, amenorrhea. A small proportion of patients develop a nephrotic syndrome, which appears to be due to chronic intravascular coagulation initiated by factors released from the tumor. The uterus is commonly enlarged, but a pregnancy test is positive in only one-third of patients, this reflecting the fact that the principal secretory product of extravillous trophoblast is human placental lactogen (HPL) rather than HCG.

The tumors tend to form tan, white or yellow masses within the myometrium, and often protrude into the endometrial cavity, sometimes forming a polypoidal mass. Histologically, the tumor replicates in an anarchic form, the appearances seen in the normal placental bed being formed principally of mononuclear cytotrophoblastic cells with an irregular and inconsistent admixture of multinucleated cells. The tumor cells infiltrate between and dissect the myometrial fibers as cords and sheets with a striking absence of necrosis and hemorrhage

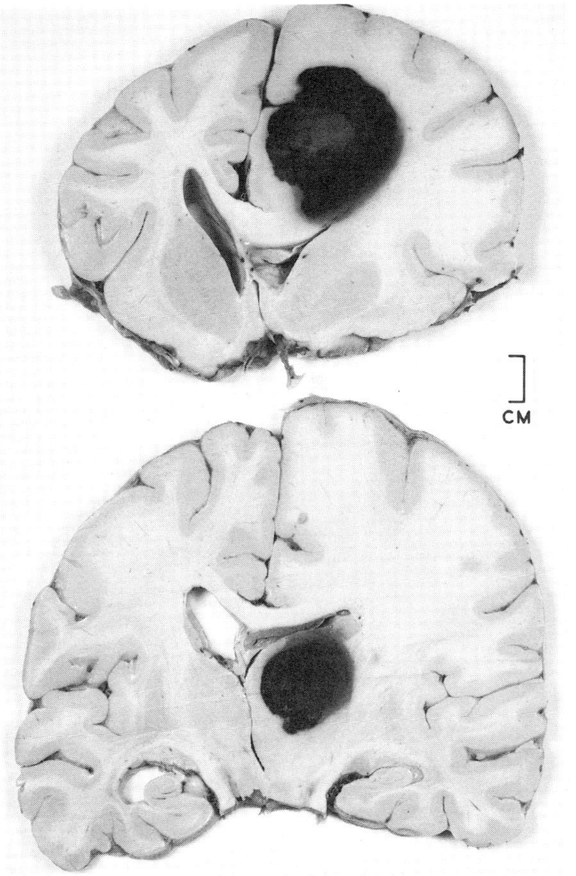

Figure 30.9. Choriocarcinoma. Metastases to the brain. The coronal section shows two spherical hemorrhagic nodules (from Elston, 1987, with permission).

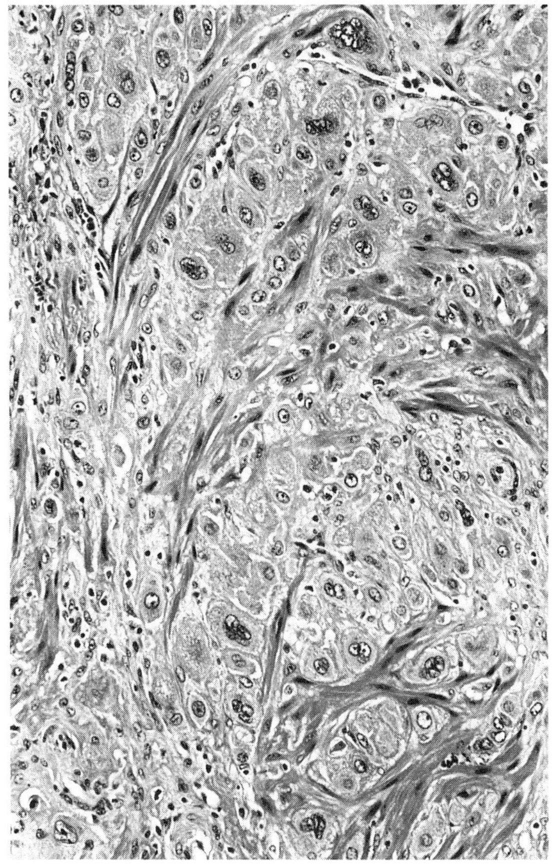

Figure 30.10. Placental site trophoblastic tumor. Cords of trophoblastic cells infiltrate between the smooth muscle bundles of the myometrium: note the occasional multinucleated trophoblastic cell.

(*Figure 30.10*). Invasion of vessels by tumor cells is common, but the massive intravascular growth that characterizes a choriocarcinoma is not seen and some vessels within the tumor are surrounded, but not invaded, by neoplastic cells. Non-infiltrated vessels often show fibrinoid necrosis of their wall, while a pseudodecidual change, and sometimes an Arias–Stella reaction, may be apparent in the adjacent endometrium.

About 15–20% of placental site trophoblastic tumors behave in a malignant fashion (Young *et al.*, 1988) and either recur locally or spread to such distant sites as the liver, lung and central nervous system. Assessment of the degree of malignancy of any individual neoplasm is, however, difficult because although those that have run a malignant course have usually had a high mitotic count, this is not an invariable rule (Eckstein *et al.*, 1982), and a low mitotic count should not necessarily engender a sense of security.

Summary of Core Information

- All moles are a form of abortion; they are not neoplasms.
- Despite their morphologic dissimilarity, there is some genetic and cytogenetic overlap between complete and partial moles.
- Normal trophoblast is invasive: an invasive mole is the molar equivalent of a placenta increta and its invasive capacity is not an indication that it is a neoplasm.
- Normal trophoblast spreads via the bloodstream to extrauterine sites. The occurrence of metastases in an invasive mole is not an indication that it is a neoplasm.
- Choriocarcinomas following a normal pregnancy are probably metastases from an unnoticed small intraplacental choriocarcinoma.
- Some postmolar choriocarcinomas are genetically identical to the previous mole; sometimes despite intervening normal pregnancies.
- Some postmolar choriocarcinomas may be metastases from intramolar choriocarcinomas.
- Some postmolar choriocarcinomas may be new pregnancies (choriocarcinomas *ab initio*).
- Placental site trophoblastic tumors are neoplasms derived from extravillous trophoblast.
- The 10–15% of placental site trophoblastic tumors that are malignant cannot be reliably identified as such histologically and these neoplasms respond poorly to chemotherapy.

References

■ Acosta-Sison H (1955) Can the implanting trophoblast of the fertilized ovum develop immediately into choriocarcinoma? *Am. J. Obstet. Gynecol.* **69:** 442–444.

Attwood HD & Park WW (1961) Embolism to the lungs by trophoblast. *J. Obstet. Gynaecol. Br. Cwlth.* **68:** 611–617.

Azuma C, Sami F, Nobunaga T *et al.* (1990) Studies of the pathogenesis of choriocarcinoma by analysis of restriction fragment length polymorphisms. *Cancer Res.* **50:** 488–491.

Bagshawe KD, Dent J & Webb J (1986) Hydatidiform mole in England and Wales 1973–83. *Lancet* **2:** 673–677.

Bagshawe KD, Lawler SD, Paradinas F, Dent J, Brown P & Boxer GM (1990) Gestational trophoblastic tumours following initial diagnosis of partial hydatidiform mole. *Lancet* **335:** 1074–1076.

Brewer JL & Mazur MT (1981) Gestational choriocarcinoma: its origin in the placenta during seemingly normal pregnancy. *Am. J. Surg. Pathol.* **5:** 267–277.

Chaganti RSK, Koduru PRK, Chakraborty R & Jones WB (1990) Genetic origin of a trophoblastic choriocarcinoma. *Cancer Res.* **50:** 6330–6333.

Cheung AN, Ngan HY, Chen WZ, Loke SL & Collins RJ (1993) The significance of proliferating cell nuclear antigen in human trophoblastic disease: an immunohistochemical study. *Histopathology* **22:** 565–568.

Christopherson WA, Kanbour A & Szulman AE (1992) Choriocarcinoma in a term placenta with maternal metastases. *Gynecol. Oncol.* **46:** 239–245.

Eckstein RP, Paradinas FJ & Bagshawe KD (1982) Placental site trophoblastic tumour (trophoblastic pseudotumour): a study of four cases requiring hysterectomy, including one fatal case. *Histopathology* **6:** 221–226.

■ Elston CW (1976) The histopathology of trophoblastic tumours. *J. Clin. Pathol.* **29 (Suppl. 19):** 11–13.

Elston CW (1987) Gestational trophoblastic disease. In: Fox H (ed) *Haines and Taylor: Obstetrical and Gynaecological Pathology* 3rd edition. pp. 1045–1078. Edinburgh: Churchill Livingstone.

Elston CW & Bagshawe KD (1972) The value of histological grading in the management of hydatidiform mole. *J. Obstet. Gynaecol. Brit. Cwlth.* **79:** 717–724.

Fisher RA, Newlands ES, Jeffreys AJ *et al.* (1992) Gestational and non-gestational trophoblastic tumors distinguished by DNA analysis. *Cancer* **69:** 839–845.

Fox H & Laurini RN (1988) Intraplacental choriocarcinoma: a report of two cases. *J. Clin. Pathol.* **42:** 1085–1088.

Fukunaga M, Ushigome S, Fukunaga M & Sugishita M (1993) Application of flow cytometry in diagnosis of hydatidiform moles. *Mod. Pathol.* **6:** 353–359.

Gardner HAR & Lage JL (1992) Choriocarcinoma following a partial mole: a case report. *Hum. Pathol.* **23:** 468–471.

Genest DG, Laborde O, Berkowitz RS *et al.* (1991) A clinical–pathologic study of 153 cases of complete hydatidiform mole (1980–1990): histologic grade lacks prognostic significance. *Obstet. Gynecol.* **77:** 111–115.

Goto S, Yamada A, Ishizuka T & Tomoda Y (1993) Development of postmolar trophoblastic disease after partial molar pregnancy. *Gynecol. Oncol.* **48:** 165–170.

Hallam LA, McLaren KM, El-Jabbour JN, Helm CW & Smart GE (1990) Intraplacental choriocarcinoma: a case report. *Placenta* **11:** 247–251.

Heifetz SA & Csaja J (1992) *In situ* choriocarcinoma arising in partial hydatidiform mole: implications for risk of persistent trophoblastic disease. *Pediat. Pathol.* **12:** 601–611.

Hemming JD, Quirke P, Womack C, Wells M & Elston CW (1987) Diagnosis of molar pregnancy and persistent trophoblastic disease by flow cytometry. *J. Clin. Pathol.* **40:** 615–620.

Hemming JD, Quirke P, Womack C, Wells M, Elston CW & Pennington GW (1988) Flow cytometry in persistent trophoblastic disease. *Placenta* **9:** 615–621.

Jacobs PA, Wilson CM, Sprenkle JA, Rosenhein NB &

Migson BR (1980) Mechanisms of origin of complete hydatidiform mole. *Nature* **286:** 714–716.

Jacobs PA, Szulman AE, Funkmouska J, Maatsura JS & Wilson CC (1982) Human triploidy: relationship between paternal origin of the additional haploid complement and development of partial hydatidiform mole. *Ann. Hum. Genet.* **46:** 223–231.

Johnson TR, Comstock CH & Anderson DG (1979) Benign gestational trophoblastic disease metastatic to pleura: unusual cause of hemothorax. *Obstet. Gynecol.* **53:** 509–511.

■ Kajii T & Ohama K (1977) Androgenetic origin of hydatidiform mole. *Nature* **268:** 633–634.

Koenig C, Demopoulos RI, Vamvakas EC, Mitial KR, Feiner HD & Espiritu B (1993) Flow cytometric DNA ploidy and quantitative histopathology in partial moles. *Int. J. Gynecol. Pathol.* **12:** 235–240.

Lage JM & Popek EJ (1993) The role of DNA flow cytometry in evaluation of partial and complete hydatidiform moles and hydropic abortions. *Sem. Diag. Pathol.* **10:** 267–274.

Lage GM & Roberts DJ (1993) Choriocarcinoma in a term placenta: pathologic diagnosis of tumor in an asymptomatic patient with metastatic disease. *Int. J. Gynecol. Pathol.* **12:** 80–85.

Lage JM & Young RH (1993) Pathology of trophoblastic disease. In: Clement PB & Young RH (eds) *Tumors and Tumorlike Lesions of the Uterine Corpus and Cervix*, pp. 419–475. New York: Churchill Livingstone.

Lage JM, Weinberg JS, Yavner DL *et al.* (1989) Tetraploid partial hydatidiform moles: histopathology, cytogenetics, and flow cytometry. *Hum. Pathol.* **20:** 419–425.

Lage JM, Berkowitz RS, Rice LW, Goldstein DP, Bernstein MR & Weinberg DS (1991) Flow cytometric analysis of DNA content in partial hydatidiform moles with persistent gestational trophoblastic tumor. *Obstet. Gynecol.* **77:** 111–115.

Lage JM, Mark SD, Roberts DJ *et al.* (1992) A flow cytometric study of 137 fresh hydropic placentas: correlation between types of hydatidiform moles and nuclear DNA ploidy. *Obstet. Gynecol.* **79:** 403–410.

Lawler SD, Fisher RA, Pickhall VJ, Povey S & Evans MW (1982) Genetic studies on hydatiform moles. I. The origin of partial moles. *Cancer Genet. Cytogenet.* **5:** 309–320.

Looi LM & Sivanesaratnam A (1981) Malignant evolution with fatal outcome in a patient with partial hydatidiform mole. *Aust. NZ J. Obstet. Gynaecol.* **21:** 51–52.

Miller D, Jackson R, Ehein T & McMuurtrie E (1993) Complete hydatidiform mole coexistent with a twin live fetus: clinical course of four cases with complete cytogenetic analysis. *Gynecol. Oncol.* **50:** 119–123.

Mueller UW, Hawes CS, Wright AE *et al.* (1990) Isolation of fetal trophoblast cells from peripheral blood of pregnant women. *Lancet* **336:** 197–200.

Mutter GL, Pomponio RJ, Berkowitz RS & Genest DR (1993) Sex chromosome composition of complete hydatidiform mole: relationship to metastasis. *Am. J. Obstet. Gynecol.* **168:** 1547–1551.

Osada H, Kawata M, Yamada M, Okumura K & Takamizawa H (1991) Genetic identification of pregnancies responsible for choriocarcinoma after multiple pregnancies by restriction fragment length polymorphism analysis. *Am. J. Obstet. Gynecol.* **165:** 682–688.

Paradinas FJ (1994) The histological diagnosis of hydatidiform moles. *Curr. Diag. Pathol.* **1:** 24–31.

Popek EJ (1994) Complete hydatidiform mole with coexistent twin. *Modern Pathol.* **7:** 7P.

Rice LW, Berkowitz RS, Lage JM, Goldstein DP & Bernstein MR (1990) Persistent gestational trophoblastic tumor after partial hydatidiform mole. *Gynecol. Oncol.* **36:** 358–362.

Ring AM (1972) The concept of benign metastasizing hydatidiform moles. *Am. J. Clin. Pathol.* **58:** 111–117.

Stellar MA, Genest DR, Bernstein MR *et al.* (1994) The natural history of twin pregnancy with complete hydatidiform mole and coexisting fetus. *Obstet. Gynecol.* **83:** 35–42.

Surti U, Szulman AE & O'Brien S (1982) Dispermic origin and clinical outcome of three complete hydatidiform moles with 46XY karotype. *Am. J. Obstet. Gynecol.* **144:** 84–87.

Surti U, Szulman AE, Wagner K, Leppert M & O'Brien SJ (1986) Tetraploid partial hydatidiform moles: two cases with a triple paternal contribution and a 92 XXXY karotype. *Hum. Genet.* **72:** 15–21.

Suzuki Y, Goto S, Nawa A, Kurauchi D, Saito M & Tomoda Y (1993) Identification of the pregnancy responsible for gestational trophoblastic disease by DNA analysis. *Obstet. Gynecol.* **82:** 629–634.

■ Szulman AE & Surti U (1978a) The syndromes of hydatidiform mole. I. Cytogenetic and morphologic correlations. *Am. J. Obstet. Gynecol.* **131:** 665–671.

■ Szulman AE & Surti U (1978b) The syndromes of hydatidiform mole. II. Morphologic evolution of the complete and partial mole. *Am. J. Obstet. Gynecol.* **132:** 20–27.

Teng NNH & Ballon SC (1984) Partial hydatidiform mole with diploid karyotype: report of three cases. *Am. J. Obstet. Gynecol.* **150:** 961–964.

Tsukamoto N, Kashimura Y, Sano M, Salto T, Kanda T & Taki I (1981) Choriocarcinoma occurring within the normal placenta with breast metastasis. *Gynecol. Oncol.* **11:** 348–363.

Vassilakos P, Riotton G & Kajii T (1977) Hydatidiform mole: two entities: a morphologic and cytogenetic study with some clinical considerations. *Am. J. Obstet. Gynecol.* **127:** 167–170.

■ Vejerslev LO, Fisher RA, Surti U & Walke N (1987) Hydatidiform mole: cytogenetically unusual cases and their implications for the present classification. *Am. J. Obstet. Gynecol.* **157:** 180 184.

Vejerslev LO, Sunde L, Hansen BF *et al.* (1991) Hydatyidiform mole and fetus with normal karotype: support of a separate entity. *Obstet. Gynecol.* **77:** 868–874.

Wake N, Fujino T, Hoshi S *et al.* (1987) The propensity to malignancy of dispermic heterozygous moles. *Placenta* **8:** 318 326.

Womack C & Elston CW (1985) Hydatidiform mole in Nottingham: a 12 year retrospective epidemiological and morphological study. *Placenta* **6:** 95–105.

Young RH, Kurman RJ & Scully RE (1988) Proliferations and tumors of the placental site. *Semin. Diagn. Pathol.* **5:** 223–237.

31 Benign Gestational Trophoblastic Neoplasia and Overall Surgical Management

J L Currie

Introduction

During the past 40 years gestational trophoblastic neoplasia (GTN), once the most feared of all gynecologic tumors, have become highly curable with appropriate surgical management and chemotherapy. Nevertheless, success in treating these neoplasms depends on accurate staging and diagnosis as well as appropriate management and follow-up. The ensuing chapter will describe the presentation of benign gestational trophoblastic disease (for the most part hydatidiform mole), address the staging and nomenclature of malignant disease and discuss surgical and multimodality therapy for both benign and malignant disease. The subsequent chapter (Chapter 32) will consider the chemotherapeutic management of malignant disease.

Technically, gestational trophoblastic disease can be divided into two broad categories: benign disease (almost always complete or partial hydatidiform mole) and malignant disease, which presents as recurrent or persistent hydatidiform mole, chorioadenoma destruens (invasive mole) or the pure epithelial tumor, choriocarcinoma. While histologic confirmation is commonly available for molar gestations, the diagnosis of malignant disease is usually rendered on the basis of plateauing or rising serum human chorionic gonadotropin (HCG) titers in patients who have previous molar disease. The most recently described variant of GTN, placental site trophoblastic tumor, can be either benign or malignant, depending on its clinical course.

Hydatidiform Mole

Hydatidiform mole is an uncommon complication of pregnancy, occurring in approximately 1 in 100 to 1 in 2000 pregnancies. This wide distribution has a remarkable geographic variance, with the lowest incidence in developed countries in the Western world and the highest in the Orient. Complete hydatidiform mole is more common than partial mole in the ratio of approximately 3:1. (Newlands *et al.*, 1992).

Accurate data for determining the actual incidence of hydatidiform mole are difficult to obtain. Many spontaneous abortions may be aborted molar or pre-molar material that resolves spontaneously without histologic confirmation. Additionally, hospital information systems used for acquiring data may be skewed without reporting the true incidence of pregnancy for any one area, and population-based studies are infrequently performed in countries that might be expected to have a high frequency of moles. Therefore, the incidence figures reported in *Table 31.1* are divided according to their methodology, and a wide range even within a country is noted.

An incidence in the Western world of 1 in 1200–1500 pregnancies is accepted by most clinicians as broadly representative of the incidence of mole in clinical practice. For the obstetrician, gynecologist or family practitioner with a reasonably busy obstetrical service, hydatidiform mole can be expected to be encountered once or twice a year. Although the incidence in the USA and UK is relatively low, the occurrence of this disease is frequent enough and the consequences of inappropriate management serious enough that obstetricians and gynecologists should always have this eventuality in mind. Additionally, the reported 1 in 600 incidence of molar material among specimens from therapeutic abortions (Cohen *et al.*, 1979) mandates careful examination of these specimens.

From epidemiologic reports it appears that certain women have an increased risk of developing a molar gestation (Buckley, 1984; Grimes, 1984; Messerli *et al.*, 1985). Although occupation, a previous history of abortions, very young age, long non-pregnant intervals and low socioeconomic status may confer increased statistical risk of molar pregnancy, these factors are of minimal significance for the clinician. In fact, the single most important risk factor is a previous molar pregnancy, and all prenatal evaluations should be cognizant of this history. The combination of recurrent spontaneous abortions, cancer, and GTN in families may impart a greater risk, suggesting major histocompatibility complex-linked genes are involved in the pathogenesis. (Ho, *et al.*, 1991). Finally, the marked increase in risk for advanced maternal age – reaching 80 times control by the age of 50 years – is an important fact for the astute physician to remember (Buckley, 1984;

Table 31.1. Worldwide incidence of hydatidiform mole (from Buckley, 1984; Grimes, 1984; Mazzanti *et al*., 1986).

Country	Hydatidiform moles/pregnancies
Hospital-based estimates	
Indonesia	1/85
Taiwan	1/120
India	1/160
Philippines	1/200
Mexico	1/200
USA (Hawaii)	1/238
Hong Kong	1/530
USA (New York)	1/1000
Italy (Lombardy)	1/1510
USA (Cook County)	1/1724
Population-based estimates	
Japan	1/522
Singapore	1/823
China	1/1290
USA (Honolulu)	1/1326
USA (Rhode Island)	1/1450
Sweden	1/1560

Table 31.2. Signs and symptoms of hydatidiform moles.

Size–date discrepancy
Sudden uterine enlargement
Uterine bleeding
Toxemia in early pregnancy
Hyperemesis
Hyperthroidism
Passage of vesicles
Development of theca lutein cysts
Human chorionic gonadotropin >200,000

Ozumba and Ofodile, 1993). There appears to be no consensus on other previously implicated risk factors such as marital status, religion, education, income and ABO blood group.

The signs and symptoms of hydatidiform mole are summarized in *Table 31.2*. In general, when any abnormality in the first trimester of pregnancy occurs, hydatidiform mole should be considered among the differential diagnoses. Approximately half the patients will present with a uterus too large for dates, and 20% will present with a uterus small for dates or with a suspicion of intrauterine fetal demise (Kohorn, 1984). Bleeding in the first trimester is a very common symptom, and even though this particular symptom is experienced in up to 25% of normal gestations, hydatidiform mole should be considered in the differential diagnosis. Hypertension and rarely eclampsia in early pregnancy may be the presenting symptom (Slattery *et al.*, 1993; Cox and Klein, 1993). As trophoblastic tissues from moles produce more isoforms of HCG with thyrotropic activity, hyperthyroidism should also prompt evaluation for GTN (Yoshimura *et al.*, 1994)

The availability of high resolution ultrasound has rendered all other means of diagnosis of hydatidiform mole obsolete (Hammond *et al.*, 1979). Continued evolution of this valuable technique has allowed even more sophisticated preoperative assessment with transvaginal color flow Doppler sonography. While the pulsatility index is strongly associated with prognosis and correlates with the HCG values (Carter *et al.*, 1993), the expense of this evaluation would limit its usefulness to high-risk cases, confusing clinical presentations, or localization and characterization of persistent disease. Similarly, computerized tomography (CT) and magnetic resonance imaging (MRI) are expensive and rarely helpful in primary diagnosis; in fact MRI in persistent GTN, incomplete abortion and ectopic pregnancy is relatively nonspecific, with actual usefulness limited to determining depth of invasion and localization of persistent disease (Barton *et al.*, 1993)

Occasionally, molar pregnancy is diagnosed by the actual passage of vesicles vaginally and the observation of hydatid degeneration of aborted material. For the majority of cases in which the suspicion arises or when there is a routine investigative ultrasound in early pregnancy, hydatidiform mole is easily observed on sonography with the characteristic intrauterine echoes. Several laboratory methods can be used to distinguish moles from hydropic degeneration in aborted tissues. Both flow histogram patterns (Bocklage *et al.*, 1994) and proliferation cell nuclear antigen immunoreactivity (Suresh *et al.*, 1993) have been described for this purpose, but their utilization in actual clinical practice has yet to be determined.

Once the diagnosis of hydatidiform mole is made, the majority of patients must be evacuated operatively. The steps in the preoperative assessment are listed in *Table 31.3*. It is important that the evacuation of even the smallest mole is taken seriously, as complications from inappropriate preoperative assessment and management are possible. In addition to history and physical examination, preoperative chest radiography and ultrasound are required; indicated laboratory tests for thyroid function, coagulation, and liver functions, along with blood type, rhesus and crossmatching are essential. For patients with large uteri, Twiggs (1984) recommends arterial blood gases preoperatively.

Occasionally, especially in the older patient for whom childbearing is no longer desired, permanent sterilization is preferred, or in patients with

Table 31.3. Preoperative assessment of hydatidiform mole.

History and physical examination
Chest radiography
Pelvic ultrasound
Type and crossmatch blood
Complete blood count with platelets
Coagulation profile
Thyroid panel
Multi-panel blood chemistries (including liver function tests)
Electrocardiogram (optional)
VDRL
Syphilis test
Indicated consultations
Arterial blood gases

gynecological problems, hysterectomy may be the method of choice for surgical treatment. For most patients, however, suction curettage is the evacuation method of choice (Schlaerth, 1984). This can be accomplished with local anesthesia in cases of normal or small uterine size using paracervical block and analgesia; when evacuating large-for-dates moles, general anesthesia is preferred. Intravenous fluids must be running continuously through a large bore catheter, and, especially for large moles, blood must be crossmatched and available for immediate transfusion. Dilatation of the cervix is easily accomplished without the use of laminaria, and a 10 mm suction curette is usually sufficient for prompt evacuation. Care should be taken to introduce the suction curette no further than just beyond the internal os, as insertion into the fundus is unnecessary and hazardous. Suction is applied at high negative pressure (70 cm Hg) and evacuation usually proceeds rapidly, as the curette is gently rotated. After the initiation of evacuation and when the uterus begins to contract, intravenous oxytocin, 20 units l^{-1} at 150 ml h^{-1}, should be administered. Once evacuation is judged complete, thoroughness can be assured with a large blunt curette, but vigorous sharp curettage is risky and can lead to uterine perforation, excessive hemorrhage or post-evacuation Asherman's syndrome. The suggestion that sharp curettage provides prognostic information in which fibrinoid deposits at the implantation site portend a greater risk of persistent GTN (Rice *et al.*, 1991) requires further investigation before such curettage can be routinely recommended. Maintenance intravenous fluids and continued intravenous pitocin are usually required for at least 6–8 hours post-evacuation. The anesthesiologist should be aware that enormous volumes of molar tissue and bloody fluid are possible, and should be prudent in the administration of replacement solutions.

Postoperatively, patients with a pre-evacuation uterus of greater than 20 weeks' size should be maintained on intravenous pitocin in an in-hospital setting for at least 24 hours post-evacuation. Those with smaller gestations can frequently be discharged on an outpatient basis depending on the availability of follow-up facilities and the patient's reliability to report symptoms. Within 24 hours of evacuation, repeat physical examination and chest radiography should be performed. In all patients, including those who have undergone hysterectomy, close post-operative monitoring of HCG titers is essential for adequate follow-up. The recommended follow-up plan post-evacuation of hydatidiform mole is given in *Table 31.4.*

Common complications of hydatidiform mole are listed in *Table 31.5.* Among the most serious is the post-evacuation pulmonary insufficiency syndrome, often called shock lung, a clinical picture of adult respiratory distress syndrome (ARDS). Although the etiology is uncertain, a possible cause is deportation of molar material through the venous sinuses to the lungs. Occasionally respiratory embarrassment can

Table 31.4. Post-evaluation follow-up of hydatidiform mole.

Postoperative physical examination and chest radiograph
Follow-up human chorionic gonadotropin (HCG) titers weekly
Confirmatory titer one month after first negative titer
HCG titers every 2–3 months for one year
Good contraception for one year
If any elevation in HCG titer occurs, or plateauing titers are noted, work up for malignant gestational trophoblastic neoplasia must be undertaken, and appropriate therapy instituted

Table 31.5. Complications of hydatidiform mole.

Perioperative
Excessive blood loss and hypovolemic shock
Disseminated intravascular coagulation
Hyperthyroidism with storm
Shock lung syndrome
Uterine perforation with hemoperitoneum or broad ligament hematoma
Rupture or torsion of theca lutein cysts
Postoperative
Delayed hemorrhage
Complications of persistent theca lutein cysts (hyperstimulation syndrome, ascites, peritonitis, torsion)
Invasive mole with uterine perforation and hemoperitoneum
Malignant gestational trophoblastic neoplasia

be sufficient to cause admission for intensive care monitoring or even rarely death (Twiggs, 1984). For this reason, patients should be carefully observed clinically during evacuation and post-evacuation, with prompt assessment of arterial gases if tachypnea or shortness of breath occur. A postoperative chest radiograph and physical examination may reveal unsuspected respiratory compromise which may not manifest itself until after discharge. Appropriate warnings should be given to patients regarding signs and symptoms of this important complication.

Additionally, although it is unusual for disseminated intravascular coagulopathy to be insidious in onset, this possibility should be considered whenever persistent bleeding occurs immediately after evacuation of hydatidiform mole. Appropriate coagulation studies and clotting factor replacement are essential for management. Uterine perforation, despite the best efforts to avoid it, is an occasional complication and must be managed initially with appropriate aggressive intravenous fluids and blood replacement. Laparoscopy is often needed to assess intra-abdominal damage, and laparotomy to repair the uterine rent or injured viscus may be necessary. If the perforation occurs in the broad ligament, the accompanying hypovolemia and clinical picture of hematoma and eventual abscess may be less apparent acutely, and careful clinical awareness is essential to make the diagnosis and effect the indicated evacuation.

The histologic confirmation and grading of hydatidiform mole after evacuation, once historically important, cannot uniformly predict trophoblastic sequelae. In fact, differentiating the partial mole from complete moles or even hydropic degeneration carries a high incidence of inter- and intra-pathologist variability (Messerli *et al.*, 1987; Howat *et al.*, 1993). Therefore, this potential uncertainty further underscores the compulsive necessity to follow all possible molar gestations with serial HCG titers. Nevertheless, histologic confirmation is often necessary to distinguish complete moles from their less common counterpart, partial mole.

Most complete moles possess two haploid sets of chromosomes, 46XX, both of which are paternally derived, whereas partial moles are most often triploid, with a contribution from both parents (Szulman and Surti, 1984; Ohama *et al.*, 1986; Berkowitz, 1992). Modern cytogenetic studies have allowed the discovery of numerous variations in karyotypes of both complete and partial moles, and isolated reports of rare presentation, including those concomitant with an intact fetus, are given in the literature (Deaton *et al.*, 1989). More sophisticated molecular biology techniques have revealed even more complex findings: a relaxation of imprinting was suggested to explain the expression of the maternally expressed H19 gene in the androgenetic tissue of complete moles (Ariel *et al.*, 1994), and mitochondrial DNA has been demonstrated to be of maternal ovum origin (Berkowitz, 1992). These studies and others clearly demonstrate that complete hydatidiform mole results from the fertilization of an anuclear empty ovum (Lawler *et al.*, 1991). However, heterozygous complete moles represent an important variant (Berkowitz *et al.*, 1991). A classification of hydatidiform moles, with the laboratory variations and clinical features is presented in *Table 31.6*. For the clinician, the separation is almost academic, for careful evacuation and appropriate follow-up with serial HCG determination remains the cornerstone of management.

The very rare occurrence of an apparently normal viable fetus with either a complete or partial mole must be managed on an individualized basis with appropriate consultation. Recently, the natural history of this eventuality was described in eight patients managed at the same institution, and compared with 14 other cases described in the literature (Steller *et al.*, 1994). Surgical management

Table 31.6. Comparison of complete and partial hydatidiform moles.

Parameter	*Complete mole*	*Partial mole*
Uterine size	Markedly enlarged or top normal	Normal to small
Bleeding	May be heavy	Usually light
Usual preoperative diagnosis	Complete mole	Missed abortion
Vesicles	Markedly hydropic, large	Small, scanty
Tissue volume	Moderate to marked	Low, scanty
Ultrasound picture	Homogeneously echogenic with varying cystic sizes	Variable gestational sac with increased transverse diameter Cystic irregularities in tissues around sac
Serum human chorionic gonadotropin	Usually very high (>100,000)	Usually low (<50,000)
Trophoblastic proliferation	May be marked	Usually low
Fetal features	Virtually absent	Varying, but present; intact fetus possible
Cytogenetics	XX, all paternal origin	XXY, paternal, maternal origin
Malignant sequelae	Relatively high (10–30%)	Relatively low (4–10%)

of the eight cases was variable, with cesarean hysterectomy, hysterotomy, vaginal delivery and suction evacuation being employed in individual cases with no surviving fetuses; four of the cases from the literature reported fetal survival. Although the prospect of fetal survival might prompt delayed surgical intervention, the risk of persistent trophoblastic disease is very high: 55% in the combined series (Steller *et al.*, 1994). With the propensity of ovulation induction and other assisted reproductive technologies for causing multiple gestation, such cases will probably increase.

Close follow-up of patients with evacuated hydatidiform moles is mandatory. Included in this follow-up is good contraception, which must usually be maintained for at least one year. Earlier data suggested that the use of oral contraceptives might lead to increased malignant sequelae, but this has not been confirmed (Morrow, 1984). A randomized prospective study by the Gynecologic Oncology Group (Curry *et al.*, 1989) confirmed that oral contraceptives do not confer increased risk, and more recently an evaluation of 299 patients suggested an actual outcome advantage for patients who used oral contraceptives for contraception after molar pregnancy (Deicas *et al.*, 1991). Therefore, most clinicians consider oral contraceptives to be the optimal means of preventing unwanted pregnancy after hydatidiform mole. Barrier contraception may be effective, but should be used fastidiously. Even with sensitive ultrasound, the confusion of an early intrauterine pregnancy with recurrent or persistent mole presents a difficult clinical dilemma and thus should therefore be avoided.

Approximately 20% of complete hydatidiform moles will fail to resolve spontaneously and become a persistent mole, develop chorioadenoma destruens (invasive mole) or evolve into choriocarcinoma. The exact figure for such malignant sequelae is difficult to determine, and varies from 10% to more than 30% in various series. However, certain patients are known to be at-risk for malignant sequelae; risk factors for malignant GTN after molar evacuation are summarized in *Table 31.7*. A worrisome symptom is persistent or unexplained vaginal bleeding in the molar follow-up period, and close observation and appropriate evaluation of these patients is essential. Patients with large theca lutein cysts (>6 cm), uteri large for dates or high initial HCG titers (>100,000) are also at increased risk. For older patients (age >40 years), the risk for persistent disease increases significantly.

With the understanding that patients with one or more high-risk factors have a risk of developing malignant GTN up to 10 times greater than that of their low-risk counterparts (Morrow, 1984), the use of prophylactic chemotherapy for this group is frequently considered. In a randomized study, Kim *et al.* (1986) found that prophylactic chemotherapy did decrease the risk of malignant sequelae in high-risk patients, but not in low-risk patients. Unfortunately, treated patients require more chemotherapy to sustain remission. Similarly, Ayhan *et al.* (1990), administering methotrexate prophylactically to both high-risk and low-risk groups, found that the development of persistent disease was not statistically different in either group when compared to that of untreated patients. Therefore, although prophylactic chemotherapy may be indicated before the actual plateauing or elevation of titers post-evacuation in high-risk patients with suspected poor follow-up potential, its routine use is not recommended.

As long as HCG titers continue to decline, intervention is unnecessary. Titers will decline quite rapidly in most patients immediately after evacuation, and will become normal by eight weeks. A reference regression curve has been established, and plotting individual cases' titers again such a standard has been recommended (Morrow, 1984). Although unnecessary in most circumstances, this approach may prove useful in patients with prolonged titer elevations or tardy regressions. It is uncertain, however, if the initial curve can be a reliable predictor for malignant sequelae. A small percentage of patients will have a very slow and gradual decline, thus provoking anxiety as to whether or not intervention is indicated. Although some clinics set arbitrary cut-off times to initiate treatment, there is no definite evidence that malignant sequelae are more likely to be unmanageable in patients who exhibit slow, but steady declines in HCG titer. Using a 95th percentile line, Yedema *et al.* (1993) identified 92% of patients who would develop persistent disease, but their methodology was difficult and the outcomes no different. Therefore, whenever problematic patients are encountered, consultation with a trophoblastic disease center is recommended in order to assure appropriate management. By definition, stabilization of three consecutive weekly titers, or elevation of two consecutive weekly titers is sufficient grounds to terminate expectant management and begin staging and treatment for malignant disease.

After the first negative titer, a confirmatory value should be determined in one month and then the

Table 31.7. Risk factors for the development of malignant gestational trophoblastic neoplasia after molar evacuation.

Delayed post-evacuation bleeding
Theca lutein cysts
Uterus pre-evacuation >20 weeks' size
Previous hydatidiform mole
Pulmonary insufficiency syndrome
Advanced maternal age
High initial human chorionic gonadotropin (>100,000)

patient should be followed for six months to one year with bi-monthly titers with good contraception. If titers continue to remain negative, pregnancy can be considered.

The risk of repeat hydatidiform mole after a previous molar pregnancy is 20–40 times greater than the primary risk (Grimes, 1984), and even greater after a second or third mole (Narayan *et al.*, 1991), but the overall incidence is sufficiently low that patients should not avoid attempting pregnancy if they desire. In numerous series there appears to be no greater risk for abortion, cesarean section or fetal anomalies in subsequent pregnancies, yet appropriate prenatal counseling is mandatory for patients who have had a previous molar pregnancy.

Diagnosis and Staging of Malignant Gestational Trophoblastic Neoplasia

Patients with documented persistent hydatidiform mole, whether determined by histologically examined tissue, or by elevating or plateauing titers after molar evacuation, must undergo immediate staging and treatment for malignant GTN. Additionally, patients who have been shown to have choriocarcinoma following a term pregnancy, or present with evidence of GTN after therapeutic abortion, tubal pregnancy or remote pregnancy should be thoroughly evaluated and prepared for chemotherapy on a somewhat emergent basis.

The issue of repeat curettage is unsettled. In situations where the patient is symptomatically bleeding or if the diagnosis is uncertain, curettage may be of both therapeutic and diagnostic benefit. However, most patients who have plateauing or rising titers after hydatidiform mole evacuation will not need repeat curettage, and its value in asymptomatic patients is questioned. In fact, the potential complications associated with unnecessary curettage, including uterine perforation, broad ligament hematoma and exacerbated hemorrhage, would suggest such repeat curettage to be meddlesome. In a retrospective study, Schlaerth *et al.* (1990) described three patients (8.1%) who suffered perforation, two of whom required hysterectomy. In addition, there is no documented evidence that 'debulking' of persistent hydatidiform mole is of therapeutic value, nor is establishing a histologic diagnosis in patients with non-metastatic disease after molar evacuation, as all such patients will be treated virtually the same.

A full metastatic work-up including a thorough history and physical examination is essential. In most modern clinics, this can be accomplished quickly and easily by enhanced CT scan of the pelvis, abdomen, lungs and brain. Certain circumstances may mitigate against 'total body' CT scan, but its role in detecting small metastases in the lungs has been established (Mutch *et al.*, 1986). Likewise, although MRI has been advocated for diagnostic purposes in GTN, the value of CT scan and its wide availability secure its role in the work-up of patients with GTN. Repeat ultrasound is useful to document uterine size and establish the presence and dimensions of theca lutein cysts. As previously stated, MRI may be useful for documenting uterine disease, but its overall role in the work-up for malignant GTN remains investigational.

After staging studies, patients are grouped for treatment planning according to one of three principal systems. The staging system advocated by Hammond *et al.* (1980), shown in *Table 31.8*, has gained wide popularity. Patients are divided into non-metastatic and metastatic groupings, and those with metastatic disease are further classified as low-risk and high-risk depending on certain prognostic factors. Alternately, the International Federation of Gynecology and Obstetrics (FIGO) staging system (see *Table 47.9*) is used in some clinics, although its usefulness is somewhat limited when planning chemotherapy. The multi-faceted prognostic scoring system popularized by Bagshawe and Wong (1986) and adopted by the World Health Organization, is very useful in establishing a medium-risk group of patients who may benefit from less intensive chemotherapy. The version of this system as modified by Lewis (1993) is shown in *Table 47.10*. That there are at least twelve variations in this system currently in use in various centers (Kohorn, 1995) clearly speaks for the need for consensus and uniformity, adds further merit to the

Table 31.8. Categorization of gestational trophoblastic disease.

Non-metastatic disease
Persistent hydatidiform mole
Chorioadenoma destruens
Choriocarcinoma
Metastatic disease
Low-risk, good prognosis
Human chorionic gonadotropin (HCG) <40,000 miu ml^{-1}
No liver or brain metastasis
Duration of disease < four months
No previous chemotherapy
High-risk, poor prognosis
HCG >40,000 miu ml^{-1}
Brain metastasis
Liver metastasis
Duration of disease >four months
Previously failed chemotherapy
Disease following term pregnancy

simplified NIH system popularized by Hammond, and explains why the latter remains the foundation for management in many centers. Chemotherapeutic management of malignant GTN is discussed in the following chapter.

The Role of Surgery

At one time, surgical management was the only hope for the treatment of persistent hydatidiform mole, chorioadenoma destruens and uterine choriocarcinoma, but total surgical management of gestational trophoblastic disease in the era of modern chemotherapy is unusual. Nevertheless, selected surgical procedures should remain in the therapeutic armoury of clinicians caring for patients with GTN. These may be used in roughly five circumstances:

- primary surgical management of hydatidiform mole;
- combined therapeutic hysterectomy and chemotherapy in the management of non-metastatic disease;
- adjunctive surgery in patients with metastatic disease;
- surgery for persistent isolated metastases;
- operative intervention for complications of GTN.

Primary Surgical Management of Hydatidiform Mole

As previously indicated, certain women may be ideal candidates for an initial management of hydatidiform mole by therapeutic hysterectomy. Since the risk of malignant sequelae is higher for women of over 40 years, in this age-group hydatidiform moles may be treated with hysterectomy and decrease the risk of malignant sequelae. If such patients have a history of gynecologic problems, such as pelvic pain, leiomyoma or another gynecologic problem for which uterine removal might be a therapeutic indication, initial hysterectomy might be the procedure of choice. It is imperative, however, that such patients are followed-up as outlined in *Table 31.2* for follow-up of hydatidiform mole.

Combined Management for Patients with Non-metastatic Disease

Patients with recurrent hydatidiform mole who have completed childbearing may undergo hysterectomy during their initial course of chemotherapy. Hammond *et al.* (1980) have shown that primary hysterectomy decreases the number of courses of chemotherapy needed to achieve remission. Usually hysterectomy is performed on the second or third day of a five-day course of single-agent chemotherapy, and with completion of chemotherapy during the immediate postoperative course. Hammond *et al.* (1980) and Lewis *et al.* (1966) reported no increased surgical complications from this combined treatment. If initial chemotherapy fails to cure stubborn foci of GTN in the uterus, hysterectomy may be necessary. Alternatively, arterial infusion chemotherapy (Maroulis *et al.*, 1975) may be attempted; this technique was successful in avoiding hysterectomy in three of seven patients in the series of Hammond *et al.* (1980).

Hysterectomy Associated with Chemotherapy Treatment of Metastatic Disease

When the bulk of the demonstrable GTN is present in the uterus, but there is metastatic disease elsewhere, hysterectomy may decrease the number of courses of chemotherapy necessary to achieve complete remission. Although 'debulking' is not typically associated with GTN, reduction of tumor volume is the goal with the additional benefits of hysterectomy being complementary. As with surgery during the therapy for non-metastatic disease, chemotherapy is administered perioperatively.

Surgical Removal of Sites of Occult or Persistent Disease

Most series on high-risk GTN report a significant number of patients needing surgical intervention to effect cure (Hammond *et al.*, 1980; Jones and Lewis, 1983; Surwit *et al.*, 1984; DuBeshter *et al.*, 1987). Resistant foci of choriocarcinoma are amenable to surgical extirpation, especially lesions in the lung, where segmental resection can be curative for patients whose only disease is a persistent nodule (Libshitz *et al.*, 1977). Occasionally surgery can remove other metastases (e.g. metastases in the liver or kidney), but it is extremely unusual for such intervention to be elective.

Surgery for Complications

Complications of therapy for GTN are numerous, especially in patients with high-risk disease (DuBeshter *et al.*, 1987). A hemoperitoneum may result from uterine perforation from chorioadenoma destruens and requires prompt surgical management. Likewise, intra-abdominal metastases, especially those in the liver, may rupture spontaneously or may begin to bleed during the initiation of chemotherapy, and surgical exploration is mandatory. For patients with brain metastases, craniotomy may be life saving, but the use of concomitant radiation has greatly reduced the need for operative intervention (Yordan *et al.,* 1987). The uncommon occurrence of hemothorax associated with the treatment of pulmonary metastases may require chest tube manipulation or even thoracotomy to stop profuse hemorrhage. Although rare, intestinal obstruction from intra-abdominal metastases from choriocarcinoma may be encountered, often requiring bowel resection to avoid disastrous consequences. Since GTN can metastasize to virtually any site, surgical intervention may be indicated for such eventualities as spinal cord compression, articular effusion and genitourinary hemorrhage.

Vaginal metastasis of GTN offers a tempting opportunity to perform biopsies. However, these lesions are extraordinarily vascular and serious hemorrhage or hematoma can result from attempts to do excisional vaginal biopsies. Only in unusual circumstances is surgery indicated to establish the diagnosis of recurrent disease, and surgical biopsy of unknown lesions may be best delayed until HCG titer observation.

Although the high incidence (25% of cases with hydatidiform mole) and occasionally enormous size of theca lutein cysts would suggest a role for frequent surgical intervention, complications requiring operative management are actually rare and primary surgical drainage is controversial. Montz *et al.* (1988), in a review of 102 patients with theca lutein cysts, noted serious complications in three cases, two of which required surgery (one for torsion, one for hemorrhage) and the third of which had ascites, which resolved with supportive care. None of their patients underwent laparoscopy for decompression. In contrast, Goldstein and Berkowitz (1982) advocated laparoscopic decompression of cysts larger than 10 cm. Thus, conservatism rather than aggressive surgical intervention seems prudent for the management of theca lutein cysts, and regression usually occurs after primary control of the trophoblastic event.

Placental Site Trophoblastic Tumor

Placental site trophoblastic tumor (PSTT) was first described by Kurman *et al.* (1976) as 'trophoblastic pseudotumor', and as awareness of this entity was diffused throughout the clinical arena, PSTT has emerged in the past decade as an unusual presentation of trophoblastic disease. In a report by Lathrop *et al.* (1988), 43 cases had been reported and these authors added five additional cases; almost concomitantly, Finkler *et al.* (1988) added seven more cases, and Funkunaga and Ushigome's report (1993) on immunohistochemical and flow cytometry of two patients brought the number of reported cases to 90. These, combined with the description of radiologic, surgical and pathologic methods of evaluating the extent of disease by Hoffman *et al.* (1993), make it apparent that this entity does not behave like traditional trophoblastic neoplasms, and the outcome may be unpredictable.

The diagnosis is most often rendered on curettage in situations of abnormal uterine bleeding, and pathologically the tumor is characterized by proliferation of the intermediate cytotrophoblast. These tumors secrete varying amounts of HCG, and titer levels may not reflect tumor volume or be indicative of persistent or recurrent disease. Human placental lactogen (HPL) is the predominant hormone marker, but does not appear to be clinically useful in monitoring therapy. Apparently, PSTT can follow any gestation, and the antecedent pregnancy may be remote.

Although originally thought to be benign, PSTT clearly has malignant potential as numerous deaths have been reported. All reports incriminate a high mitotic count in the curettage specimen as being an ominous prognostic sign. The optimal management of these patients is unknown, as curettage alone is therapeutic in some incidences. However, prompt hysterectomy in patients with non-metastatic disease would seem prudent management unless there are overwhelming reasons to preserve the uterus.

Unfortunately, for patients with metastatic disease or recurrent disease after hysterectomy, chemotherapy has proved less effective than in other trophoblastic diseases. Experience continues to accumulate with this problematic entity. The most efficacious chemotherapy regimen has yet to be elucidated, therefore aggressive early surgical management is preferred. At the time of writing it is uncertain which regimen is the most preferred for metastatic disease.

Conclusion

The next chapter describes the chemotherapeutic management of patients with malignant GTN. Prompt diagnosis and proper management of patients with benign lesions as well as thorough staging and categorization of malignant disease can lead to continued improvement in the survival of all patients with this group of neoplasms.

Summary of Management Options

- The single most important risk factor for hydatidiform moles is previous molar pregnancy, and all prenatal evaluations should be cognizant of this history. The combination of recurrent spontaneous abortions, cancer, and gestational trophoblastic neoplasia (GTN) in families may impart a greater risk as does advanced maternal age.
- The availability of high resolution ultrasound has rendered all other means of diagnosis of hydatidiform mole obsolete.
- For most patients, suction curettage is the evacuation method of choice.
- Among the most serious post-evacuation complications is the pulmonary insufficiency syndrome, often called shock lung, or a clinical picture of adult respiratory distress syndrome.
- Uterine perforation, despite the best efforts to avoid it, is an occasional complication. Laparoscopy is often needed to assess intra-abdominal damage, and laparotomy to repair the uterine rent or injured viscus may be necessary.
- Histologic grading of hydatidiform mole cannot uniformly predict trophoblastic sequelae. In fact, differentiating the partial mole from complete moles or even hydropic degeneration carries a high incidence of inter- and intra-pathologist variability.
- Careful evacuation and appropriate follow-up with serial human chorionic gonadotropin determinations remain the cornerstone of management.
- The use of prophylactic chemotherapy in high-risk patients with suspected poor follow-up potential is not recommended based on current information.
- Since the risk of malignant sequelae is higher for women over 40 years, hydatidiform moles in this age-group may be treated with hysterectomy and decrease the risk of malignant sequelae.
- Patients with recurrent hydatidiform mole who have completed childbearing may undergo hysterectomy during their initial course of chemotherapy.
- When the bulk of the demonstrable GTN is present in the uterus, but there is metastatic disease elsewhere, hysterectomy may decrease the number of courses of chemotherapy necessary to achieve complete remission.
- Resistant foci of choriocarcinoma are amenable to surgical extirpation, especially lesions in the lung, where segmental resection can be curative for patients whose only disease is a persistent nodule.
- Conservatism rather than aggressive surgical intervention seems prudent for the management of theca lutein cysts, and regression usually occurs after primary control of the trophoblastic event.

References

Ariel I, Lustig O, Oyer CE *et al.* (1994) Relaxation of imprinting in trophoblastic disease. *Gynecol. Oncol.* **53:** 212–219.

Ayhan A, Ergeneli MH, Yuce K *et al.* (1990) Effects of prophylactic chemotherapy for postmolar trophoblastic disease in patients with complete hydatidiform mole. *Int. J. Gynecol. Obstet.* **32:** 39–41.

Barton JW, McCarthy SM, Kohorn EI *et al.* (1993) Pelvic MR imaging findings in gestational trophoblastic disease, incomplete abortion, and ectopic pregnancy: Are they specific? *Radiology* **186:** 163–168.

■ Berkowitz RS (1992) Gestational trophoblastic disease: Recent advances in the understanding of cytogenetics, histopathology, and natural history. *Curr. Opin. Obstet. Gynecol.* **4:** 616–620.

Berkowitz RS, Goldstein DP & Bernstein MR (1991) Evolving concepts of molar pregnancy. *J. Reprod. Med.* **36(1):** 40–44.

Bocklage TJ, Smith HO & Bartow SA (1994) Distinctive flow histiogram pattern in molar pregnancies with elevated maternal serum human chorionic gonadotropin levels. *Cancer* **73:** 2782–2790.

Buckley JD (1984) The epidemiology of molar pregnancy and choriocarcinoma. *Clin. Obstet. Gynecol.* **28:** 153–159.

Carter J, Fowler J, Carlson J *et al.* (1993) Transvaginal color flow Doppler sonography in the assessment of gestational trophoblastic disease. *J. Ultrasound Med.* **12:** 595–599.

Cohen BA, Burkman RT, Rosenshein NB *et al.* (1979) Gestational trophoblastic disease within an elective abortion population. *Am. J. Obstet. Gynecol.* **135:** 452–454.

Cox SM & Klein VR (1993) Partial molar pregnancy associated with severe pregnancy-induced hypertension. *J. Perinatol.* **XIII(2):** 103–106.

■ Curry SL, Schlaerth JB, Kohorn EI *et al.* (1989) Hormonal contraception and trophoblastic sequelae after hydatidiform mole; a Gynecologic Oncology Group study. *Am. J. Obstet. Gynecol.* **160:** 5–11.

Deaton JL, Hoffman JS, Saal H *et al.* (1989) Molar pregnancy coexisting with a normal fetus: A case report. *Gynecol. Oncol.* **32:** 394–397.

Deicas RD, Miller DS, Rademaker AW & Lurain JR (1991) The role of contraception in the development of postmolar gestational trophoblastic tumor. *Obstet. Gynecol.* **78:** 221.

DuBeshter B, Berkowitz RS, Goldstein DP *et al.* (1987)

Metastatic gestational trophoblastic disease: Experience at the New England Trophoblastic Disease Center, 1965 to 1985. *Obstet. Gynecol.* **69:** 390–395.

Finkler NJ, Berkowitz RS, Driscoll SG *et al.* (1988) Clinical experience with placental site trophoblastic tumors at the New England Trophoblastic Disease Center. *Obstet. Gynecol.* **71:** 854–857.

Fukunaga M & Ushigome S (1993) Metastasizing placental site trophoblastic tumor: An immunohistochemical and flow cytometric study of two cases. *Am. J. Surg. Path.* **17(10):** 1003–1010.

Goldstein DP & Berkowitz RS (1982) *Gestational Trophoblastic Neoplasms,* pp. 106–108. Philadelphia: WB Saunders.

■ Grimes DA (1984) Epidemiology of gestational trophoblastic disease. *Am. J. Obstet. Gynecol.* **150:** 309–318.

Grumbine FC, Rosenshein NB, Brereton HD & Kaufman SL (1980) Management of liver metastasis from gestational trophoblastic neoplasia. *Am. J. Obstet. Gynecol.* **137:** 959–961.

Hammond CB, Haney AF & Currie JL (1979) The role of diagnostic tests in gestational trophoblastic disease. *Am. J. Diag. Obstet. Gynecol.* **1:** 319–330.

■ Hammond CB, Weed JC Jr & Currie JL (1980) The role of operation in the current therapy of gestational trophoblastic disease. *Am. J. Obstet. Gynecol.* **136:** 844–858.

Ho HN, Gill TJ, Hsieh CY *et al.* (1991) The prevalence of recurrent spontaneous abortions, cancer, and congenital anomalies in the families of couples with recurrent spontaneous abortions or gestational trophoblastic tumors. *Am. J. Obstet. Gynecol.* **165:** 461–466.

■ Hoffman JS, Silverman AD, Gelber J & Cartun R (1993) Placental site trophoblastic tumor: A report of radiologic, surgical, and pathologic methods of evaluating the extent of disease. *Gynecol. Oncol.* **50:** 110–114.

Howat AJ, Beck S, Fox H *et al.* (1993) Can histopathologists reliably diagnose molar pregnancy? *J. Clin. Pathol.* **46:** 599–602.

Jones WB & Lewis JL Jr (1983) Late recurrence of gestational trophoblastic disease. *Gynecol. Oncol.* **20:** 83–91.

Kim DS, Moon H, Kim KT *et al.* (1986) Effects of prophylactic chemotherapy for persistent trophoblastic disease in patients with complete hydatidiform mole. *Obstet. Gynecol.* **67:** 690–694.

Kohorn EI (1984) Molar pregnancy: Presentation and diagnosis. *Clin. Obstet. Gynecol.* **27:** 181–191.

■ Kohorn EI (1995) The trophoblastic tower of Babel: Classification systems for metastatic gestational trophoblastic neoplasia. *Gynecol. Oncol.* **56:** 280–288.

Kurman RJ, Scully RE & Norris NJ (1976) Trophoblastic pseudotumor of the uterus. *Cancer* **38:** 1214.

Lathrop JC, Lauchlan S, Ramakrisna N & Ambler M (1988) Clinical characteristics of placental site trophoblastic tumor (PSTT). *Gynecol. Oncol.* **31:** 32–42.

Lawler SD, Fisher RA & Dent J (1991) A prospective genetic study of complete and partial hydatidiform moles. *Am. J. Obstet. Gynecol.* **164:** 1270–1277.

■ Lewis JL (1993) Diagnosis and management of gestational trophoblastic disease. *Cancer* **71(Suppl. 4):** 1639–1647.

Lewis JL Jr, Ketcham AS & Hertz R (1966) Surgical intervention during chemotherapy of gestational trophoblastic neoplasms. *Cancer* **19:** 1517.

Libshitz HI, Barber CE & Hammond CB (1977) The pulmonary metastases of choriocarcinoma. *Obstet. Gynecol.* **49:** 412–416.

Lurain JR, Sand PK & Brewer JI (1986) Choriocarcinoma associated with ectopic pregnancy. *Obstet. Gynecol.* **68:** 286–287.

Maroulis GB, Hammond CB, Johnsrude IS *et al.* (1975) Arteriography and infusional chemotherapy in localized trophoblastic disease. *Obstet. Gynecol.* **45:** 397–406.

Mazzanti P, La Vecchia C, Parazzini F & Bolis G (1986) Pregnancy of hydatidiform mole in Lombardy, Northern Italy. *Gynecol. Oncol.* **24:** 337–342.

Messerli ML, Parmley TH, Woodruff JD *et al.* (1987) Inter- and intra-pathologist variability in the diagnosis of gestational trophoblastic neoplasia. *Obstet. Gynecol.* **69:** 622–626.

Montz FJ, Schlaerth JB & Morrow CP (1988) The natural history of theca lutein cysts. *Obstet. Gynecol.* **72:** 247–251.

Morrow CP (1984) Post molar trophoblastic disease: Diagnosis, management and prognosis. *Clin. Obstet. Gynecol.* **27:** 211–220.

Mutch DG, Soper JT, Baker ME *et al.* (1986) Role of computed axial tomography of the chest in staging patients with nonmetastatic gestational trophoblastic disease. *Obstet. Gynecol.* **68:** 348–352.

Narayan H, Mansour P & McDougall WW (1992) Recurrent consecutive partial molar pregnancy. *Gynecol. Oncol.* **46:** 122–127.

Newlands ES, Fisher RA & Searle F (1992) The immune system in disease: Gestational trophoblastic tumours. *Baillière's Clin. Obstet. Gynaecol.* **6(3):** 519–539.

Ohama K, Ueda K, Okamoto E *et al.* (1986) Cytogenetic and clinicopathogic studies of partial moles. *Obstet. Gynecol.* **68:** 259–262.

Ozumba BC & Ofodile A (1994) Twin pregnancy involving complete hydatidiform mole and partial mole after five years of amenorrhoea. *Eur. J. Obstet. Gynecol. Repro. Biol.* **53:** 217–218.

Rice LW, Genest DR, Gerkowitz RS *et al.* (1991) Pathologic features of sharp curettings in complete hydatidiform mole: Predictors of persistent gestational trophoblastic disease. *J. Reprod. Med.* **36(1):** 17–20.

Schlaerth JB (1984) Methodology of molar pregnancy termination. *Clin. Obstet. Gynecol.* **27:** 192–198.

■ Schlaerth JB, Morrow CP & Rodriguez M (1990) Diagnostic and therapeutic curettage in gestational trophoblastic disaese. *Am. J. Obstet. Gynecol.* **162:** 1465–1471.

Slattery MA, Khong TY, Dawkins RR *et al.* (1993) Eclampsia in association with partial molar pregnancy and congenital abnormalities. *Am. J. Obstet. Gynecol.* **169:** 1625–1627.

Soper JR, Clarke-Pearson D & Hammond CB (1988) Metastatic gestational trophoblastic disease: Prognostic factors in previously untreated patients. *Obstet. Gynecol.* **71:** 338–343.

Steller MA, Genest DR, Bernstein MR *et al.* (1994) Natural history of twin pregnancy with complete hydatidiform mole and coexisting fetus. *Obstet. Gynecol.* **83:** 35–42.

Suresh UR, Hale RJ, Fox H & Buckley CH (1993) Use of proliferation cell nuclear antigen immunoreactivity for distinguishing hydropic abortions from partial hydatidiform moles. *J. Clin. Pathol.* **46:** 48–50.

Surwit EA, Alberts DS, Christian CD & Graham VE (1984) Poor-prognosis gestational trophoblastic disease: An update. *Obstet. Gynecol.* **64:** 21–26.

Szulman AE & Surti U (1984) The syndromes of partial and complete molar gestation. *Clin. Obstet. Gynecol.* **27:** 172–180.

Twiggs LB (1984) Nonneoplastic complications of molar pregnancy. *Clin. Obstet. Gynecol.* **27:** 199–210.

Wong LC, Choo YC & Ma HK (1986) Primary oral etoposide therapy in gestational trophoblastic disease. *Cancer* **58:** 14–17.

Yedema KA, Verheijen RH, Kenemans P *et al.* (1993) Identification of patients with persistent trophoblastic disease by means of a normal human chorionic gonadotropin regressive curve. *Am. J. Obstet. Gynecol.* **168:** 787–792.

Yordan EL Jr, Schlaerth J, Gaddis O & Morris CP (1987) Radiation therapy in the management of gestational choriocarcinoma metastatic to the central nervous system. *Obstet. Gynecol.* **69:** 627–630.

Yoshimura M, Pekary E, Pang XP *et al.* (1994) Thyrotropic activity of basic isoelectric forms of human chorionic gonadotropin extracted from hydatidiform mole tissues. *J. Clin. Endocrinol. Metab.* **78:** 862–866.

32 Malignant Gestational Trophoblastic Neoplasia

E S Newlands

Tumor Markers and Hydatidiform Mole Follow-up

Gestational trophoblastic neoplasms (GTN) can arise after any form of normal and abnormal conception (*Table 32.1*). The most common antecedent pregnancy to a GTN is a patient presenting with a hydatidiform mole (HM), which may be either a complete HM (CHM) or a partial HM (PHM). A patient presenting with an HM can usually be identified by ultrasound, and following evacuation of the uterine cavity and histologic confirmation of the diagnosis, these patients need to be registered for regular follow-up. It is well recognized that HM is a premalignant condition and can modulate to either persistent gestational trophoblastic disease (GTD) or histologic choriocarcinoma. The incidence of patients needing chemotherapy following an HM varies from approximately 15% in patients with CHM (Paradinas, 1994) to 3.4% in patients with PHM (Berkowitz *et al.*, 1994).

In the UK all patients presenting with an HM are registered for follow-up at one of three monitoring centers located at Dundee, Sheffield and the Charing Cross Hospital in London. Approximately 1200 patients are registered each year at these three centers where they are monitored by serum human chorionic gonadotropin (HCG) estimations. GTNs produce a range of pregnancy hormones including estrogens and progesterones, but the critical clinical tumor marker remains a sensitive assay for HCG. It has not been recorded that a GTN will grow clinically without producing varying amounts of serologically detectable HCG. Of the 1200 patients registered each year in the UK, who are a mixture of CHM and PHM and patients with doubtful histology such as hydropic abortions, operating on the basis of serial HCG estimations, around 8% of this population will need chemotherapy. This results in approximately 100 UK patients per annum treated at the two treatment centers, the Charing Cross Hospital and Sheffield.

Patients registered for follow-up are selected for treatment by criteria that have been established for many years (*Table 32.2*). The first decade of this registration scheme was reviewed in 1986 (Bagshawe *et al.*, 1986) when over 8000 patients had been registered. In those patients whose HCG concentrations reach the normal range within 56 days of evacuation of the HM, the risk of persistent trophoblastic disease and choriocarcinoma is very low and their follow-up has been shortened to six months. With a further eight years' experience, this policy is clinically safe. For those patients whose HCG falls more slowly and is still abnormal eight weeks post-evacuation, we have continued follow-up for two years. It is important to recognize that the risk of a second HM is increased in patients who have had a previous HM. The incidence of second HM in these patients is approximately 1 in 76 and the risk of a third HM in these patients is 1 in 6.5 (Bagshawe *et al.*, 1986). It should also be recognized that patients who become pregnant after any form of trophoblastic disease have an increased risk of disease reactivation and need HCG estimations six and 12-weeks post-delivery to confirm that their HCG has returned to normal.

Table 32.1. Gestational trophoblastic neoplasms.

Antecedent pregnancy	*Outcome*
Hydatidiform mole	→ Spontaneous regression
	→ Persistent trophoblastic disease
	→ Choriocarcinoma
Normal pregnancy Ectopic pregnancy Stillbirth Spontaneous abortion	→ Choriocarcinoma Placental site trophoblastic tumor

Table 32.2. Indications for chemotherapy.

Serum human chorionic gonadotropin (HCG) above 20,000 iu l^{-1} more than four weeks after evacuation because of the risk of uterine perforation
Histologic evidence of choriocarcinoma
Evidence of metastases in brain, liver or gastrointestinal tract, or radiologic opacities greater than two cm on chest radiography
Long-lasting uterine hemorrhage
Rising HCG values
HCG in body fluids 4–6 months after evacuation

Although the most common antecedent pregnancy to a GTN is a patient presenting with an HM, a GTN can occur after any pregnancy. Choriocarcinoma can occur after a full-term pregnancy with an incidence of between 1 in 40,000–50,000 deliveries. A GTN can occur many years after the last recognized pregnancy and in these patients the diagnosis can be very difficult. Awareness of a possible GTN in a young woman of childbearing age is important and easy to confirm since a clearly elevated HCG estimation in the absence of an intra- or extrauterine pregnancy is highly suggestive of a GTN.

Prognostic Factors

GTNs form a wide spectrum of disease biologically, ranging from disease that can be eliminated by minimally toxic chemotherapy to highly aggressive tumors where the risk of development of drug resistance remains a major problem. The main prognostic variables that have been identified in these patients are shown in *Table 32.3*. This is based on the original analysis of the Charing Cross series (Bagshawe, 1976). The most important variables in this table are:

- the duration the disease has been present in the body since a GTN develops progressive drug resistance the longer it has been present since the antecedent pregnancy;
- an HCG higher than 100,000 iu l^{-1} broadly correlates the advanced disease and the tendency to develop drug resistance;
- failure of previous chemotherapy to eliminate the disease.

Since GTNs are usually very chemosensitive, the stratification of patients into risk groups allows the selection of the least toxic and safest treatment to be selected for each patient, depending on their prognostic score.

Other scoring systems are also used and include the International Federation of Gynecology and Obstetrics (FIGO) staging system. Originally this was primarily anatomic, but more recently has allowed the inclusion of the risk factors of an HCG higher than 100,000 iu l^{-1} and a duration of disease over 6 months. We recently performed a comparative analysis of the Charing Cross prognostic scoring system with the clinically-based part of the FIGO system. Using the anatomic staging system alone, there was a potential risk of undertreating 17 (8.2%) and overtreating 9 (4.3%) of 207 patients. The main variables that need to be considered in addition to the anatomic distribution of the disease are the HCG concentration of over 100,000 iu l^{-1}, interval from the antecedent pregnancy and term delivery (Smith *et al.*, 1993a). The Charing Cross scoring system relies primarily on the history, examination and the quantitative HCG estimation and does not therefore involve any high technology investigations such as computerized tomography (CT) scanning. The World Health Organization grading system is also used by some centers and is similar to the Charing Cross prognostic scoring system.

Treatment by Risk Group

Low-risk Patients

The majority of these patients have had an HM and have been registered for follow-up. Most are selected

Table 32.3. Charing Cross Hospital (CXH) scoring system for gestational trophoblastic disease (modified from Bagshawe, 1976 in 1983). Low risk=0–5; medium risk=6–9; high risk >9.

Variable	*Charing Cross scoring system* 0	1	2	6
Age (years)	<39	>39		
Antecedent pregnancy (AP)	Mole	Abortion or unknown	Term	
Interval (end to AP to chemotherapy at CXH) (months)	<4	4–7	7–12	>12
Human chorionic gonadotropin (iu l^{-1})	1000–100,000	<1000	10,000–100,000	>100,000
ABO (female x male)		A x O O x A O or A x unknown	B x A or O AB x A or O	
Number of metastases	Nil	1–4	4–8	>8
Site of metastases	Not detected, lungs, vagina	Spleen, kidney	Gastrointestinal tract, liver	Brain
Largest tumor mass	<3 cm	3–5 cm	>5 cm	
Previous chemotherapy	Nil	Nil	Single drug	Two or more drugs

Table 32.4. Charing Cross Hospital treatment schedules for gestational trophoblastic disease.

Low risk: Methotrexate/folinic acid

Day 1 Methotrexate 50 mg im at 12 noon
Day 2 Folinic acid 6 mg im at 6 p.m.
Day 3 Methotrexate 50 mg im at 12 noon
Day 4 Folinic acid 6 mg im at 6 p.m.
Day 5 Methotrexate 50 mg im at 12 noon
Day 6 Folinic acid 6 mg im at 6 p.m.
Day 7 Methotrexate 50 mg im at 12 noon
Day 8 Folinic acid 6 mg im at 6 p.m.

Cycles are repeated after a six-day drug-free interval

Medium risk

1. Treatment a: Etoposide
   Day 1 Etoposide 250 mg m^{-2} iv in 500 ml Nsaline over 1 h
   Day 2 No treatment
   Day 3 Etoposide 250 mg m^{-2} iv in 500 ml Nsaline over 1 h
2. Treatment b: HuMMP
   Day 1 Hydroxyurea 500 mg oral 12 hourly $\times 2$ doses
   Day 2 Methotrexate 50 mg im at noon
   Day 3 6-Mercaptopurine 75 mg oral at noon
   Folinic acid 6 mg im at 6 p.m.
   Day 4 Methotrexate 50 mg im at noon
   Day 5 6-Mercaptopurine 75 mg oral at noon
   Folinic acid 6 mg im at 6 p.m.
   Day 6 Methotrexate 50 mg im at noon
   Day 7 6-Mercaptopurine 75 mg oral at noon
   Folinic acid 6 mg im at 6 p.m.
   Day 8 Methotrexate 50 mg im at noon
   Day 9 6-Mercaptopurine 75 mg oral at noon
   Folinic acid 6 mg im at 6 p.m.
3. Treatment c: Actinomycin D
   Actinomycin D 0.5 mg iv days 1–5 inclusive
   Sequence: a, b, c, b, a, b, c, b, with six-day intervals between courses.

High risk

EMA/CO

Week 1

Day 1 Actinomycin D 0.5 mg iv bolus
Etoposide 100 mg m^{-2} iv in 500 ml Nsaline over 30 min
Methotrexate 300 mg m^{-2} iv in one litre Nsaline over 12 h

Day 2 Actinomycin D 0.5 mg iv bolus
Etoposide 100 mg m^{-2} iv in 500 ml Nsaline over 30 min
Folinic acid 15 mg oral/im 12 hourly $\times 4$ doses starting 24 h after commencing methotrexate.

Week 2 Vincristine 1.4 mg m^{-2} iv bolus (max. 2 mg).
Cyclophosphamide 600 mg m^{-2} iv in 500 ml Nsaline over 30 min

for treatment before any adverse prognostic variable can develop except on occasion of an HCG over 100,000 iu l^{-1}. They form the largest group treated at the Charing Cross Hospital and accounted for 984 (62%) of 1596 patients treated between 1958 and 1994. Patients in the low-risk category are treated with methotrexate and folinic acid on a schedule that has been widely used over many years (*Table 32.4*). An illustration of the use of serial HCG estimations as a tumor marker monitoring response to treatment, and the way methotrexate and folinic acid are administered is shown in *Figure 32.1*. Once the HCG concentrations have reached the undetectable level, methotrexate is continued for a further 6–8 weeks to minimize the risk of relapse. The current sensitivity of HCG assays can miss up to approximately 100,000 tumor cells by extrapolation from HCG production by choriocarcinoma cell lines in culture.

The methotrexate and folinic acid schedule is relatively non-toxic. It does not induce any major alopecia, but some patients will get varying amounts of mucositis, which can be minimized by a high fluid intake, and in a small number of patients, by increasing the dose of folinic acid to 9 or 12 mg per dose. Pleuritic chest pain can also develop in some patients and is probably related to a chemically-induced pleurisy induced by methotrexate when used in this schedule. Rising transaminases can also occur and occasionally the therapy needs to be changed from methotrexate. Up to 5% of patients will need to change from methotrexate and folinic acid because of intolerance to these side-effects.

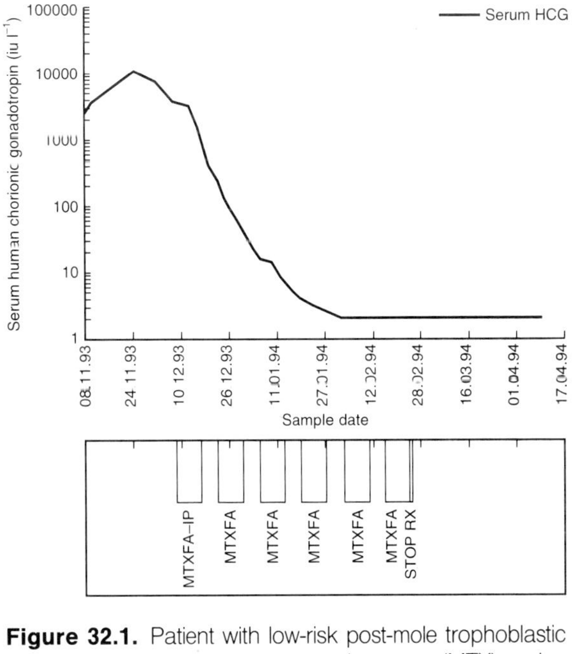

Figure 32.1. Patient with low-risk post-mole trophoblastic disease achieving remission on methotrexate (MTX) and folinic acid (FA).

Approximately 20% of low-risk patients develop drug resistance to methotrexate and need chemotherapy with alternative agents. This tendency for drug resistance to develop increases with increasing uterine volume on ultrasound (*Figure 32.2*). This means that a total of 25% of patients in the low-risk group will need to change from methotrexate and folinic acid to alternative chemotherapy (Bagshawe *et al.*, 1989). Despite this failure rate on methotrexate and folinic acid, we still regard this schedule as the treatment of choice for low-risk patients with a GTN since the long-term toxicity profile with this schedule is excellent and no evidence of carcinogenicity has yet been identified. In addition, all patients who need to change to more intensive chemotherapy can be salvaged and therefore the disease-specific survival in the low-risk patients remains 100% (Bagshawe *et al.*, 1989).

Our current policy for patients who develop drug resistance to methotrexate and folinic acid is adjusted to the concentration of HCG at which drug resistance is detected. If the HCG is approaching normal (<1000 iu l^{-1}), patients can usually achieve remission either with repeated courses of actinomycin D (see *Table 32.4* medium-risk schedules) or actinomycin D alternating with etoposide as a single agent (see *Table 32.4*). For those patients whose HCG plateaus at higher levels or who relapse after methotrexate and folinic acid, we have increasingly used the EMA/CO schedule shown in *Table 32.4* (*Figure 32.3*), which was devised for high-risk patients. Although intensive, this schedule rapidly induces remission in these patients, thereby shortening their treatment, and only requires one overnight stay in hospital every two weeks. This policy has been adopted as we have become more confident about the long-term safety profile of the EMA/CO schedule.

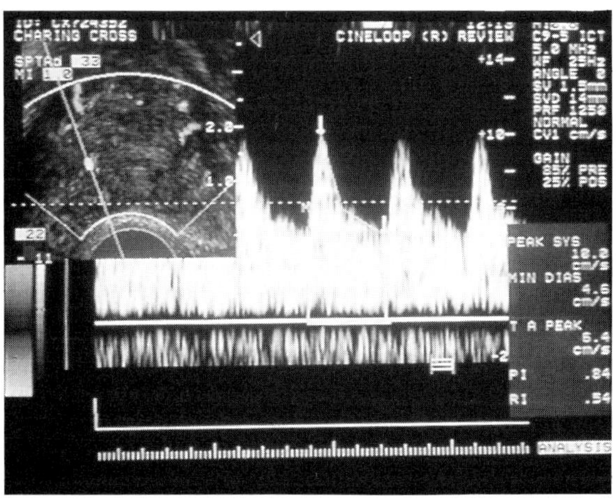

Figure 32.2. Doppler ultrasound of a patient admitted with PTD showing a large uterus with greatly increased blood flow and markedly decreased pulsatility index in the uterine arteries.

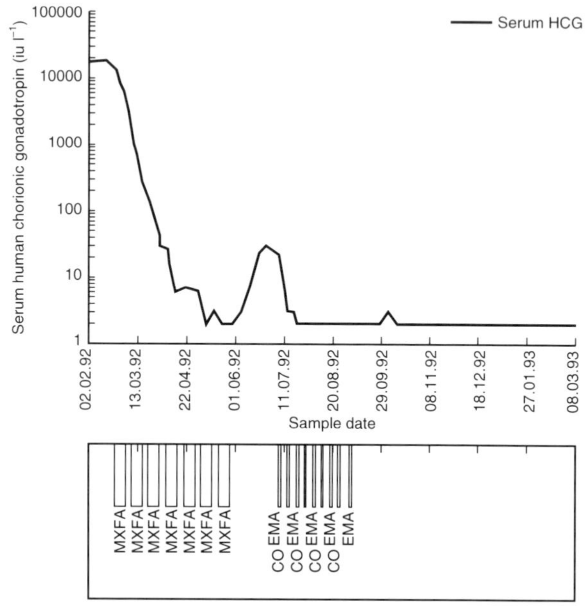

Figure 32.3. Low-risk post-mole patient responding to methotrexate (MX) and promptly relapsing, then requiring more intensive chemotherapy with EMA/CO. The current overall risk of relapse after chemotherapy is 4%. For details of EMA/CO, see *Table 32.4*.

Medium-risk Patients

Patients with a prognostic score on the Charing Cross system of 6–9 commonly develop drug resistance if they are treated with methotrexate and folinic acid (Bagshawe *et al.*, 1989). These patients need at least multiple drugs used in sequence, as in our traditional medium-risk schedule (see *Table 32.4*). This group of patients comprised 350 (22%) of 1596 patients treated at the Charing Cross Hospital between 1958 and 1994. Before the introduction of etoposide in the 1970s we had two patients who died from drug-resistant disease in the medium-risk category. Since the introduction of etoposide as one of the first-line agents for patients with medium- and high-risk GTNs, there have been no deaths in the medium-risk category of patients and the schedule we have used is shown in *Figure 32.4*. The advantage of this schedule is that it allows assessment of a new drug such as etoposide in a patient category with a survival of 100% (Newlands *et al.*, 1986). Clearly in the long term we need better and less toxic agents than those currently in use. The disadvantage of the traditional medium-risk schedule is the number of days the patient needs to spend at the Trophoblastic Disease Centre. Increasingly we have tended to treat these patients with the EMA/CO schedule because of its ease of administration and many fewer days spent by the patient at the Trophoblastic Disease Centre, with

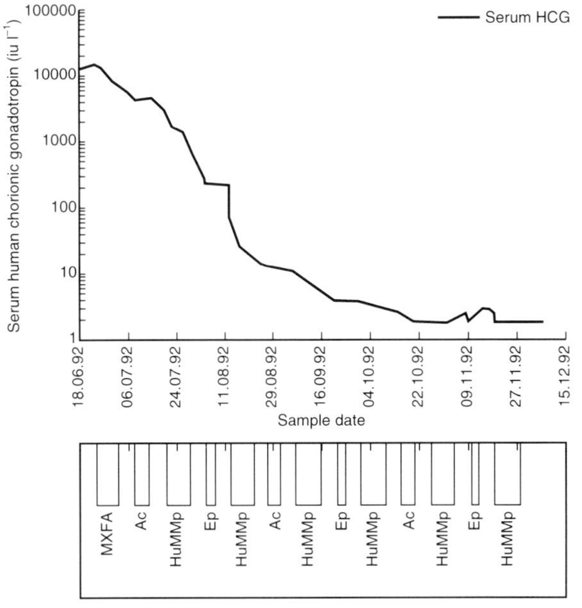

Figure 32.4. Patient with a medium-risk gestational trophoblastic neoplasm treated on the EMA/CO schedule (see *Table 32.4*). (Mx, M, methotrexate; FA, folinic acid; Ac, actinomycin D; Hu, hydroxyurea; Mp, 6-mercaptopurine; Ep, etoposide.)

one overnight stay per two weeks with the EMA schedule.

High-risk Patients

By definition, high-risk patients can present a range of clinical problems. In our series, this group accounts for 262 (16%) of 1596 patients treated between 1958 and 1994. Clinical experience over many years has indicated that high-risk GTNs will commonly regrow during the intervals between conventional chemotherapy cycles which are spaced at either three- or four-week intervals. The ability to be able to see the tumor regrowth on the basis of a rise in HCG estimation has emphasized the need for a different approach in the treatment of this category of patients. To address this problem, we developed a weekly intensive schedule, the EMA/CO regimen, which we have used in the high-risk category of patients since 1979 (*Figure 32.5*). We reported the first decade of its use in 1991 (Newlands *et al.*, 1991). The schedule is devised to give intensive weekly chemotherapy to minimize the risk of development of drug resistance. The introduction of granulocyte colony stimulating factor (neupogen) reduces the leukopenia, which is commonly the dose-limiting toxicity requiring treatment delay, and can assist in maintaining the relative dose intensity of this schedule. In addition the introduction of the 5HT3 antagonist antiemetics (ondansetron, granisetron and tropisetron) used either alone or with the addition of dexamethasone (Smith *et al.*, 1991) can minimize or eliminate the nausea and vomiting associated with the chemotherapy.

In our analysis (Newlands *et al.*, 1991), there were 76 patients who had received no previous chemotherapy and 62 (82%) of these patients are in remission. However, ten of the 14 deaths occurred within three weeks of the initiation of treatment. These patients died from disease extent involving lung (five patients), brain (three patients) and liver (one patient) and a single patient died of pulmonary embolus. In the patients who were evaluable for response beyond the three weeks cut-off, 62 (94%) of 66 patients are in remission on the EMA/CO schedule. In contrast, 72 patients who had received previous chemotherapy were treated with the EMA/CO schedule and 64 (89%) are in remission. This better survival in patients who had relapsed after previous treatment was due to less extensive disease since these patients were on regular HCG follow-up. The main cause of death in this category of patients was the development of drug resistance. Using the EMA/CO schedule, our overall survival is 85%. The EMA/CO schedule has been widely adopted in other trophoblastic disease centers worldwide.

However, patients who develop resistant disease to the EMA/CO schedule need alternative treatment. The main chemotherapeutic agent not included in

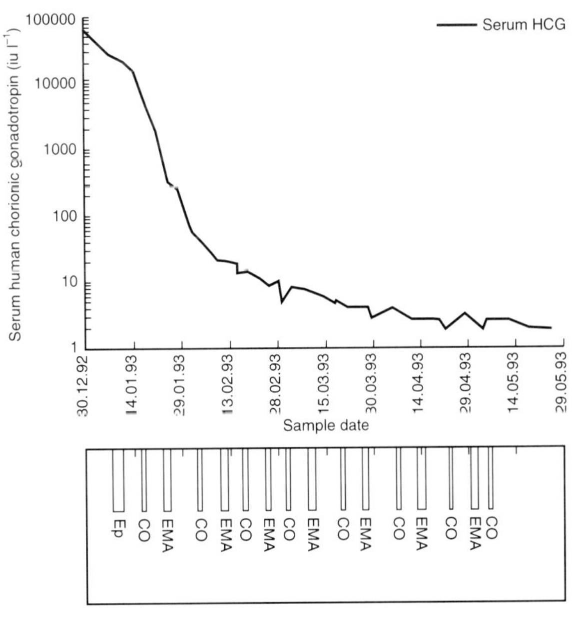

Figure 32.5. Patient with a high-risk gestational trophoblastic neoplasm. (Ep, E, etoposide; C, cyclophosphamide; O, vincristine (Oncovin); M, methotrexate; A, actinomycin D.)

the EMA/CO schedule is cis-platinum. Cis-platinum clearly has significant activity against GTNs (Newlands, 1982). Mainly we have integrated cis-platinum into salvage therapy by combining it in the EP schedule (etoposide 150 mg m^{-2} given together with cis-platinum 75 mg m^{-2}). In most cases we have alternated this with the EMA schedule shown in *Table 32.4*. However, this schedule is fraught with clinical difficulties since it is alternating a nephrotoxic drug, cis-platinum, with a renally excreted drug, methotrexate. Great care needs to be taken in monitoring renal function if major methotrexate toxicity is not going to develop after several cycles. However, by using this approach we have salvaged nine (82%) out of 11 patients who had developed drug resistance to EMA/CO and they did not require surgery (Newlands *et al.*, 1991).

The alternative approach to introducing cis-platinum is surgery to remove the site of drug-resistant disease. Unlike most other aggressive tumors, salvage surgery when combined with additional chemotherapy produces very gratifying results. In the 1979–1991 analysis, salvage surgery was important in inducing the long-term remission of 21 (75%) of 28 patients. However, the site of successful surgery was surprising in that hysterectomy was clinically useful in only two (15%) of 13 patients; thoracotomy was successful in six (43%) of 14 patients; and craniotomy was successful in five (71%) of seven patients. The developments in computerized tomography (CT) and magnetic resonance imaging (MRI) scanning has greatly helped the localization of sites of residual active disease. In addition anti-HCG scanning can be useful in patients where multiple radiologic abnormalities persist and the biologically active focus of disease is difficult to identify (Begent *et al.*, 1987).

Central Nervous System Prophylaxis and Metastases

GTNs are extremely vascular and readily metastasize via the venous system to the lungs, brain, liver and other sites. Potentially brain metastases are a sanctuary site for tumors since the majority of chemotherapeutic agents are water-soluble and poorly penetrate the blood–brain barrier. Identification of cerebral metastases is now much easier with the aid of both CT and MRI scanning. It continues to be our policy to give central nervous system (CNS) prophylaxis in patients with pulmonary metastases, and this consists of intrathecal methotrexate in a dose of 12.5 mg (total dose) either on the same day as the methotrexate dose on the methotrexate and folinic acid schedule or with the CO of the EMA/CO treatment. For prophylaxis we have reduced the number of intrathecal injections, usually to three, as we have become more confident that isolated relapse in the brain is rare.

For patients with established cerebral metastases our policy has been to consider surgery at the outset if the metastasis is isolated and superficial and if surgery is not going to induce a major neurologic deficit. Since these tumors are extremely vascular, the risk of hemorrhage at the initiation of chemotherapy is real. We have modified the EMA/CO schedule to deal with established cerebral metastases by increasing the dose of methotrexate to 1 g m^{-2} given as a 24-hour infusion, followed by folinic acid 15 mg eight-hourly for 72 hours, starting 32 hours after the beginning of the methotrexate infusion. At this dose of methotrexate, renal function needs to be monitored carefully to adjust the dose of folinic acid required. High-dose methotrexate from the systemic circulation is one way of penetrating the relative blood–brain barrier. The other modification of the treatment is to give intrathecal methotrexate 12.5 mg (total dose) with the CO part of the EMA/CO schedule. In patients with established brain disease, both the high-dose systemic methotrexate and the intrathecal methotrexate is continued until the HCG is normal in both the serum and cerebrospinal fluid (CSF). In our last analysis of 23 consecutive patients with established brain disease treated with this schedule, the survival was 15 (65%) (Rustin *et al.*, 1989). The role of CSF monitoring of HCG is still relevant in patients at risk of CNS involvement from a GTN. Normally the serum : CSF ratio should be higher than 65:1. Where this ratio is less than 65:1, patients clearly have a major risk of involvement of the CNS by a GTN. Occasionally the CSF HCG can pick up CNS involvement that is not readily identifiable on either CT or MRI scanning.

The role of radiotherapy in patients with established CNS metastases from a GTN is uncertain. We have not used it in our series and isolated drug-resistant brain disease is rarely the cause of death in these patients. Recently one patient with a deep isolated, but small, recurrence in the optic radiation was treated with a combination of the EMA/CO schedule adjusted for CNS disease and a single fraction of stereotactic radiotherapy to the metastasis. This patient remains in remission two years after completing treatment and this approach needs to be assessed in other patients with comparable localized deep CNS disease.

Reasons for Treatment Failure and Potential New Approaches

There are several reasons why treatment failure can occur in patients with a GTN. Failure to register a patient at risk of developing a GTN following an

HM can allow the development of advanced disease with drug-resistant tumor a long time after the initial pregnancy. The registration scheme in the UK minimizes this problem. Failure to stratify patients by prognostic factors can result in initial treatment failure and the induction of drug resistance. An obscure obstetric history can fail to raise the suspicion of the presence of a GTN, resulting in patients presenting with organ failure at the time of initiating chemotherapy so that patients die from cerebral, pulmonary and other fatal events before adequate treatment can be given (Newlands *et al.*, 1991). Individual very large tumor masses are probably best excised surgically at the end of chemotherapy in case a focus of viable tumor remains within the mass.

Placental site trophoblastic tumors (PSTT) present a particular management problem. These are predominantly cytotrophoblastic tumors and can occur after either an HM or a full-term pregnancy (Fisher *et al.*, 1992). PSSTs tend to be locally infiltrating, but can metastasize both through the lymphatic system and to the lungs. When localized to the uterus, the treatment of choice is surgery. While some PSTTs can respond well to intensive chemotherapy such as the EMA/CO schedule, drug resistance can occur quite rapidly and unfortunately several patients with advanced disease died from their tumor (Dessau *et al.*, 1990). Clearly the development of different chemotherapy for this rare variant of GTN is required.

Since the survival in patients with GTN is already extremely good, few patients are entered on experimental protocols. Some tumors that are resistant to conventional-dose chemotherapy respond well to high-dose chemotherapy with autologous bone marrow transplantation. At present few patients have been treated with this approach and while it needs to be studied in more patients, the initial results are not very encouraging. However, a range of new therapeutic agents have entered or are entering the clinic and these will need to be assessed in patients with drug-resistant disease. They include the taxanes, taxol and taxotere; the camptothecans, topotecan and irinatecan; temozolomide; and the thymidylate synthetase inhibitor, tomudex.

Follow-up and Subsequent Fertility

After completing their chemotherapy for their GTN, patients are followed by serial HCG estimations (*Table 32.5*). If there is a clinical abnormality that needs to be rechecked, our policy is to see the patients for one follow-up appointment six weeks after completing treatment. Apart from this single clinical check-up, the follow-up is initially on serum and urine HCG estimations and finally on urine estimations alone. Our policy is to continue follow-up for life on patients who have received chemotherapy, which allows us to reassure them that their disease is in remission and to confirm that there are few, if any, late sequelae from their chemotherapy.

Our policy is to advise patients not to become pregnant for 12 months after completing chemotherapy:

- to confirm that their tumor has been eliminated with a high degree of probability;
- to minimize the potential teratogenicity of the chemotherapy.

The post-chemotherapy fertility from five different centers has recently been summarized (Berkowitz *et al.*, 1994); 77.5% of the patients had live births and only 2% had fetal abnormalities. These figures indicate that patients can be reassured that their fertility is not normally going to be impaired by even quite intensive chemotherapy. Intensive chemotherapy in patients approaching the menopause may induce sufficient ovarian suppression to result in an early menopause.

Second Tumor Incidence

We have previously reported our results (Rustin *et al.*, 1983) showing no increase in second tumors after chemotherapy in patients with GTN. We are currently re-analysing the whole series to 1990. There are four patients who have developed acute myeloid leukemia (AML) and one patient developed chronic myeloid leukemia (CML). Three of these patients received intensive chemotherapy, one on relapse after previous chemotherapy and two on the EMA/CO schedule as their initial treatment. The two other patients (one with AML, one with CML) were treated on the medium-risk schedule (see *Table 32.4*). We think that the four patients probably developed

Table 32.5. Follow-up for gestational trophoblastic neoplasm patients who have received chemotherapy.

Time after treatment	*Human chorionic gonadotropin estimations*
Year 1	Weekly SERUM and URINE for six weeks
	SERUM and URINE every two weeks until six months post-treatment
	URINE ONLY every two weeks until one year post-treatment
Year 2	URINE sample every four weeks
Year 3	URINE sample every eight weeks
Year 4	URINE sample every 12 weeks
Year 5	URINE sample every 16 weeks
Subsequently every six months INDEFINITELY	

AML from their intensive chemotherapy, in particular etoposide, which is known to be one of the agents that can initiate AML (Smith *et al.*, 1993b). We have analysed the second tumor incidence with age-matched controls and the relative risks of developing a second tumor were: myeloid leukemia (16.6:1; p=0.0005); colon carcinoma (4.5:1; p=0.005); melanoma 3.4:1; p=0.031); a late increase (>25 years) in breast carcinoma (5.7:1; p=0.016). There was no increase in carcinoma of the lung or cervix, or non-melanoma of the skin. While the increase in myeloid leukemia is likely to be therapy related, it is possible that the increase in incidence of the other tumors may reflect a constitutional predisposition to cancer in patients who develop GTN. It is clear that we need to develop better and less toxic chemotherapeutic agents in the future.

Conclusion

We have recently analyzed the whole Charing Cross series of patients treated from 1958 up to 1992 (*Figure 32.6*). The initial cohort of patients treated during the development of effective chemotherapy for GTN produced a survival that was already quite good, with chemotherapy primarily based on methotrexate, actinomycin D, cyclophosphamide and vincristine. The cohort between 1974 and 1979 was stratified by the prognostic factors introduced in 1974 (see *Table 32.3*). Clearly the more systematic management of these patients resulted in a further improvement in survival. In the late 1970s and 1980s the introduction of etoposide and cis-platinum (Newlands, 1982) and the introduction of CT and MRI scanning have resulted in a further improvement in survival so that for patients treated between 1979 and 1992 the survival was 94% in 994 patients, with a maximum follow-up of 15 years.

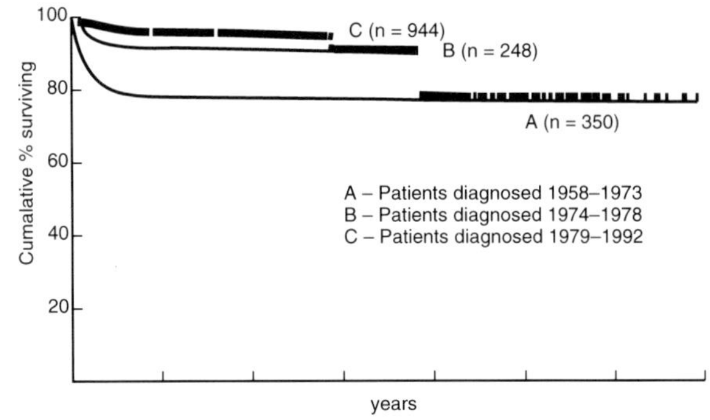

Figure 32.6. Cumulative percentage survival of all patients with gestational trophoblastic disease treated at Charing Cross Hospital from 1958 up to 1992.

Summary of Management Options

- Patients at risk of developing a gestational trophoblastic neoplasm (GTN) (those with hydatidiform mole and partial hydatidiform mole) should be registered for regular human chorionic gonadotropin (HCG) follow-up so as to identify those who will need further treatment.
- Awareness of a potential GTN in a patient of childbearing age with evidence of malignancy should be considered, and physicians and gynecologists should have a low threshold for obtaining a quantitative HCG where the diagnosis is not clearcut.
- Patients with GTN form a heterogeneous group and their treatement should be stratified according to recognized prognostic variables.
- Treatment of these patients should be in Trophoblastic Disease Centers where patients are managed by staff with experience of this rare, but very treatable, tumor.
- Trophoblastic Disease Centers need to integrate the full range of currently available therapy and imaging technology to optimize their patients' treatment and to systematically develop new and better chemotherapeutic agents, which hopefully will have a better long-term toxicity profile than the agents currently in the clinic.

References

Bagshawe KD (1976) Risk and prognostic factors in trophoblastic neoplasia. *Cancer* **38:** 1373–1385.

■ Bagshawe KD, Dent J & Webb J (1986) Occasional survey: hydatidiform mole in England and Wales 1973–83. *Lancet* **ii:** 673–677.

■ Bagshawe KD, Dent J, Newlands ES *et al.* (1989) The role of low dose methotrexate and folinic acid in gestational trophoblastic tumours (GTT). *Br. J. Obstet. Gynaecol.* **96:** 795–802.

Begent RHJ, Bagshawe KD, Green AJ *et al.* (1987) The clinical value of imaging with antibody to human chorionic gonadotrophin in the detection of residual choriocarcinoma. *Br. J. Cancer* **55:** 657–660.

■ Berkowitz RS, Bernstein MR, Laborde O *et al.* (1994) Subsequent pregnancy experiences in patients with gestational trophoblastic disease. *J. Reprod. Med.* **39:** 228–232.

Dessau R, Rustin GJS, Dent J *et al.* (1990) Surgery and chemotherapy in the management of placental site tumour. *Gynecol. Oncol.* **339:** 56–59.

Fisher RA, Paradinas FJ, Newlands ES *et al.* (1992) Genetic evidence that placental site trophoblastic tumours can originate from a hydatidiform mole or a normal conceptus. *Br. J. Cancer* **65:** 355–358.

Newlands ES (1982) New chemotherapeutic agents in the management of gestational trophoblastic disease. *Semin. Oncol.* **9:** 239–243.

Newlands ES (1991) Gestational trophoblastic tumors. In: Blackledge GRP, Jordan JA & Shingleton HM (eds) *Textbook of Gynecologic Oncology,* pp. 464–473.

■ Newlands ES, Bagshawe KD, Begent RHJ *et al.* (1986) Developments in chemotherapy for medium and high risk patients with gestational trophoblastic tumours (1974–84). *Br. J. Obstet. Gynaecol.* **93:** 63–69.

■ Newlands ES, Bagshawe KD, Begent RHJ *et al.* (1991) Results with the EMA/CO (etoposide, methotrexate, actinomycin D, cyclophosphamide, vincristine) regime in high risk gestational trophoblastic tumours, 1979 to 1989. *Br. J. Obstet. Gynaecol.* **98:** 550–557.

Paradinas FJ (1994) The histological diagnosis of hydatidiform moles. *Curr. Diagn. Pathol.* **1:** 24–31.

Rustin GJS, Rustin F, Dent J *et al.* (1983) No increase in second tumours after cytotoxic chemotherapy for gestational trophoblastic tumours. *New Eng. J. Medicine* **308:** 473–476.

Rustin GJS, Newlands ES, Begent RHJ *et al.* (1989) Weekly alternating etoposide, methotrexate and actinomycin/vincristine and cyclophosphamide chemotherapy for the treatment of CNS metastases of choriocarcinoma. *J. Clin. Oncology* **7:** 7, 900–903.

Smith DB, Newlands ES, Rustin GJS *et al.* (1991) Comparison of ondansetron and ondansetron plus dexamethasone as antiemetic prophylaxis during cisplatin-containing chemotherapy. *Lancet* **338:** 487–490.

Smith DB, Newlands ES & Bagshawe ES (1993a) Correlation between clinical staging (FIGO) and prognostic groups with gestational trophoblastic disease. *Br. J. Obstet. Gynaecol.* **100:** 157–160.

Smith MA, Rubinstein L, Cazenave L *et al.* (1993b) Report of the Cancer Therapy Evaluation Program Monitoring Plan for Secondary Acute Myeloid Leukaemia following Treatment with Epipodophyllotoxins. *J. Natl. Cancer Inst.* **85:** 7, 558–553.

33 Screening for Common Cancers in Women

J R van Nagell Jr
P D DePriest

Introduction

The value of early detection of most malignancies affecting women has been clearly established. Generally, early stage cancers are curable by surgery alone, whereas more advanced lesions often persist despite combined therapy. In order to determine the efficacy of screening in a particular disease, it is important to understand:

- the definition of screening;
- the characteristics of diseases that benefit from screening.

Screening can be defined as the testing of apparently healthy volunteers from the population in order to separate them into groups with high and low probabilities for a given disease (Prorok, 1984). Since there is an implicit promise that those who volunteer to be screened will benefit from screening, it is essential that screening programs are not undertaken unless certain guidelines are met.

For screening to be effective, a disease should:

- be a major cause of mortality or morbidity in the screened population;
- have a reasonably high prevalence in the screened population;
- have a preclinical phase during which screening can detect the disease while it is still curable;
- be amenable to therapy such that the survival rate of patients with early stage disease is significantly higher than that of patients with advanced disease.

An optimal screening test should be safe, time-efficient, easy to apply and acceptable to the patients being screened. It should also have a high sensitivity, specificity, positive predictive value and negative predictive value (*Table 33.1*). When applied to a population, an effective cancer screening test should produce:

- a decrease in stage at detection;
- a decrease in case-specific mortality;
- a decrease in the site-specific mortality from the disease in the screened population (Hulka, 1988).

If all these criteria are met, the test should be cost-effective so that its use will decrease the overall health care costs of those receiving screening.

Cervical Cancer

Cervical cancer is the prototype of a disease that has been controlled by screening. In the countries of the developing world where cervical cytologic screening is often unavailable, cervical cancer remains the leading cause of cancer mortality. This year, it is estimated that there will be 340,000 new cases of invasive cervical cancer in developing countries and that 160,000 women will die of disease. The exact prevalence rates of cervical intraepithelial neoplasia (CIN) in the USA are unknown. However, a survey by the American College Health Association, the parent organization for college-based health clinics, reported a prevalence rate of abnormal cervical cytology of 4–15% (Richart and Wright, 1993). In the USA this year, 600,000 new cases of CIN will be detected, and 15,000 women will be diagnosed with invasive cervical cancer. The incidence rates of carcinoma *in situ* and invasive cervical cancer for women aged 25–35 years in this country are 130/100,000 and 20/100,000, respectively (Cramer, 1993). Although CIN is viewed as a biologic precursor of invasive cancer, the duration of the preclinical phase in cervical cancer may vary widely from months to years depending upon a number of factors including the biologic aggressiveness of the tumor and the immune status of the host. Cervical cytologic screening is highly accurate in detecting CIN, and most patients can be treated by

Table 33.1. Statistical definitions in cancer screening.

Term	*Screen*	*Findings*
True positive (TP)	Positive	Cancer
True negative (TN)	Negative	No cancer
False positive (FP)	Positive	No cancer
False negative (FN)	Negative	Cancer

Sensitivity = TP/(TP + FN)
Specificity = TN/(TN + FP)
Positive predictive value = TP/(TP + FP)
Negative predictive value = TN/(TN + FN)
Accuracy = TP + TN/(TP + FP + TN + FN)

conservative measures. Since the cure rate of CIN is extremely high, very few adequately screened patients experience progression of their disease to invasive cancer.

Cervical cytology fulfills the prerequisites of an effective screening test. A Papanicolaou (Pap) smear is well-accepted by patients, takes very little time to perform; and is cost-effective. A properly obtained cytology specimen includes both exocervical cells obtained by scraping the cervix with an Ayre spatula and cells from the endocervical canal. A widely accepted technique that enhances the collection of endocervical cells is the use of an endocervical brush (Cytobrush). The use of the Cytobrush has been shown to increase retrieval of cells from the squamo–columnar junction from 88% to 98% (Taylor *et al.*, 1987). The cytology specimen is applied immediately to a glass slide and placed in fixative (*Figure 33.1*).

The accuracy of a Pap smear in predicting cervical neoplasia varies according to the experience of the clinician who is taking it, and the expertise of the cytotechnologist who is interpreting it. Sedlis *et al.* (1974) simultaneously obtained paired Pap smear on

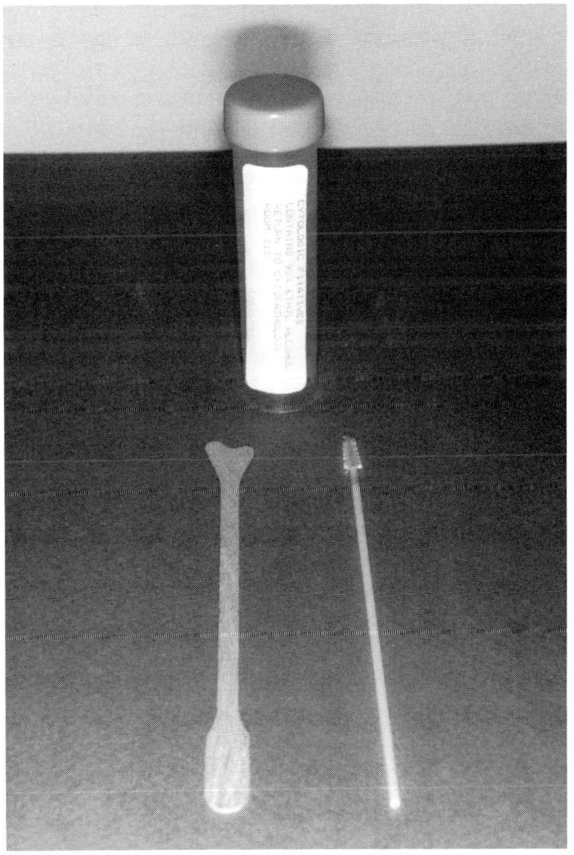

Figure 33.1. Materials for cervical cytology. Ayre spatula for exocervical sampling; Cytobrush for endocervical sampling; and fixative with slide in place.

17,737 patients. They found a sampling error of 9.3% (dysplasia confirmed on only one of the paired Pap smears), and a laboratory interpretive error of 0.06% (one of the paired slides erroneously read as negative). The authors reported that cervical cytology had an overall sensitivity of 90.6% in this study. Recently, Koss (1993) reported the results of a prospective targeted rescreening study at a large New York cytopathology laboratory. Over a three-year period from 1989–1991, 43,121 smears were screened and reported as negative by the cytotechnologist. A total of 10,374 (24%) of these negative smears were rescreened by a cytopathologist. Of these, 1693 smears were found to contain neoplastic changes missed by the first screener for an average false negative primary screening rate of 3.9%. In a follow-up study, a retrospective review of previously negative smears in women returning with an abnormal smear was undertaken for the first two years of the study period (1989 and 1990). An additional 20 false negative smears were found due to interpretive error. This increased the average false negative rate to 5%, with annual false negative rates of 4.4% for 1989, 5.5% for 1990, and 5.1% for 1991.

Women at high risk for cervical cancer include those less than 18 years of age at the time of first coitus, those with multiple sexual partners, and those with a documented human papillomavirus (HPV) infection. Annual Pap smear screening should be initiated at the age of first intercourse or routinely after the age of 18 years. Annual screening should be continued throughout life, although a woman's physician may recommend less frequent screening in patients who have undergone hysterectomy for benign disease. Patients with abnormal Pap smears should be contacted immediately and evaluated by colposcopy and directed biopsies. It should be noted that the false negative rate of cervical cytology in the presence of clinically apparent invasive cervical cancer may be as high as 20% (Gay *et al.*, 1985). For this reason, any visible cervical lesion should be biopsied at the time of clinical examination even if the Pap smear has been reported to be normal.

The effect of annual Pap smear screening on cervical cancer mortality has been most significant. Specifically, with the introduction of cervical cytologic screening in British Columbia, the mortality rate from cervical cancer fell from 13.5/100,000 in 1958 to 11.7/100,000 in 1966 to 5.8/10,000 in 1974 (Boyes *et al.*, 1977). In the USA, the widespread use of Pap smear screening has resulted in a 70% decline in the age-adjusted cancer death rate for cervical cancer during the last 30 years (White, 1993). As a result of cervical cytologic screening, over 97% of patients with cervical neoplasia are detected and treated before invasion has occurred, and are cured with minimal cost and discomfort to the patient. Most importantly, only 4400 women will die of cervical cancer in the USA this year (Boring *et al.*, 1994).

Endometrial Cancer

Endometrial cancer does not meet the criteria of a disease that should benefit significantly from screening. The prevalence of endometrial cancer is not high in the general population. Also, endometrial cancer causes abnormal uterine bleeding early in the disease process. As a result, over three-fourths of women with endometrial cancer present initially with Stage I disease. Since Stage I endometrial cancer is highly curable, only about 3000 women will die from endometrial cancer in the USA this year (Boring *et al.*, 1994).

Nevertheless, there are certain women who have a high risk for endometrial cancer in whom screening should be considered. The frequency of endometrial adenocarcinoma is related directly to obesity, and women who are overweight are at risk of developing this disease (Porazzini *et al.*, 1991). Henderson *et al.* (1988), for example, reported that women weighing 190 lbs and over had a relative risk for endometrial cancer of 17.7 compared to women weighing 130 lbs or under. For this reason, some authors advocate annual endometrial sampling in this high-risk population even in the absence of symptoms.

Endometrial sampling is optimally performed with a Pipelle biopsy (*Figure 33.2*). This screening method can be performed on an outpatient basis, and is well accepted by patients. Most importantly, the results of Pipelle biopsy correlate closely with those obtained by formal curettage of the uterus. Goldschmidt *et al.* (1993), for example, noted that Pipelle histology agreed with that obtained by curettage in 90% of cases sampled. Pipelle aspiration was even more accurate when used in patients with an endometrial thickness of at least 5 mm as determined by vaginal sonography. No cases of endometrial cancer were missed using this technique.

A second population at high risk for endometrial cancer is postmenopausal women with confirmed endometrial cells on Pap smear. Less than 1% of postmenopausal women will have this finding, but the presence of endometrial cells on a cytologic specimen is very suggestive of a histologic abnormality in the endometrium. Yancy *et al.* (1990) reported that 5% of asymptomatic postmenopausal women with typical endometrial cells on Pap smear had endometrial hyperplasia or cancer. In postmenopausal women with atypical endometrial cells on Pap smear, 22% had endometrial adenocarcinoma. For this reason, women with typical or atypical endometrial cells on Pap smear should undergo screening with Pipelle endometrial biopsies.

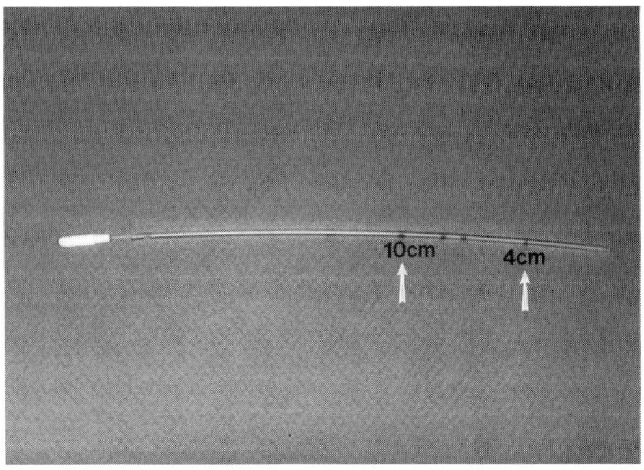

Figure 33.2. Pipelle for endometrial sampling. Marks are placed at 4 cm and 10 cm depths (note the arrows).

Women with histologically confirmed adenomatous hyperplasia who are being treated medically should also undergo screening with endometrial sampling. Although the frequency of co-existing endometrial cancer in patients with simple or complex endometrial hyperplasia without atypia is low, periodic endometrial sampling every six months is indicated to ensure that progression to atypical hyperplasia or adenocarcinoma has not occurred.

Finally, there is an increased risk for endometrial cancer in women taking tamoxifen. Patients with breast cancer also have a higher risk for developing endometrial carcinoma. Adami *et al.* (1987) evaluated 60,063 women with primary breast cancer and found that 260 of these patients also developed endometrial neoplasia. This reflected a calculated relative risk ratio of 1.7. Other authors have found that tamoxifen therapy in patients with breast carcinoma predisposes a woman to endometrial hyperplasia and cancer (Mathew *et al.*, 1990; Neven and DeMuyleder, 1990; Gal *et al.*, 1991). For these reasons, endometrial sampling should be performed every 6–12 months in breast cancer patients who are taking tamoxifen.

Ovarian Cancer

Ovarian cancer fulfills the criteria of a disease that should be amenable to screening. First, it is a major cause of mortality and morbidity. It is estimated that there will be over 24,000 new cases of ovarian cancer in the USA this year, and that 13,000 women will die of disease (Boring *et al.*, 1994). Ovarian cancer now ranks as the fourth leading cause of cancer death among women in this country. Although ovarian cancer is not prevalent in the general population, it is more common in women over the age of 50 years and in those with a family history of the disease. The prevalence of ovarian cancer in women over the age of 50 years is approximately 50/100,000, and increases to 390/100,000 in women with a documented first- or second-degree relative with the disease (Bourne *et al.*, 1991).

The existence and duration of a preclinical phase in ovarian cancer has not been fully defined. However, there is increasing circumstantial evidence to suggest that a preclinical phase does exist in ovarian cancer. Puls *et al.* (1992) examined histologic material from 96 serous and mucinous ovarian cystadenocarcinomas. They observed benign epithelium adjacent to malignant epithelium in 79% of cases. The precise area of histologic transition from benign to malignant epithelium was identified in 40% of patients without taking additional sections of the ovarian tumors. The site of histologic transition from benign to malignant epithelium has also been confirmed in serous ovarian tumors using scanning electron microscopy (Stenback, 1981). Also, Bourne *et al.* (1991) reported that there was a significant increase in the frequency of benign epithelial ovarian tumors in women with a confirmed family history of ovarian cancer. These authors concluded that their data were consistent with the hypothesis that certain benign or borderline ovarian neoplasms undergo malignant transformation. Studies are in progress to determine if there are molecular genetic changes present in selected benign or borderline epithelial ovarian tumors that would predispose them to malignant change. If these tumors could be detected by a screening test and removed surgically, the subsequent occurrence of ovarian cancer in the screened population would be reduced.

Finally, there is little doubt that early-stage ovarian cancer is significantly more curable than the late-stage disease. The reported five-year survival rates of patients with Stage I ovarian cancer treated with surgery and platinum-based chemotherapy is approximately 90% (Young *et al.*, 1990). In contrast, the survival rate of patients with Stages III or IV ovarian cancer is only 10–15% despite aggressive tumor debulking and appropriate combination chemotherapy.

The two methods of ovarian cancer screening that have been evaluated most extensively are serum CA-125 and transvaginal sonography (TVS). CA-125 is an antigenic determinant on a high molecular weight glycoprotein that is recognized by a monoclonal antibody, OC-125 (Bast *et al.*, 1983). CA-125 is expressed by epithelial ovarian malignancies and is present in highest concentrations on the surface of tumor cells (Kabawat *et al.*, 1983). Although this antigen is elevated (>35 u/ml) in the sera of 80% of ovarian cancer patients, it is abnormal in approximately only one-third of women with Stage I disease (Bourne *et al.*, 1994). In addition, CA-125 is elevated in the sera of patients with a number of benign gynecologic conditions such as endometriosis, pelvic inflammatory disease and benign ovarian tumors. The lack of sensitivity of CA-125 in patients with early-stage disease has severely limited its effectiveness as a screening method for ovarian cancer. When CA-125 was used as the initial screening method, early-stage ovarian cancers were missed and the stage at detection was not significantly decreased.

The TVS is performed using a standard ultrasound unit with a 5.0 Mhz vaginal transducer (*Figure 33.3*). The test is painless and is best performed with an empty bladder. It takes approximately five minutes to complete, and a permanent hard copy of each sonogram is generated for inclusion in the patient record. Each ovary is measured in three dimensions, and ovarian volume is calculated using the prolate ellipsoid formula ($L \times H \times W \times 0.523$). An ovarian volume of 20 cm^3 or more in premenopausal women and 10 cm^3 or more in postmenopausal women is considered abnormal (van Nagell *et al.*, 1990). These values are two standard deviations above the published values for normal ovarian volumes in premenopausal and postmenopausal women. In addition, any papillary projection from the tumor wall is considered abnormal. In the University of Kentucky Ovarian Cancer Screening Project, women with an abnormal screen are asked to have a repeat sonogram in 4–6 weeks. If the repeat sonogram is abnormal, the patient undergoes Doppler assessment of tumor blood flow, a serum CA-125 determination, and morphologic indexing of the tumor. The patient then undergoes operative removal of the ovarian tumor by laparoscopy or laparotomy (DePriest *et al.*, 1993). If the screen is normal, as evidenced by normal

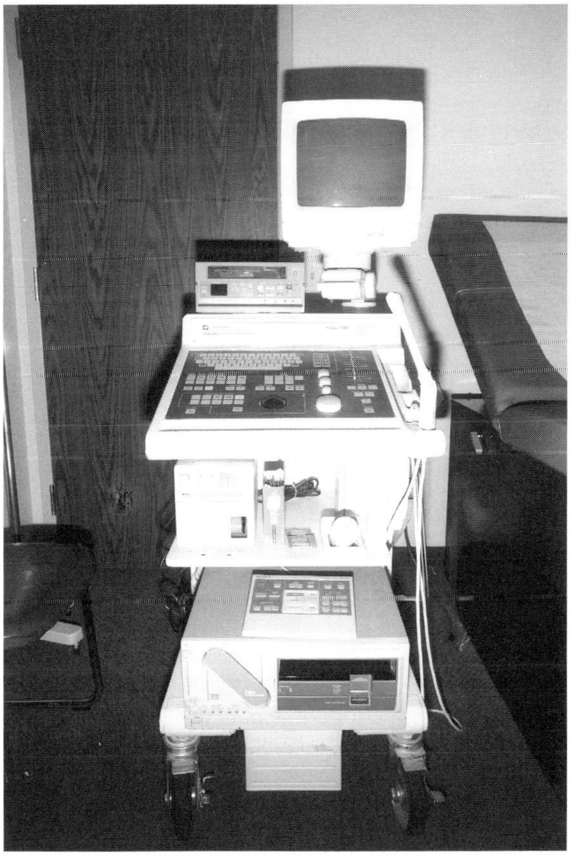

Figure 33.3. Ultrasound machine with vaginal transducer used for ovarian cancer screening.

ovarian volume and morphology, the patient is asked to return for a repeat screen in one year.

There are two populations of women in which ovarian cancer screening has been evaluated. The first is postmenopausal women over the age of 50 years. Since physiologic variation in ovarian volume occurs before the menopause, TVS has been shown to be most effective in postmenopausal women. Also, the prevalence of ovarian cancer is highest in women over the age of 50. In the University of Kentucky Screening Project, approximately 5000 asymptomatic postmenopausal women have been screened using the aforementioned protocol. Five ovarian cancers have been detected: 4 Stage IA, and 1 Stage IIIB. All patients with Stage I ovarian cancer had normal pelvic examinations and normal serum CA-125 values. These patients are all alive with no evidence of disease 1–5 years after conventional treatment. At present, there have been approximately 20,000 screening years of follow-up, and there have been no ovarian cancer deaths in the screened population. The second population in which ovarian cancer screening has been evaluated is in women of 30 years of age and over in whom there is a documented history of ovarian cancer in a primary or secondary relative. Bourne *et al.* (1991) screened 776 such patients with TVS and detected three primary ovarian cancers. All patients had Stage I tumors and are presently cured of disease. The prevalence of ovarian cancer in this population was 390/100,000 or approximately nine-fold higher than that in the general population.

Although sonographic screening has been extremely sensitive in detecting ovarian cancer, its specificity and positive predictive value have only been moderate. The reported specificity of TVS screening is 0.987, and its positive predictive value is 0.07 (van Nagell *et al.*, 1991). As a result, approximately ten patients with ovarian tumors are operated upon in order to detect one ovarian cancer. In an effort to increase the positive predictive value of TVS, DePriest *et al.* (1993) developed a morphology index based upon sonographic findings in ovarian tumors. The morphology index was constructed using three basic categories – tumor volume, wall structure and septal structure. A point scale (0–4) was developed within each category according to specific criteria (*Figure 33.4*) with the total points per evaluation varying from 0–12. Using this morphology index 121 ovarian tumors were evaluated before surgical removal; 80 had a morphology index score less than five and all were benign. In postmenopausal patients, a morphology index value of five and over had a positive predictive value for ovarian malignancy of 0.47. All ovarian malignancies had significant abnormalities in wall structure and had total volumes in excess of 10 cm^3.

Doppler flow sonography has also been proposed as an adjunctive method to differentiate between benign and malignant ovarian tumors. This method is based on the observation that the walls of blood vessels within ovarian malignancies have a reduced medial thickness and therefore a lower resistance to flow than vessels supplying benign ovarian tumors. Transvaginal color Doppler can be used to study blood flow patterns within ovarian vessels, and resistance to flow can be quantitated. Using this technology, Weiner *et al.* (1992) studied the blood flow patterns of 53 ovarian tumors before laparotomy. These investigators reported that there was a low impedance to flow (pulsatility index <1.0) in 16 of 17 malignant ovarian tumors. In contrast, the pulsatility index was higher than 1.0 in 35 of 36 benign ovarian tumors. Unfortunately, not all ovarian tumors have evaluable blood flow, and there are still insufficient data concerning the blood flow characteristics of small early-stage ovarian cancers.

To date, TVS screening has produced a decrease in stage at detection and a decrease in case-specific ovarian cancer mortality. Approximately 13,000 women have been screened and 15 ovarian cancers have been detected. The stage distribution of these tumors is as follows: Stage IA, 12; Stage IIA, 1; and Stage IIIB, 2. These patients are all alive and well after conventional therapy. At present, the case-

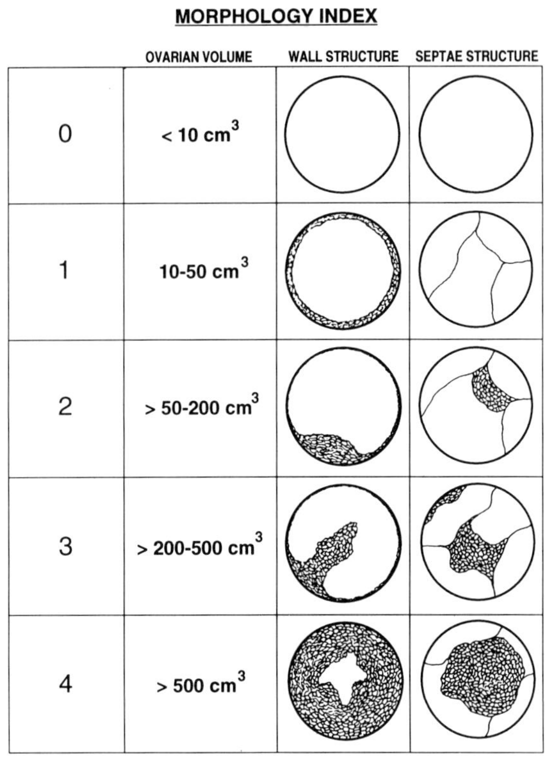

Figure 33.4. Morphology index used in association with transvaginal sonography as a screening method for ovarian cancer (reprinted with permission from DePriest *et al.* (1993) *Gynecol. Oncol.* **51:** 7–11).

specific mortality rate for ovarian cancers detected by screening is 0%.

A multi-institutional trial enrolling a large number of patients is required to determine if ovarian cancer screening will produce a significant reduction in site-specific ovarian cancer mortality in the screened population. Until such a trial is complete, ovarian cancer screening should be provided at no cost to the patient as part of well-designed clinical investigations.

Breast Cancer

Breast cancer is the most common cancer in women in this country. Approximately 183,000 new cases of breast cancer will be detected in 1995 in the USA, and 46,000 women will die of the disease (Boring *et al.*, 1994). As such, breast cancer ranks as the second leading cause of cancer death in American women. Breast cancer incidence rates have increased approximately 2% per year from 84/100,000 in 1980 to 108/100,000 in 1994 (Boring *et al.*, 1994). The five-year survival of patients with localized breast cancer is 93% compared to only 18% in patients with advanced disease. As a result, breast cancer is a disease that should benefit from early detection through screening.

The two screening methods that have proven effective in the detection of breast cancer are clinical examination and mammography. Clinical examination is relatively inexpensive and may detect cancers that are not evident on mammography. In 1988, consensus guidelines for breast cancer screening were developed by the American Cancer Society, the National Cancer Institute and ten other medical organizations (Dodd, 1992). It was recommended that annual clinical examination of the breast be performed beginning at 40 years of age. Although the efficacy of breast self-examination has not been demonstrated by a prospective randomized trial, it is generally acknowledged that the majority of clinically-detectable breast cancers are diagnosed by the patient herself. For this reason, most physicians recommend breast self-examination at monthly intervals beginning as early as 20 years of age.

The most effective screening method for detecting early-stage breast cancer is mammography. The mean radiation glandular dose for a two-view per breast grid study using a modern mammographic unit is approximately 2.5 mGy (Feig and Hendrick, 1993). Using this dose, the risk of mammographic radiation actually causing breast cancer is negligible (five excess cancers per one million women aged 45 years or over receiving yearly mammograms). There are now sound scientific data to suggest that breast cancer screening reduces the number of deaths from breast cancer. The Health Insurance Plan (HIP) of Greater New York initiated a randomized controlled trial in 1963 to evaluate the effect of annual mammographic screening on breast cancer mortality. The data from this trial demonstrated a reduction in breast cancer mortality of 40% in women over 50 years of age who received annual mammographic screening compared to those who did not have mammography (Thier and Loeb, 1978). More recently, analysis of data from randomized trials in 282,717 Swedish women followed 5–13 years demonstrated a 24% reduction in breast cancer mortality in women in the screening arm versus those in the control arm (Nystrom *et al.*, 1993). The largest reduction in breast cancer mortality occurred in women of 50–69 years of age at the time of randomization.

The American Cancer Society recommends that asymptomatic women of 40–49 years of age have a screening mammogram at 1–2-year intervals. A mammogram should be performed annually in women of 50 years of age and over (*Table 33.2*). Women with symptoms suggestive of breast cancer should consult their personal physician for recommendations concerning the optimal frequency of mammography.

Colorectal Cancer

Colorectal carcinoma is the second most common cancer in American women and is the third leading cause of cancer death in the USA population. In the USA, over 74,000 new cases of colorectal cancer will be detected in women during the present year, and over 28,000 women will die of the disease (Boring *et al.*, 1994). Symptoms of colon cancer include rectal bleeding, blood in the stool, and a change in bowel habits. Recent evidence would suggest that there is a stepwise evolution from normal epithelium to hyperprolific epithelium, to adenomatous polyps and finally to invasive cancer (Fearon and Vogelstein, 1990). The majority of adenomatous polyps are detectable endoscopically, and can be removed before neoplastic transformation. In addition, the five-year survival of localized colon cancer is 92% as opposed to only 7% when there are distant metastases. For this reason, there has been increased interest in the screening of high-risk populations for colorectal carcinoma.

Table 33.2. American Cancer Society recommendations for breast cancer screening in asymptomatic women.

Age (yrs)	*Screening test*
40	Baseline mammogram
40–49	Annual clinical examination
	Screening mammogram every 1–2 yrs
$\geqslant$50	Annual clinical examination
	Annual screening mammogram

Table 33.3. American Cancer Society recommendations for colorectal cancer screening.

Age (yrs)	*Screening test*
>39	Annual digital rectal examination
⩾50	Annual stool guaiac
⩾50	Sigmoidoscopy every 3–5 years

Digital rectal examination, occult blood testing and sigmoidoscopy have all been evaluated as screening methods for colorectal carcinoma. Data concerning the efficacy of these methods as screening tests for colorectal carcinoma are limited. However, in a controlled screening trial conducted by the Kaiser Foundation, a group of 5000 patients were offered annual digital rectal examination, occult blood testing and sigmoidoscopy. A similar control group was followed without these tests (Dales *et al.*, 1979). During 11 years of follow-up, the screened group experienced a statistically significant ($p<0.005$) reduction in death rate (1.0 per 1000 versus 3.3 per 1000) from colorectal cancer (Friedman *et al.*, 1986). In an additional study, 21,000 subjects in Minnesota underwent an annual physical examination that included sigmoidoscopy. Any polyps detected by sigmoidoscopy were then removed. The number of colon cancers detected in the screened population was only 15% of the number of expected cases, and all were localized. No cancer deaths occurred in the screened population (Gilbertsen, 1974). These data suggest that sigmoidoscopy is effective in detecting colonic polyps, which can then be removed before malignant transformation occurs.

The efficacy of the occult blood test as a means of detecting colon cancer has been evaluated in a number of studies. A stool sample is obtained by the patient or by a physician at the time of a digital rectal examination. This sample is then tested for the presence of occult blood. In a randomized trial conducted in the UK, approximately 10,000 individuals received periodic testing for occult blood in the stool. They were compared to a similar group of patients who were not screened: 13 colon cancers were detected in the screened group, nine of which were Duke's A and two Duke's B, whereas ten colon cancers were diagnosed in the control group, but only four were Duke's B and the remainder were more advanced (Hardcastle *et al.*, 1983). Similar results were reported in another randomized trial performed at the University of Minnesota. Approximately 16,000 persons received annual screening for occult blood in the stool. An equal number of persons received biennial screening, and a third group received no screening at all. Preliminary data from this trial indicate a trend toward earlier stage at detection in the two screening arms of the study (Gilbertsen *et al.*, 1980). Despite these data, the specificity of testing for occult blood in the stool is not high and several recent reviews have indicated the need for additional testing (Simon, 1985). The American Cancer Society and the NCI have recommended an annual digital rectal examination over the age of 39 years, an annual stool guaiac test beginning at the age of 50 years, and sigmoidoscopy every 3–5 years beginning at the age of 50 years (*Table 33.3*).

Lung Cancer

Lung cancer is now the leading cause of cancer deaths in American women. During 1995, over 62,000 new cases of lung cancer will be diagnosed in females in the USA, and over 59,000 will die of the disease (Boring *et al.*, 1994). Unfortunately, early lung cancer produces no symptoms, and there is very little evidence to suggest that screening has any effect on mortality. Both chest radiography and sputum cytology as screening methods for lung cancer have been evaluated in randomized trials. The combination of annual chest radiography and sputum cytology was evaluated both at the Johns Hopkins University Hospital (Levin *et al.*, 1982) and the Memorial Sloan–Kettering Cancer Center (Melamed *et al.*, 1981). At these two institutions, patients in the study group received annual chest radiography and sputum cytology every four months, whereas those in the control group had only an annual chest radiograph. Screening with chest radiography and sputum cytology was shown to produce a decrease in stage at detection. However, there was no effect of screening on lung cancer mortality (Melamed *et al.*, 1984).

The best way to reduce lung cancer mortality is to avoid the most important risk factor for the disease, cigarette smoking. It has been estimated that cigarette smoking is responsible for 80% of lung cancer deaths in women (Lung Cancer. ACS Cancer Facts & Figures, 1994). Women who smoke cigarettes are 12 times more likely to die from lung cancer than those who have never smoked. Therefore, all women should be cautioned not to smoke and those who do should be encouraged to stop smoking as soon as possible.

Summary of Core Information

- For screening to be effective, a disease should be a major cause of mortality and morbidity in the screened population, have a reasonably high prevalence in the screened population, have a preclinical phase during which screening could detect the disease while it is still curable, and be amenable to therapy such that the survival rate of patients with early stage disease is significantly higher than that of patients with advanced disease.
- An optimal screening test should be safe, time-efficient, easy to apply and acceptable to the patients being screened. It should also be highly sensitive and specific.
- When applied to a population, an effective cancer screening test should produce a decrease in stage at detection, a decrease in case-specific mortality, and a decrease in the site-specific mortality from the disease in the screened population.
- Cervical cytology is the prototype of an effective screening method. Annual Papanicolaou (Pap) smear screening has produced a significant reduction in cervical cancer mortality, and is recommended for all women after the onset of sexual activity.
- Endometrial sampling is recommended in women with endometrial cells on Pap smear or adenomatous endometrial hyperplasia who are being treated medically.
- Transvaginal sonography is the most effective screening method for ovarian cancer and has produced a decrease in stage at detection and case-specific mortality from ovarian cancer.
- Annual screening mammography and breast clinical examination are recommended in all women over the age of 50 years.
- Stool guaiac testing should be performed annually and sigmoidoscopy every 3–5 years in women over the age of 50 years.
- Since there is no effective screening method for lung cancer, women should be encouraged to avoid smoking.

References

Adami HO, Krusemo UB, Bergkvist L *et al.* (1987) On the age-dependent associations between cancer of the breast and of the endometrium: a nationwide cohort study. *Br. J. Cancer* **47:** 77.

Bast RC, Klug TL & John ER *et al.* (1983) A radioimmunoassay using a monoclonal antibody to monitor the course of epithelial ovarian cancer. *New Engl. J. Med.* **308:** 883–887.

Boring CC, Squires TS, Tong T & Montgomery S (1994) Cancer statistics. *CA* **44:** 7.

■ Bourne TH, Campbell J, Reynolds K *et al.* (1994) The potential role of serum CA-125 in an ultrasound-based screening program for familial ovarian cancer. *Gynecol. Oncol.* **52:** 379–385.

Bourne TH, Whitehead M, Campbell S *et al.* (1991) Ultrasound screening for familial ovarian cancer. *Gynecol. Oncol.* **43:** 92–97.

Boyes DA, Nichols TM, Milner AM & Worth AJ (1977) Recent results from the British Columbia Screening Program for Cervical Cancer. *Am. J. Obstet. Gynecol.* **128:** 692–693.

Cramer DW (1993) Epidemiologic aspects of gynecologic oncology. In: Knapp RC and Berkowitz RS (eds) *Gynecologic Oncology*, pp. 139–150. New York: McGraw–Hill.

Dales LG, Friedman GD & Collen MF (1979) Evaluating periodic multiphasic health check-up: A controlled trial. *J. Chronic Dis.* **32:** 385–404.

■ DePriest PD, Shenson D, Fried A *et al.* (1993) A morphology index based on sonographic findings in ovarian tumors. *Gynecol. Oncol.* **51:** 7–11.

DePriest PD, van Nagell JR, Gallion HH *et al.* (1993) Ovarian cancer screening in asymptomatic post-menopausal women. *Gynecol. Oncol.* **51:** 205–209.

Dodd GD (1992) American Cancer Society guidelines on screening for breast cancer: An overview. *CA* **42:** 177–180.

Fearon ER & Vogelstein B (1990) A genetic model for colorectal tumorigenesis. *Cell* **61:** 759–767.

■ Feig SA & Hendrick RE (1993) *Risk, Benefit, and Controversies in Mammographic Screening*, pp. 77–93. Society of Breast Imaging.

Feig SA & Hendrick RE (1994) Syllabus – A categorical course in physics. Technical aspects of breast imaging. Updated by Haus AG and Yaffe MJ (eds) Chicago, Illinois. *Radiol. Soc. of N. Amer.* 3rd edition, pp. 121–138.

Friedman GD, Collen MF & Fireman BH (1986) Multiphasic health checkup evaluation: a 16-year follow-up. *J. Chronic Dis.* **6:** 453–463.

Gal D, Kopel S, Bashevkin M *et al.* (1991) Oncogenic potential of Tamoxifen on endometria of postmenopausal women with breast cancer – preliminary report. *Gynecol. Oncol.* **42:** 120–123.

Gay JD, Donaldson LD & Goellner JR (1985) False-negative results in cervical cytologic studies. *Acta Cytol.* **20:** 203–206.

Gilbertsen VA (1974) Proctosigmoidoscopy and polypectomy in reducing the incidence of rectal cancer. *Cancer* **4:** 936–939.

Gilbertsen VA, McHugh RB, Schuman LM *et al.* (1980) Colon cancer control study: an interim report. In: Winawer S, Schottenfeld D & Sherlock P (eds) *Progress in Cancer Research and Treatment. Colorectal Cancer*

Prevention and Screening, **13,** pp. 261–266. New York: Raven Press.

Goldschmidt R, Katz Z, Blickstein I, Caspi B & Dgani R (1993) The accuracy of endometrial Pipelle sampling with and without sonographic measurement of endometrial thickness. *Obstet. Gynecol.* **82:** 727–730.

Hardcastle JD, Farrands PA, Balfour TW *et al.* (1983) Controlled trial of fecal occult blood testing in the detection of colorectal cancer. *Lancet* **ii:** 1–4.

Henderson BE, Pike M, Ross RK, Mack TM & Lobo RH (1988) Re-evaluating the role of progestogen therapy after the menopause. *Fertil. Steril.* **49 (Suppl.)** 9S–15S.

Hulka BS (1988) Cancer Screening: degrees of proof and practical application. *Cancer* **62:** 1776–1789.

Kabawat SE, Bast RC, Bahan AK *et al.* (1983) Tissue distribution of a coelomic epithelium-related antigen recognized by the monoclonal antibody OC-125. *Lab. Invest.* **48:** 42A.

Koss LG (1993) Cervical Pap smear. *Cancer* **71:** 1405–1412.

Levin ML, Tockman MS, Frost JK *et al.* (1982) Lung cancer mortality in males screened by chest x-ray and cytologic sputum examination: A preliminary report. *Rec. Res. Cancer Res.* **82:** 138–146.

Lung cancer. *ACS Cancer Facts & Figures – 1994,* p. 9. Atlanta, Georgia: American Cancer Society.

Mathew A, Chabon AB, Kabakow B, Drucker M & Hirschman RJ (1990) Endometrial carcinoma in five patients with breast cancer on Tamoxifen therapy. *N.Y. J. Med.* **90:** 207–208.

Melamed MR, Flehinger BJ, Zaman MB *et al.* (1981) Detection of true pathologic stage I lung cancer in a screening program and the effect on survival. *Cancer* **47:** 1182–1187.

Melamed MR, Flehinger BJ, Zaman MB *et al.* (1984) Screening for lung cancer. Results of the Memorial Sloan–Kettering study in New York. *Chest* **86:** 44–53.

Neven P & DeMuyleder X (1990) Hysteroscopic follow-up during Tamoxifen treatment. *Eur. J. Obstet. Gynecol.* **35:** 235–238.

Nystrom L, Rutqvist L, Wall S *et al.* (1993) Breast cancer screening with mammography: Overview of Swedish randomised trials. *Lancet* **341:** 973–978.

Porazzini F, LaVecchia C, Bocciolone L & Franceschi S (1991) The epidemiology of endometrial cancer. *Gynecol. Oncol.* **41:** 1–16.

■ Prorok C (1984) Evaluation of screening programs for the early detection of cancer. *Statistical Textbooks Monograph* **51:** 267–238.

■ Puls LE, Powell DE, DePriest PD & van Nagell JR (1992) Transition from benign to malignant epithelium in mucinous and serous ovarian cystadenocarcinoma. *Gynecol. Oncol.* **47:** 53–57.

Richart R & Wright T (1993) Controversies in the management of low-grade cervical intraepithelial neoplasia. *Cancer* **71:** 1413–1421.

Sedlis A, Walters AT, Balin W, Hontz A & Sciuto L (1974) Evaluation of two simultaneously obtained cervical cytological studies. *Acta Cytol.* **18:** 291–296.

Simon JB (1985) Occult blood screening for colorectal carcinoma: A critical review. *Gastroenterology* **88:** 820–837.

Stenback F (1981) Benign, borderline and malignant serous cystadenomas of the ovary. *Pathol. Res. Pract.* **172:** 58–72.

Taylor PT, Anderson WA, Barber SR *et al.* (1987) The screening Pap smear: contribution of the endocervical brush. *Obstet. Gynecol.* **70:** 734–738.

Thier S & Loeb V (1992) Meeting on breast cancer screening: Issues and recommendations. National Institutes of Health/National Cancer Institute Consensus Development. *J. Natl. Cancer Inst.* **60:** 1519–1521.

van Nagell JR, DePriest PD, Puls LE *et al.* (1991) Ovarian cancer screening in asymptomatic postmenopausal women by transvaginal sonography. *Cancer* **68:** 458–462.

■ van Nagell JR, Higgins RV, Donaldson ES *et al.* (1990) Transvaginal sonography as a screening method for ovarian cancer: A report of the first 1000 cases screened. *Cancer* **65:** 573–577.

Weiner Z, Thaler I, Beck D *et al.* (1992) Differentiating malignant from benign ovarian tumors with transvaginal color flow imaging. *Obstet. Gynecol.* **79:** 159–162.

White L (1993) An overview of screening and early detection of gynecologic malignancies. *Cancer* **71:** 1400–1405.

Yancy M, Magelssen D & DeMaurez A (1990) Classification of endometrial cells on cervical cancer. *Obstet. Gynecol.* **76:** 1000–1005.

Young RC, Walton LA & Ellenberg SS (1990) Adjuvant therapy in stage I and stage II epithelial ovarian cancer. *New Engl. J. Med.* **311:** 1021–1027.

34 Advanced Cancer: The Hospice Approach

C F B Regnard
M C Comiskey

Palliative medicine is concerned with the study and care of patients with advanced disease in whom the prognosis is limited and the focus of care is the quality of life (Calman *et al.*, 1989). Although now recognized as a full speciality of medicine in the UK, this does not imply the restriction of this care to specialist teams. Palliative medicine can be successfully practised wherever there is a team with sufficient interest, expertise and understanding to create an environment where patients feel safe to express their distress safely and constructively. The fact that hospices are only one of many settings is why 'hospice care' was rejected as the name for this new speciality. 'Terminal care' was felt to be too restrictive, suggesting the care of patients only in their last days and weeks. Indeed 'terminal' as an adjective can imply loss, failure; "I'm sorry, she's terminal, there's nothing more we can do." Palliative medicine concerns rehabilitation, relief and comfort with the likelihood of success in the face of the probable death of the patient.

The Problems

Patients with advanced cancer experience a wide variety of physical symptoms (*Table 34.1*). These combine with psychologic and social problems to spill over to affect family, friends and care givers. Relatively straightforward problems can be submerged in such situations and seen as more complex than they really are. Conversely, there is the temptation to treat complex problems superficially as if they were straightforward. This may partly explain the reasons for the surprisingly large proportion of unrelieved symptoms in advanced disease.

Wilkes (1984) looked at 262 deaths in a UK city excluding hospice patients and those suffering traumatic or sudden death. One-third had cancer. The proportion of patients with unrelieved symptoms was 67% of those with pain, 74% of those with constipation and 80% of those with vomiting. In another study Twycross and Fairfield (1982) found that 73 of 100 patients admitted to a hospice had suffered pain for more than two months, and 57 for more than four months. More than 75% of these patients described the pain as severe, very severe or excruciating.

Pain Control

Principles

Pain should not be seen as an inevitable accompaniment to malignancy. Overall, 30% of patients with malignancies of the genitourinary tract have little or no pain (Foley, 1979). The prevalence of pain increases with disease progression. In women with carcinoma of uterine cervix 38% suffered moderate to severe pain within six months of diagnosis (Greenwald *et al.*, 1987) rising to a mean prevalence of 75% in those with advanced disease (Bonica, 1990). Even in those with pain, malignancy is not always the cause and nearly one-quarter of pains in cancer patients are unrelated to malignancy.

Table 34.1. Common symptoms in 6677 patients admitted to St Christopher's Hospice, 1975–1984 (from Annual reports: St Christopher's Hospice – Details of admissions and discharges).

Symptom	*Frequency (%)*
Weight loss	77
Pain	71
Anorexia	67
Dyspnea	51
Cough	50
Constipation	47
Weakness	47
Nausea/vomiting	40
Edema/ascites/effusion	31
Insomnia	29
Urinary problems	23
Pressure sore	19
Hemorrhage	14
Drowsiness	10
Paralysis	8
Jaundice	6
Colostomy	5
Diarrhea	4
Fistula	1

Accurate diagnosis of the cause of pain is essential (*Table 34.2*). Half of cancer patients in one series had three or more different pains, some as many as eight (Twycross and Fairfield, 1982). Different pains require different therapeutic approaches (*Table 34.3*). Diagnosis is the vital first step to successful treatment, yet it is surprising how often this stage is glossed over.

It is necessary to ask about pain rather than waiting for the patient to complain. Many patients are stoical or see pain as inevitable and unavoidable. Such patients also need to be observed for the effects of pain such as reduced mobility, apathy or irritability.

A clear explanation of the cause of pain(s) and proposed treatment plan can help many patients to cope and adopt reasonable expectations of treatment. Realistic goals are useful markers for both patient and clinician. Initially a pain-free, full night's sleep should be the aim, followed by relief during the day. Freedom from pain at rest during the day should be the next step, followed by reduced pain on movement. Being pain-free on movement and indeed at all times is the final aim, but it may not be possible to achieve this in all cases.

The use of primary and secondary analgesics should be well understood. An appropriate analgesic should be used regularly, in doses titrated to each individual so that pain is prevented from returning. There should be a realistic attitude to the risks and myths of opioids in cancer patients in order to prevent both underuse and overuse. At all stages of disease it is important to consider the likely benefits of disease-modifying treatments such as radiotherapy, chemotherapy, hormone therapy and surgery.

Patients should be assessed repeatedly and regularly. This allows adequate analgesic titration

Table 34.2. Diagnosing the cause of pain – clinical decision checklist (adapted with permission from Regnard and Tempest, 1992, and Regnard, 1995).

Is pain related to movement?
- Worsened by the slightest passive movement?
  - Consider: skeletal instability due to pathologic fracture, nerve compression/soft tissue inflammation or infiltration
- Worsened by bone strain during passive movement on examination?
  - Consider: bone metastasis/intermittent nerve compression due to skeletal instability
- Worsened by active movement only (i.e. movement against resistance)?
  - Consider: myofascial pain/skeletal muscle strain or spasm
- Worsened by inspiration?
  - Consider: rib metastases/pleuritic pain (inflammation, tumor, infection, embolus)/peritoneal inflammation/liver capsule stretch or inflammation
- Worsened by joint movement?
  - Consider: arthritis (inflammation, infection, metastasis)
- Cause still uncertain?
  - Consider: organ distension (tumor infiltration, hemorrhage)/soft tissue inflammation or tumor infiltration

Is pain periodic?
- Related to bowel?
  - Consider: constipation/bowel irritation (drugs, radiotherapy, chemotherapy, bile, infection)/bowel obstruction
- Related to bladder?
  - Consider: infection/outflow obstruction/unstable bladder/irritation by tumor
- Related to ureter?
  - Consider: infection/obstruction

Is pain related to eating?
- Consider: mucosal problems in mouth, esophagus, stomach, bowel/distension of stomach or bowel

Are there associated skin changes?
- Consider: trauma/pressure damage/infiltration/infection/irritation/skin disease/sympathetically-maintained pain

Are unpleasant sensory changes present at rest?
- Consider: neuropathic pain (deafferentation pain, sympathetically-maintained pain, painful peripheral neuropathies, peripheral neuralgias)/soft tissue inflammation

Is pain in an area supplied by a peripheral nerve?
- Consider: dermatomal nerve compression, peripheral neuropathy (e.g. compression, B12 neuropathy, paraneoplastic)

Do signs and symptoms suggest a central nervous system lesion?
- Consider: cord compression/cranial nerve damage or compression/thalamic pain/meningeal distension or irritation

Is cause of pain still uncertain?
- Consider: vascular disease/infection

Table 34.3. Suggestions for the treatment of cancer pain depending on the causes (adapted with permission from Regnard and Tempest, 1992, and Regnard and Stedeford, 1995) (TENS, transcutaneous electrical nerve stimulation; NSAID, non-steroidal anti-inflammatory drug.)

Cause of pain	*First-line treatment*	*Second-line treatment*	*To consider*
Pain worsened by movement			
Pathologic fracture	Immobilization Morphine	Spinal analgesia	Orthopedic surgery
Bone metastasis	Morphine Radiotherapy	Ibuprofen	Orthopedic surgery Bisphosphonates
Myofascial pain	Injection of trigger point with local anesthetic	Transcutaneous nerve stimulation	Baclofen or low-dose diazepam at night
Skeletal muscle spasm pain	Treat cause if possible	TENS Oral baclofen	Spinal baclofen Phenol block
Pleuritic pain	Treat cause if possible	Intercostal nerve block	Morphine $\pm$ NSAID
Peritoneal pain	Treat cause if possible	Morphine	If noninfective consider dexamethasone
Liver distension pain	Morphine	Low-dose dexamethasone (4 mg daily)	High-dose dexamethasone
Gastric distension pain	Metoclopramide or domperidone	If obstruction: high-dose dexamethasone	Nasogastric suction Gastrostomy
Bowel distension pain	Remove cause if possible	Hyoscine butylbromide	Obstruction: surgery or dexamethasone
Rectal distension pain	Empty rectum of stool	If local tumor: high-dose dexamethasone	Consider nerve block
Inflammatory pain	Exclude and treat infection	Dexamethasone	Ibuprofen Heat or cold
Periodic pain			
Bowel colic	Remove cause if possible	Hyoscine butylbromide	Obstruction: surgery or dexamethasone
Bladder spasm	Remove cause if possible	Hyoscine butylbromide	Irritation by tumor: instill 0.25% bupivacaine
Ureteric colic	Diclofenac 75 mg IM or 100 mg PR	Hyoscine butylbromide	Obstruction: stent or dexamethasone
Other pains			
Skin damage pain	Remove or treat cause	Topical benzydamine cream	If inflammatory: topical corticosteroid
Soft tissue infiltration	Morphine	Topical benzydamine cream	Radiotherapy or chemotherapy
Deafferentation pain	Morphine	Low-dose amitriptyline $\pm$ carbamazepine Contact pain specialist	Other secondary analgesic, nerve block or spinal drugs
Sympathetic dependent pain	Amitriptyline $\pm$ carbamazepine	TENS (place over artery in hypoactive type)	If hyperactive type: chemical sympathectomy
Nerve root compression	Morphine	Radiotherapy $\pm$ high-dose dexamethasone	TENS Nerve block
Thalamic pain	Amitriptyline	Amitriptyline + carbamazepine	Naloxone infusion

to the pain expressed by the patient. It also prevents premature withdrawal of an analgesic because of treatable adverse effects, and increases the patient's confidence in both the treatment and the clinician.

Finally, empathy, understanding, diversion and elevation of mood must be seen as essential adjuncts to analgesia. Drugs are only part of pain control.

Diagnosis

Pain in cancer may be:

- caused directly by the cancer;
- related to the cancer;
- related to treatment;
- unrelated to the cancer or treatment.

Pain caused directly by tumor involvement (e.g. bone metastases, nerve compression, soft tissue infiltration or visceral involvement) is the commonest cause accounting for 67% of pains, while 33% of pains in patients with cancer are not directly caused by the cancer. These may be related to treatment (e.g. postoperative pain, opioid-induced constipation), associated with the condition (e.g. zoster neuralgia, pressure sores) or unrelated to the disease or treatment (e.g. osteoarthritis). These causes may require very different approaches such that an incorrect approach will fail (see *Table 34.3*).

Correct diagnosis of the pain consequently requires a careful history and examination, together with information of past and recent investigations. Some pains are characteristic. Bowel colic is easily recognized, although the radiation is not typical. Thigh pain on standing, which is less painful when sitting or fully upright, is suggestive of a femoral metastasis eroding a significant proportion of the cortex. Many other pains present only as a dull ache and are differentiated by their site, such as right hypochondrial pain in the presence of hepatic metastases. Pain from bone metastases is usually well localized, although muscle spasm of nearby muscles can cause a more diffuse pattern. This is most commonly seen in the paraspinal muscles associated with a lumbar vertebral metastasis. Nerve compression pain usually has a dermatomal pattern, although the site of compression may be uncertain. Thus L1 dermatomal pain may be due to compression of the genitofemoral nerve along the pelvic brim, the L1 root at the intervertebral foramen, or in the vertebral canal. Nerve damage may result in pain with altered sensation – anesthesia, paresthesia or even hyperesthesia. This is known as neuropathic pain.

Case history

A 52-year-old woman with advanced ovarian carcinoma was referred for treatment of abdominal pain unrelieved by four-hourly intramuscular injections of 30 mg diamorphine. Her description of the pain strongly suggested bowel colic, although it radiated to her back. Treatment of her constipation resolved her pain and all analgesia was stopped.

Choice of Primary Analgesic

Since estimating pain severity is highly subjective this should not be the basis for choosing a primary analgesic. The World Health Organization analgesic staircase (*Figure 34.1*) bases the choice on the patient's response to the analgesic. If pain fails to respond to a non-opioid then a weak opioid is the next step. If a weak opioid fails then a strong opioid is the next logical step rather than an alternative weak opioid of similar efficacy. As codeine is basically a prodrug for morphine one may theoretically skip the second step and prescribe low-doses of a strong opioid instead. This has practical application where compliance or limiting the actual numbers of tablets is an issue. Use of this staircase assumes the pain is likely to be opioid responsive. Belief that all pains will respond to an opioid is incorrect, and this must be taken into account (*Table 34.4*). Pains unresponsive to opioid will require different approaches (see below).

The choice of primary analgesics is wide, but only a few are needed (*Table 34.5*). Diamorphine is

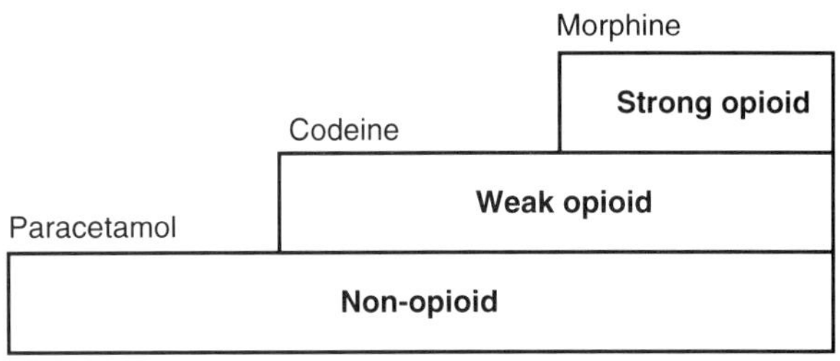

Figure 34.1. The analgesic staircase allows for the titration of the analgesic to the patient's pain. The use of the opioid steps assumes the pain is opioid-responsive. The middle step (weak opioids) can be missed by changing to low doses of strong opioids.

Table 34.4. Opioid-responsive pain in advanced cancer.

Complete or partial response	*Partial response or unresponsive*
Soft tissue infiltration	Lymphedema
Organ compression	Nerve destruction
Bone involvement	Colic
Nerve compression	Skin pressure
	Tenesmus
	Ischemia

Table 34.5. Choice of primary analgesics.

Analgesic class	*First choice*	*Second choice*
Non-opioid	Paracetamol (acetaminophen)	Non-steroidal anti-inflammatory drugs Aspirin
Weak opioid agonist	Codeine	Dihydrocodeine Dextropropoxyphene (propoxyphene)
Strong opioid agonist	Morphine	Hydromorphone Diamorphine Methadone Oxycodone

Table 34.6. Approximate equivalents of oral opioids (adapted with permission from Regnard and Tempest, 1992).

Opioid	*Conversion factor to oral morphine*[†]
Pentazocine	0.06
Codeine	0.08
Dihydrocodeine	0.1
Dextropropoxyphene[‡]	0.16
Pethidine	0.125
Dipipanone (in Diconal)	0.5
Diamorphine (oral)	1.0
Methadone[‡]	1–4
Oxycodone	1.3
Dextromoramide	2
Morphine (parenteral)	2
Diamorphine (parenteral)	3
Phenazocine	5
Levorphanol	5
Hydromorphone (oral)	7.5
Hydromorphone (parenteral)	15
Buprenorphine	60
Fentanyl (transdermal) (for 72-hour dose)	50

[†]Example of conversion: diamorphine 20 mg parenterally daily. Conversion factor is ×3. Patient is on equivalent of 60 mg oral morphine daily.
[‡]Methadone and dextropropoxyphene have prolonged half-lives resulting in accumulation with repeated doses.

rapidly metabolized to morphine and can therefore be considered as a prodrug for morphine. It is no more effective than morphine by oral or intramuscular routes (Twycross, 1977; Inturrisi *et al.*, 1984). Diamorphine and hydromorphone are both more soluble than morphine making them common choices for parenteral use. Methadone, oxycodone and levorphanol are useful alternative strong opioids with differing opioid receptor selectivity in morphine intolerant patients. Pethidine (Meperidine) and dextromoramide are too short-acting for use in chronic pain – both give only 2–3 hours' relief. Transdermal fentanyl patches are useful in patients on a stable opioid dose unable to take oral medication. Buprenorphine's adverse effects are similar to morphine although it is less constipating. It is a potent analgesic (each tablet of 0.2 mg is approximately equivalent to 12 mg oral morphine) and is an alternative to morphine in the lower morphine dose range. However, a practical ceiling in terms of the number of sublingual tablets patients can manage and the likelihood of future need for morphine limit its usefulness in cancer pain. Tramadol is a centrally acting opioid and monoamine re-uptake blocker recently licensed in the UK for the treatment of moderate to severe pain. Results of studies comparing the efficacy of oral tramadol and morphine in cancer patients with severe chronic pain are conflicting (Osipova *et al.*, 1991; Wilder–Smith *et al.*, 1994). It may cause less constipation. There is no clinical evidence for the claim that it has a 'dual action' (Anonymous, 1994).

Use of Strong Opioids

Dosage

Analgesics should be given regularly and the dose titrated until pain relief is constant. In this situation the aim is to prevent the pain returning. Timing depends on the typical length of action of the preparation – thus, experience has shown that morphine sulphate solution can be given every four hours, while controlled-release morphine (MST, MS Contin) can be given every 12 hours. PRN (i.e. as required) prescribing should never be used as a sole basis for analgesia, although it has a place in addition to a regular regimen.

The starting dose depends on several factors. Previous analgesic requirements are important since analgesics vary in their potency compared with morphine (*Table 34.6*). A typical starting dose when converting from 60 mg dihydrocodeine four-hourly would be 10 mg morphine four-hourly. Patients converting to morphine from buprenorphine require a higher equivalent dose ratio of 100:1 if pain was poorly controlled (Twycross, 1994a). These rules can be safely followed for those with reduced hepatic function since, excluding hepatic failure, such patients probably metabolize morphine normally (Patwardhan *et al.*, 1981). For those with poor renal function (and therefore some elderly patients) these rules still apply, but titration will have to be slower because morphine is metabolized to an active metabolite that acts centrally, morphine-6-glucuronide (M6G), and is excreted via the kidney (Hanks and Hoskin, 1987). Weight, height and surface area correlate poorly with the amount of opioid needed (Kaiko *et al.*, 1982).

Myths of strong opioids

Fear of strong opioids by patients and doctors alike has been a major factor in the slow acceptance and inappropriate use of such drugs over the past 20 years.

Opioids show the remarkable property of selective tolerance. There is no evidence of tolerance to opioid analgesia and if it exists it is slow to develop and easily matched by dose increases. In fact the main reason for dose increase is not tolerance, but progression of the disease (Twycross, 1994b). In contrast, tolerance to euphoria is rapid, which makes their use as euphoriants illogical. Patients much prefer to remain fully alert while on an opioid and this is usually possible. Any mild sedation during titration settles within five days at the same dose. Many patients do not develop nausea on opioids. If it occurs, control is achieved in most with low dose haloperidol 1.5–3.0 mg at night for 10–14 days. There is no observable tolerance to constipation, and so prophylactic laxatives are *de rigueur* with opioids. Respiratory depression is not a problem in patients on long-term oral morphine (Walsh, 1984). The exception is if pain is suddenly relieved by another method (e.g. nerve block), in which case respiratory depression may occur if the opioid dose has not been reduced.

Physical dependence does occur, but clinical experience shows that when pain settles, such as after radiotherapy, opioid doses can often be reduced over 5–10 days without precipitating withdrawal symptoms. Psychologic dependence is not observed in advanced cancer patients on opioids. Patients given insufficient or infrequent analgesics will ask for more, but this is not psychologic dependence, simply an appropriate demand for adequate pain relief.

Non-oral routes

There are few indications for parenteral analgesics in cancer patients and 66% of patients can remain on oral medication on the last day of their lives (Lombard and Oliver, 1989), but indications include the last hours or days of life, vomiting, severe dysphagia and occasionally an acute exacerbation of pain. Small-volume injections are kinder in these patients, and the high solubility of diamorphine hydrochloride (1 g in 1.6 ml) or hydromorphone (1 g in 3 ml) are useful. When changing from the oral to parenteral route the following approximate dose equivalents apply: 3 mg oral morphine = 3 mg oral diamorphine = 1 mg subcutaneous or intramuscular diamorphine = 1.5 mg subcutaneous or intramuscular morphine = 0.2 mg subcutaneous or intramuscular hydromorphone.

If the parenteral route is indicated subcutaneous injections through a fine 25 g needle or where repeated doses are required, through an indwelling 25 g subcutaneous canula are kinder. Continuous subcutaneous infusions can be given using small battery-driven portable pumps. Continuous intravenous infusions are unnecessary and there is no evidence that this route has any advantage over other routes. If there is already a permanent indwelling central venous catheter in place, intravenous infusion is preferable to bolus injections since the latter appears to encourage rapid analgesic tolerance (Hanks & Hoskin, 1987).

Many opioids can be given by the buccal route (buprenorphine, diamorphine, morphine, dextromoramide and phenazocine), but high doses are impractical. The rectal route is always worth considering. Morphine and hydromorphone can both be given rectally in the same doses as oral medication.

Spinal analgesia should be considered in the minority of patients with opioid-sensitive pain who are troubled by adverse effects. Effective analgesia can be achieved with low doses (e.g. morphine 2–20 mg/24 hours) (Regnard and Tempest, 1992). In patients with pain refractory to systemic opioid, a spinal infusion of low-dose opioid and local anesthetic is valuable (Sjõberg *et al.*, 1991).

Adverse effects

Constipation affects virtually all patients on strong opioids, but should not prevent their use. Treatment is discussed later. Troublesome nausea with low-volume vomiting will usually respond to 1.5–3 mg haloperidol at bedtime. Intermittent large-volume vomiting with little nausea suggests gastric stasis and is occasionally caused by opioids. It will respond to metoclopramide or domperidone 10 mg eight-hourly.

Drowsiness may occur on the initial introduction of morphine and with subsequent dose increases, settling within 5–7 days each time. Impairment of cognitive function was found in patients whose opioid dosage had increased by 30% within the previous three days, but not in those on a stable dose (Bruera *et al.*, 1989). It appears that the cancer itself also impairs cognitive function (Clemons, 1990). Dysphoria is uncommon with appropriate doses and titration. Euphoria is rarely seen, but confusion occasionally occurs and appears to be dose-related. If dysphoria or confusion persist despite opioid dose reduction and withdrawal of other offending agents an alternative strong opioid or method of pain relief may be necessary.

Persistent Pain

When pain is still present despite an appropriate use of analgesics the checklist in *Table 34.7* should be used. The possibility of a new pain should always be considered. Poor compliance may be due to a fear of opioids, which will require informed explanation.

Secondary analgesics, also termed 'co-analgesics' or adjuvant analgesics produce pain relief through an indirect mechanism. They may be used as adjuncts or replacements for primary analgesics (see *Table 34.3*). Corticosteroids will reduce the peri-tumor edema of cerebral metastases, but the same principle applies to nerve compression pain in pelvic or retroperitoneal tumors. Doses of 16 mg dexamethasone daily for one week gradually reducing to a maintenance dose of 2–4 mg once daily, is an appropriate regimen. Neuropathic pain can be particularly difficult to treat. Low-dose tricyclic antidepressants (TCAs) and anticonvulsants either alone or in combination are the mainstay of treatment. Mexilitene, flecainide and clonidine are also used. As TCAs and antiarrhythmics can cause arrhythmias, they should not be given simultaneously and a washout period of at least three days is recommended (Twycross, 1994c).

Non-steroidal anti-inflammatory drugs (NSAIDs) are used for mild to moderate cancer pain including painful bone metastases. Either diclofenac or naproxen are suitable first-line agents and should be interchanged if patients are intolerant or refractory (Rawlins, 1993). Adverse effects, particularly of the gastrointestinal tract, can be a problem.

Radiotherapy for localized metastatic bone pain achieves worthwhile analgesia in 80% of patients and complete pain relief in many (Hoskin, 1993). Approximately 15% of patients will respond within five days of treatment and 66% within three weeks. It is also helpful for pain due to local recurrence of carcinoma of cervix, ovary, uterus and vagina.

Other modes of therapy include nerve blocks (Wells, 1989), transcutaneous electrical nerve stimulation (TENS), acupuncture (Thompson and Filshie, 1993) and hypnosis.

Finally it must be remembered that fear, anxiety or depression will prevent adequate pain control. Explanation and empathy are the most effective secondary analgesics.

Table 34.7. Checklist for persistent pain.

Is the diagnosis correct?
Are the analgesics appropriate?
Is there a new pain?
Have the basic principles been followed?
Does the patient understand the purpose, timings and doses of drugs?
Is a secondary analgesic needed?
Are other treatment options needed?
Is there fear, anxiety or depression?

Control of Other Symptoms

Principles

As with pain it is essential to diagnose carefully, set realistic goals and titrate drug doses to the individual patient.

Constipation

Constipation is defined as the infrequent uncomfortable passage of hard stool. It is a major problem and almost 80% of hospice cancer patients require laxatives (Sykes, 1993). Patients with advanced malignancy have many predisposing factors. Drugs, particularly opioids and those with anticholinergic activity, are the major cause, but reduced mobility, dehydration, low roughage diet, the presence of intra-abdominal and pelvic tumor and hypercalcemia also contribute. Constipation causes abdominal masses, anorexia, nausea, vomiting, pain, diarrhea and confusion and may therefore be misdiagnosed as disease progression.

Management depends on the clinical findings. If the rectum is full of hard stool, softening with a glycerine suppository or oil enema may suffice; however, manual evacuation under sedative cover may be necessary. If soft stool is present a stimulant laxative (e.g. bisacodyl) may be given orally or rectally ensuring contact with the rectal mucosa. If the colon is loaded, rectal measures using bisacodyl suppository or mini-enema may be used. In addition an oral contact (stimulant) laxative such as danthron or senna, which acts on the colon, should be started and titrated every third day. The contact laxative is best used with a wetting agent – docusate or poloxamer – either in combination (UK: CO-danthrusate, CO-danthramer) or prescribed concurrently. If doses of nine CO-danthrusate capsules per day (danthron and docusate) or six senna tablets per day are ineffective, then patients will be helped by the addition of an osmotic laxative, which acts on both the small and large bowel.

Nausea and Vomiting

Commonly overlooked causes in advanced cancer are constipation, hypercalcemia, pharyngeal stimulation by copious sputum, gastric stasis and emetic drugs other than opioids such as metronidazole. These and more obvious causes must be differentiated before starting treatment, particularly if the cause is reversible as in hypercalcemia (Regnard and Comiskey 1995).

In choosing an antiemetic it is helpful to consider which receptors are being stimulated and then choose appropriate blocking agents (Peroutka and Snyder, 1982; Allan, 1988). Chemical causes of nausea and vomiting (e.g. opioids, hypercalcemia, uremia, toxins) act via the chemoreceptor trigger zone (CTZ), which in animals has a preponderance of dopamine receptors (Stefanni and Clement–Cormier, 1981). It is therefore logical to use a potent dopamine antagonist such as haloperidol. Haloperidol is superior to prochlorperazine and its 15–25-hour half-life allows a single night-time dose of 1.5–3 mg – a dose unlikely to cause extrapyramidal problems.

Stimulation of the vomiting centres may occur directly (radiotherapy to head, raised intracranial pressure) via vestibular pathways or via vagal and sympathetic afferents from the pharynx, liver capsule (liver metastases), bowel wall (constipation, bowel obstruction) or urinary tract (ureteric obstruction). Palacios *et al.* (1981) identified a predominance of histamine receptors in brainstem centers that process emetic sensory information. This makes the antihistamine cyclizine a logical choice. Cholinergic receptors are also prominent on the vagal pathway, hence hyoscine hydrobromide, a potent anticholinergic agent is a useful second-line agent.

Antiemetics acting on the upper gastrointestinal tract are useful in gastric stasis when due to reduced motility. Metoclopramide is the first choice with domperidone as an alternative if extrapyramidal problems are a risk. Cisapride is a useful second-line treatment for gastric stasis and also stimulates the intestine. Metoclopramide acts on the CTZ only at high doses when it is probably acting as a $5HT_3$ (5 hydroxytryptamine-3) antagonist. Specific $5HT_3$ antagonists (ondansetron, granisetron) are more effective in chemotherapy-induced emesis; however, there is no evidence they are useful in palliative care.

The non-oral route for antiemetics is often needed. Haloperidol, cyclizine and metoclopramide can all be given subcutaneously including by continuous infusion. Domperidone is available in suppository form. Cyclizine will precipitate with diamorphine if the concentration of either exceeds 25 mg ml^{-1} (Regnard *et al.*, 1986).

Bowel Obstruction

Obstruction here is defined as any process preventing the movement of bowel contents distally. The reported incidence in patients with ovarian cancer is 25–42% (Tunca *et al.*, 1981; Beattie *et al.*, 1989) and 3% of all those with advanced cancer (Baines *et al.*, 1985). Obstruction may be due to extramural compression, intraluminal tumor, peristaltic failure or blockage by bowel contents. Diagnosis is mainly by history, observation and radiology. Treatment is outlined in *Figure 34.2.*

Nausea usually settles with cyclizine 25–50 mg subcutaneously (SC) eight-hourly or 75–100 mg by SC infusion. In patients with distended colons, the addition of haloperidol 3–5 mg d^{-1} abolishes chemically-mediated nausea secondary to absorption of colonic bacterial toxins (see section on nausea and vomiting). Methotrimeprazine 25–150 mg d^{-1} or hyoscine hydrobromide 0.6–1.2 mg d^{-1} are useful second-line agents, but have more adverse effects. Metoclopramide 60–240 mg d^{-1} has been used with success (Isbister, 1990), but may cause colic. The somatostatin analog, octreotide, effectively controlled nausea and reduced gastrointestinal secretions in obstructed patients (Mercadente and Maddaloni, 1992; Khoo *et al.*, 1994). The recommended dose is 100–600 μg d^{-1} by SC infusion. The majority of patients continue to vomit not more than once daily, but their most distressing symptom, nausea, is under control (Baines *et al.*, 1985).

Parenteral hydration is only occasionally necessary. If symptomatic dehydration occurs, fluids may be administered by intravenous or preferably SC infusion (Fainsinger *et al.*, 1994). Nasogastric suction is rarely required except in proximal intestinal obstruction to prevent distressing distension and vomiting. A venting gastrostomy is more acceptable to patients who require continued nasogastric suction and is easily inserted endoscopically (Ashby *et al.*, 1991; Adelson and Kasowitz, 1993).

Treating colic in complete inoperable obstruction is straightforward. All laxatives should be stopped and an ileus created using hyoscine butylbromide (Buscopan) 60–180 mg d^{-1} by SC infusion. In partial obstruction an ileus must be avoided and a balance struck between promoting the distal movement of feces and preventing colic. Strong stimulant and osmotic laxatives should be stopped. Docusate is a wetting agent with weak stimulant activity and in doses of 100–600 mg daily does not usually precipitate colic while promoting the continued production of soft stool. Intermittent colic can be treated with the judicious use of sublingual hyoscine hydrobromide (Kwells in the UK). Patients are instructed to take 300 μg sublingually, repeated, if necessary, after 30 minutes, with a limit of 1200 μg d^{-1}. Continuing and distressing colic can herald a complete obstruction, which may warrant surgical intervention. Corticosteroids may relieve

Is there doubt this is obstruction? History, observation, clinical examination, radiology

→ **Yes:** Consider other cause of:
- Nausea and vomiting
- Abdominal distension (e.g. ascites)
- Colic (e.g. contact laxatives)
- Altered bowel habit (e.g. constipation)

↓ **No**

Is constipation the sole cause?

→ **Yes:** Clear rectum and commence laxative (then return to "Is constipation the sole cause?")

↓ **No**

Is a physical blockage absent?

→ **Yes:** Peristaltic failure (absent bowel sounds, distension, little vomiting):
- Exclude peritonitis/septicemia/recent spinal cord compression
- Stop antiperistatic drugs (e.g. anticholinergics, loperamide, osmotic laxatives
- Start docusate 100 mg eight hourly
- Consider cisapride 10–20 mg eight-hourly and bisacodyl 10–20 mg 12-hourly

↓ **No**

Is severe thirst present?

→ **Yes:** Parenterally hydrate (usually intravenously, but up to one litre can be infused into inner aspect of each thigh subcutaneously) (then continue to next step)

↓ **No**

Operable obstruction and fit for surgery?

→ **Yes:** Indicators of a good prognosis
- No ascites or abdominal masses
- No previous radiotherapy
- Large bowel blockage
- Single blockage
- Good nutritional and medical condition
- Contact surgeon to consider surgical exploration

Note: 10% of obstructions in malignancy are due to adhesions; some palliative surgical procedures are simple and straightforward (then continue to next step)

↓ **No**

Nausea and /or vomiting present?

→ **Yes:**
- Start cyclizine 50 mg orally eight-hourly or 150 mg d^{-1} by continuous subcutaneous infusion (reduce these doses by 50% if over 70 years age)
- If nausea is still present and colon is distended
  - Add haloperidol 5 mg orally or subcutaneously once at night
- If no improvement, consider replacing above with:
  - Methotrimeprazine 25–75 mg per 24 hours subcutaneous infusion (may cause drowsiness)
  - or Octreotide 300–600 mg per 24 hours subcutaneous infusion
- If vomiting persistent feculant or fecal, consider nasogastric tube

↓ **No**

Is obstruction complete and continuous?

→ **Yes:**
- Stop all laxatives. Treat dry mouth
- If colic present: commence hyoscine butylbromide 30 mg d^{-1} by continuous subcutaneous infusion (up to 180 mg)
- Hydrate and feed orally in occasional snacks
- Consider high-dose dexamethasone (see text)

↓ **No**

- Stop osmotic and strong contact laxatives. Treat dry mouth
- Start docusate 100 mg eight hourly and titrate dose
- Intermittent colic: hyoscine hydrobromide 300 µg sublingually (max. 1200 µg in 24 hours)
- Treat other pain
- Hydrate and feed orally in small frequent snacks

↓ **No**

Return to beginning

Figure 34.2. Flow diagram on the medical management of bowel obstruction (adapted with permission from Regnard, 1995).

obstruction by reducing peritumor edema although their role in obstruction has yet to be established.

Patients may manage small frequent snacks of low fiber foods. Enteral or parenteral feeding are rarely needed in advanced gynecologic cancer.

This scheme of management has now been used successfully in many palliative care centres in the UK. It enables nearly all obstructed patients with advanced cancer to be managed without nasogastric suction or intravenous hydration, promotes comfort and even allows some patients to be managed in their own homes.

Anorexia

It is normal for reduced activity to result in smaller energy needs, and no treatment is needed in asymptomatic patients. Reversible causes of anorexia include constipation, pain, nausea, vomiting, anxiety, depression, body odors, oral problems, drugs, unappetizing food and food odors. Small, attractively presented meals, perhaps preceded by an alcoholic drink, are more likely to be eaten. Corticosteroids promote appetite and wellbeing, but their effects are shortlived and merely symptomatic (Bruera and Fainsinger, 1993). Megestrol is preferable in patients expected to live longer and promotes weight gain as well as appetite.

Ascites

Ovarian carcinoma is a common cause of malignant ascites. When disease control is no longer possible, symptomatic treatment of ascites may be necessary (Regnard and Mannix, 1995). If the patient is very ill due to the cancer and the ascites is causing no symptoms, then no action is necessary. If troublesome symptoms are present in such an ill patient then paracentesis alone is the option. This is best done in the left iliac fossa or midline suprapubically (making sure of an empty bladder) using a peritoneal dialysis catheter. The lateral approach is preferable in patients with distended bowel. The use of 0.5% bupivicaine at the puncture site allows pain-free drainage for 8–10 hours. Two liters should be drained for immediate comfort, followed by drainage to dryness over the ensuing ten hours. A colostomy bag can be placed over the puncture site for a few days until the site heals.

In active asymptomatic patients diuretic therapy may prevent or reduce further fluid accumulation. This is based on the finding of increased plasma renin in malignant ascites (Greenway *et al.*, 1982) and the value of a combination of spironolactone and a loop diuretic (Fogel *et al.*, 1981). The starting dose is spironolactone 100 mg and frusemide 40 mg daily and it may be doubled. Active, but symptomatic patients should undergo paracentesis, as above, before commencing diuretic therapy.

If the ascites recurs, the insertion of a peritoneovenous shunt may help. There is no evidence that increased metastatic disease occurs (Tarin *et al.*, 1984), but loss of patency, disseminated intravascular coagulation, thromboembolism, sepsis and pulmonary edema are potential problems. Occasionally viscous ascites is encountered due to mucin production by the tumor. Such mucinous ascites can be removed from a small incision using suction, and the procedure repeated if necessary.

Oral Problems

Cancer patients are more commonly troubled with dirty mouths, dryness (Regnard and Fitton, 1995) and *Candida* infection and management will depend on the cause. Debility often results in poor oral hygiene due to reduced oral intake. Chlorhexidine, 0.2% mouthwash, reduces dental plaque formation and the build-up of oral debris. Coated tongues and mucosal surfaces are helped by chewing tinned pineapple chunks, which contain the proteolytic enzyme annanase or rinsing with an effervescent solution of vitamin C.

Reduced fluid intake in the last days of life does not usually cause problems with thirst, but patients may complain of a dry mouth. Local measures can be helpful such as petroleum jelly to the lips, sucking frozen drinks (tonic water, whisky and lemonade, fruit juices) or chewing pineapple chunks. The use of lemon juice or other acidic preparations can rapidly exhaust the salivary glands. Methylcellulose artificial salivas can be helpful, but some patients complain of their ‘oily’ taste. Porcine mucin spray (Saliva Orthana) is a well-tolerated alternative. Glycerol has a dehydrating effect on the oral mucosa unless it is diluted to at least a 30% solution.

Hematuria

Blood loss from urinary tract invasion by a pelvic tumor is not usually severe. Often it is the patient’s anxiety that is uppermost and skillful reassurance may be the most effective treatment. Infection should be treated, if present. Repeated infection with coliforms suggests a vesicocolic fistula, which may require surgical intervention.

Palliative radiotherapy can reduce troublesome hematuria arising from a bleeding malignant lesion of the urinary tract. Bleeding from the bladder can be reduced by instillation of a 1% alum solution for 30 minutes, 1–5 times daily in moderate hemorrhage or by continuous irrigation for 24–72 hours in severe hemorrhage. This acts by precipitating exposed protein and has no local or systemic toxicity (Bullock and Whitaker, 1985). Ethamsylate by mouth is a useful alternative or maintenance therapy. Tranexamic acid may cause the formation of hard clots and should be avoided.

Bronchial Secretions

At the end of life bronchial secretions can produce a 'death rattle,' which although not apparently distressing to the patient who is often comatose, can be distressing to both relatives and staff. Some conscious, but very debilitated patients are too weak to cough and are also troubled with secretions.

Treatment is with hyoscine hydrobromide (scopolamine), 300–800 μg four-hourly SC as required. This drug is sedative, but preferable to atropine, which can cause agitation. A few patients will be precipitated into ventricular failure by their prone position despite the normal dehydration that occurs at the end of life. Therefore, some cases of bronchial secretions resistant to hyoscine hydrobromide may respond to a loop diuretic such as frusemide (furosemide) or bumetanide given intramuscularly.

Fistulae

Fistulae present special problems that can be particularly distressing to the patient, family and care-givers.

Vesicocolic fistulae result in frequency, dysuria and painful bladder spasm through bladder irritability caused by persistent infection. Pneumaturia is unusual, but strongly suggests an enterovesical fistula. A rectovaginal fistula causes distressing fecal incontinence, sometimes accompanied by a malodorous discharge. Fashioning a simple loop colostomy should always be considered, even in a patient with only a few weeks to live, since the procedure is straightforward in most cases and the symptomatic relief is profound. Even if the fistula is more proximal, the problems of an ileostomy may be less than the distress of the fistula. Use of a transverse colon conduit for a vesicovaginal fistula has been described in advanced cervical carcinoma (Kisner and Kesner, 1987), but is limited by the more complex nature of the procedure. For some patients, however, surgery is not an option because they are too ill, their tumor too extensive or they do not wish further intervention. Such patients can be difficult to treat symptomatically.

Urinary incontinence from a small vesicovaginal fistula can be helped with vaginal tampons. Urinary leakage from larger fistulae has been managed using a urinary catheter placed intravaginally inside a vaginal prosthesis made from methylmethacrylate (Green and Phillips, 1986). Softer and more comfortable prostheses can be made from alginate. Persistent leakage can be markedly reduced at night to allow sleep by the use of desmopressin. This synthetic analog of antidiuretic hormone reduces urinary output overnight in a dose of 5–20 μg intranasally at bedtime. A check on fluid balance must ensure a good daytime output to prevent water intoxication.

In small bowel fistulae, output and enzymatic content may be significantly reduced by octreotide, 100–600 μg d^{-1} by subcutaneous infusion. It is a somatostatin analog that reduces intestinal secretions and suppresses the release of gut peptide hormones.

Fecal leakage from a small rectovaginal fistula is helped by keeping the stool well formed by reducing laxatives or the judicious use of loperamide, and by the use of vaginal tampons. Leakage from larger fistulae may be reduced by using alginate intravaginal plugs formed by using a condom placed within the vagina to prevent leakage of the alginate through the fistula. Fortunately, as a patient deteriorates, fecal output often trails off.

Discharges and Odors

Discharges can be due to mucous discharge or infection or both. Discharges of watery mucus with minimal infection from advanced cervical or vaginal carcinomas can sometimes be reduced using 400 μg hyoscine hydrobromide diluted in 5 ml 0.9% sodium chloride solution and administered intravaginally. Some discharges are caused by inflammation surrounding the local tumor and respond well to corticosteroids administered topically to the tumor. Malodorous thick discharges imply infection, and foul-smelling discharges suggest anaerobic infection. Metronidazole, 200–500 mg twice daily, is the treatment of choice for anaerobic infections. Some patients are nauseated on metronidazole when it can be given topically to the tumor surface. Aerobic infections alone usually respond partially to antibiotics, but this may be sufficient to at least temporarily reduce discharge. Debulking of the tumor with radiotherapy, cryotherapy, diathermy or laser may be a suitable option that can reduce discharge and odor.

Attempts to mask a smell with other odors such as perfumes usually fail since patient and staff come to associate the new odor with the unpleasant one, and soon it too becomes intolerable. Having attempted to reduce the discharge volume and treated anaerobic infection, it may be possible to mask the odor using adsorbents such as charcoal dressings. Oxychlorodene (Ostobon) is a chlorine-releasing powder that cannot be applied directly to tissues, but has no inherent odor and can be sprinkled between dressings to further reduce odor.

Hypercalcemia

Hypercalcemia occurs in 10% of patients with advanced cancer (Kaye and Oliver, 1985). Malignancies of epithelial origin are the usual primary, with gynecologic cancers accounting for 6% (Fisken *et al.*, 1980); 20% of patients with hypercalcemia do not have bone metastases. The mechanism is through increased bone resorption in all cases, due either to local production of cytokines and prostaglandins by tumor metastases in bone or humoral factors in those without bone metastases. In addition, renal clearance of calcium is reduced.

Hypercalcemia may cause drowsiness, nausea, vomiting, thirst, polyuria, anorexia, constipation and confusional states, but it is usual for only one or two symptoms to be present, drowsiness occurring in over half of patients. Since such symptoms mimic those of advanced cancer it is all too easy for them to be ascribed to an irreversible deterioration. Diagnosis, therefore, is often made on suspicion of hypercalcemia. Unless ionized calcium is measured, the total serum calcium should always be corrected according to the serum albumin: serum calcium = measured calcium + 0.025 × (40 − albumin) (Selby *et al.*, 1984).

There will always be occasions when a patient is already profoundly ill due to the malignancy, and if the symptoms of hypercalcemia are not distressing there is no reason to treat. In such cases, there will be no reason to confirm the clinical suspicion biochemically. In many cases, however, it is appropriate to treat hypercalcemia in advanced cancer to relieve its distressing effects.

Hypercalcemia is readily treated by rehydration and administration of bisphosphonates, which inhibit osteoclastic resorption. Dietary restriction of calcium is unnecessary, loop diuretics are not indicated, and corticosteroids are useful for hematologic malignancies only. There are three commercially available bisphosphonates: etidronate, clodronate and pamidronate in ascending order of potency. Pamidronate and, more recently, clodronate, are licensed for use as a single intravenous infusion (O'Rourke *et al.*, 1993) whereas etidronate requires repeated infusions. The onset of effect is 1–3 days with maximal effect on day 5–6 (Ralston, 1992). Duration of action is greatest with pamidronate (20–30 days) and retreatment may be required every 3–4 weeks unless disease-modifying treatment is instituted. Oral clodronate and etidronate are marketed as maintenance therapy to prevent or retard recurrence of hypercalcemia. Their low bioavailability and gastrointestinal side-effects limit their usefulness.

Lymphedema

Lymphedema due to lymphatic obstruction is a treatable condition, and legs should never be allowed to increase to a disabling and distressing size on the assumption that nothing can be done. Management consists of truncal massage, containment bandaging or hosiery, exercises and skin care (Regnard *et al.*, 1988; Badger and Regnard, 1989).

Since lymphedema is a high-protein edema, the use of compression alone simply encourages water to return into the circulation, leaving an even higher concentration of protein, which strongly attracts the return of the water on removal of the compression. In addition, the tissues around the limb root of many patients are already edematous, thereby compounding the problem. If the protein can be removed, the water will follow. The large protein molecules can only be removed through the lymphatics, and although major lymphatic trunks are blocked, minor lymphatics in the tissues around the hips and buttocks are usually intact. Massage encourages lymph drainage and should be started in the trunk quadrant furthest away from the affected limb, gradually moving towards the limb, and finally including the limb itself. The massage is most easily done by the patient using a handheld, electrical body massager in gentle strokes and without oil or talc. The function of containment bandaging or hosiery is to prevent the protein and water returning. Bandaging is used if the limb is too large to fit hosiery (>30% above normal limb), for deep skin folds (>1 cm), if the skin is broken or fragile, or if the limb is too painful to allow the fitting of hosiery. Bandaging should use a combination of padding and low elasticity bandages (Twycross and Badger, 1988). The most comfortable elastic hosiery is readymade from nylon and lycra (e.g. Medi Forte, Duomed). Normal use should be made of the limb in addition to exercises, which are best completed after massage and while wearing containment bandaging or hosiery. Skin care is essential to prevent entry of infection and consequent cellulitis, and the simplest measure is moisturizing the skin at night.

Lumbosacral Plexopathy

Lumbosacral plexopathy in patients with gynecologic malignancy usually occurs due to compression or infiltration of the lower lumbosacral plexus (L4–S1) by direct extension from intrapelvic tumor, although the entire plexus (L1–S3) may be affected (Jaeckle *et al.*, 1985).

The malignant psoas syndrome is characterized by lumbosacral plexopathy, ipsilateral hip pain and a positive psoas muscle test due to neoplastic involvement of adjacent psoas muscle (Stevens and Gonet, 1990). Radiation-induced plexopathy is rare and may occur 1–30 years following radiotherapy. Intracavitary radium implants for carcinoma of cervix may increase the risk. Pain is the earliest and commonest symptom in malignant lumbosacral plexopathy. It is characteristically aching or stabbing in nature and felt in the buttock, pelvis, perineum and leg. Dysesthesia indicates nerve damage rather than compression. There may be associated muscle weakness, sensory loss, tenesmus, sphincter disturbance, bladder spasm and lymphedema as disease progresses.

High-dose dexamethasone may reduce peritumor edema sufficiently to relieve compressive symptoms. We suggest a starting dose of 16–24 mg d^{-1}, reducing gradually after one week to the lowest dose that controls symptoms. Radiotherapy or chemotherapy should be considered. Surgical debulking is not usually possible and will not relieve symptoms due to nerve damage.

Pain can be dealt with as described earlier. In addition to opioids those patients with neuropathic pain are likely to require an anticonvulsant (e.g. sodium valproate) or a low-dose tricyclic antidepressant (e.g. 15–50 mg amitriptyline at night) or both. Motor weakness and sensory symptoms will lessen only if they are due to tumor compression and if it is possible to reduce tumor bulk or peritumor edema. Tenesmus is an unpleasant sensation of a full rectum, which is often resistant to analgesic therapy, but may respond to chemical sympathectomy (Bristow and Foster, 1988) or to oral nifedipine. Bladder irritability has many causes including infection, irritation by catheter or tumor, sacral nerve damage (neuropathic bladder) and anxiety. It may be eased by drugs with anticholinergic activity such as amitriptyline, flavoxate, propantheline and belladonna alkaloids. If still troublesome, the twice daily bladder instillation of 10 ml 0.5% bupivicaine can be effective. Spinal analgesia or nerve block may be required for persistent neuropathic pain due to lumbosacral plexopathy.

Hydration and Feeding in the Very Ill

In the very ill patient there is sometimes a strong need among relatives and staff to provide the patient with water and food, but this natural feeling must not override the patient's need for comfort. Intravenous hydration and nasogastric feeding can be distressing to the patient in their last days. Indeed, dehydration can improve comfort: urinary output drops so reducing the need for catheterization, bronchial secretions lessen, and in bowel obstruction vomiting reduces and may stop. On the other hand dehydration can cause confusion, discomfort, lethargy, accumulation of toxic drug metabolites, increased risk of pressure sores and constipation. The traditional medical and surgical approach has been to maintain hydration and feeding while the early hospice movement advised against non-oral hydration and feeding in such patients. Good palliative care lies somewhere between these two viewpoints, tailoring treatment to the individual patient's needs. Where hydration is indicated, hypodermoclysis (i.e. subcutaneous infusion of fluid) offers advantages over the intravenous route (Fainsinger *et al.*, 1994). Saline or saline–dextrose solutions may be infused through an indwelling subcutaneous cannula or needle at a rate of 80–500 ml h^{-1}. Although many centres add hyaluronidase to the infusion, it confers little benefit (Constans *et al.*, 1991). A dry mouth can be treated with local measures (see above). Energy requirements are usually low so that feeding is unnecessary. As deterioration continues, the aim of feeding is for pleasure, not survival. Families and staff, as well as patients, need to understand this.

Psychologic Problems

Patients do not work through an orderly sequence of stages of denial, bargaining, anger, guilt and finally acceptance. More often they oscillate between various stages, sometimes missing one or more stages altogether, sometimes becoming stuck at one stage. It is normal that patients and their families should feel anxious, frightened, angry or sad at what is happening to them. It is therefore essential to provide an environment where it is safe for that patient and family to express their distress in a constructive way (Stedeford, 1987). Patients and families may or may not be willing to discuss the cancer, but staff being prepared to offer open honest discussion with adequate information is a prerequisite for such an environment (Vachon, 1988).

The question is often asked "Should we tell the patient?" This implies that the patient has no suspicion of what is happening. And yet it is surprising how easily patients pick up clues from care-givers that all is not well – the concerned frown, the unexpected physical contact, the whispers at the foot of the bed, our discomfort. If patients are unaware of their diagnosis they soon come to suspect that something is seriously wrong. Consequently, in our need to protect the patient from the truth there is a danger that we may be leaving them alone with the truth. This conspiracy of silence spreads fear and distrust between patient, care-givers and the family.

A more appropriate question to ask, therefore, is "How much does the patient want to know now?", which implies more listening than telling. It also implies that some patients prefer not to discuss their diagnosis. Open questions such as "Are you worried about your illness?" can often allow patients to express their fears. A direct answer such as "I've got cancer, haven't I?" needs to be answered honestly. Such a conversation is never comfortable, but can be made easier by giving the facts in stages: "We found a lump;" "The lump was abnormal;" "Tests showed the abnormality was cancer;" "We took out the lump, but we couldn't take out all the cancer." Patients who deny their diagnosis will often make this clear when responding to an open question: "Oh, I don't want to talk about THAT!" This is an acceptable way of coping and can be effective, but it is never acceptable to lie to such patients that they are cured, particularly as they may later wish to discuss their diagnosis. Staff skills vary and there is no shame in finding such situations too uncomfortable; the shame comes in not admitting the fact and refusing to allow colleagues to help. Despite the discomfort felt during such discussions, they are often made easier by the patient and can form a basis of trust between the patient and care-giver.

Anxiety

Drugs can never substitute for empathetic explanation. True anxiolytics that 'lyse' anxiety do not exist. It is important to distinguish between moderate anxiety (i.e. predictable anxiety occurring as a reaction to the diagnosis) and a clinical anxiety state (Maguire *et al.*, 1995). Moderate anxiety generally responds to psychologic measures whereas an anxiety state requires an active drug regimen.

For many patients, exploring their fears (e.g. of mode of death, physical suffering, uncertainty about the future, loss of role or independence, spiritual and practical issues), allowing them to voice their concerns and giving appropriate information and assurance will reduce the anxiety significantly. Muscle relaxation and autogenic relaxation techniques will also help. When a clinical anxiety state is present, with a loss of ability to function on an everyday basis, a major tranquillizer such as haloperidol or thioridazine should be started immediately to control the anxiety and a benzodiazepine prescribed on a PRN basis as maintenance therapy. The tricyclic antidepressant clomipramine is used for panic and phobic disorders. Some patients will have mixed anxiety and depression and require treatment for both. Specialist advice from a psychiatrist, psychologist, counselor or social worker should be sought if there has been no response in one week.

Depression

Sadness is a normal feature of advanced cancer and should not be mistaken for depression. The diagnosis of depression is difficult in these patients, but is strongly suggested by the presence of feelings of guilt, low self-esteem, early morning wakening with no other disturbance of sleep and loss of interest (Stedeford, 1994a). Loss of weight, libido and appetite, constipation and sleep disturbance may be due to the primary illness and are not helpful in making the diagnosis. Suicidal thoughts should never be discounted, but in cancer patients such thoughts may reflect a wish to regain control over life or a wish to be less of a burden.

Patients with mild or moderate depression may respond to psychosocial measures alone (Stedeford, 1994b). For moderate to severe depression, a tricyclic antidepressant such as amitriptyline or lofepramine (which has less antimuscarinic effects) should be started. A few patients respond rapidly, but it may take six weeks or more to see an improvement, with care-givers usually noticing an improvement before the patient.

Confusional States

A useful concept in confusional states is that confusion makes it difficult for environmental stimuli to get through and lets more stimuli through from the body and memory, while making it difficult to differentiate the sources of the stimuli (Stedeford, 1994b). The implication is that self-awareness is at least partly intact and while this is probably why many such patients are very frightened, it does allow a means to treat the confusion. A further implication is that sedative drugs will simply reduce what awareness is present. Confusion may therefore present with disorientation, misinterpretation, short-term memory loss, and occasionally, hallucinations. Attempts to 'escape' by insisting on returning home, or paranoid thoughts when these attempts are blocked, become understandable. Common causes include drugs (sedatives, opioids, corticosteroids), infection, metabolic disturbances, and cardiac or respiratory failure. Stedeford (1994b) offers valuable advice on how to manage such patients. Guidelines are given in *Figure 34.3*.

Palliative Care Services

In one series of 612 interviews, 55% of patients expressed a preference to die at home in the week before death (Hinton, 1994). In the UK, only 26% actually achieve this wish (Hanks, 1994). In another series of patients referred to a home palliative care service, patients were more likely to die at home compared to those referred to other services (Dunphy and Amesbury, 1990). There is, therefore, a need for both a range of palliative care services in the hospital, hospice and home and for cooperation between such services.

In the UK there is now a wide range of palliative services available to the patient with advanced cancer, both within and outside the National Health Service (NHS) (*Table 34.8*). It should never be the intention of any service to provide care to the exclusion of another. The advent of palliative care units and teams in the past 20 years has been seen as a threat by some care-givers, but no palliative team can or should replace existing services – the aim must always be to act as a resource for existing services. Because many palliative services are funded from voluntary sources, they have had to act independently and have not always been included in local NHS plans. While this can cause difficulties, there is no reason why established teams cannot use the resources and expertise available in such teams for the benefit of their patients.

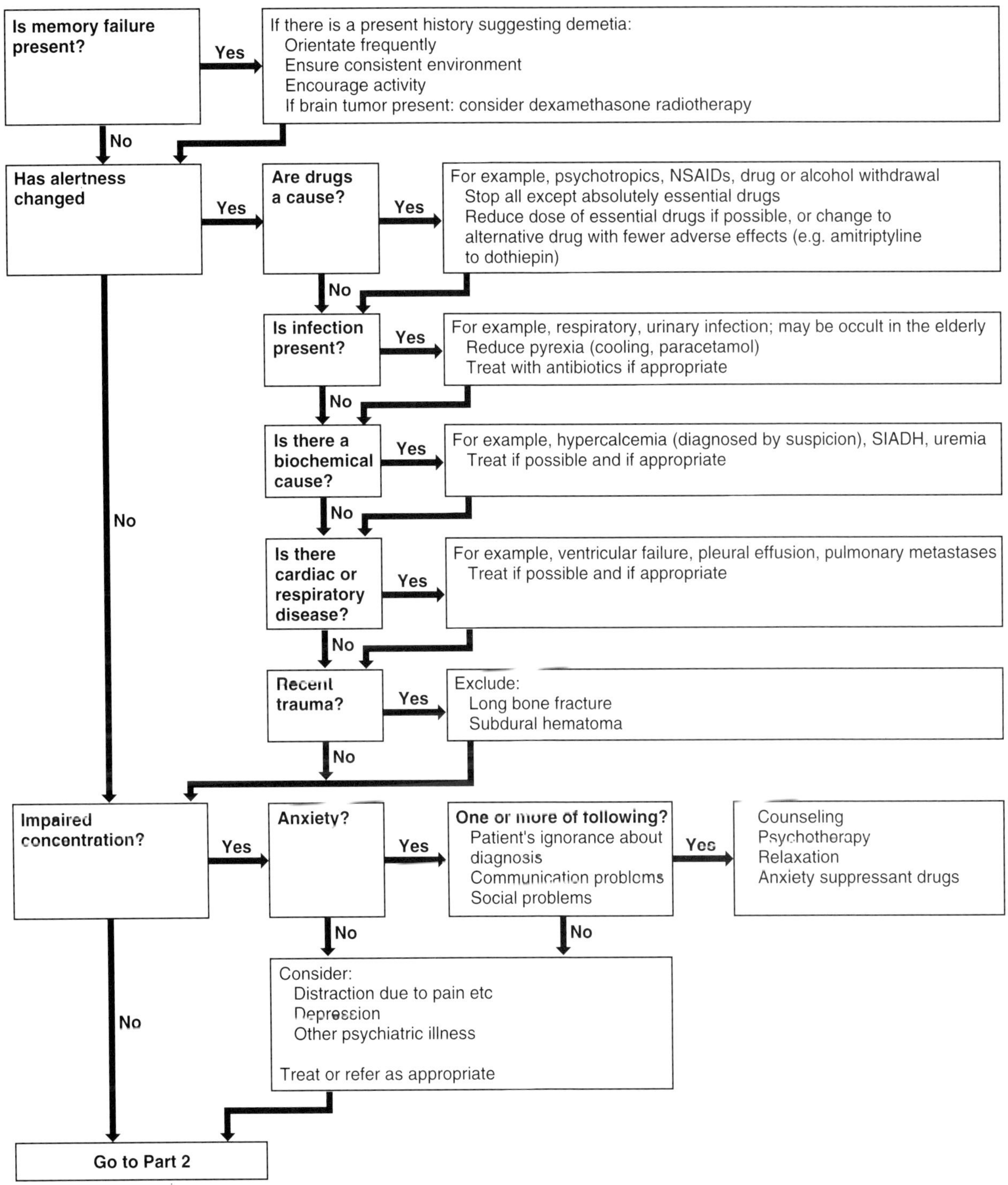

Figure 34.3. Flow diagram on the management of confusional states (adapted with permission from Regnard and Hockley, 1995). (NSAIDs, non-steroidal anti-inflammatory drugs; SIADH, syndrome of inappropriate antidiuretic hormone secretion.)

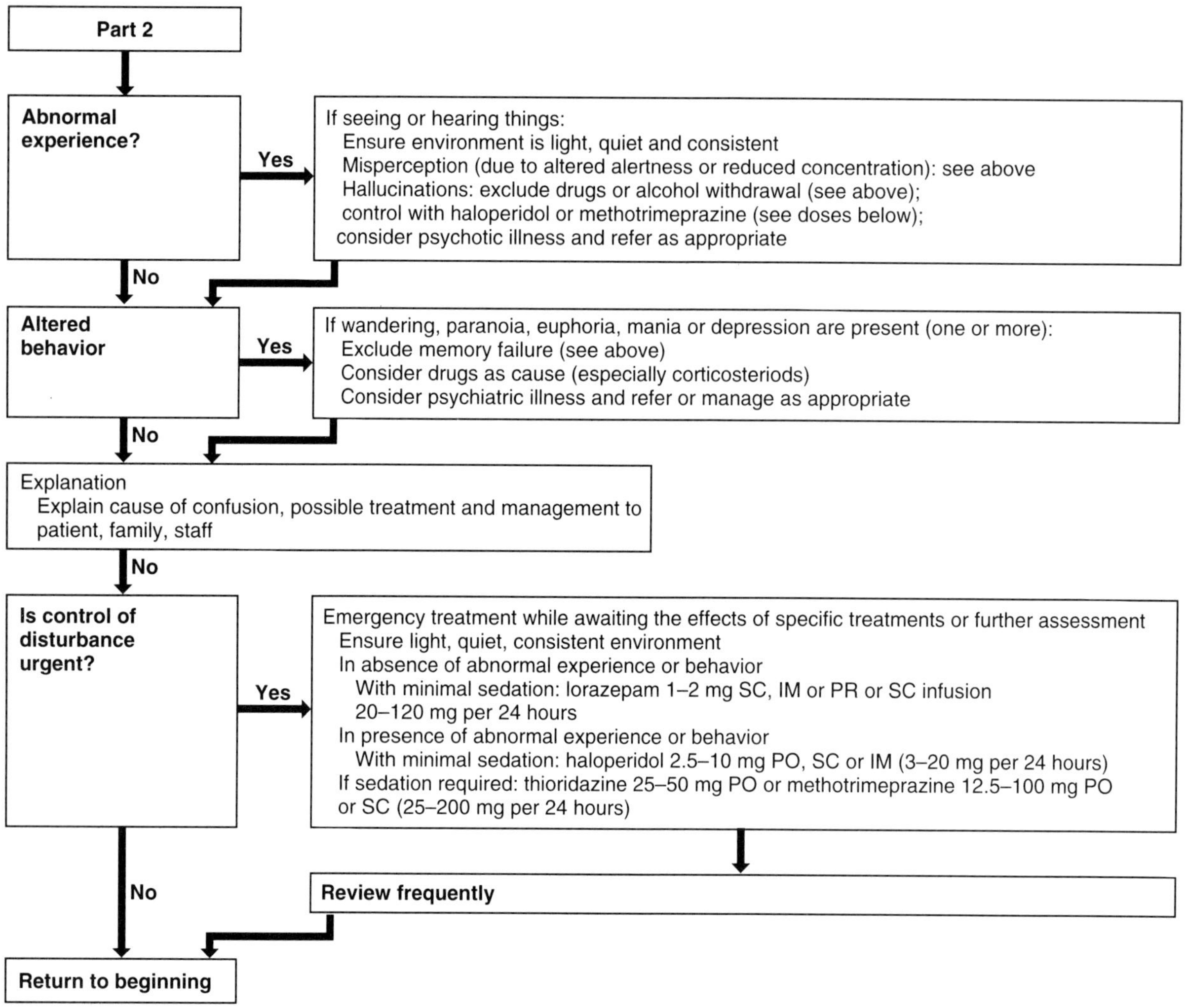

Figure 34.3. *continued*

Table 34.8. Palliative care services available in the UK.

Hospital
- Oncology teams, including chaplain and social worker
- Nurse specialists: breast counseling; chemotherapy; palliative care ('Macmillan,' 'terminal,' 'Support')
- Support/terminal care team (doctor, nurse specialist(s), chaplain, social worker)
- Psychologists/psychiatrists

Community
- General Practitioner
- Community nurses
- Community nurse specialists: palliative care ('Macmillan,' 'Special Care')
- Social Services
- Day hospice/hospice outpatients

Palliative care units

Chronic palliative care units Acute palliative care units	Hospice, Continuing care unit, Macmillan Unit, Marie Curie Home, Sue Ryder Home

Palliative care units offer in-patient care together with one or more of the following: day care, outpatient care, palliative nurse specialist community support, hospital support, telephone advisory service, bereavement service, palliative information service, higher specialist training in palliative medicine, educational services and resources

Summary of Core Information

- Despite the resources and care spent on women with gynecologic malignancies, it remains a sobering fact that at least half will die from their disease.
- For many women, palliation of their physical, psychologic and social difficulties becomes of paramount importance.
- Diagnosing the cause of pain is an essential requisite to choosing an appropriate analgesic treatment, as well as understanding analgesics, including the strong opioids.
- The management of constipation, nausea, vomiting, bowel obstruction and a range of other symptoms is of great importance to the very ill patient.
- Psychologic support of the anxious, depressed, or confused patient is required as is the range of palliative care services available.
- Effective palliative care demands adequate knowledge, anticipation of problems, and an empathetic approach that enables treatment choices to be made that are appropriate to the individual woman.

References

Adelson MD & Kasowitz MH (1993) Percutaneous endoscopic drainage gastrostomy in the treatment of gastrointestinal obstruction from intraperitoneal malignancy. *Obstet. Gynecol.* **81:** 467–741.

Allan SG (1988) Emesis in the patient with advanced cancer. *Pall. Med.* **2(2):** 89–100.

■ Anonymous (1994) Tramadol – a new analgesic. *Drug Ther. Bull.* **32:** 85–87.

Ashby MA, Game PA, Devitt P *et al.* (1991) Percutaneous gastrostomy as a venting procedure in palliative medicine. *Pall. Med.* **5:** 147–150.

Badger C & Regnard C (1989) Oedema in advanced disease – a flow diagram. *Pall. Med.* **3(3):** 213–215.

Baines MJ, Oliver DJ & Carter RL (1985) Medical management of intestinal obstruction in patients with advanced malignant disease: a clinical and pathological study. *Lancet* **ii:** 90–93.

Beattie GJ, Leonard RCF & Smyth JF (1989) Bowel obstruction in ovarian carcinoma: a retrospective study and review of the literature. *Pall. Med.* **3:** 275–280.

Bonica JJ (1990) Cancer pain: current status and future needs. In: Bonica JJ (ed) *The Management of Pain*, 2nd ed, pp. 400–445. Philadelphia: Lea and Febiger.

Bristow A & Foster SMG (1988) Lumbar sympathectomy in the management of rectal tenesmoid pain. *Ann. R. Coll. Surg. Engl.* **70:** 38–39.

Bruera E, Macmillan K, Hanson J & MacDonald N (1989) The cognitive effects of the administration of narcotic analgesics in patients with cancer pain. *Pain* **39:** 13–16.

Bruera E & Fainsinger RL (1993) Clinical management of cachexia and anorexia. In: Doyle D, Hanks GW & MacDonald N (eds) *Oxford Textbook of Palliative Medicine*, pp. 330–337. Oxford: Oxford University Press.

Bullock N & Whitaker RH (1985) Massive bladder haemorrhage. *Br. Med. J.* **291:** 1522–1523.

Calman KC, Benton TF, Berkley TF *et al.* (1989) *Teaching and Learning in Palliative Medicine. Report of Working Party*. Edinburgh: St Oswald's Hospice, Newcastle upon Tyne, UK.

Clemons, M (1990) *Alertness and Morphine in Patients with Advanced Cancer*. BMSc. Thesis. Newcastle: University of Newcastle upon Tyne.

Constans T, Dutertre J & Froge E (1991) Hypodermoclysis in dehydrated elderly patients – local effects with and without hyaluronidase. *J. Pall. Care* **7:** 10–12.

■ Doyle D, Hanks GWC & McDonald N (eds) (1993) *Oxford Textbook of Palliative Medicine*. Oxford: Oxford Medical Publications. A Guide to Symptom Relief.

Dunphy KP & Amesbury BDW (1990) A comparison of hospice and home care patients: patterns of referral, patient characteristics and predictions of place of death. *Pall. Med.* **4:** 105–111.

Fainsinger RL, MacEachern T, Miller MJ *et al.* (1994) The use of hypodermoclysis for rehydration in terminally ill cancer patients. *J. Pain Sympt. Manag.* **9:** 298–302.

Fisken RA, Heath DA & Bold AM (1980) Hypercalcaemia: a hospital survey. *Q. J. Med.* **49:** 405–418.

Fogel MR *et al.* (1981) Diuresis in the ascitic patient: a randomised controlled trial of three regimens. *J. Clin. Gastroenterol.* **3(Suppl. 1):** 73–80.

Foley KM (1979) Pain syndromes in patients with cancer. In: Bonica JJ & Ventrafridda V (eds) *Advances in Pain Research and Therapy*, Vol. 2, pp. 59–75. New York: Raven Press.

Green DE & Phillips GL (1986) Vaginal prosthesis for control of vesicovaginal fistula. *Gynecol. Oncol.* **23:** 119–123.

Greenwald HP, Bonica JJ & Bergner M (1987) The prevalence of pain in four cancers. *Cancer* **60:** 2563–2569.

Greenway B, Johnson PJ & Williams R (1982) Control of malignant ascites with spironolactone. *Br. J. Surg.* **69:** 441–442.

Hanks GW (1994) Hospital palliative care teams and the disadvantaged dying. *Eur. J. Pall. Care* **1:** 112.

Hanks G & Hoskin PJ (1987) Opioid analgesics in the management of pain in patients with advanced cancer: a review. *Pall. Med.* **1(1):** 1025.

Hinton J (1994) Can home care maintain an acceptable quality of life for patients with terminal cancer and their relatives? *Pall. Med.* **8:** 183–196.

Hoskin PJ (1993) Radiotherapy in symptom management. In: Doyle D, Hanks GW & MacDonald N (eds) *Oxford Textbook of Palliative Medicine*, pp. 117–129. Oxford: Oxford University Press.

Inturrisi CE, Max MB, Foley KM *et al.* (1984) The pharmacokinetics of heroin in patients with chronic pain. *New Engl. J. Med.* **310:** 1213–1217.

Isbister WH, Elder P & Symons L (1990) Non-operative

management of malignant intestinal obstruction. *J. Roy. Coll. Surg.* **35:** 369–372.

Jaeckle KA, Young DF & Foley KM (1985) The natural history of lumbosacral plexopathy in cancer. *Neurology* **35:** 8–15.

Kaiko RF *et al.* (1982) Narcotics in the elderly. *Med. Clin. N. Am.* **66**(5): 1079–1089.

Kaye PM & Oliver DJ (1985) Hypercalcaemia in advanced malignancy. *Lancet* **i:** 512.

Khoo D, Hall E & Motson R (1994) Palliation of malignant intestinal obstruction using octreotide. *Eur. J. Cancer* **30A:** 28–30.

Kisner CD & Kesner KM (1987) Use of the transverse colon conduit for vesicovaginal fistula in late stage carcinoma of cervix. *Br. J. Urol.* **59:** 234–238.

Librach SL & Rapson LM (1988) The use of transcutaneous electric nerve stimulation (TENS) for the relief of pain in palliative care. *Pall. Med.* **2**(1): 15–20.

Lombard DJ & Oliver DJ (1989) The use of opioid analgesics in the last 24 hours of life of patients with advanced cancer. *Pall. Med.* **3**(1): 27–29.

Maguire P, Faulkner A & Regnard C (1995) The anxious person. In: Regnard CFB & Hockley J (eds) *Flow Diagrams in Advanced Cancer and other Diseases.*, pp. 73–76. London: Edward Arnold.

Mercadente S & Maddaloni S (1992) Octreotide in the management of inoperable gastrointestinal obstruction in terminal cancer patients. *J. Pain Sympt. Manag.* **7:** 496–498.

■ Open Learning Series in Palliative Care. Modules on pain control, controlling symptoms, psychological needs, caring for the carers, bereavement and lymphoedema. Information from St. Oswald's Hospice, Regent Avenue, Gosforth, Newcastle upon Tyne, NE3 1EE.

O'Rourke NP, McCloskey EV, Vasikaran S *et al.* (1993) Effective treatment of malignant hypercalcaemia with a single intravenous infusion of clodronate. *Br. J. Cancer***67:** 560–563.

Osipova NA, Novikov GA, Beresnev VA & Loseva NA (1991) Analgesic effect of tramadol in cancer patients with chronic pain: a comparison with prolonged-action morphine sulfate. *Curr. Ther. Res.* **50:** 812–821.

Palacios JM, Wamsley JK & Kuhar MJ (1981) The distribution of histamine H_1-receptors in the rat brain: an autoradiographic study. *Neuroscience* **6:** 15–17.

Patwardhan RV *et al.* (1981) Normal metabolism of morphine in cirrhosis. *Gastroenterology* **81:** 1006–1011.

Peroutka SJ & Snyder SH (1982) Antiemetics neurotransmitter receptor binding predicts therapeutic actions. *Lancet* **i:** 658–659.

Ralston SH (1992) Medical management of hypercalcaemia. *Br. J. Clin. Pharmacol.* **34:** 11–20.

Rawlins MD (1993) Non-opioid analgesics. In: Doyle D, Hanks GW & MacDonald N (eds) *Oxford Textbook of Palliative Medicine*, pp. 182–187. Oxford: Oxford University Press.

Regnard CFB (1995) Bowel obstruction. In: Regnard CFB & Hockley J (eds) *Flow Diagrams in Advanced Cancer and Other Diseases*, pp. 29–31. London: Edward Arnold.

Regnard CFB & Comiskey M (1995) Nausea and vomiting. In: Regnard CFB and Hockley J (eds) *Flow Diagrams in Advanced Cancer and Other Diseases.* pp. 14–18. London: Edward Arnold.

Regnard C & Fitton S (1995) Mouth care. In: Regnard C, Hockley (eds) *Flow Diagrams in Advanced Cancer and Other Diseases*, pp. 22–24. London: Edward Arnold.

■ Regnard C & Hockley J (eds) (1995) *Flow Diagrams in Advanced Cancer and Other Diseases.* London: Edward Arnold.

Regnard CFB & Mannix KA (1995) Ascites. In: Regnard CFB and Hockley J (eds) *Flow Diagrams in Advanced Cancer and Other Diseases*, pp. 36–38. London: Edward Arnold.

Regnard CFB & Stedeford A (1995) Confusion. In: Regnard CFB and Hockley J (eds) *Flow Diagrams in Advanced Cancer and Other Diseases*, pp. 68–72. London: Edward Arnold.

Regnard CFB & Tempest S (1992) *A Guide to Symptom Relief in Advanced Cancer.* Manchester: Haigh & Hochland.

Regnard CFB, Pashley S & Westrope F (1986) Antiemetic/ diamorphine compatability in infusion pumps. *Br. J. Pharmaceut. Pract.* **8**(8): 218–220.

Regnard C, Badger C & Mortimer P (1988) *Lymphoedema: Advice on Treatment.* Beaconsfield, Beaconsfield Publishers.

Selby PC, Peacock M & Marshall DH (1984) Hypercalcaemia: management. *Br. J. Hosp. Med.* **March:** 186–197.

Sjõberg M, Appelgren L, Einarsson S *et al.* (1991) Long-term intrathecal morphine and bupivicaine in "refractory" cancer pain. 1. Results from the first series of 52 patients. *Acta Anaesthesiol. Scand.* **35:** 30–43.

Stedeford A (1987) Hospice: a safe place to suffer? *Pall. Med.* **1:** 73–74.

■ Stedeford A (1994) *Facing Death: Patients, Families and Professionals*, 2nd Edition. Oxford: Sobell Publications.

Stedeford A (1994a) Depression, requests for euthanasia and related problems. In: *Facing Death: Patients, Families and Professionals*, pp. 129–147. Oxford: Sobell Publications.

Stedeford A (1994b) Confusion. In: *Facing Death: Patients, Families and Professionals*, pp. 149–163. Oxford: Sobell Publications.

Stevens MJ & Gonet YM (1990) Malignant psoas syndrome: recognition of an oncologic entity. *Australas. Radiol.* **34:** 150–154.

Stefanni E & Clement–Cormier Y (1981) Detection of dopamine receptors in the area postrema. *Eur. J. Pharmacol.* **74:** 257–260.

Sykes NP (1993) Constipation and diarrhoea. In: Doyle D, Hanks GW & MacDonald N (eds) *Oxford Textbook of Palliative Medicine*, pp. 299–310. Oxford: Oxford University Press.

Tarin D, Price JE, Kettlewell MGW *et al.* (1984) Clinicopathological observations on metastases in man studied in patients with peritoneovenous shunts. *Br. Med. J.* **288:** 749–751.

Thompson JW & Filshie J (1993) Transcutaneous electrical nerve stimulation (TENS) and acupuncture. In: Doyle D, Hanks GW & MacDonald N (eds) *Oxford Textbook of Palliative Medicine*, pp. 229–244. Oxford: Oxford University Press.

Tunca JC, Buchler DA, Mack EA *et al.* (1981) The management of ovarian cancer-caused bowel obstruction. *Gynecol. Oncol.* **12:** 186–192.

Twycross RG (1977) Choice of strong analgesic in terminal cancer: diamorphine or morphine? *Pain* **3:** 93–104.

■ Twycross R (1994) *Pain Relief in Advanced Camcer.* Edinburgh: Churchill Livingstone.

Twycross R (1994a) Strong opioids II. In: *Pain Relief in Advanced Cancer*, pp. 277–305. Edinburgh: Churchill Livingstone.

Twycross R (1994b) Misunderstandings about morphine. In: *Pain Relief in Advanced Cancer*, pp. 333–347. Edinburgh: Churchill Livingstone.

Twycross R (1994c) Miscellaneous drug. In: *Pain Relief in*

Advanced Cancer, pp. 455–486. Edinburgh: Churchill Livingstone.

Twycross RG & Badger C (1988) *Management of Lymphoedema: Guidelines*. Oxford: Sir Michael Sobell House, Churchill Hospital.

Twycross RG & Fairfield S (1982) Pain in far-advanced cancer. *Pain* **14:** 303–310.

Vachon MLS (1988) Counselling and psychotherapy in palliative/hospice care: a review. *Pall. Med.* **2:** 36–50.

Walsh TD (1984) Opiates and respiratory function in advanced cancer. *Rec. Res. Cancer Res.* **89:** 115–117.

Wells JCD (1989) The use of nerve destruction for relief of pain in cancer: a review. *Pall. Med.* **3:** 239–247.

Wilder-Smith CH, Schimke J, Osterwalder B & Senn H-J (1994) Oral tramadol, a μ-opioid agonist and monoamine reuptake-blocker and morphine for strong cancer-related pain. *Ann. Oncol.* **5:** 141–146.

Wilkes E (1984) Dying now. *Lancet* **i:** 950–952.

35 Hormone Replacement Therapy After the Diagnosis and Treatment of Hormone Sensitive Tumors

R Sands
J Studd

Introduction

Hormone-related cancers such as breast and endometrial cancer account for more than 40% of all newly diagnosed malignancies in women in developed countries. The notion that the use of hormone replacement therapy (HRT) is likely to increase the incidence of these tumors and promote their growth seems logical, but is probably too simplistic as epidemiologic studies have consistently reported a survival advantage for those women who have used HRT compared to non-users.

The prognosis of women with hormone-related cancers has improved due to early screening and modern therapy, resulting in an increase in the prevalence of women treated for cancer. Unfortunately this gain in longevity is not necessarily complemented by an improvement in quality of life since the majority of premenopausal women are rendered menopausal and estrogen-deficient either due to their primary surgery or adjuvant therapy. Women who have undergone ovarian ablation also lose the ongoing production of ovarian androgens. The treatment of menopausal symptoms with estrogens in women with hormone-sensitive cancers has traditionally been contraindicated whether the cancer was diagnosed pre- or postmenopausally because of the theoretic risk of hastening the overt appearance of dormant metastases or increasing the risk of a new growth in a high-risk patient. This prohibition has been challenged by recent clinical reviews and prescribing practice has become less dogmatic

In addressing the subject of HRT in malignancy it would be appropriate to review the following:

- the benefits of estrogen replacement therapy (ERT), and progestogen and androgen replacement;
- the data gleaned from 'natural experiments;'
- retrospective data regarding the use of HRT in women following treatment for cancer and their outcome;
- the application of this information to women with cancer of the breast, endometrium, ovary, cervix and melanoma.

Benefits of Hormone Replacement Therapy

The decline in ovarian function that produces the menopause gives rise to an endocrinopathy, which leads to multisystem changes. Vasomotor symptoms affect 75% of postmenopausal women and are subjectively debilitating in 30% of cases. They persist for longer than five years in 25% and may be lifelong in a small minority (Studd *et al.*, 1977). The quality of life of menopausal women is further influenced by insomnia and symptoms of depression, anxiety and irritability, which may occur in up to 30% of climacteric women (Montgomery *et al.*, 1987). The estrogen deficiency also causes atrophic changes to end-organs, particularly the genitourinary systems with the sequelae of dyspareonia or apareunia and urinary symptoms of frequency, voiding difficulties and urgency. These genitourinary symptoms compound the loss of sexuality and may be very disturbing to women who already have had an altered body image because of the diagnosis and treatment of cancer. Similarly any feelings of depression can be aggravated by the sex hormone deficient state associated with the menopause (Studd, 1992).

Generalized atrophy of the connective tissue manifests as skin thinning, brittle nails, loss of hair and osteoporosis. A major impact of decreased estrogens on long-term health is the progressive increase in cardiovascular disease, with myocardial infarction constituting the leading cause of death in the elderly. This is probably mediated through increased arterial impedance as well as adverse lipid changes. Osteoporosis with its attendant risk of fracture is an important consequence of estrogen deficiency. It has been calculated that one in four women at the age of 70 years will have one or more osteoporotic fractures and for women treated for cancer with chemotherapy premenopausally this risk is increased. Estrogen therapy not only prevents bone loss, but can produce a substantial increase in bone density, particularly using percutaneous estrogen when higher levels of estrogen are achieved (Studd *et al.*, 1994). (*Table 35.1*).

Table 35.1. Life-time risks of disease for a 50-year-old Caucasian woman (from Grady *et al.*, 1992).

	Probability of developing (%)	*Probability of dying (%)*	*Median age (yrs)*
Coronary heart disease	46	31	74
Stroke	20	8	83
Osteoporotic fracture	15	1.5	79
Breast cancer	10	3	68
Endometrial cancer	2.6	0.3	69

The benefits of ERT are well established. Administration of ERT alleviates vasomotor symptoms in nearly all women and reduces menopausal-related psychogenic problems, and ERT is the most effective treatment for atrophic vaginitis and estrogen deficiency-related urinary symptoms. It reduces the risk of coronary artery disease by 40%, decreases the incidence of significant coronary atherosclerosis and prolongs survival in those with established coronary disease (Stampfer and Colditz, 1991). Morbidity is further substantially reduced by the bone sparing/replacing effect of estrogen and it has been calculated that five years of HRT halves the lifetime risk of a hip fracture (Lindsay, 1988). There is evidence that the sex hormones are involved in cognitive functioning, mood and probably play a preventive role in Alzheimer's disease (Holloway, 1992).

Cyclical progestogen is used in conjunction with ERT for its antiproliferative effect on the endometrium. Unopposed estrogen results in a 15% incidence of endometrial hyperplasia, which is reduced to 0% by the concurrent use of 12 days of progestogen (Sturdee *et al.*, 1977). Because of the dose-dependent side-effects including depression, irritability, loss of energy, loss of libido and mastalgia in up to 30% of women, it is unnecessary in women who have had a hysterectomy. However, progestogen administration (at variable dosages) may be valuable for the treatment of some tumors or the alleviation of vasomotor symptoms in those very few cases where estrogen is thought to be contraindicated.

Women who have had a medical or surgical ovarian ablation loose not only production of ovarian estrogens, but also androgens. This 'andropause' can lead to multiple changes affecting the skin and muscle, and symptoms of loss of energy, depression and sexual dysfunction, which respond well to a combination of ERT and androgen replacement therapy (Brincat *et al.*, 1984). Furthermore there is some evidence that androgens may protect against neoplasia and enhance immune surveillance (Gordon *et al.*, 1987). It may prove to be a valuable adjunct to ERT.

It is possible that HRT is the most important advance in preventive medicine in developed countries in the last half-century (Studd, 1992); it contributes significantly to enhancing the quality of life of many postmenopausal women. However, there is uncertainty as to whether this therapy is responsible for any increase in malignancy in estrogen-sensitive organs; the mortality from breast and endometrial cancer in estrogen users is no greater than for non-users. There is even debate as to whether ERT is contraindicated in women with a past history of these cancers.

Breast Cancer

Breast cancer is the most common malignancy in women in the UK with 25,000 new cases diagnosed each year, resulting in 15,000 deaths per annum. Despite this mortality rate the number of women with a near normal life expectancy following the diagnosis of localized breast cancer is ever increasing due to early detection and improved therapy (Kelsey and Gammon, 1990). This associated increase in survival is not necessarily complemented by an increase in quality of life since women successfully treated for breast cancer may face several decades of estrogen deficiency postmenopausally and the treatment modalities used may also cause a premature menopause. These women are usually denied HRT because of the prevailing view that breast cancer is an unequivocal contraindication to HRT.

A recent survey of 174 women with breast cancer revealed that 40% of menopausal and 59% of premenopausal women were prepared to consider taking estrogen replacement therapy under close medical supervision (Vassilopoulou–Sellin and Zoninski, 1992). Their concerns about heart disease and osteoporosis together with distress about the vasomotor and other physical symptoms would seem to be equipoised with the theoretic risk of precipitating recurrence of the tumor. The fear of recurrence among clinicians treating breast cancer is based on epidemiologic, biologic and clinical data.

Arguments Against the Use of Hormone Replacement Therapy

Many of the epidemiologic risk factors for breast cancer have an endocrinologic component. Prolonged endogenous hormone production is associated with early menarche, late menopause, large number of menstrual cycles (Brinton *et al.*, 1988), and obesity (Lupin *et al.*, 1985). All these factors increase the relative risk of primary breast cancer. Conversely hormone deprivation caused either by a premature oophorectomy and early menopause (Negri *et al.*, 1988) are associated with a decreased risk (*Table 35.2*).

A number of laboratory studies have demonstrated the ability of estrogens to generate mammary tumors in animals (Jordan, 1976) and act as a growth factor for established breast cancer cell lines (Darbre and King, 1988). In clinical practice it has long been recognized that depriving breast cancer lines of estrogen, either by oophorectomy or by competitive binding of estrogen receptors (e.g. tamoxifen), thereby decreasing estrogen at a cellular level, are effective treatments producing remission in 30% of women with advanced breast cancer (Early Breast Cancer Trialists' Collaborative Group, 1992). However, there is growing evidence that women with breast cancer when exposed to endogenous or exogenous estrogen do not have a real increased risk of cancer recurrence and high estrogen doses may sometimes be used for therapy.

Endogenous Estrogen

There is very little correlation between endogenous levels of estradiol and initiation and promotion of breast cancer growth. On the other hand premenopausal women with estradiol levels more than ten times higher than postmenopausal women have a better prognosis when matched for stage at diagnosis (Adami *et al.*, 1987). Premenopausal women with breast cancer who subsequent to chemotherapy return to cyclical ovarian function and renew menstruation have no significant difference in outcome compared to those who do not (Sacks *et al.*, 1993). Furthermore, treatment with tamoxifen, which is effective against breast cancer, results in a significant rise in serum estradiol levels in premenopausal women from a range of 296–367 pmol l^{-1} during the follicular phase to a mean value of 1800 pmol l^{-1} after two months of tamoxifen treatment (Neven *et al.*, 1993).

Table 35.2. Risk factors for breast cancer (includes all variables except nulliparous women; from Negri *et al.*, 1988). (*Reference category.)

Variable		*Relative risk*	*Confidence intervals*
Age at menarche	>15*	1	
(yrs)	12–14	1.32	1.15–1.52
Age at menopause	>50*	1	
(yrs)	45–49	0.77	0.67–0.90
	<45	0.73	0.61–0.88
Parity	1*	1	
	2	0.99	0.87–1.12
	3–4	0.99	0.86–1.15
	>5	0.62	0.50–0.76
Body mass index	<20*	1	—
in menopausal	25–29	1.3	—
women	>30	1.6	—

Although a number of studies have implicated that increased levels of plasma-free estradiol are seen in women with breast cancer when compared with matched controls without breast cancer, these results are not consistent, possibly because of small sample size and incomplete matching for age, weight and stage distribution, all of which may represent sources of bias between case and control populations.

It is possible to examine the effect of increased endogenous hormones on breast cancer since 3% of patients diagnosed with breast cancer are either pregnant or lactating, and 7% of women who are fertile postmastectomy will go on to have children. Early investigators believed that gestational breast cancer was a more aggressive tumor than non-pregnancy breast cancer and 50 years ago it was declared incurable and attempts at surgery futile (Haagensen, 1943). The popular opinion was that the increase in estradiol levels was responsible for this and the logical extension of this theory was that methods aimed at decreasing hormone levels (termination of pregnancy and oophorectomy) would be beneficial. This rational therapy was not helpful. More recent studies reveal that the outcome in women, when matched for age and stage of disease, is no different than the results in non-pregnant women (Petrek *et al.*, 1991), and that the additional factor of pregnancy does not confer a worse prognosis. This is further supported by the evidence that attempts at decreasing endogenous levels of estrogen with oophorectomy or termination of pregnancy have not been shown in prospective studies to improve the outcome of pregnant woman with breast cancer (Hoover, 1990), and women who become pregnant after treatment for breast cancer have similar or better overall survival when controlled for age and stage (Donegan, 1977).

This discrepancy between the traditional teaching and the current analysis can be partly explained. A breast lump in pregnancy is difficult to detect due to physiologic hypertrophy. Definitive histologic investigations on new masses are often deferred until the end of the pregnancy with the mistaken belief that it is a normal consequence of pregnancy. Mammography is perceived as harmful to the fetus and when performed has a poor diagnostic yield because of increased density associated with pregnancy. Consequently the diagnosis is made at a later stage and more advanced disease is being treated (Peters, 1968). The pathology is identical to that found in non-pregnant women and in common with premenopausal women, most of the cancers are estrogen receptor and progestogen receptor negative (Nugent and O'Connell, 1985).

Exogenous Estrogen

The epidemiologic evidence does not support the view that the oral contraceptive pill (OCP) increases the risk of primary breast cancer (FDA Drug Bulletin, 1984). Furthermore, females with breast cancer who have been exposed to the OCP during the evolution phase of the tumor do not have an inferior prognosis when matched for age and parity with a control group without a history of OCP exposure (Rosner and Lane, 1986).

The use of HRT does not incur a major increase in the risk of breast cancer in the normal population. The conclusions of all the observational and case-controlled studies of HRT use and breast cancer are contradictory. However two of the four meta-analyses published to date show a duration exposure risk of about 25–30% above controls after 15 years of use (Steinberg *et al.*, 1991; Grady and Ernster, 1991) (*Table 35.3*). The two other studies showed no significant increase in breast cancer risk with HRT and no effect of duration, dosage, or type of estrogen (Dupont and Page, 1991; Armstrong, 1988). There is the confounding factor that the theoretic increase in risk of breast cancer in HRT-users may be confined to women with a modest alcohol consumption (Colditz *et al.*, 1990).

There is a clear correlation between a family history (on the maternal side) and an increased risk of breast cancer at a young age. This increased risk is mainly for premenopausal cancer and after the menopause the risk for most women reverts back to the risk for their age group. This risk of breast cancer in women with a family history does not appear to be altered by HRT use, possibly because HRT is being used at a time when these women no longer have an increased risk.

The slight excess observed with prolonged use can be explained by the increased surveillance these patients received, which would result in a greater proportion of early-stage tumors (Studd, 1989). This view is supported by the significantly decreased mortality from breast cancer in patients receiving estrogen therapy (Bergkvist *et al.*, 1989; Hunt *et al.*, 1987).

In women with benign breast disease, HRT seems to be protective in those with atypical hyperplasia and proliferative disease without atypia. A large study demonstrated that HRT lowered the relative risk of breast cancer in patients with atypical hyperplasia from 4.5 to 3 (Dupont, 1989). There is a view that the factors operative in the increase of endometrial carcinoma of better prognosis in the 1970s (more screening, difficulty in distinguishing between borderline atypical hyperplasia and invasive carcinoma and biologically less invasive tumor) may explain the apparent increase in breast cancer or may partly reflect the unique biologic characteristics of estrogen-associated tumors (Studd, 1989). It is notable that at the time of writing there is not a sentence in the literature indicating an increase in mortality from breast cancer in estrogen users compared with a matched population of non-users.

Hormone Replacement Therapy After Breast Cancer

There is a paucity of published data on the use of HRT in women treated for breast cancer. *Table 35.4* summarizes the outcome in the five series published to date. Although these studies report on only a total of 277 women followed up for a relatively short period and used various formulations and dosages

Table 35.3. Meta-analyses of breast cancer incidence among hormone replacement therapy users versus non-users. (RR, relative risk; CI, confidence interval.)

Authors	*Effects of ever use RR (95% CI)*	*Use more than 15 years RR (95% CI)*	*Special risk group RR (95% CI)*
Armstrong, 1988	0.96 (0.98–1.05)	1.04 (0.88–1.24)	Nil identified
Dupont and Page, 1991	1.08 (0.96–1.2)	No conclusion	Nil identified
Steinberg *et al.*, 1991	1.0	1.3 (1.2–1.6)	Family history 3.4
Grady and Ernster, 1991	No increase	1.25	Nil identified

Table 35.4. Hormone replacement therapy (HRT) in women with a history of breast cancer. (NED, no evidence of disease; REL, relapse; IS, *in situ*; CONJ, conjugated; NORG, norgestrol (0–15 mg.)

Authors	HRT	No.	Median age (yrs)	Stage IS	I	II	III	IV	Follow-up (months)	Outcome
Wile *et al.*, 1993	Varied	25	51	2	13	7	1	2	35	88% NED 12% REL
DiSaia, 1993	Varied	77	50	6	43	17	5	6	59	92% NED 8% REL
Stoll and Parbhoo, 1988	CONJ 0.625 NORG	50	?			—			24	100% NED
Powles *et al.*, 1993	Varied	35	51		12	14	9		43	94% NED 6% REL
Eden *et al.*, 1995	Varied	90	?			—			>72	93% NED 7% REL

of HRT with various stages of breast cancer, none showed an increased risk of relapse.

Eden *et al.* (1995) treated 90 women who previously had cancer and complained of distressing symptoms of estrogen deficiency with HRT. In 1992 each of these women was matched with two control patients who also had breast cancer but did not receive HRT. Mean tumor size and follow-up period (>6 years) were similar between these two groups. Breast cancer recurred in 7% of HRT users with no deaths recorded and in 17% of non-users with 6% deaths. Although these figures represent a small number of patients, these results are encouraging.

Tamoxifen

Adjuvant tamoxifen produces a highly significant decrease in the annual rate of recurrence and death and risk of developing contralateral cancer (Jones and Powles, 1993). This decrease in mortality is maintained for 10 years although it may have been used for only two years. It is of particular use in postmenopausal women. Tamoxifen is not essentially an estrogen antagonist, but rather a partial estrogen agonist that acts by competitive binding to estrogen receptors. Its mechanism of action in the treatment of breast cancer is still unknown (Neven *et al.*, 1993) since estradiol levels in females receiving tamoxifen are substantially raised and patients with estrogen receptor-negative tumors also respond to tamoxifen. There is evidence that tamoxifen stimulates stromal cells to secrete growth inhibiting factors for neighboring breast cancer cells, thus acting indirectly in its anti-tumor effect (Benson and Baum, 1993). Tamoxifen decreases the risk of osteoporosis (Love *et al.*, 1992) and has a favorable estrogenic effect on the lipid profile (Love *et al.*, 1990), but it can produce debilitating vasomotor symptoms. Irregular periods and vaginal dryness or discharge occur in 15–20% of women. There are also concerns regarding its possible role in inducing other endometrial (Fornander *et al.*, 1989) or hepatic tumors after long-term use.

Progestogens

The effect of progestogens on the breast is confusing. Megestrol acetate, a progestogen, has been found to be an effective treatment for hot flushes, but the effect of progestogens on breast tissue is uncertain. Laboratory studies have demonstrated that both progesterone agonists and antagonists have an anti-tumor effect on breast cancer cells (Bakker *et al.*, 1989). Although early clinical studies suggested that progestogens are protective against the development of breast cancer (Gambrell *et al.*, 1993), recent studies have not confirmed this finding (UK National Case Control Study, 1989). This subject, as well as the possible different influence of androgenic progestogens, still needs clarification.

Recommendations

A prospective randomized trial is needed to study the effect of HRT on women who have been treated for breast cancer.

Until the dilemma is resolved it would seem acceptable to offer HRT:

- to women who were treated for cancer premenopausally and who were subsequently stimulated by their own endogenous estrogens with resumption of their periods without any adverse effect;

- where it would improve the quality of life significantly;
- to patients with a low bone density;
- in conjunction with tamoxifen for the relief of vasomotor symptoms.

Endometrial Cancer

The knowledge of a hormone-tumor relationship has evolved largely from our understanding of the effect of steroid hormones on the uterus, an organ of clearly defined endocrine effects and furthermore easily accessible for tissue sampling. It has long been observed that obesity, infertility due to failure of ovulation, dysfunctional bleeding in the perimenopausal years, theca–granulosa cell tumors and the Stein–Leventhal syndrome are all associated with endometrial cancer. It was noted that prolonged stimulation of the uterus by estrogen without progestational modification produced an endometrial cancer precursor, adenomatous hyperplasia (Gusberg, 1947). In 1948, Novak and Rutledge distinguished this type of hyperplasia from cystic glandular hyperplasia, and soon after Hertig *et al.* (1949) confirmed this entity as a cancer precursor and called its extreme form carcinoma *in situ*. With the acceptance of this precursor concept the search in the 1950s was for an estrogen antidote. Such an antagonist was provided by the studies that described control of some metastatic lesions with large doses of progestin (Kelley and Baker, 1960).

The development of steroid receptor science in the 1960s helped characterize these estrogen-related tumors; namely slow growing, well-differentiated, relatively benign cancers sharing the biologic properties of their host tissues.

The concept that hormonally-dependent tumors are highly curable has become well-known and is illustrated by the relative stability of the incidence rate of endometrial cancer from 1950–1970, after which a significant rise occurred. The overall rate rose from 23.2 per 100,000 in 1950 to 33.2 per 100,000 in 1975, a rise of 43%. There was a decline thereafter to a rate of 23.4 per 100,000 in 1985, not significantly different from the 1950 figure (Gusberg, 1989). The mortality rate was unchanged during this time. In the late 1970s several gynecologic studies revealed an increase in endometrial cancer in women taking unapposed estrogen (Ziel and Finkle, 1975; Smith *et al.*, 1975). The protective effects of progestogen were soon appreciated and it has now become routine to give at least ten days of progesterone per cycle (Studd and Thom, 1981). Overall this combination therapy does not increase the incidence of endometrial cancer and those women who develop endometrial cancer secondary to its use have a better prognosis compared to non-HRT related cancers; the five-year survival is 92% compared to 68% in non-users with endometrial cancer (Collins *et al.*, 1980).

The use of sequential and cyclical regimens are increasingly being replaced by continuous estrogen/progestogen therapies that do not produce bleeding. However, it is not clear whether the latter is as effective as sequential regimens in reducing the risk of endometrial cancer (Leather *et al.*, 1991; Woodruff and Pickar, 1994).

Estrogen Replacement Therapy After Endometrial Cancer

It is not surprising that estrogen replacement has been contraindicated in women cured of endometrial cancer, whether pre- or postmenopausal and that progestogens are given liberally.

Although endometrial cancer is usually a disease of postmenopausal women, at least 25% of cases occur in women aged 40–50 years. About 65% of these women are cured of their disease, but all are either menopausal or rendered menopausal as a result of their treatment. Many who are several years postmenopausal will also develop vasomotor symptoms because of the removal of the androgens produced by the ovarian stroma, which are converted peripherally to estrogens. Progestogens can eliminate vasomotor symptoms, but have a significant side-effect profile. In view of all these symptoms, some women treated for early endometrial cancer were treated with estrogens and several non-randomized series have been reported. The estrogen users have had no adverse effects (*Table 35.5, Figure 35.1*). Creaseman *et al.* (1986) compared 47 women with Stage IA and B against 174 controls and found a significant survival advantage for ERT users over controls and furthermore found that estrogen protected against recurrence. These findings are consistent with Lee (1990) in his series of 44 HRT users versus 99 controls.

Table 35.5. Hormone replacement therapy (HRT) in women treated for endometrial cancer.

Authors	HRT	No.	Median age (yrs)	Stage IA	IB	Follow-up (months)	Outcome (recurrence)
Creaseman *et al.*, 1986	Vaginal and oral	47	57	30	17	32	2.1%
Lee *et al.*, 1990	Oral	44	57	24	20	87	Nil
Woolas, 1994	Oral	4	<35	2	2	84	Nil

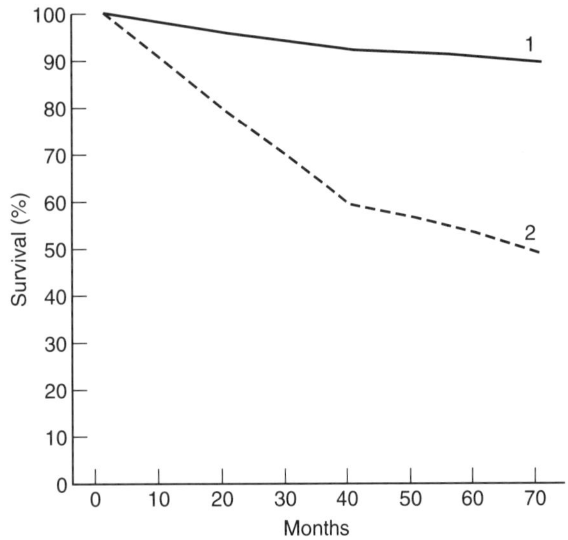

Figure 35.1. Endometrial cancer (Stage I, Grade III) survival (from Creaseman *et al.*, 1986). (1, E2 users; 2, non-users.)

These findings have challenged our understanding of hormone–tumor biology and hinted at the possible role of the immune system in affecting the tumor–host relationship.

The current recommendations for endometrial cancer patients are that estrogen replacement can be considered in those "selected candidates ... based on prognostic indicators and the risk the patient is willing to assume" (American College of Obstetricians and Gynecologists, Committee on Gynecologic Practice, 1990) and we suggest the following two groups.

- Women with Stage I endometrial cancer who have been appropriately managed. The chance of complete cure is very high and there should be no reason why combined HRT should not be commenced shortly after surgery. This may be one example where progestogen would be used in a woman without a uterus in addition to estrogen.
- Women with endometrial cancer with nodal involvement for whom ERT should not be used may be considered for treatment after three years providing there has been no recurrence.

Ovarian Cancer

Despite all the advances in diagnostic and therapeutic modalities in the management of ovarian cancer over the last 20 years, the overall five-year survival rate has remained at about 30%. A large number of women treated for ovarian cancer would benefit from HRT if it was shown not to increase the risk of recurrence. Understandably with the knowledge that ovarian tumor cells contain estrogen and progesterone receptors, coupled with early epidemiologic studies that showed an increased risk of ovarian cancer in women who received HRT (La Vecchia *et al.*, 1982), there has been some reluctance to prescribe HRT to women treated for ovarian cancer.

More recently, however, studies have demonstrated that HRT has a protective effect against ovarian cancer with risk ratios of 0.6–0.9 (Hunt *et al.*, 1987). This is supported by a retrospective analysis of woman with ovarian cancer who had received HRT and concluded that there was no evidence that HRT was detrimental to disease-free and overall survival (Eeles *et al.*, 1991).

The recommendation would be that since there is no risk HRT should be given to women with ovarian cancer. Administration could be commenced shortly after surgery for all stages with the possible exception of endometrioid tumors.

Cervical Cancer

The interplay of host–tumor defence mechanisms is partly illustrated in cancer of the cervix since it has been established that women who have human immunodeficiency virus or who are taking immunosuppressive treatment following transplants or who smoke have an increased incidence of cervical dysplasia. However, there is no evidence to implicate HRT in the etiology of cervical cancer, but it may theoretically stimulate adenocarcinoma of the cervix (Brinton, 1991). This issue still needs to be resolved, but a previously abnormal cervical smear, once appropriately managed, should be no contraindication to HRT. It has also been reported that women exposed to exogenous estrogens who subsequently develop cervical cancer have a lower than expected mortality (Hunt *et al.*, 1987). Therefore a good case could be made for ERT in premenopausal women following a radical hysterectomy or radiation since many will experience a premature menopause and run the risk of prolonged estrogen deficiency. A good proportion of women with cervical cancer are young and subsequent to adjuvant therapy experience a loss of libido due to androgen deficiency. By administering hormone implants (50 mg of estradiol and 100 mg testosterone) subcutaneously both osteoporosis and sexual dysfunction are treated and this should be regarded as the preferred method of treatment.

Melanoma

There is a view that the sex hormones are involved in the growth of melanoma. This belief is based upon anecdotal reports relating rapid growth of melanoma in pregnancy and the alleged increased risk of melanoma in women on the OCP (Beral *et al.*, 1977). However, recent reviews challenge this

Table 35.6. Hormonal and non-hormonal options for the treatment of complications of the menopause. (ERT, estrogen replacement therapy; PRT, progesterone replacement therapy; ART, androgen replacement therapy; ↓, decrease; ↑, increase; S/E, side effects.)

	Recurrence	*Cardiovascular disease*	*Bone density*	*Hot flushes*	*Vaginitis*	*Other*
ERT	?	↓	↑	↓	↓	
Topical ERT	?				↓	
PRT	?	?	↑	↓		S/E
ART	?	?	↑	↓	↓	S/E
Bisphosphonates			↑			
Tamoxifen	↓	↓	↑	↑	↑	Other cancer
Clonidine				↓		S/E

Table 35.7. An approach to women with cancer: considerations.

- Recurrence risk
  - Histopathology
  - Size of tumor
  - Nodal involvement
  - Type of therapy
  - Time elapsed since diagnosis
- Cardiovascular disease
  - Family history
  - Life-style
  - Metabolic profile
- Osteoporosis
  - Family history
  - Life-style
  - Drug history
  - Bone mineral density
- Menopausal symptoms
  - Vasomotor
  - Genitourinary symptoms
  - Quality of life

assertion and show no evidence to implicate exogenous estrogen, be it the OCP or HRT in the pathogenesis of melanoma. Furthermore contradictary evidence exists (Franceschi *et al.*, 1990); endogenous estrogens seem to have a beneficial effect since women have a better prognosis than men (Shaw *et al.*, 1980) and melanomas diagnosed premenopausally are more likely to metastasize many years later in the postmenopausal period (Raderman *et al.*, 1986). Further support is the fact that survival in premenopausal women is significantly better than that in postmenopausal women. Similarly exogenous oestrogens do not promote progression of the disease as women who have taken either the OCP or HRT coincidently to having undiagnosed melanoma do not have a worse prognosis, and pregnancy subsequent to the diagnosis of melanoma does not increase the risk of recurrence (MacKie *et al.*, 1991).

The growing evidence would suggest that estrogen may have an indirect beneficial effect on melanoma that still needs to be elucidated, but there would seem to be no reason not to offer these women HRT under medical supervision (Jatoi and Gore, 1993).

Other Malignancies

Other malignancies that may be theoretically affected by HRT are those of the lung, liver, kidney and bowel. However, there is no available clinical evidence to substantiate this concern (Bergkvist, 1989), and considering all the proven benefits, HRT should be offered to all these patients. A reassuring note is found in the Hunt study (1990) showing an overall decrease in deaths from any malignancy of 50% in women taking HRT. There would seem to be an urgent need to study the effect of HRT on the immune system and the host response to tumors.

Treatment

Although non-hormonal alternatives are available for the relief and treatment of menopausal symptoms, HRT remains the only comprehensive inexpensive and safe treatment. Estrogen may be administered orally, transvaginally or through the skin as a percutaneous cream or skin patch or as implants. The pharmacodynamic properties of exogenous oestrogens vary markedly with different routes of administration. Oral estrogens are the most widely used and convenient form of treatment. It may not be the best route because of the first-pass effect. Vaginal estrogen creams are valuable, but should not be used under the misapprehension that they are only effective locally. Percutaneous estrogen cream is popular in continental countries, and as with other parenteral routes of administration, the liver is bypassed. The cream needs to be applied on a daily basis to maintain estradiol levels. Transdermal patches are a convenient mode of hormone administration with a high patient acceptability because the gastrointestinal side-effects of oral therapy are avoided. Troublesome skin reactions are rare. Hormone implant therapy has been used for many years and avoids the need for daily compliance, gives good symptomatic relief and has few side-effects. Testosterone pellets (100 mg) may be added to estrogen implants and provide patients with greater relief of the symptoms of lethargy and loss of libido.

Conclusion

Implicit in the philosophy of holistic care for patients with cancer is their involvement in management decisions. After all, it is only by focusing in on subjective perceptions that progress can be achieved in quality of life issues. Counseling women treated for hormone-sensitive tumors about HRT in all its forms (estrogen and androgen replacement) has been made more complex with the new evidence that women given HRT not only gain from an improvement in quality of life, but may also not have an increased risk of recurrence. It is our responsibility to convey the updated information, be it yet untested by controlled trials, in order to enable a complete and fair assessment of the risk–benefit balance (*Table 35.6*).

The relationship between HRT and cancer risk could be modified by patient characteristics and perhaps the future lies with the creation of individual risk profiles that embody both epidemiologic components (e.g. family history, life-style, diet, smoking, alcohol, stature) and molecular components (e.g. metabolic genotype, altered oncogenes, tumor suppressor genes). This would enable not only primary and secondary cancer prevention, but optimal safe HRT for those women at risk of osteoporosis and cardiovascular disease (*Table 35.7*).

There is already considerable evidence that the immune system is regulated in part by sex steroids and the exploitation of these qualities as a therapeutic tool for the chemoprevention and treatment of cancers could be a possibility in the future.

Summary of Management Options

- Hormone replacement therapy (HRT) contributes significantly to enhancing the quality of life of many postmenopausal women.
- There is growing evidence that women with breast cancer do not have an increased risk of cancer recurrence when exposed to endogenous or exogenous estrogen.
- A prospective randomized trial is needed to study the effect of HRT on women who have been treated for breast cancer.
- Tamoxifen decreases the risk of osteoporosis and has a favorable estrogenic effect on the lipid profile, but it can produce debilitating vasomotor symptoms.
- There are concerns regarding tamoxifen's possible role in inducing other tumors such as endometrial or hepatic tumors after long-term use.
- It would seem acceptable to offer HRT to those women who were treated for breast cancer premenopausally and who subsequently resumed their periods without any adverse effect and in conjunction with tamoxifen for the relief of vasomotor symptoms.
- The current recommendations for endometrial cancer patients are that estrogen replacement can be considered in some women based on prognostic indicators and the risk the patient is willing to assume.
- With Stage I endometrial cancer combined estrogen–progesterone therapy could begin shortly after surgery. This may be one example where progestogen might be beneficial to a woman without a uterus.
- In endometrial cancer where there is nodal involvement, ERT should not be used, but may be considered after three years providing there has been no recurrence.
- Since there is no known risk, HRT should be given to women with ovarian cancer. Administration can be commenced shortly after surgery.
- In cervical cancer, estrogen replacement therapy should be given to premenopausal women following a radical hysterectomy or radiation.
- There seems to be no reason not to offer women with melanoma HRT under medical supervision.
- HRT should be offered to all patients with lung, liver, renal and bowel tumors as there is no good evidence that it is harmful.

References

Adami HO, Holmberg L, Malker B (1987) Survival and age at diagnosis in breast cancer. *New Engl. J. Med.* **316:** 752.

■ American College of Obstetricians and Gynecologists, Committee on Gynecologic Practice (1990) Estrogen replacement therapy and endometrial cancer. *ACOG Committee Opinion No. 80*. Washington DC: American College of Obstetricians and Gynecologists.

Armstrong BK (1988) Oestrogen therapy after the menopause – boon or bane? *Med. J. Aust.* **148:** 213–214.

Bakker GH, Setyono–Han B, Portengen H *et al.* (1989) Endocrine and antitumour effects of combined treatment with an antiprogestin and antioestrogen or luteinizing hormone-releasing hormone agonist in female rats bearing mammary tumours. *Endocrinology* **125:** 1593–1598.

Benson JR & Baum M (1993) Breast cancer, desmoid tumours, and familial adenomatous polyposis – a unifying hypothesis. *Lancet* **342:** 848–850.

Beral V, Ramcharan S & Faris R (1977) Malignant melanoma and oral contraceptive use among women in California. *Br. J. Cancer* **36:** 804–809.

Bergkvist L (1989) Risk of cancer in women receiving hormonal replacement therapy. *Int. J. Cancer* **44:** 833–839.

Brincat M, Magos AL, Studd JWW *et al.* (1984) Subcutaneous implants for the control of climacteric symptoms: A prospective study. *Lancet* **1:** 16–18.

Brinton LA, Hoover R & Fraumeni JF Jr (1986) Menopausal oestrogens and breast cancer: an expanded case–control study. *Br. J. Cancer* **54:** 825–832.

Brinton LA, Schairer C, Hoover RN & Fraumeni JF (1988) Menstrual factors and risk of breast cancer. *Cancer Invest.* **6:** 245–254.

Brinton LA (1991) Oral contraceptives and cervical neoplasia. *Contraception* **43:** 581–595.

Colditz GA, Stampfer MJ, Willet WC *et al.* (1990) Prospective study of estrogen replacement therapy and risk of breast cancer in postmenopausal women. *JAMA* **264:** 2648–2653.

Collins J, Allen L, Donner A *et al.* (1980) Oestrogen therapy and the menopausal syndrome. *Lancet* **ii:** 961–963.

Creaseman WT, Henderson D, Hinshaw W *et al.* (1986) Estrogen replacement therapy in the patient treated for endometrial cancer. *Obstet. Gynecol.* **67:** 326–330.

Darbre PD & King RJB (1988) Steroid hormone regulation of cultured breast cancer cells. In: Lippman ME, Dickson RB (eds) *Breast Cancer: Cellular and Molecular Biology*, pp. 307–341. Boston: Kluwer Academic Publishers.

■ DiSaia PJ (1993) Hormone-replacement therapy in patients with breast cancer. *Cancer* **71(Suppl.):** 1490–1500.

Donegan WL (1977) Breast cancer and pregnancy. *Obstet. Gynecol.* **50:** 244–252.

Dupont WD (1989) Influence of exogenous oestrogens, proliferative breast disease and other variables on breast cancer risk. *Cancer* **63:** 948–957.

Dupont WD & Page DL (1991) Therapy and breast cancer. *Arch. Intern. Med.* **151:** 67–72.

■ Early Breast Cancer Trialists' Collaborative Group (1992) Systemic treatment of early breast cancer by hormonal, cytotoxic, or immune therapy. *Lancet* **339:** 1–15, 71–85.

Eden JA, Bush T, Nand S & Wren BG (1995) A case-control study of combined continuous estrogen-progestin replacement therapy among women with a personal history of breast cancer. *Menopause* **2:** 67–72.

■ Eeles RA, Tan S, Wiltshaw E *et al.* (1991) Hormone replacement therapy and survival after surgery for ovarian cancer. *Br. Med. J.* **302:** 259–262.

FDA Drug Bulletin (1984) Oral contraceptives and cancer. *FDA Drug Bull.* **14:** 2–3.

Fornander T, Rutqvist LE, Cedermark B *et al.* (1989) Adjuvant tamoxifen in early breast cancer: occurrence of new primary cancers. *Lancet* **i:** 117–120.

Franceschi S, Baron AE & La Vecchia C (1990) The influence of female hormones on malignant melanoma. *Tumori* **76:** 439–449.

Gambrell RD Jr, Maier RC & Sanders BI (1993) Decreased incidence of breast cancer in postmenopausal oestrogen–progestogen users. *Obstet. Gynecol.* **62:** 435–443.

Gordon GB, Shantz LM & Talalay P (1987) Modulation of growth, differentiation and carcinogenesis by dehydroepiandrosterone. *Adv. Enzyme Regu.* **26:** 355–382.

Grady PD & King RJB (1988) Steroid hormone regulation of cultured breast cancer cells. In: Lippman ME & Dickson RB (eds) *Breast Cancer: Cellular and Molecular Biology* pp. 307–341. Boston: Kluwer Academic Publishers.

Grady D & Ernster V (1991) Invited commentary: does postmenopausal hormone therapy cause breast cancer? *Am. J. Epidemiol.* **134:** 1396–1400.

Gusberg SB (1947) Precursors of corpus carcinoma-estrogens and adenomatous hyperplasia. *Am. J. Obstet. Gynecol.* **54:** 905.

Gusberg SB (1989) The rise and fall of endometrial cancer. *Gynecol. Oncol.* **35:** 124.

Haagensen CD & Stout AP (1943) Carcinoma of the breast. *Ann. Surg.* **118:** 859–870.

Hertig AT & Sommers SC (1949) Genesis of endometrial carcinoma . *Cancer* **2:** 946.

Holloway M (1992) The estrogen factor. *Scient. Am.* **266(6):** 26.

Hoover HC (1990) Breast cancer during pregnancy and lactation. *Surg. Clin. North Am.* **70:** 1151–1163.

■ Hunt K, Vessey M, McPherson K & Coleman M (1987) Long term surveillance of mortality and cancer incidence in women receiving hormone replacement therapy. *Br. J. Obstet. Gynaecol.* **94:** 620–634.

Jatoi I & Gore ME (1993) Sex, pregnancy, hormones and melanoma. *Br. Med. J.* **307:** 2–3.

Jones AL & Powles TJ (1993) Chemoprevention of breast cancer. *Rev. Endo-Rel. Cancer* **43:** 33–42.

Jordan VC (1976) Effect of tamoxifen (IC 16474) on initiation and growth of DMBA-induced rat mammary carcinomata. *Eur. J. Cancer* **12:** 419–424.

Kelley RM & Baker WH (1960) Progestational agents in treatment of carcinoma of the endometrium. *Proc. Am. Cancer Res.* **3:** 125.

Kelsey JL & Gammon MD (1990) Epidemiology of breast cancer. *Epidemiol. Revs.* **12:** 228–240.

La Vecchia C, Liberati A & Franceshi S (1986) Noncontraceptive estrogen use and the occurrence of ovarian cancer. *J. Natl. Cancer Inst.* **69:** 1207.

Leather AT, Savvas M & Studd JWW (1991) Endometrial histology and bleeding patterns after 8 years of continuous combined oestrogen and progestogen therapy in postmenopausal women. *Obstet. Gynecol.* **78:** 1008–1010.

Lee RB, Burke TW & Park RC (1990) Estrogen replacement therapy following treatment for Stage I endometrial carcinoma. *Gynecol. Oncol.* **36:** 189–191.

Linsay R (1988) Pathogenesis, detection and prevention of postmenopausal osteoporosis. In: Studd JWW & Whitehead MI (eds). *The Menopause*, pp. 156–157. Oxford: Blackwell Scientific.

Love RR, Mazess RB, Barden HS *et al.* (1992) Effects of tamoxifen on bone mineral density in postmenopausal women with breast cancer. *New Engl. J. Med.* **13:** 852–857.

Love RR, Newcombe PA, Wiebe DA *et al.* (1990) Effects of tamoxifen on lipid and lipoprotein levels in postmenopausal patients with node-negative breast cancer. *J. Natl. Cancer Inst.* **82:** 1327–1332.

Lupin F, Ruder AM, Wax T & Modan B (1985) Overweight and changes in weight throughout adult life in breast cancer etiology. *Am. J. Epidemiol.* **122:** 579.

MacKie RM, Bufalino R, Morabito A *et al.* (1991) Lack of effect of pregnancy on outcome of melanoma. *Lancet* **337:** 653–655.

Montgomery JC, Appleby L, Brincat M *et al.* (1987) Effects of oestrogen and testosterone implants on psychological disorders in the climacteric. *Lancet* **i:** 297–299.

Negri E, La Vecchia C, Bruzzi P, Dardanoni G *et al.* (1988) Risk factors for breast cancer: pooled results from three Italian case-control studies. *Am. J. Epidemiol.* **128:** 1207–1215.

Neven P, Shepherd JH & Lowe DG (1993) Tamoxifen and the Gynaecologist. *Brit. J. Obstet. Gynaecol.* **100:** 893–897.

Novak E & Rutledge F (1948) Atypical endometrial simulating adenocarcinoma. *Am. J. Obstet. Gynecol.* **55:** 46.

Nugent P & O'Connell TX (1985) Breast cancer and pregnancy. *Arch. Surg.* **120:** 1221–1224.

Peters MV (1986) The effect of pregnancy in breast cancer. In: Forrest APM & Kunkler PB (eds) *Prognostic Factors in Breast Cancer,* pp. 65–89. Baltimore: Williams.

Petrek JA, Dukoff R & Rogatko A (1991) Prognosis of pregnancy-associated breast cancer. *Cancer* **67(4):** 867–872.

Powles TJ, Hickish T & Casey S (1993) Hormone replacement after breast cancer. *Lancet* **342:** 60–61.

Raderman D, Giler S, Rothem A *et al.* (1986) Late metastases (beyond ten years) of cutaneous malignant melanoma. *J. Am. Acad. Dermatol.* **15:** 374–378.

Rosner D & Lane WW (1986) Oral contraceptive use has no adverse effect on the prognosis of breast cancer. *Cancer* **57:** 591–596.

Sacks NPM *et al.* (1993) How much of the effect of chemotherapy is due to hormonal manipulation? In: Fletcher GH & Levitt SH (eds) *Controversial Issues in the Management of Apparently Non-disseminated Breast Cancer.* New York: Springer-Verlag.

Shaw HM, McGovern VJ, Milton GW *et al.* (1980) Malignant melanoma: influence of site of lesion and age of patient in the female superiority in survival. *Cancer* **46:** 2731–2735.

Smith DC, Prentice R, Thompson DJ *et al.* (1975) Association of exogenous estrogens and endometrial carcinoma. *N. Engl. J. Med.* **293:** 1164–1167.

Stampfer MJ & Colditz GA (1991) Estrogen replacement therapy and coronary heart disease: a quantitative assessment of the epidemiologic evidence. *Prev. Med.* **20:** 47–63.

Steinberg KK, Thacker SB, Smith SJ *et al.* (1991) A meta-analysis of the effect of estrogen replacement therapy on the risk of breast cancer. *JAMA* **265:** 1985–1990.

Stoll BA & Parbhoo SC (1988) Treatment of menopausal symptoms in breast cancer patients. *Lancet* **i:** 1278–1279.

Strudee DW, Wade-Evans T, Paterson MEL, Thom NH & Studd JWW (1978) Relations between bleeding pattern, endometrial histology and oestrogen treatment in menopausal women. *Br. Med. J.* **1:** 1575–1577.

Studd JWW, Chakravarti S & Oram D (1977) The climacteric and the menopause. In: Greenblatt RB & Studd JWW (eds) *Clinics in Obstetrics and Gynaecology,* Vol. 4, pp. 3–29. Philadelphia: WB Saunders.

Studd JWW & Thom M (1981) Oestrogens and endometrial cancer. In: Studd JWW (ed) *Progress in Obstetrics and Gynaecology,* Vol. 1, pp. 182–189. Edinburgh: Churchill Livingstone.

Studd JWW (1989) HRT & breast cancer (letter): Hormone replacement therapy and breast cancer. *Lancet* **ii:** 1164.

Studd JWW & Baber R (1992) The menopause. In: Shaw R, Soutter P & Stanton S (eds) *Gynaecology,* pp. 341–354. London: Churchill Livingstone.

Studd JWW (1992) Oestrogens and depression in women *Br. J. Hosp. Med.* **48:** 211–213.

Studd JWW, Holland EFN, Leather AT & Smith RNJ (1994) The dose–response of percutaneous oestradiol implants on the skeleton of post-menopausal women. *Br. J. Obstet. Gynecol.* **101:** 787–791.

UK National Case–Control Study Group (1989) Oral contraceptive use and breast cancer risk in young women. *Lancet* **i:** 973–982.

Vassilopoulou-Sellin R & Zolinski C (1992) Estrogen replacement therapy in women with breast cancer: A survey of patient attitudes. *Am. J. Med. Sci.* **304:** 145–149.

Wile AG, Opfell RW & Margileth DA (1993) Hormone replacement therapy in previously treated breast cancer patients. *Am. J. Surg.* **165:** 372–375.

Woodruff JD & Pickar JH (1994) Incidence of endometrial hyperplasia in postmenopausal women taking conjugated estrogens (Premarin) with medroxyprogesterone acetate or conjugated estrogens alone. *Am. J. Obstet. Gynecol.* **170:** 1213–1223.

Woolas R (1994) Abstract from British Menopause Society Meeting July 1994, York, UK.

Ziel HK & Finkle WD (1975) Increased risk of endometrial carcinoma among users of conjugated estrogens. *N. Engl. J. Med.* **293:** 1167–1170.

36 Care of the Critically Ill Cancer Patient

Y Kim
S Menda
AC Casey
R Farias–Eisner

Introduction

Critical care when applied to oncology patients encompasses a wide range of conditions. Most oncology patients are in an older age group and as such are at risk for the usual cardiac, pulmonary, infectious, electrolyte, acid–base and renal complications after surgery. In addition, gynecologic oncology patients have a number of more specific problems that make postoperative intensive care unit (ICU) management a challenge: rapid accumulation of ascites or massive third-space fluid loss, high risk for thromboembolic disease and an immunocompromised state. Advances in treatment, aggressive surgical management, and postoperative support have prolonged the survival of many oncology patients. This chapter discusses the usual as well as the special critical care issues that arise when dealing with the gynecologic oncology patient.

Preoperative Assessment

The purpose of the initial preoperative assessment of the gynecologic oncology patient is to identify surgical risk factors and to anticipate any perioperative or postoperative complications that may arise. The preoperative evaluation, in addition to the routine history and physical examination, should specifically include information about the age, nutritional status, medical illnesses, and past surgeries of the patient.

The American Society of Anesthesiologists (ASA) has developed a classification system to preoperatively assess the risks of surgery and general anesthesia: Class I, normal; Class II, mild disease; Class III, severe disease that is activity limiting, but not incapacitating; Class IV, disease that is severe, incapacitating and a constant threat to life; and Class V, terminal illness from which the patient is expected to die within 24 hours (Saklad, 1941). The ASA system is one of the best predictors of operative mortality. In a study of 500 surgical patients older than 80 years, the operative mortality was 6.2%. Most deaths occurred in patients classified as ASA Class III or IV. Age itself, however, was not a significant risk factor, except in cases of emergency intraabdominal or intrathoracic procedures.

Cardiac Care and Complications

Surgery can pose severe stress on the cardiovascular system of a patient by several mechanisms: decreased myocardial contractility, changes in vascular tone induced by anesthesia, and changes in intravascular volume status because of hemorrhage or third-space fluid losses. The danger of a postoperative myocardial infarction (MI) is approximately 0.2% in patients undergoing surgery and general anesthesia. However, the risk increases to 5–10% in patients with a history of a previous MI, with an associated mortality rate of up to 50%. Hence, the importance of preventing a postoperative MI cannot be overemphasized. Goldman *et al.* (1977) established a multifactorial cardiac risk index, which lists nine factors that help identify patients at risk for a perioperative MI and given below in descending order of importance.

- Third heart sound or jugular venous distension.
- MI within preceding six months.
- Greater than five premature ventricular contractions per minute on preoperative electrocardiogram (ECG).
- Rhythm other than sinus or presence of premature atrial contractions on last preoperative ECG.
- Age greater than 70 years.
- Emergency operation.
- Intraperitoneal, intrathoracic or aortic surgery.
- Significant aortic valvular stenosis.
- Poor general medical condition (P_{O_2} <60 mm Hg, P_{CO_2} >50 mm Hg, potassium <3.0 mEq l^{-1}, bicarbonate <20 mEq l^{-1}), acute or chronic renal failure (blood urea nitrogen >50 mg dl^{-1} or creatinine >3.0 mg dl^{-1}, hepatic dysfunction, or chronically bed-ridden state.

Accurate assessment of cardiac risk factors may allow appropriate institution of preoperative interventions aimed at decreasing cardiac complications (i.e. delaying elective surgery for six months after a

MI, or treating arrhythmias, congestive heart failure and aortic stenosis). During surgery, patients with cardiac risk factors should be maintained in a normotensive state because intraoperative hypotension (a decrease in systolic blood pressure of 40% or more for more than 15 minutes) increases the risk of MI. Postoperatively, hypertension, arrhythmias, and heart failure commonly occur in the first 2–3 days after surgery, but the risk of MI persists for at least five days and peaks on the third postoperative day. Therefore, ECGs should be ordered, especially in the first five days, following surgery. For high-risk cases, serial cardiac enzymes should be obtained, even in the absence of chest pain, since postoperative MI is often painless (Tarhan *et al.*, 1972).

Hypertension

According to Goldman (1983), mild to moderate preoperative hypertension does not increase the incidence of postoperative MI, even in patients taking antihypertensive medications. Patients on beta-blocker medication should continue their medication up to, during, and after the surgical procedure since sudden discontinuation can cause a rebound phenomenon resulting in acute hypertension, arrhythmias and angina, which peaks 4–7 days after discontinuation of the drug (Goldman, 1981). Generally, hypertensive patients are more prone to develop blood pressure fluctuations; most commonly, intraoperative hypotension and postoperative hypertension. Therefore, blood pressure should be closely regulated in these patients. Postoperative hypertension, if severe and lasting longer than one hour can be managed by pain management (i.e. narcotics), decreased carbon dioxide via adjustment of ventilator settings, diminishing sensory stimulation during the postanesthesia recovery period, and with the use of vasodilators such as nitroprusside titrated to a diastolic blood pressure of 90 mm Hg.

Congestive Heart Failure

Patients with congestive heart failure should have medical optimization of their condition before surgery. In patients with a third heart sound, jugular venous distension, or severe cardiac decompensation, hemodynamic monitoring via a perioperative pulmonary artery (Swan–Ganz) catheter can help to manage intravascular volume, blood pressure and cardiac output. Patients taking digitalis for congestive heart failure should have close monitoring of drug levels because of the narrow therapeutic range of digitalis. Since postoperative patients are often dependent on intravenous replacement of fluids and electrolytes, they are particularly prone to digitalis toxicity.

Heart Block

In cases of second- and third-degree heart block, surgery should not be attempted without medical clearance. Patients with third-degree heart block without a pacemaker should be considered for preoperative placement of a pacemaker. These patients have an increased risk of cardiac arrest during surgery because of an inability to adequately increase their heart rate and hence maintain an adequate cardiac output in response to the stress of surgery. Patients with milder degrees of heart block, such as bifascicular heart block, usually do not require a pacemaker during surgery (Goldman *et al.*, 1978; Pastore *et al.*, 1978). However, patients developing a new bifascicular block postoperatively, in association with an acute MI, have a higher risk of progressing to complete heart block. These patients should be managed by placement of temporary pacemakers and cardiology evaluation (Rooney *et al.*, 1976).

Of note, patients with pacemakers should undergo three precautionary measures before abdominal surgery. First, patient should have a preoperative cardiologic evaluation to check pacemaker function to prevent back-up demand pacemaker failure during anesthesia. Second, the use of electrocautery should be minimized during surgery and the electrocautery grounding electrode should be placed as far as possible from the chest area since electromagnetic impulses from cauterization may interfere with pacemaker function. Finally, a magnet should be available in the operating room to convert the pacemaker from demand to fixed pacing mode if necessary (Simon, 1977).

Pulmonary Care

In managing the acutely ill cancer patient, postoperative pulmonary complications such as atelectasis, pneumonia and respiratory failure contribute to morbidity and mortality. Surgery and general anesthesia cause changes in lung volumes, ventilatory patterns (decreased sighing and coughing) and defense mechanisms. Following lower abdominal surgery, a 25–30% decrease in vital capacity is frequently observed (Jackson, 1988) in association with a decline in the arterial saturation of oxygen. Decreased coughing and sighing, secondary to anesthesia and postoperative sedation, predispose patients to pneumonia due to diminished mucociliary clearance of bacteria and atelectasis.

Preoperative Evaluation

Factors predisposing patients to pulmonary complications include chronic obstructive pulmonary disease (COPD), smoking, obesity, advanced age, anesthesia time greater than three hours, a thoracic or abdominal incision, and rhonchi or wheezing on physical examination (Jackson, 1988). Preoperative evaluation for high-risk patients should include arterial blood gases and pulmonary function tests (spirometry) to allow for optimization of perioperative pulmonary care. The following test result parameters are associated with an increased risk of postoperative pulmonary complications.

- A forced expiratory time longer than four seconds.
- An inspiratory to expiratory (I/E) ratio of 1/4–1/6, indicating lung disease such as emphysema (normal I/E ratio is 1/2 or 1/3).
- Hypercarbia ($P_{CO_2}>45$ mm Hg).
- Hypoxemia.

Hypercarbia poses a significant risk for pulmonary decompensation and isolated hypoxemia may also significantly increase pulmonary risk (Tisi, 1979; Gass and Olsen, 1986).

Pulmonary function testing, although somewhat controversial because of the variability of flow rates in normal people, can be helpful in evaluating pulmonary disease. A forced expiratory volume in one second (FEV1) of less than one liter indicates high risk and an FEV1 of 1–2 liters indicates medium risk of pulmonary complications. The forced expiratory volume in one second/forced vital capacity (FEV1/FVC) ratio may also be used to determine risk. However, this ratio is frequently no more sensitive than a history and physical examination (Zibrak *et al.*, 1990).

Preoperative Pulmonary Care

Patients at high risk for postoperative pulmonary complications should be advised to stop smoking for at least two weeks (preferably six months) before surgery, to use deep breathing, and to use incentive spirometry. The effects of smoking on anesthesia and surgery are substantial. Smokers have 2–6 times the risk of non-smokers for pulmonary complications. Smokers have an increased level of carboxyhemoglobin in their blood, which may cause tissue hypoxia by affecting oxygen transport to the myocardium and other tissues. Smoking also increases pulmonary secretions, promotes atelectasis, and decreases mucocilary defense mechanisms in the lung (Pearce and Jones, 1984).

Studies have shown that the clearance of carboxyhemoglobin occurs within 48 hours of cessation of smoking, while improvements in pulmonary clearance and sputum production require 2–6 weeks. Abstinence from smoking for six months before surgery virtually eliminates any increased risk of pulmonary complications that smokers have over nonsmokers.

Other preventive measures include chest physiotherapy, bronchodilators, antibiotics and early postoperative ambulation. Studies on the relative benefits of incentive spirometry, deep breathing, or chest physical therapy have not been done; however, the use of these measures appears beneficial. Intermittent positive pressure breathing (IPPB) should not be used in place of incentive spirometry because IPPB may increase the risk of pneumonia and bronchitis, especially in the high-risk pulmonary patient (Dahi and Gold, 1978).

Respiratory Failure

By definition, respiratory failure is the failure of the respiratory system to accomplish adequate ventilation and perfusion. In gynecologic oncology patients, respiratory failure may be caused by many factors:

- nervous system depression (narcotic overdose);
- bronchospasm;
- pneumonia;
- pulmonary edema;
- septicemia;
- disseminated intravascular coagulation (DIC);
- pulmonary embolism;
- prolonged hypotension (shock lung);
- lymphangitic spread of cancer;
- massive intraabdominal ascites.

Adult respiratory distress syndrome (ARDS) is a severe and frequently fatal form of respiratory failure presenting as severe hypoxemia unresponsive to oxygen supplementation, decreased lung compliance, bilateral diffuse pulmonary infiltrates and the presence of rales with normal or decreased pulmonary capillary wedge pressures (PCWP < 18). ARDS occurs when an insult to the lung results in increased pulmonary capillary permeability and leakage of water into the pulmonary extravascular space with the development of noncardiogenic pulmonary edema. Early recognition of patients with pulmonary problems postoperatively may help to prevent ARDS. Patients with respiratory failure may show signs of altered mental status, hypertension, diaphoresis and cyanosis. The presence of hypoxemia or hypercapnia in arterial blood gas analysis confirms the presence of respiratory failure, especially if baseline preoperative arterial blood gases were normal. A reliable measure of gas exchange and pulmonary function (not influenced by the inspired oxygen concentrations or hyperventilation) is the alveolar–arterial oxygen gradient (A–a gradient) which can be calculated using the following equations: A–a gradient $= P_{A_{O_2}} - Pa_{O_2}$, and $P_{A_{O_2}} = (F_{I_{O_2}} \times 760 \text{ mm Hg}) - (Pa_{CO_2} \times 1.2)$, where $F_{I_{O_2}}$ = fraction of oxygen in the inspired air (at sea level this value is approximately 0.21 on room air), $P_{A_{O_2}}$ = alveolar tension of oxygen, Pa_{CO_2} = arterial tension of carbon dioxide, Pa_{O_2} = arterial tension of oxygen.

The treatment of respiratory failure is endotracheal intubation and mechanical ventilation. But, the decision of when to initiate mechanical ventilation is based on clinical judgement. The presence of acute respiratory acidosis, progressive hypoxemia unresponsive to oxygen, and ARDS are all indications for ventilatory support. Additional indications for mechanical ventilation are the following:

- Respiratory rate >35 respirations min^{-1}.
- Pa_{O_2} <55 mm Hg.
- P_{CO_2} >55 mm Hg.
- Negative inspiratory force (NIF) < −20 mm Hg.
- Vital capacity <10 ml kg^{-1} of body weight.
- Minute ventilation <3 l min^{-1} or >20 l min^{-1}.
- An A–a oxygen gradient with 100% oxygen >450 mm Hg.

Before initiating ventilatory support, the patient must be endotracheally intubated, orally or using the nasotracheal approach. Oral intubation is preferred in patients who are comatose or not spontaneously ventilating. Patients who are awake may require sedation with a barbiturate such as Brevital (methohexital) or an opiate (morphine sulfate) before orotracheal intubation or may undergo nasotracheal intubation. Following intubation, the physician must choose the type of ventilation system to be used, either the assist-control mode (AC) or intermittent mandatory ventilation (IMV) (*Figure 36.1*).

The AC method is the standard mode in most ICUs. In the AC mode, the ventilator delivers a preset tidal volume at a backup ventilatory rate. The ventilator will provide assistance to any breaths initiated by the patient by delivering the predetermined tidal volume as well as uninitiated inspriations to ensure minimum ventilation at the back-up rate. In contrast, the IMV mode does not assist any spontaneous respiratory efforts by the patient, but provides a fixed number of breaths. Possible, but as yet unproven, advantages of IMV over AC ventilation include a decreased weaning time, a decreased need for patient sedation, fewer complications, fewer cardiovascular effects from positive end-expiratory pressure (PEEP) and decreased need for monitoring (Grum and Chauncey, 1988). IMV is also more useful for patients who hyperventilate. Patients receiving ventilatory support for acute respiratory failure should have initial ventilator settings with an FI_{O_2} of 100%, a tidal volume of 12 ml kg^{-1} a backup rate of 12 breaths min^{-1}, a flow rate of 40 l min^{-1}, and an I/E ratio of 1:3 (Grum and Chauncey, 1988).

Following repeat arterial blood gas measurements demonstrating adequate oxygenation, the FI_{O_2} can be titrated down to maintain a Pa_{O_2} of 60–80 mm Hg and a Pa_{CO_2} of 35–40 mm Hg. In patients with persistent hypoxemia despite high FI_{O_2} concentrations and the presence of rales with normal or low left atrial pressures, ARDS must be suspected. Patients with ARDS frequently respond to PEEP as tolerated by blood pressure and mechanical ventilation. The underlying cause of ARDS (e.g. infection, pulmonary embolism) must be treated while fluid status/pressures are optimized. The use of a Swan–Ganz catheter allows pulmonary capillary wedge pressures to be kept as low as possible. Diuretics can be used to minimize filling pressures. The use of PEEP during mechanical ventilation has certain benefits over volume-cycled ventilators. PEEP allows a reduction in the FI_{O_2} necessary to maintain adequate oxygen saturations and thus minimizes oxygen toxicity. However, because of high ventilatory pressures, complications of PEEP include barotrauma, pneumothorax, subcutaneous emphysema, depressed cardiac output, increased work of breathing and complications with pulmonary catheters (Grum and Chauncey, 1988).

Most patients on ventilatory support can be extubated within 3–7 days. A study of 100 patients

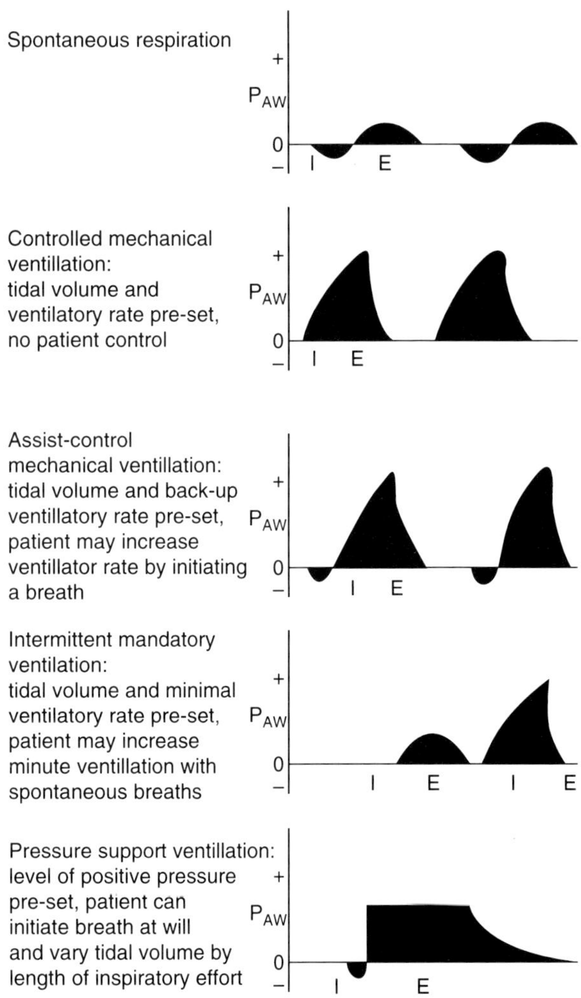

Figure 36.1. Airway pressure profiles in spontaneous respiration and with various modes of mechanical ventilation.

revealed that respiratory parameters help to predict successful extubation of patients. Patients with a resting minute ventilation of less than 10 l min^{-1}, a maximum voluntary ventilation two times greater than the minute ventilation, and a maximal inspiratory pressure of less than −30 cm H_2O were successfully extubated (Sahn and Lakshminarayan, 1973).

Shock

Shock is a clinical syndrome resulting in decreased tissue perfusion and end-organ damage because of inadequate delivery of oxygen to cells or inability of cells to utilize oxygen. Three shock states frequently found in the practice of gynecologic oncology are hemorrhagic, septic and cardiogenic shock. The pathophysiology and management of each of the three shock states will be discussed.

Hemorrhagic Shock (Hypovolemic Shock)

In gynecologic oncology patients, hemorrhagic shock is a problem seen frequently after radical pelvic surgery. In hemorrhagic shock, patients will present with decreased cardiac output, blood pressure, and oxygen transport due to fluid loss. Sympathetic stimulation will result in compensatory tachycardia, increased cardiac contractility, and increased peripheral vascular resistance to preserve blood flow to the heart and the brain. Because of these compensatory mechanisms, a patient may even appear normotensive despite their shock state. Classically, the patient will appear hypotensive, tachycardic, tachypneic, anxious, or frankly comatose, with pale, cool skin and delayed capillary refill. In the case of active bleeding, the hemoglobin and hematocrit may not immediately reflect the amount of blood lost. Delay in recognizing early shock may be detrimental to the patient's survival. The clinical manifestations of acute hemorrhage depend on the amount and rate of blood loss. Patient's with mild hemorrhage (<750 ml) develop tachycardia without hypotension. Moderate hemorrhage (<1500 ml) causes tachycardia and hypotension (decreased systolic blood pressure) and severe hemorrhage (>1500 ml or 30% of the cardiac output) produces hypotension, oliguria and mental status changes (Lucas and Ledgerwood, 1983).

The diagnosis of intraperitoneal bleeding postoperatively should be suspected in the patient who is hemodynamically unstable. Retroperitoneal bleeding may present more subtly as a patient who requires multiple transfusions postoperatively with a progressively decreasing hematocrit level. In either case, the immediate goal of treatment is to restore adequate circulating fluid volume to a mean arterial pressure above 80 mm Hg and adequate urine output (>50 ml h^{-1}). Urine output is a very sensitive indicator of adequate resuscitation. Immediate volume replacement with crystalloid or colloid solutions (albumin, plasma protein fraction) is as important as replacement of blood (Shoemaker, 1976). Until blood is available, Ringer's lactate or normal saline can be infused via two large-bore intravenous lines in a 3 to 1 ratio (for every ml of blood loss, 3 ml of crystalloid is required) (Lowery *et al.*, 1971). Ringer's lactate is preferable to normal saline, because normal saline can produce hyperchloremic acidosis. Massive hemorrhage should also be treated with fresh red blood cells rather than blood products stored for longer than one week because of the improved oxygen-carrying capacity of fresh products.

Colloid versus crystalloid

There is considerable debate regarding the advantages of either colloid or crystalloid solutions in treating hypovolemic shock and preventing pulmonary complications. Several clinical studies comparing colloid versus crystalloid preparations in volume resuscitation show no clear advantage of either solution (Skillman *et al.*, 1975; Lowe *et al.*, 1977; Weil *et al.*, 1979; Jelenko *et al.*, 1979). Colloid solutions are more efficient, since they are initially distributed to the intravascular space, and half the volume is required for resuscitation compared to crystalloid solutions. Crystalloid solutions, however, cost less and are more easily available. Regardless of which solution is used, the ultimate goal is adequate volume replacement titrated to blood pressure measurements and urine output. The use of sodium bicarbonate and osmotic diuretics has no clear benefit. Vascoconstrictive agents should also be avoided. After volume resuscitation, the most important goal is to arrest hemorrhage. If the patient is unstable following transfusion, then operative intervention for surgical hemostasis is critical to prevent irreversible end-organ damage. Following radical pelvic surgery, with reoperation for bleeding, the surgeon should isolate and ligate the hypogastric arteries and then search for other sources of bleeding outside the pelvis such as omental vessels, splenic or liver capsules, and mesenteric vessels.

Postoperatively, coagulation studies should be carefully monitored and normalized with appropriate blood products. Common problems include dilutional thrombocytopenia (following a transfusion of more than ten units of blood), clotting factor deficiencies, platelet dysfunction, and hemolytic transfusion reactions. If bleeding persists despite the above therapeutic measures, then military antishock trousers for 24–48 hours may be used, except in patients with congestive heart failure or cardiomyopathy (Johnson *et al.*, 1987). Military antishock trousers redistribute venous blood from the abdomen and lower extremities to the heart and the brain and increase peripheral vascular resistance.

Septic Shock

Septic shock is the second most common cause of shock in surgical patients and probably the most common cause of shock in cancer patients. Septic shock is caused by infection with gram-negative or gram-positive organisms or fungi with activation of the complement cascade, intrinsic clotting factors, vasodilator substances (bradykinin), histamine and thrombolytic factors with subsequent bleeding.

Early septic shock (warm shock) is characterized by peripheral vasodilation and decreased oxygen consumption despite a normal or increased cardiac output and oxygen delivery to tissues. Patients in early septic shock present clinically with fever, mental status changes, oliguria, tachycardia, and low systolic blood pressure, but a relatively normal pulse pressure and cardiac output. Arterial blood gases show mild hypoxemia and respiratory alkalosis due to ventilation perfusion mismatch. Serum lactate levels are normal or mildly elevated. The afebrile patient in early septic shock has a higher mortality rate than the febrile patient. Mortality from septic shock has been shown to be directly proportional to the serum lactate levels which should be closely monitored in these patients (Blair, 1971; Weil and Nishijima, 1978; Iverson, 1988).

The late phase of septic shock (cold shock) represents a progressive deterioration leading to a decline in cardiac function. Cardiac index falls, lactate levels rise, and the patient becomes severely acidotic. The patient's skin will become cold, clammy, cyanotic and mottled because of peripheral vascoconstriction and tissue hypoperfusion. Some investigators have postulated the existence of a 'cardiac depressant factor' that causes the progression to late shock (Love *et al.*, 1971) and eventual multisystem organ failure.

The cornerstone of the treatment of sepsis is early recognition, drainage of septic collections, immediate initiation of antibiotics, and vigorous fluid replacement. The following steps are involved in the management of patients in septic shock.

- Transfer to ICU.
- Swan–Ganz and arterial catheter placement for hemodynamic monitoring and to confirm sepsis.
- Fluid resuscitation.
- Broad-spectrum antibiotics including gram-negative and anaerobic coverage.
- Surgical drainage of septic collections (abscess) or removal of any source of infection.
- Cultures taken from all potential sites of infection.
- Scans if necessary to rule out septic collections.
- Vasopressor and inotropic drugs as necessary to improve cardiac output and tissue perfusion.

If, despite aggressive fluid resuscitation and optimal pulmonary capillary wedge pressures, hypotension still persists, then vasopressors such as dopamine can be implemented. One of the complications of septic shock is the development of ARDS, which increases the mortality rate of septic shock (Bernsten and Sibbald, 1989).

Postulated, but as yet unproven, aspects of therapy for septic shock include corticosteroids, the opiate antagonist naloxone, and ibuprofen. Corticosteroid therapy was initially thought to improve the course of septic shock because of its antiinflammatory effects. However, two large randomized clinical trials showed that corticosteroids neither prevent sepsis nor improve mortality rates of septic patients (Lucas and Ledgerwood, 1983; Methylprednisolone Severe Sepsis Study Group, 1987; Nicholson, 1989).

The opiate antagonist naloxone, through an unknown mechanism, has proven useful in patients and in animals with septic shock. A study by Roberts *et al.* (1988) showed that continuous infusion of naloxone reduced the heart rate and improved stroke volume, thereby diminishing the vasopressor and inotrope requirements of patients in septic shock. Other studies have shown no hemodynamic improvement in patients in septic shock who were given boluses of naloxone rather than continuous infusions (Bonnet *et al.*, 1985; Rock *et al.*, 1985). Further investigation is warranted as to the mechanism and the role of this drug in treating septic shock.

Cyclooxygenase inhibitors such as ibuprofen or indomethacin have proven useful in the treatment of gram-negative shock caused by the release of endotoxin from gram-negative bacteria. In a study of dogs, ibuprofen reduced thrombocytopenia and hemodynamically improved endotoxic shock in these animals (Almqvist *et al.*, 1984). However, in a study of rabbits with gram-positive sepsis (Peevy *et al.*, 1988), ibuprofen had no effect in improving survival or preventing sepsis. Because of the high mortality rate associated with septic shock (up to 75%), more investigation into treatments and early recognition and prevention of sepsis is critical for patient survival.

Cardiogenic Shock and Hemodynamic Monitoring

Cardiogenic shock is tissue hypoperfusion from cardiac pump failure due to various causes such as ischemic heart disease, valvular heart disease, arrhythmias or trauma. Patients in cardiogenic shock present with hypotension, tachycardia, decreased cardiac output, and decreased oxygen delivery with high pulmonary capillary wedge pressures (PCWP). On physical examination, the patient will present with jugular venous distension, rales, wheezes and an S3 (third heart sound) gallop. The goal of the treatment is improvement of cardiac output without increasing myocardial demand (with risk of ischemia) or pulmonary congestion. Thus, a precarious balance must be obtained between volume replacement, the use of chronotropic/inotropic agents, and vasopressor therapy to prevent volume overload and pulmonary edema. With cardiogenic shock, the use of hemodynamic monitoring is critical to allow monitoring of pressure, volume and cardiac function indices. A patient presumed to be in cardiogenic shock who has evidence of pulmonary edema on examination (rales or hypoxemia) requires invasive monitoring.

The Swan–Ganz catheter is a flow-directed balloon-tipped pulmonary artery catheter that has revolutionized ICU hemodynamic monitoring of critically ill patients. It is indicated if there is underlying heart disease or pulmonary edema or in any patient requiring fluid/pressure management. The Swan–Ganz catheter measures the PCWP, which is an approximation of left atrial pressure and left ventricular end-diastolic pressure or 'preload' in the absence of cardiac valvular disease. From catheter measurements, cardiac output, systemic vascular resistance and mean arterial pressures can be calculated.

Complications from insertion of the Swan–Ganz catheter include, but are not limited to, pneumothorax, arterial puncture, air embolism, hemorrhage, misplacement, arrhythmias, and valvular damage. Many of these complications can be prevented by the use of fluoroscopy for difficult insertions, the use of the internal jugular vein to reduce the incidence of pneumothorax (Elliott *et al.*, 1979), and follow-up chest radiographs to detect pneumothorax. Complications from the presence of a Swan–Ganz catheter are infection, thrombosis, pulmonary infarction and rupture of the pulmonary artery. Many of these complications can be prevented by changing or removing the catheters after 72 hours, keeping a syringe in the balloon port, continuous monitoring, careful positioning of catheter, and daily chest radiographs to determine catheter position. Normal hemodynamic parameters for Swan–Ganz catheters are as follows (Sibbald *et al.*, 1983):

- mean arterial pressure, 95 mm Hg;
- pulmonary artery wedge pressure, 20/10 mm Hg;
- PCWP, 8–12 mm Hg;
- cardiac index, 2.5–3.5 ml m^{-2};
- systemic vascular resistance, 1760–2600 dyn . sec. cm^{-5} m^{-2};
- O_2 delivery, 520–720 ml min^{-1} m^{-2};
- O_2 extraction, 22–32%.

In managing any patient with hypotension, the initial treatment is volume replacement to increase preload. Following volume infusion, three conditions may occur (*Table 36.1*). First, the patient may develop a large increase in PCWP with a small volume load and increased systemic vascular resistance (blood pressure). In this case nitroprusside and other vasodilators may reduce PCWP and systemic resistance (afterload). Phentolamine, an alpha-blocker, may reduce systemic resistance, but not PCWP (Sibbald *et al.*, 1983). Second, if after a given volume load, there is a fall in both PCWP and systemic resistance, slow careful fluid infusion is needed to optimize PCWP between 15–18 mm Hg and to avoid pulmonary congestion. Third, if a rise in PCWP and a fall in systemic resistance occurs, the use of an inotropic agent such as dopamine or dobutamine is preferred. Pulmonary edema in the critically ill patient may also be treated with mechanical ventilation and PEEP.

In the management of cardiogenic shock, PCWP should be optimized. Chronotropic drugs such as dopamine or dobutamine may be used to improve cardiac output without increasing myocardial ischemia. Chronotropic drugs such as isoproterenol and norepinephrine are of little benefit because they increase myocardial oxygen consumption. Some studies recommend the use of an inotropic agent (dopamine or dobutamine) with a vasodilator (nitroprusside) to improve overall cardiac output in cardiogenic shock (Shoemaker, 1982; Chatterjee,

Table 36.1. Hemodynamic parameters in various shock states. (Reproduced with permission from Lawrence (1992) *Essentials of General Surgery*, 2nd ed., p. 109. Maryland MA: Williams and Wilkins.) (BD, arterial blood pressure; P, pulse; PCWP, pulmonary capillary wedge pressure; CI, cardiac index; SVR, systemic vascular resistance; O_2D, oxygen delivery; O_2C, oxygen consumption).

Condition	BP (mm Hg)	P	PCWP (mm Hg)	CI ($l\ min^{-1}\ m^{-2}$)	SVR ($dyn.sec.cm^{-5}\ m^{-2}$)	O_2D $ml\ mm^{-1}$	O_2C $ml\ mm^{-1}$
Normal N	120/70	80	5–15	2.5–3.5	1000–1500	900–1200	200–300
Hypovolemia	↓	↑	↓	↓	↑	↓	↓
Congestive heart failure	↑	↑	↑	↓	↑	↓	↓
Cardiogenic shock	↓	↑	↑	↓↓	↑↑	↓↓	↓↓
Sepsis	↓	↑	↓ or N	↑	↓	↑	↑ or N
Neurogenic	↓	↑ or N	↓ or N	↑ or N	↓	↑ or N	N

1982). Dopamine and dobutamine increase cardiac output and reduce ventricular filling pressures. Nitroprusside improves cardiac performance by diminishing the afterload, but may contribute to hypotension. As a last resort, intraaortic balloon counterpulsation may decrease myocardial work, improve coronary perfusion, and decrease afterload (Berger and Merin, 1982).

Although perioperative hemodynamic monitoring of gynecologic oncology patients is rare, studies by Orr *et al.* (1983) of 31 patients undergoing pelvic exenteration for recurrent cancer demonstrated the benefits of invasive monitoring. Invasive monitoring permitted individualized volume resuscitation of these patients titrated to their pressure and cardiac function levels. Orr *et al.* found that pressure measurements such as mean arterial pressures did not correlate with cardiac index. Eisner *et al.* (1990) demonstrated that patients undergoing cytoreductive surgery for ovarian cancer with mild cardiopulmonary disease or ascites benefitted from postoperative hemodynamic monitoring. Of 128 patients who underwent invasive monitoring, 23 demonstrated rapid acute changes in their hemodynamic profile during the immediate postoperative period. Within 24 hours postoperatively, the cardiac output rose from 4.5 to 7.0 $l\ min^{-1}$, PCWP rose from 7 to more than 10 mm Hg, systemic vascular resistance decreased from 1400 to 860 $dyn.sec.cm^{-5}\ m^{-2}$ and fluid requirements dropped from 19.0 to 2.5 $ml\ kg^{-1}\ h^{-1}$. This study reported no significant complications from hemodynamic monitoring. With invasive hemodynamic monitoring, many patients at risk for postoperative cardiopulmonary complications may have early recognition and treatment of their problems.

Multisystem Organ Failure

Shock, if left untreated may progress to multisystem organ failure. In postoperative patients with chronic illness, any number of complications may result in respiratory, renal or cardiovascular failure. Mortality rates in multisystem organ failure are related to the number of systems that fail. With failure of two or more organ systems, the mortality rate is 75% (Fry, 1988). However, with concomitant renal failure, the mortality rate increases to 98%. Septic shock is very similar to multisystem organ failure because both states are characterized by elevated cardiac output with peripheral vasodilation, hypoxemia and lactic acidosis. Various immunologic factors such as interleukin-1 (IL-1), thromboxane, hormones (cortisone), oxygen radicals and complement factors may all contribute to multisystem organ failure and sepsis. Treatment consists of ventilatory support, treatment of renal failure (possibly via hemodialysis), nutritional support, avoidance of fluid overload, antibiotics and early detection of sepsis.

Volume and Electrolyte Abnormalities

Volume Disturbances

Management of water and electrolyte therapy is an important part of critical care of the gynecologic oncology patient. The normal adult female loses three liters of water per day, two liters in urine and the remaining one liter in perspiration, respiration and feces. Thus, in a patient undergoing minor abdominal surgery with an anesthesia time of less than four hours and little blood loss, a reasonable maintenance fluid management would be three liters per day of half normal saline in a 5% dextrose solution with 20 meq of potassium chloride per liter. However, patients undergoing more extensive surgery or with ascites should have replacement of volume losses by the use of balanced crystalloid or colloid solutions. Volume replacement should adequately replace all fluid losses including those from vomiting, diarrhea, fever or nasogastric suction (*Table 36.2*).

Patients with hypovolemia may have different presentations, depending on the degree of intravascular depletion. With mild hypovolemia, the patient will demonstrate thirst. Moderate to severe fluid losses may cause orthostatic changes in blood pressure, tachycardia, urine output higher than 30 $ml\ h^{-1}$ and an increased blood urea nitrogen (BUN)/creatinine ratio. The rate of volume replacement depends on the patient's ability to receive fluid loads without developing pulmonary edema or congestive heart failure. Severe hypovolemia may require rapid infusion or one or more liters over 15–30 minutes and then completion of fluid replacement over the next 24 hours. In less severe cases, fluids may be replaced over 24 hours. Indications of adequate fluid replacement are a urine output greater than 40 $ml\ h^{-1}$, normal BUN/creatinine ratios, normalized blood pressure and pulse rates.

Volume overload, often seen in cases of congestive heart failure, cirrhosis or nephrotic syndrome, may be treated by fluid/salt restriction and if severe, with diuretics such as furosemide administered parenterally.

Sodium Disturbances

Sodium is the principal ion determining osmolarity in extracellular fluid compartments. Both hyponatremia and hypernatremia can produce neurologic signs including changing mental status, fasciculations, seizures and even coma.

Clinically, hyponatremia is significant when sodium levels are less than 130 $mEq\ l^{-1}$. However, the rate of change of sodium levels is more reflective

Table 36.2. Electrolyte content of sweat and gastrointestinal secretions. (5% D/W, 5% dextrose; KCl, potassium chloride; $NaHCO_3$, sodium bicarbonate.)

Sweat or gastrointestinal secretion	**Electrolyte concentration ($mEq\ l^{-1}$)** *Na^+*	*K^+*	*H^+*	*Cl^-*	*HCO_3^-*	**Replacement amount for each liter lost** *Isotonic saline (ml)*	*5% D/W (ml)*	*KCl[a] (mEq)*	*$NaHCO_3$[b] (mEq)*
Sweat	30–50	5		45–55		300	700	5	
Gastric secretions	40–65	10	90[c]	100–140		300	700	20[d]	
Pancreatic fistula	135–155	5		55–75	70–90	250	750	5	90
Biliary fistula	135–155	5		80–100	35–50	750	250	5	45
Ileostomy fluid	120–130	10		50–60	50–70	300	700	10	67.6
Diarrhea fluid	25–50	35–60		20–40	30–45		1000	35	45

[a]Caution should be used in administering potassium faster than 10 mEq h^{-1}.
[b]One ampule of 7.5% $NaHCO_3$ contains 45 mEq HCO_3^-.
[c]Variable (e.g. achlorhydria).
[d]Administration of more than the observed gastric loss of potassium is often required because of enhanced urinary potassium excretion in alkalosis.

of neurologic complications than the absolute level. Hyponatremia may be classified in three ways according to Berl *et al.* (1976).

- Hyponatremia associated with extracellular volume depletion. In these patients the urine sodium may be low (<10 mEq l^{-1}) and the patient may appear dehydrated. The body, in response to hypovolemia or surgical stress, has blocked free water excretion by increasing antidiuretic hormone production, producing a dilutional hyponatremia. Replacement of fluid losses with hypotonic fluids may contribute to this syndrome. The treatment of these patients is normal saline volume repletion. In life-threatening cases of hyponatremia with neurologic manifestations, hypertonic saline may be infused. The amount of sodium required can be calculated by the following equation: Na^+ needed = (140 serum Na^+) $\times$ (0.6 $\times$ weight in kg). No more than one half of the total amount of sodium should be given over the first 12 hours and the remainder should be given over the next 24–48 hours.
- Hyponatremia with normal extracellular volumes may be caused by the syndrome of inappropriate antidiuretic hormone production. This syndrome is frequently seen in patients with cancer or hypothroidism. Urinary sodium levels may be high or low. The treatment consists of restricting free water intake and, if persistent, a trial of demeclocycline.
- Hyponatremia in edematous patients with increased extracellular volume. This is found most commonly in patients with congestive heart failure, nephrotic syndrome, or cirrhosis. Urinary sodium is usually low. Therapy involves furosemide and replacement of urine output with normal saline.

In addition to the above, a 'false' state of hyponatremia may be due to elevated blood glucose, serum lipids or proteins.

Hypernatremia (Na >150 mEq l^{-1}) is usually due to hypotonic fluid losses, limited intake of water or decreased excretion of sodium due to diabetes insipidus or adrenal hyperfunction. For each liter of water deficit, the serum sodium will rise by 3 mEq above normal. The treatment of hypernatremia is slow fluid replacement with a 5% dextrose solution. Ideally, the plasma osmolality should not be corrected at a rate greater than 2 mOsm $kg^{-1}\ h^{-1}$ or a sodium concentration change of greater than 1 mEq $l^{-1}\ h^{-1}$. This can be accomplished by administering one-half of the calculated water deficit over the first 24 hours, followed by continued correction of the water deficit over the ensuing 1–2 days. If fluid replacement is too rapid, lethargy, seizures and cerebral edema may occur.

Potassium Disturbance

Potassium is normally excreted by the kidney. Approximately 98% of total body potassium is intracellular. Therefore, a small decrease in serum potassium concentration reflects a large total body deficit of potassium. Serum potassium levels also vary with acidosis and alkalosis. Acidosis causes a redistribution of potassium from the intracellular to the extracellular space due to exchange of hydrogen and potassium ions. Alkalosis causes an opposite shift of potassium ions from the extracellular to the intracellular space.

Hypokalemia becomes clinically significant when potassium levels fall to less than 3.0 mEq l^{-1}. At levels of 2.5 mEq l^{-1} patients may experience muscle weakness, which can progress to paralytic ileus and paralysis. ECG changes may demonstrate arrhythmias, prominent U waves, flat T waves, prolonged PR interval, and a widened QRS complex. Therapy of hypokalemia preferably involves oral potassium supplementation. If parenteral potassium replacement is necessary then close monitoring is required to prevent hyperkalemia.

Hyperkalemia in the gynecologic oncology patient is most often due to renal failure or massive hemolysis. Other causes include acidosis, adrenal insufficiency, and overzealous potassium supplementation. Hyperkalemia affects the heart and nervous system causing weakness, paresthesias, paralysis and eventual ventricular fibrillation and cardiac arrest. The majority of patients, however, have no symptoms. Evaluation of hyperkalemia includes an immediate ECG. Emergent treatment of hyperkalemia in patients who are hypotensive or have prolonged QRS intervals involves:

- calcium gluconate to stabilize the cardiac membrane potential;
- intravenous glucose and insulin (50 ml of 50% glucose solution and one unit of intravenous regular insulin for each 10 g of glucose);
- sodium bicarbonate (both insulin and bicarbonate stimulate potassium uptake by cells);
- in patients with potassium levels higher than 6.5 mEq l^{-1} and widened QRS complexes, kayexylate (sodium polystyrene sulfonate, potassium exchange resins) can be given every four hours along with a loop diuretic such as furosemide.

Patients with mild hyperkalemia may be carefully monitored by ECG.

Hypercalcemia

The two most common causes of hypercalcemia are malignancy and hyperparathyroidism. In gynecologic oncology patients with ovarian carcinoma, tumor secretion of substances such as parathormone-like factors, prostaglandins, or other humoral substances increases osteoclastic bone resorption, causing hypercalcemia. The clinical manifestations of hypercalcemia are lethargy, confusion, nausea and vomiting, polyuria, polydipsia, and abdominal pain. Electrocardiographically, shorted QT intervals, prolonged PR interval and a widened T-wave may be noted.

Treatment of hypercalcemia begins with restricting calcium intake, intravenous hydration with normal saline, and furosemide to increase renal excretion of calcium. Intravenous phosphate has also been used to lower serum calcium by complexing calcium. However, if phosphate is given at a rate greater than 50 mM per 12 hours or for more than 48 hours it may precipitate hypocalcemia. Contraindications to phosphate therapy include renal failure or hyperphosphatemia. Although the use of high-dose corticosteroids reduced calcium levels in patients with breast cancer and leukemia, gynecologic patients may not respond to corticosteroids. In urgent circumstances, mithramycin, a cytotoxic drug with renal and hematologic toxic effects, has been very successful in treating hypercalcemia. Mithramycin inhibits bone resorption by suppressing osteoclasts. It can be infused at a dose of 2 $\mu g\ kg^{-1}\ d^{-1}$ for up to three days.

Acid–base Disturbances

Both the lungs and the kidneys participate in the acid–base balance of the body. While the lungs regulate the level of carbon dioxide in the body by controlling ventilation, the kidneys control reabsorption of bicarbonate. The balance between bicarbonate (a plasma buffer) and carbon dioxide (a volatile acid) determines the pH. There are four basic acid–base disturbances: metabolic acidosis, metabolic alkalosis, respiratory acidosis and respiratory alkalosis.

Metabolic Acidosis

Metabolic acidosis is defined by a decrease in bicarbonate level and a reduced pH. The first step in evaluating the cause of metabolic acidosis is to calculate the anion gap: anion gap $= (Na^+ + K^+) - (Cl^- + HCO_3^-)$. A normal anion gap is 10–14 mEq l^{-1}. Retention of acid produces an increased anion gap and a loss of alkali (HCO_3) produces a non-anion gap acidosis. Causes of an increased anion gap acidosis include renal failure, lactic acidosis, ketoacidosis, uremia, salicylates and alcohol, whereas, a normal anion gap acidosis is caused by diarrhea, renal tubular acidosis, ureteral fistulas and post-hypocapnia (*Table 36.3*). Treatment of metabolic acidosis should be considered when pH is less than 7.20 and/or HCO_3 is less than 10 mEq l^{-1}, in which case intravenous bicarbonate should be infused (one ampoule of sodium bicarbonate in one liter of half normal saline over 24–48 hours). Complications from bicarbonate infusion, including hypokalemia, hypocalcemia and metabolic alkalosis should be corrected immediately.

Metabolic Alkalosis

Metabolic alkalosis is defined as an increase in pH caused by a retention of bicarbonate. Metabolic alkalosis may be stimulated by volume depletion and reabsorption of sodium and chloride ions. However, when urinary chloride is depleted, sodium is reabsorbed with bicarbonate ions, producing alkalosis. Metabolic alkalosis may be chlorine sensitive (usually due to vomiting, diarrhea, and other gastrointestinal losses, diuretics and chronic

Table 36.3. Causes of metabolic acidosis (derived from Leonard (1993) *Clinician's Pocket Reference*, 7th ed., p. 139. Connecticut: Appleton & Lange).

- Normal anion gap
  - Gut
    - Diarrhea
    - Fistulae
    - Ileal loop
  - Renal
    - Renal tubular acidosis
    - Carbonic anhydrase inhibitor
    - Post-hypocapnia
- Increased anion gap
  - Exogenous
    - Salicylates
    - Methanol
    - Paraldehyde
    - Ethylene glycol
    - Hyperalimentation
    - Ketoacidosis
    - Ethanol
  - Endogenous
    - Lactic acidosis
    - Ketoacidosis
      - a. Diabetic
      - b. Starvation
    - Uremia

Table 36.4. Causes of metabolic alkalosis (derived from Leonard (1993) *Clinician's Pocket Reference*, 7th ed., p. 141. Connecticut: Appleton & Lange).

- Urine chloride less than 10 mEq l^{-1} (chloride-responsive)
  - Renal loss of chloride
    - Diuretics
    - Miscellaneous
      - Cystic fibrosis
    - Post-hypercapnia
- Gastrointestinal loss of hydrogen and chloride ions
    - Nasogastric suctioning
    - Vomiting
    - Chloride-wasting diarrhea
      - Congenital in children
      - Villous adenoma
- Urine higher than 10 mEq l^{-1} (chloride-resistant)
  - Excess mineralocorticoid
    - Adrenal
      - Cushing's syndrome
      - Hyperaldosteronism (Conn's syndrome)
    - Exogenous steroid administration
    - Bartter's syndrome

hypercapnia) with a urine chloride level of less than 10 mmol l^{-1}. The treatment for this condition is normal saline fluids. Chloride-resistant metabolic alkalosis is characterized by high levels of urinary chloride (>20 mmol l^{-1}) with treatment directed at the underlying cause (*Table 36.4*).

Respiratory Acidosis

Primary respiratory acidosis is identified by an increased carbon dioxide level with an associated fall in pH and is usually due to hypoventilation. Renal compensation of respiratory acidosis consists of retention of bicarbonate, which occurs over a few days. Treatment is directed at eliminating narcotics, which suppress respiratory drive, and using methods to improve ventilation (i.e. mechanical ventilation, if necessary).

Respiratory Alkalosis

Respiratory alkalosis is characterized by an increase in serum pH with a decrease in P_{CO_2} concentration, usually caused by hyperventilation. A simple way to treat hyperventilation is breathing into a paper bag.

If a mixed metabolic and respiratory acid–base disorder is suspected, the expected P_{CO_2} can be calculated from the following equation: expected $P_{CO_2} = 1.5$ (measured HCO_3^-) ± 2.

In a patient with metabolic acidosis, if the P_{CO_2} levels are higher than expected, then a concomitant respiratory acidosis exists. If the P_{CO_2} is lower than expected, a respiratory alkalosis is present.

Renal Failure

Preoperative renal failure in gynecologic oncology patients is often due to ureteral or bladder obstruction secondary to invasive cancer, nephrotoxic chemotherapy, antibiotics, contrast agents or pre-existing medical conditions. Nonetheless, finding the cause and treating renal failure before surgery may prevent unnecessary postoperative complications such as bleeding, volume overload, hyperkalemia, metabolic acidosis and infection. Preoperative evaluation may include renal ultrasound, retrograde pyelography and renal biopsy, if necessary.

Patients with mild to moderate renal failure (creatinine clearance >20 ml min^{-1}) should be managed by avoiding radiologic contrast, avoiding nephrotoxic antibiotics and strict maintenance of fluid/electrolyte balance.

Acute renal failure in the surgical patient may be due to prerenal, postrenal (obstructive) or renal causes. Acute renal failure in the critical care setting may present as oliguria and azotemia (a rising serum creatinine) as well as a retention of nitrogenous wastes secondary to an impairment in renal function. Oliguria is often seen postoperatively, but creatinine levels usually remain stable in patients with normal renal function. Postoperatively, surgical trauma, pain and peripheral vasodilation from anesthetic agents may increase antidiuretic hormone levels and produce sympathetic vasoconstriction of renal blood flow. Thus, a temporary decrease in urine output is expected.

Acute renal failure may progress through three phases: oliguria (few hours to six weeks), diuresis (with reduction and stabilization of BUN and creatinine levels) and return to near normal or normal renal function. Pathologically, renal failure may be caused by acute tubular necrosis, interstitial nephritis and papillary necrosis (Handa and Morrin, 1967; Light *et al.*, 1989). Urinalysis may help to differentiate between these diseases. Red blood cell casts are found with glomerulonephritis, renal tubular casts with acute tubular necrosis, and eosinophils in the urine are diagnostic of drug-induced interstitial nephritis. Prerenal and postrenal causes of renal failure are most common in gynecologic oncology patients.

Prerenal and Renal Causes

Adequate blood flow to the kidney is critical for maintenance of glomerular filtration rate and renal function (Light *et al.*, 1989). Hence, correction of any postoperative volume depletion may prevent acute tubular necrosis. Oliguria, or a urine output of less than 400 ml d^{-1} is one of the most common critical care problems. Evaluation of the oliguric patient includes looking for evidence of orthostatic blood pressure changes, hypovolemia, liver disease and a palpable bladder. Urine and serum electrolytes, osmolality, and BUN/creatinine levels are necessary to determine the cause of renal failure. Hypovolemia, congestive heart failure and liver disease may cause similar renal findings as they all produce prerenal azotemia. Prerenal azotemia is associated with a high urine osmolality ($>$350–500 mOsm kg^{-1}), a low urinary sodium ($<$20 mEq l^{-1}), an elevated BUN/creatinine ratio, and most importantly, a fractional excretion of sodium (FENA) of less than 1%. Acute renal failure or obstruction typically presents with a FENA of more than 1% (Miller *et al.*, 1978).

The treatment of prerenal renal failure in the absence of congestive heart failure, is adequate volume replacement with monitoring of urine output. A fluid challenge of 500–1000 ml given within 10–15 minutes should increase urine output. If urine output does not respond after sufficient fluid challenge, then 40 mg of furosemide should be given and steadily increased to 400 mg if no improvement in urine output is seen. If the loop diuretic fails, then low-dose dopamine may improve glomerular filtration rate and renal perfusion (Handa and Morrin, 1967; Levinsky and Bernard, 1988). If all these measures fail, then the patient may have acute tubular necrosis and should be treated by fluid restriction and maintenance of electrolyte balance. Indications for dialysis include:

- BUN over 100 mg dl^{-1};
- severe uncontrolled hyperkalemia or acidosis;
- volume overload;
- uremia with evidence of pericarditis;
- coagulopathy (Hakim and Lazarus, 1988).

Much debate has centered around the advantages of converting oliguric renal failure to the nonoliguric form via infusion of furosemide with mannitol. Infusion should be discontinued if urine output does not increase within 12 hours. Some experts feel nonoliguria may improve prognosis with little or no toxicity to the kidney.

Obstructive Causes of Renal Failure

Although most postoperative renal failure is due to hypovolemia, anuria, uncorrectable by volume loading, may be indicative of obstruction. Obstruction presents as hydronephrosis (dilation of renal calyces) on renal ultrasound within 24 hours of obstruction (Light *et al.*, 1989). After the diagnosis of obstruction, surgical correction, placement of a stent, or placement of a percutaneous nephrostomy should be performed to bypass the site of obstruction.

Renal Causes of Renal Failure

Nephrotoxic agents such as aminoglycoside antibiotics and radiographic contrast media may cause intrinsic renal failure. When used judiciously, renal failure is preventable. The aminoglycoside antibiotics may produce a nonoliguric renal failure. Within a two-week period, significant azotemia develops. Even after cessation of antibiotics, it can take months for renal function to return to normal (Handa and Morrin, 1967). In high-risk elderly patients, with preexisting renal disease, aminoglycosides should be avoided, if possible. When used in this population, dose monitoring of peak and trough drug levels and adequate hydration may reduce the high incidence (7–20%) of nephrotoxicity (Handa and Morrin, 1967; Fang, 1989). The contrast media used for radiologic studies frequently produces an oliguric renal failure that appears clinically identical to prerenal failure. Renal failure develops within 24 hours after the contrast is used and continues for the next 7–10 days. Prevention of contrast-induced nephrotoxicity is by adequate hydration before the study, mannitol and furosemide diuresis following the study, and monitoring of urine output for the subsequent 24 hours after the study. Treatment involves discontinuation of all contrast agents and other nephrotoxic drugs. Of note, clinicians often mistakenly volume overload these patients because of a low urinary sodium and the characteristic 'prerenal' picture of contrast-induced renal failure.

Rare causes of renal failure in cancer patients include tumor lysis syndrome and thrombotic thrombocytopenic purpura, a paraneoplastic syndrome. Tumor lysis syndrome occurs with massive lysis and death of tumor cells due to chemotherapy, producing hyperphosphatemic oliguric renal failure. Although rare in gynecologic malignancies, tumor lysis syndrome is an indication for dialysis. Thrombotic thrombocytopenic purpura (TTP) is renal failure associated with changes in mental status, hemolytic anemia, and thrombocytopenia. Treatment for TTP is plasmapheresis and fresh frozen plasma.

Special Critical Care Issues

Deep Venous Thrombosis and Pulmonary Emboli

Gynecologic oncology patients have an increased risk of developing deep venous thrombosis (DVT) in the calf veins following surgery because of postoperative immobilization and the hypercoagulable state of malignancy. The incidence of DVT after major gynecologic surgery has been estimated at 7–45% (Walsh *et al.*, 1974; Clarke–Pearson *et al.*, 1984). In a study by Clarke–Pearson *et al.* (1983), approximately 50% of DVTs were detected within 48 hours of surgery; 92% of the DVTs observed either spontaneously lysed (27%) or remained stable (65%). Prophylactic measures for DVT include heparin, warfarin, graded elastic compression stockings, and external pneumatic compression. Low-dose heparin, which facilitates the action of antithrombin III, given as 5000 units subcutaneously every 12 hours before surgery has reduced the risk of DVT in surgery patients over 40 years of age (Salzman and Davies, 1980). However, low-dose heparin, when given after major surgery for gynecologic malignancies was ineffective. External pneumatic calf compression boots are the most effective method of DVT prophylaxis when used during the first five postoperative days.

A DVT presents with clinical signs such as calf tenderness, swelling in the leg, or palpable venous cords only 50% of the time. Venography is the most accurate test for confirming the diagnosis. Alternative tests include thromboscintigraphy, which is most sensitive in the lower leg, and impedance plethysmography with highest sensitivity in the proximal veins. Doppler ultrasound is a noninvasive and relatively new diagnostic modality that appears to have excellent sensitivity and specificity for DVT. The treatment for DVT is aimed at preventing propagation of the clot and causing a life-threatening pulmonary embolism. Intravenous heparin is given with a 5000 unit bolus plus 10–15 units kg^{-1} h^{-1} until the activated partial thromboplastin time (aPTT) is approximately 2–3 times the control aPTT. Following therapeutic aPTT levels, warfarin (coumadin) may be started and the dose adjusted until the prothrombin time (PT) level is 1.5–2.5 times the normal control value. Patients should receive warfarin for 3–6 months.

Pulmonary embolism postoperatively presents as sudden onset of pleuritic chest pain, shortness of breath, cough, hemoptysis and signs of tachycardia, tachypnea, hypotension, right-sided congestive heart failure and a pleural friction rub. Arterial blood gases may show an increased alveolar–arterial gradient and a profile consistent with a respiratory alkalosis. The diagnosis of pulmonary embolism must be confirmed by a ventilation–perfusion scan. A normal scan rules out a pulmonary embolus. A high-probability scan has a 96% diagnostic accuracy and justifies full anticoagulation therapy. An intermediate- or low-probability scan mandates a pulmonary angiogram for confirmation of this diagnosis if clinical suspicion is high before treatment is begun. After diagnosis of a pulmonary embolism, treatment with heparin and subsequently coumadin is recommended. If acute hemorrhage develops, the heparin should be discontinued and protamine sulfate (heparin antagonist) administered. In pulmonary embolus less than one week old, thrombolytic therapy with streptokinase or urokinase is useful in clot lysis. Thrombolytic therapy is contraindicated in patients at risk for hemorrhage, for example patients who:

- have had major surgery within last ten days;
- have a history of gastrointestinal bleeding;
- have left atrial thrombosis;
- are aged over 75 years;
- are pregnant;
- have diabetic retinopathy;
- have bacterial endocarditis (National Institutes of Health Consensus Development Conference, 1980).

Another treatment option, if a patient cannot tolerate heparin, is insertion of a venocaval filter through the internal jugular vein. This treatment does not prevent emboli from the heart and other extremities, but is a useful alternative for the immediate postoperative patient.

Postoperative Ascites

Patients with ovarian carcinoma may experience large third-space fluid losses because of radical pelvic surgery. Rapid accumulation of ascites postoperatively may contribute to hypovolemia, respiratory complications and delayed wound healing because of fluid leakage from the abdominal incision. Patients on mechanical ventilation who develop ascites may be more difficult to wean. In patients with massive ascites, aggressive postoperative fluid replacement with crystalloids and colloids must be performed to avoid hypovolemia and resultant acute tubular necrosis. Central venous/Swan–Ganz catheters are helpful in assessing the fluid status in these patients perioperatively. The placement of an intraperitoneal catheter during the surgery may permit drainage of ascites through the catheter. In one institution, thiotepa has been used to treat ascites in a 45 mg intravenous dose following surgery. Thiotepa appeared to minimize the complications of ascites, although no controlled studies have been conducted to assess its actual efficacy, and placement of intraperitoneal catheters is not commonplace.

Nonsurgical Treatment of Pelvic Hemorrhage

Postoperative hemorrhage following radical pelvic surgery is usually managed by reoperation and fluid replacement; however, in critically ill patients other options for hemostasis are now available. Percutaneous angiographic embolization of the bleeding vessel can be performed under local anesthesia with cannulation of the femoral artery. The active bleeding site is localized through angiography. Embolic agents, including short- or long-term occluders such as Gelfoam (short-term) or coils (long-term), are then injected into the bleeding vessel(s) (Schwartz, 1982). Gelfoam has several advantages including low tissue reactivity and a long-lasting effect of 20–50 days. Long-term occluders such as Gianturco–Anderson–Wallace stainless steel or cryoacrylate are used for aneurysms and shunts. Vasopressin is not as effective as short or long-term occluders in controlling hemorrhage from malignant neovasculature. In the clinical trials carried out by Mann *et al.* (1980) all 13 patients had their hemorrhage successfully controlled by angiographic embolization without reoperation. Complication of this procedure include embolization and ischemia to the lower extremeties.

Nonsurgical Treatment of Abdominal Abcess

Before the advent of computed tomography (CT) scans, intra-abdominal abcess was treated by incision and drainage of the fluid collections with the associated morbidity and mortality of a second surgery. With the use of CT-guided localization and percutaneous drainage of intra-abdominal abcesses, there is an 85–96% success rate when used to treat a single well-defined abcess (Brolin *et al.*, 1981). Catheters must be frequently irrigated and a repeat scan should confirm drainage of abcess. A complication rate of 15% or less primarily involves infection from manipulation of catheters (Gerzof *et al.*, 1981; Pruett and Simmons, 1988).

Summary of Management Options

Postoperative hypertension

- For severe postoperative hypertension lasting longer than one hour, options include pain management, decreased carbon dioxide via adjustment of ventilatory settings and decreased sensory stimulation in recovery room.
- Medical management of blood pressure includes vasodilators such as nitroprusside to a diastolic blood pressure of 90 mm Hg.

Respiratory failure and adult respiratory distress syndrome (ARDS)

- Endotracheal intubation.
- Mechanical ventilation can be initiated, particularly in the presence of acute respiratory acidosis, progressive hypoxemia and ARDS with initial ventilator setting at F_{IO_2} of 100%.
- Intermittent mandatory ventilation is preferred for patients who hyperventilate.
- If repeat arterial blood gas measurements show adequate oxygenation, F_{IO_2} can be titrated to maintain Pa_{O_2} of 60–80 mm Hg and Pa_{CO_2} of 35–40 mm Hg.
- Patients with ARDS often respond to positive end-expiratory pressure (PEEP) and mechanical ventilation.
- Treat underlying cause of ARDS (e.g. infection, embolism, disseminated intravascular coagulation).
- In patients with ARDS, optimize fluid pressure status via invasive hemodynamic monitoring. The goal is to keep pulmonary capillary wedge pressure (PCWP) as low as possible with diuretics.

Hemorrhagic shock

- Early recognition of hemorrhagic shock is critical to patient survival.
- Goal is to restore circulating fluid volume in a 3:1 ratio (3 ml fluid/1 ml of blood loss) to mean arterial pressure of over 80 mm Hg and urine output over 50 ml h^{-1}. Use Ringer's lactate preferably for volume replacement.
- Massive hemorrhage should be treated with transfusion of fresh red blood cells.
- If patient is still unstable, immediate operative intervention for surgical hemostasis is recommended. Isolate and ligate hypogastric arteries and search for other non-pelvic sources of bleeding.
- Postoperatively, monitor coagulation studies and normalize with blood products.

Septic shock

- Transfer to intensive care unit; Swan–Ganz placement with fluid resuscitation.
- Broad-spectrum antibiotics including gram-negative bacteria/anaerobic coverage.
- Cultures from all sites and scans to rule out septic collections.
- Surgical drainage of abscess and removal of source of infection.
- Vasopressor/inotropic drugs.
- Postulated, but as yet unproven, therapeutic agents include corticosteroids, naloxone, ibuprofen.

Cardiogenic shock

- Invasive hemodynamic monitoring.
- If patient is hypotensive, volume placement is recommended to increase preload.
- If after volume load, there is a large increase in PCWP and increased systemic vascular resistance (SVR), then give nitroprusside and vasodilators to diminish afterload. If after volume load PCWP is decreased and SVR is decreased, continue slow-volume infusion to optimal PCWP of 15–18 mm Hg.
- If after volume load both PCWP and SVR are increased, dopamine or dobutamine should be given.
- Pulmonary edema is treated with mechanical ventilation and PEEP.

Hypercalcemia

- Restrict calcium intake.
- Intravenous hydration with saline and furosemide.
- Intravenous phosphate can lower calcium (contraindications are renal failure and hyperphosphatemia).
- In emergency cases, mithramycin can be infused for up to three days.

Renal failure

- To determine the cause of renal failure: urinalysis, urine and serum electrolytes, osmolality, blood urea nitrogen (BUN)/creatinine levels, and possibly a renal untrasound.
- Prerenal failure without congestive heart failure: treatment begins with adequate volume replacement with urine output monitored. If urine does not increase, then add furosemide. If the above measures fail, then low-dose dopamine can improve glomerular filtration rate.
- Obstructive renal failure: place a stent, percutaneous nephrostomy, or surgical correction to relieve obstruction.
- Intrinsic causes of renal failure: renal failure may be improved by discontinuation of nephrotoxic antibiotics, hydration and diuresis (furosemide or mannitol) before radiographic studies with contrast.

Deep venous thrombosis (DVT)

- Prophylaxis for DVT includes heparin, warfarin, pneumatic compression boots, elastic compression stockings.
- Treatment for DVT is heparin 5000 unit bolus + 10–15 U kg^{-1} h^{-1} until activated partial thromboplastin time (aPTT) is 2–3 times normal control value.
- Following therapeutic aPTT levels, warfarin should be started until the prothrombin time (PT) is 1.5–2.5 times normal control value. Continue warfarin for 3–6 months.

References

Almqvist PM, Kueazig M & Schwartz SI (1984) Treatment of experimental canine endotoxin shock with ibuprofen, a cyclooxygenase inhibitor. *Circ. Shock* **13:** 227.

Berger RB & Merin G (1982) Mechanical support of the failing left ventricle. In: Berk JL & Sampliner JE (eds) *Handbook of Critical Care,* 2nd ed, p. 285. Boston: Little Brown.

■ Berl T, Anderson RJ, McDonald KM *et al.* (1976) Clinical disorders of water metabolism. *Kidney Int.* **10:** 117.

Bernsten A & Sibbald W (1989) Acute lung injury in septic shock. *Crit. Care Clin.* **5:** 49.

Blair E (1971) Acid base balance in bacteremic shock. *Arch. Intern. Med.* **127:** 731.

Bonnet F, Bilaine J, Lhoste F *et al.* (1985) Naloxone therapy of human septic shock. *Crit. Care Med.* **13:** 972.

Brolin RE, Nosher JL & Leiman S (1981) Percutaneous catheter versus open surgical drainage of abdominal abscesses. *New Engl. H. Med.* **305:** 653.

Chatterjee K (1982) Acute heart failure. In: Berk JL & Sampliner JE (eds) *Handbook of Critical Care,* 2nd ed, p. 203. Boston: Little Brown.

Clarke–Pearson DL, Jelovesk FR & Creasman WT (1983) Thromboembolism complicating surgery for cervical and uterine malignancy: Incidence, risk factors, and prophylaxis. *Obstet. Gynecol.* **61:** 87.

Clarke–Pearson DL, Synan IS, Coleman E *et al.* (1984) The natural history of postoperative venous thromboemboli in gynecologic oncology: A prospective study of 382 patients. *Am. J. Obstet. Gynecol.* **148:** 1051.

Dahi S & Gold MI (1978) Comparison of two methods of postoperative respiratory care. *Chest* **73:** 592.

■ Eisner FR, Montz FJ & Berek JS (1990) Cytoreductive surgery for advanced ovarian cancer: Cardiovascular evaluation with pulmonary artery catheters. *Gynecol. Oncol.* **37:** 11.

Elliott CG, Zimmerman GA & Clemmer TP (1979) Complications of pulmonary artery catheterization in the case of critically ill patients: A prospective study. *Chest* **76:** 647.

Fang LS (1989) Therapy of renal diseases. In: Larson EB & Ramsey PG (eds) *Medical Therapeutics,* p. 183. Philadelphia: WB Saunders.

Fry DE (1988) Multiple system organ failure. *Surg. Clin. North Am.* **68:** 107.

Gass GD & Olsen GN (1986) Preoperative pulmonary function testing to predict postoperative morbidity and mortality. *Chest* **89:** 127.

Gerzof SG, Robbins AH & Johnson WC (1981) Percutaneous catheter drainage of abdominal abscesses. *New Engl. J. Med.* **305:** 653.

Goldman L (1981) Noncardiac surgery in patients receiving propranolol. Case reports and a recommended aproach. *Arch. Intern. Med.* **141:** 193.

Goldman L (1983) Cardiac risks and complications of noncardiac surgery. *Ann. Intern. Med.* **98:** 504.

■ Goldman L, Caldera DL, Southwick FS *et al.* (1977) Multifactorial index of cardiac risk in noncardiac procedures. *N. Engl. J. Med.* **297:** 845.

Goldman L, Caldera DL, Southwick FS *et al.* (1978) Cardiac risk factors and complications in non-cardiac surgery. *Medicine* **57:** 357.

■ Grum CM & Chauncey JB (1988) Conventional mechanical ventilation. *Clin. Chest Med.* **9:** 37.

Hakim RM & Lazarus JM (1988) Hemodialysis in acute renal failure. In: Brenner BM & Lazarus JM (eds) *Acute Renal Failure,* 2nd ed, p. 767. New York: Churchill Livinstone.

Handa SR & Morrin PA (1967) Diagnostic indices in acute renal failure. *Can. Med. Assoc. J.* **96:** 78.

Iverson RL (1988) Septic shock: A clinical perspective. *Crit. Care Clin.* **4:** 215.

Jackson MCV (1988) Preoperative pulmonary evaluation. *Arch. Intern. Med.* **148:** 2120.

Jelenko C III, Williams JB, Wheeler MC *et al.* (1979) Studies in shock and resuscitation: I. Uses of a hypertonic, albumin-containing, fluid demand regimen (HALFD) in resuscitation. *Crit. Care Med.* **7:** 157.

Johnson G, Bond FF, Stack LB, Class CA & Hardebeck JR (1987) Efficacy of military antishock trousers in compensatory and decompensatory hemorrhagic hypotension. *Circ. Shock* **21:** 233.

Lawrence PF (1992) *Essentials of General Surgery,* 2nd ed, p. 109. Baltimore: MA: Williams & Wilkins.

Levinsky NG & Bernard DB (1988) Mannitol and loop diuretics in acute renal failure. In: Brenner BM & Lazarus JM (eds) *Acute Renal Failure,* 2nd ed, p. 841. New York: Churchill Livingstone.

■ Light PD, Spar BM & Moran MT (1989) Renal assessment and management. In: Wolfsthal SD (ed) *Medical Perioperative Management,* p. 150. Norwalk: Appleton and Lange.

Love HW, Wangensteen S & Glenn T (1980) Presence of a myocardial depressant factor in patients in circulatory shock. *Surgery* **70:** 223.

Lowe RJ, Moss GS, Jilak J & Levine HD (1977) Crystalloid vs colloid in the etiology of patient failure after trauma: a randomized trial in man. *Surgery* **81:** 676.

Lowery BD, Cloutier CT & Carcy LC (1971) Electrolyte solutions in resuscitation in human hemorrhagic shock. *Surg. Gynecol. Oncol.* **133:** 273.

Lucas CE & Ledgerwood AM (1983) The fluid problem in the critically ill. *Surg. Clin. North Am.* **63:** 439.

Mann WJ, Jander HP, Partridge EE *et al.* (1980) Selective arterial embolization for control of bleeding in gynecologic malignancy. *Gynecol. Oncol.* **10:** 279.

Methylprednisolone Severe Sepsis Study Group (1987) A controlled clinical trial of high-dose methylprednisolone in the treatment of severe sepsis and septic shock. *N. Engl. J. Med.* **317:** 659.

Miller TR, Anderson RJ, Linas SC *et al.* (1978) Urinary diagnostic indices in acute renal failure: a prospective study. *Ann. Int. Med.* **89:** 47.

National Institutes of Health Consensus Development Conference (1980) Thrombolytic therapy in thrombosis. *Ann. Int. Med.* **93:** 141.

Nicholson DP (1989) Review of corticosteroid treatment in sepsis and septic shock: Pro or con. *Crit. Care Clin.* **5:** 151.

Orr JW, Shingleton HM, Soong SJ *et al.* (1983) Hemodynamic parameters following pelvic exenteration. *Am. J. Obstet. Gynecol.* **146:** 882.

Pastore JO, Yurchak PM, Janis KM *et al.* (1978) The risk of advanced branch block in surgical patients with right bundle branch block and left axis deviation. *Circulation* **57:** 677.

Pearce AC & Jones RM (1984) Smoking and anesthesia: Preoperative abstinence and perioperative morbidity. *Anesthesiology* **61:** 576.

Peevy KJ, Ronnlund RD, Chartarand SA *et al.* (1988) Ibuprofen in experimental group B streptococcal shock. *Circ. Shock* **24:** 35.

Pruett TL & Simmons RL (1988) Status of percutaneous catheter drainage of abscesses. *Surg. Clin. North Am.* **68:** 89.

Roberts DE, Dobson KE, Hall DW & Light RB (1988) Effects of prolonged naloxone infusion in septic shock. *Lancet* **24:** 700.

Rock P, Silverman H & Plump D (1985) Efficacy and safety of naloxone in septic shock. *Crit. Care Med.* **13:** 28.

Rooney SM, Goldiner PL & Muss E (1976) Relationship of right bundle branch block and left axis deviation to complete heart block during general anesthesia. *Anesthesiology* **44:** 64.

Sahn SA & Lakshminarayan S (1973) Bedside criteria for discontinuation of mechanical ventilation. *Chest* **63:** 1002.

Saklad M (1941) Grading of patients for surgical procedures. *Anesthesiology* **2:** 281.

Salzman E & Davies G (1980) Prophylaxis of venous thromboembolism. *Ann. Surg.* **191:** 207.

Schwartz PE (1982) Arterial hemorrhage in gynecologic malignancies. In: Delgado G & Smith P (eds) *Management of Complications in Gynecologic Oncology*, p. 35. New York: John Wiley & Sons.

Shoemaker WC (1976) Comparison of the relative effectiveness of whole blood transfusions and various types of fluid therapy in resuscitation. *Crit. Care Med.* **4:** 71.

Shoemaker WC (1982) Pathophysiology and therapy of shock states. In: Berk JL & Sampliner JE (eds) *Handbook of Critical Care*, 2nd ed, p. 253. Boston: Little Brown.

■ Sibbald WJ, Calvin JE, Holliday RL & Driedger AA (1983) Concepts in the pharmacologic and nonpharmacologic support of cardiovascular function in critically ill surgical patients. *Surg. Clin. North Am.* **63:** 455.

Simon AB (1977) Perioperative management of the pacemaker patient. *Anesthesiology* **46:** 127.

Skillman JS, Restal DS & Salzman EW (1975) Randomized trial of albumin vs electrolyte solutions during abdominal aortic operations. *Surgery* **78:** 291.

Tarhan S, Moffitt RA, Taylor WF & Giulian ER (1972) Myocardial infarction after general anesthesia. *JAMA* **220:** 1451.

Tisi GM (1979) Preoperative evaluation of pulmonary function: Validity, indications, and benefits. *Am. Rev. Respir. Dis.* **119:** 293.

Walsh JJ, Bonnar J & Wright FW (1974) A study of pulmonary embolism and deep leg thrombosis after major gynecologic surgery using labeled fibrinogen, phlebography and lung scanning. *J. Obstet. Gynecol. Br. Cwlth.* **81:** 311.

Weil MH, Henning RS & Puri VK (1979) Colloid oncotic pressure: clinical significance. *Crit. Care Med.* **7:** 113.

Weil MH & Nishijima H (1978) Cardiac output in bacterial shock. *Am. J. Med.* **64:** 920.

Zibrak JD, O'Donnell CR & Marton KL (1990) Indications for pulmonary function testing. *Ann. Intern. Med.* **112:** 7636.

37 Imaging Techniques in the Evaluation of Patients with Gynecologic Malignancies

J T Lomerci
C D Runowicz
A Frost

Introduction

Technologic advances in radiology have resulted in improved imaging techniques, which have the potential to facilitate the diagnosis and treatment of diseases. The cross-sectional imaging modalities, such as ultrasound (US), computed tomography (CT), and magnetic resonance imaging (MRI) have largely replaced conventional radiographic techniques. This chapter will focus on the roles of US, CT, MRI and radioimmunoscintigraphy (RIS) in the pre-treatment evaluation and post-treatment monitoring of patients with gynecologic malignancies. Positron emission tomography (PET) is a new form of computer-assisted imaging. The preliminary studies addressing its role in ovarian cancer will be discussed.

Imaging Modalities

Modern ultrasound diagnostics use real-time B-picture machines. The frequencies emitted are 3.5–5 MHz for transabdominal sonography, and up to 10 MHz for endovaginal sonography. In combination with transvaginal sonography, color-coded Doppler imaging and spectral analysis assess blood flow in pelvic organs. Ultrasonic images are created by taking advantage of differences in acoustic impedance between tissues. Echo-free cysts and cystic–solid masses can be distinguished by their sonographic characteristics (Goodsitt, 1993). Ultrasound examination provides important information about the structure and the borders of tumors. With pulsed Doppler, a sample volume can be selected and a spectral wave form recorded. The wave form is an indication of the relative resistance to flow within an organ. The spectral wave form can be quantified using indexes such as the pulsatility (PI) and resistivity (RI) indexes.

Advantages of ultrasonography include:

- the ability to scan rapidly in multiple planes;
- low cost;
- wide availability;
- the lack of ionizing radiation.

Disadvantages include:

- the requirement of a full urinary bladder to visualize pelvic structures transabdominally;
- difficulty in consistently visualizing the retroperitoneum, peritoneal tumor nodules and the pelvic side walls.

Doppler evaluation is being increasingly used in an attempt to improve the specificity of transabdominal and transvaginal sonography. Transvaginal US improves the spatial resolution of structures located near the transducer and does not require a full bladder; however, the field of view is limited. Placement of the vaginal probe may be difficult in premenarchal and postmenopausal women.

A CT image is an X-ray-generated imaging modality. A computer is used to analyze the attenuation of each X-ray beam that passes through the patient. Images of transverse sections of the body are subsequently reconstructed using a filtered back projection technique and displayed using a grey scale series of attenuation units (Pelc and Colsher, 1993). Tissue differentiation can be enhanced by intravenous contrast medium, which opacifies the bladder and ureters, and distinguishes between contrast-filled blood vessels and adjacent lymph nodes. For visualization of small and large bowel, oral contrast enhancement is also necessary. If rectal involvement is suspected, a dilute water-soluble contrast enema with air insufflation can be administered.

CT advantages include:

- intravenous contrast enhancement of blood vessels;
- oral contrast enhancement of the gastrointestinal (GT) tract;
- quick scan times;
- high spatial resolution.

CT limitations include:

- an inability to image in sagittal planes without a computed reconstruction;
- high cost;
- the risk of intravenous contrast allergy;
- image degradation from metal hip prostheses;
- its use of ionizing radiation.

Tissues that are markedly different in density such as calcium, water, fat and air are clearly distinguishable by CT examination. A significant limitation of CT is its poor soft tissue resolution because soft tissue structures have only minimal density differences (Fritzsche *et al.*, 1989).

MRI is a non-ionizing, computer-based technique that provides cross-sectional images. MRI relies on differences in specific tissue parameters in order to produce images. These tissue parameters include the hydrogen content of fat or water (proton density), blood flow, and T1/T2 tissue magnetic relaxation times (Brant–Zawadzki, 1987). T1 and T2 magnetic relaxation times reflect the rates at which protons emit their signals after excitation by a radiofrequency (RF) pulse and are inherent characteristics of a particular tissue. Differences in these tissue dependent variable (i.e. proton density, blood flow, and T1 and T2 relaxation times) are greater than differences obtainable with radiographic contrast (i.e. electron density). Hence, more soft tissue contrast can be demonstrated with MRI as compared to CT (Brant-Zawadzki, 1987).

All MR imaging systems are based on either resistive or superconducting magnets with field strengths that vary from 0.08 to 2.0 Telso. Increasing magnetic field strength results in enhanced resolution and a reduction in scan time. Partial distension of the bladder is preferred during MR imaging as it displaces small bowel loops from the pelvis. Glucagon (1 mg intravenously or intramuscularly) can be administered to reduce motion artifact produced by bowel peristalsis (Olson *et al.*, 1992). A complete examination requires both T1 and T2 weighted pulse sequences. T2 weighted MR images delineate the internal anatomy of the uterus, cervix, and vagina. T1 weighted images are useful in detecting tumor extension into retroperitoneal fat and in detecting lymph node enlargement (Olson *et al.*, 1992).

In addition to its excellent soft tissue contrast resolution and multi-planar imaging capabilities, advantages of MRI include:

- an ability to visualize blood vessels without IV contrast agents;
- biological safety;
- no special patient preparation.

Limitations of MRI include:

- cost;
- relatively long scan time;
- poorer spatial resolution as compared to CT;
- image degradation from motion;
- patient claustrophobia and poor patient tolerance;
- an inability to image patients with cardiac pacemakers or cerebral vascular clips (Fritzsche *et al.*, 1989).

Radioimmunoscintigraphy (RIS) uses radiolabeled monoclonal antibodies (MoAbs) specific for a tumor antigen to visualize tumors with a gamma camera. RIS is a functional or biologic imaging modality. Successful radioimmunodetection of tumors requires:

- antibody stability;
- optimal antibody specificity to reduce radiation to nontargeted tissues and to reduce background radioactivity;
- a radiolabel half-life long enough to image the tumor site, but short enough to reduce radiation to surrounding normal tissues;
- antibody characteristics that maximize tumor targeting and minimize the formation of human anti-mouse antibody complexes (Kim and Kasi, 1993).

Scintigraphic display of the *in vivo* biodistribution of intravenously administered radioactive MoAb is performed using a gamma camera with a large field of view and equipped with a low–medium energy collimator. A whole body planar scintigraphy can be enhanced by a single-photon emission computed tomography (SPECT), which allows three-dimensional display of the activity distribution in the patient after performing a 360° rotation around the body.

The number of radionuclides that are suitable for immunoscintigraphy is limited. At present, the radiolabel most suitable for imaging ovarian cancer is indium-111 (^{111}In), a gamma-emitting isotope. It has a long half-life, which permits imaging up to 10–14 days after injection, dual photon peaks which allow superior planar and tomographic imaging, easy preparation in a kit form, and a lack of beta emission. The major limitation of ^{111}In is its tendency to accumulate in the liver and spleen (Neal *et al.*, 1993). Technetium-99m (^{99m}Tc) is also a suitable radiolabel due to its low cost, ease of handling, favorable gamma emissions, and low radiation to normal tissue (Neal *et al.*, 1993). However, it has a relatively short physical half-life.

It is possible to detect tumors immunoscintigraphically even when CT, MRI and sonography are normal. It is also possible to detect recurrences in patients with normal tumor markers. However, its clinical usefulness in the detection of small (<1 cm) tumor nodules awaits further clinical investigation.

Since the radiolabeled MoAbs are murine in origin, patients may develop anti-mouse antibodies. The production of human anti-mouse antibodies (HAMA) can result in very high false-positive CA-125 values in patients with elevated HAMA titers (Halpern, 1992; Neal *et al.*, 1993). Because of the development of HAMA, RIS is usually used only once in each patient.

Cervical Cancer

To conform with the International Federation of Gynecology and Obstetrics (FIGO), patients with cervical cancer are clinically staged. The clinical staging includes a bimanual pelvic examination, chest radiography, excretory urography (IVP), barium enema, cystoscopy and sigmoidoscopy. Clinical staging is accurate in only 65–70% of patients when compared to surgical staging (van Nagell *et al.*, 1971; Averette *et al.*, 1975). Clinical examination is limited to estimating the size of the tumor, parametrial spread and pelvic sidewall involvement. Since approximately 7.3% of cervical cancer patients will have hydronephrosis or nonvisualization of the kidneys, IVP will be normal in the majority of patients. Similarly, barium enema is not a useful test in that only 3.4% of patients will have an abnormal result (Griffin *et al.*, 1976). Therefore, the clinical stage of the disease is no longer the exclusive parameter in the selection of therapy.

Computed Tomography

The reported overall accuracy of CT in the staging of cervical carcinoma ranges from 58–88% (Lee and Marx, 1989; Kim *et al.*, 1993). In patients with clinical Stage IIB–IIIB, CT understages 12–33% of patients due to microscopic tumor involvement of the pelvic sidewall, bladder, lymph nodes or omentum (Kilcheski *et al.*, 1981; Walsh *et al.*, 1981; Villasanta *et al.*, 1983). CT relies on lymph node size as the only criteria for possible tumor involvement. Nodes larger than 1.0–1.5 cm are considered abnormal. Whitely *et al.* (1982) and Walsh *et al.* (1980) reported accuracies for the detection of pelvic lymph node metastases between 74–83%. CT has a higher rate of accuracy in evaluating paraaortic lymph node metastases, with a sensitivity of 67–77%, a specificity of 86–100% and an overall accuracy of 80–98% (Kilcheski *et al.*, 1981; Villasanta *et al.*, 1983; Bandy *et al.*, 1985; Camilien *et al.*, 1988). Involvement of paraaortic nodes is identified more readily than that of pelvic nodes due to the surrounding retroperitoneal fat.

Because surgery is reserved for patients with tumor confined to the cervix, accurate assessment of parametrial tumor extension is a crucial point in the preoperative staging of cervical cancer. Tumor invasion of the parametrium is seen as poor definition or irregularity of the lateral cervical margins or prominent parametrial soft tissue strands on CT (*Figure 37.1*). A definitive CT diagnosis of parametrial tumor extension requires demonstration of a parametrial soft tissue mass and loss of the periureteral fat plane. Enhanced blood vessels, the ovaries, and round, broad and uterosacral ligaments can be misinterpreted as lateral tumor extension (Kim *et al.*, 1990). Confluent, irregular, linear parametrial soft tissue strands extending to the obturator internus muscle laterally or pyriformis muscle posterolaterally indicate true pelvic sidewall extension (Lee and Marx, 1989). The accuracy of CT in determining parametrial status ranges from 30–70% (Grumbine *et al.*, 1981; Walsh *et al.*, 1981; Whitely *et al.*, 1982; Vick *et al.*, 1984; Worthington *et al.*, 1986; Kim *et al.*, 1990). In patients with clinical Stage IB lesions, CT has an error rate of 42–70% in accurately diagnosing parametrial tumor extension (Grumbine *et al.*, 1981; Kilcheski *et al.*, 1981; Walsh *et al.*, 1981; Villasanta *et al.*, 1983). Thus, for documenting parametrial involvement by tumor, CT scans have not been found to be clinically useful. A careful examination by an experienced gynecologic or radiation oncologist is more accurate in determining parametrial spread.

CT scans can enhance clinical staging in advanced staged disease, particularly in the detection of enlarged lymph nodes. With invasive radiology and the ability to perform diagnostic needle aspirations, metastatic spread to lymph nodes, liver and lung

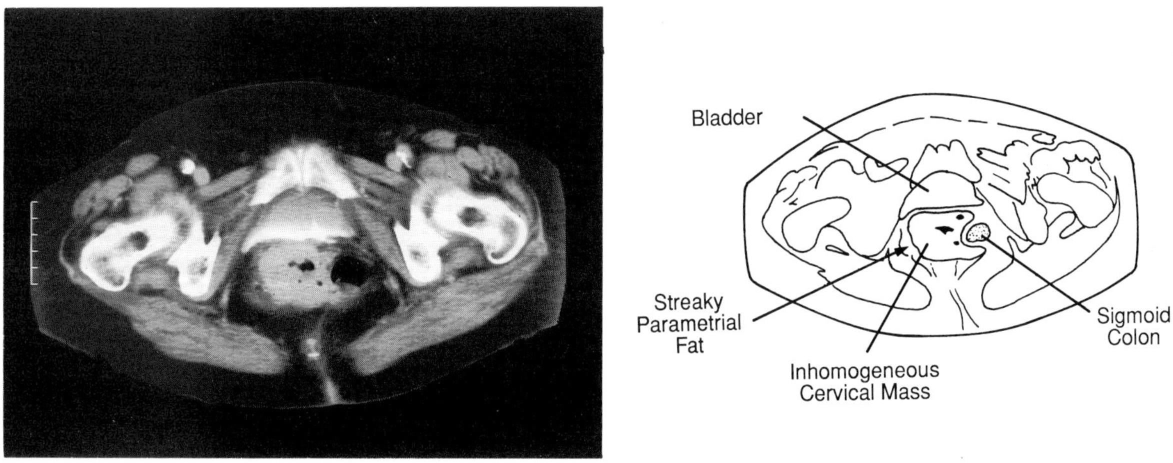

Figure 37.1 left & right. Stage IIB cervical cancer. CT scan through a contrast-filled bladder shows gas bubbles and hypodense cervical cancer highlighted by intravenous contrast-enhancement of the cervical stroma. Streaking of the parametrial fat is consistent with tumor infiltration.

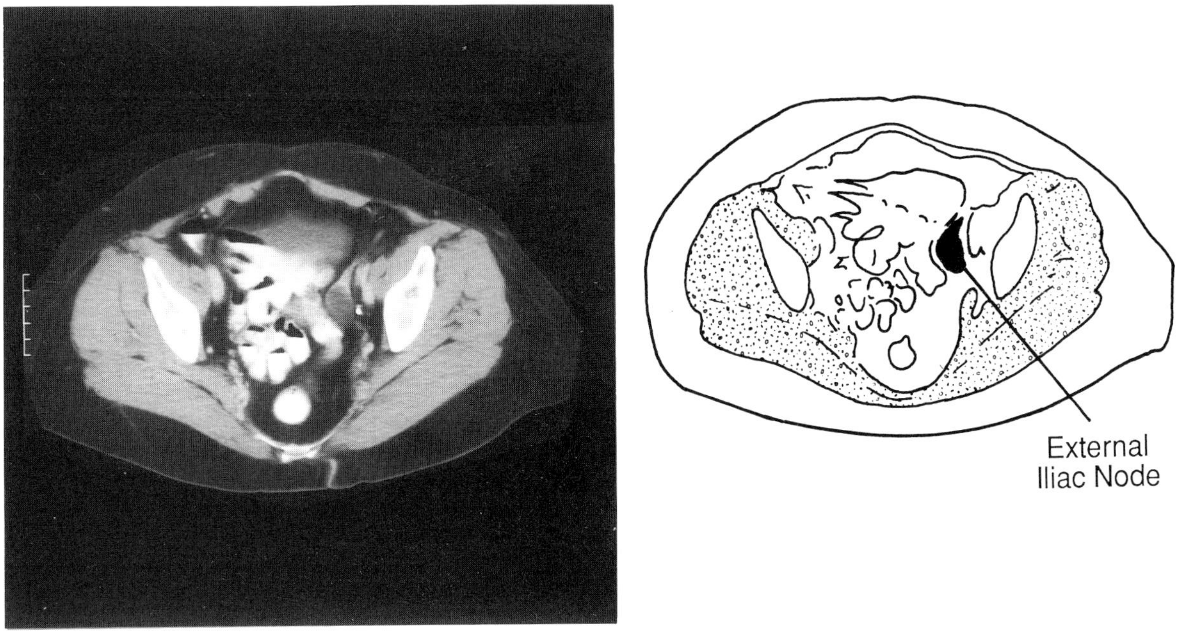

Figure 37.2 left & right. Recurrent cervical cancer. CT scan shows a 1.6 × 2.8 cm hypodense left external iliac lymph node metastasis.

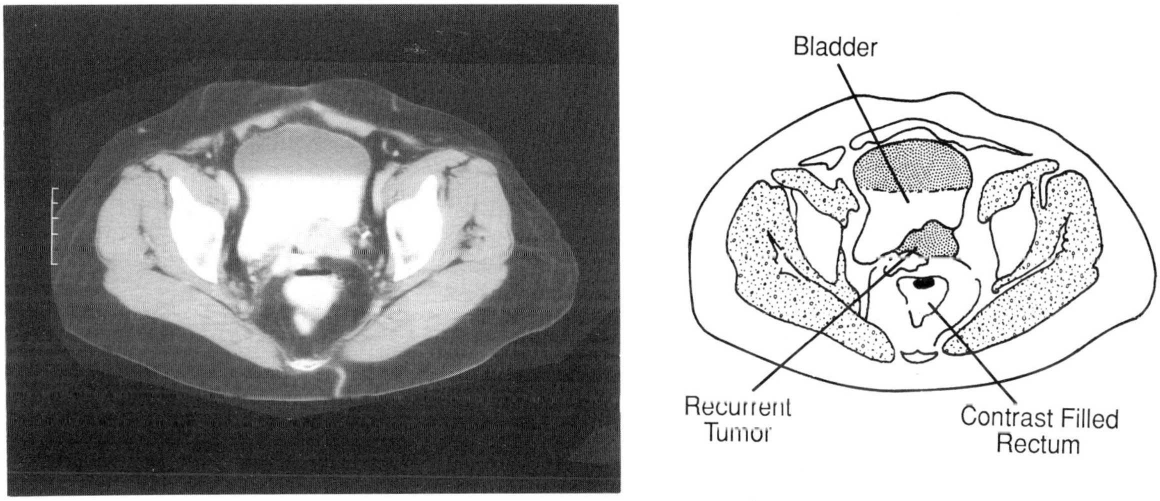

Figure 37.3 left & right. Recurrent cervical cancer. CT scan through bladder shows a 2.5 × 4.2 cm hypodense recurrent tumor as a slightly lobulated density adjacent to the vaginal vault between the contrast-filled rectum and the bladder.

can be cytopathologically documented, thus eliminating the need for surgery. CT scans of the abdomen and pelvis are also useful in monitoring patients for recurrent disease following treatment (*Figures 37.2 and 37.3*). Radiation-induced changes on CT include a thickened bladder and rectal wall, thickened perirectal fascia, and widening of the presacral space (Doubleday and Bernardino, 1980).

The accuracy of CT in the detection of local recurrences is approximately 80–85% (Walsh *et al.*, 1981; Heron *et al.*, 1988). The primary limitation of CT is the inability to differentiate fibrotic changes from tumor (*Figure 37.4*).

Magnetic Resonance Imaging

MRI identifies carcinoma of the cervix as a relatively high signal intensity lesion on T2-weighted images. MRI cannot distinguish between carcinoma *in situ*, microinvasive disease, or small (<0.5 cm) superficially invasive tumors (Togashi *et al.*, 1986; Togashi *et al.*, 1989). This insensitivity is due to poor contrast between the relatively high signal intensity tumor and the high signal intensity normal epithelium (Togashi *et al.*, 1989). MRI has a high predictive value for identifying invasive tumor confined to the cervix. The accuracy of MRI in demonstrating

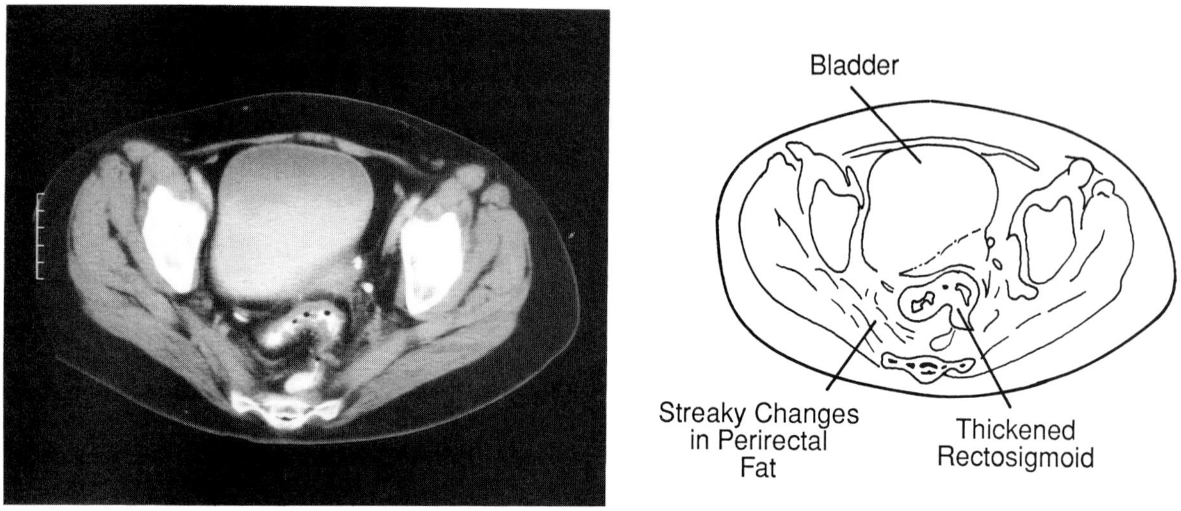

Figure 37.4 left & right. Radiation therapy changes. CT scan through bladder shows a thick-walled rectosigmoid as well as streaky changes in the perirectal fat.

invasive disease (stromal invasion) approaches 85% (Sironi *et al.*, 1993). Because low signal intensity cervical stroma provides excellent contrast to hyperintense tumor, deep stromal invasion is clearly identified by MRI (Hricak *et al.*, 1988). Intravenous gadolinium-diethylenetriamine-pentaacetate (Gd-DTPA)-enhanced MRI renders the tumor equal in tissue density to the surrounding normal tissue and is not advantageous (Sironi *et al.*, 1993). Contrast enhancement is useful in the detection of bladder wall and rectal invasion (Bragg and Hricak, 1993).

MRI has a reported accuracy of 86–100% in predicting endometrial extension and approximately 100% in predicting vaginal extension (Hricak *et al.*, 1988; Sironi *et al.*, 1993). On axial T2-weighted images, preservation of the low signal intensity ring of cervical stroma is a reliable indicator of the absence of full-thickness stromal or parametrial invasion. Lesions with full-thickness stromal invasion show a relatively high incidence of microscopic parametrial involvement, which is not detectable by MRI (Togashi *et al.*, 1989). If a full-thickness lesion exhibits poorly defined margins or protrudes through a defect in the stromal ring, macroscopic parametrial invasion is possible (Togashi *et al.*, 1986; Hricak *et al.*, 1988; Togashi *et al.*, 1989; Kim *et al.*, 1990). MRI has been reported to predict parametrial extension with an accuracy of 85–88%, with a false-positive rate of 8–15% (Hricak *et al.*, 1988; Greco *et al.*, 1989; Sironi *et al.*, 1993). Morphologic and signal intensity alterations indicating parametrial tumor spread (Stage IIB) include an irregular lateral margin, prominent parametrial strands, eccentric parametrial enlargement, and loss of periparametrial fat planes on T1-weighted images and/or an abnormally high intensity signal in the involved parametrium on T2-weighted images (Togashi *et al.*, 1986; Hricak *et al.*, 1988; Kim *et al.*, 1990). In the largest series with surgical correlation, the negative predictive value of MRI for parametrial extension was 94% (Hricak *et al.*, 1988). A comparative study of CT and MRI reported that the overall accuracy for parametrial evaluation was 78% for clinical evaluation, 70% for CT, and 92% for MRI (Kim *et al.*, 1990).

Discussion of radiologic criteria for pelvic sidewall involvement is difficult because histologic confirmation is not usually obtained. Frequently, a clinical diagnosis of Stage IIIB lesions will fail to show radiographic evidence of disease extension to the pelvic musculature. The suspicion of pelvic sidewall involvement in T1-weighted images is raised when an ill-defined lesion exhibits unusually prominent strands extending to the pelvic sidewall or when an ill-defined lesion completely obliterates normal vascular structures within the cardinal ligament (Togashi *et al.*, 1986; Togashi and Konishi, 1989).

In Stage IVA disease, sagittal images facilitate clear visualization of the relationship of the posterior bladder wall and tumor. Segmental disruption of the low signal intensity wall is a reliable indicator that the lesion involves the muscular layer (Togashi *et al.*, 1986; Togashi and Kanishi, 1990). Direct rectal involvement is indicated by segmental loss of fat or unusually prominent strands between the tumor and rectum, as well as segmental thickening or loss of the anterior rectal wall (Hricak *et al.*, 1988).

There is debate as to which modality, CT or MRI, is better in assessing lymph node involvement since both modalities are dependent on lymph node size. Some investigators argue that the two imaging modalities are equivalent (Kim *et al.*, 1994), while others argue that MRI is better in detecting regional lymph node involvement (Hricak *et al.*, 1991).

Approximately 35% of patients treated for

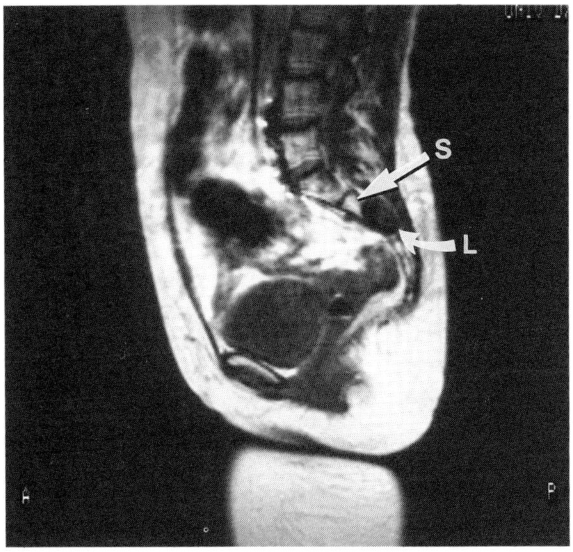

(A)

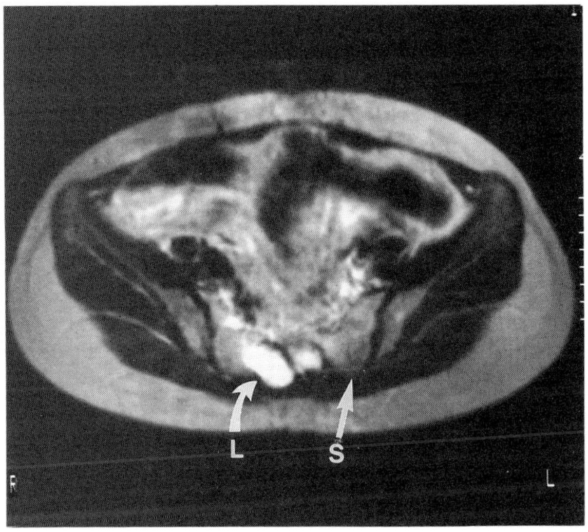

(B)

Figure 37.5. Recurrent cervical carcinoma. (**A**) A sagittal T1-weighted image through the pelvis showing a 1.2 × 3 cm hypointense lesion (L) at the right aspect of sacrum (S). (**B**) An axial T2-weighted image through the sacrum shows the same lesion as hyperintense.

invasive cervical cancer develop recurrent disease, and 80% of recurrences develop within the first two years after treatment (Montana *et al.*, 1985; Montana *et al.*, 1986). When compared to physical examination or CT, MRI is superior in its ability to differentiate between residual tumor and fibrosis (*Figure* 37.5). Radiation therapy leads to progressive replacement of tumor by scar tissue resulting in reduced signal intensity (Flueckiger *et al.*, 1992). Flueckiger *et al.* (1992) found that tumors that demonstrated complete regression following radiation therapy showed a marked decline in relative signal intensity, which was most pronounced during the first three months and was complete at six months. The declining, but still relatively high, signal intensity in irradiated cervical cancers within three months of radiation therapy was due to the presence of residual, but devitalized tumor tissue, necrosis, edema, bleeding and/or inflammatory reactions. Within this series 7 patients with persistent tumor at six months by MRI still had subsequent cure, suggesting that a decision based on MRI findings regarding persistent disease cannot be made until nine months following radiation therapy.

Parametrial or lateral pelvic recurrence is a common pattern of failure of patients with advanced disease (Jampolis *et al.*, 1975; Bachaud *et al.*, 1991). Inadequate radiation field size may be a contributing factor. MRI appears useful in optimizing radiation port placement and determining optimum field size. Mayr *et al.* (1993) evaluated the use of MRI in radiation treatment planning. Adjustments in radiation fields were made due to more extensive tumor involvement as demonstrated by MRI in 53%

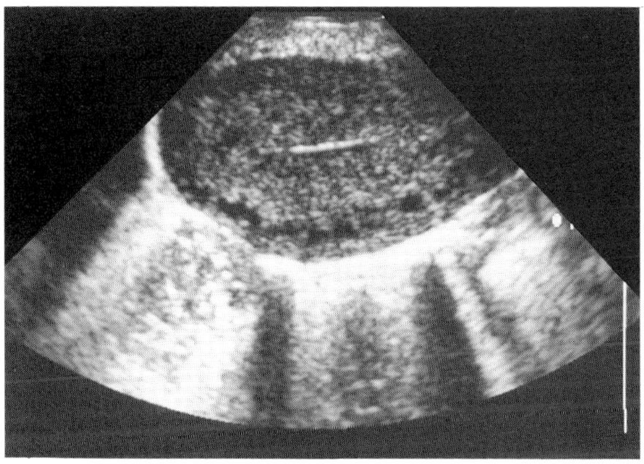

(A)

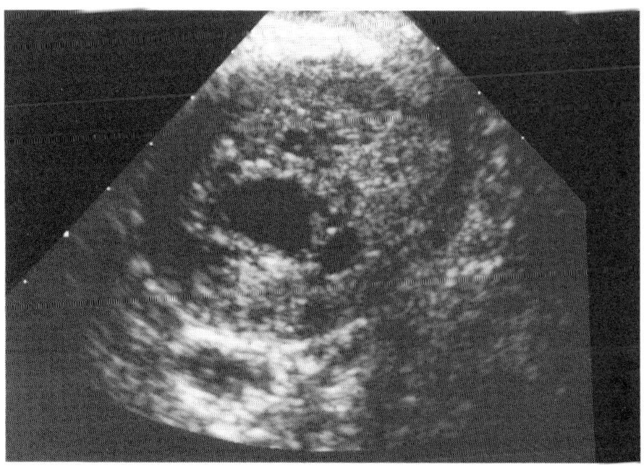

(B)

Figure 37.6. (**A**) Transvaginal ultrasound of normal endometrium showing thin endometrial echo. (**B**) Thickened endometrium with cystic areas consistent with endometrial hyperplasia/carcinoma.

of patients. A significant number of port misplacements were due to underestimates of the extent of parametrial and vaginal tumor involvement.

Endometrial Cancer

Although endometrial cancer is surgically staged, preoperative evaluation to determine the extent of disease may be helpful in the preparation of the patient for surgery and in determining if a pelvic and paraaortic lymphadenectomy is necessary.

Ultrasonography

The uterine cavity appears on ultrasound as an echo-dense line, which represents the endometrium, surrounded by a halo of low level echoes. Following menopause, the endometrium is usually less than 5 mm (*Figure 37.6A*). If the endometrial stripe is larger than 5 mm, a histopathologic diagnosis by endometrial sampling is required (*Figure 37.6B*). Transvaginal color flow Doppler has been used successfully in differentiating benign from malignant endometrial lesions based on flow impedance characteristics (Bourne *et al.*, 1991) and may improve the detection of smaller endometrial tumors. However, it must be remembered that sonography provides morphologic and not histologic data.

Ultrasound has a reported accuracy of 80–90% in distinguishing deep from superficial myometrial tumor invasion (Fleischer *et al.*, 1987; Cacciatore *et al.*, 1989; Shipley *et al.*, 1992). Intrauterine probes (7.5 MHz) have also been developed to evaluate the depth of invasion (Hoetzinger, 1991). Use of an intrauterine probe may avoid the limitations of US, such as its tendency to understage myometrial invasion when the tumor is exophytic and has a significant intraluminal polypoid component, in addition to myometrial invasion.

Computed Tomography

Without contrast media, CT scans demonstrate only focal or diffuse enlargement of the uterine body. Following administration of contrast media, the tumor mass can be visualized because of the lower attenuation of the tumor compared to the surrounding myometrium. Tumor may be confined to the endometrial cavity and appear as a hypodense polypoid mass surrounded by less dense endometrial fluid or may focally invade the myometrium and be highlighted by adjacent normal enhanced myometrium (Lee *et al.*, 1989).

The overall accuracy of CT staging in endometrial carcinoma is reported to be 84–88% (Hricak, 1991). Accuracy in Stage I or II disease is 83% and 92% respectively, and in Stage III or IV disease, the accuracy is 83% and 86% respectively (Walsh and Goplerud, 1982; Balfe *et al.*, 1983). The depth of myometrial invasion can be determined with an overall accuracy of approximately 76% (Hamlin *et al.*, 1987). Angio-CT, which provides enhanced tumor definition due to the higher concentration of contrast media obtained adjacent to the tumor, has been used to successfully delineate the extent of invasion (Hirai *et al.*, 1989). Endometrial tumor involvement of the cervix is characterized by cervical enlargement (>3.5 cm) with hypodense areas within the fibromuscular stroma. The appearance of parametrial and pelvic sidewall extension and detection of lymph node involvement is similar to that of cervical carcinoma (Lee *et al.*, 1989).

Franchi *et al.* (1989) found that the overall diagnostic accuracy in determining recurrent disease was 92%. CT was found to be particularly advantageous with a 100% diagnostic accuracy in those patients where symptomatology (i.e. deteriorating performance status, weight loss, lumbar pain, and intestinal obstruction) was suggestive of recurrent tumor. As with recurrent cervical cancer, the main disadvantage of CT is the difficulty in distinguishing inflammation and extensive post-surgical and/or radiation fibrosis from recurrent tumor (Walsh and Goplerud, 1982).

Magnetic Resonance Imaging

Uterine zonal anatomy is appreciated on T2-weighted images with three discernible signal intensities. The endometrium has a high signal intensity similar to or greater than that of fat. The myometrium has a medium signal intensity. Between these two signal intensities is a third, low intensity junctional zone that is thought to correspond to the innermost portion of the myometrium. If this zone is intact, myometrial invasion is essentially excluded (Olson *et al.*, 1992). The junctional zone may not be visible as a distinct structure in premenarchal and postmenopausal women and therefore assessment of depth of invasion may be difficult in these patients (Togashi and Tonishi, 1990).

Endometrial carcinoma is identified as abnormal thickening of the central high intensity zone or may be depicted as a change of signal intensity (Togashi and Konishi, 1990). A central high intensity area in the uterus with a thickness greater than 1 cm in the reproductive years or greater than 3–5 mm in the postmenopausal age group is suggestive of an endometrial carcinoma. Because diagnosis of endometrial carcinoma depends on the measured thickness of the central high intensity zone, superficial or small lesions may be missed (Togashi and Konishi, 1990). In addition, other conditions such as endometrial hyperplasia, fluid retention or blood may also exhibit varied signal intensities or thickening of the central high intensity zone.

Following Gd-DTPA contrast media administration, endometrial carcinoma demonstrates enhancement. Unlike MRI contrast enhancement of the cervix, the distinction between tumor and normal endometrium is accentuated and it becomes possible to identify small tumors confined to the endometrium. Intravenous contrast also improves assessment of myometrial invasion and tumor location, and can help differentiate between retained debris and tumor (Hricak *et al.*, 1991).

Differentiation between Stage IIA and Stage IIB is made by assessment of the cervical stroma. Uninvolved stroma is of low signal intensity on T2-weighted images (Hricak, 1991). MRI may also be used to evaluate extrauterine tumor spread. The bladder or rectum is considered to be involved when the wall of the respective organ demonstrates focal loss of normal low signal intensity on T2-weighted images (Hricak, 1991).

Leiomyosarcoma presents as a sharply marginated low intensity mass with or without the speckled high intensity area, which is characteristic of leiomyoma (Worthington *et al.*, 1986). Stromal sarcoma and mixed müllerian tumors usually manifest as large ill-defined masses, which develop from the endometrium and deeply invade the myometrium. On T2-weighted images, the lesions display a heterogeneous appearance consisting of medium and high signal intensities (Shapero and Hricak, 1989). Since these findings are nonspecific, sarcomas cannot be differentiated from advanced endometrial carcinoma.

MRI has been shown to be useful in staging endometrial carcinoma, with an overall accuracy of approximately 82–92% (Olson *et al.*, 1992). This is largely due to the greater soft tissue contrast between tumor and surrounding normal tissue. Lien *et al.* (1991) found the overall accuracy of MRI in assessing depth of myometrial invasion to be 82%. False-positive results with respect to deep myometrial invasion were found on histologic examination to be due to large polypoid tumors distending the uterus. Sironi *et al.* (1992) found the sensitivity and specificity of MRI in the assessment of deep myometrial invasion to be 88% and 85% respectively. Errors in MRI interpretation were more frequently overestimates rather than underestimates secondary to the presence of polypoid tumors that induced marked distortion of the uterine cavity. MRI has not replaced CT for staging because it is less sensitive in detecting extrauterine metastases, more expensive, requires a longer time and is less acceptable to patients (Lee *et al.*, 1989).

Ovarian Cancer

The role of imaging and tumor markers in the early detection of ovarian cancer remains under investigation. Because the majority of patients with ovarian cancer are detected when they have Stage III or IV disease, studies addressing refinements and advances in screening modalities are crucial to define a role for these procedures in the early detection of ovarian cancer. Much better defined is the clinical usefulness of imaging in the preoperative assessment of patients with a pelvic/abdominal mass and in the follow-up of patients with ovarian cancer. Treatment response and disease status can be monitored by non-invasive imaging techniques.

Ultrasonography

Although US has been recommended for ovarian cancer screening (van Nagell *et al.*, 1991; Bourne *et al.*, 1994), it currently does not play a routine role in the detection of ovarian cancer in low-risk groups due to the lack of specificity. Refinements in assessing morphologic criteria, vascular characteristics and flow may improve the specificity and positive predictive value of US. Until such time, sonography should not be used in the detection of ovarian cancer outside of a clinical trial. The National Institutes of Health held a consensus conference on ovarian cancer in April, 1994 which supported this view.

When an ovarian lesion is clinically suspected, US can be used to confirm the presence or absence of a lesion and can be helpful in characterizing the mass. Sonographic criteria used in distinguishing benign from malignant masses include:

- the amount of echogenicity or solid material within the mass;
- size and thickness of the septa;
- wall structure;
- tumor size (DePriest *et al.*, 1993).

The accuracy of US in the diagnosis of pelvic masses ranges from 42–92% (Benacerraf *et al.*, 1990). The introduction of transvaginal Doppler US has allowed detailed hemodynamic assessment of ovarian tumors. The diagnostic accuracy of color Doppler sonography in distinguishing benign from malignant lesions ranges from 70 90% (Fleischer and Jones, 1993). The lack of universally applied specific 'cut-off values' for benign versus malignant hemodynamic values, such as pulsality index (PI) or resistive index (RI), probably accounts for the wide variation in diagnostic accuracy. Rather than trying to determine a specific cut-off level for benign versus malignant lesions based on flow impedance, Kurjak *et al.* (1993) suggested employing a multiparameter ultrasonographic analysis of ovarian tumors. In addition to examining pulsed Doppler waveform characteristics, vessel location and arrangement were also used to distinguish benign from malignant tumors. Results demonstrated that benign ovarian masses were associated with peripheral and pericystic vessel location coupled with a single vessel arrangement and RI greater than 0.41. Vessels

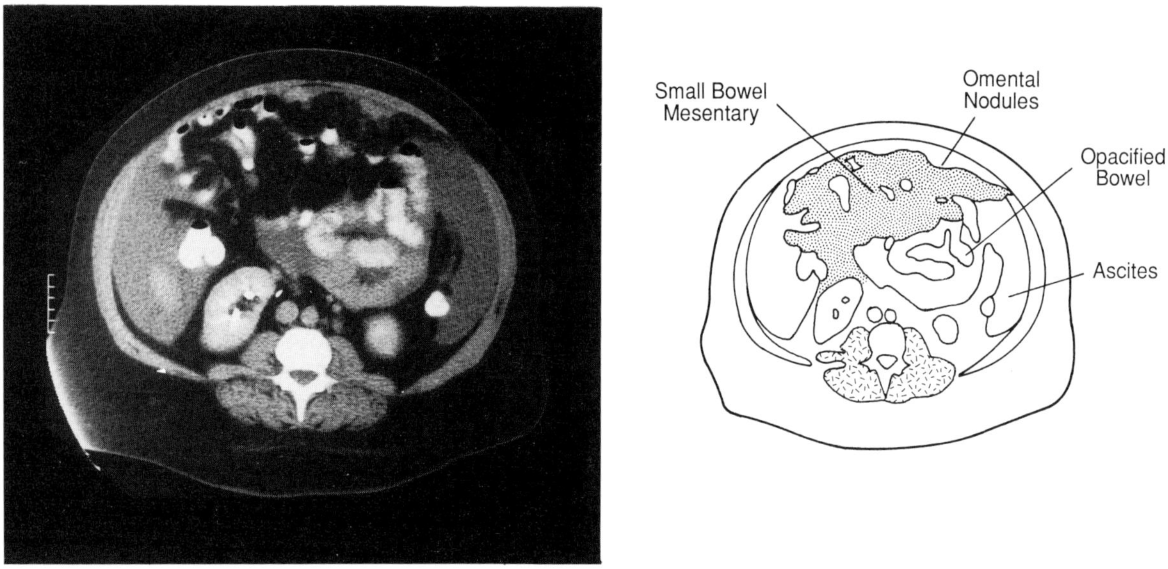

Figure 37.7 left & right. Papillary serous adenocarcinoma of the ovary. CT scan through the right kidney shows omental nodules, nodules in the small bowel mesentery, opacified small bowel and ascites.

located in the center or septum and with a diffuse or dispersed vascular arrangement, RI below 0.40, and associated with a papillary projection of the tumor were highly correlated with malignancy.

With respect to staging or in the follow-up of patients with ovarian cancer, ultrasound is limited by its ability to detect peritoneal or omental metastatic disease if the lesions are less than 1–2 cm, or to detect plaque-like lesions of the pelvic peritoneum (Murolo *et al.*, 1989). Requard *et al.* (1981) found that US correctly staged only 48% of patients, and detected only 20% of omental and peritoneal metastases and 25% of lymph node metastases. US has been shown to accurately identify clinically suspected recurrent disease larger than 2 cm (Murolo *et al.*, 1989). Ultrasound also has the greatest sensitivity in detecting recurrent tumor in the pelvis or around the liver and right hemidiaphragm in the presence of ascites (Pussell *et al.*, 1980; Murolo *et al.*, 1989).

Computed Tomography

With the current use of high resolution scanners, CT has become the preoperative imaging modality of choice for ovarian carcinoma. CT is capable of defining the nature of the primary ovarian lesion by detecting fat, calcifications, cystic or solid masses and septations. Mesenteric metastases are represented by round or poorly defined masses adjacent to contrast-enhanced loops of small bowel and mesenteric fat or by thickened leaves of mesentery (*Figure 37.7*). An omental cake may appear as an irregular sheet of nodular soft tissue densities beneath the anterior abdominal wall. Peritoneal and omental

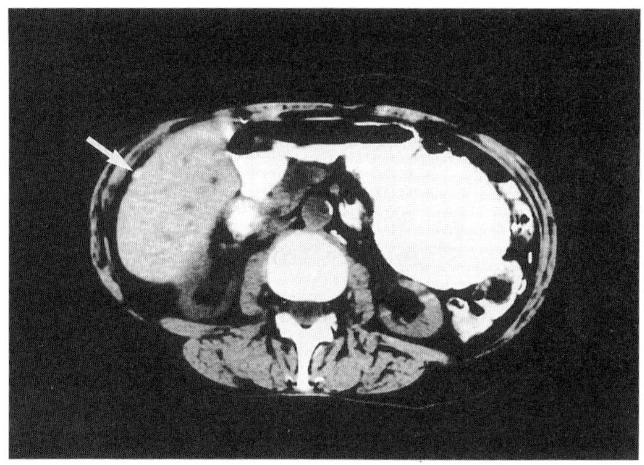

(A)

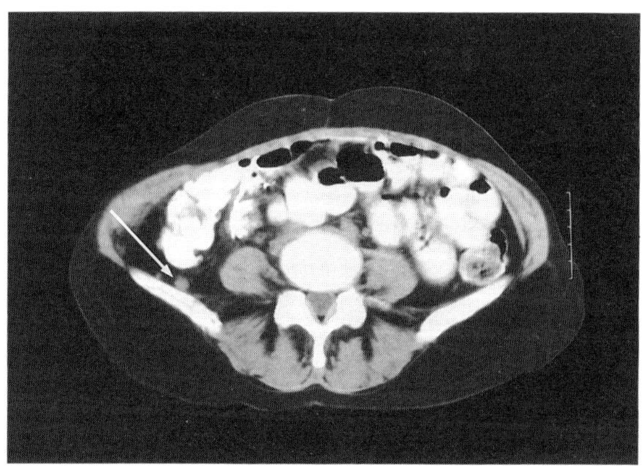

(B)

Figure 37.8. Papillary serous adenocarcinoma of the ovary. (**A**) CT scan through the right lobe of the liver shows tumor implants on the liver surface. (**B**) CT scan through the iliac crests shows a peritoneal implant 8 mm in size anterior to the right ilium in the right paracolic gutter (arrow).

metastases larger than 2 cm can be demonstrated by CT (Walsh *et al.*, 1978) and current high resolution scanners can detect peritoneal implants as small as 5 mm (Buy *et al.*, 1988) (*Figure 37.8*). Loculated malignant ascites can be detected with an accuracy of 90% (Dunnick *et al.*, 1979). Staging by CT has been found to correlate with surgical staging in approximately 70% of cases (Sanders *et al.*, 1983; Shiels *et al.*, 1985). Its greatest advantage is its ability to detect disease within the pelvis as well as extrapelvic disease in the liver, retroperitoneum and omentum.

In advanced stage disease, CT can assist in planning the optimal extent of tumor cytoreductive surgery. Nelson *et al.* (1993) demonstrated the ability of CT to predict the likelihood of optimal tumor cytoreduction. CT findings accurately predicted surgical outcome with a sensitivity of 92.3% and specificity of 79.3%. The study concluded that preoperative CT scanning may be useful in defining those patients in whom a laparotomy would not successfully result in residual disease less than 1 cm and could potentially result in significant operative morbidity. They suggest that these patients be offered neo-adjuvant chemotherapy followed by cytoreduction after completing several cycles of chemotherapy.

In studies designed to evaluate the potential usefulness of CT as an alternative to second-look laparotomy, the percentage of false-negative CT examinations has ranged from 15–64% (Calkins *et al.*, 1987; Silverman *et al.*, 1988). A more recent study by Reuter *et al.* (1989) demonstrated more favorable results for CT in determining tumor status with a sensitivity of 84%, specificity of 88%, and an 86% correlation between CT and surgical findings (*Figure 37.9*). The primary weakness of CT is its inability to consistently detect disease less than 1 cm in the omentum, peritoneum, mesentery and visceral surfaces (Brenner *et al.*, 1985). Frasci *et al.* (1994) evaluated the use of intraperitoneal contrast and CT imaging (IPC-CT) of the abdomen and pelvis in patients with advanced ovarian carcinoma who had normal conventional CT scans. Compared to conventional CT, IPC-CT was superior in detecting nodules less than 2 cm in diameter, but failed to detect solitary nodules measuring 0.5 cm or less. IPC-CT missed macroscopic disease in 12% of cases.

At the present time, a negative CT cannot replace second-look laparotomy in the assessment of disease status following first-line chemotherapy. In conjunction with serum tumor markers, a CT scan may be useful in monitoring patients with ovarian cancer during or following therapy.

Magnetic Resonance Imaging

MRI can be helpful in distinguishing a pedunculated leiomyoma from an adnexal mass. MRI may demonstrate feeding vessels originating from the uterus, suggesting a uterine rather than adnexal origin of the mass (Togashi and Konishi, 1990).

MRI features suggestive of ovarian malignancy include the detection of a lesion with a wall thickness greater than 3 mm or wall nodularity (Bragg and Hricak, 1993). Technical advances such as the use of

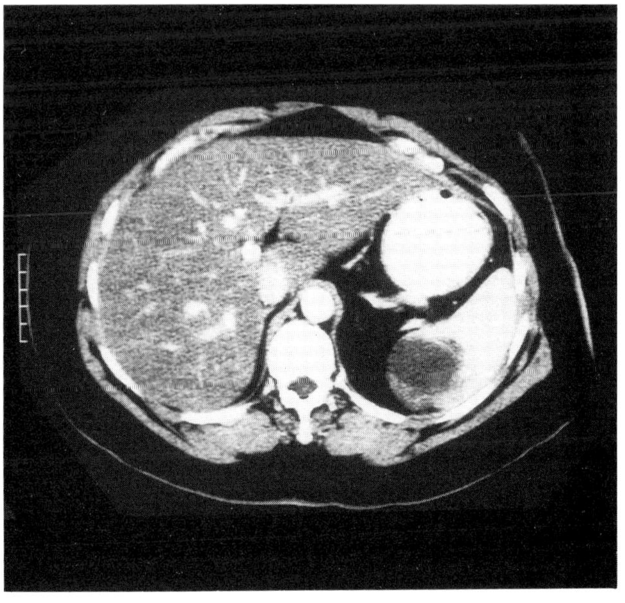

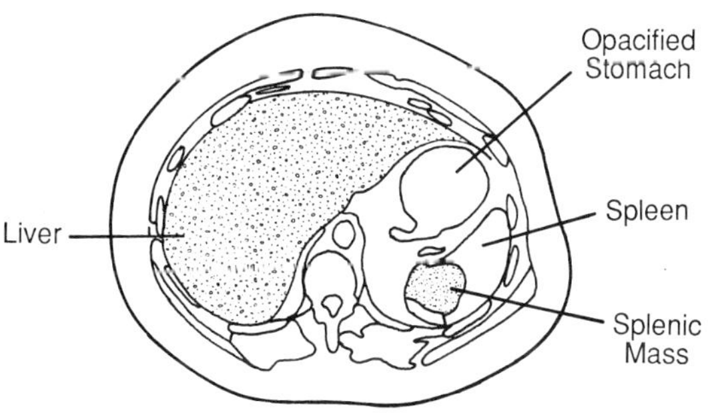

Figure 37.9 left & right. Recurrent papillary serous adenocarcinoma of the ovary in a 55-year-old female with an increasing CA-125. An exploratory laparotomy revealed an isolated focus of adenocarcinoma within the spleen without other evidence of intra-abdominal disease.

intravenously administered paramagnetic contrast agents such as Gd-DTPA and superparamagnetic particle oral contrast media have improved the specificity of MRI in detecting ovarian cancer. Thurnher (1992) reported that intravenous contrast media resulted in an MRI accuracy of 95% in distinguishing benign from malignant neoplasms. Compared to T2-weighted images, post-contrast T1-weighted images demonstrated superior overall tumor delineation, assessment of intratumoral architecture and definition of tumor origin. Mesenteric and omental metastases also enhance after Gd-DTPA injection. Semelka *et al.* (1993) used intravenously administered Gd-DTPA in the assessment of ovarian tumors and the extent of intraperitoneal disease. Due to higher contrast resolution, small ($\leqslant$1 cm) peritoneal metastases were more readily seen on contrast MRI as compared to noncontrast imaging.

The inability to reliably distinguish bowel loops from pathologic solid tissue is one of the major limitations of MRI of the abdomen and pelvis. Signal intensity of bowel contents vary over a wide range and consequently delineation of the gastrointestinal tract is insufficient in many patients. Prayer *et al.* (1993) completed a prospective study to determine the diagnostic value of MRI before and after ingestion of superparamagnetic oral contrast media in patients with treated ovarian cancer. Depiction of bowel loops was judged sufficient in 47% of plain scans and in 85% of enhanced scans. Diagnostic information obtained after contrast enhancement was estimated to be superior to that of plain MRI in 20% of patients.

MRI has not made a major impact on staging in ovarian carcinoma. Because it requires a relatively long examination time and exhibits image degradation from respiratory and bowel movement, it is less advantageous than CT or US (Jain *et al.*, 1993; Buist *et al.*, 1994).

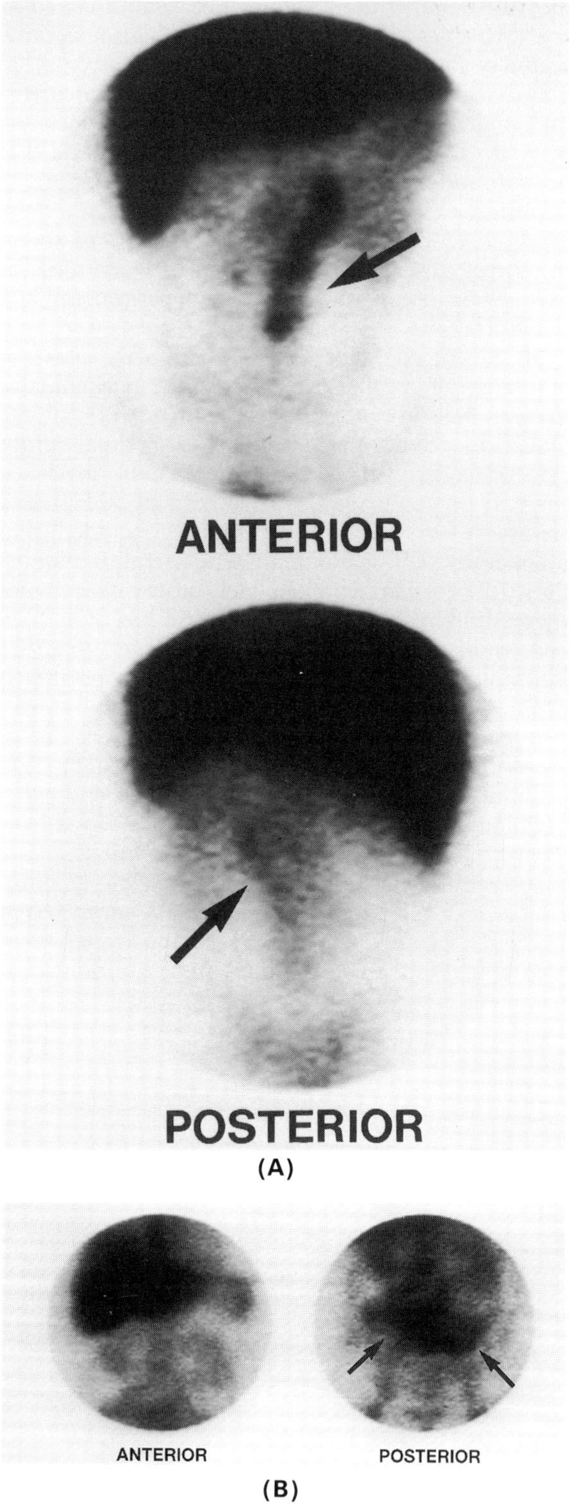

Figure 37.10. ^{111}In-CYT-103 immunoscintigraphy of recurrent ovarian carcinoma. (**A**) Anterior and posterior planar gamma camera images show abnormal radiolocalization consistent with paraaortic lymph node metastases (arrow). (**B**) Images show diffuse radiolocalization in the lower abdomen and pelvis consistent with peritoneal carcinomatosis (arrows, posterior view).

Immunoscintigraphy

Presently, US, CT, and MRI lack sufficient sensitivity and/or specificity to serve as definitive diagnostic tests for ovarian cancer or to rule out recurrent/persistent disease. Over the past decade, numerous radiolabeled MoAbs and their fragments have been evaluated for their diagnostic, staging and postoperative monitoring capabilities (Neal *et al.*, 1993).

OV-TL3 is a murine MoAb that recognizes a cell surface antigenic determinant, OA_3, found in immunohistochemical studies in over 90% of ovarian carcinomas (Boerman *et al.*, 1990). Massuger *et al.* (1990) examined the safety and diagnostic accuracy of ^{111}In-labeled OV-TL3 $F(ab')_2$. Both planar CT and SPECT scintigraphy were performed up to four days after intravenous injection of the labeled MoAb fragments. Ovarian carcinoma was accurately identified in 94% of cases. Because of its high sensitivity for ovarian cancer, high tumor uptake, and absence of a serum antigen, OV-TL3 is a strong candidate for immunodetection of ovarian carcinoma.

Intraperitoneal administration of radiolabeled MoAbs has been shown to have a high sensitivity in the detection of carcinomatosis (Carrasquillo *et al.*, 1988; Crippa *et al.*, 1991). However, benefits of the intraperitoneal route such as higher tumor uptake and a more favorable tumor to background ratio can be canceled by nonspecific accumulations of the antibody within the pelvis.

^{111}In-CYT-103, which reacts with TAG-72, an antigen reportedly expressed in up to 100% of ovarian adenocarcinomas (Thor *et al.*, 1986) has undergone a multicenter trial described by Gallup (1992) involving 108 patients at 18 study sites. Planar images were obtained at two sessions 2–7 days after injection. Antibody imaging performance based on prospective interpretations demonstrated a sensitivity of 68%. RIS using ^{111}In-CYT-103 detected occult tumor in 20 of 71 patients (28%) with ovarian cancer, including six patients with normal CA-125 levels and negative preoperative work-ups. Higher sensitivity was noted in patients with primary as compared with recurrent disease (95% versus 59%). This was thought to be related to larger tumor size. A comparison of CT and ^{111}In-CYT-103 images in 101 patients revealed that the sensitivity for CYT-103 imaging (69%) was greater than that of CT imaging (44%). However, the per patient specificity of CT (79%) was higher than that of antibody imaging (54%). Of 70 patients with surgically confirmed ovarian carcinoma who were evaluated by both CT and ^{111}In-CYT-103 imaging, lesions were correctly identified by both modalities in 29 patients. ^{111}In-CYT-103 imaging correctly detected lesions in an additional 29 patients who had negative CT scans. CT identified lesions in only two patients with negative antibody images. Overall detection rate for carcinomatosis by ^{111}In-CYT-103 imaging and CT was 71% and 45%, respectively.

Following therapy, ^{111}In-CYT-103 immunoscintigraphy may be a valuable whole-body presurgical diagnostic imaging test for complete clinical responders and in the follow-up of patients (*Figure 37.10*). Although the initial reports are encouraging, more data are needed to determine the place of ^{111}In-CYT-103 in the management of patients with known or suspected ovarian cancer.

Positron Emission Tomography

PET is a form of computer-assisted imaging that uses radiopharmaceuticals labeled with positron-emitting isotopes. With emission, positrons undergo annihilation with electrons, which results in two oppositely directed photons (Correia, 1993). These photons are then detected by sensors in a circular array around the patient. Computer-generated tomographic images are then constructed. The images are reflective of the biochemistry of the tissues rather than their physical characteristics.

PET imaging with the positron-emitting glucose analog 2-[18F]-fluoro-2-deoxy-D-glucose (FDG) exploits the accelerated rate of glycolysis, characteristic of malignant tissue, to image tumors. Karlan *et al.* (1993) evaluated 13 patients before planned surgical exploration. In the six complete clinical responders, five were found to have microscopic disease. Unfortunately, the PET FDG did not detect this disease. In the seven patients clinically suspected of having recurrent disease, which was confirmed at laparotomy, the PET FDG detected the presence of disease. The authors conclude that PET could not detect tumors of 1.0 cm or less in diameter. Hubner *et al.* (1993) assessed PET FDG and CT scans in patients with suspected ovarian cancer or for follow-up for suspected recurrent or metastatic tumor. Their results revealed that the positive predictive value for ovarian cancer was 86% and the negative predictive value was 76%. However, combining PET and CT resulted in a negative predictive value approaching 100%. Rubin *et al.* (1993) have coupled immunologic targeting with PET scanning by using the ^{124}I-labeled antibodies MX35 and MH99. ^{124}I is a positron-emitting radionuclide with a half-life of 4.2 days. PET calculation of isotope uptake ratios demonstrated specific localization of the antibodies in tumor within nude rats. Subcutaneous ovarian cancer nodules as small as 7 mm were identified. These preliminary data suggest that PET scanning may effectively supplement clinical evaluation and CT information in the preoperative evaluation of patients. However, more studies are needed to define its role.

Summary of Management Options

- Magnetic resonance imaging (MRI) has a higher accuracy in detecting cancer confined to the cervix than computed tomography (CT). However, in the case of full-thickness cervical stromal invasion, parametrial tumor extension is difficult to exclude on the basis of MRI scans.
- MRI is superior to physical examination or CT in its ability to differentiate between residual or recurrent disease and fibrosis.
- In endometrial cancer, MRI is useful in the patient who is difficult to examine (e.g. due to obesity). MRI with contrast enhancement makes it possible to differentiate the tumor margin from the normal endometrium and allows for evaluation of the depth of myometrial invasion.
- Transvaginal ultrasound (US) is effective in distinguishing deep from superficial myometrial invasion and is well tolerated by most patients. When inaccuracies with US occur, they most often result from the presence of intraluminal polypoid tumors, which cause distortion of the endometrial cavity.
- US and, in particular, color flow Doppler are highly accurate in distinguishing benign from malignant adnexal masses.
- The use of US for preoperative staging in ovarian cancer is limited due to its inability to consistently detect lesions of 2 cm or less in size or plaque-like intraperitoneal disease.
- CT is the imaging modality of choice in the preoperative and post-treatment evaluation of ovarian cancer. Although high resolution scanners may depict peritoneal implants as small as 5 mm, the primary weakness of CT is its inability to consistently detect disease less than 1 cm in diameter.
- CT cannot replace second-look laparotomy in the assessment of disease status, but can, in conjunction with serum tumor markers, provide useful information in monitoring patients.
- Radioimmunoscintigraphy (RIS) may be a valuable presurgical diagnostic test for patients with suspected or persistent/recurrent ovarian carcinoma and may be particularly advantageous in the subgroup of patients with negative tumor markers and CT evaluation. More clinical experience is needed to define the role of RIS in the management of patients with ovarian cancer.
- Currently available imaging modalities are not sensitive or specific enough to use in screening the population at large for ovarian cancer.

References

Averette HE, Ford JH, Dudan RC *et al.* (1975) Staging of cervical cancer. *Clin. Obstet. Gynecol.* **98:** 215–232.

Bachaud JM, Fu RC, Delannes M *et al.* (1991) Non-randomized comparative study of irradiation alone or in combination with surgery in stage IB, IIA and "proximal" IIB carcinoma of the cervix. *Radiother. Oncol.* **22:** 104–110.

Balfe DM, van Dyke JW, Lee JKT *et al.* (1983) Computed tomography in malignant endometrial neoplasms. *J. Comput. Assist. Tomogr.* **7:** 677–681.

Bandy LC, Clarke–Pearson DL, Silverman PM *et al.* (1985) Computed tomography in evaluation of extrapelvic lymphadenopathy in carcinoma of the cervix. *Obstet. Gynecol.* **65:** 73–76.

Bennacerraf BR, Finkler NJ, Wojciechowski C *et al.* (1990) Sonographic accuracy in the diagnosis of ovarian masses. *J. Reprod. Med.* **35:** 491–495.

Boerman O, Massuger L, Makkink K *et al.* (1990) Comparative *in vitro* binding characteristics and biodistribution in tumor-bearing athymic mice of anti-ovarian carcinoma monoclonal antibodies. *Anticancer Res.* **10:** 1289–1296.

Bourne TH, Campbell S, Steer CV *et al.* (1991) Detection of endometrial cancer by transvaginal ultrasonography with color flow imaging and blood flow analysis: A preliminary report. *Gynecol. Oncol.* **40:** 253–259.

Bourne TH, Campbell S, Reynolds K *et al.* (1994) The potential role of serum CA125 in an ultrasound-based screening program for familial ovarian cancer. *Gynecol. Oncol.* **52:** 379–385.

■ Bragg DG & Hricak H (1993) Imaging in gynecologic malignancies. *Cancer* **71:** 1648–1651.

Brant–Zawadzki MB (1987) Magnetic resonance imaging principles: Part 1. *MRI decisions* **Nov/Dec:** 11–15.

Brenner DE, Shaff MI, Jones HW *et al.* (1985) Abdomino-pelvic computed tomography evaluation in patients undergoing second-look laparotomy for ovarian carcinoma. *Obstet. Gynecol.* **65:** 715–719.

Buist MR, Golding RP, Burger CW *et al.* (1994) Comparative evaluation of diagnostic methods in ovarian carcinoma with emphasis on CT and MRI. *Gynecol. Oncol.* **52:** 191–198.

Buy JN, Moss AA, Ghossain MA *et al.* (1988) Peritoneal implants from ovarian tumors: CT findings. *Radiology* **169:** 691–694.

Cacciatore B, Lehtovirta P, Wahlstrom T *et al.* (1989)

Preoperative sonographic evaluation of endometrial cancer. *Am. J. Obstet. Gynecol.* **160:** 133–137.

Calkins AR, Stehman FB, Wass JC *et al.* (1987) Pitfalls in interpretation of computed tomography prior to second-look laparotomy in patients with ovarian cancer. *Br. J. Radiol.* **60:** 975–979.

Camilien L, Gordon D, Fruchter RG *et al.* (1988) Predictive value of computerized tomography in the presurgical evaluation of primary carcinoma of the cervix. *Gynecol. Oncol.* **30:** 209–215.

Carrasquillo JA, Sugarbaker P, Colcher D *et al.* (1988) Peritoneal carcinomatosis: Imaging with intraperitoneal injection of I^{131} labeled B72.3 monoclonal antibody. *Radiology* **167:** 35–40.

Correia JA (1993) Physical aspects of positron emission tomography (PET). In: Travers JM & Ferrucci JT (eds) *Radiology Diagnostic-Imaging-Intervention*, pp. 1–5. Philadelphia: JB Lippincott.

Crippa F, Buraggi GL, Di Re E *et al.* (1991) Radioimmunoscintigraphy of ovarian cancer with the Mov18 monoclonal antibody. *Eur. J. Cancer* **27:** 724–729.

DePriest PD, Shenson D, Fried A *et al.* (1993) A morphology index based on sonographic findings in ovarian cancer. *Gynecol. Oncol.* **51:** 7–11.

Doubleday LC & Bernardino ME (1980) CT findings in the perirectal area following radiation therapy. *J. Comput. Assist. Tomogr.* **4:** 634.

Dunnick NR, Jones RB, Doppmen JL *et al.* (1979) Intraperitoneal contrast infusion for assessment of intraperitoneal fluid dynamics. *Am. J. Radiol.* **133:** 221–223.

Fleischer AC & Jones HW (1993) Color Doppler sonography of ovarian masses: The importance of a multiparameter approach. *Gynecol. Oncol.* **50:** 1–2.

Fleischer AC, Dudley BS, Entman SS *et al.* (1987) Myometrial invasion by endometrial carcinoma: Sonographic assessment. *Radiology* **162:** 307–310.

Flueckiger F, Ebner F, Poschauko H *et al.* (1992) Cervical cancer: Serial MR imaging before and after primary radiation therapy – A two year follow-up study. *Radiology* **184:** 89–93.

Franchi M, LaFianza A, Babilonti L *et al.* (1989) Clinical value of computerized tomography (CT) in assessment of recurrent uterine cancers. *Gynecol. Oncol.* **35:** 31–37.

Frasci G, Contino A, Iaffaioli RV *et al.* (1994) Computerized tomography of the abdomen and pelvis with peritoneal administration of soluble contrast (IPC-CT) in detection of residual disease for patients with ovarian cancer. *Gynecol. Oncol.* **52:** 154–160.

Fritzsche P, McCarthy S & Winkle L (1989) Gynecologic radiology: Malignant disorders. In: Travers JM & Ferrucci JT (eds) *Radiology Diagnosis-Imaging-Intervention*, pp. 1–12. Philadelphia: JB Lippincott.

Gallup DG (1992) Multicenter clinical trial of ^{111}In-CYT-103 in patients with ovarian cancer. In: Maguire RT & van Norstrand D (eds) *Diagnosis of Colorectal and Ovarian Carcinoma. Application of Immunoscintigraphic Technology*, pp. 111–124. New York: Marcel Dekker.

Goodsitt JA (1993) The basic physics of ultrasound imaging. In: Travers JM & Ferrucci JT (eds) *Radiology Diagnosis-Imaging-Intervention*, pp. 1–15. Philadelphia: JB Lippincott.

Greco A, Mason P, Leong AWC *et al.* (1989) Staging of carcinoma of uterine cervix: MRI – surgical correlation. *Clin. Radiol.* **40:** 401–405.

Griffin TW, Parker RG & Tyler WJ (1976) An evaluation of procedures used in staging carcinoma of the cervix. *Am. J. Radiol.* **127:** 825–827.

Grumbine FC, Rosenshein NB & Zerhouni EA (1981) Abdominopelvic computed tomography in the preoperative evaluation of early cervical cancer. *Gynecol. Oncol.* **12:** 286–290.

Halpern SE (1992) An overview of radioimmunoimaging. In: Maguire RT & van Nostrand D (eds) *Diagnosis of Colorectal and Ovarian Carcinoma. Application of Immuno-Scintigraphic Technology*, pp. 10–11. New York: Marcel Dekker.

Hamlin DJ, Burgener FA & Beechum JB (1987) CT of intraluminal endometrial carcinoma: Contrast enhancement is essential. *Am. J. Radiol.* **137:** 551–554.

Heron CW, Husband JE, Williams MP *et al.* (1988) The value of CT in the diagnosis of recurrent carcinoma of the cervix. *Clin. Radiol.* **39:** 496–501.

Hirai Y, Kaku S, Teshima H *et al.* (1989) Use of angio-computed tomography to evaluate extent of endometrial carcinoma. *Gynecol. Oncol.* **33:** 372–375.

Hoetzinger H (1991) Hysterosonography and hysterography in benign and malignant diseases of the uterus. *J. Ultrasound Med.* **10:** 259–263.

■ Hricak H (1991) Carcinoma of the female reproductive organs. Value of cross-sectional imaging. *Cancer* **67:** 1209–1218.

Hricak H, Lacy CG, Sandles LG *et al.* (1988) Invasive cervical carcinoma: Comparison of MR imaging and surgical findings. *Radiology* **166:** 623–631.

Hricak H, Hamm B, Semelka RC *et al.* (1991) Carcinoma of the uterus: Use of Gadopentetate Dimeglumine in MR imaging. *Radiology* **181:** 95–106.

Hubner KF, McDonald TW, Niethammer JG *et al.* (1993) Assessment of primary and metastatic ovarian cancer by positron emission tomography (PET) using 2-[^{18}F]deoxy-glucose (2-[^{18}F] FDG). *Gynecol. Oncol.* **51:** 192–204.

Jain KA, Friedman DL, Pettinger TW *et al.* (1993) Adnexal masses: Comparison of specificity of endovaginal US and pelvic MR imaging. *Radiology* **186:** 697–704.

Jampolis S, Andras J & Fletcher GH (1975) Analysis of sites and causes of failures of irradiation in invasive squamous cell carcinoma of the intact uterine cervix. *Radiology* **115:** 681–685.

Karlan BY, Hawkin SR, Hoh C *et al.* (1993) Whole-body positron emission tomography with 2-[^{18}F]-Fluoro-2-deoxy-D-glucose can detect recurrent ovarian carcinoma. *Gynecol. Oncol.* **51:** 175–181.

Kilcheski TS, Ager PH, Mulhern CB *et al.* (1981) Role of computed tomography in the presurgical evaluation of carcinoma of the cervix. *J. Comput. Assist. Tomogr.* **5:** 378.

Kim EE & Kasi LP (1993) Challenges in immunoscintigraphy of ovarian cancer. *Gynecol. Oncol.* **48:** 283–284.

Kim SH, Choi BI, Lee HP *et al.* (1990) Uterine cervical carcinoma: comparison of CT and MRI findings. *Radiology* **175:** 45–51.

Kim SH, Choi BI, Hank JK *et al.* (1993) Preoperative staging of uterine cervical carcinoma: comparison of CT and MRI in 99 patients. *J. Comput. Assist. Tomogr.* **17:** 633–640.

Kim SH, Kim SC, Choi BI *et al.* (1994) Uterine cervical carcinoma: evaluation of pelvic lymph node metastasis with MR imaging. *Radiology* **990:** 807–811.

Kurjak A, Predanic M, Kupesic–Urek S *et al.* (1993) Transvaginal color and pulsed doppler assessment of adnexal tumor vascularity. *Gynecol. Oncol.* **50:** 3–9.

Lee JKT & Marx MV (1989) Pelvis. In: Lee JKT, Sagel SS & Stanley RJ (eds) *Computed Body Tomography with MRI Correlation*, pp. 851–897. New York: Raven Press.

Lien HH, Blomlie V, Trope C *et al.* (1991) Cancer of the endometrium: Value of MR imaging in determining depth of invasion into the myometrium. *Am. J. Radiol.* **157:** 1227–1233.

Massuger LFAG, Kennemans P, Claessens RAMJ *et al.* (1990) Immunoscintigraphy of ovarian cancer with indium-111 labeled OV-TL 3 $(ab')_2$ monoclonal antibody. *J. Nucl. Med.* **31:** 1802–1810.

■ Mayr NA, Tali ET, Yuh WTC *et al.* (1993) Cervical cancer: Application of MR imaging in radiation therapy. *Radiology* **189:** 601–608.

Montana GS, Fowler WC, Varia MA *et al.* (1985) Analysis of results of radiation therapy for stage II carcinoma of the cervix. *Cancer* **55:** 956–962.

Montana GS, Fowler WC, Varia MA *et al.* (1986) Carcinoma of the cervix, stage III: results of radiation therapy. *Cancer* **57:** 148–154.

Murolo C, Constantini S, Foglia G *et al.* (1989) Ultrasound examination in ovarian cancer patients. A comparison with second look laparotomy. *J. Ultrasound Med.* **8:** 441–443.

National Institute of Health (1995) National Institute of Health Consensus Conference on Ovarian Cancer, Screening, treatment and follow-up. *JAMA* **273:** 491–497.

■ Neal CE, Swenson LC, Fanning J *et al.* (1993) Monoclonal antibodies in ovarian and prostate cancer. *Semin. Nucl. Med.* **23:** 114–126.

■ Nelson BE, Rosenfield AT & Schwartz PE (1993) Preoperative abdominopelvic computed tomographic prediction of optimal cytoreduction in epithelial ovarian carcinoma. *J. Clin. Oncol.* **11:** 166–172.

Olson MC, Posniak HV, Tempany CM *et al.* (1992) MR imaging of the female pelvic region. *Radiographics* **12:** 445–465.

Pelc NJ & Colsher JG (1993) Principles of X-ray computed tomography. In: Travers JM & Ferrucci JT (eds) *Radiology Diagnosis-Imaging-Intervention*, pp. 1–11. Philadelphia: JB Lippincott.

Prayer L, Stiglbauer R, Kramer J *et al.* (1993) Superparamagnetic particles as oral contrast medium in magnetic resonance imaging of patients with treated ovarian cancer – comparison with plain MRI. *Br. J. Radiol.* **66:** 416–419.

Pussell SJ, Cosgrove DO, Hinton J *et al.* (1980) Carcinoma of the ovary – correlation of ultrasound with second-look laparotomy. *Br. J. Obstet. Gynaecol.* **87:** 1140–1144.

Requard CK, Mettler FA & Wieks JD (1981) Preoperative sonography of malignant ovarian neoplasms. *Am. J. Radiol.* **137:** 79–82.

Reuter KL, Griffin T & Hunter RE (1989) Comparison of abdominopelvic computed tomography results and findings at second-look laparotomy in ovarian cancer patients. *Cancer* **63:** 1123–1128.

Rubin SC, Kairemo KJA, Brownell A *et al.* (1993) High resolution positron emission tomography of human ovarian cancer in nude rats using ^{124}I-labeled monoclonal antibodies. *Gynecol. Oncol.* **48:** 61–67.

Sanders RC, McNeil BJ, Finberg HJ *et al.* (1983) A prospective study of computed tomography and ultrasound in the detection and staging of pelvic masses. *Radiology* **146:** 439–442.

Semelka RC, Lawrence PH, Shoenut JP *et al.* (1993) Primary ovarian cancer: Prospective comparison of contrast-enhanced CT and pre- and post-contrast, fat-suppressed MR imaging, with histologic correlation. *J. Magn. Reson. Imaging* **3:** 99–106.

Shapero LG & Hricak H (1989) Mixed müllerian sarcoma of the uterus: MR findings. *Am. J. Radiol.* **153:** 317–319.

Shiels RA, Peel KR, MacDonald HN *et al.* (1985) A prospective trial of computed tomography in the staging of ovarian malignancy. *Br. J. Obstet. Gynaecol.* **92:** 407–412.

Shipley CF, Smith ST, Dennis EJ *et al.* (1992) Evaluation of pretreatment transvaginal ultrasonography in the management of patients with endometrial carcinoma. *Am. J. Obstet. Gynecol.* **167:** 406–412.

Silverman PM, Osborne M, Dunnick NR *et al.* (1988) CT prior to second-look operation in ovarian cancer. *Am. J. Radiol.* **150:** 829–832.

Sironi S, Taccagni G, Garancini P *et al.* (1992) Myometrial invasion by endometrial carcinoma. Assessment by MR imaging. *Am. J. Radiol.* **158:** 565–569.

Sironi S, De Cobelli F, Scarfone G *et al.* (1993) Carcinoma of the cervix: Value of plain and gadolinium-enhanced MR imaging in assessing degree of invasiveness. *Radiology* **188:** 797–801.

Thor A, Obuchi AN, Szpak CA *et al.* (1986) Distribution of oncofetal antigen tumor-associated glycoprotein-72 defined by monoclonal antibody B72.3. *Cancer Res.* **42:** 3118–3124.

Thurnher SA (1992) MR imaging of pelvic masses in women: Contrast-enhanced versus unenhanced images. *Am. J. Radiol.* **159:** 1243–1250.

Togashi K, Nishimura K, Itoh K *et al.* (1986) Uterine cervical cancer: Assessment with high-field MR imaging. *Radiology* **160:** 431–435.

Togashi K, Nishimura K, Sagoh T *et al.* (1989) Carcinoma of the cervix: Staging with MR imaging. *Radiology* **171:** 245–251.

■ Togashi K & Konishi J (1990) Magnetic resonance imaging in the evaluation of gynecologic malignancy. *Magn. Reson. Q.* **6:** 250–275.

van Nagell JR, Roddick JW & Lown DM (1971) The staging of cervical cancer: inevitable discrepancies between clinical stage and pathologic findings. *Am. J. Obstet. Gynecol.* **110:** 973–978.

van Nagell JR, DePriest PD, Puls LE *et al.* (1991) Ovarian cancer screening in asymptomatic postmenopausal women by transvaginal sonography. *Cancer* **68:** 458–462.

Vick CW, Walsh JW, Wheelock JB *et al.* (1984) CT of the normal and abnormal parametria in cervical cancer. *Am. J. Radiol.* **143:** 597–603.

Villasanta U, Whitley NO, Haney PJ *et al.* (1983) Computed tomography in invasive carcinoma of the cervix: An appraisal. *Obstet. Gynecol.* **62:** 218–224.

Walsh JW, Rosenfield AT, Jaffe CC *et al.* (1978) Prospective comparison of ultrasound and computed tomography in the evaluation of gynecologic pelvic masses. *Am. J. Radiol.* **131:** 955–960.

Walsh JW, Amendola MA, Konerding KF *et al.* (1980) Computed tomographic detection of pelvic and inguinal lymph-node metastases from primary and recurrent pelvic malignant disease. *Radiology* **137:** 157–166.

Walsh JW & Goplerud DR (1981) Prospective comparison between clinical and CT staging in primary cervical carcinoma. *Am. J. Radiol.* **137:** 997–1003.

Walsh JW, Amendola MA, Hall DJ *et al.* (1981) Recurrent carcinoma of the cervix: CT diagnosis. *Am. J. Radiol.* **136:** 117–122.

Walsh JW & Goplerud DR (1981) Computed tomography of primary, persistent, and recurrent endometrial malignancy. *Am. J. Radiol.* **139:** 1149–1154.

Whitely NO, Brenner DE, Francis A *et al.* (1982) Computed tomographic evaluation of carcinoma of the cervix. *Radiology* **142:** 439–446.

Worthington JL, Balfe DM, Lee JKT *et al.* (1986) Uterine neoplasms: MR imaging. *Radiology* **159:** 725–730.

38 Vascular and Peritoneal Access

P S Braly

Introduction

With the increasing use of multiagent chemotherapeutic regimens as well as the supportive therapies of parenteral nutrition and long-term antibiotic administration, the need for consistent and safe access to the vascular system and peritoneal cavity has become critical to the management of patients with gynecologic malignancies. The development of central venous catheters and, more recently, implantable subcutaneous ports, has had an enormous impact on the care of these patients. In 1986 approximately 2.75 million central venous catheters were placed and 500,000 patients received total parenteral nutrition (Lowell and Bothe, 1991). The recent trend toward ambulatory chemotherapy and home delivery of parenteral nutrition, antibiotics and analgesia has been associated with a continued dramatic increase in the use of these devices. The use of intraperitoneal chemotherapy regimens has been dependent on (and limited by) the systems developed for reliable access of the peritoneal cavity. Despite the critical importance of methods to access the peritoneal cavity, the great majority of information in the literature is related to drug regimens and pharmacokinetic studies with little available data for optimizing these peritoneal access systems. In this chapter, the current aspects of intravascular and intraperitoneal access devices will be discussed.

History of Central Venous Access Systems

The first reported use of central venous catheters was by Aubaniac in 1952 when he described his ten-year experience with the infraclavicular subclavian vein catheterization for the rapid infusion of fluids during the resuscitation of military casualties. The next major contribution occurred in 1960 when Quinton *et al.* described the first long-term access to the vascular system for chronic hemodialysis. The introduction of the concept of total parenteral-nutrition (TPN) in 1968 by Dudrick *et al.* led to the development and widespread use of central venous catheters. Broviac *et al.* (1973) developed a soft silicone rubber catheter, the Silastic catheter, which incorporated a Dacron cuff and a relatively long subcutaneous tunnel. In 1973, Hickman *et al.* described the use of a similar catheter with a slightly thicker wall and a larger internal diameter for use in bone marrow transplant patients. This larger lumen allowed for the drawing of blood and the transfusion of blood products. Because of the need in oncology patients to simultaneously administer antibiotics, hyperalimentation and blood products, the double-lumen Hickman catheter was introduced in 1982 (Sanders *et al.*, 1982). In the early 1980s, both Bothe *et al.* (1984) and Neiderhuber *et al.* (1982) described the development of totally implantable central venous access systems that include a subcutaneous injection port and catheter. A more recent modification in catheter design (the Groshong catheter) involves a two-way slit valve that minimizes clotting by preventing blood from returning retrograde into the lumen of the catheter when not in use (Delmor *et al.*, 1989). With the dramatic increase in home intravenous therapy, a new peripherally inserted central catheter (PICC) has been developed to combine more reliable central vascular access with the possibility of bedside insertion by trained nurses (Brown, 1989). The risk of central catheter insertion such as pneumothorax or injury to great vessels is eliminated by this approach. Recently, a modification of the Hickman catheter was reported for use in bone marrow transplant recipients and other critically ill oncology patients (the Hickman–Crawford catheter) that permits passage of a 5-Fr pulmonary artery catheter through the larger of the two lumens (Crawford *et al.*, 1994). There are also at least two catheters available that can be used for long-term venous access and have plasmapheresis and hemodialysis capabilities (Hickman *et al.*, 1991).

Preoperative Considerations

Many factors including patient considerations and catheter selection must be taken into account before placement of long-term central venous access. Common indications for central venous catheterization include poor or inadequate peripheral venous access, rapid large volume transfusion requirements, administration of sclerosing agents such as TPN or chemotherapy, emergency access for resuscitation, and when central venous pressure monitoring is necessary. Permanent central venous access should be considered for any patient who requires chronic administration of antibiotics, TPN or chemotherapy.

Permanent lines provide secure access and decrease the possibility of extravasation and patient discomfort and anxiety from repeated venepunctures. Permanent central venous catheters are also very useful for home and hospice care, providing reliable access for the administration of pain medications. Other factors, including the ability of the patient to care for an external cathether or implantable port, the support group available to the patient, and the potential for the catheter to be used for non-medical uses (i.e. illicit drug use) should also be considered before insertion of a permanent central venous access system.

Patient Characteristics

Knowledge of the patient's general condition and previous procedures that the patient has undergone is critical to minimize the potential for catheter-related complications (Alexander, 1994). A previous history of thoracic surgical procedures, the presence of active mediastinal disease such as Hodgkin's disease or bulky metastatic disease, previous chest radiation, or multiple previous bilateral central lines increase the likelihood that the venous anatomy of the chest may be abnormal. In these cases, preoperative evaluation of the venous patency with ultrasound or digital subtraction angiography may be useful in selecting the most appropriate site of catheter insertion. Knowledge of the patient's pulmonary status including the presence and extent of pleural effusions, previous pulmonary resection and extent of pulmonary metastatic disease may guide the surgeon in selection of the side and site of insertion. The presence of a tracheostomy increases the risk of infection with external or internal jugular vein placement. The insertion of a catheter into an area of extensive scarring or through irradiated skin should also be avoided secondary to the increased risk of infectious complications.

Recently administered chemotherapeutic agents are often associated with neutropenia and/or thrombocytopenia. Since the timing of placement of most long-term venous access devices is elective, this procedure should be performed when conditions are optimal for the patient. Since patients whose catheters are placed during episodes of neutropenia are more likely to develop sepsis compared to those patients without neutropenia (Hartman and Schochat, 1987), it is usually prudent to postpone catheter replacement until recovery of the neutrophil count to 1500 mm^{-3}. Patients with infection should not undergo catheter placement until appropriate antibiotic treatment has been initiated and clinical evidence of infection has resolved. Thrombocytopenia is a frequently encountered situation in cancer patients and secondary platelet dysfunction problems may exacerbate an already low platelet count. Even with thrombocytopenia, long-term venous access devices can usually be placed safely without significant bleeding problems with perioperative platelet transfusions to a platelet count of 50,000 ml^{-1} or by using a venous cutdown approach to the external or internal jugular, cephalic or saphenous vein (Thompson *et al.*, 1985).

Catheter Selection

Selection of the type of venous access device depends on many factors, including the planned treatment regimen, patient preference and habitus, and the institutional and surgeon experience and preference

Table 38.1. Chronic venous access devices: selection criteria.

Access device	*Advantages*	*Disadvantages*
Percutaneous catheters (e.g. Hickman, Broviac, Groshong catheters)	Easily inserted Easy to remove Lower initial cost Most reliable for continuous intravenous therapy and blood sampling	Regular maintenance required Higher maintenance costs Visible catheter Restricts some activities
Implantable port systems	Cosmetically superior Minimal interference with life style Lower maintenance costs Ideal for intermittent therapy	Higher initial cost Port (especially for double-lumen catheter) is large Requires non-coring needling for access Requires second surgery to remove device Extravasation difficult to identify

(*Table 38.1*). There are, in general, two types of permanent central lines: the external catheter (e.g. Broviac, Hickman and Groshong catheters) and the subcutaneous port systems (e.g. Port-A-Cath, Mediport, Infus-a-Port, and the peripherally implanted PAS Port). Advantages of the external catheters include lower cost, ease of access that does not require special needles, ability to handle rapid high volume infusions and exchanges, and availability for immediate use. Oncology patients will often benefit from the placement of a double-lumen or triple-lumen catheter because of their requirements for concurrent hydration, TPN, chemotherapeutic agents, antibiotics and pain medications. Occasionally patients will require either hemodialysis or plasmapheresis during their therapy; in these cases, consideration should be given to placement of the shorter, large-bore plasmapheresis-type catheters (e.g. Quinton catheter). Disadvantages of these devices include the requirement for frequent maintenance, interference with certain patient activities such as swimming and hot tub usage and the fact that the catheters are visible, even when not in use. There is some evidence that the double- and triple-lumen catheters are associated with an increased incidence of thrombotic and infectious complications. The subcutaneous port systems are ideal for the patient receiving infrequent infusions over a long period of time, and have several advantages over the external devices, including improved body image, ease of care and possibly a decreased risk of infection. Disadvantages of these systems include a higher cost, the risk of the needle dislodging with resulting drug extravasation, the requirement for special non-coring needles and the development of subcutaneous 'pocket' infection around the port. Although the initial cost of insertion of subcutaneous port systems is higher than for external catheters, the cost of maintenance is also lower for the ports, so that after approximately six months, the expense of the two is comparable (Ross *et al.*, 1988).

Intraoperative Considerations

Complications

The most important predictor of complications associated with insertion of central venous catheters, especially pneumothorax, is the experience of the physician placing the catheter (Lowell and Bothe, 1991). In a study by Bernard and Stahl (1971), all complications associated with catheter placement occurred in those placed by the group of physicians who had placed fewer than 50 catheters. This study also reported that physicians with less experience had more than twice the rate of catheter sepsis. Another study (Nelson, 1986) noted that 50% of the complications occurred in only 2.5% of the patients, with the highest complication rate in the patients who required emergency placement of central venous catheters. Because of this, long-term vascular access devices should rarely be placed emergently, especially by inexperienced surgeons.

The majority of acute complications related to central venous catheter placement are related to the percutaneous approach. In a study by Scott (1989) there were approximately 1800 major complications that occurred during placement of an estimated 2.5 million central venous catheters. There were 32 resulting deaths, most being related to physician error in technique. In this study all the deaths occurred in patients undergoing percutaneous catheter placement and were associated with pneumothorax, hemothorax, air embolus, pericardial tamponade, hydromediastinum and cerebral infarction. Pneumothorax occurs in 1–3% of all percutaneous procedures and can usually, but not always, be predicted by the appearance of air in the syringe during needle entry. Acute tension pneumothorax will present with respiratory distress, chest pain and a drop in P_{O2}, often requiring immediate chest tube placement for relief. Other patients, however, remain asymptomatic, especially if the pneumothorax is less than 15%. Most authors recommend chest tube placement for any pneumothorax larger than 15%, especially if associated with symptoms. Under no circumstances should bilateral attempts at percutaneous placement of subclavian vein catheters be made until a pneumothorax is ruled out on the side first used.

One of the most frequently encountered complications at the time of catheter placement is arrhythmia, with one study (Stuart *et al.*, 1990) reporting an incidence of atrial arrhythmia of 41% and significant ventricular arrhythmia of 11%. In a series of 300 patients who underwent placement of implantable infusion ports (Brothers *et al.*, 1988), the incidence of arrhythmia that required cardioversion was 0.9%. Both of these studies concluded that arrhythmia associated with the placement of central venous catheters is a result of overinsertion of either the guidewire or the catheter, and is most likely to occur in patients with a history of cardiac arrhythmia or who have electrolyte abnormalities. When the vein dilator is used, care must be taken to pass it only a short distance into the subclavian vein because passing it too far has been associated with puncture of the myocardium with resulting cardiac tamponade and, rarely, death.

Surgical Technique

Placement of long-term venous access systems may be accomplished using a surgical cutdown approach or by a percutaneous approach using the modified

Seldinger technique using a peel-away sheath and a vein dilator (Hickman *et al.*, 1991). The choice of the vessel used for the surgical cutdown technique is limited only by the skill of the surgeon, but usually involves either the external or internal jugular vein, the brachiocephalic vein at the deltopectoral groove, or the saphenous or femoral vein. When none of these are available, brachial, intrathoracic, mammary and azygous veins have all been successfully used for placement of central venous catheters. Using the percutaneous approach, subclavian veins, internal and external jugular veins and femoral veins have been cannulated. The percutaneous approach to the subclavian vein can be via either the supraclavicular or the infraclavicular approach, with the latter being the most popular with most surgeons. Takasugi and O'Connell (1988) reported that the failure rate for the percutaneous subclavian vein approach was 10% compared to 15% for the cephalic vein cutdown, and 4% for both the internal and external jugular vein cutdown.

There continues to be no consensus regarding which basic surgical approach is the best. Most procedures can be performed safely on an outpatient basis, typically in the operating room to optimize sterile conditions. Ideally, fluoroscopy or X-ray facilities will be available for catheter localization. Most surgeons believe that the patient should be in a slight Trendelenburg position with the head turned to the opposite side and the arms at the sides. There is some debate as to whether a rolled towel or blanket should be placed down the middle of the back; it is designed to allow the shoulders to fall back and facilitate access to the subclavian vein, but this technique has also been shown to decrease the caliber of the subclavian vein (Lechner *et al.*, 1989). If the internal or external jugular vein is being used, it is helpful to place a 'roll' under the shoulders to extend the neck and improve the definition of the anatomy of the triangle made by the two heads of the sternocleidomastoid muscle and the clavicle (Hickman *et al.*, 1991).

With the exception of extensive thrombosis of the superior vena cava (SVC), there are few significant contraindications to central venous catheter placement (Seewaldt and Greer, 1994). Even in situations where the subclavian veins, jugular veins and SVC are occluded, alternative access routes are available and have been the topic of numerous surgical and radiologic publications. In this situation where the upper central vessels are obliterated, femoral vein catheterization is the most common route. This approach is probably the safest way to achieve central access in patients with bleeding disorders or who are receiving thrombolytic therapy. Disadvantages of this approach include a higher rate of infection and thrombosis compared with catheterization at other sites (Seewaldt and Greer, 1994).

Percutaneous catheterization of the inferior vena cava (IVC) by a translumbar approach using radiographic guidance has also been described (Kenney *et al.*, 1985). The translumbar approach is from a point over the right iliac crest at a cephalad oblique angle entering the IVC below the renal veins at the L2–L3 level. The catheter is tunneled with an exit site in the flank or anterolateral right chest below the breast. Alternatively, a transhepatic route to the IVC or via a hepatic vein using an approach analogous to that of transhepatic cholangiography has been reported with few complications and good long-term results (Azizkhan *et al.*, 1992). Another technique involving combined venographic and operative approaches uses a Dormier basket to pull a catheter into the appropriate position distal to a thrombus through a patent collateral vein (Torosian *et al.*, 1986).

Even though tunneled Silastic catheters and subcutaneous port systems have been designed for long-term use, there are many reasons why these systems may need to be removed despite the continued need for central venous access. The main indications for removal include irreparable damage to the Silastic catheter, erosion of the port, an infected subcutaneous port or exit site or thrombotic occlusion of the catheter. A recently described technique (Lowell and Bothe, 1991) permits replacement of the central venous catheter using a new tunnel without the inherent risks of repeat venepuncture.

Postoperative Considerations

Catheter Maintenance

Careful attention to maintenance of line patency and care of the exit site clearly prolong the useful life of the central venous catheter. There is no consensus related to the optimal catheter maintenance regimen with considerable variability being found between institutions in the recommended frequency of flushes and the concentration of heparin in the flush solution. Typically, if external catheters are not being used, they are flushed every one or two days with a dilute heparin solution with subcutaneous ports being flushed less often (e.g. once a month) or not at all. One study reported that only 15% of Hickman catheters became occluded without any routine flushing (Gilles *et al.*, 1985). Optimal care of the exit site for external catheters is also not clear (Ledgerwood *et al.*, 1993). Hickman *et al.* (1979) recommended daily cleansing of the site with povidone–iodine and hydrogen peroxide followed by the application of povidone–iodine ointment at the exit site. Broviac *et al.* (1973) recommended a dry dressing after cleansing. Others use water-tight occlusive dressings (e.g. Op-site).

Complications of Catheter Use

Catheter occlusion

The majority of postoperative complications related to long-term central venous access systems are occlusive, thrombotic or infectious in nature. Catheter occlusion, defined as the inability to infuse fluids or withdraw blood, can be the result of catheter tip malposition, catheter kinking, fibrin sheath formation around the catheter, luminal occlusion due to blood clot or precipitation of solution compounds, or catheter tip abutment against the vein wall (Alexander, 1994). Most catheter malfunctions are manifest by the inability to withdraw blood, usually related to fibrin sheath formation (Hickman *et al.*, 1991). If luminal occlusion occurs and fluid cannot be infused through the catheter, a chest radiograph should be obtained to rule out catheter malposition or kinking. The ability to infuse, but not aspirate, from the catheter is called withdrawal occlusion and is usually attributable to the development of a fibrin sheath around the tip of the catheter. The incidence of fibrin sheath formation in subclavian venous catheters has been reported to be as high as 80% (Alexander, 1994). Fibrin sheath development appears to be associated with local extravasation of infusate. This syndrome consists of pain and tenderness following an infusion, typically with resolution when the infusion is discontinued. When this diagnosis is suspected, a radiographic contrast dye study should be performed; confirmation of this diagnosis is made if the contrast flows retrograde into the subcutaneous tissues. Catheters can often be salvaged with the use of thrombolytic agents. Administration of urokinase (250,000 U in 150 ml D_5W) infused over 90 minutes can correct withdrawal occlusion in more than 90% of catheters (Alexander, 1994). For catheter luminal occlusion, 2 ml of urokinase (2500–5000 U/ml), infused and left in the catheter for 30–120 minutes is effective.

Blood clots within the catheter lumen are uncommon, but occlusion by precipitation of calcium salts and Intralipid is possible. If catheter blockage is suspected to be related to calcium salt precipitation, ammonium chloride or 0.1N hydrogen chloride has been efficacious in dissolving the precipitate (Hickman *et al.*, 1991). If this therapy does not work, treatment of the catheter with a 70% ethanol lock for one hour may dissolve Intralipid precipitates.

Catheter-related thrombosis

Central venous catheter-related thrombosis was first described in 1971 (McDonough and Altemeier, 1971) and is often associated with thrombophlebitis of the cannulated central vein. Important factors that might contribute to thrombus formation include traumatic insertion, duration of use, and the composition, size and flexibility of the catheter itself, as well as venous stasis and hypercoagulability. The infusion of sclerosing compounds and solutions with extremes of pH and osmolarity is also associated with an increase in thrombosis. A frequent association between catheter-related infection and thrombosis has been described (Lowell and Bothe, 1991). The reported incidence of catheter-related thrombosis ranges from 3–70%, which reflects the difficulty in accurately defining and diagnosing this complication (Lowell and Bothe, 1991). Incidences vary greatly depending on whether the diagnosis is made on clinical grounds or as the result of various diagnostic tests, done either prospectively or as indicated because of clinical findings. Clinical signs and symptoms of catheter-related thrombosis include ipsilateral swelling of the arm or neck, collateral venous distension, and nonspecific pain in the neck and anterior chest wall. Despite the fact that clinically apparent catheter-related thrombosis occurs in only 0–4.8% of patients, several prospective studies have demonstrated partial or complete venous thrombosis by venography in 28–54% of patients (Lowell and Bothe, 1991).

Treatment of patients with catheter-related thrombosis includes local thrombolytic therapy, systemic anticoagulation and catheter removal, depending on the severity of symptoms and the need for continued venous access. In patients with long-term needs for central vascular access, systemic heparinization followed by warfarin therapy while the catheter is left in place is recommended. Early identification and treatment of catheter-related infection is also important to control thrombosis. In patients receiving TPN, the addition of heparin (3000 U/l) to the TPN solution can significantly decrease the risk of thrombosis formation, in one study going from 32% to 8% in the group receiving continuous heparin infusion (Kunkel and Machleder, 1989). Another method to decrease catheter-related thrombosis is the administration of low-dose warfarin (1 mg/d), starting three days before catheter placement. In one prospective study using digital subtraction angiography, catheter-related thrombosis was diagnosed in 50% of the control patients at three months whereas only 11% of the patients on low-dose warfarin developed thromboses (Bern *et al.*, 1986).

Catheter-related infection

Catheter-related infection has been one of the most common complications associated with the use of long-term vascular access devices, accounting for approximately half of all complications. Reported overall infection rates range from 3–60%, with a widely accepted complication rate being approximately 0.3 per 100 catheter days (Press *et al.*, 1984). The risk of developing septic complications is higher in patients with prolonged neutropenia, in patients under two years of age, and possibly with external catheters compared with subcutaneous port systems (Alexander, 1994). The two most important factors increasing the risk of infection, however, are the experience of the personnel inserting and using the catheters, and the care that the catheters receive during use (Hickman *et al.*, 1991). Other reported risk factors include the presence of venous thrombosis and the use of multiple-lumen catheters, but distant sites of infection, fever, and neutropenia at the time of catheter insertion do not appear to significantly increase the risk of catheter-related infection. Uncontrolled bacteremia is the only infectious contraindication to catheter placement.

Catheter-related infections can be divided into four categories: exit site functions; tunnel or pocket infection; line sepsis or catheter-related bacteremia; and septic thrombophlebitis. Exit site infections are the most common, accounting for approximately 50% of all catheter-related infectious complications. Septicemia alone without specific catheter-associated signs is the second most common infection, accounting for approximately 30% of these complications. Tunnel infections account for approximately 20% of reported cases of infection, and septic thrombophlebitis is uncommon, occurring in less than 5% of all cases (Seewaldt and Greer, 1994). Approximately half of the catheter-related infections are associated with bacteremia, with exit site infection being less likely than tunnel infections to have a concurrent diagnosis of bacteremia (Hickman *et al.*, 1991).

Exit site infections are defined as the development of erythema, tenderness, induration and purulent drainage within 2 cm of the catheter exit site without systemic signs of infection. Most exit site infections are caused by *Staphylococcus epidermidis*, and respond to local wound care and oral antibiotics, with or without a short course of parenteral antibiotics. In most instances, the catheter does not need to be removed unless these therapies fail to clear the infection. There are some data that other etiologic organisms, especially *Staph. aureus*, are more virulent, are associated with a higher mortality rate, and may require catheter removal more frequently as part of the management of these infections.

The second type of infection related to long-term central venous access systems is a tunnel or pocket infection. By definition, a tunnel infection is characterized by the development of erythema, tenderness, and induration along the subcutaneous catheter tunnel at a distance of more than 2 cm from the exit site, whether or not the exit site is also involved or involving the subcutaneous port pocket. Frequently, it is possible to aspirate purulent fluid from the involved tunnel or port pocket. Because these infections involve a foreign body, are suppurative and are associated with cellulitis, it is usually necessary to remove the catheter and implanted port in order to adequately treat the infection (Alexander, 1994).

Line sepsis or catheter-related bacteremia is the most serious and potentially life-threatening infection related to indwelling central venous catheters. The incidence of this infectious complication varies greatly with the definition being used. The clinical definition of catheter-related sepsis is fever, with or without leukocytosis, without any other obvious source, that resolves after removal of the central venous catheter. With the use of clinical criteria alone to identify and treat patients with line sepsis as many as 85% of the catheters would be removed unnecessarily (Lowell and Bothe, 1991). A qualitative bacteriologic definition of catheter-related sepsis is infection in which identical organisms are cultured from both a peripheral site as well as from the tip of the central venous catheter without other identified sources of infection. The cause of line sepsis is unknown, but may be related to chronic colonization of the intravascular portion of the catheter from external sites. A quantitative Gram's stain method has been proposed to define catheter-related infection, which is diagnosed if a culture of the catheter tip shows over 15 colonies per blood agar plate (Cooper and Hopkins, 1985). In many instances, however, it is preferable to confirm the diagnosis of catheter-related sepsis with the catheter *in situ* so that unnecessary line removal can be avoided. If positive blood cultures collected through the catheter show a 5- to 10-fold increase in colony count compared with peripheral quantitative blood cultures, or if peripheral blood cultures are not collected, 100 colony-forming units per ml or more from the indwelling catheter are identified, line sepsis can be confirmed (Alexander, 1994). Another study evaluated the importance of exit site and catheter hub cultures and found that if these superficial cultures were negative, the diagnosis of line sepsis was unlikely because no catheter tip cultures were positive with negative external cultures (Cercenado *et al.*, 1990).

The most common pathogen found in Hickman catheter-related sepsis is *Staph. epidermidis*, accounting for approximately 40% of isolates from positive blood cultures, and it has emerged as a major cause of sepsis in neutropenic patients. Other organisms associated with catheter-related sepsis include *Staph. aureus, Candida* species, diphtheroids, *Pseudomonas aeruginosa*, and other aerobic gram-negative rods. Polymicrobial infections are often encountered in immunocompromised patients, but it is not clear whether these are related to the catheter or to other etiologies.

There are no prospective controlled clinical trials available to document the best method for treating catheter-related sepsis and no clear consensus on which catheters can be safely left *in situ* during treatment. Most studies have documented that in cases of catheter-related sepsis secondary to *Candida* or *Staph. aureus*, early catheter removal should be performed along with appropriate antibiotic treatment. In patients with other organisms, the decision to remove the catheter should be individualized depending on the clinical situation and response to initial antibiotic therapy (Alexander, 1994). If catheter removal and replacement appear to be indicated, replacement of infected catheters can be performed on the contralateral side within 24–72 hours after removal with appropriate antibiotic coverage, resulting in little risk of repeat infection.

Patients with catheter-related sepsis whose infection does not respond promptly to appropriate antibiotic therapy may have unrecognized septic thrombophlebitis. In this situation, a contrast dye study through the catheter should be considered and if catheter thrombosis is identified, the addition of thrombolytic therapy may be successful (Lowell and Bothe, 1991).

Peritoneal Access Systems

Despite the widespread use of aggressive surgical debulking followed by combination systemic chemotherapy, epithelial ovarian cancer continues to be the leading cause of death from gynecologic malignancies, with an estimated 24,000 new cases and 13,600 deaths in 1994 (Boring *et al.*, 1994). Since the majority of patients originally present and recur with disease largely confined in the peritoneal cavity, there has been significant interest in the development of intraperitoneal (IP) chemotherapy regimens for primary treatment, consolidation therapy and for the treatment of recurrent disease. Dedrick *et al.* (1978) at the National Cancer Institute first reported that the peritoneal clearance of certain neoplastic drugs was much lower than the serum clearance. Because the peritoneal administration of drugs was associated with a significant increase in the concentration difference between the peritoneal cavity and the systemic circulation, the IP instillation of neoplastic agents was thought to be a logical form of therapy for ovarian and other tumors primarily confined to the peritoneal cavity.

During the last 15 years, numerous papers dealing with IP chemotherapy have been published describing both theoretic considerations and therapeutic regimens. Despite this widespread interest in and use of IP chemotherapy, very little information is available regarding the methodology of peritoneal cavity access and other technical aspects of this therapy. Since there are no randomized prospective trials evaluating peritoneal cavity access devices, there is no widespread consensus regarding these and other theoretic considerations.

There are three principle methods of accessing the peritoneal cavity for the administration of chemotherapeutic agents. The first is a temporary indwelling catheter placed percutaneously before each IP treatment administration The second method uses a semipermanent indwelling Tenckhoff catheter, in a manner similar to the access used for peritoneal dialysis. The third method uses a totally implanted port and catheter system (e.g. Port-A-Cath) in an attempt to increase patient acceptance and decrease the risk of infection.

Before the use of IP chemotherapy, the majority of information regarding the technical aspects of peritoneal cavity access and the related complications was found in the peritoneal dialysis literature. Reported complications have included peritonitis, infections involving the catheter itself, failure of the catheter to infuse or drain, leakage of dialysate, displacement of the catheter, and hernia formation; and it is logical to expect similar complications in patients receiving IP chemotherapy (Davidson *et al.*, 1991). However, as first pointed out by Piccart *et al.* (1985), there are several basic differences between these patients with IP malignancy and those on chronic ambulatory peritoneal dialysis (CAPD) for renal failure: a higher incidence of previous laparotomies, known malignant disease in the peritoneal cavity, less frequent access to the peritoneal cavity, and the unknown effect of cytotoxic agents on the peritoneal membrane and cells. These variables will obviously affect the type and rate of complications associated with IP chemotherapy.

Even though the technique of peritoneal dialysis was first described in 1923, it was not until 1968 when Tenckhoff and Schecter reported the development of a peritoneal access device suitable for long-term use that peritoneal dialysis began to be widely used for maintenance therapy. This device consists of a Silastic catheter modified by the addition of Dacron felt cuffs intended to seal the sinus tract around the catheter and therefore decrease bacterial access to the peritoneal cavity. The widely accepted contraindications to peritoneal dialysis include the presence of some type of abdominal pathology, including loss of peritoneal surface area, recent abdominal surgery, and a history of extensive abdominal surgery as well as intra-abdominal or abdominal wall infection. Obviously, many of these factors are present in the typical patient with advanced ovarian cancer being considered for IP chemotherapy, thereby limiting the usefulness of studies involving CAPD patients to aid in the development of appropriate access techniques and regimens for IP chemotherapy patients.

Several studies have reported on peritoneal access-related complications and other technical aspects of IP chemotherapy, but since all of these suffer the limitations of retrospective studies, there is little consensus on some of the basic and important aspects of these systems (Piccart *et al.*, 1985; Braly *et al.*, 1986; Runowicz *et al.*, 1986; de Graaf *et al.*, 1988; Pfeiffer *et al.*, 1989; Davidson *et al.*, 1991).

Table 38.2. Complications of peritoneal access systems.

Complication	*Tenckhoff catheter*	*Port-catheter system*	*Single-use catheter*
Inflow obstruction	1/12[a]	3/145[c]	0/21[a]
	1/59[b]	0/33[e]	1/22[d]
	6/143[c]	20/227[f]	
Intestinal perforation	0/12[a]	3/145[c]	0/21[a]
	2/59[b]	1/33[e]	0/22[d]
	5/143[c]	8/227[f]	
Infections			
Abdominal wall	0/12[a]	0/145[c]	0/21[a]
	0/59[b]	2/33[e]	0/22[d]
	9/143[c]	10/227[f]	
	3/12[a]	12/145[c]	
Peritonitis	6/59[b]	5/33[e]	0/21[a]
	8/143[c]	2/227[f]	0/22[d]

[a]Runowicz *et al.*, 1986
[b]de Graaf *et al.*, 1988
[c]Piccart *et al.*, 1985
[d]Pfeiffer *et al.*, 1989
[e]Braly *et al.*, 1986
[f]Davidson *et al.*, 1991
[g]Kaplan *et al.*, 1985

Table 38.2 describes some of the reported complications related to peritoneal access systems. Davidson *et al.* suggest that implantation of a subcutaneous port and catheter system be delayed for 1–2 weeks if large bowel surgery is performed during laparotomy and tumor debulking, but no study has documented a statistically significant increase in infectious complications if a catheter is placed at the time of this procedure. Despite the fact that all these studies have reported adhesion formation and catheter inflow obstruction rates of 2.1–8.8%, there is no uniform recommendation on timing of catheter use after implantation or the use of flushing or irrigation protocols in an attempt to minimize these complications. It has been clearly established, however, that radiographic catheter dye studies should be liberally performed when there is a question of catheter obstruction, disconnection of the port and catheter, or the possibility of catheter erosion into bowel. If catheter erosion into bowel has been documented, it appears safe to remove the catheter without laparotomy and treat with antibiotics. One group (de Graaf *et al.*, 1988) has suggested that the combination of reassessment laparotomy with peritoneal catheter placement leads to a 'rather high complication rate,' presumably related to the extensive adhesiolysis that often accompanies these procedures. These authors do state, however, that no directions for patient selection and for pre- and postoperative management can be given. This does not agree with data from other studies, including Braly *et al.* (1986), who found that laparotomy with lysis of adhesions improved peritoneal fluid distribution as measured by IP contrast CT scan.

Infectious complications related to peritoneal catheter systems include both abdominal wall (cellulitis or pocket/tunnel) infections and peritonitis. In agreement with what has been previously described for central venous catheter systems, subcutaneous infections including exit site and tunnel or pocket infections usually require catheter removal for adequate treatment. Kaplan *et al.* (1985) reported on 32 episodes of infectious peritonitis in 90 patients receiving IP chemotherapy. In this series, *Staph. epidermidis* was the most commonly cultured organism, being identified in 65% of the isolates. It is important to note that the initial Gram's stain of the peritoneal fluid was positive in only 35% of cases, while the development of fever and abdominal pain, as well as rising peripheral and peritoneal fluid white blood cell counts, was helpful in making the appropriate diagnosis. In this study, 75% of the episodes of infectious peritonitis could be cleared with antibiotics alone and 25% required catheter removal for persistent or recurrent infection with the same organism within four weeks.

Summary of Management Options

- During the last two decades, there has been a dramatic increase in the use of long-term central venous access devices with an associated marked improvement in quality of life for patients with gynecologic malignancies and other disorders requiring reliable venous access.
- Continued improvement in techniques for catheter placement and care as well as modifications in these systems will be associated with fewer complications and clear benefits.
- For intraperitoneal chemotherapy regimens to be optimal, additional attention to the technical aspects of delivery and fluid distribution is necessary.
- Common indications for central venous catheterization include poor or inadequate peripheral venous access, rapid large volume transfusion requirements, administration of sclerosing agents such as total parenteral nutrition or chemotherapy, emergency access for resuscitation, and when central venous pressure monitoring is necessary.
- A previous history of thoracic surgical procedures, the presence of active mediastinal disease such as Hodgkin's disease or bulky metastatic disease, previous chest radiation, or multiple previous bilateral central lines increase the likelihood that the venous anatomy of the chest may be abnormal.
- There are, in general, two types of permanent central lines: the external catheter (e.g. Broviac, Hickman and Groshong catheters) and the subcutaneous port systems (e.g. Port-a-Cath, Mediport, Infus-a-Port, and the peripherally-implanted PAS Port). Advantages of the external catheters include lower cost, ease of access that does not require special needles, ability to handle rapid high-volume infusions and exchanges, and availability for immediate use.

References

■ Alexander HA (1994) Vascular access and other specialized techniques of drug delivery. In: De Vita VT, Hellman S & Rosenberg SA (eds) *Cancer: Principles and Practice of Oncology*, pp. 556–564. Philadelphia: JB Lippincott Co.

Aubaniac R (1952) L'injection intraveineuse sous-claviculaire: Avantages et technique. *Press. Med.* **60:** 1456.

Azizkhan RG, Taylor LA, Jaques PF, Mauro MA & Lacey SR (1992) Percutaneous translumbar and transhepatic inferior vena caval catheters for prolonged venous access in children. *J. Pediat. Surg.* **27:** 165–169.

Bern M, Lokich J, Wallach S *et al.* (1986) Very low-dose warfarin prevents thrombosis of central vein catheters. *Proc. Am. Soc. Clin. Oncol.* **5:** 254.

Bernard RW & Stahl WM (1971) Subclavian vein catheterization: A prospective study. *Ann. Surg.* **173:** 184–190.

Boring CC, Squires TS, Tong T & Montgomery S (1994) Cancer statistics, 1994. *CA – A Cancer Journal for Clinicians* **44:** 7–26.

Bothe A, Piccione W, Ambrosino JJ *et al.* (1984) Implantable central venous access system. *Am. J. Surg.* **147:** 565–569.

Braly P, Doroshow J & Hoff S (1986) Technical aspects of intraperitoneal chemotherapy in abdominal carcinomatosis. *Gynecol. Oncol.* **25:** 319–333.

Brothers TE, Von Moll LK, Niederhuber JE *et al.* (1988) Experience with subcutaneous infusion ports in three hundred patients. *Surg. Gynecol. Obstet.* **166:** 295–301.

Broviac JW, Cole JJ & Scribner GH (1973) A silicone rubber atrial catheter for prolonged parenteral alimentation. *Surg. Gynecol. Obstet.* **136:** 602–606.

Brown JM (1989) Peripherally inserted central catheters: Use in home care. *Intraven. Nurs.* **12:** 144–000.

Cercenado E, Ena J, Rodriguez–Crexems M, Romeo I & Bouza E (1990) A conservative procedure for the diagnosis of catheter-related infections. *Arch. Intern. Med.* **150:** 1417–1420.

Cooper GL & Hopkins CC (1985) Rapid diagnosis of intravascular catheter-associated infection by direct Gram staining of catheter segments. *New Engl. J. Med.* **312:** 1142–1147.

Crawford SW, Hickman RO, Ulz L *et al.* (1994) Use of the Hickman–Crawford critical care catheter in marrow transplant recipients: A pulmonary artery catheter–adaptable central venous access. *Critical Care Med.* **22:** 347–352.

Davidson SA, Rubin SC, Markman M *et al.* (1991) Intraperitoneal chemotherapy: Analysis of complications with an implanted subcutaneous port and catheter system. *Gynecol. Oncol.* **41:** 101–106.

Dedrick RL, Myers CE, Bungay PM & DeVita VT (1978) Pharmacokinetic rationale for peritoneal drug administration in the treatment of ovarian cancer. *Cancer Treat. Rep.* **62:** 1–11.

de Graaf PW, Mellema MM, ten Bokkel Huinink WW *et al.* (1988) Complications of Tenckhoff catheter implantation in patients with multiple previous intraabdominal procedures for ovarian carcinoma. *Gynecol. Oncol.* **29:** 43–49.

Delmor JE, Horbelt DV, Jack BL *et al.* (1989) Experience with the Groshong long term central venous catheter. *Gynecol. Oncol.* **34:** 216–218.

Denny DF (1993) Placement and management of long-term central venous access catheters and ports. *Am. J. Radiol.* **161:** 385–393.

Dudrick SJ & Wilmore DW (1968) Long-term parenteral feeding. *Hosp. Pract.* **3:** 65–78.

Dudrick SJ, Wilmore DW, Vars HM *et al.* (1968) Long-term

total parenteral nutrition with growth, development, and positive nitrogen balance. *Surgery* **64:** 134–142.

Gilles H, Rogers HJ, Johnston J, Harper PG & Rudge CJ (1985) Is repeated flushing of Hickman catheters necessary? *Br. Med. J.* **290:** 1708.

Hartman GE & Shochat SJ (1987) Management of septic complications associated with Silastic catheters in childhood malignancy. *Pediatr. Infect. Dis. J.* **6:** 1042–1047.

Hickman RO, Buckner CD, Clift RA *et al.* (1979) A modified right atrial catheter for access to the venous system in marrow transplant recipients. *Surg. Gynecol. Obstet.* **148:** 871–875.

■ Hickman RO, Ramsey PG & Tapper D (1991) Central venous access. In: Greer BE & Berek JS (eds) *Current Topics in Obstetrics and Gynecology. Gynecologic Oncology: Treatment Rationale and Techniques*, pp. 286–308. New York: Elsevier.

Hill SL & Berry RE (1990) Subclavian vein thrombosis: A continuing challenge. *Surgery* **108:** 1–9.

Kaplan RA, Markman M, Lucas WE, Pfeifle C & Howell SB (1985) Infectious peritonitis in patients receiving intraperitoneal chemotherapy. *Am. J. Med.* **78:** 49–53.

Kenney PR, Dorfman GS & Denny DF (1985) Percutaneous inferior vena cava cannulation for long term parenteral access. *Surgery* **97:** 602–605.

Kunkel JM & Machleder HI (1989) Treatment of Paget–Schroetter syndrome: A staged, multidisciplinary approach. *Arch. Surg.* **124:** 1153–1157.

Lechner P, Anderhuber F & Tesch NP (1989) Anatomical bases for a safe method of subclavian venipuncture: Clinical experience in 350 cases. *Surg. Radiol. Anat.* **11:** 91–95.

Ledgerwood AM, Saxe JM & Lucas CE (1993) Venous access devices: A review. *Surg. Annual* **25:** 45–57.

■ Lowell JA & Bothe A (1991) Venous access: Preoperative, operative, and postoperative dilemmas. *Surg. Clin. NA* **71:** 1231–1246.

McDonough JJ & Altemeier WA (1971) Subclavian venous thrombosis secondary to indwelling catheters. *Surg. Gynecol. Obstet.* **133:** 397–400.

Neiderhuber JE, Ensminger W, Gyves JW *et al.* (1982) Totally implanted venous and arterial access system to replace external catheters in cancer treatment. *Surgery* **92:** 706–712.

Nelson EW (1986) Venous access techniques. *Urol. Clin. North Amer.* **13:** 475–487.

Pfeiffer P, Asmussen L, Kvist–Poulsen H & Bertelsen K (1989) Intraperitoneal chemotherapy: Introduction of a new "single use" delivery system – A preliminary report. *Gynecol. Oncol.* **35:** 47–49.

Piccart MJ, Speyer JL, Markman M *et al.* (1985) Intraperitoneal chemotherapy: Technical experience at five institutions. *Semin. Oncol.* **12:** 90–96.

Press OW, Ramsey PG, Larson EB *et al.* (1984) Hickman catheter infections in patients with malignancies. *Medicine* **63:** 189–200.

Quinton W, Dillard D & Scribner BH (1960) Cannulation of blood vessels for prolonged hemodialysis. *Trans. Am. Soc. Artif. Intern. Organs* **6:** 1043.

Ross MN, Haase GM, Poole MA, Burrington JD & Odom LF (1988) Comparison of totally implanted reservoirs with external catheters as venous access devices in pediatric oncology patients. *Surg. Gynecol. Obstet.* **167:** 141–144.

Runowicz CD, Dottino PR, Shafir MK, Mark MA & Cohen CJ (1986) Catheter complications associated with intraperitoneal chemotherapy. *Gynecol. Oncol.* **24:** 41–50.

Salem RR, Ward BA & Ravikumar TS (1993) A new peripherally implanted subcutaneous permanent central venous access device for patients requiring chemotherapy. *J. Clin. Oncol.* **11:** 2181–2185.

Sanders JE, Hickman RO, Aker BS *et al.* (1982) Experience with double lumen right atrial catheters. *J. Parenter. Enter. Nutr.* **6:** 95.

Sariego J, Bootorabi B, Mastumoto T & Kerstein M (1993) Major long-term complications in 1,422 permanent venous access devices. *Am. J. Surg.* **165:** 249–251.

Scott WL (1989) Complications associated with central venous catheters. A survey. *Chest* **94:** 1221–1224.

■ Seewaldt VL & Greer BE (1994) Vascular Access. In: Orr JW & Shingleton HM (eds) *Complications in Gynecologic Surgery: Prevention, Recognition and Management*, pp. 189–204. Philadelphia: JB Lippincott.

Seigel EL, Jew AC, Delcore R *et al.* (1993) Thrombolytic therapy for catheter-related thrombosis. *Am. J. Surg.* **166:** 716–719.

Stuart RK, Shikora SA, Akerman P *et al.* (1990) Incidence of arrhythmia with central venous catheter insertion and exchange. *J. Parenter. Enter. Nutr.* **14:** 152–155.

Tenckhoff H & Schecter H (1968) A bacteriologically safe peritoneal access device. *Trans. Amer. Soc. Artif. Intern. Org.* **14:** 181–187.

Thompson WR, Alexander HR, Martin AJ, Fletcher JR & Ghosh BC (1985) Percutaneous subclavian catheterization for prolonged systemic chemotherapy. *J. Surg. Oncol.* **29:** 184–189.

Torosian MH, Meranze S, McLean G *et al.* (1986) Central venous access with occlusive central venous thrombosis. *Ann. Surg.* **203:** 30–33.

39 The Lymphatic System and Lymphadenectomy in Gynecologic Malignancy

P J MacKoul
W C Fowler Jr
W A Marston

Introduction

Metastasis to the lymphatic system plays a crucial role in the management of gynecologic malignancy. The lymphatic system is a major pathway for the spread of gynecologic cancer, especially those that spread regionally. Surgical evaluation of the pelvic and paraaortic nodes is required for the precise management of cervical, endometrial and ovarian carcinoma, and often changes the diagnosis, prognosis and management of these patients if metastases are discovered.

Aortic and pelvic lymphadenectomy is the most complex retroperitoneal procedure in gynecologic oncology, and requires a thorough knowledge of the vascular and lymphatic anatomy of these areas, both normal and aberrent. Expert surgical technique is necessary, and surgeons must be well versed in the many different approaches to lymphadenectomy to optimize patient care. Extensive lymph node dissection increases the risk of complications, both intraoperative and postoperative, and a rational knowledgeable approach to handling these problems is essential.

This chapter is devoted exclusively to lymphadenectomy in gynecologic malignancy. Transperitoneal and extraperitoneal approaches to pelvic and paraaortic lymphadenectomy are reviewed, including indications and operative technique. Sections on laparoscopic pelvic and paraaortic lymphadenectomy, as well as inguinal node dissection and scalene node dissection, are also included. This chapter will also discuss the normal anatomy, anatomic abnormalities, and complications encountered during these procedures.

Anatomy

The major nodal groups of concern in gynecologic malignancy include the lumbar or aortic nodes, the pelvic nodes, and the inguinal nodes (*Figure 39.1*). The supraclavicular nodes are of importance mainly in cervical cancer, and are discussed later.

Pelvic Lymphatics

The pelvic lymphatics are comprised of six nodal systems. These include the common, external and internal iliac nodes, as well as the obturator nodes. Presacral and parametrial nodes are also included.

External iliac nodes

This group consists of approximately 8–10 nodes that are located on the lateral and posteromedial aspect of the external iliac artery and vein, with the lower posteromedial nodes continuous with the deep nodes of the femoral canal. Lateral nodes are often between the external iliac artery and the psoas

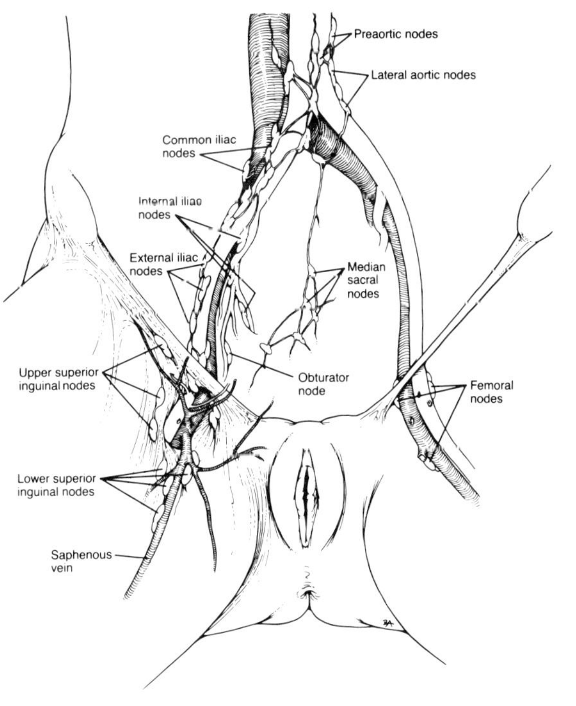

Figure 39.1. Lymph nodes of the lower paraaortic, iliac, and inguinal-femoral vessels. (Permission from Gershenson DM, DeCherney AH & Curry SL *et al.* (1993).)

muscle. The medial chain is located between the external iliac and internal iliac vessels, and these nodes are sometimes called the interiliac nodes, as described by Plentl and Friedman (1971).

The entire nodal group receives drainage from the superficial and deep inguinal nodes, as well as the anterior abdominal wall below the umbilicus. The medial segment of nodes receives drainage from the bladder and urethra, as well as from the uterus, vagina and fallopian tube. This nodal group discharges to the common and internal iliac nodes (Woodburne, 1983).

Internal iliac nodes

The internal iliac nodes are from 4–8 in number, and lie on top of and medial to all branches of the internal iliac vessels. This includes both the anterior and posterior divisions of the internal iliac artery. The posterior division gives rise to the superior gluteal, lateral sacral and iliolumbar vessels. The anterior division divides to form the inferior gluteal, obturator, internal pudendal, uterine, superior vesical, vaginal and middle rectal vessels. Plentl and Friedman originally described the internal iliac nodes as the superior and inferior gluteal nodes.

These nodes receive drainage from many pelvic organs – the bladder, urethra, uterus, vagina and rectum, as well as from the gluteal region and thigh. Internal iliac nodes drain to the external and common nodes.

Common iliac nodes

Six nodes are present that lie laterally, medially and posteriorly along the common iliac artery and vein. The lateral and posterior nodes continue from the external iliac nodes, and the medial nodes are located over the sacral promontory below the bifurcation of the aorta. Only 1–2 nodes are present over the common iliac artery, with most nodes located deep and posterior to the vessel. Panici *et al.* (1992) describe dissection of the posterior chain with 4–5 nodes identified and removed after isolation of the iliolumbar veins and the obturator and ischiadic nerves.

Since these nodes receive drainage from the external and internal iliac groups, they receive lymph from the pelvic wall and viscera, as well as from the lower limb, perineum, and lower abdominal wall. Drainage from these nodes is to the lumbar chain.

Obturator nodes

The obturator fossa contains approximately 15 nodes, 11 located superficially above the obturator nerve, and an additional 4–5 located deep in the fossa below the nerve. Lymphatic drainage to these nodes is similar to that of the internal iliac nodes. The obturator nodes in particular play an important role in the lymphatic drainage of the cervix and lower uterine segment of the uterus, since drainage from the parametrial nodes is often directly to the obturator nodes.

Parametrial nodes

The lateral parametrial tissue contains nodes ranging in number from 4–8, and receive drainage directly from the cervix and lower uterine segment. Drainage from these nodes is to the obturator, internal iliac, external iliac, sacral and median common iliac nodes.

Sacral nodes

Two or three sacral nodes are located along the lateral sacral arteries opposite the second and third sacral foramina. They receive drainage from the uterus, vagina, rectum and posterior pelvic wall, and drain to the medial common iliac nodes.

The Lumbar (Aortic) Lymphatics

The lumbar nodal chain extends from the aortic bifurcation to the aortic hiatus of the diaphragm, and there are more than 50 in number. Nodes are present on both the left and right side of the aorta. On the left, they lie between the aorta and the psoas, while on the right they lie in front of the vena cava and behind it on the psoas muscle. Drainage to these nodes is from the following structures:

- the common iliac nodes;
- lympatics from the ovary, fallopian tube and uterine fundus;
- the kidneys, suprarenal glands, and abdominal surface of the diaphragm;
- the lumbar arteries of the lateral abdominal wall.

Inferior mesenteric nodes also drain toward the left lumbar chain.

The Inguinal Nodes

Superficial inguinal nodes

Approximately 20 nodes are present, ten on each side, and are arranged in the form of a T in the subcutaneous tissue of the groin. Anatomically, the superficial nodes are located beneath Camper's fascia, but above the cribriform fascia. These nodes can be separated into four groups: the great saphenous vein group, the superficial circumflex iliac and external pudendal vein groups, and the superficial epigastric vein group. The horizontal part of the T is composed of most of the nodes, and is located in a chain parallel to and 1–2 cm below the inguinal ligament. Drainage to these nodes is from the lower abdominal wall, buttocks, labia majora and minora, and perineum. The vertical position of the T lies along the greater saphenous vein, and is composed of fewer nodes. These drain the superficial lymphatics of the lower limb, and some vessels of the labia majora and minora, as well as the perineum. Drainage from these nodes is to the deep inguinal or femoral nodes.

Deep inguinal or femoral nodes

Only 2–3 nodes comprise this group, and are located on the medial side of the femoral vein. One node is usually at the femoral canal, one at the upper end of the femoral ring, and the third below the junction of the saphenous and femoral veins. Cloquet's node, or the node of Rosenmüller, is the highest deep inguinal node before the external iliac nodes. They receive drainage from the limb and perineum, and discharge to the external iliac nodes.

Surgical Technique

Surgical evaluation of the lymph nodes is limited to either selective lymphadenectomy or systematic lymphadenectomy, and can be performed through a transperitoneal, extraperitoneal or laparoscopic approach.

Selective lymphadenectomy, often referred to as lymph node sampling, is the removal of individual lymph nodes or enlarged nodes. The lymph nodes to be removed are grasped and dissected free from the vessel one by one until an adequate number of nodes have been obtained. In ovarian cancer, for example, complete lymphadenectomy of the pelvic and paraaortic nodes is not indicated or required for staging purposes or for therapy, and lymph node sampling is the procedure of choice. Sampling of the pelvic and paraaortic nodes is performed for endometrial, ovarian and fallopian tube carcinomas.

Systematic lymphadenectomy, or complete node dissection, is the removal of all lymphatic tissue that is accessible, including the lymph nodes and the lymphatic channels between them. Adequate systematic lymphadenectomy requires incising the perivascular sheath overlying the vessels, and removal of all fibrofatty and lymphatic tissue around and between the vessels. Systematic pelvic lymphadenectomy during radical hysterectomy, for example, refers to complete removal of the external and internal iliac nodes, as well as the common nodes and obturator nodes as a diagnostic and therapeutic procedure. The inferior gluteal nodes are not accessible and cannot be removed. The use of lymphadenectomy in gynecologic oncology is generally limited to vulvar and cervical cancer. Supraclavicular (scalene) node dissection may be indicated in some patients. The following descriptions of pelvic and paraaortic node dissection refer to systematic lymphadenectomy.

Transperitoneal Pelvic Lymphadenectomy

Technique

The abdominal cavity is entered through either a transverse or vertical abdominal incision, depending upon the indication for the procedure. After a self-retaining retractor has been placed, and the bowels packed away, the surgeon can proceed with lymphadenectomy. Two approaches are presented here, the standard approach performed at most institutions, and the 'stripping' technique as described by Yong–Liang.

Standard approach

The retroperitoneal space is opened to expose the iliac vessels, and the paravesical and pararectal spaces are developed (*Figure 39.2*). The anatomy of the pelvic sidewall is completely identified, with particular attention directed to isolation of the ureter. The psoas muscle, genitofemoral nerve, external and internal iliac arteries and veins, common iliac artery, and cardinal ligament or 'web' are easily identified. The superior vesical artery and uterine artery are visualized as well.

Exposure to the vessels and lymphatics of the retroperitoneal space is the most important component to successful pelvic lymph node dissection. Proper development of anatomic spaces of the pelvis combined with the use of Deaver retractors will adequately expose the vessels and retract the ureter without difficulty. The iliac vessels and their divisions can now be completely defined, and the pelvic node dissection can begin. Clinically, we

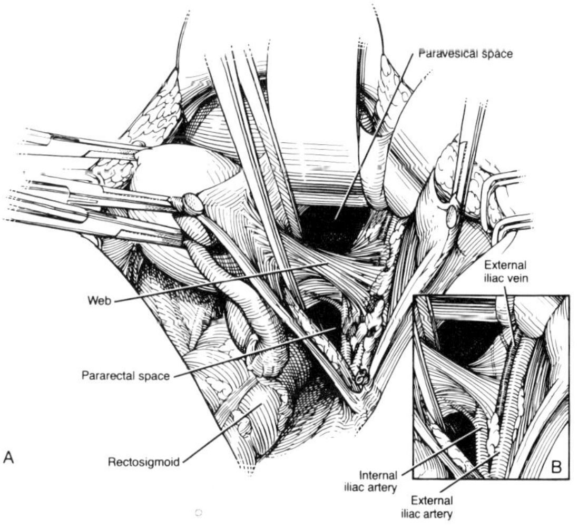

Figure 39.2. Pelvic node dissection. Development of the paravesical and pararectal spaces allows mobilization of the ureter and adequate exposure to the illac and obturator nodes. (By permission of Mayo foundation, Lee RA (1992a).)

describe the external iliac lymph nodes as all lymphatic tissue lateral to the external iliac artery, extending from the bifurcation of the common iliac artery to the circumflex iliac vein. Nodes between the artery and the psoas muscle are also labeled as external iliac nodes. The internal iliac nodes represent all lymphatic tissue between the external and internal iliac artery, from the bifurcation to the pelvic wall. Lymphatic tissue obtained from the obturator fossa is labeled as obturator nodes.

Pelvic node dissection usually begins with dissection of the external iliac nodes. The perivascular sheath that overlies the external iliac artery is incised from the bifurcation of the common iliac artery to the crossover point of the circumflex iliac vein to completely expose the vessel. The genitofemoral nerve is identified lateral to the artery on the psoas muscle. In some cases the nerve is in close proximity to the lymphatic tissue and must be dissected free to avoid injury. The lymphatic tissue is then transected at the level of the bifurcation, and all fibroareolar and lymophatic tissue lateral to the external iliac artery and caudad to the circumflex iliac vein is removed using surgical clips as needed for hemostasis.

Before proceeding with dissection of the internal and obturator nodes (*Figure 39.3*), the obturator space can be developed from above. This will allow removal of nodes between the psoas muscle and the artery and vein, and will aid in dissection of the internal iliac nodes and the obturator fossa. Using blunt dissection, the external iliac artery is separated from the psoas muscle, and the artery is retracted medially. Lymph nodes in this space can now be removed, and further gentle blunt dissection between the psoas muscle and the external iliac vein will expose the obturator space and the nerve.

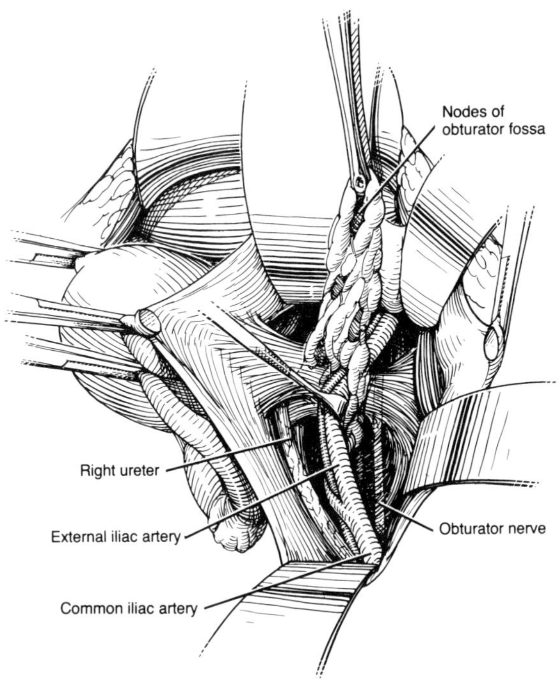

Figure 39.3. Pelvic node dissection. After the obturator nerve has been identified, the internal iliac and obturator nodes can be easily removed *en bloc*. The external iliac node dissection has already been accomplished. (Permission from Lee RA (1992b).)

The internal iliac and obturator node dissection is begun by exposing the external iliac vein. After the perivascular sheath surrounding the vein has been dissected free, gentle traction can be used to elevate the vein and expose the obturator fossa and the obturator nerve. Note that the obturator nerve has already been freed of nodal tissue from above. The internal and obturator lymphatic tissue is now grasped, and sharp dissection is used to free this tissue from the internal iliac artery and the external iliac vein, and from the obturator fossa. Nodal and fatty tissue can be dissected free from the superior vesical artery in a lateral and caudad direction. At this point in the dissection, the nodal bundle including internal iliac and obturator nodes has been freed from the external iliac vein, the bifurcation and the internal iliac vein, the superior vesical artery, and from the obturator nerve and fossa. Dissection of the bundle from the pelvic wall will allow removal of the nodes from the operative field.

Care should be taken when dissecting at the bifurcation of the common iliac artery since a small vessel usually exits from this area to the nodal bundle. If transected, the vessel may retract and bleeding may be difficult to control. Particular care must also be taken when working in the obturator fossa to avoid trauma to the obturator nerve and vessels. Nodal tissue is not removed beneath the obturator nerve since the obturator vein forms a rich anastomotic network with the internal iliac vein, and bleeding in this area is difficult to control. If nodal tissue must be removed in this region, the obturatory veins should be clipped before dissection starts. Bleeding in this area is best controlled with pressure hemostasis and packs.

Removal of the common iliac nodes requires extension of the peritoneal incision cephalad and replacement of the Deaver retractor. Starting at the bifurcation of the iliac vessels, the perivascular sheath overlying the common iliac artery is grasped and incised. The incision is continued towards the bifurcation of the aorta. Nodal tissue lateral and medial to the common iliac artery is removed. Posterior nodal tissue can also be removed, with care to avoid lumbar branches. Pelvic lymphadenectomy to the common, external and internal iliac vessels, and the obturator fossa is now complete.

The stripping technique

This is a technique developed by Gao Yong–liang (1992) of the Zhejiang Cancer Hospital in China that makes use of blunt dissection, or 'stripping', to obtain lymph nodes in patients with cervical cancer. The iliac vessels are exposed in the standard fashion. At a point 2–3 cm above the common iliac bifurcation, the lymphatic bundle overlying the common iliac artery is ligated and transected, and a Kelly clamp is used to grasp the proximal pedicle. In a direction cephalad to caudad, the common and external iliac nodes are bluntly stripped along the surface of the vessel in one piece until the inguinal ligament is reached. The entire bundle is elevated, clipped and transected, and removed *en bloc* as external and common iliac nodes.

The obturator space is now opened from above, and blunt dissection of the obturator nodes from the pelvic wall is performed. The obturator nerve is identified. The paravesical space is also developed. The obturator nerve is now grasped between the index and middle fingers, and the nodes are stripped away from the nerve in a caudad to cephalad direction, thereby bluntly dissecting the obturator and internal iliac nodes. Yong–liang claims that the procedure, when compared to the standard approach to pelvic lymphadenectomy, is as complete in the number of nodes removed, but is associated with less complications and bleeding, and is easier to perform, and also that the procedure is not indicated when large metastatic nodes are encountered or when there are adhesive lesions to the vessels.

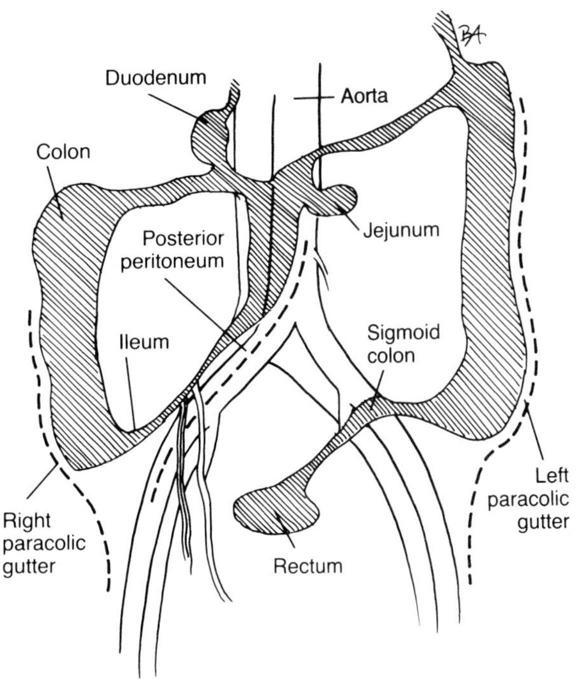

Figure 39.4. Paraaortic node dissection. Three approaches are illustrated here. **1.** Left paracolic. The peritoneum of the left paracolic gutter is incised and the descending and sigmoid colon are molbilized medially to expose the aorta and vena cava. Care must be taken to avoid injury to the ureter and inferior mesenteric artery during mobilization and retraction. **2.** Right paracolic. In a similar approach, the peritoneum along the right gutter is incised and the ascending colon is mobilized medially to expose the vessels. In both of these approaches, the duodenum can be freed cephalad to obtain higher access to the large vessels. **3.** Direct approach. This involves incising the peritoneum directly above the right common iliac artery and aorta to obtain access to the left- and right-sided lymph nodes. The bowel is either exteriorized or packed away to obtain exposure. (Permission from Gershenson DM, DeCherney AH & Curry SL (1993b).)

Transperitoneal Paraaortic Lymphadenectomy

Technique

Several different approaches have been advocated transperitoneally for lymph node dissection of the aortacaval region (*Figure 39.4*). All of these approaches make use of a midline skin incision with extension above the umbilicus, with different peritoneal incisions to expose the paraaortic and common iliac nodes. The standard approach uses a peritoneal incision directly over the common iliac artery and aorta to expose the lymph nodes. The left and right paracolic approaches both involve incising the peritoneum along the white line of Toldt on either side, with reflection of the peritoneum and bowel medially to expose the vessels and nodes.

Standard approach

The omentum, transverse colon, and small bowel are packed in the upper abdomen or the small bowel is placed in a bowel isolation bag and then exteriorized with the patient in deep Trendelenburg's position to obtain maximum exposure. The common iliac arteries and the bifurcation of the aorta are identified, as well as the right ureter.

The right paraaortic nodes are removed first (*Figure 39.5*). The posterior peritoneum over the common iliac artery on the right is incised, and the incision is carried to approximately 6 cm above the bifurcation of the aorta. Traction sutures can be used on the peritoneal edges to aid in exposure. Deaver retractors are then placed, one in the midline and the other on the right, to retract the peritoneum and bowel from the field, and to isolate the right ureter. After adequate exposure has been obtained, the lymph node dissection begins on the patient's right. The perivascular sheath overlying the right common iliac artery is incised and extended cephalad as far as needed. The nodal bundle just below the bifurcation is transected, and gentle blunt and sharp dissection is used to free the node-containing fat pad from the vena cava and aorta. Care should be taken

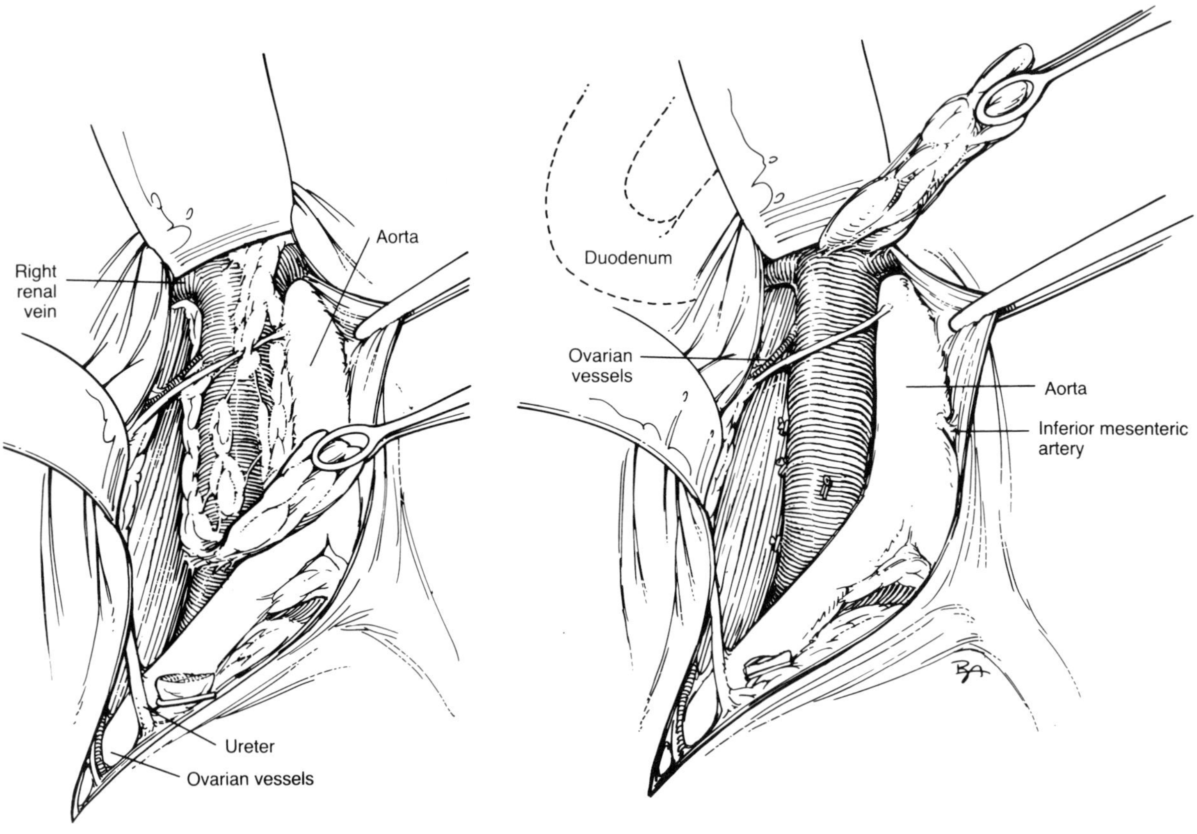

Figure 39.5. Paraaortic node dissection. Access to the precaval and aortic nodes has been obtained via the direct approach. The nodes are dissected free from caudad to cephalad using gentle blunt dissection and sharp dissection, with liberal use of surgical clips as needed to control bleeding. Note the location of the inferior mesenteric artery and the outline of the duodenum. The right ureter is retracted away from the field of dissection. (Permission from Gershenson DM, DeCherney AH & Curry SL (1993c).)

during the dissection to clip and cut small vessels running from the vena cava to the nodal bundle just above the bifurcation of the aorta, and small arteries running from the aorta to the nodal bundle should be carefully identified and clipped as well. The use of hemoclips allows for faster dissection, and also marks the area of nodal dissection for the radiation therapist if adjuvant radiation therapy is necessary. This dissection may continue cephalad to the third portion of the duodenum. If dissection above the duodenum is indicated, this structure can be retracted for further exposure.

To begin removal of lymph nodes from the left side of the aorta, the left common iliac vessels and left ureter are identified. The perivascular sheath above the left common iliac artery is incised, and adequate exposure is now developed by placing a Deaver retractor beneath the mesentery of the left colon to retract both the peritoneum and the bowel, as well as the left ureter. The inferior mesenteric artery is easily visualized, and care must be taken to avoid avulsing this structure during retraction. The nodal bundle to the left common iliac vessel is transected, and the nodes are removed with careful dissection. A vein retractor can be placed to retract the aorta toward the right side to aid in the dissection. Care to avoid laceration to the perilumbar vessels is essential since the lymph nodes are more posterior on the left side.

Dissection continues to the inferior mesenteric artery (IMA). In general, this is the most cephalad point of dissection. If indicated, dissection can continue above the inferior mesenteric artery by replacing the Deaver retractor above the IMA to retract the bowel, peritoneum, and ureter. In the event of laceration or avulsion of the IMA, ligation of the artery and the aortic stump is performed as long as backflow from the artery is seen, indicating an intact marginal artery of Drummond. If backflow is not present, reimplantation of the artery is necessary.

Right-sided approach

A transperitoneal right-sided approach to the paraaortic nodes was first reported in the literature by Lubicz (1985) (*Figure 39.6*). The ascending colon and cecum are identified, and an incision is made

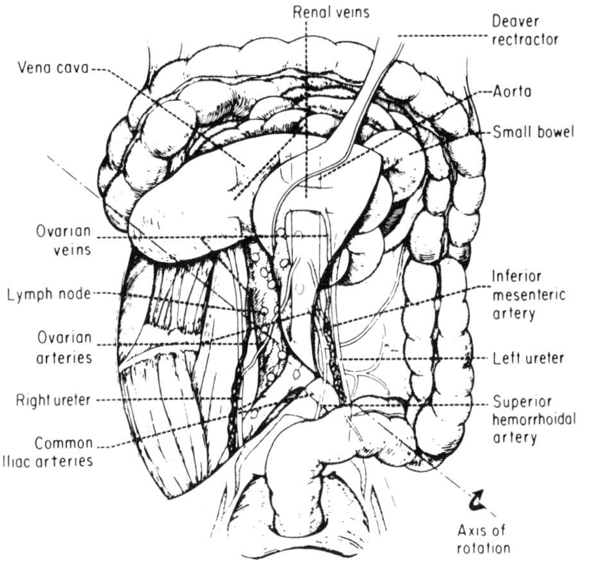

Figure 39.6. Transperitoneal right-sided approach. Complete mobilization of the right-sided bowel and ureter allows excellent exposure to the retroperitoneal space. (Permission from Lubicz S (1985).)

in the peritoneum starting 2 cm caudad and lateral to the cecum and extended cephalad along the white line of Toldt parallel to the colon to the level of the hepatic flexure. The right ureter must be identified at all times. Blunt dissection can be used to help elevate the peritoneum off the psoas muscle. The peritoneal incision is now extended horizontally and medially starting from the initial incision made near the cecum toward the sacral promontory. The right common iliac vessels are identified as well as the ureter, and the incision should overlie the common iliac artery. Exposure can now be gained to the aortocaval area and to the right common iliac artery and bifurcation after the ascending colon, small bowel, and their mesenteries are mobilized. This is done with sharp and blunt dissection from right to left until eventually the vena cava and aorta are unroofed and exposed. Greater exposure is obtained by dissecting the ovarian vessels and ureter from the peritoneum. If oophorectomy is to be done, the ovarian vessels should be ligated at the aorta and vena cava to gain further exposure. The retroperitoneal space can be further developed cephalad as far as needed, eventually revealing the entire kidney, duodenum, and pancreas. The entire retroperitoneal floor is exposed, with the ureter and ovarian vessels freed from the peritoneum for optimal exposure. With the ascending colon and mesentery being retracted with a Deaver and rotated toward the midline, the vena cava, aorta, and right common iliac vessels are exposed for lymphadenectomy.

Lymph node dissection is performed as mentioned previously. After completion, the peritoneum of the colon is reattached to the lateral abdominal peritoneum. Drains can be placed if necessary. The main advantage to this approach is better exposure, allowing for an easier, less complicated, and faster node dissection. Less retraction is required, thereby minimizing trauma to the colon and small bowel, as well as the spleen. The main disadvantage to this approach is poor access to the left-sided aortic nodes, since these nodes are lateral and posterior to the aorta.

Left-sided approach

A similar approach originating from the left side has been described more recently by Beneditti–Panici *et al.* (1994) with excellent exposure to the lymph nodes left of the aorta. Dissection of the right aortocaval nodes from the left side is also possible.

The left colon is identified and retracted medially to expose the peritoneum of the left paracolic gutter. The peritoneal incision is made from the round ligament to the splenic flexure of the left colon along the white line of Toldt. Blunt and sharp dissection is used to free the colon from its attachments. The ureter and ovarian vessels can be freed from the peritoneum for greater exposure if needed. Exposure to the level of the renal vessels is obtained easily, with complete visualization of the inferior mesenteric artery, left ovarian artery and the insertion of the left ovarian vein to the left renal vein. During retraction, care must be taken to avoid extensive medial retraction and damage to the inferior mesenteric artery. Lymphadenectomy can now be performed to the left and right sides of the aorta. Note that with dissection on the left side, lumbar vessels are frequently encountered and must be carefully avoided or ligated and cut. Dissection of the left side requires mobilizing the lymphatic tissue from the lateral side of the aorta initially.

Extraperitoneal Pelvic and Paraaortic Lymphadenectomy

Incision

The incision used greatly depends upon which nodal groups are to be evaluated. If only the pelvic nodes are to be sampled, bilateral groin incisions or the OIPE incision (one incision, pararectal, extraperitoneal) should be used. Paraaortic nodes are easily sampled through the upper abdominal or sunrise incisions. All of these incisions can be extended, if necessary, to include the pelvic or paraaortic nodes. Midline and J incisions can be used for both node groups.

The following sections on technique describe each incision and the approach to develop exposure of the retroperitoneal space during extraperitoneal lymphadenectomy.

Extraperitoneal paraaortic lymphadenectomy and bilateral pelvic lymphadenectomy

Midline incision

The use of a midline incision for pelvic and paraaortic lymph node dissection is well described by Gallup *et al.* (1986). A vertical incision is made extending from the symphysis to the umbilicus, and the fascia is incised down to the level of the symphysis. The incision is extended to the left above the umbilicus to allow exposure to the paraaortic nodes.

The rectus muscles are identified and bluntly dissected from the peritoneum. The midline raphe between the pyramidalis muscles is separated to obtain maximum exposure distally. The peritoneum is grasped and pulled forward with one hand while the other hand is used to develop the space of Retzius. Again using blunt dissection with either the hand or a spongestick, the peritoneum is freed from iliac vessels and Cooper's ligament. Dissection is continued until the obturator nerve is clearly visible to the sidewall of the pelvis. The round ligament is then transected and ligated, and the hand is now used to pull the peritoneum toward the opposite side, exposing the pelvic sidewall and vessels. The ureter is easily visible on the peritoneum. A retractor can be placed over the peritoneum and the patient can be tilted toward the opposite side to aid further exposure. The pelvic vessels are now completely exposed, and the lymph node dissection can begin. The same technique is used to expose the pelvic vessels on the opposite side.

Access to the paraortic nodes is accomplished by extending the incision and mobilizing the peritoneum from the left or right side. This will require transecting the transverse abdominus muscle on each side to gain access to the peritoneum on the left and right. After the peritoneum has been bluntly dissected from the retroperitoneal floor and mobilized medially, retractors are used to maintain exposure to the common iliac vessels and the aorta, and the lymphadenectomy is performed in the standard fashion. Note that a self-retaining retractor can be used for further assistance with exposure if needed. This may be especially helpful in obese patients. This incision provides the best exposure to both the left and right pelvic and paraaortic nodes, and can also be used for transperitoneal radical hysterectomy after node dissection is completed.

Left- or right-sided J-shaped vertical incision

Bergman *et al.* (1977) described the use of a left-sided J-shaped incision to gain access to the pelvic and paraaortic nodes bilaterally (*Figure 39.7*). A left-sided incision is made starting above the symphysis and parallel to the inguinal ligament, continuing vertically 3 cm medial to the iliac crest, and extending above the umbilicus. The incision continues through the fascia of the external oblique muscle, and then the internal oblique and transversalis muscles are transected using cautery to expose the peritoneum. The peritoneum is then dissected off the pelvic wall, and the round ligament and inferior epigastric vessels are transected to provide better exposure. The peritoneum is further mobilized, exposing the aorta and common iliac vessels, as well as the pelvic vessels. Left paraaortic lymph node dissection is performed initially, followed by pelvic lymphadenectomy.

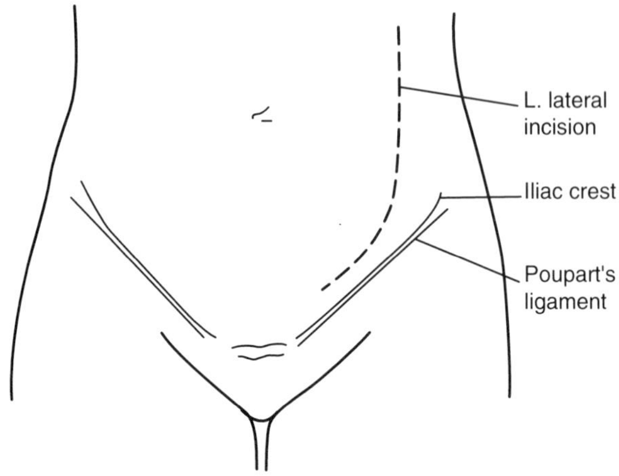

Figure 39.7. Left-sided J-shaped incision. Extraperitoneal pelvic and paraaortic node dissection can be performed to the left side without difficulty. Right-sided node dissection can also be accomplished through this incision, but care must be taken to avoid avulsion of the inferior mesenteric artery through excessive retraction. (Permission from Bergman ML, Lagasse LD & Atring WG (1977).)

After the left side is complete, the peritoneum is further dissected free from the aorta, vena cava and pelvic vessels on the right. Retractors are placed beneath the peritoneum to elevate it, with the operating room table being tilted to the right to optimize exposure. Dissection of the right paraaortic and pelvic nodes is then carried out, with the surgeons performing the entire procedure from the left side. Care must be taken to avoid injury to the inferior mesenteric artery secondary to excessive traction. Ballon *et al.* (1981) have reported avulsion of the inferior mesenteric artery through this approach.

A right-sided incision is performed in a similar fashion, and will allow greater access to the right-sided aortocaval nodes, but difficult access to the left-sided aortic nodes since they lie lateral and posterior to the aorta. The left-sided incision does allow access to all nodal groups, although exposure of the aortocaval nodes is not optimal. In general, with both approaches the ipsilateral node dissection is excellent, but the contralateral exposure to paraaortic nodes may be compromised.

Extraperitoneal pelvic lymphadenectomy

Bilateral groin incisions

Groin incisions are used exclusively for pelvic lymph node dissection. Paraaortic node exposure is possible only if the incisions are extended significantly, usually requiring the conversion of the left incision into a modified J-type incision. Bilateral incisions are made parallel to the inguinal ligament and 3 cm above the ligament. The fascia is transected, and the internal and transversalis muscles are divided, and then bluntly dissected away from the peritoneum. The peritoneum is then mobilized medially, exposing the round ligament, which is transected, as well as the inferior epigastric vessels. Further mobilization of the peritoneum reveals the pelvic vessels, and the node dissection is then started after adequate exposure is obtained with retractors.

OIPE incision (one incision pararectal extraperitoneal)

The OIPE incision was originally described by Kelami (1980), and is similar to an extended Maylard incision. The incision extends in a horizontal, semilunar fashion from left anterior iliac spine to the right anterior iliac spine. The incision is placed 3 cm above the symphysis and 2 cm above the inguinal ligament. The rectus abdominus muscles are initially transected, followed by the external, transverse, and internal abdominus muscles in a lateral direction. The peritoneum is now visible, and in order to reflect it superiorly and medially, the inferior epigastric artery and vein, the round ligament, and the obliterated hypogastric artery are clamped and ligated.

After complete reflection of the peritoneum, the entire pelvic sidewall is exposed, and the lymph node dissection to the common iliac, external and internal iliac vessels is accomplished easily. The main disadvantage to this procedure is limited access to the paraortic nodes.

Extraperitoneal paraaortic lymphadenectomy

Sunrise incision

Gallup *et al.* (1991) described the use of this incision for paraaortic lymphadenectomy in the staging of cervical cancer as a new approach to prevent delays in beginning radiation therapy. This approach provides good exposure to the aortocaval nodes, but poor exposure to the pelvis, and requires caudad extension of the incision for pelvic lymph node dissection. The incision is made 6 cm above the umbilicus in the center, and is extended laterally and downward towards the iliac crests on both sides. If necessary, the incision can be extended parallel to the inguinal ligament for evaluation of the pelvic nodes.

Upper abdominal vertical incision

Schellhas (1975) proposed this incision as a method of sampling paraaortic nodes in patients with cervical cancer to avoid gastrointestinal complications with the transperitoneal approach. An incision is made approximately 7.5 cm in length at the midpoint of the rectus muscle on the right side beginning at the level of the umbilicus. This incision allows better exposure to the left paraaortic nodes than does the right-sided J-incision. Pelvic nodes are difficult to remove with the vertical incision, although extension caudad will allow better access to this area.

Laparascopic Pelvic and Paraaortic Lymphadenectomy

The use of the laparoscope in gynecologic oncology is relatively new. Over the past five years, laparoscopic procedures in benign gynecology have become part of the repertoire of many surgeons, including such procedures as tubal ligation, ovarian cystectomy, salpingectomy and salpingostomy for ectopic gestation, and salpingoophorectomy and hysterectomy as well. General surgeons are now routinely performing laparoscopic cholecystectomy and appendectomy, as well as numerous other pulmonary, chest, and abdominal procedures. Gynecologic oncologists are now beginning to use the laparoscope to perform pelvic and paraaortic lymphadenectomy for a variety of indications. Controversy exists, however, as to whether these procedures are safe in the hands of inexperienced laparoscopists, whether they are truly indicated in some instances, whether they are more often node sampling rather than lymphadenectomy *per se,* and also whether they do present a cost/benefit advantage.

Technique

All patients should have a thorough bowel preparation before the procedure. This allows maximal decompression of the bowel for easier packing into the upper abdomen and greater exposure. A clear liquid diet several days before the procedure along with either magnesium citrate or GoLYTLEY as an osmotic bowel agent will give adequate preparation. A Fleet enema can be given before the procedure as well to fully evacuate the rectum and sigmoid.

In the operating room, one or both arms should be tucked to the side of the patient to allow easier access by the surgeon. General anesthesia is used, and the patient is placed either supine for procedures limited to lymphadenectomy alone, or in dorsal lithotomy position if vaginal hysterectomy is to follow. Standard equipment for laparoscopy is used.

After a pneumoperitoneum has been established, four ports are placed into the abdomen. If there is no previous incision, or if a previous incision does not extend to the umbilicus, a 10 mm trochar and sleeve is placed through the umbilicus for the camera. If a previous incision is present through the umbilicus, a 5 mm trochar can be placed in the left upper quadrant 2 cm below the costal margin in the midclavicular line. A 5 mm laparoscope can then be used through this trochar to assess the abdominal cavity. An umbilical port can then be placed for the camera, or the left upper quadrant port can be used. Additional ports are placed on either side halfway between the umbilicus and anterior superior iliac spine. If a surgical stapling device is to be used 12 mm ports can be placed, otherwise standard 5 mm ports can be placed. The fourth port is placed in the midline above the symphysis.

The first step is to assess the abdomen and pelvis. A systematic, organized approach should be used starting in the pelvis and moving from the right side of the abdomen to the left, with complete visualization of all structures, including the diaphragm and gutters. Washings are taken as indicated.

Pelvic lymphadenectomy is performed by the surgeon on the opposite side. Using the lateral port on that side and the lower midline port, the peritoneum over the external iliac artery is incised. If a laparoscopically-assisted vaginal hysterectomy is to be performed, the round ligament can be incised and the peritoneum opened. The external and internal iliac artery and vein are identified, as well as the genitofemoral nerve. The adventitia overlying the external iliac artery near the bifurcation is grasped and incised up to the circumflex iliac vein. The nodal dissection then proceeds with the monopolar cautery scissors, using coagulation for small blood vessels. Visualization with the laparoscope is excellent, and careful dissection using cautery when needed results in a clean dissection. After the entire bundle of lymphatic tissue is removed from the artery and psoas muscle, a clip or coagulation can be used before amputating the bundle. The lymph nodes are then removed from the abdomen using spoon forceps.

Dissection of the internal iliac nodes begins with sharp and blunt dissection of the adventitial tissue from the external iliac vein over the entire length of this vessel. Coagulation is used as needed for small vessels. This frees the nodal bundle from its superior attachment. The obturator nerve is then identified, and nodal tissue cleaned from the nerve using sharp and blunt dissection. The attachment of the nodal bundle to the pelvic wall is then dissected free using cautery. The final point of attachment of the nodal bundle to the internal iliac artery is dissected free using blunt and sharp dissection with cautery, and the tissue is then removed from the operative field.

Paraaortic lymphadenectomy can be performed on the right or left side of the aorta. The surgeon performs the procedure from the contralateral side. Dissection on the right side is begun by incising the peritoneum over the right common iliac artery and extending the incision over the aorta. The right ureter is identified and dissected free from the underlying areolar tissue. The assistant then retracts the ureter from the operative field by placing the grasper located in the right lateral port under the ureter and retracting laterally. In addition to moving the ureter out of the way, small bowel is also kept from the operative field. The surgeon then uses the left lateral port and midline port to perform the lymph node dissection. Using similar techniques described in the pelvic dissection, the adventitia overlying the aorta is grasped and incised. Lateral dissection is then performed to expose the vena cavae, using cautery as needed for small blood vessels. Surgical clips can also be used as indicated, especially for perforating vessels from the vena cava and aorta. The caudad end of the nodal bundle is transected, and the bundle is then elevated with continued dissection laterally in a cephalad direction. The cephalad end is then transected when indicated, and the nodal tissue removed from the operative field. Left-sided dissection is performed in a similar fashion, with care taken to avoid injury to the inferior mesenteric artery and left ureter. Exposure may be more difficult on the left side since the nodes lie lateral and posterior to the aorta. After all dissections have been completed, the operative field is thoroughly irrigated and inspected for hemostasis.

Excellent detailed descriptions of laparoscopic nodal dissection can be found in several articles and reviews by the authors referenced above, including a more recent review of paraaortic lymphadenectomy by Childers *et al.* (1993).

Inguinal Lymphadenectomy

Technique

Inguinal lymphadenectomy is performed with the classic *en bloc* radical vulvectomy, or through separate incisions in the modified technique. The modified approach makes use of three incisions, one for groin dissection on each side, and a separate vulvectomy incision. This approach is currently favored, since primary wound healing is greatly improved, thereby reducing breakdown of the incision and reducing both morbidity and time in the hospital. Hacker *et al.* (1981) evaluated this technique, and found that none of the patients treated this way had recurrence of disease to the skin bridge above the symphysis, and wound breakdown was reduced from 40–80% in the *en bloc* approach to 14% with the three-incision approach. Lymphedema is a major complication, regardless of which approach is used. This is especially true if the nodes below the cribriform fascia are removed.

The patient is placed on the operating room table in the modified dorsal lithotomy position using Allen stirrups. The hips are abducted 30 degrees and extended 10 degrees, while the knees are flexed 90 degrees. This allows good access to the groin area and the perineum. The incision is made 2 cm below and parallel to the inguinal ligament, extending from the medial border of the Sartorius muscle to the lateral border of the adductor longus muscle (*Figure 39.8*). Some prefer to extend the incision from the anterior superior iliac spine to 4 cm lateral to the pubic tubercle.

The incision is then carried down to Camper's fascia. The superficial node dissection includes removal of all lymphatic and fatty tissue between Camper's fascia and the cribriform fascia. This fascial plane is easily identified by dissecting bluntly below the inguinal ligament near the saphenous opening. Note that the cribriform fascia is contiguous with the fascia lata. The term cribriform refers to holes in the fascia, namely the saphenous opening, through which vessels travel.

Dissection of all fatty and lymphatic tissue between Camper's fascia and the cribriform fascia is performed from the following points: superiorly from 2 cm above the inguinal ligament to a point inferiorly 2 cm above the adductor or Hunter's canal. Hunter's canal is the aponeurotic space in the middle third of the thigh that contains the femoral artery and vein. The lateral point of dissection is the medial edge of the sartorius muscle and the medial border is the fascia overlying the adductor longus muscle. Vessels are ligated and cauterized as needed during the dissection. The mobilized fat pad containing the superficial inguinal nodes is now turned medially, and the saphenous vein can be identified at the lower end of the incision. This vessel is ligated at this point, and then traced upward to the saphenofemoral junction where it is again clamped and ligated, thereby freeing the nodal bundle.

If a femoral node dissection is to be performed, the femoral triangle is identified, and the fascia lata overlying the femoral vessels is incised longitudinally. The perivascular sheath surrounding the vessels is opened, and fatty tissue medial to femoral vein containing the lymph nodes if removed. Note that only 2–3 nodes are present in this area.

Superficial inguinal and deep femoral node dissection is now complete. Transposition of the sartorius muscle is often used to protect the vessels. A closed suction drain is placed in the groin, the incision is closed in layers, and bed rest is maintained for four days after the procedure.

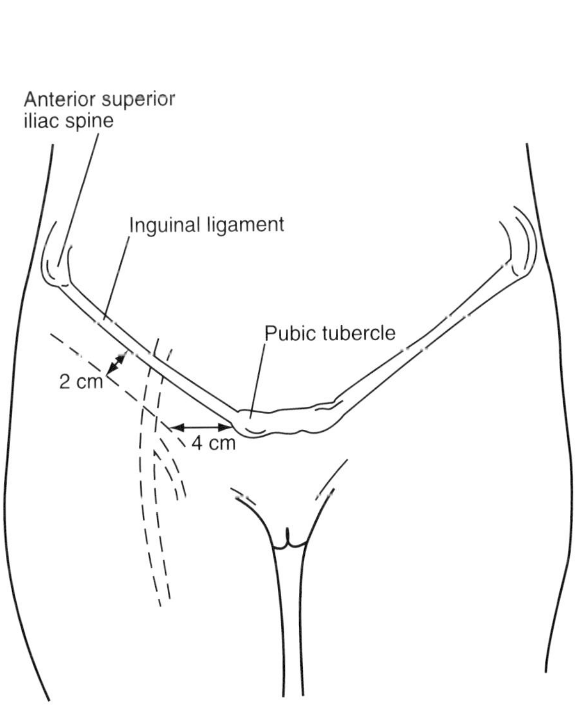

Figure 39.8. Inguinal node dissection. The groin incision is placed 4 cm lateral to the pubic tubercle and 2 cm below the inguinal ligmanent. (Permission from Gallup GD & Talledo OE (1994a).)

Scalene Node Dissection

Anatomy

The supraclavicular triangle is a division of the posterior triangle of the neck. The muscular and bony boundaries of the triangle include the sternocleidomastoid muscle anteriorly, and omohyoid muscle posteriorly, and the clavicle as the base of the triangle. The vascular boundaries include the internal jugular vein anteriorly behind the sternocleidomastoid, and the subclavian vein behind the clavicle. The phrenic nerve is located on the floor of the triangle on top of the scalenus anterior muscle, and the thoracic duct which overlies the phrenic nerve at the anterior base of the triangle, between the internal jugular and subclavian veins. The left scalene area is dissected since the thoracic duct empties into the left innominate vein, and is in close association with the scalene nodes on this side of the neck. Approximately 8–10 scalene nodes are located in the fat pad overlying the scalenus anterior muscle. The transverse cervical artery courses across the scalenus anterior muscle, and can be ligated if necessary without complications.

Technique

The technique of scalene node biopsy presented here is a modification of that reported by Ashbaugh

(1969). The patient is placed on the operating room table in the supine position with the head turned to the right side to expose the left supraclavicular triangle. The neck is supported, and then prepped. An incision is made 2–3 cm above the middle third of the clavicle, at the anterior border of the clavicular head of the sternocleidomastoid muscle, and extended laterally for 5 cm (*Figure 39.9*). The incision extends down through the skin and fascia, transecting the platysma muscle to expose the supraclavicular triangle. The sternocleidomastoid muscle and external jugular vein are seen initially. With retraction of the sternocleidomastoid and the skin and fascia superiorly, the internal jugular vein and omohyoid muscle come into view. The fat pad lying between the clavicle, sternocleidomastoid muscle and omohyoid contains the scalene lymph nodes.

The fat pad is then mobilized and transected near the clavicle. Elevating the fat pad superiorly, the lymph nodes and fat are then dissected bluntly from the fascia of the scalenus anterior muscle. Very careful attention must be taken to avoid injury to the phrenic nerve and thoracic duct, both of which lie over the scalenus anterior muscle beneath the fascia of this muscle. After the dissection is complete, a drain can be placed, and the muscle and skin closed.

Anatomic Abnormalities of the Retroperitoneum

Abnormalities encountered during lymphadenectomy are usually limited to the vascular and urinary systems. Vascular anomalies are much more frequent, and are present throughout the vascular system of the retroperitoneum. An excellent review of anomalies of the vascular and urinary system in relation to retroperitoneal surgery is presented by

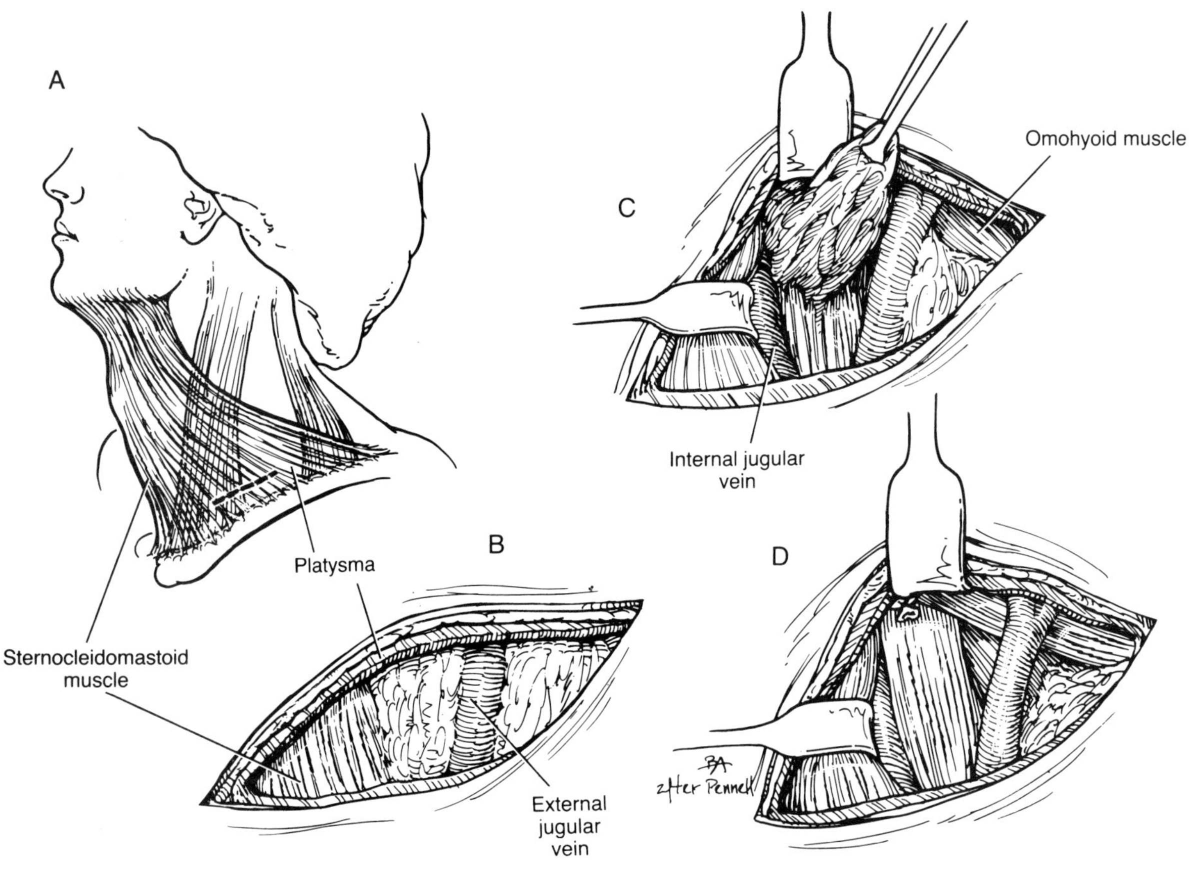

Figure 39.9. Scalene node dissection. **A.** The initial incision is made 2 cm above the clavicle at the middle third and extended anterior to posterior for 5 cm. **B.** The platysma muscle and fascia are transected revealing the sternocleidomastoid muscle and the external jugular vein. **C.** Retraction of the sternocleidomastoid muscle reveals the internal jugular vein. The scalene lymph nodes are bordered by the clavicle, the internal jugular vein and sternocleidomastoid, and by the omohyoid muscle. **D.** After the nodes are removed, the scalenus anterior muscle can be seen. The phrenic nerve and thoracic duct lie under the fascia of this muscle, and must be identified during dissection to avoid injury. (Permission from Gallup GD & Talledo OE (1994b).)

Panici *et al.* (1994). Clinically significant abnormal findings to the large vessels of the abdomen and pelvis and the urinary system as related to lymphadenectomy are listed below. A thorough knowledge of the most common of these anomalies will allow easier identification and help avoid damage to the vascular and urinary systems during lymphadenectomy, thereby decreasing hemorrhage and morbidity.

Vascular Anomalies

Renal artery

Accessory renal arteries occur in about 20% of patients, and are usually more common on the left side (Anson *et al.*, 1942). These vessels often arise directly from the aorta, and may also derive from the common iliac and internal iliac vessels. During dissection of the aortocaval nodes near the renal vessels, close attention is necessary to define accessory arteries extending toward the renal artery from the aorta to avoid injury and hemorrhage.

Renal vein

A second retroaortic renal vein on the left side has been described in the literature (Reis and Esenther, 1959). Normally, a single renal vein extending from the vena cava and crossing over the aorta drains the left kidney. Note that the left ovarian vein can join either limb. Anomalies of the right renal venous system are more common than the left. Multiple right renal veins have been described, as well as independent renal veins draining the pole of the right kidney to the vena cava.

Ovarian artery and vein

Multiple anomalies of the ovarian artery have been described, including double arteries, arteries originating from the renal artery on the left or right side instead of the aorta, and ovarian arteries from anomalous vessels.

The right ovarian vein has been described emptying into the vena cava above the renal vein and also into the right renal vein itself. The left ovarian vein may join the second lumbar vein or the lumbar vein and the left ovarian vein can enter the renal vein together.

Vena cava

Complete inversion of the vena cava and aorta has been reported, with the vena cava on the left and the aorta on the right side, usually associated with inversion of the abdominal and thoracic organs. Other anomalies in the length, caliber, and number of vessels are also possible.

Iliac vessels

Common iliac anomalies are unusual. Absence of the common iliac trunk as well as anomalies in the take-off points of the internal iliac artery and veins are possible. The anatomy of the branching system of the internal iliac artery and vein is variable. The obturator artery is anomalous in as many as 30% of patients. Normally, this artery is the initial branch of the anterior division of the internal iliac artery, but may take its origin from the deep epigastric artery or, in some cases, the external iliac artery, and pass downward across the brim of the pelvis to the obturator foramen. An anomalous obturator vein may also enter the external iliac vein as well, and must be identified and ligated during lymphadenectomy.

Urinary Anomalies

Urinary anomalies are less frequent than vascular, and are limited to duplication of the ureter, with unilateral duplication occurring more frequently, and kidney malformations. The most frequently diagnosed kidney anomaly is horseshoe kidney, and is found in 0.25% of the population. Ectopic kidneys are found more frequently than other anomalies such as supernumerary kidneys, unilateral agenesia, and anomalies of rotation, form, and fusion (Perlmutter *et al.*, 1986).

Complications of Lymphadenectomy

The most common intraoperative injuries during pelvic and aortocaval lymphadenectomy are those to the vascular system. Injury to the genitofemoral and obturator nerves, the urinary system, or to the gastrointestinal system are much less common. Common sites of injury to the large vessels of the pelvis and abdomen have been described previously in the sections on pelvic and paraaortic lymphadenectomy, and are summarized here. The surgical management of injuries to the aortocaval area and a brief review of postoperative complications is also presented.

Vascular Injuries

In general, the injury of thin-walled veins in the pelvis and abdomen is much more common than to the thick-walled arteries, and the repair of venous injuries is more difficult. Adequate exposure and a thorough knowledge of vascular anatomy, both normal and abnormal, is the best method to avoid injury.

Management

The majority of vascular injuries occurring during operative procedures in close proximity to the inferior vena cava (IVC) and aorta are limited injuries such as division of a small aortic or caval branch, or a small injury to one of the major vessels during close dissection. The majority of these injuries can be handled expeditiously with good exposure and assistance. Small injuries to veins can be managed initially with pressure hemostasis, remembering that the venous system is a low pressure system and does not require a great deal of external pressure to occlude the vessel. If bleeding does not stop, hemostatic clips may be used to repair the injury, or fine suture may be necessary. The primary goal, however, must be to avoid exacerbation of a minor injury by attempting a hasty repair without adequate exposure. Blind clamping or stitching of vessels should always be avoided. These 'minor' injuries can bleed quite profusely and secure control of the hemorrhage is the first priority, followed by assessment of the exposure and level of assistance available, and finally, controlled repair of the injury.

Control of hemorrhage

When an injury to the aorta or IVC occurs, the surgeon must obviously first control the hemorrhage. Digital pressure or packing with laparotomy pads may adequately stem the blood flow from the injury site. One or two sponge sticks can be gently placed on the IVC proximal and distal to the injury to control bleeding and allow good visualization for repair. Occasionally, these maneuvers will not control the hemorrhage, usually due to persistent lumbar branches near the injury site. In this situation, the arteriotomy or venotomy may be controlled by placing the curve of a Satinsky or Cooley–Derra vascular clamp around the injured site if the area can be adequately visualized (Blaisdell and Trunkey, 1982).

Also, inflatable Fogarty balloon occlusion catheters may be helpful in severe injuries that are difficult to control. These are inserted through the injury site into the vessel lumen and passed proximal and distal to the injury where they are inflated, isolating the injury site from blood flow. The sutures to repair the injury may be placed in a bloodless field and the balloons deflated and removed before the last few sutures are tied down, closing the injury. Foley catheters with 5 ml balloons may be used with good results if these specialized catheters are not available. Blind clamping of vessels should be avoided as this frequently worsens the situation by injuring the vessel at another site.

Before attempting repair of the injury, the surgeon must assess the adequacy of the exposure, and should not hesitate to increase the length of the incision to allow optimal access. Further retroperitoneal dissection, including mobilization of the colon or duodenum may be necessary to expose the injured area for adequate vessel control. Self-retaining retractors or additional assistants should be used as needed to allow the surgeon and first assistant to be completely free of retracting or exposing duties during the repair. If the patient has lost a large volume of blood leading to hypotension or hemodynamic instability, pressure should be maintained on the injury to allow the anesthesiologist to resuscitate the patient before proceeding with repair, which may result in further blood loss.

Once the surgeon is prepared to repair the injury, the pressure on the site should be released with suction available. The site and type of injury should be noted if possible. Injuries to the IVC can often be controlled for repair using sponge sticks as described above. If the injury is to a branch of the aorta or IVC, this can often be controlled under direct vision with a right angle clamp and sutured. Small injuries to the wall of the aorta or IVC should be sutured using interrupted or continuous permanent monofilament sutures. This can usually be done without placing clamps on the vessel or encircling it. It is best to avoid encircling the aorta or IVC as this requires posterior dissection, which may result in injury to the lumbar vessels or other posterior branches. If the injury is larger, control of the vessel with a curved vascular clamp (Satinsky or Cooley–Derra) or with balloon occlusion catheters will allow a more involved repair. If this is not possible, two straight vascular clamps may be placed across the aorta vertically in the anterior to posterior direction without dissecting behind these vessels for control. This is usually effective, but carries some risk of avulsion of a posterior lumbar branch. Vascular clamps are rarely needed to control the IVC and may cause tears to the vessel, so they should be avoided if possible.

Posterior injuries or branch avulsions are very challenging to repair as they require mobilization of the vessel and rotation to visualize the posterior wall of the IVC or aorta. The assistance of an experienced vascular surgeon should be obtained if possible.

All repairs should be performed with permanent monofilament suture. For IVC injuries, we prefer to use 4-0 Prolene with felt or Teflon pledglets in an interrupted horizontal mattress. The thin wall of the IVC may tear easily, particularly if sutured under tension. Tension should therefore be removed from the area as described above, and pledglets may be used to prevent the thin monofilament suture from tearing the IVC wall. One may use a continuous suture without pledglets with good results, however. Aortic repairs require a stronger suture such as 2-0 or 3-0 Prolene due to the higher pressures and frequent presence of plaque in the aortic wall. Pledglets may be used in aortic repairs if the aorta is particularly artherosclerotic. There are really no disadvantages to using pledglets other than the time needed to place them on each stitch. When repairing the IVC, the surgeon should attempt to evert the intima to avoid exposing the lumen to a thrombogenic surface such as the adventitia.

After completing the repair, the area should be examined for continued bleeding. Extravasation through suture holes can usually be controlled with Surgical or Gelfoam and several minutes of gentle compression unless a coagulopathy is present. Heparin need not be given unless a complex venous repair or prolonged vessel occlusion is required. After completing the node dissection, the area around the repair should be carefully covered with retroperitoneal tissue to reduce the potential for adhesion or fistula development between the repair site and the duodenum or small bowel.

Nerve Injuries

Genitofemoral nerve

This nerve arises from the anterior branches of the first and second lumbar nerves, and passes over the psoas muscle underneath the peritoneum. The nerve divides into femoral and genital branches at varying levels, sometimes with both divisions being visible overlying the psoas. The genital branch enters the inguinal canal through the deep ring and supplies the cremaster and labium majus. The femoral branch enters the femoral sheath, supplying the skin of the femoral triangle and a portion of the anterior medial thigh. Transection of the nerve does not require repair, and results in loss of sensation or paresthesia to the skin over the medial aspect of the thigh.

Obturator nerve

The obturator nerve originates from L2–L4, and emerges from the medial side of the psoas to enter the thigh through the obturator foramen. This nerve supplies the adductor muscles, gracilis, skin of the medial side of the thigh, and the hip and knee joints. The obturator nerve lies in extraperitoneal fat and can be injured during removal of the obturator nodes. Transection or injury will result in loss of adduction of the thigh on the ipsilateral side, with some sensory loss to the skin on the medial side of the thigh. Repair should be attempted, but is not mandatory since a significant number of patients will regain adductor function with physical therapy and time.

Postoperative Complications

Lymphocyst formation after pelvic node dissection

Lymphocysts are collections of retroperitoneal fluid occurring mostly in the pelvis at the site of pelvic lymphadenectomy. True lymphocysts of the para-aortic area are unusual, with only a few cases reported in the literature (Helmkamp *et al.*, 1980). A specific case for lymphocyst formation has not been described, but several risk factors have been proposed. Extensive lymphadenectomy is the cause most often reported. Theoretically, extensive removal of lymph nodes and obstruction of the lymphatic system will result in significant leakage of lymph fluid in the area of dissection, with a greater incidence of lymphocyst formation. Radiation therapy before pelvic node dissection is also thought to be a cause (McDonald *et al.*, 1983).

Management of lymphocysts depends on the size. Small cysts do not cause symptoms, and do not usually require treatment. Larger lymphocysts cause symptoms due to compression of adjacent structures, such as the ureter, bowel, bladder or pelvic veins. Patients generally present 2–3 weeks after the surgery with abdominal pain, constipation or urinary frequency. Rarely, compression of the ureter can cause hydronephrosis and back pain, as well as pyelonephritis. Pelvic vein compression may cause deep venous thrombosis and lower extremity edema, but this is very unusual. Computed tomography or ultrasound are used to diagnose lymphocysts, and percutaneous drainage is the primary form of therapy, allowing continuous drainage of the lymphocyst over a period of time. Larger cysts require longer drainage times, often beyond the normal requirement of 2–3 weeks, and catheters can eventually be removed with decreasing drainage. If percutaneous drainage fails, sclerosis of the cyst using tetracycline can be performed (Mann *et al.*, 1986), or the anterior wall of the cyst can be surgically removed to allow drainage of the lymph fluid into the peritoneal cavity.

Lymphocyst formation can probably be prevented to a large extent by not reapproximating the peritoneum after lymph node dissection, and employing good surgical techniques during the procedure. The use of closed suction drains does not prevent lymphocyst formation, and should probably not be used (Ilancheran and Monaghan, 1988).

Seroma formation after groin dissection

Seromas can develop in up to 20% of patients undergoing inguinal lymphadenectomy, and form due to blockage of lymphatic channels and the development of dead space under the skin after the procedure. The use of suction drains after groin dissection for 5–7 days until drainage has stopped decreases the formation of seromas. External pressure to the groins in the form of sandbags or pressure dressings postoperatively is not recommended since this may interrupt blood supply to the skin edges, causing necrosis. If seromas do form, needle aspiration is used as needed under sterile conditions.

Lymphedema

Edema of the lower extremity is common after groin dissection, and less frequent after pelvic node dissection. Acute lymphedema occurs more commonly than chronic edema, and is also related to the extensiveness of the node dissection. The incidence of lymphedema is higher if groin irradiation follows groin dissection. Most cases are mild and limited and can be managed with bed rest, the use of stockings or pneumatic compression devices, elevation of the leg, and treatment of cellulitis with antibiotics. Surgical therapy has not been successful.

Summary of Management Options

- Lymphadenectomy in gynecologic malignancy is a complex procedure that involves the selective or systematic removal of lymph nodes to the pelvic, paraaortic, inguinal, or scalene areas.
- Lymphadenectomy is accomplished through either a transperitoneal or extraperitoneal approach.
- Laparoscopic pelvic and paraaortic lymphadenectomy is now being used more frequently for endometrial and cervical cancer, as well as for early-stage ovarian cancer.
- A clear understanding of anatomic abnormalities associated with the retroperitoneal space simplifies lymphadenectomy and decreases morbidity.
- The most common complications of lymphadenectomy are vascular or nerve injuries.
- Injuries to the vascular system during lymphadenectomy require a systematic approach to repair. After hemorrhage has been controlled, adequate exposure is developed, additional assistance is called for if needed, and surgical repair is then performed.

References

Anson BJ, Pick JW & Cauldwell EW (1942) The anatomy of commoner renal anomalies, ectopic and horseshoe kidneys. *J. Urol.* **47:** 112.

■ Ashbaugh DG (1969) Scalene node lymph node biopsy. *Surg. Clin. North Amer.* **49(6):** 1385–1389.

Ballon SC, Berman ML, Lagasse LD *et al.* (1981) Survival after paraaortic lymphadenectomy and radiation therapy in cervical cancer. *Obstet. Gynecol.* **57:** 90.

Benedetti–Panici P, Maneschi F, Scambia G *et al.* (1994) A new transabdominal approach to the left retroperitoneum for systematic removal of lymph nodes left of the aorta in gynecologic malignancies. *Obstet. Gynecol.* **83:** 1060–1064.

Bergman ML, Lagasse LD & Atring WG (1977) The operative evaluation of patients with cervical carinoma by an extraperitoneal approach. *Obstet. Gynecol.* **50:** 659.

■ Blaisdell FW & Trunkey DD (1982) *Abdominal Trauma,* pp. 270–274. New York: Thieme–Stratton.

■ Childers JM, Hatch KD & Tran AN (1993) Laparoscopic paraaortic lymphadenectomy in gynecologic malignancies. *Obstet. Gynecol.* **82:** 741–747.

Gallup DG, Jordan GH & Talledo OE (1986) Extraperitoneal lymph node dissections with use of a midline incision in patients with female genital cancer. *Am. J. Obstet. Gynecol.* **155:** 559–564.

Gallup DG, King LA, Messing MJ *et al.* (1991) Paraaortic lymph node sampling using an extraperitoneal approach with a supraumbilical transverse "sunrise" incision. Abstract at the Twentieth Annual Meeting Society of Pelvic Surgeons, Scotsdale, AZ.

Gallup DG & Talledo OE (1994a) *Surgical Atlas of Gynecologic Oncology,* p. 127. Philadelphia: WB Saunders.

Gallup DG & Talledo PE (1994b) *Surgical Atlas of Gynecologic Oncology,* p. 228. Philadelphia: WB Saunders.

Gao Y (1992) Pelvic lymphadenectomy with stripping technique in 43 cases. *Chin. Med. J.* **105(3):** 251–255.

Gershenson DM, DeCherney AH & Curry SL (1993a) *Operative Gynecology,* p. 175. Philadelphia: WB Saunders.

Gershenson DM, DeCherney AH & Curry SL (1993b) *Operative Gynecology,* p. 384. Philadelphia: WB Saunders.

Gershenson DM, DeCherney AH & Curry SL (1993c) *Operative Gynecology,* p. 385. Philadelphia: WB Saunders.

Hacker NF, Leuchter RS, Berek JS *et al.* (1981) Radical vulvectomy and bilateral inguinal lymphadenectomy through separate groin incisions. *Obstet. Gynecol.* **58:** 574.

Helmkamp BF, Krebs HB, Jsikoff MB *et al.* (1980) Para-aortic lymphocyst. *Am. J. Obstet. Gynecol.* **138:** 395.

Ilancheran A & Monaghan JM (1988) Pelvic lymphocyst, a 10 year experience. *Gynecol. Oncol.* **29:** 333.

Kelami A (1980) One incision, pararectal, extraperitoneal (OIPE) approach for bilateral procedures on lower two thirds of ureters. *Urology* **15:** 296–297.

Lee RA (1992a) *Atlas of Gynecologic Surgery,* p. 783. Philadelphia: WB Saunders.

Lee RA (1992b) *Atlas of Gynecologic Surgery,* p. 184. Philadelphia: WB Saunders.

■ Lubicz S (1985) Approach to the abdominal retroperitoneum in patients with gynecologic malignancies. *Gynecol. Oncol.* **22:** 32–39.

Mann WJ, Vogel F, Pastner B & Chalas E (1986)

Management of lymphocysts after radical gynecologic surgery. *Gynecol. Oncol.* **24:** 309.
McDonald TW, Morley GW, Choo YC *et al.* (1983) Fine needle aspiration of paraaortic and pelvic lymph nodes showing lymphographic abnormalities. *Obstet. Gynecol.* **61:** 383.
Panici PB, Maneschi F, Scambia G *et al.* (1994) Anatomic abnormalities of the retroperitoneum encountered during aortic and pelvic lymphadenectomy. *Am. J. Obstet. Gynecol.* **170:** 111–116.
Panici PB, Scambia G, Baiocchi G *et al.* (1992) Anatomical study of para-aortic and pelvic lymph nodes in gynecologic malignancy. *Obstet. Gynecol.* **79:** 498–502.
Perlmutter AD, Retik AB & Bauer SB (1986) Anomalies of the upper urinary tract. *Campbells Urology,* 5th ed., pp 1665–1725 Philadelphia: WB Saunders.
■ Plentl AA & Friedman EA (1971) *Lymphatic System of the Female Genitalia,* pp. 170–173. Philadelphia: WB Saunders.
Reis RH & Esenther G (1959) Variation in the pattern of renal vessels and their relation to the type of posterior vena cava in man. *Am. J. Anat.* **104:** 295–317.
■ Schellhas HF 1975) Extraperitoneal paraaortic node dissection through an upper abdominal incision. *Obstet. Gynecol.* **46:** 444–447.
Woodburne RT (1983) *Essentials of Human Anatomy.* New York: Oxford University Press, pp. 508–509.

40 Pelvic Reconstructive Surgery

D L Doering
J R Bosscher
G R Tobin

Dedication

The authors dedicate this chapter to the memory of Thomas G Day Jr MD, our colleague and friend.

Introduction

Therapy of gynecologic malignancies often involves radical or ultraradical resection of the female reproductive organs and adjacent structures. Radiation therapy can also cause injury to these same structures. When this occurs, patients may experience anatomic disfigurement, resulting in loss of function and diminished self-image. Women with newly diagnosed gynecologic cancer already have significantly decreased sexual activity and satisfaction (Harris *et al.*, 1982). In addition, radical pelvic or genital surgery is known to be a prominent cause of sexual dysfunction (Schover and Fife, 1985). The prospect of disfiguring therapy and loss of normal sexual, urinary, or gastrointestinal function can adversely impact the quality of life of the gynecologic cancer patient.

As gynecologic oncologists seek to combine an enhanced quality of life with attainment of clinical cure, attention will be focused upon surgical reconstruction of those organs removed or damaged by therapy, and restoration of function whenever possible. This chapter will review the techniques of vaginal and vulvar reconstruction, urinary tract reconstruction and preservation of rectal function. Attention will be focused on new and innovative techniques that can restore or approximate normal anatomy and function.

Vaginal Reconstruction

Fortunately, vaginectomy is rarely necessary in the primary therapy of gynecologic malignancies. However, injury or destruction of normal vaginal anatomy and function may occur as a result of therapy for several gynecologic cancers. Most patients with vaginal cancer receive radiation therapy, and virtually all patients with cervical cancer beyond Stage IIA will receive whole pelvis irradiation. Women with early-stage cervical cancer who are not operative candidates are also treated with radiation. Radiotherapy causes fibrosis of the vaginal walls, with stenosis of the vault. Loss of elasticity and lubrication occur, and mucosal ulceration may also result. These changes can result in marked impairment of sexual function and diminished self esteem.

Pelvic exenteration requires ultraradical resection of the pelvic viscera. Unless reconstructive procedures are employed, these patients lose vaginal function, as well as bladder and/or rectal function. Even among exenteration patients who are asymptomatic and clinically free of disease, sexual functioning continues as the area of greatest disruption in their lives (Andersen and Hacker, 1983).

Anatomic considerations in the reconstruction of pelvic oncologic resections go beyond the repair or reconstruction of the specific organs excised. Exenterations and abdominoperineal resections leave large endopelvic dead spaces within rigid walls that increase the risk of postoperative infection and invite migration of intestines from the abdominal cavity with the associated complications of obstruction and fistulae. These extensive resections place the patient at unusually high risk for the development of wound infection and healing complications because of this endopelvic dead space in combination with the magnitude of the operations, the frequent history of previous radiation therapy, and the regional bacterial flora of the colon, vagina, and perineal skin.

The anatomic needs of reconstruction for radical pelvic surgery therefore require exceptionally large volumes of well-vascularized tissue. Flaps that are capable of meeting these reconstructive challenges have been developed only within the past few years with the definition of compound muscle–skin (musculocutaneous or myocutaneous) flaps provided by regional muscle pedicles that include large paddles of well-vascularized skin and subcutaneous tissue, principally the rectus abdominis (Tobin and Day Jr, 1988; Shepherd *et al.*, 1990) and gracilis (McCraw *et al.*, 1976) muscle–skin flaps.

Indications for vaginal reconstruction fall into two groups. The first group includes patients who require repair or reconstruction of only the vagina, without the need to fill spaces created by excision of adjacent structures. This group includes agenesis, vaginectomy, partial vaginectomy and repair of vaginal stenosis. These reconstructions can be satisfactorily addressed by a wide variety of described techniques that include skin grafts, large or small bowel segments, and regional skin flaps from the groin, lower abdomen, perineum and thigh.

The second group of indications for vaginal reconstruction also includes the need to fill endopelvic dead space left by resection of structures adjacent to the vagina. This group includes pelvic exenterations and abdominoperineal resections that include the vagina. Nearly all women who have pelvic exenterations or abdominoperineal resections with vaginal excision for pelvic carcinoma originating in the cervix, vagina, or rectum benefit from vaginal reconstruction with large muscle–skin flaps for wound management purposes. These flaps block the entry of bowel into the pelvis from the abdomen, revascularize irradiated pelvic cavity walls, and lessen the incidence of pelvic infection, fistulae, and chronically open perineal wounds, in addition to restoring sexual capacity. Reconstruction is best done at the time of tumor resection to obtain the benefits of bowel exclusion and wound revascularization.

The introduction of gracilis muscle–skin flap vaginal reconstructions in 1976 provided the first satisfactory technique of vaginal reconstruction for the exenteration patient and simultaneously initiated the modern era of muscle–skin flap reconstruction (McCraw *et al.*, 1976). Although this method of reconstruction substantially improved results compared to previous reconstructive methods, it does not completely block the entry of bowel into the pelvis; it is associated with a high incidence of partial paddle loss (McCraw *et al.*, 1976; Heath *et al.*, 1984) and its passage around the retained distal vagina in supralevator exenterations can be difficult. Because of these problems, we developed a vaginal reconstruction technique based on the rectus abdominis muscle–skin unit (Tobin and Day Jr, 1988) that is substantially free of the disadvantages associated with gracilis flaps. The rectus abdominis flap has become the preferred choice for vaginal reconstruction of defects created by radical pelvic surgery. The techniques of rectus abdominis, gracilis and other methods of vaginal reconstruction will be described below.

Rectus Abdominis Flap Vaginal Reconstruction

Rectus abdominis muscle–skin flaps are taken from the ventral abdominal wall and are supplied by the deep inferior epigastric vessels to the distally-based rectus abdominis muscle. The paired rectus abdominis muscles provide the ventral abdominal wall musculature and lie on either side of the linea alba. They originate on the most caudal ribs of the ventral thorax, and insert on the parasymphyseal region of the pubic bone. The anterior and posterior rectus sheath encase the upper two-thirds of the muscle, but the posterior rectus sheath is absent behind the distal muscle caudal to the linea arcuata. The upper muscle is supplied by the superior epigastric vessels, which are a continuation of the internal mammary vessels, and run on the deep surface of the muscle. The overlying epigastric skin is supplied by cutaneous perforators from the muscle, which pass through the anterior rectus sheath. The blood supply to the distal muscle is the deep inferior epigastric vessels, which originate from the external iliac vessels near the inguinal ligament and run on the deep surface of the muscle (*Figure 40.1*). The skin of the lower abdomen is supplied by cutaneous perforators from this vascular trunk, as well as the superficial inferior epigastric vessels, which run cephalad from the groin in the subcutaneous tissue. The deep inferior and superior epigastric vascular systems are joined by anastomotic vessels across a vascular watershed in the mid-portion of the muscle near the umbilicus, which allows vascular supply to the entire muscle from the source on either end. The muscle also receives a secondary vascular supply, whoch accompanies the motor nerves entering its lateral border in a segmental manner.

The optimal time for rectus abdominis vaginal reconstruction is at the time of the radical pelvic surgery. If the reconstruction is carried out later the benefits of bowel exclusion and wound healing to the first operation are lost and a dissection of the intestines in the pelvis is required to allow placement of the flap.

When reconstruction is performed during radical pelvic surgery, the flap is designed and elevated after removal of the pelvic organs. One must be sure that the inferior epigastric vascular pedicle was not divided during the current or previous pelvic resection. If this has happened, the contralateral rectus abdominis flap is used. If both inferior epigastric vessels have been divided, then another reconstruction technique is performed.

The cutaneous paddle is designed as a wide vertical ellipse centered over the upper one-half of the muscle, extending from the costal margin to just below the umbilicus and marked 12–15 cm wide (see *Figure 40.1*). Flaps of this width provide a neovagina of about 4 cm in diameter when inversely tubed. Following incision of the skin paddle, a corresponding island of the underlying anterior rectus sheath is incised. This fascial island can be made narrower than the overlying skin paddle to permit direct closure of the residual anterior rectus sheath. A strip of medial anterior rectus sheath adjacent to the linea alba and another strip of lateral anterior rectus sheath 3–4 cm adjacent to the external oblique aponeurosis are left *in situ* if direct closure of the fascial layer is intended (*Figure 40.2*).

The muscle is transected at the level of the costal margin near the apex of the skin paddle, and the superior epigastric vessels are divided. The skin

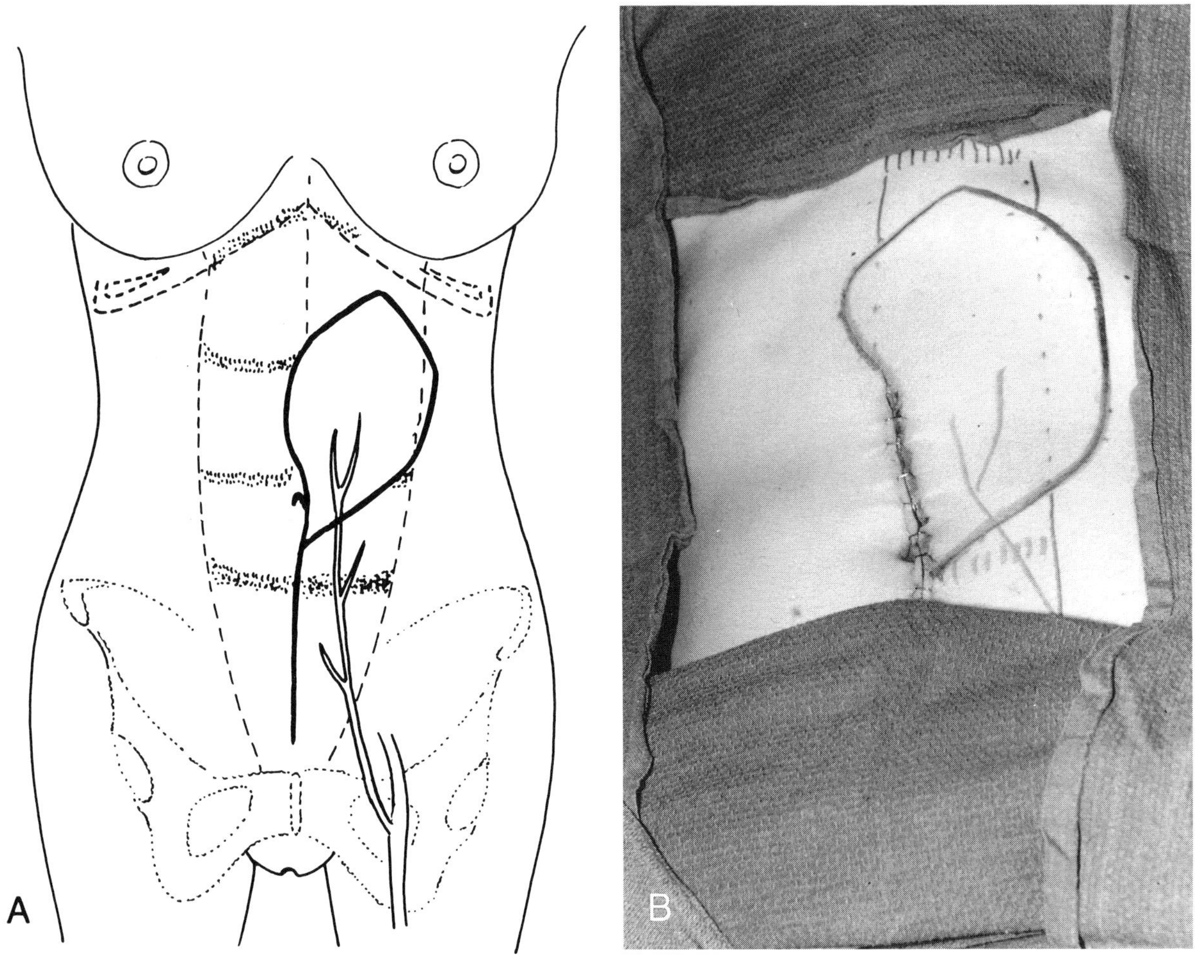

Figure 40.1. (**A**) Cutaneous paddle design of rectusabdominis flaps for vaginal and pelvic reconstruction showing the relationship of the paddle to the muscle, vascular pedicle, laparotomy incision and surface landmarks. (**B**) Marking of the paddle on a patient undergoing vaginal reconstruction at the time of pelvic exenteration. (From Tobin GR & Day TG (1988) Vaginal and pelvic reconstruction with distally based rectus abdominis myocutaneous flaps. *Plast. Reconstr. Surg.* **81:** 62–69, with permission.)

paddle and muscle pedicle are then elevated from the underlying posterior rectus fascia by sequential division of the segmental neurovascular pedicles that enter the lateral muscle border. This is continued only until the flap is sufficiently mobilized to reach the recipient site (see *Figure 40.2*). Distal to the skin paddle, the anterior rectus sheath is left *in situ* with the overlying hypogastric skin and subcutaneous tissue to provide abdominal wall structure following flap transfer.

Following elevation, the flap is transposed distally onto the groin region surface for formation of the vaginal pouch by inverse tubing of the skin paddle. This allows a second surgical team to construct the urinary conduit and colostomy while the vagina is simultaneously being formed. The vaginal pouch is formed by inversely tubing the skin paddle to place the skin on the inside. The lateral margins and distal apex are sutured to each other to form a blind pouch (*Figure 40.3*). The flap is then passed through the distal midline peritoneal incision into the pelvis behind the pubis, and the open end of the vaginal pouch is inset into the perineal defect to form a neo-introitus (*Figure 40.4*).

Following placement of the colostomy and urinary conduit stomas, the abdominal wall donor site is reconstructed and the abdomen closed. In the skin–fascial paddle donor site, the lateral and medial remnants of the anterior rectus sheath may be sutured together to provide a second layer of fascial closure over the posterior rectus sheath (*Figure 40.5*). Occasionally, the fascial margins cannot be approximated due to excess tension, and the distal anterior rectus sheath is simply inset into the posterior rectus sheath just above the linea arcuata. This method of fascial closure was performed in our initial experience with this flap (Tobin and Day Jr, 1988), and no fascial donor site hernias have occurred in

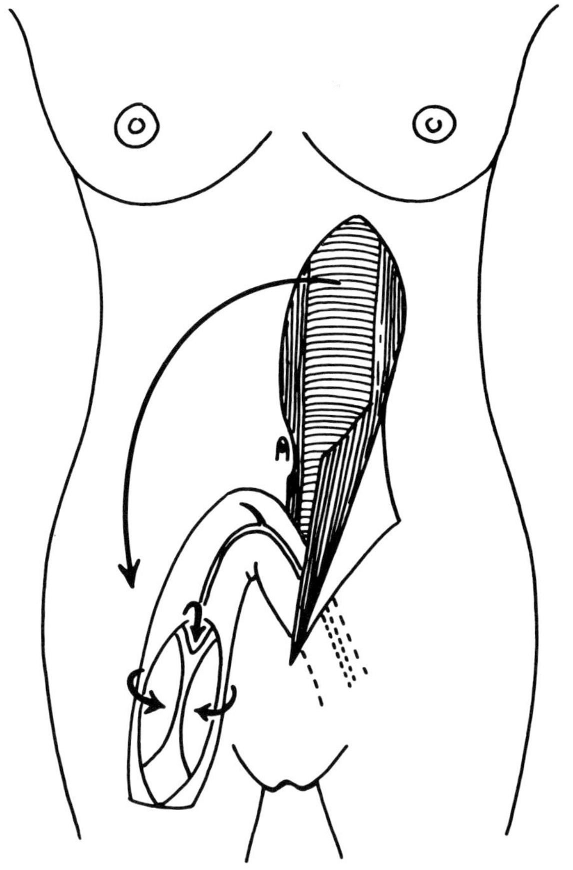

Figure 40.2. Transposition of the flap from the abdominal field to the groin surface for formation of the vaginal pouch, which allows simultaneous construction of the urinary conduit and colostomy. (From Tobin GR & Day TG (1988) Vaginal and pelvic reconstruction with distally based rectus abdominis myocutaneous flaps. *Plast. Reconstr. Surg.* **81:** 62–69, with permission.)

these patients to date. However, the theoretic potential for herniation led us to close the anterior rectus sheath when possible in recent years (Tobin *et al.*, 1990; Tobin, 1994).

Distal to the umbilicus, the midline anterior rectus sheath incision is closed by suturing it to the linea alba over the flap pedicle. The cutaneous paddle donor defect is closed directly in continuity with the laparotomy incision by direct approximation of the elliptical margins (*Figure 40.6*). Closed suction drains are used in both the donor and recipient sites. Stents or dilations of the neovagina are not required postoperatively (*Figure 40.7*).

Rectus abdominis flaps have now been used in radical pelvic surgery for ten years (Tobin and Day Jr, 1988; Tobin *et al.*, 1990; Tobin, 1994). Our experience with rectus abdominis vaginal reconstruction has been substantially more favorable than with previously used methods such as gracilis flaps. The advantages of the rectus abdominis reconstructions are numerous. First, obliteration of residual endopelvic space and exclusion of bowel created by the bulk of the rectus abdominis flap is far superior to that of any other flap. Rectus abdominis flaps are also far more reliable than gracilis flaps, which have a high incidence of partial paddle loss (McCraw *et al.*, 1976; Heath *et al.*, 1984). The gracilis flap has one of the highest incidences of flap loss and the rectus abdominis has one of the

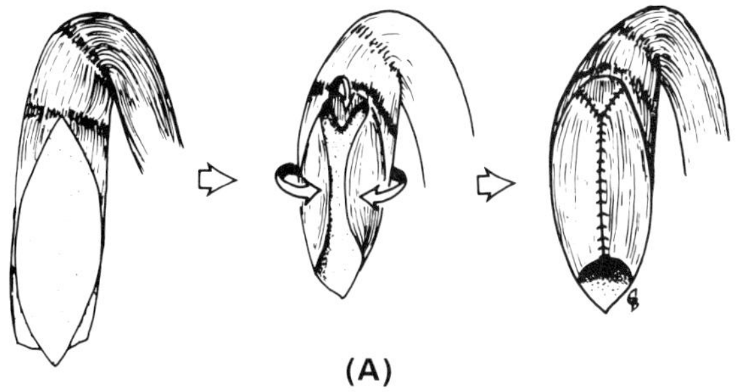

(A)

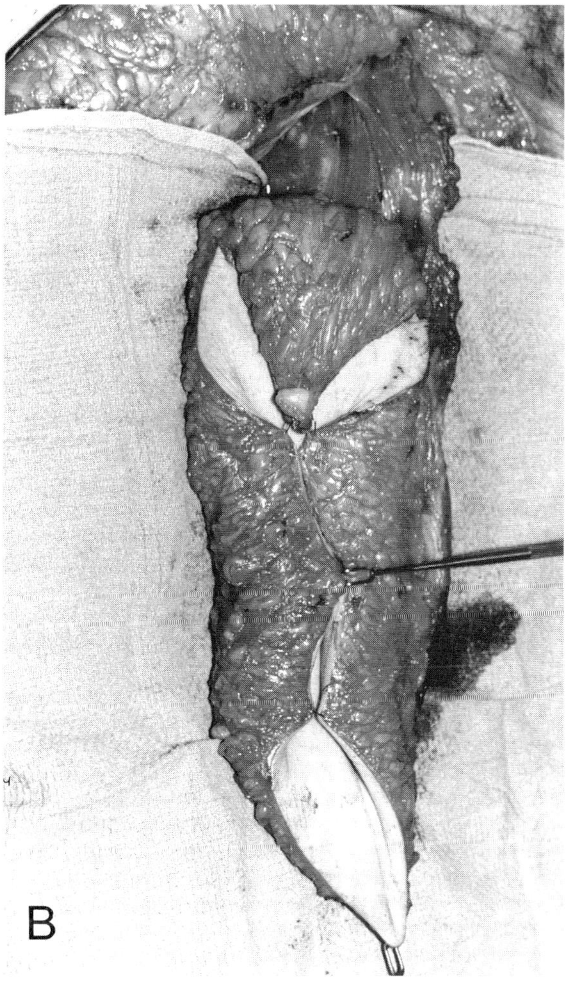

B

Figure 40.3. (**A**) The inverse tubing method of the skin paddle to create a vaginal pouch. Curved arrows indicate infolding. (**B**) Execution of this maneuver in a patient undergoing vaginal reconstruction. (From Tobin GR & Day TG (1988) Vaginal and pelvic reconstruction with distally based rectus abdominis flaps. *Plast. Reconstr. Surg.* **81:** 62–69, with permission.)

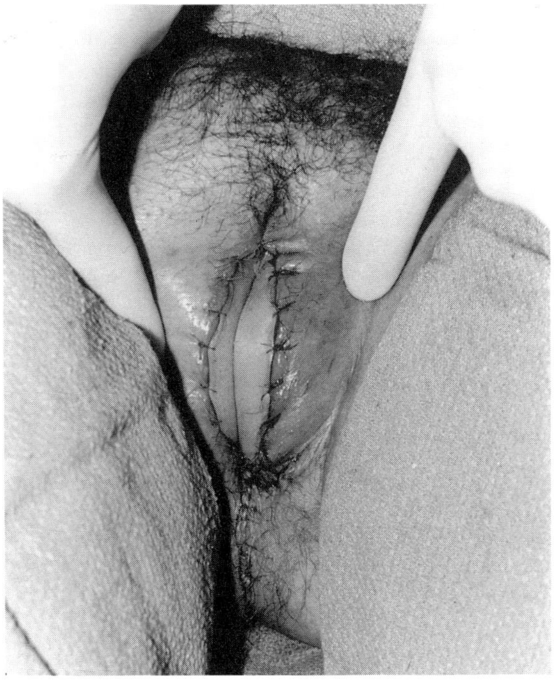

Figure 40.4. Inset of the reconstructed vaginal pouch in the perineal defect. (From Tobin GR & Day TG (1988) Vaginal and pelvic reconstruction with distally based rectus abdominis myocutaneous flaps. *Plast. Reconstr. Surg.* **81:** 62–69, with permission.)

lowest (Mathes and Nashai, 1984). Third, a single flap restores the vaginal pouch, compared with the bilateral flaps that are required of gracilis and other flap reconstructions. Fourth, when a distal vaginal cuff is retained, as in supralevator exenterations, rectus abdominis reconstructions remain technically straightforward. This is in contrast to gracilis and other flaps from the thigh, which are difficult to pass around the retained vaginal cuff. A fifth advantage is that the rectus abdominis donor site closes in continuity with the laparotomy incision and avoids additional donor sites on the thighs, which are occasionally sensitive (Massey, 1986). Sixth, surface quality restoration is excellent with rectus abdominis flaps and stents or dilators are not required to maintain luminal dimensions in vaginal reconstruction. Finally, revascularization of irradiated pelvic wounds is provided by the excellent vascularity of this flap, and the incidence of infection after radical pelvic surgery when this flap is used has fallen dramatically from that occurring before its introduction.

Gracilis Flap Vaginal Reconstruction

Gracilis muscle–skin flaps originate from the medial thigh and are supplied by the medial femoral circumflex artery to the proximally-based gracilis muscle. This muscle is the most superficial of the adductors, and is located near the medial thigh midline. Originating on the pubis, the muscle inserts on the medial aspect of the tibia. Cutaneous perforators from the muscle supply a narrow corridor of overlying skin along the medial thigh. These perforators are few and are narrowly arranged compared with broader muscles (i.e. the rectus abdominis, latissimus dorsi, pectoralis major). This accounts for the higher incidence of gracilis skin paddle losses compared with that of other muscle–skin units (Mathes and Nashai, 1984). Also, the narrow corridor of supplied skin shifts posteriorly in the lithotomy position, and the skin paddle must be carefully placed to avoid complete paddle loss. Blood supply is variable to the distal portion of the gracilis muscle, accounting for the variability in survival of the distal flap.

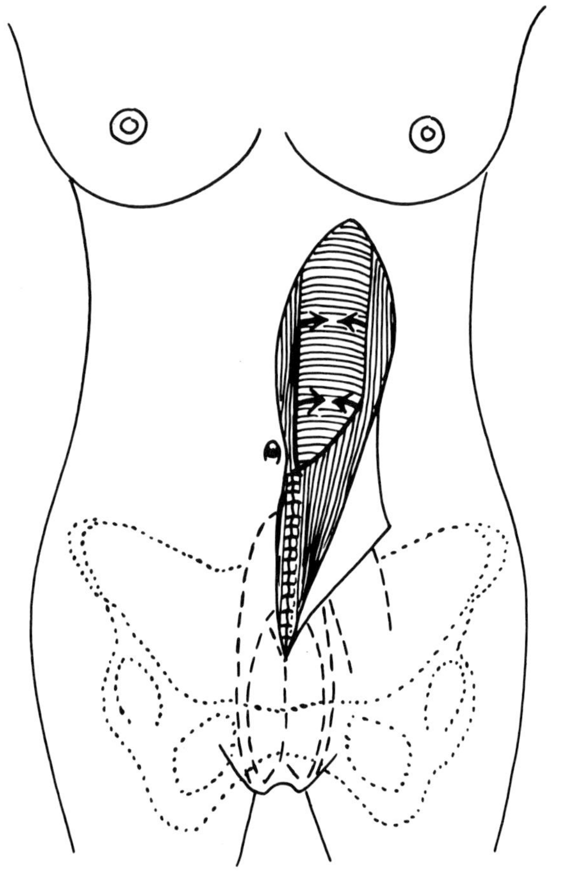

Figure 40.5. Closure of the donor defect and reconstruction of the abdominal wall by suture of the anterior rectus fascia to the linea alba below the umbilicus and direct closure of the anterior rectus fascia remnants over the posterior rectus fascia above the umbilicus (arrows). Complete fascial reconstruction of the abdominal wall results. (From Tobin GR, Pursell SH & Day TG (1990) Refinements in vaginal and pelvic reconstruction using rectus abdominis flaps. *Clin. Plast. Surg.* **117:** 705–712, with permission.)

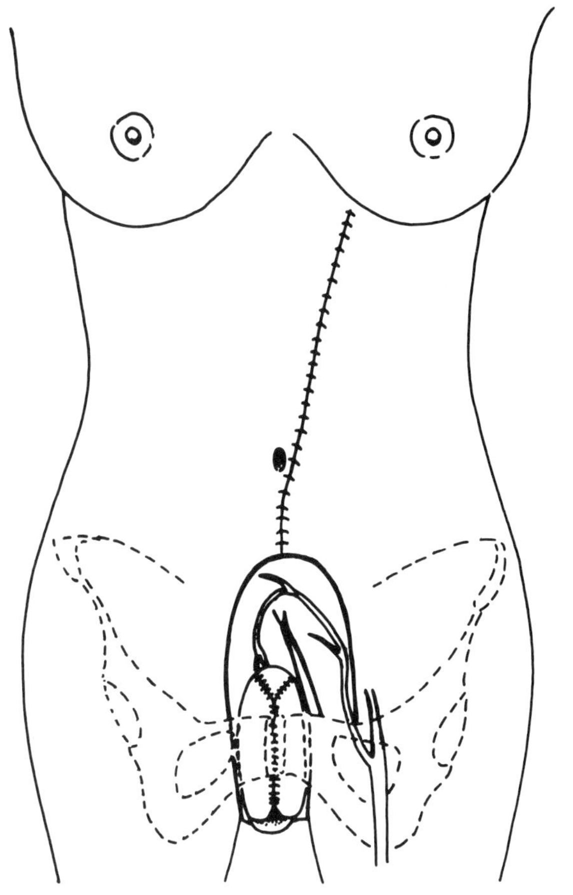

Figure 40.6. The directly closed cutaneous donor site is in continuity with the laparotomy incision following perineal inset of the flap. (From Tobin GR and Day TG (1988) Vaginal and pelvic reconstruction with distally based rectus abdominis myocutaneous flaps. *Plast. Reconstr. Surg.* **81:** 62–69, with permission.)

Gracilis vaginal reconstruction is performed with bilateral flaps taken from each medial thigh (*Figure 40.8*). Placement of the skin paddles is critical for lessening the incidence of partial, and occasionally total, loss of the neovagina. The paddle is always marked posterior and parallel to a line joining the adductor tubercle and the semitendinosus tendon (McCraw *et al.*, 1976; Massey, 1986). If the paddle is extended into the distal third of the thigh, the risk of skin loss increases because of a variable segmental blood supply to the underlying muscle. Once marked, the anterior margin of the paddle is incised, its relationship to the underlying muscle is confirmed, and the neurovascular pedicle is identified. To lessen the risk of paddle necrosis the skin paddle is sutured to the gracilis epimysium during the dissection and transfer to protect the sparse population of cutaneous perforators, because the paddle could easily be sheared from the underlying muscle. Once the skin paddles are incised, the muscle and its neurovascular supply are dissected free from surrounding tissues and the insertion tendon is transected. Broad subcutaneous tunnels are made over the muscle origin and beneath the labia to pass the flaps from their donor site into the pelvis. Once passed through these tunnels, the flaps are joined into a pouch with the skin side facing inward, and then they are inserted into the pelvic defect (*Figure 40.8B*). Suspension of the cephalic end of the pouch from the sacral prominence or pubic symphysis is done to lessen the incidence of prolapse, which is a moderately frequent complication of gracilis vaginal reconstruction. Both donor and recipient sites are drained, the neo-introitus is sutured to the labia, and donor sites are closed.

Gracilis flaps have now been used for over 18 years in radical pelvic surgery (McCraw *et al.*, 1976). Before the introduction of the distally-based rectus abdominis flap, gracilis flaps were the mainstay for vaginal reconstruction in radical pelvic surgery. Because gracilis flaps do not fill the pelvic inlet or block the entry of bowel into the pelvis as well as rectus abdominis flaps, and have a higher risk of necrosis and prolapse, they now have a backup role, and are used when rectus abdominis flaps are not available. They remain exceptionally valuable, however, for perineal resurfacing and fistula repair.

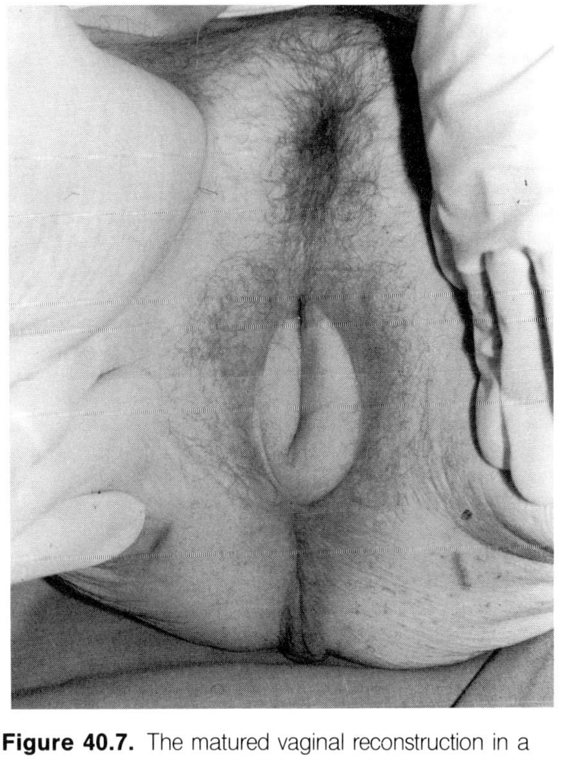

Figure 40.7. The matured vaginal reconstruction in a patient several months following pelvic exenteration. (From Tobin GR and Day TG (1988) Vaginal and pelvic reconstruction with distally based rectus abdominis myocutaneous flaps. *Plast. Reconstr. Surg.* **81:** 62–69, with permission.)

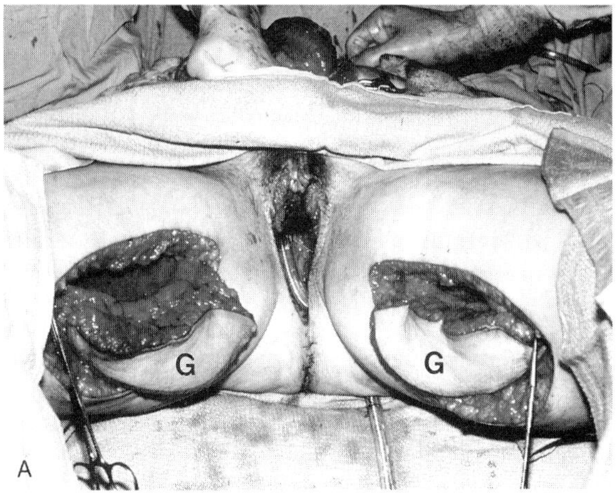

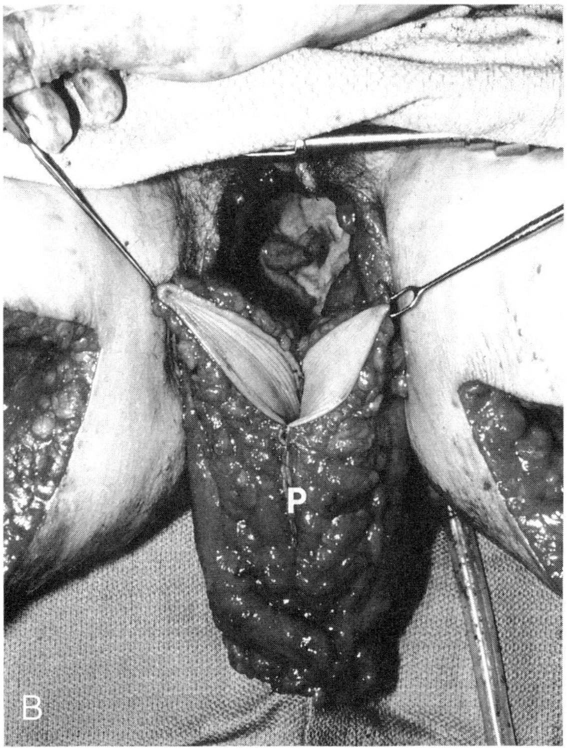

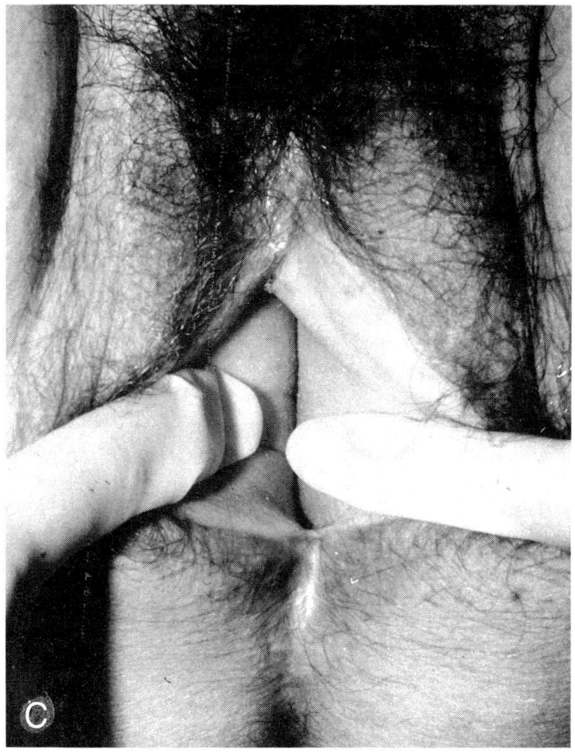

Figure 40.8. (**A**) Vaginal reconstruction with gracilis myocutaneous flaps. Bilateral gracilis myocutaneous flaps (G) are raised from each thigh. (**B**) Inverse tubing of flaps sutured together creates a vaginal pouch (P), shown here before inset into defect created by pelvic exenteration. (**C**) The flaps provide a vagina adequate for sexual function. (From Tobin GR (1984) Myocutaneous and muscle flaps. *Surg. Clin. North Am.* 64–667, with permission.)

Other Methods of Vaginal Reconstruction

A wide variety of vaginal reconstruction techniques have been described over the years using skin grafts, bowel and axial skin flaps from the groin, perineum, lower abdomen and thigh. The historic development and applications of these methods have been reviewed elsewhere (Goldwyn, 1977; Tobin, 1989). A common feature is their lack of bulk, which makes them most suitable for agenesis, repair of stenosis, and reconstruction of partial or total vaginectomy where adjacent structures are preserved. This same feature makes them less suitable for exenteration defects, where endopelvic dead space requires the bulk of compound muscle–skin flaps such as the rectus abdominis.

Skin Grafts

Vaginal reconstruction with a skin-grafted perineal pouch was introduced by Abbe (1898) and popularized by McIndoe (1950). This technique has been the procedure of choice for the reconstruction of congenital absence, and is also used to restore lining if flap reconstructions suffer partial loss. Skin grafts do not provide a satisfactory vaginal reconstruction for pelvic exenteration defects because of the inadequate bed and lack of bulk. Skin grafts must be immobilized by stents during the first 5–7 days postoperatively to take, and postoperative dilatation or stenting is required to maintain luminal diameter.

Bowel Segments

Both ileal and sigmoid colon segments have been transposed on mesenteric vascular pedicles for vaginal replacement (Pratt, 1972). Because of a fragile lining and excessive secretions, ileal segment use has been abandoned. Sigmoid colon epithelium is more durable and less secretory, and a sigmoid colon segment can provide a vaginal reconstruction, although skin grafts for congenital defects and myocutaneous flaps for acquired defects are preferred.

Regional Skin Flaps

A number of skin flaps for vaginal reconstruction based on regional axial or fasciocutaneous vascular supplies have been described. All of these are similar in concept, but are each based on different branches of the groin, perineal and thigh vessels. In general, they are less suited for reconstruction of exenteration defects, but are preferred for simple vaginectomy or stenosis repair.

The regional flaps and their vascular supplies fall into four major groups, based upon the origin of the vascular supply:

- axial flaps from branches of the common femoral vessels in the groin;
- axial flaps from the internal pudendal vessels;
- axial flaps from the posterior thigh;
- fasciocutaneous flaps from the medial thigh.

Vaginal reconstructions from axial flaps based on common femoral vessel branches in the groin include the groin and extended groin flaps based on the superficial circumflex iliac vessels (McGregor and Jackson, 1972; Bertani *et al.*, 1990), the superficial inferior epigastric vessel flap (Shaw and Payne, 1946), and the Beijing method, based on the confluence of both of the above vascular branches (Tobin, 1988; Zhou and Qiano, 1988). These methods provide skin flaps from the lower abdomen and lateral groin.

Axial branches of the internal pudendal vessels supply the Singapore flap (Wee and Joseph, 1989; Woods *et al.*, 1992) and the vulvobulbocavernosus or Martius flap methods (Martius, 1928; Hatch, 1984). These methods provide skin flaps from the vulva and uppermost medial thigh.

The axial descending branch of the inferior gluteal artery and the cruciate anastomosis supply the gluteal–thigh flap (Hurwitz and Dweibel, 1985). This flap provides skin from the posterior thigh surface for vaginal and perineal reconstruction.

Fasciocutaneous flaps from the medial thigh are supplied by terminal branches of the obturator, medial femoral circumflex and internal pudendal vessels forming a plexus running at the level of the deep fascia (Pakiam, 1980; Wang *et al.*, 1987). This is also the blood supply to 'short' gracilis flap vaginal reconstruction (Soper *et al.*, 1989), since the primary blood supply to the gracilis muscle is divided in this method.

Vulvar Reconstruction

Therapy of vulvar cancer almost always involves some degree of injury to the external genitalia. Despite trends toward less extensive resection for early lesions, many patients with vulvar malignancies are best treated by radical vulvectomy with bilateral inguinal lymphadenectomy. This disfiguring procedure results in loss of the external genitalia and has a high incidence of wound infection and breakdown, resulting in delayed healing or requiring additional surgical procedures or skin grafting. Reports of the incidence of wound breakdown are as high as 80–95%, and management of this complication results in extended hospital stays for these patients (Chafe *et al.*, 1983). Wound healing by secondary intention or split-thickness skin grafting directly over the surgical defect can result in severe perineal contractions, which interfere with sexual and urinary function.

Many radical vulvectomy wounds can be closed primarily without undue tension on the skin edges. Others require full-thickness rotational skin flaps such as the Z-plasty (Julian *et al.*, 1971) or rhomboid flap (Barnhill *et al.*, 1983) in order to achieve tension-free closure. Moderately large defects can be closed using these techniques; however, careful flap design is important. Flap thickness should include the skin and subcutaneous fat, and flap length should not exceed twice the width. Flaps may be unilateral or bilateral, and care must be exercised to avoid tension on the suture lines. Certain perineal resections, however, are so extensive that primary closure is not possible, even using rotational skin flaps. In these patients, cutaneous or myocutaneous flaps will be necessary for wound closure and healing.

A variety of rotational flaps based upon branches of the thigh, groin and abdominal vasculature have been described for vulvar reconstruction (Tobin, 1994). Ideally, myocutaneous flap vulvar reconstruction should provide functional, cosmetic and anatomic restoration of the vulva. The flaps should be expendable at the donor site, and should be mobilized with minimal patient morbidity. In addition, the donor site scar must be acceptable to the patient. The gracilis myocutaneous flap was first used for vaginal reconstruction (McCraw *et al.*, 1976); however, the same technique can be modified to provide resurfacing for the vulva and perineum (Ballon *et al.*, 1979). A recent modification of the gracilis myocutaneous flap, the gracilis V–Y advancement flap, provides excellent results and has a more reliable vascular supply than the classical rotational flap (Peled, 1990; Tobin *et al.*, 1990). Another recently described technique, the superficial external pudendal artery flap, also provides superior restoration of anatomy and function while limiting the donor site scar to the lower abdomen (Mayer and Rodriguez, 1991). The rectus abdominis flap can provide a large area of well-vascularized skin for coverage of large defects (Tobin, 1994); however, the donor site requires an upper abdominal incision. Tensor fascia lata flaps from the lateral thigh are another source of coverage for the perineum, although skin grafts are sometimes necessary for donor site closure (Chafe *et al.*, 1983). These techniques are described below.

Gracilis Flap Vulvar Reconstruction

Since the demonstration that the viability of the isolated gracilis muscle with overlying skin and subcutaneous tissue could be maintained by preservation of its vascular pedicle, the gracilis myocutaneous flap has been widely used for reconstruction of vaginal, groin and vulvar defect (McCraw *et al.*, 1976; Ballon *et al.*, 1979). Only slight modifications of McCraw's original technique are necessary to provide a flap for resurfacing the vulva after radical vulvectomy. As described for gracilis flap vaginal reconstruction, the flap is outlined posterior to a line from the pubic tubercle to the medial condyle of the tibia, with its base at the lateral edge of the perineal defect (*Figure 40.9*). The skin and subcutaneous tissue are incised down to the adductor longus fascia, and the dominant vascular pedicle is identified approximately 8 cm from the pubic ramus. The gracilis muscle is transected distally, and may be transected at its insertion on the pubis or left attached. Caution must be exercised to avoid confusing the gracilis and sartorius muscles distally. Once the flaps are elevated, they are rotated into position over the vulva and sutured in place. The donor sites are closed primarily. Closed suction drains are placed under the flaps as well as the donor sites. In obese patients, the subcutaneous fat overlying the gracilis muscle may be too bulky to properly reconstruct the vulva. A more satisfactory result can be achieved in these patients by rotating the gracilis muscle alone, without the overlying skin and subcutaneous tissue. A split-thickness skin graft is used to cover the muscle (Kaplan, 1985).

Gracilis V–Y Advancement Flap Vulvar Reconstruction

Recently, the gracilis island pedicle flap has been modified to provide a more reliable vascular supply and lessen the incidence of partial or complete paddle loss (Peled, 1990 and Tobin *et al.*, 1990). The gracilis V–Y advancement flap is a composite graft, which relies upon the vascular pedicle from the medial femoral circumflex vessels as well as a cutaneous pedicle for additional circulation (Tobin *et al.*, 1990). The flap is outlined as described previously, with its base at the lateral edge of the perineal defect. A broader flap may be advanced than the gracilis island transposition flaps used for vaginal reconstruction (*Figure 40.10*). A lateral cutaneous pedicle is left either anteriorly or posteriorly, depending upon the anatomy of the defect to be reconstructed. Distally, the muscle is transected near the musculotendinous junction so that the flap can be advanced and rotated

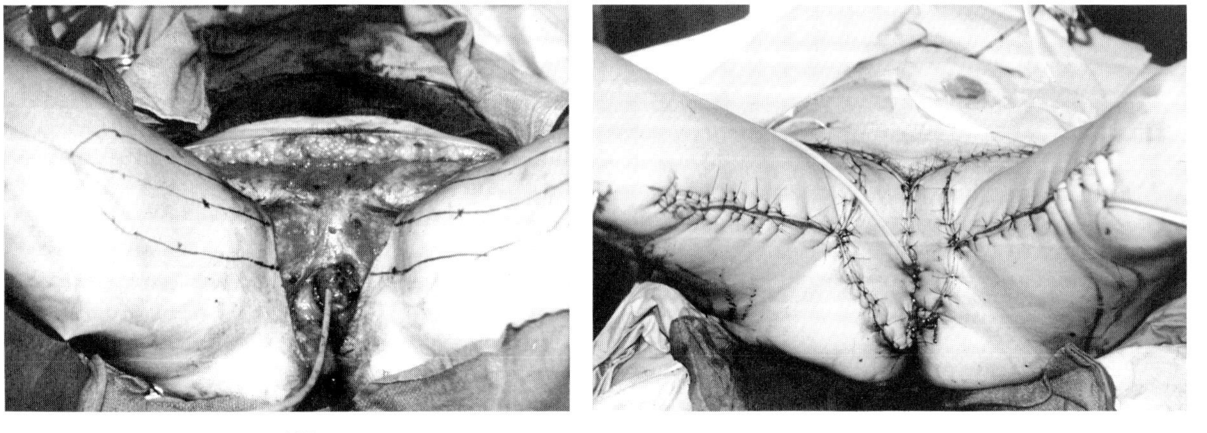

(A) (B)

Figure 40.9. (**A**) Radical vulvectomy defect with bilateral gracilis flaps outlined on the medial thighs. (**B**) Completed vulvar reconstruction.

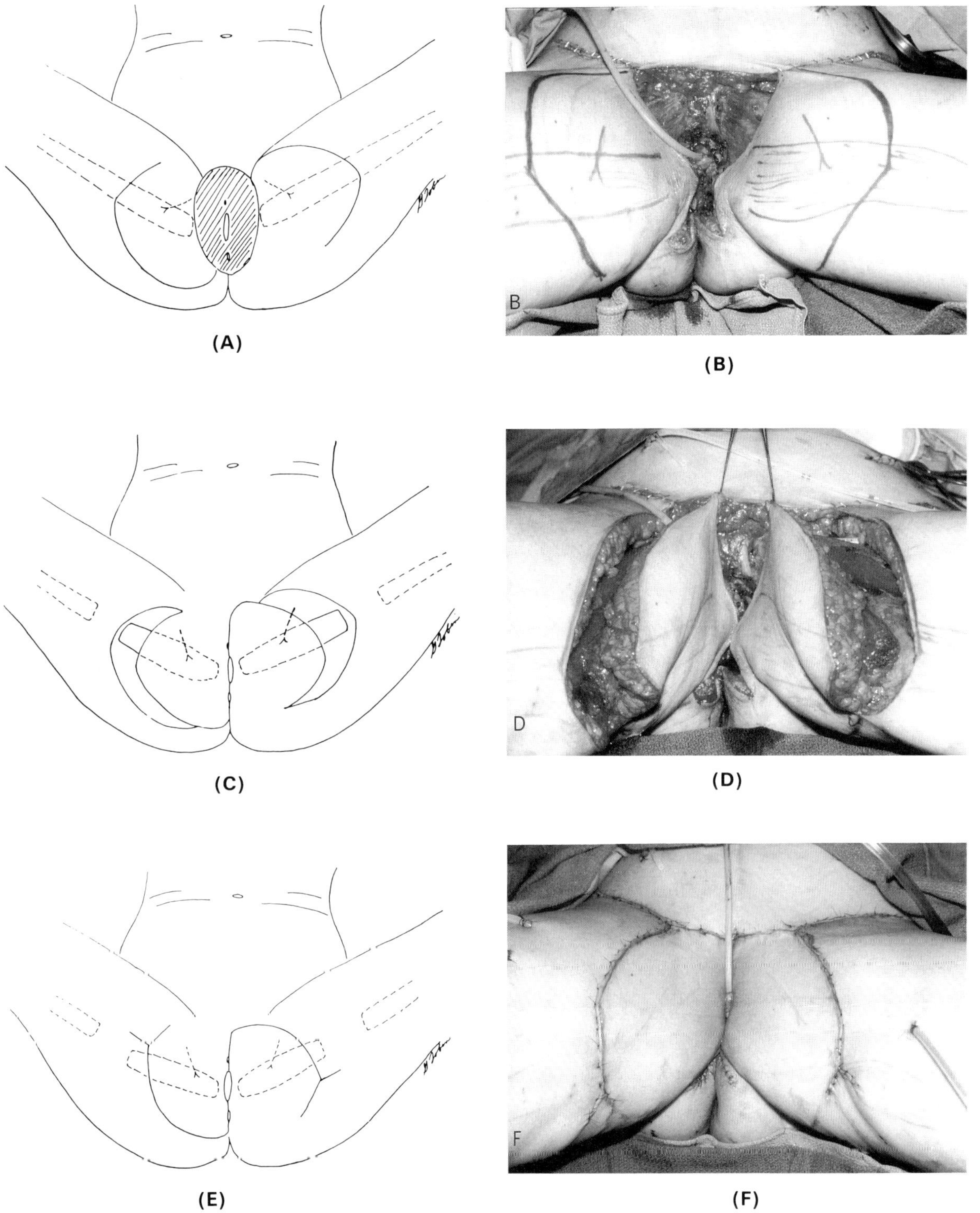

Figure 40.10. (**A**) Gracilis V–Y advancement flaps used for a large perineal defect (shaded). The flaps illustrated have a dorsal cutaneous pedicle on the left leg, and a ventral cutaneous pedicle on the right leg (**B**) Gracilis V–Y advancement flaps outlined on a patient undergoing vulvar reconstruction her both have dorsal cutaneous pedicles. (**C**) The flaps and their vascularized muscle pedicles are advanced into the perineal defect. (**D**) Execution of this maneuver in a patient undergoing vulvar reconstruction. (**E**) V–Y closure of the thigh donor defects. (**F**) Completed gracilis V–Y advancement flap vulvar reconstruction. (From Tobin GR (1994) Pelvic, vaginal, and perineal reconstruction in radical pelvic surgery. *Surg. Oncol. Clin. North Am.* **3:** 397–413, with permission.)

into the wound; the muscle origin on the pubis may be transected if necessary. Care must be taken to preserve the vascular pedicle. A back-cut is used to allow optimal advancement. The leading edge of the flap is inset first, so that there is no tension from closure of the trailing edge and donor site. Donor site closure is accomplished in a V–Y fashion.

Superior External Pudendal Artery Flap Vulvar Reconstruction

The superficial external pudendal artery arises from the femoral artery at the saphenofemoral junction and courses cephalad, piercing the cribriform fascia and crossing over the inguinal ring (*Figure 40.11*).

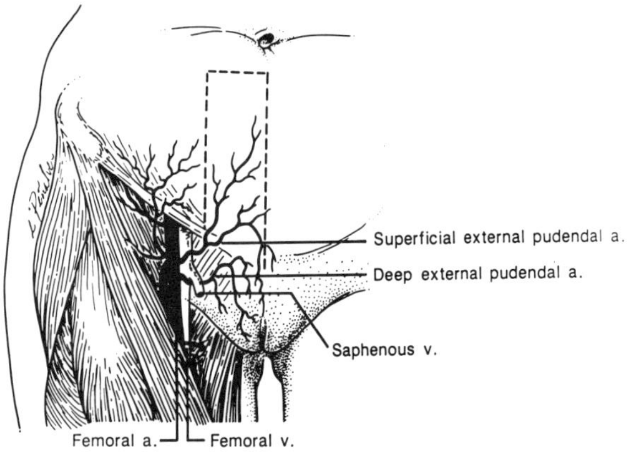

Figure 40.11. The anatomic course of the superficial external pudendal artery and outline of the flap (dotted line). (a, artery; v, vein.) (Reprinted from Mayer AR & Rodriguez RL (1991) *Obstet. Gynecol.* **78:** 964–968, with permission from The American College of Obstetricians and Gynecologists.)

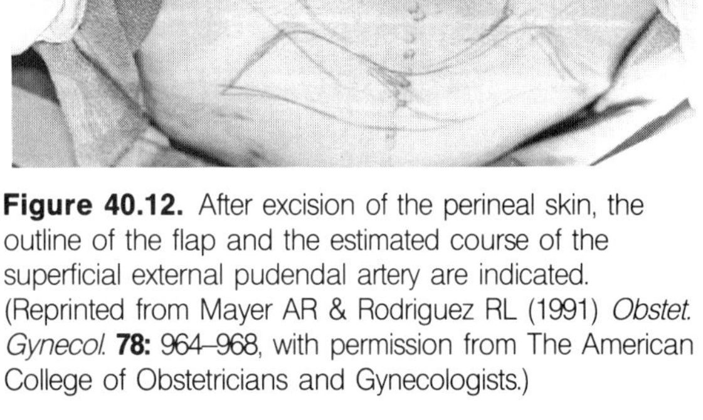

Figure 40.12. After excision of the perineal skin, the outline of the flap and the estimated course of the superficial external pudendal artery are indicated. (Reprinted from Mayer AR & Rodriguez RL (1991) *Obstet. Gynecol.* **78:** 964–968, with permission from The American College of Obstetricians and Gynecologists.)

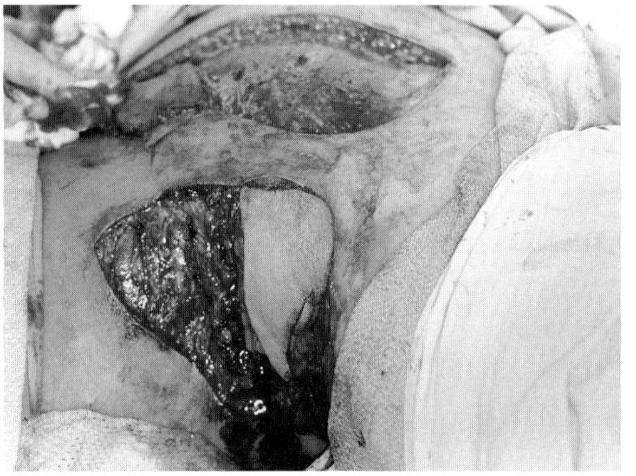

Figure 40.13. With the flap raised, the tissues are rotated onto the perineum. (Reprinted from Mayer AR & Rodriguez RL. (1991) *Obstet. Gynecol.* **78:** 964–968, with permission from The American College of Obstetricians and Gynecologists.)

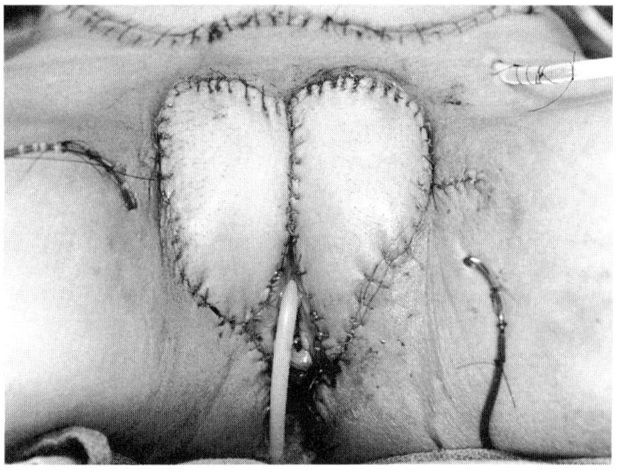

Figure 40.14. The flaps are secured, and closed suction drainage is placed. (Reprinted from Mayer AR & Rodriguez RL (1991) *Obstet. Gynecol.* **78:** 964–968, with permission from The American College of Obstetricians and Gynecologists.)

It travels through Camper's fascia toward the midline of the abdomen to the level of the umbilicus (Dias, 1984). An axial pedicle skin flap measuring 4.5 cm (9 cm when used bilaterally) can be raised around the superficial external pudendal artery and rotated onto the perineum (Mayer and Rodriguez, 1991). After measuring the perineal defect, the flap is outlined on the anterior abdominal wall (*Figure 40.12*). The skin is incised, and the superficial external pudendal artery is identified midway between the pubic tubercle and the anterior superior iliac spine. The flap is raised sharply off the underlying rectus fascia (*Figure 40.13*). Once mobilized, the flap is rotated and tunneled beneath the mons pubis, placed over the perineal defect, and sutured into place (*Figure 40.14*). Closed suction drainage is used beneath the flap. The anterior abdominal wall incision can be closed either transversely or vertically. This technique provides a very acceptable cosmetic and functional reconstruction (*Figure 40.15*).

Superficial external pudendal artery axial–cutaneous flaps have a number of advantages over other techniques of vulvar reconstruction. The thickness of the flap closely approximates that of the recipient site. In addition, the donor site can be closed transversely, resulting in a well-concealed lower abdominal scar.

Rectus Abdominis Flap Vulvar Reconstruction

The distally-based rectus abdominis myocutaneous flap provides an extremely reliable flap, which can be used to resurface large perineal defects. As described for rectus abdominis flap vaginal reconstruction, the flap is outlined on the anterior abdominal wall above the umbilicus. Once mobilized, the flap is rotated inferiorly and tunneled beneath the mons pubis to the perineum, where it is sutured into place. A single rectus flap may be split centrally to encompass the introitus and reconstruct bilateral vulvar defects (Tobin, 1994).

Tensor Fascia Lata Vulvar Reconstruction

The tensor fascia lata is a broad short muscle that originates from the anterior aspect of the iliac crest and inserts into the fascia lata at the mid-thigh. It is supplied by a terminal branch of the lateral circumflex femoral artery, which enters the muscle approximately 6–8 cm below the anterior superior iliac spine. Perforators from the muscle supply the skin overlying it as well as the fascia lata to within 6–8 cm from the knee (Kaplan, 1985). This muscle can therefore support an area of skin up to 15 cm in width and 40 cm in length, which is suitable for resurfacing the groin and perineum after radical resection (Chafe *et al.*, 1983).

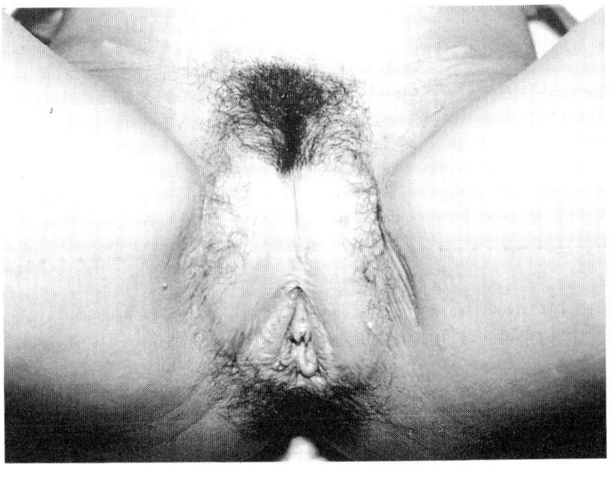

Figure 40.15. The reconstructed area one year after surgery. (Reprinted from Mayer AR & Rodriguez RL (1991) *Obstet. Gynecol.* **78:** 964–958, with permission from The American College of Obstetricians and Gynecologists.)

The surgical defect is carefully measured, as is the distance from the vascular supply of the flap (6–8 cm below the anterior superior iliac spine) to the most inferior aspect of the vulvectomy wound. Anteriorly, the flap is bordered by a line drawn from the superior iliac spine to the lateral condyle of the tibia. The posterior border extends along a line from the greater trochanter of the hip to the knee (Chafe *et al.*, 1983). Flap length and width are determined by the dimensions of the wound. The skin, subcutaneous fat and fascia are incised, and the flap is elevated from the distal end in the subfascial plane, temporarily suturing the fascia to the dermis to prevent avulsion of the cutaneous perforating vessels. Once the vascular pedicle is identified, dissection is carried superiorly as far as necessary to obtain an adequate arc of rotation. The flaps are then rotated anteriorly and sutured into place. Closed suction drains are placed beneath the flaps. Ambulation is begun on the second postoperative day. The donor site can generally be closed primarily; however, split-thickness skin grafts are sometimes necessary.

Urinary Tract Reconstruction

Recently, interest has been renewed in continent urinary diversions for gynecologic oncology patients. Patients with recurrent gynecologic malignancies undergoing pelvic exenteration will require urinary diversion. Cystectomy or supravesical urinary diversion may also be necessary in the management of radiation injury to the bladder or of certain urinary fistulae. The development of continent diversion procedures has allowed many patients to avoid the inconvenience and negative changes in body image associated with a urinary appliance.

Kock *et al.* (1982) introduced the continent ileal conduit, which used ileoileal intussusceptions for its efferent and afferent nipples, creating a nonreflux ureteral anastomosis and a continence mechanism, respectively. Low pressure was maintained in the reservoir by detubularizing the ileum. In 1985 the Mainz pouch was developed using an ileoileal intussusception for an efferent catheterizing channel in the cutaneous diversion and a spherical pouch constructed from cecum and two-folded and detubularized limbs of attached terminal ileum (Thuroff *et al.*, 1985). Both these procedures were technically difficult and time-intensive to construct. Follow-up studies have shown that the Kock's pouch has a failure rate of 10–20% in the efferent nipple and a 1% afferent nipple failure. Efforts to replace the intussuscepted intestinal valves with another continent outlet mechanism led to various procedures incorporating a detubularized segment of cecum and ascending colon forming the low pressure reservoir, with the ileocecal valve and plicated terminal ileum supplying the continence mechanism. Various improvements in these procedures continue to simplify their construction and reduce the risk of complications (Penalver *et al.*, 1994).

Patient selection is critical for the success of the procedure. The ideal candidate has the desire, the dexterity and the willingness to take on the responsibility of performing the clean intermittent catheterization and irrigation necessary with a continent urinary reservoir. Patients who are morbidly obese, have a serious concomitant medical illness, are psychologically unstable or have poor compliance with medical treatment regimens should not have the procedure. These patients should be considered for the technically less difficult and faster ileal or transverse colon conduit.

The continent urinary reservoir used at the University of Louisville is a modification of previously described ileocolonic techniques. The procedure is quick and technically simple to construct. Preoperatively, the patient should undergo a barium enema to assess the competence of the ileocecal valve and ensure there is no colonic pathology. A mechanical and antibiotic bowel preparation is routinely given. After completion of the anterior or total pelvic exenteration, a frozen section of the ureteral margin should be obtained to be certain there is no malignancy at the anastomotic site.

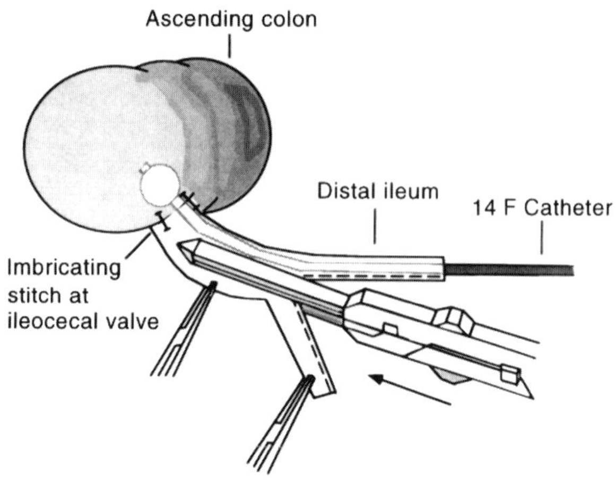

Figure 40.17. The terminal ileum is tapered using an intestinal dividing and stapling device. The ileocecal valve may be plicated if necessary.

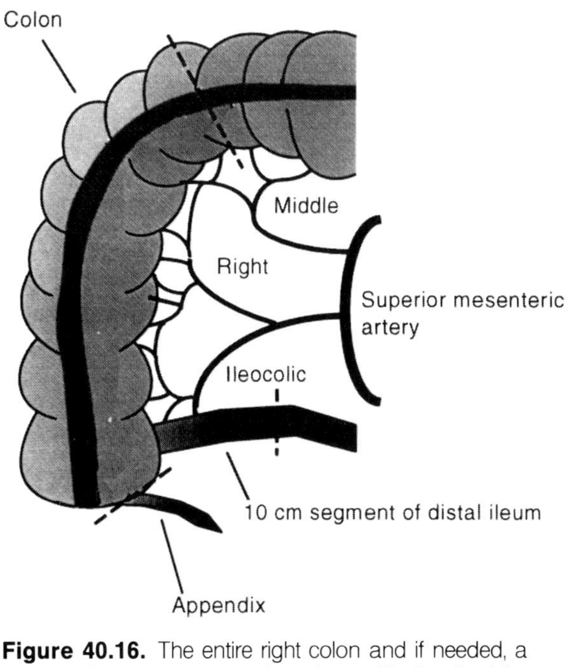

Figure 40.16. The entire right colon and if needed, a portion of the transverse colon along with the distal ileum are used for the continent urinary pouch. The appendix is removed if present.

The reservoir is constructed from 10 cm of distal ileum, the ascending colon and about 5 cm of transverse colon. The entire right colon to the junction of the right and middle colic blood supply is used (*Figure 40.16*). The colon is mobilized by opening the peritoneum along the white line of Toldt at the base of the mesentery. Before transecting the bowel one should ensure that the colon and distal ileum have enough mobilization to reach from the ureteral anastomosis in the pelvis to the anterior abdominal wall where the ileal stoma is constructed. Bowel continuity is restored with GIA and TA staplers, using a side-to-side, functional end-to-end anastomotic technique. The continence mechanism is created by plicating the ileum with a GIA stapler over a 14 F catheter inserted through the ileum into the cecum (*Figure 40.17*). Continence is tested by instilling about 100 ml of fluid into the cecum. If leakage occurs, several ileocecal imbricating stitches can be placed. The colon is next detubularized to create the low-pressure reservoir. Several techniques have been described. As originally described by Heineke–Mikulicz (Rowland *et al.*, 1987), the bowel is irrigated and opened along the taenia on its antimesenteric border. The appendix should be removed if present. One side of the reservoir is stapled using a TA or GIA stapler. The ureters are anastomosed by a direct non-tunneled mucosa-to-mucosa technique. Both ureters are spatulated 0.5 cm and secured with interrupted 4-0 polyglycolic suture. A 7F ureteral stent is passed up each ureter and sutured to the mucosa of the colon near the orifice with 3-0 chromic suture. The stents and a 22 F Malecot cecostomy tube are passed through the anterior wall of the reservoir. The remainder of the reservoir is then closed with staples.

Recently, a new technique of reservoir construction has been described (Dottino *et al.*, 1994). The colon is folded on itself, aligning the distal opened end with a previously made cecostomy. One side of a GIA polysorb stapler is inserted in the distal opening and the other through the cecostomy (*Figure 40.18*). The stapler is then fired along the antimesenteric aspect of the folded bowel. The bowel is inverted with Babcock clamps to continue the stapling (*Figure 40.19*). Three or four firings are required and the last application transfixes the apex of the fold of bowel. A figure eight suture of 2-0 chromic is applied to each small area between staple applications not included in the closure. The ureters are anastomosed as previously described. A purse-string suture is placed around the Malecot drain to minimize leakage. The coalesced distal colon and cecostomy are closed with a TA stapler or a running 2-0 polyglycolic suture (*Fiure 40.20*). After creation of the reservoir, the Malecot catheter and the ureteral stents are passed through the anterior abdominal wall and the reservoir is secured to the anterior abdomen with permanent suture. The ileal stoma is then sutured flush with the skin, making sure not to kink the small bowel and allowing a catheter to pass into the reservoir with little difficulty. Finally, a suction drain should be placed beneath the pouch.

Postoperatively, the pouch is irrigated with 60 ml of saline every 4–6 hours to prevent mucus plugs from forming. Some authors have stopped this practice with no apparent complication (Rowland *et al.*, 1987). The ureteral stents are removed in approximately two weeks. If minimal drainage is obtained, the drain is also removed. Radiography of the pouch is performed 2–4 weeks postoperatively and if no leaks are present the cecostomy tube is clamped and the patient can begin intermittent catheterizations. Post-void residuals are monitored through the cecostomy tube and if minimal, the Malecot catheter is also removed. Follow-up should include an outpatient examination

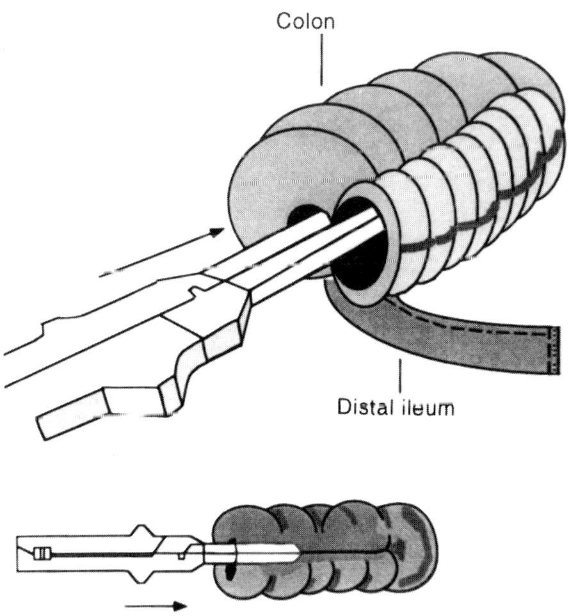

Figure 40.18. The divided colon is folded on itself, aligning the proximal transverse colon with the cecum along the antimesenteric line.

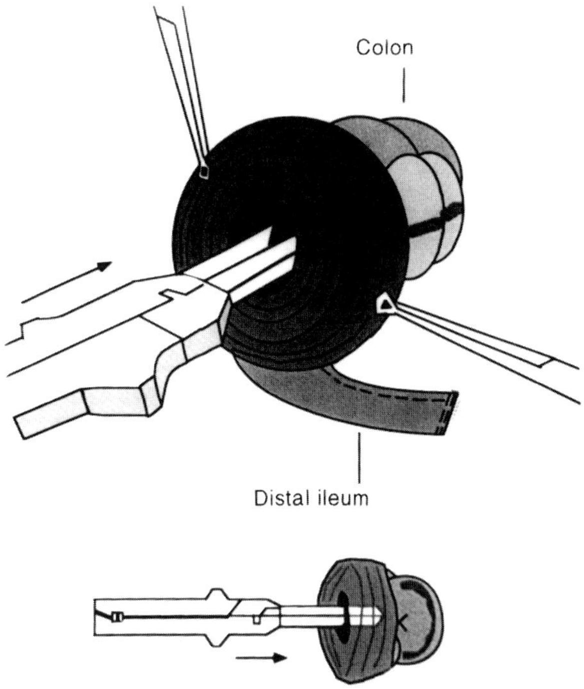

Figure 40.19. The bowel is inverted to allow multiple staple applications in order to create a detubularized reservoir.

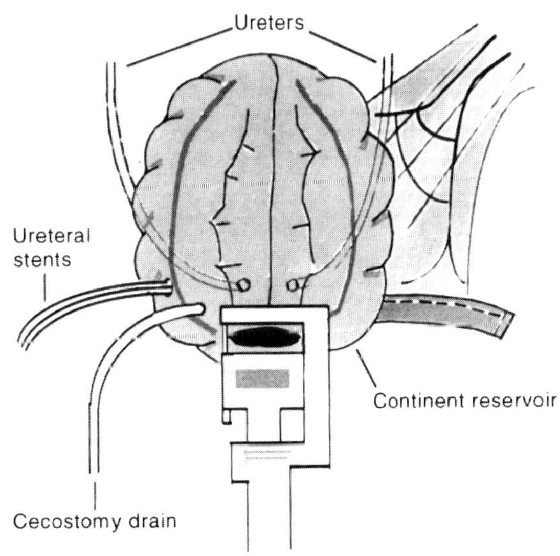

Figure 40.20. After completion of the ureteral anastomosis, the cecostomy is closed with a linear stapling device.

every three months. Routine labs including serum electrolytes and creatinine are obtained each visit. An intravenous pyelogram should be performed every six months to detect ureteral obstruction or retrograde flow of urine.

The incidence of complications is no greater than occurs with ileal or colonic conduits (Benson *et al.*, 1992). Ureteral obstruction occurs in less than 7% of the ureterocolonic anastomoses. Reflux occurs in approximately 8% of these units, but is not commonly associated with renal deterioration. Anastomotic leaks are found in only 5% of cases. Leakage from the site of the Malecot catheter develops in 5% of patients. (However, a recent report (Penalver *et al.*, 1994) suggests that the drain may not be necessary.) Although hyperchloremia can occur, it is usually not associated with acidosis (Mitchell, 1990). The bowel mucosa loses most of its villi and crypts with time, thus reducing its surface area (Carlen *et al.*, 1990). Both active and passive fluid and electrolyte absorption as well as secretion are reduced, thereby decreasing the incidence of hyperchloremic acidosis. Difficulty in catheterization is another problem encountered and may be secondary to reservoir overdistension. Patients should be instructed to catheterize themselves every 6–8 hours to avoid this complication. In spite of these problems, continence is achieved in over 90% of cases. A properly functioning continent reservoir results in the absence of a urinary drainage appliance, thus enhancing patient satisfaction and self-esteem. In addition, the construction of a low-pressure reservoir may result in less upper tract deterioration over time.

Preservation of Rectal Function

Introduction of the end-to-end anastomosis (EEA) stapling device simplified the surgical technique for low rectal anastomoses (Ravitch and Steichen, 1979). Certain gynecologic cancer patients who require rectosigmoid resection can now be spared a permanent colostomy. Frequently, total pelvic exenteration for recurrent cervical carcinoma can be performed using the supralevator technique, allowing preservation of the distal anus and rectal sphincter. Low rectal anastomosis in these patients can be performed successfully with acceptable morbidity and is facilitated by use of the EEA stapler; however, there is a high incidence of tenesmus and fecal frequency, especially in patients who have undergone total pelvic irradiation (Wheeless Jr, 1987). Restoration of rectal reservoir function via construction of a J-shaped colonic reservoir increases the capacity of the rectum and decreases the number of bowel movements per day (Lazorthes *et al.*, 1986; Parc *et al.*, 1986; Wheeless Jr, and Hempling, 1989).

After resection of the rectosigmoid colon, a reservoir is constructed from the terminal colon in a J configuration. The arms of a GIA stapling device are inserted through a colostomy incision into the two limbs of the J. Activating the stapler creates the reservoir. A low coloanal anastomosis is then performed with the EEA stapler. In irradiated patients, a diverting loop colostomy is performed to protect the anastomosis. The diverting colostomy is closed using an extraperitoneal technique 6–8 weeks after the primary procedure.

Summary of Management Options

- Vaginal reconstruction for agenesis or surgical loss without ultraradical pelvic resection can be readily accomplished via a variety of techniques, including skin grafts, regional skin flaps, or the use of bowel segments. These techniques do not fill endopelvic dead space or provide adequate vascularization to the pelvis.
- After pelvic exenteration, a large volume of well-vascularized tissue is necessary for vaginal reconstruction in order to fill the pelvis and prevent the migration of bowel loops into the pelvis. Revascularization also facilitates wound healing and decreases the incidence of postoperative infection. The rectus abdominus myocutaneous flap is ideally suited for these purposes.
- Vulvar reconstruction after radical vulvectomy enhances wound healing and improves cosmetic and functional results. Gracilis myocutaneous flaps from the medial thighs or superficial external pudendal artery cutaneous flaps from the lower abdomen can accomplish these surgical goals.
- Continent urinary diversion allows patients who require urinary diversion to avoid the necessity of an external applicance. These low-pressure reservoirs may also prevent upper urinary tract damage.
- Resection of the distal rectum and anus is generally not necessary in the management of gynecologic malignancies. Low colorectal anastomosis avoids colostomy in these patients. Creation of a 'J' pouch restores rectal reservoir capacity and prevents tenesmus and fecal frequency.

References

Abbe R (1986) New method of creating a vagina in a case of congenital absence. *Med. Rec.* **54:** 836–838.

Andersen BL & Hacker NF (1983) Psychosexual adjustment following pelvic exenteration. *Obstet. Gynecol.* **61(3):** 331–338.

Ballon SC, Donaldson RC, Roberts JA & Lagasse LD (1979) Reconstruction of the vulva using a myocutaneous graft. *Gynecol. Oncol.* **7:** 123–127.

Barnhill DR, Hoskins WJ & Metz P (1983) Use of the rhomboid flap after partial vulvectomy. *Obstet. Gynecol.* **62(4):** 444–447.

Benson MC, Slawin KM, Wechsler MH & Olsson CA (1992) Analysis of continent versus standard urinary diversion. *Br. J. Urol.* **69(2):** 156–162.

Bertani A, Riccio M & Belligolli A (1990) Vulval reconstruction after cancer excision: the island groin flap technique. *Br. J. Plast. Surg.* **43(2):** 159–161.

Carlen B, Willen R & Mansson W (1990) Mucosal ultrastructure of continent cecal reservoir for urine and its ileal nipple valve 2–9 years after construction. *J. Urol.* **143(2):** 372–376.

Chafe W, Fowler WC, Walton LA & Currie JL (1983) Radical vulvectomy with use of tensor fascia lata myocutaneous flap. *Am. J. Obstet. Gynecol.* **145:** 207–213.

Dias AD (1984) The superficial external pudendal artery (S.E.P.A.) axial–pattern flap. *Br. J. Plast. Surg.* **37:** 256–261.

■ Dottino PR, Segna RA, Jennings TS, Beddoe AM & Cohen CJ (1994) The stapled continent ileocecal urinary reservoir in the surgical management of gynecologic malignancy. *Gynecol. Oncol.* **55(2):** 185–189.

Goldwyn RM (1977) History of attempts to form a vagina. *Plast. Reconstr. Surg.* **59:** 319–329.

Harris R, Good R & Pollack L (1982) Sexual behavior of gynecologic cancer patients. *Arch. Sex. Behav.* **11:** 503–510.

Hatch KD (1984) Construction of a neovagina after exenteration using the vulvobulbocavernosus myoutaneous graft. *Obstet. Gynecol.* **63:** 110–114.

Heath PM, Wood JE, Podratz KC, Arnold PG & Irons GB Jr (1984) Gracilis myocutaneous vaginal recontruction. *Mayo Clin. Proc.* **59(1):** 21–24.

Hurwitz DJ & Dweibel PC (1985) Gluteal thigh flap repair of chronic perineal wounds. *Am. J. Surg.* **150:** 386–391.

Julian CG, Callison J & Woodruff JD (1971) Plastic management of extensive vulvar defects. *Obstet. Gynecol.* **38(2):** 193–198.

Kaplan AL (1985) Vulvar reconstruction. *Clin. Obstet. Gynecol.* **28(1):** 211–219.

Kock NG, Nilson AE, Nilsson LO, Norlen LJ & Philipson BM (1982) Urinary diversion via a continent ileal reservoir: clinical results in 12 patients. *J. Urol.* **128(3):** 469–475.

Lazorthes F, Fages P, Chiotasso P, Lemozy J & Bloom E (1986) Resection of the rectum with construction of a colonic reservoir and colo-anal anastomosis for carcinoma of the rectum. *Br. J. Surg.* **73:** 136–138.

Martius H (1928) Die operative wiederherstellung der volkommen fehlenden harnrohre und des schiesmuskels derelben. *Zentralbl. Gunak.* **52:** 480–486.

Massey F (1986) Vulvovaginal reconstruction following radical resections. *Clin. Obstet. Gynecol.* **29(3):** 617–627.

Mathes S & Nashai F (1984) Muscle and myocutaneous flaps. In: Goldwyn RM (ed) *The Unfavorable Result in Plastic Surgery: Avoidance and Treatment,* 2nd ed. pp. 91–122. Boston: Little, Brown & Co.

■ Mayer AR & Rodriguez RL (1991) Vulvar reconstruction using a pedicle flap based on the superficial external pudendal artery. *Obstet. Gynecol.* **78:** 964–968.

■ McCraw JB, Massey FM, Shanklin KD & Horton CE (1976) Vaginal reconstruction with gracilis myocutanous flaps. *Plast. Reconstr. Surg.* **58(2):** 176–183.

McGregor IA & Jackson IT (1972) The groin flap. *Br. J. Plast. Surg.* **25:** 3–16.

McIndoe A (1950) Treatment of congenital absence and obliterative conditions of the vagina. *Br. J. Plast. Surg.* **2:** 254–267.

Mitchell ME (1990) This month in Investigative Urology: long-term prospects and problems of continent urinary diversions (comment). *J. Urol.* **143(2):** 370–371.

Pakiam AI (1980) Repair of posttraumatic vaginal stenosis using local thigh flaps. *Br. J. Plast. Surg.* **33(1):** 54–55.

Parc R, Tiret E, Frileux P, Moszkowski E & Loygue J (1986) Resection and colo-anal anastomosis with colonic reservoir for rectal carcinoma. *Br. J. Surg.* **73:** 139–141.

Peled IJ (1990) Reconstruction of the vulva with V–Y advanced myocutaneous gracilis flap. *Plast. Reconstr. Surg.* **86(5):** 1014–1016.

Penalver M, Donato D, Sevin BU *et al.* (1994) Complications of the ileocolonic continent urinary reservoir (Miami pouch). *Gynecol. Oncol.* **52(3):** 360–364.

Pratt JH (1972) Vaginal atresia corrected by use of small and large bowel. *Clin. Obstet. Gynecol.* **15:** 639–649.

Ravitch MM & Steichen FM (1979) A stapling instrument for end-to-end inverting anastomoses in the gastroinestinal tract. *Ann. Surg.* **189(6):** 791–797.

Rowland RG, Mitchell ME, Bihrle R, Kahnoski RJ & Piser JE (1987) Indiana continent urinary reservoir. *J. Urol.* **137(6):** 1136–1139.

Schover LR & Fife M (1985) Sexual counseling of patients undergoing radical surgery for pelvic or genital cancer. *J. Psychosoc. Oncol.* **3:** 21–41.

Shaw OT & Payne RL (1946) One-staged tubed abdominal flaps: single pedicle tubes. *Surg. Gynecol. Obstet.* **83:** 205–209.

Shepherd JH, Van Dam PA, Jobling TW & Breach N (1990) The use of rectus abdominis myocutaneous flaps following excision of vulvar cancer. *Br. J. Obstet. Gynaecol.* **97:** 1020–1025.

Soper JT, Larson D, Hunter VJ, Berchuck A & Clarke–Pearson DL (1989) Short gracilis myocutaneous flaps for vulvovaginal reconstruction after radical pelvic surgery. *Obstet. Gynecol.* **74(5):** 823–827.

Thuroff JW, Alekn P, Riedmiller H *et al.* (1985) The Mainz pouch for bladder augmentation and continent diversion. *World J. Urol.* **3:** 179.

Tobin GR (1988) Dermal flaps to reconstruct the vagina: Reply (Letter). *Plast. Reconstr. Surg.* **82:** 727.

Tobin GR (1989) Vaginal reconstruction. In: Marsh JL (ed) *Current Therapy in Plastic and Reconstructive Surgery,* pp. 122–126. Toronto: BC Decker.

Tobin GR (1994) Pelvic, vaginal and perineal reconstruction in radical pelvic surgery. *Surg. Oncol. Clin. North Am.* **3:** 397–412.

Tobin GR, Brown GL, Derr JW, Barker JH & Weiner LJ (1990) V–Y advancement flaps: reusable flaps for pressure ulcer repair. *Clin. Plast. Surg.* **17(4):** 727–732.

■ Tobin GR & Day TG Jr (1988) Vaginal and pelvic reconstruction with distally based rectus abdominis myocutaneous flaps. *Plast. Reconstr. Surg.* **81(1):** 62–70.

Tobin GR, Pursell SH & Day TG Jr (1990) Refinements in vaginal reconstruction using rectus abdominis flaps. *Clin. Plast. Surg.* **17(4):** 705–712.

Wang T, Whetzel T, Mathes SJ & Vasconez LO (1987)

A fasciocutaneous flap for vaginal and perineal reconstruction. *Plast. Reconstr. Surg.* **80(1):** 95–102.
Wee JTK & Joseph VT (1989) A new technique of vaginal reconstruction using neurovascular pudendal–thigh flaps: a preliminary report. *Plast. Reconstr. Surg.* **83(4):** 701–709.
Wheeless CR Jr (1987) Incidence of fecal incontinence after coloproctostomy below five centimeters in the rectum. *Gynecol. Oncol.* **27:** 373–379.
■ Wheeless CR Jr & Hempling RE (1989) Rectal J pouch reservoir to decrease the frequency of tenesmus and defecation in low coloproctostomy. *Gynecol. Oncol.* **35:** 136–138.
Woods JE, Alter G, Meland B & Podratz K (1992) Experience with vaginal reconstruction utilizing the modified Singapore flap. *Plast. Reconstr. Surg.* **90(2):** 270–274.
Zhou G & Qiano O (1988) Dermal flaps to reconstruct the vagina (Letter). *Plast. Reconstr. Surg.* **82:** 726–727.

41 Fine Needle Aspiration Biopsy of the Female Genital Tract and Breast

W H Rodgers
R D Alvarez

Introduction

Fine needle aspiration (FNA) is a biopsy technique where tissues are sampled for the purpose of cytologic diagnosis using a relatively thin needle, typically attached to a syringe (*Figure 41.1*). It was originally developed as a rapid relatively noninvasive method for the diagnosis of palpable masses (reviewed in Koss *et al.*, 1992). It has also acquired wide acceptance as a method of diagnosis of deeper lesions identified by ultrasound or other imaging techniques (reviewed in Ell, 1991). Diagnosis is based on the examination of aspirated material spread directly on glass slides after brief fixation and staining. The biopsy procedure is brief and virtually free of discomfort for the patient. The specimen can be interpreted immediately – yielding a diagnosis in less than ten minutes. These advantages have made it a safe and simple alternative to traditional biopsies in an increasing number of clinical circumstances, particularly in situations where rapidity of diagnosis and minimal trauma to the biopsy site, as well as minimal expense, are desirable. This chapter will discuss the application of FNA in the management of patients with a known or suspected gynecologic or mammary malignancy.

FNA Biopsy in Clinical Practice

With the exception of the ovary and fallopian tubes, gynecologic tumors are readily accessible by relatively noninvasive traditional histologic biopsy techniques. FNA biopsy is therefore rarely used for the primary diagnosis of tumors of the female genital tract. FNA is, however, is a useful approach to the diagnosis of recurrent gynecologic tumors, and to the clinical staging of primary or metastatic tumors.

Cervical Cancer

Patients with advanced or bulky early-stage cervical cancer have a higher incidence of pelvic and paraaortic nodal metastasis than patients with small-volume early-stage disease. These patients are often initially evaluated by computed tomography (CT), magnetic resonance imaging (MRI) or lymphangiogram to detect nodal metastasis, which may consequently alter treatment strategy. Evaluation of paraaortic metastasis, which may lie beyond the borders of standard pelvic radiation ports, is particularly important. Without FNA, verification of nodal metastasis requires surgical exploration via a transperitoneal or retroperitoneal approach. Under radiographic imaging guidance, percutaneous FNA of paraaortic adenopathy can confirm the presence of metastasis with high sensitivity and specificity (Zornoza J *et al.*, 1977; Dolan and McIntosh, 1981; Ewing *et al.*, 1982; McDonald *et al.*, 1987). In patients who are explored and who are found to have unresectable adenopathy, intraoperative FNA may be used to confirm the metastasis.

For suspected recurrent cervical cancer in the absence of a cervical lesion, suspicious parametrial or pelvic masses can be evaluated by transvaginal, transrectal or percutaneous FNA. Confirmation of recurrence in patients with a non-palpable pelvic

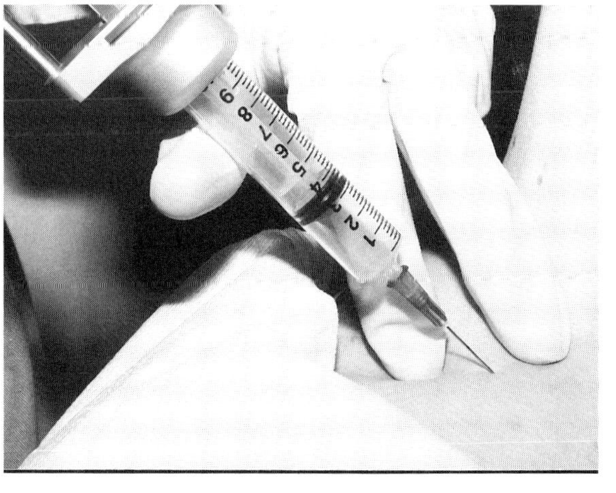

Figure 41.1. Fine needle aspiration of a cervical lymph node using a syringe holder and 1.5 in. 22 gauge needle. The needle is inserted into the center of the target and the syringe is retracted to 3 ml (see text). Note the bracing of the syringe barrel by the fingers of the palpating hand.

mass or with suspicious pelvic or paraaortic adenopathy is achieved using radiographic-guided FNA. Several authors have documented the excellent diagnostic yield of FNA in these clinical situations (*Table 41.1*).

Adnexal Masses and Ovarian Cancer

The role of FNA in the management of the patient with an adnexal mass or ovarian neoplasm remains controversial due to concern regarding the potential risk of tumor implantation with rupture of a malignant ovarian mass and the accuracy of the method (Kjellgren *et al.*, 1971). The former concern is not supported by recent data suggesting that tumor rupture is not an independent predictor of poor outcome in early-stage ovarian cancer (Purola and Neeminen, 1968; Grogan, 1987; Dembo *et al.*, 1990). The latter concern is addressed by studies demonstrating ovarian FNA as both diagnostic and therapeutic in selected patients (Granberg *et al.*, 1989; Bret *et al.*, 1992; Zanetta *et al.*, 1993).

Patients should be selected for ovarian FNA using strict sonographic criteria (DePriest *et al.*, 1993). Cysts with non-malignant sonographic characteristics (i.e. <10 cm in diameter, unilocular, with one or less smooth septation, and no solid components) are biopsied under radiographic imaging guidance only if a patient is symptomatic. A normal CA-125 improves the accuracy of a benign diagnosis of an ovarian mass with these sonographic findings (Parker and Berek, 1990). Clear fluid with few non-atypical cells confirms the diagnosis of a benign lesion in symptomatic patients. This approach offers an intermediate step between medical management and invasive surgery, avoiding unnecessary laparotomy. The fluid within a benign ovarian cyst may reaccumulate in up to 60% of patients, many of whom, however, will be asymptomatic (Bret *et al.*, 1992; Zanetta *et al.*, 1993). Conservative management with observation alone for a selected period of time is appropriate for the asymptomatic premenopausal patient with a cyst less than 8 cm in size or postmenopausal patient with a cyst less than 4 cm, provided they meet the previously described criteria for a benign process.

FNA of an adnexal mass with sonographic characteristics suggesting malignancy (multiseptated,

Table 41.1. Fine needle aspiration in the evaluation of recurrence in cervical cancer patients.

Authors	*No. of patients*	*Accuracy (%)*
Sevin *et al.*, 1980	58	93
Bottles and Cohen, 1991	30	93
Lopez *et al.*, 1988	76	89

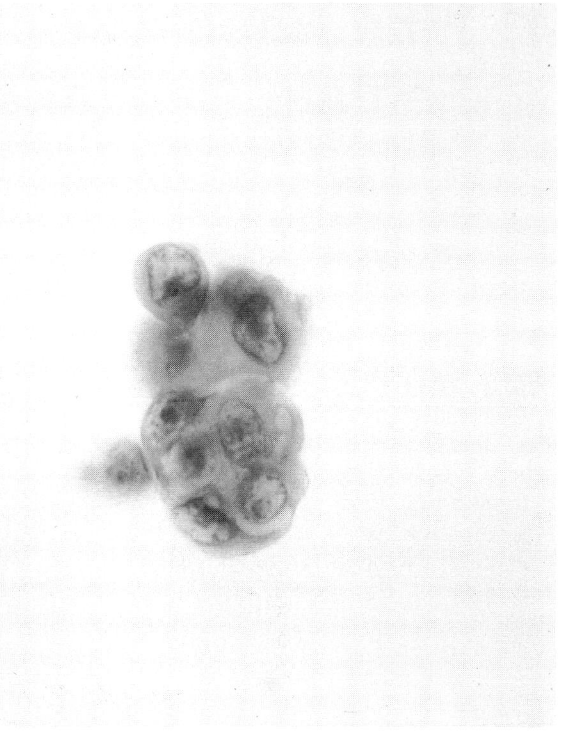

(A)

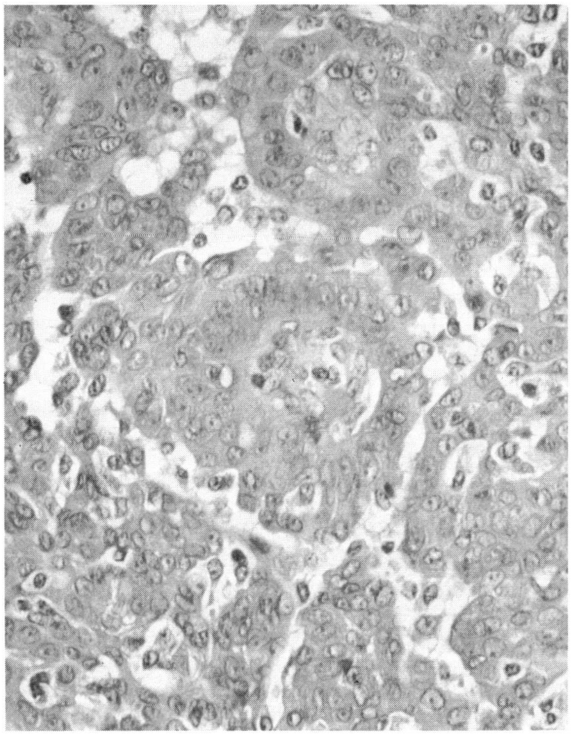

(B)

Figure 41.2. Fine needle aspiration (FNA) and biopsy of recurrent ovarian carcinoma. (**A**) Transvaginal FNA of adnexal mass showing metastatic papillary serous carcinoma (Papanicolaou ×100). (**B**) Primary ovarian serous papillary carcinoma (hematoxylin and eosin ×40).

solid or complex) is highly accurate, but rarely necessary since most of these patients require surgical exploration. For those patients deemed inoperable, however, FNA of a ovarian mass can confirm the diagnosis of malignancy. FNA of a pleural effusion, hepatic mass or suspicious supraclavicular or inguinal adenopathy is helpful in assigning the clinical stage of the tumor (*Figure 41.2*). Patients with advanced-stage ovarian cancer who are unsuitable candidates for debulking may have the diagnosis confirmed by analysis of ascitic fluid or FNA of the ovarian mass with minimal morbidity before the institution of chemotherapy.

Endometrial Cancer

Most patients with endometrial cancer present with clinical Stage I disease and undergo surgical staging. Occasionally, a patient presents with clinically detectable tumor extension or metastasis. Transvaginal FNA can be used to identify parametrial extension. This is most useful when cervical extension is suspected and when therapeutic intervention (i.e. preoperative radiation or chemotherapy) may depend on the results. FNA may also be used to confirm nodal metastasis preoperatively or intraoperatively (in patients who are explored and found to have unresectable adenopathy).

Vulvar Cancer

FNA is generally not required in most patients with vulvar cancer even those with late-stage disease. Confirmation of nodal metastasis in patients with suspicious inguinal adenopathy can be easily achieved using percutaneous FNA. The accuracy of FNA of suspicious inguinal adenopathy has been demonstrated to be as high as 93% (Crosby *et al.*, 1989). Patients with inguinal nodal metastasis may be candidates for neoadjuvant therapy or multi modality protocols, particularly when inguinal adenopathy is deemed unresectable.

Enlarged Lymph Nodes

Metastatic tumors, particularly those with a known primary site, are easily and accurately diagnosed by FNA biopsy, with a diagnostic accuracy better than 90% (Betsill and Hajdu, 1980; Kline, 1988; Das, 1991). As alluded to in previous sections, metastases to lymph nodes occur frequently in gynecologic malignancies. Metastases to lymph nodes are generally readily identified, either clinically or radiographically, and easily sampled. The aspirates are very cellular, usually without identifiable normal lymphoid elements (*Figure 41.3*). Preoperative evaluation of pelvic lymph node metastases in gynecologic malignancies has been shown to accurately predict nodal involvement, thereby avoid-

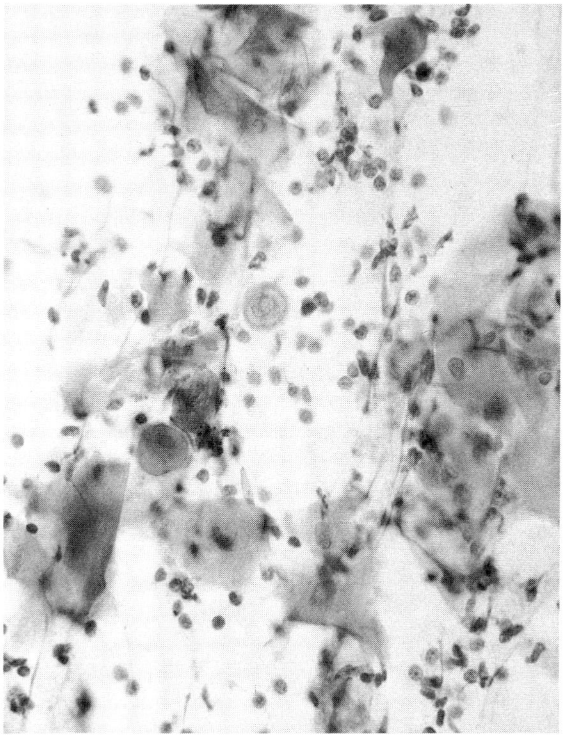

(A)

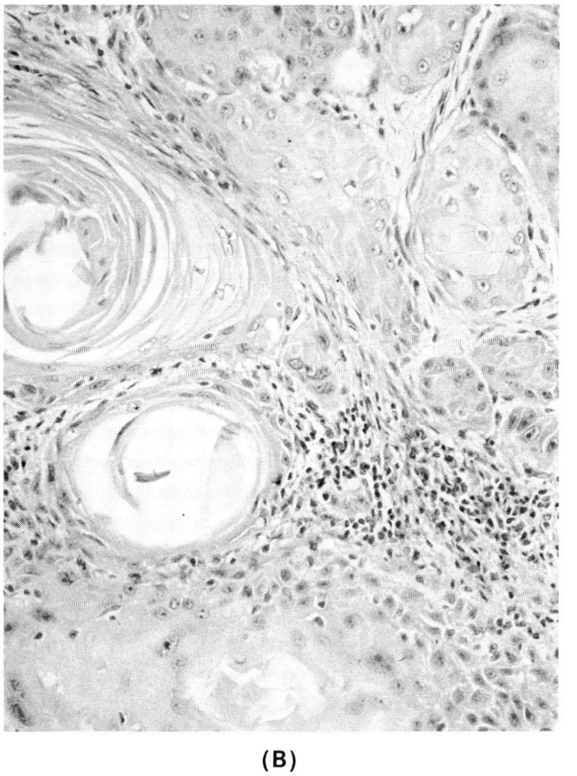

(B)

Figure 41.3. Fine needle aspiration (FNA) and biopsy of cervical carcinoma metastatic to inguinal lymph node. (**A**) FNA of inguinal lymph node showing keratinizing squamous cell carcinoma (Papanicolaou ×40). (**B**) Biopsy of cervical primary keratinizing squamous cell carcinoma (H and E ×40).

Table 41.2. Accuracy of fine needle aspiration of adenopathy in gynecologic malignancies.

Authors	*No. of patients*	*Nodal site*	*Accuracy (%)*
Zornoza J, 1977	17	Pelvic	100
Dolan and McIntosh, 1981	50	Pelvic/PAN*	86
Ewing *et al.*, 1982	61	Pelvic/PAN	NA**
McDonald *et al.*, 1983	50	Pelvic/PAN	74
Crosby *et al.*, 1989	48	Inguinal	93

*Paraaortic lymph nodes.
**Not analyzed.

Table 41.3. Accuracy of fine needle aspiration in gynecologic oncology.

Authors	*No. of patients*	*Accuracy (%)*
Belinson *et al.*, 1981	90	96
Flint *et al.*, 1982	48	96
Fortier *et al.*, 1985	82	93
Imachi *et al.*, 1992	287	95
Jacques *et al.*, 1978	17	71
Layfield *et al.*, 1991	59	85
McDonald *et al.*, 1987	138	89
Moriarty *et al.*, 1986	259	92
Nadji *et al.*, 1994	209	97
Nash *et al.*, 1988	139	73
Nordqvist *et al.*, 1979	74	97
Sevin *et al.*, 1979	124	97
Wojcik and Selvaggi, 1992	95	97

ing staging lymph node procedures and more radical surgical procedures (*Table 41.2*).

Diagnostic Accuracy in Gynecologic Oncology

The accuracy of a positive FNA diagnosis is comparable to traditional biopsy methods when performed and interpreted by experienced personnel (Palombini *et al.*, 1988). The interpretation of negative FNA results is somewhat problematic, being strongly influenced by the possibility of sampling error and the specific clinical situation. The accuracy of FNA is best in centers with a multidisciplinary approach to FNA and with experienced cytopathologists. In a recent review of the results of FNA diagnosis of 232 palpable lesions of the vulva, vagina, inguinal area and perineum in one center, Nadji *et al.* (1994) obtained a specificity of 100% (0% false positives, 4.6% false negatives) based on the correct identification of 87 malignant tumors. All false negatives were due to failure to sample the lesion; 140 nonmalignant FNA diagnoses were obtained, with 20% of them attributable to specific benign processes (i.e. endometriosis, abscess). The identity of the other lesions was not determined. Therefore, the specificity of the test for malignancy, based on the known false negatives in this series is 92.5%. In a separate study, Wojcik and Selvaggi (1992) demonstrated that a precise cytologic diagnosis as to tumor cell type could be made in 75% of patients with a positive FNA. These results are comparable to the success rates for more traditional biopsy methods and are typical of published results from centers with experienced aspirators and cytopathologists (*Table 41.3*).

Breast

Palpable lesions of the breast are readily accessible for FNA. Despite concern in the literature over dissemination of tumor by FNA diagnosis, no case of dissemination has been documented. The survival of women with breast cancer diagnosed by aspiration is the same as those diagnosed by other means (Berg and Robbins, 1962). These advantages have made FNA evaluation of breast masses a valuable, accurate and cost-effective diagnostic procedure (Silverman *et al.*, 1986), particularly in making the distinction between benign and malignant lesions (Bauermeister, 1980).

FNA provides a rapid and accurate means of distinguishing cystic lesions from solid lesions, obviating the need for additional studies such as ultrasound or mammography. Aspiration of cystic fluid, associated with the disappearance of the palpable mammary mass, is both diagnostic of non-neoplastic processes, and potentially therapeutic. Bloody fluids and those associated with residual masses should be submitted for cytologic analysis (Takeda *et al.*, 1982; Ciatto *et al.*, 1987).

The diagnosis of solid mammary lesions by FNA has been extensively used and analyzed (reviewed in Silverman, 1991). The diagnosis of malignancy is typically highly accurate (*Figure 41.4A&B*). In a recent statistical review of the literature of over 3000 mammary FNAs followed up by histologic biopsy, an average sensitivity of 87% (range 72–99%), specificity and positive predictive values of over 98%, and a negative predictive value of over 87% were

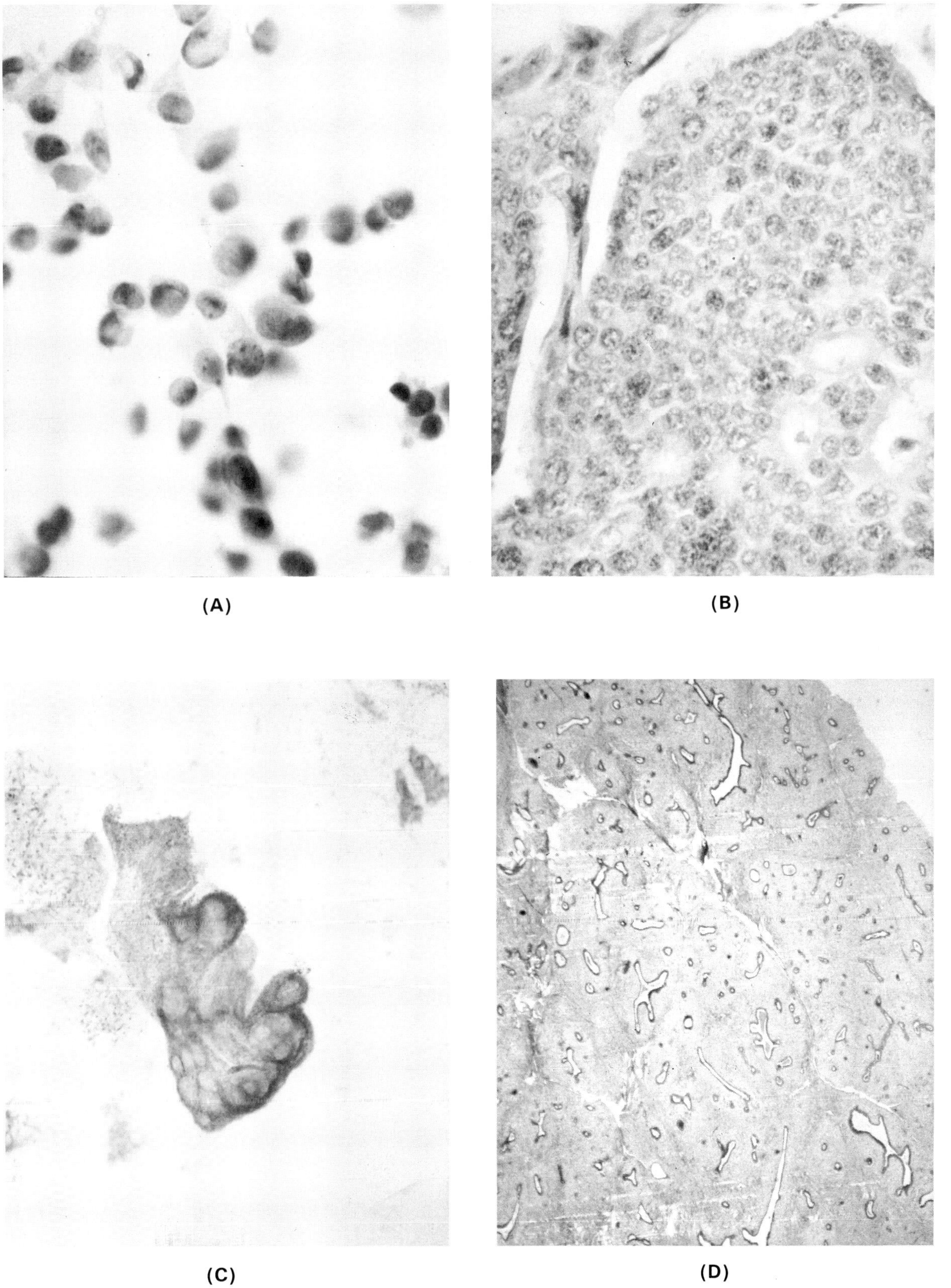

(A) (B) (C) (D)

Figure 41.4. Fine needle aspiration (FNA) and biopsies of mammary carcinoma and fibroadenoma. (**A**) FNA of mammary carcinoma (H and E ×40). (**B**) Biopsy of mammary carcinoma (H and E ×40). (**C**) FNA of fibroadenoma (H and E ×20). (**D**) Biopsy of fibroadenoma seen in C (H and E ×20).

found for the procedure (Hammond *et al.*, 1987). The best results, comparable to excisional biopsy results, are obtained in centers with personnel experienced in mammary biopsy and smear interpretation. Excellent results for the specific diagnosis of benign lesions (*Figure 41.4C&D*) as well as for the determination of malignancy, can also be obtained in specialized centers (Maygarden *et al.*, 1994).

Mammary FNA biopsy has excellent patient acceptance and virtually no associated morbidity. Complications are rare, except for local hematoma. Although pneumothorax is a reported complication of mammary aspiration, it is exceedingly rare, and can be avoided by using an oblique approach to lesions abutting the chest wall.

The Method of FNA

Principles and Technique

Consistently successful results with FNA technique require attention to specific aspects of sampling, smear preparation and microscopic interpretation (Silverman, 1991; Koss and Zajicek, 1992). Depending on local custom, the preparation and interpretation of FNA slides involves the participation of clinicians, pathologists, cytotechnologists, and, in the case of non-palpable lesions, radiologists or ultrasonographers. The microscopic interpretation of FNA specimens is best provided by a pathologist with a special interest and experience in FNA interpretation. Sample quality and smear preparation contribute significantly to the accuracy of the diagnoses (reviewed in Ljung, 1992) – the chances of obtaining a definitive diagnosis are greatest with high quality specimens. Experience and training in the aspiration and sample preparation techniques are major factors in the accuracy of the method. It is beyond the scope of this chapter to fully discuss technical aspects of FNA or the advantages or disadvantages of particular institutional organizations for aspiration diagnosis. The reader is referred to Ljung (1992) and Koss and Zajicek (1992) for excellent detailed discussions of practical aspects of FNA aspiration technique and slide preparation. What is presented here is an outline of a basic FNA diagnostic approach that can be easily used by physicians in their offices or clinics to provide good specimens for cytologic interpretation.

Instrumentation and Procedure

Aspiration

Aspiration of palpable masses is done with a standard disposable 21 to 26 gauge 1.5 in. beveled needle attached to a disposable syringe. Various syringe holders are available to facilitate sampling of masses requiring more than one free hand. Local anesthesia is not generally needed or recommended – the pain of two to three aspiration procedures is comparable to the pain of anesthesia, and the anesthesia can interfere with the palpation of the lesion (by causing swelling) and can diminish the quality of the cytologic sample (if infiltrated anesthesia is recovered by the aspiration or if the anesthesia infiltration causes hemorrhage).

The target lesion is palpated and immobilized with the non-dominant hand. Without moving the palpating hand, the skin is cleansed with an alcohol swab using the other hand. The syringe is picked up and the needle inserted into the center of the target. Usually a tactile sensation of the needle moving into a lesion will be felt as the needle moves into the tissues at a depth expected for the palpated target. If this does not occur the needle may be partially withdrawn and redirected, using the needle as a palpating probe until the needle has met its mark. Once the needle is within the target, suction is applied, by pulling the plunger of the syringe approximately to the 1–3 ml mark, and maintained until the syringe is withdrawn. Without the aid of a syringe holder this may be accomplished by grasping the barrel of the syringe with the palm and four fingers of the hand (needle side away from the thumb) and using the thumb to push the plunger up and out of the syringe barrel. Alternatively, once the needle is positioned in the target, the plunger of the syringe may be grasped with the second through fourth fingers of the hand and pulled away from the barrel by using the index finger to brace the syringe barrel, preventing it from moving while the plunger is pulled. While maintaining the vacuum, the needle tip is moved back and forth within the lesion (not in and out of the lesion) 5–20 times in approximately the same needle tract, or until material appears in the needle hub or syringe. *The suction is released before removing the needle.* The needle is withdrawn from the target. Slides are prepared (see below). After slide preparation, the needle and syringe may be rinsed in saline or another suitable transport fluid for recovery of material remaining in the syringe. A second aspiration is typically performed in a different area if the lesion is sufficiently large. Multiple aspirations increase the diagnostic yield, provide for a more representative sample of the mass, and increase the probability that the lesion has been successfully sampled.

Slide Preparation

The object of slide preparation is to gently distribute tissue fragments and cells in a thin film that will yield a well-preserved and stained specimen. There are a variety of specific slide preparation techniques. What is described here are two simple methods of slide preparation which generally give good results.

After the needle is withdrawn from the patient, the needle is removed, the syringe plunger is pulled back and the needle is replaced. With the tip of the needle bevel touching and facing the slide, the specimen is expelled by forcing air gently into the needle with the syringe. A *small* droplet of material is placed on each slide and smeared between the slides by pressing a second slide directly on top of the droplet. The second slide is pulled straight up and away from the first slide. Alternatively, the two slides may be gently separated by pulling them in opposite directions causing their flat surfaces to slide against each other until they slide apart, gently smearing the sample between the slides. The edges and flat surfaces of the slides in either method should not scrape each other. This first method is best for small specimens, the latter method for more abundant or bloody specimens. Once smeared the sample must be either air dried or *immediately* fixed in 95% alcohol or with spray fixative in the method used for Papanicolaou smears – the method determined by the staining procedure preferred by the pathologist. Air drying of alcohol-fixed material and overly thick smears should be avoided.

Comments and Recommendations

The appearance of blood in the hub of the needle during aspiration usually indicates that hemorrhage is occurring. In most instances it is best to stop sampling immediately as continued aspiration serves to dilute the diagnosable sample with blood, which often results in inferior cellular preparations. Many of the best specimens are obtained from aspirations that do not yield visible material in the syringe hub before ceasing aspiration. The relatively small amount of material present within the needle is sufficient for diagnoses. Movement of the needle throughout the target while aspirating by redirecting the action of the needle may in some circumstances increase the yield of diagnostic tissue; however, it most often results in increased hemorrhage and dilution of the specimen, giving the aspirator a false impression of successful sampling.

The purpose of the syringe is to provide a slight vacuum, it is not meant to contain the specimen (except in the case of cystic lesions). If the vacuum is released before the needle is removed from the target the sample will be drawn into the syringe from which it will be difficult to expel onto slides. The size of the syringe is unimportant; indeed, entirely adequate biopsies may be obtained using a bare needle without attached syringe. In general, smaller needles provide better samples from hard fibrotic lesions and lesions prone to hemorrhage; larger needles are used for deeper lesions, particularly deep FNAs directed by radiologic techniques, and transrectal or transvaginal aspirates of the ovary and adnexa. In these circumstances, the increased rigidity of the larger needles aids in directing the needle to the target.

Feedback on the quality of the preparations from the pathologist is valuable when learning the method. In clinical situations where experience with slide preparation or materials for slide preparation is lacking, good results can often be obtained by injecting the specimen into buffered saline or tissue culture medium and submitting the specimen to a cytopathologist.

Summary of Management Options

- Fine needle aspiration (FNA) is a useful approach to the clinical staging of primary or metastatic tumors through the evaluation of enlarged lymph nodes or a suspicious mass and to the diagnosis of recurrent gynecologic tumors.
- Aspiration of small ovarian cysts with benign clinical characteristics can be safely performed for selected symptomatic patients as an intermediate step between medical management and invasive surgery.
- Patients suspected of having advanced-stage ovarian cancer who are unsuitable candidates for debulking may have the diagnosis confirmed by analysis of ascitic fluid or FNA of the ovarian mass to confirm the diagnosis before the institution of chemotherapy.
- Patients with bulky early-stage cervical cancer or with advanced-stage cervical cancer who have suspicious paraaortic adenopathy on radiographic imaging can have percutaneous FNA performed to confirm the presence of metastasis.
- Metastases to lymph nodes other than the paraaortic region occur not infrequently in gynecologic malignancies and are generally readily identified, either clinically or radiographically, and easily sampled with FNA.
- FNA provides a rapid and accurate means of distinguishing cystic breast lesions from solid ones, obviating the need for additional studies such as ultrasound or mammography. Aspiration of cystic fluid associated with the disappearance of the palpable mammary mass is both diagnostic of non-neoplastic processes and potentially therapeutic. Bloody fluids and those associated with residual masses should be submitted for cytologic analysis.

References

Bauermeister D (1980) The role and limitation of frozen section and needle aspiration biopsy in breast cancer diagnosis. *Cancer* **46:** 947–949.

Belinson J, Lynn J, Papillo J *et al.* (1981) Fine-needle aspiration cytology in the management of gynecologic cancer. *Am. J. Obstet. Gynecol.* **139:** 148–153.

Berg J & Robbins G (1962) A late look at safety of aspiration biopsy. *Cancer* **15:** 826–827.

Betsill W & Hajdu S (1980) Percutaneous aspiration biopsy of lymph nodes. *Am. J. Clin. Pathol.* **73:** 471–479.

Bottles K & Cohen M (1991) An approach to fine-needle aspiration biopsy diagnosis of hepatic masses. *Diagn. Cytopathol.* **7:** 204–210.

■ Bret P, Guibaud L, Atri M *et al.* (1992) Transvaginal US-guided aspiration of ovarian cysts and solid pelvic masses. *Radiology* **185:** 377–380.

Ciatto S, Cariaggi P & Bulgaresi P (1987) The value of routine cytologic examination of breast cyst fluids. *Acta Cytol.* **31:** 301–304.

Crosby J, Bryan A, Gallup D & Talledo O (1989) Fine-needle aspiration of inguinal lymph nodes in gynecologic practice. *Obstet. Gynecol.* **73:** 281–284.

Das D (1991) Lymph nodes. In: Bibbo M (ed) *Comprehensive Cytopathology*, pp. 671–702. Philadelphia: WB Saunders.

Dembo A, Davy M, Stenwig A *et al.* (1990) Prognostic factors in patients with Stage I epithelial ovarian cancer. *Obstet. Gynecol.* **75:** 263–272.

DePriest PD, Shenson D, Fried A *et al.* (1993) A morphologic index based on sonographic findings in ovarian cancer. *Gynecol. Oncol.* **51:** 7–11.

Dolan T & McIntosh P (1981) Percutaneous retroperitoneal lymph node biopsy: an appraisal for a substitute to laparotomy in far advanced metastatic carcinoma. *Gynecol. Oncol.* **11:** 364–370.

Ell SR (1991) Imaging techniques. In: Bibbo M (ed). *Comprehensive Cytopathology*, pp. 615–620. Philadelphia: WB Saunders.

Ewing T, Buchler D, Hoogerland D *et al.* (1982) Percutaneous lymph node aspiration in patients with gynecologic tumors. *Am. J. Obstet. Gynecol.* **143:** 824–828.

Flint A, Terhart K, Mura T & Taylor P (1982) Confirmation of metastases by fine needle aspiration biopsy in patients with gynecologic malignancies. *Gynecol. Oncol.* **14:** 382–391.

Fortier K, Clarke–Pearson D, Creasman W & Johnston W (1985) Fine-needle aspiration in gynecology: evaluation of extrapelvic lesions in patients with gynecologic malignancy. *Obstet. Gynecol.* **65:** 67–72.

Granberg S, Wikland M & Jansson I (1989) Macroscopic characterization of ovarian tumors and the relation to the histological diagnosis: criteria to be used for ultrasound evaluation. *Gynecol. Oncol.* **35:** 139–144.

Grogan R (1987) Accidental rupture of malignant ovarian cysts during surgical removal. *Obstet. Gynecol.* **30:** 718–720.

Hammond S, Keyhani–Rofagha S & O'Toole R (1987) Statistical analysis of fine needle aspiration cytology of the breast: A review of 678 cases plus 4265 cases from the literature. *Acta Cytol.* **31:** 276–280.

Imachi M, Tsukamoto N, Shigematsu T *et al.* (1992) Fine-needle aspiration cytology in patients with gynecologic malignancies. *Gynecol. Oncol.* **46:** 309–312.

Jacques P, Staab E, Richey W *et al.* (1978) CT assisted pelvic and abdominal aspiration biopsies in gynecological malignancy. *Radiology* **128:** 651–655.

Kjellgren O, Angstrom T, Bergman F & Wiklund D (1971) Fine needle aspiration biopsy in diagnosis and classification of ovarian carcinoma. *Cancer* **28:** 967–976.

Kline T (1988) *Aspiration Biopsy Cytology*, pp. 199–252. New York: Churchill Livingstone.

Koss L, Woyke S & Olszewski W (1992) Principles of aspiration biopsy: Part 1 Historical developments and basic principles. In: Koss L and Woyke (eds) *Aspiration Biopsy. Cytologic Interpretation and Histologic Bases*, pp. 3–5. New York & Tokyo: Igaku–Shoin.

Koss L & Zajicek J (1992) Aspiration biopsy. Part I: Introduction to techniques and interpretation. In: Koss L (ed) *Diagnostic Cytology and its Histopathologic Bases*. pp. 1234–1250. Philadelphia: JB Lippincott.

Layfield L, Heaps J & Berek J (1991) Fine-needle aspiration cytology accuracy with palpable gynecologic neoplasms. *Gynecol. Oncol.* **40:** 70–73.

■ Ljung B–M (1992) Principles of aspiration biopsy: Part II Techniques of aspiration and smear preparation. In: Olszewiski W (ed) *Aspiration Biopsy. Cytologic Interpretation and Histologic Bases*. pp. 12–38. New York & Tokyo: Igaku–Shoin.

Lopez M, Kraybill W, Fuchs G *et al.* (1988) Transvaginal parametrial needle biopsy for detection of postirradiation recurrent cancer of the cervix. *Cancer* **61:** 275–278.

Maygarden S, Novotny D, Johnson D & Frable W (1994) Subclassification of benign breast disease by fine needle aspiration cytology: comparison of cytologic and histologic findings in 265 palpable breast masses. *Acta Pathol.* **38:** 115–129.

McDonald T, Morley G, Choo Y *et al.* (1983) Fine needle aspiration of para-aortic and pelvic lymph nodes showing lymphangiographic abnormalities. *Obstet. Gynecol.* **61:** 383–388.

McDonald T, Shepherd J, Morley G *et al.* (1987) Role of needle biopsy in the investigation of gynecologic malignancy. *J. Reprod. Med.* **32:** 287–292.

Moriarty A, Glant M & Stehman F (1986) The role of fine needle aspiration cytology in the management of gynecologic malignancies. *Acta Cytol.* **30:** 59–64.

Nadji M, Defortuna S, Sevin B & Ganjei P (1994) Fine needle aspiration cytology of palpable lesions of the lower female genital tract. *Int. J. Gynecol. Pathol.* **13:** 54–61.

Nash J, Burke T, Woodward JE *et al.* (1988) Diagnosis of recurrent gynecologic malignancy with fine-needle aspiration cytology. *Obstet. Gynecol.* **71:** 333–337.

Nordqvist SRB, Sevin B–U, Nadji M *et al.* (1979) Fine needle aspiration cytological and gynecologic oncology I. Diagnostic accuracy. *Obstet. Gynecol.* **54:** 719–724.

Palombini L, Fulcinitti F & Vetrani A (1988) Fine needle aspiration biopsies of breast masses: a critical analysis of 1956 cases in 8 years (1976–1984). *Cancer* **61:** 2273–2277.

Parker WH & Berek JS (1990) Management of selected cystic adnexal masses in postmenopausal women by operative laparoscopy: A pilot study. *Am. J. Obstet. Gynecol.* **163:** 1574–1577.

Purola A & Neeminen V (1968) Does rupture of cystic carcinoma during operation influence the prognosis? *Ann. Chir. Gynaecol.* **57:** 615–617.

Sevin B, Greening S, Nadji M *et al.* (1979) Fine needle aspiration cytology in gynecologic oncology. Part I: Clinical aspects. *Acta Cytol.* **23:** 277–281.

Sevin B, Nadji M, Greening S *et al.* (1980) Fine-needle-aspiration in gynecologic oncology: "Early detection of occult persistent, or recurrent cancer after radiation therapy". *Gynecol. Oncol.* **9:** 351–360.

■ Silverman J. (1991) Breast. In: Bibbo M (ed) *Comprehensive Cytopathology*, pp. 703–770. Philadephia: WB Saunders.

Silverman J, Lannin D, O'Brien K & Norris H (1986) The triage role of fine needle aspiration biopsy of palpable breast masses: Diagnostic accuracy and cost effectiveness. *Acta Cytol.* **31:** 731–735.

Takeda T, Suzuki M, Sato Y *et al.* (1982) Aspiration cytology of breast cysts. *Acta Cytol.* **26:** 37–43.

■ Wojcik E & Selvaggi S (1992) Diagnostic accuracy of fine-needle aspiration cytology in persistent or recurrent gynecologic malignancies. *Diagn. Cytopathol.* **8:** 322–326.

■ Zanetta G, Trio D & Lissoni A (1993) Early and short-term complications after US-guided puncture of gynecologic lesions: evaluation after 1000 consecutive cases. *Radiology* **189:** 161–164.

Zornoza J LJ, Jing BS, Wharton JT & Wallace S (1977) Percutaneous retroperitoneal lymph node biopsy in carcinoma of the cervix. *Gynecol. Oncol.* **5:** 43–51.

42 Radiation Therapy for Gynecologic Malignancies

M J Solan
L W Brady

Introduction

Ionizing radiation has been employed in the management of gynecologic malignancies since the early 1900s. Progress in the field of radiation therapy has resulted in improvement both in disease control and in quality of life. The development of megavoltage treatment equipment and afterloading brachytherapy applicators, and the technologic advances allowing computerized tomography (CT) (Sewchand *et al.*, 1982; Yu *et al.*, 1982; Ling *et al.*, 1987) and computer-assisted treatment planning (Sherouse *et al.*, 1987), have contributed greatly to improved quality of care. Ongoing technologic advances offer the prospect of further refinement of treatment planning and optimal dose delivery. The availability of high-dose rate (HDR) remote afterloading brachytherapy is rapidly changing the approach to gynecologic implants. The advent of three-dimensional (3D) conformal treatment planning allows optimal dose delivery with maximal normal tissue sparing. Promising research is directed at the use of combined chemotherapy/radiotherapy protocols, hyperthermia, and altered dose/fractionation schedules.

Radiation therapy may be the sole treatment or may be part of a multidisciplinary treatment plan together with surgery and/or chemotherapy. The optimal approach to the patient with a gynecologic tumor therefore requires a cooperative and systematic effort by the gynecologic surgeon, the medical and radiation oncologist, the pathologist and the diagnostic radiologist. With modern treatment planning and brachytherapy techniques, the radiation physicist has become an increasingly important member of this management team as has the oncology nurse.

Pre-treatment Evaluation

The treatment approach selected will depend upon the extent of disease at presentation so the initial evaluation must be comprehensive. Most pelvic 'recurrences' result from persistent disease at the primary site, pointing to the importance of accurate definition of initial disease extent (Brady *et al.*, 1987a). A complete history and physical examination is performed. The patient's performance status and complicating medical factors (i.e. cardiac, pulmonary) will indicate her ability to undergo general anesthesia or tolerate an intracavitary application. A history of previous abdominal or pelvic surgery or of chronic bowel or urologic disease (i.e. colitis, diverticulitis, nephritis, cystitis, neurogenic bladder) may impact on the patient's propensity for late normal tissue complications of therapy. Obesity, hypertension, diabetes mellitus and anemia may also hamper the ability to deliver optimal radiation treatment. Routine laboratory tests should include complete blood count (CBC), biochemical profile, urinalysis and chest radiography.

A thorough physical examination must be performed. Careful attention should be paid to the presence of scalene, inguinal or abdominal adenopathy, and to the presence of hepatomegaly and/or ascites. Rectovaginal examination under anesthesia (EUA), with appropriate biopsies, allows the best clinical evaluation of local disease extent. The full circumference and length of the vagina must be visualized and palpated to assess tumor extension. The size, shape and appearance of the uterine cervix must be noted and the uterine cavity sounded for size. Careful bimanual abdominovaginal examination is necessary to assess the degree of parametrial involvement, and the recotovaginal septum must be assessed for posterior tumor extension. A fractional dilatation and curettage (D&C) differentiates uterine and cervical origin of tumor cells.

Cystoscopy is employed to rule out bladder extension, and any suspicious site of bladder involvement must be confirmed by biopsy. Proctoscopy and barium enema may be helpful in advanced stages to assess tumor extension into the rectum or large bowel. While bipedal lymphangiography has been recommended for evaluating pelvic and paraaortic lymph node metastases, the use of this modality has markedly declined with the advant of improved resolution CT scanners, magnetic resonance imaging (MRI) and laparoscopic nodal sampling techniques. CT is also useful in evaluation for liver metastases, extrapelvic disease extension and hydronephrosis, and for delineating the location of critical normal tissues such as the kidney for radiation treatment planning.

Only after a complete staging work-up can an optimal treatment plan be devised (Brady *et al.*, 1987b). Management with radiation therapy may involve external beam irradiation and/or intracavitary or interstitial insertion of radioisotopes. In the patient with a small tumor burden without evidence of local extension or metastases, the treatment is primarily by intracavitary irradiation with external beam playing the lesser role of boosting the dose received by the pelvic lymph nodes. The more locally extensive or bulky the disease within the pelvis, the greater the emphasis on external beam irradiation.

External Beam Irradiation

Treatment planning

External beam irradiation of the pelvis directs treatment to the primary tumor as well as to sites of local extension and potential lymphatic spread. Treatment planning is performed with the aid of a simulator reproducing the geometry of the treatment machine, but allowing fluoroscopic visualization of critical structures, and radiography of diagnostic quality. A modern simulator can be linked to a dedicated CT scanner for increased accuracy in defining patient anatomy. CT cuts can be digitized onto treatment planning computers and isodose distributions then superimposed for visualization of doses that will be received by all pelvic structures.

It is essential that the radiation oncologist has a full understanding of the anatomic relationships within the pelvis and is well-acquainted with the patterns of spread and failure of the tumor in question. Treatment should be directed to sites of known tumor extension with a margin of normal tissue, and may involve prophylactic irradiation of sites of potential subclinical nodal involvement. The tolerance of normal surrounding tissue must be appreciated and all efforts made to reduce the late complications to these tissues by limiting the radiation dose that they receive.

The pelvic structures to be included in the treatment volume usually include the uterus, cervix, a variable length of vagina, and regional lymph nodes. The common iliac nodes extend from the top of L5 and bifurcate to form the external and internal iliac (hypogastric) chains. The external iliac chain spreads laterally along the pelvic wall and anteriorly. The obturator nodes form the medial group of external iliac nodes and lie along the lateral pelvic wall at about the level of the acetabulum. The internal iliac chain extends medial and posterior to the obturator nodes, while the presacral lymph nodes are located just anterior to the first through third sacral segments. The paraaortic lymph nodes extend caudally from the level of the diaphragm to L4–L5 where they bifurcate to the left and right common iliac chains. Known paraaortic or common iliac node involvement may indicate treatment to the paraaortic nodes.

The superior margin of the pelvic fields extends to L4–L5 if the common iliac nodes are to be included, or else to L5–S1 as shown in *Figure 42.1*. The inferior margin is determined by the length of vagina to be included and should give at least a 3–4 cm margin on the cervix or the most distal point of vaginal tumor extension. A radiopaque clip or marker is placed at the vaginal apex or cervical os, and under fluoroscopic visualization the inferior field margin is determined, as shown in *Figure 42.2*. Lateral field boundaries include a 1–2 cm margin at the widest portion of the bony pelvic inlet on anteroposterior (AP) and posteroanterior (PA) projection.

When lateral pelvic fields are employed, the superior and inferior borders are the same as those used for the anterior and posterior fields (*Figure 42.3*). Rectal contrast material is inserted for simulation of the lateral fields, and the posterior field edge should bisect the rectum in order to include the cervix, vagina, internal iliac and presacral nodes. The anterior field edge extends 1–2 cm anterior to the pubic symphysis for inclusion of the external iliac lymph nodes.

Oral contrast may be employed for visualization of the small bowel within the pelvis during simulation. Bladder contrast, with distension, may be employed in an attempt to push loops of small bowel out of the treatment field.

Ideal treatment employs megavoltage photon beams. Linear accelerators capable of generating beam energies from 4 to over 40 million volts (MV) allow the treatment of deep pelvic structures with

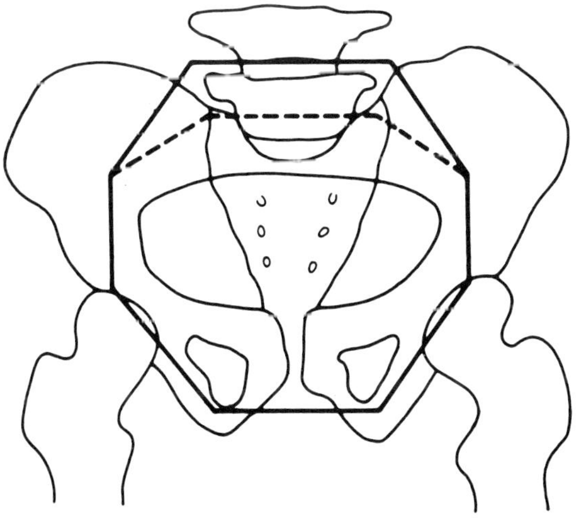

Figure 42.1. Anteroposterior portals employed in external beam irradiation. The superior field margin extends to the L4–L5 interspace for inclusion of the common iliac lymph nodes. If common iliac node coverage is not indicated, the superior field margin is reduced (broken line).

maximal sparing of skin and superficial tissue. With cobalt-60 (^{60}Co) or linear accelerators in the low-energy range of 4–10 MV, optimal dose distribution is usually attained by a four-field technique employing opposed anteroposterior and right and left lateral fields. This technique results in a uniform box-shaped, high-dose region within the treatment volume (*Figure 42.4*). High-energy linear accelerators with more penetrating beams of 18–25 MV or greater allow simpler treatment plans with parallel opposed anterior and posterior fields only. Whichever technique is used, all fields are treated daily (Wilson and Hall, 1971), usually with conventional doses of 1.8–2.0 Gy.

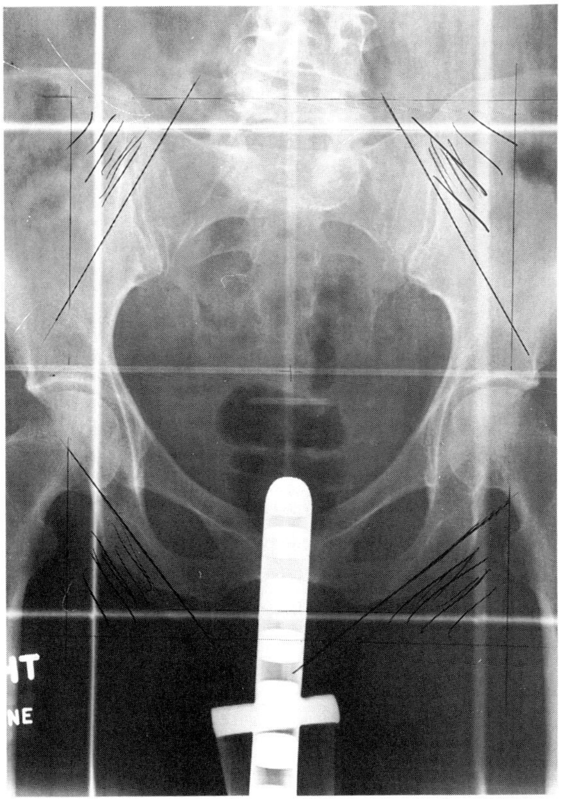

Figure 42.2. Anteroposterior simulation film showing treatment portal employed for postoperative external beam irradiation in a patient with Stage I adenocarcinoma of the endometrium. Vaginal marker localizes the vaginal apex allowing inclusion of an adequate length of vagina in the treatment portal.

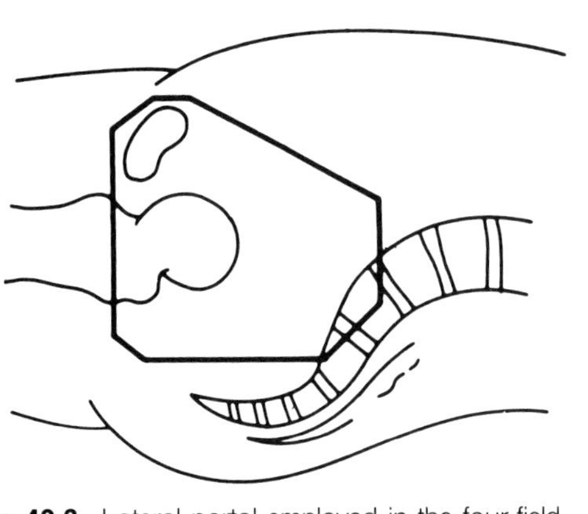

Figure 42.3. Lateral portal employed in the four-field technique.

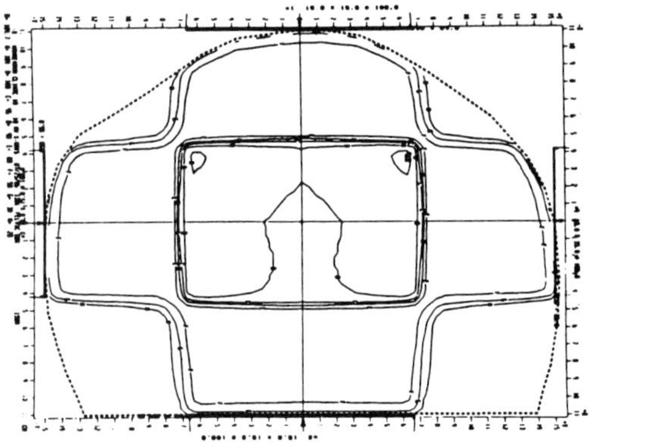

Figure 42.4. Isodose distribution for four-field 'box' pelvic irradiation employing 10 MV photons.

Low melting point bismuth alloys may be employed to form beam-shaping blocks designed to further shield normal tissue. By this means, a considerable portion of the small bowel and bladder can be eliminated from the lateral fields, and the femoral heads and a considerable proportion of the bone marrow can be shielded in the anterior and posterior fields.

The treatment of carcinoma of the vagina usually involves a target volume similar to that employed for cancer of the cervix or uterus, but longer lengths of vagina are included. For distal vaginal lesions, the inguinal lymph nodes may be treated as well. The development of treatment machines capable of generating electron beams with limited and controled depth–dose characteristics allows a boost to these superficial nodes with limited toxicity to deeper structures (Henderson *et al.*, 1984). In the treatment of ovarian cancer, the whole abdomen is often included in the irradiated volume.

When external beam irradiation is given in conjunction with intracavitary brachytherapy, it may be used to supplement the dose received by the parametrial tissue and lateral pelvic lymph nodes. For this 'parametrial boost,' a midline 5HVL (half value layer) block is inserted into the anterior and posterior opposed fields to shield the central area that has received high-dose treatment from brachytherapy (*Figure 42.5*).

Brachytherapy

Brachytherapy, or the placement of radioactive gamma-ray sources directly into or next to tumor-bearing structures, permits delivery of high doses of radiation over a short period of time to limited volumes of tissue. It may be the sole treatment mode for small carcinomas of the cervix that have little potential for nodal spread, or part of an integrated plan that includes external beam irradiation for more extensive disease. The anatomy of the uterus, cervix and vagina provides an ideal situation for insertion of radioactive sources. Very high dose rates are achieved close to the sources with rapid fall-off of dose over a short distance, thus resulting in considerable sparing of normal tissue.

Traditional brachytherapy systems for gynecologic application have been low-dose rate (LDR) systems as defined by the International Commission on Radiation Units and Measurements (ICRU) report #38 (1985) delivering 0.4–2 Gy h^{-1}, and typical implants have been of 24–72 hours' duration. Over the past two decades, HDR brachtherapy systems have gained increasing acceptance with the ability to deliver dose rates over 0.2 Gy min^{-1}, thereby allowing treatments of only several minutes' duration.

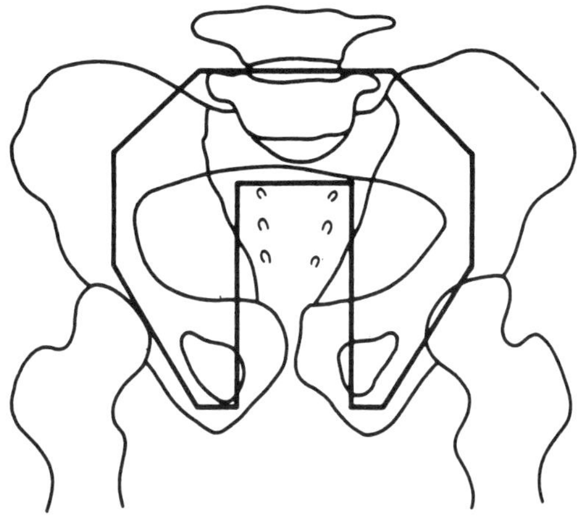

Figure 42.5. Portals employed for parametrial boost after completion of whole pelvis external beam and intracavitary irradiation. The central block shields the tissue that has received high-dose irradiation from the intracavitary insertion. Unilateral parametrial involvement may indicate treatment to only the involved half of this pelvic field.

Low-Dose Rate Brachytherapy

Historically, radium-226 (^{226}Ra) has been the radioisotope most frequently used in gynecologic brachytherapy systems. It has widely been replaced by cesium-137 (^{137}Cs) because of inherent problems with shielding and radiation protection. Sources are contained in inert tubes, which fiter out the non-therapeutic alpha radiations of ^{226}Ra and beta radiations of ^{137}Cs.

One mg of ^{226}Ra encapsulated in 0.5 mm platinum emits 8.25 R h^{-1} at a distance of 1 cm from the source. The activity of radioactive sources used in gynecologic brachytherapy is expressed in milligram radium equivalent (mg Ra eq). This is the amount of isotope that will deliver a dose rate equivalent to the specified amount of radium. Standard ^{137}Cs sources contain 5, 10, 15, 20 or 25 mg Ra eq.

The isotope sources are designed to fit into holding devices, which are inserted into the uterus, cervix or vagina. The holding apparatus is usually

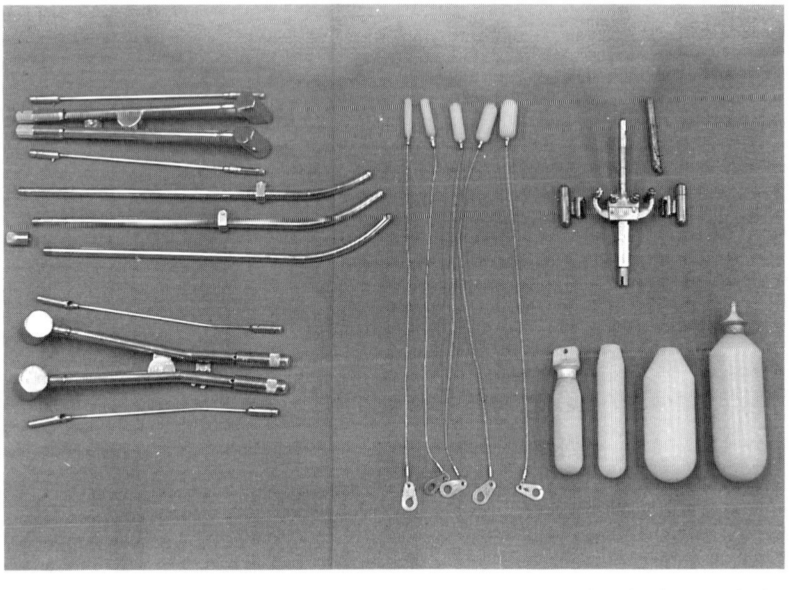

Figure 42.6. Some intracavitary applicators frequently employed in gynecologic brachytherapy. Left, top to bottom: miniovoids designed to fit a small vaginal apex; intrauterine tandems of varying curvature; Fletcher–Suit afterloading apparatus. Center: Holter–Heyman uterine capsules. Right, top to bottom: Ernst applicator; Burnett vaginal cylinders of varying diameter.

inserted in the operating room under general anesthesia, and radiopaque 'dummy' sources employed to confirm adequate placement of the apparatus on orthogonal radiographs. The actual radioactive sources are inserted or afterloaded in the patient's room. Afterloading techniques cut down considerably on radiation exposure to hospital personnel. The use of remote afterloading brachytherapy devices for low dose rate (LDR) brachytherapy even further reduces the radiation exposure of hospital personnel (Grigsby *et al.*, 1991). In addition, multiple isodose plans can be computer-generated, showing the effect of varying the activity, spacing or number of sources. This 'preplanning' allows the radiation oncologist to select the optimal source loading in terms of dose distribution to the target structures and critical normal tissues before any sources are actually placed in the patient.

Over the years, many different applicators have been designed for administration of gynecologic brachytherapy. Some commonly used LDR brachytherapy applicators are shown in *Figure 42.6*. Each is different in geometry, and therefore each offers unique dosimetric considerations. The radiation oncologist must be thoroughly familiar with the system with which he/she is working and employ the techniques and dosimetry calculations specific to that system (Delclos *et al.*, 1978; Haas *et al.*, 1985). The risk of failing to do so is overdosage of critical pelvic structures, with increased late complications, or underdosage of disease.

The most commonly used afterloading apparatus is the Fletcher–Suit–Delclos. It consists of an intrauterine tandem and vaginal colpostats modified for afterloading. The tandem is a curved hollow steel tube, about 6 mm in diameter, which is inserted into the uterine cavity. Various curvatures are available, the choice depending on the patient's anatomy. A tandem of greater curvature is generally employed in treating larger uterine cavities. Ideal placement of the tandem is in the sagittal plane of the pelvis midway between the pelvic side-walls, laterally and between the pubic symphysis anteriorly and sacral promontory posteriorly. This geometry results in symmetric dose distribution to each pelvic side-wall. The longer the tandem, the better the dose distribution laterally to the parametria and pelvic side-walls, and the tandem is therefore inserted to the full length of the uterine cavity for maximal source loading.

Radioactive sources contained in nylon or plastic tubing are afterloaded into the tandem. The tandem is held in place by a keeled flange, which is placed against the external os of the cervix. Further stabilization is achieved by gauze packing around the flange.

Afterloading colpostats, or ovoids, are inserted into each vaginal fornix. The long axis of the ovoid and the radioactive source it contains lie in the anteroposterior plane. An ideal placement geometry has the colpostats perpendicular to the axis of the tandem and bisected by the tandem, as depicted in

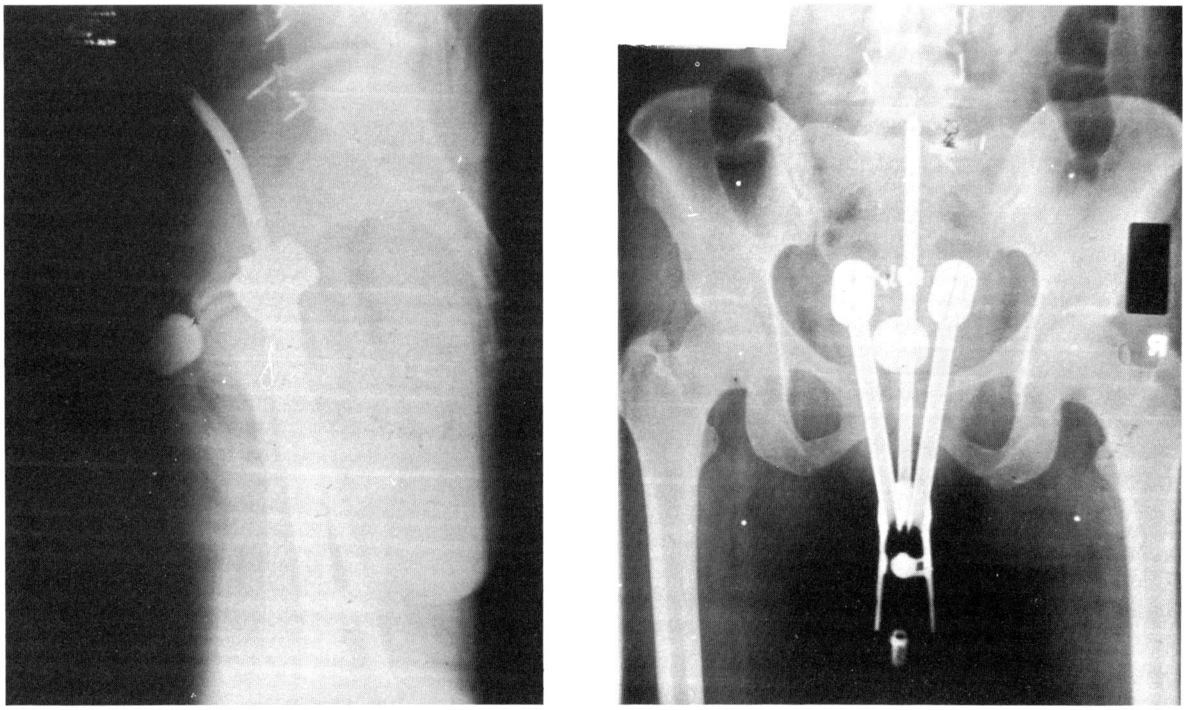

Figure 42.7. Lateral and anteroposterior views of a Fletcher–Suit brachytherapy application in a patient with carcinoma of the cervix.

Figure 42.7. This geometry is most readily maintained by employing a yoke to hold the tandem and ovoid handles in alignment with one another as they protrude from the vaginal introitus.

Colpostats may contain lead or tungsten shielding medially at each end to lessen the dose received by the bladder and rectum. Further protection of the bladder and rectum is accomplished by careful packing of gauze above and below the colpostats, thereby increasing the distance between the sources and these structures.

Variously sized colpostats are available, and generally the largest pair that can be inserted comfortably with good geometric placement is employed. This takes advantage of the inverse square law, which states that for a point source, the intensity of radiation at any distance from the source varies inversely with the square of the distance. This results in a higher depth dose for a given mucosal dose. Minicolpostats are available for use in very narrow vaginas, but often do not contain protective lead shielding. Once inserted, the colpostats are spread out for maximal separation in order to improve lateral dose distribution. This further decreases the bladder and rectal dose.

Improved dose distribution to the uterine body in patients with inoperable endometrial carcinoma can be achieved through the use of stainless steel capsules containing radioactive sources (Heyman *et al.*, 1941). The capsules are inserted into the uterine cavity, stretching the uterus to attain a more homogeneous dose across the myometrium to the serosa. The use of a tandem along with the capsules improves the dose distribution in the lower uterine segment and the parametrium. Capsules are available in varying diameters and are typically loaded with 5 mg Ra eq for capsules of smaller diameter and up to 10 mg Ra eq for larger diameters. The classic Heyman capsules have been modified for afterloading.

The uterus should be large enough to accommodate a minimum of six capsules for this technique. Care must be taken not to perforate the uterine wall on insertion. The capsules must be numbered and should be removed in the reverse sequence from their insertion.

Vaginal lesions are treated with intravaginal hollow cylinders afterloaded with radioactive sources. The dose is prescribed both to the vaginal mucosa and to a specified depth. Cylinders are available in a variety of diameters and may contain lead shielding to protect the bladder, rectum and select portions of the vaginal wall. Sources are loaded into the hollow central core of the cylinder and lie along the long axis of the vagina. Newer cylinders have been developed that place a single source at the vaginal apex perpendicular to the long axis of the vagina, improving the dose distribution at the apex.

Interstitial implants or radioactive material inserted directly into the vagina, cervix or parametria, are sometimes employed instead of, or in addition to, external beam or intracavitary techniques (Prempree, 1983). Various isotopes have been used including ^{226}Ra, ^{137}Cs, and iridium-192 (^{192}Ir). Most commonly, ^{226}Ra and ^{137}Cs are contained in metallic needles and ^{192}Ir wire or seeds are contained within plastic tubing. ^{192}Ir has gained favor over the years because of its afterloading capability and greater flexibility of use.

Needles are inserted into the cervix along its long axis or into the parametria through the vaginal fornices. Single or double plane implants may be used depending on the volume of tissue to be irradiated. Interstitial implants employing perineal templates have also been used (Aristizabel *et al.*, 1983; Martinez *et al.*, 1985; Syed and Puthwala, 1987).

High-Dose Rate Brachytherapy

HDR remote afterloading brachytherapy systems are gaining wide acceptance and changing the traditional approach to gynecologic brachytherapy. These systems have been used extensively in Japan and Europe over the past two decades (Inoue *et al.*, 1978; Shigematsu *et al.*, 1983; Teshima *et al.*, 1987; Shu–Mo *et al.*, 1991; Chen *et al.*, 1991; Arai *et al.*, 1992), and are now increasingly available in the USA. They employ single very high activity ^{60}Co or ^{192}Ir sources, which are driven into the brachytherapy applicator by remote control through hollow tubes connecting the applicator to the treatment unit. *Figure 42.8* shows a widely used HDR treatment unit. Treatment is delivered in a matter of minutes as the source is placed through programmed stops and dwell times in the applicator device before being automatically retracted back into the machine safe.

Advantages of this technique are many. There is the complete elimination of radiation exposure to all personnel. Short treatment time allows most patients to be treated on an outpatient basis, thus increasing patient convenience and reducing hospital costs. The geometry of the applicator is fixed within the patient during treatment, and patient movement is an unlikely problem with such short treatment times. There is much greater flexibility for optimization of the computer-generated treatment plan because of the infinite possible manipulations of source dwell times and stopping positions (Houdek *et al.*, 1991). Medical complications from prolonged bed rest necessary with LDR applications, such as deep vein thrombosis and pulmonary embolus, are essentially eliminated.

Initial experiences with HDR brachytherapy saw unacceptably high late complication rates (Shigematsu *et al.*, 1983; Shu–Mo *et al.*, 1989), and much work has been done to define HDR protocols that result in equivalent tumor control rates and comparable complication rates to the conventional LDR regimens (Gupta *et al.*, 1989; Fu and Phillips, 1990; Brenner *et al.*, 1991; Roman *et al.*, 1991; Patel *et al.*, 1994). Modifications in technique and treatment planning are still evolving. This evolution has seen wide variations in technique, dose fractionation and delivery, leading to the formulation of consensus guidelines for HDR brachytherapy by the Clinical Research Committee of the American Endocuriertherapy Society (Nag *et al.*, 1993). Even so, wide variation from institution to institution still exists, making data comparison difficult.

Careful consideration of time–dose–fractionation is critical to HDR treatment. Basic radiobiology relates late tissue complications to total dose delivered and dose per fraction. With treatment delivered at high dose rates, normal tissue repair of sublethal damage is hampered (Stitt *et al.*, 1992). Improving the therapeutic ratio in HDR brachytherapy compared to traditional LDR treatment requires a greater number of HDR treatment fractions and a reduction in dose delivered for an equivalent effect on the tumor and on late reacting tissues (Warmelink *et al.*, 1989; Fowler, 1990; Orton *et al.*, 1991). The relative radiobiologic disadvantage to late reacting tissues with fewer and larger HDR fractions may be offset to a certain degree by meticulous attention to techniques such as rectal retraction and packing of the rectum and bladder away from the sources (Fowler, 1990).

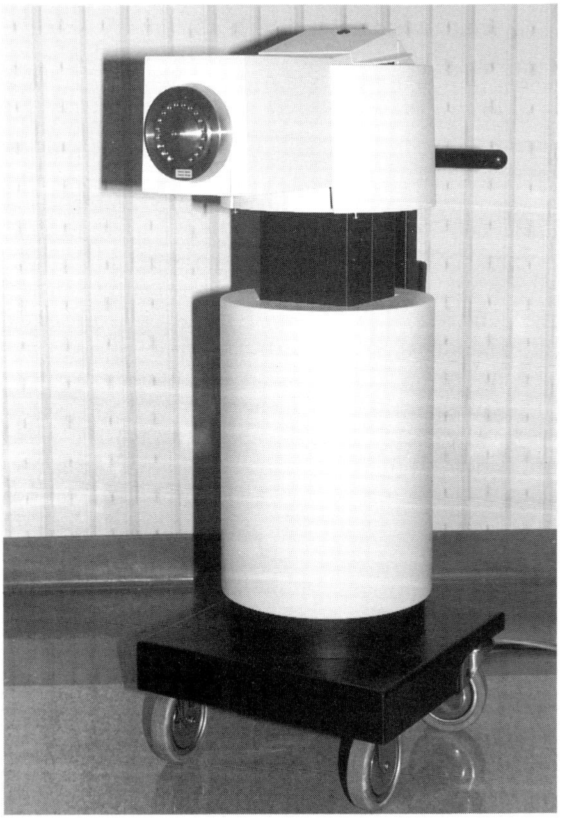

Figure 42.8. High dose rate treatment unit widely used in gynecologic brachytherapy.

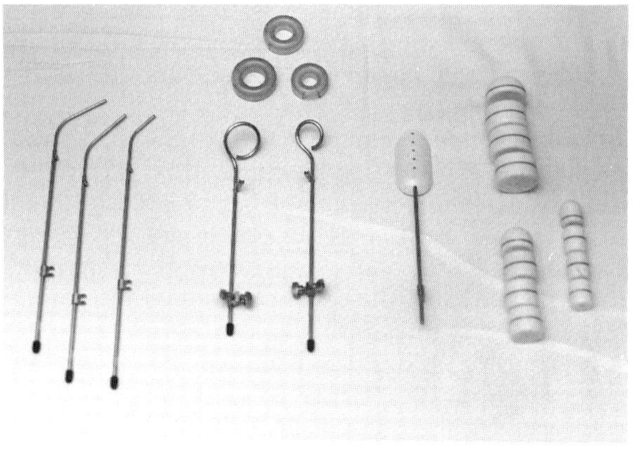

Figure 42.9. Commonly used high dose rate gynecologic applicators.

Modifications of the traditional LDR Fletcher–Suit applicator and vaginal cylinders have been developed for use in HDR brachytherapy. A ring applicator has been developed to replace the Fletcher ovoids improving the ease of applicator insertion and dosimetry. *Figure 42.9* shows some commonly used HDR gynecologic applicators.

HDR gynecologic applications can often be performed in the Radiation Oncology Department on an outpatient basis. The uterine tandem and ovoids or ring applicator are inserted under intravenous sedation, and once positioned, the applicator apparatus is locked in place to the treatment table, limiting patient movement. The very small diameter of the HDR tandem makes cervix dilatation unnecessary, and some departments insert a plastic sleeve into the cervix, which remains in place between applications and facilitates reinsertion of the tandem before each treatment fraction. A rectal retractor is attached to the applicator, and packing is inserted into the vagina to further displace the bladder and rectum from the HDR source. Orthogonal radiographs are taken from which computer dosimetry is performed.

Treatment Planning – Low Dose Rate Brachtherapy

The Paris (Baud, 1948), Stockholm (Heyman, 1935) and Manchester (Tod and Meredith, 1938) systems of intracavitary treatment planning form the historic basis for modern-day LDR brachytherapy methods. Individualized treatment plans patterned after the Manchester system prescribe to specific points of interest within the pelvis and are guided by tolerance of critical structures within the target volume.

The activity of the sources loaded into the tandem and ovoids and the duration of the application are determined by the geometry of the placement, the extent and location of disease, and the tolerance of the bladder and rectum. Isodose distributions from a typical LDR intracavitary application are depicted in *Figure 42.10*. With the aid of computer planning systems, the isodose distributions attained from various loadings can be predetermined and the doses to specific points of interest in the pelvis can be calculated (Maruyama *et al.*, 1976; Fletcher, 1980). Various loading possibilities can be tried by computer before deciding on the optimal source strength, distribution and time of application. When this is accomplished, the actual source strengths decided upon are loaded into the applicator.

In the commonly employed Manchester system, the points of interest within the pelvis important to treatment planning are designated A (right and left), B (right and left), P (right and left), bladder and rectum. Point A represents the paracervical triangle or the crossing point of the uterine artery with the ureter. By definition, it is located 2 cm above either the vaginal fornix or the cervical os and 2 cm lateral to the central uterine canal, following the axis of the uterus. Point B represents the obturator nodes and lies 2 cm cephalad from the cervical os and 5 cm to the right or left of midline. Thus the position of point B does not vary with displacement of the uterine body off the midline axis as with Point A. Point P represents the nodal chains at each pelvic side-wall and is located at the most lateral extent of the pelvic brim.

'Classic' loading of the Fletcher–Suit apparatus uses three sources of 15, 10, and 10 mg Ra eq in the uterine tandem and a 15 mg Ra eq source in each vaginal ovoid. This loading achieves a dose rate of 0.42 Gy h^{-1} at each Point A. The dose achieved at each Point B (right and left) is then approximately 25–33% of the dose received at each Point A, and the dose at each Point P (right and left) about 10–15% of the dose at each Point A. Care must be taken to ensure that the dose to the bladder or rectum from each brachytherapy application does not exceed about 80% of the dose to Point A and that the tolerance of these structures is not exceeded by

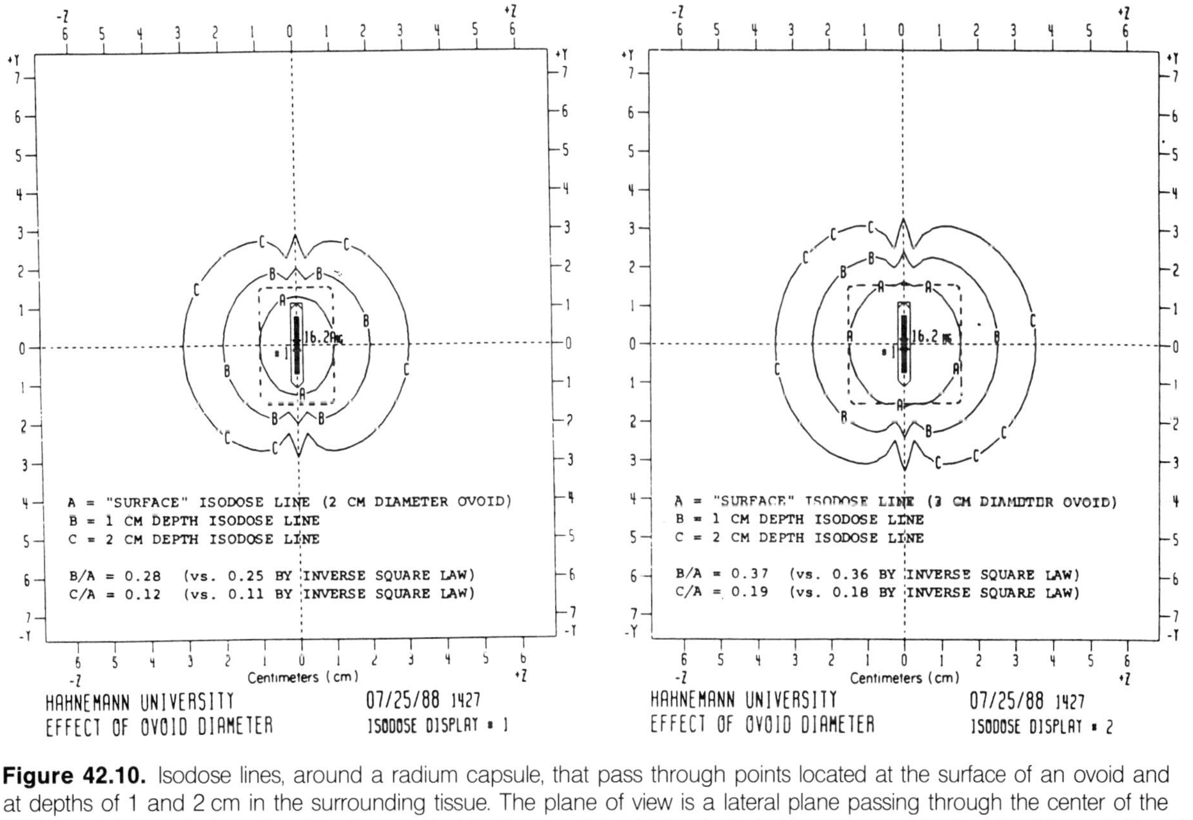

Figure 42.10. Isodose lines, around a radium capsule, that pass through points located at the surface of an ovoid and at depths of 1 and 2 cm in the surrounding tissue. The plane of view is a lateral plane passing through the center of the ovoid and does not show the distortion created by the special shielding included in some ovoids. Ovoids of 2 cm (left) and 3 cm (right) are depicted by dashed lines. The dose at depth is a higher percentage of the surface dose for a 3 cm diameter ovoid than for a 2 cm diameter ovoid. This is due to the effect of the inverse square law. The exact ratios are slightly different to those that would be obtained from simple inverse square law calculations because the source has a finite length. This illustrates the principle of achieving a more effective depth of treatment by increasing the ovoid diameter and using a stronger source or longer placement time. A = 'Surface' isodose line (2 cm diameter ovoid); B = 1 cm depth isodose line; C = 2 depth isodose line.

the combined contributions from brachytherapy and external beam treatment. The total bladder dose should not exceed 65–68 Gy, and the total rectal dose should be kept below 68–70 Gy.

The dose to Point A is determined primarily by the loading of the tandem sources, with bladder and rectal doses affected most by loading in the ovoids and distal tandem. Care should be taken to limit the duration of any single application to a maximum of 72 hours and the dose to the rectum to under 15 Gy and that to the bladder to 15–20 Gy.

Treatment Planning – High Dose Rate Brachytherapy

Most institutions using HDR brachytherapy have continued to prescribe treatment based on the traditional Manchester system using the same prescription points A, B and P. Differences in applicator geometry, isotope source and dose distribution between HDR and LDR systems have prompted some investigators to suggest modifications in the traditional LDR prescribing practice based on dose to Point A (Thomadsen *et al.*, 1992). In the Madison system, dose is prescribed instead to a Point M located 2 cm lateral to the uterine canal and 2 cm cephalad to a line joining the center dwell position of the vaginal colpostat or ring sources. Point E (right and left), the lateral pelvic wall, is located at the intersection of a horizontal line tangential to the most cephalad point of the acetabulae and a perpendicular line passing through the most medial aspect of the acetabulae. Bladder and rectal points are similarly redefined as in the location of the vaginal surface dose (SD). Dose fractionation and integration with external beam are determined by the extent of disease.

The single HDR source delivers the treatment by occupying multiple dwell positions within the applicator system for varying increments of 0.1 sec. By adjusting dwell positions employed and time the source spends at each selected position, the dosimetry can be optimized to a degree not possible with traditional LDR systems that use a much more limited choice of source activities, numbers and positions.

The Madison system developed by Stitt *et al.* (1992) employs about five weekly HDR applications, limiting the dose to the bladder and rectal points to no more than 83% Point M dose. As with LDR, the reliance on external beam irradiation increases with higher disease stage while the corresponding dose contribution from HDR brachytherapy decreases. Other institutions vary widely in their prescription points, dose specification and fractionation.

While there is still no consensus regarding actual treatment prescription, what has evolved are consensus guidelines for the development of a controlled and consistent policy within each individual institution calling for careful documentation of all treatment data and strict quality control (Nag *et al.*, 1993). Wherever possible, multiple HDR fractions are advisable. Localization films and dosimetry calculations are recommended for each fraction delivered as patient anatomy/applicator geometry can change significantly between applications. Doses to regions of interest as well as to critical structures should be recorded accurately with each application. Careful attention to applicator placement and normal tissue retraction are perhaps more important with HDR than with LDR applications. Policies and procedures are advised for all aspects of HDR brachytherapy including nursing care and sedation. Quality assurance programs are mandatory with documentation of daily machine and source checks as well as implementation of an emergency procedures program.

Sequelae of Radiation Therapy

The most frequent major complications of radiation therapy of gynecologic malignancies involved damage to the bowel and bladder. Complications have been graded according to severity (*Table 42.1*). Grade 1 complications are minor and self-limiting, responding to outpatient management. Grade 2 complications are often recurrent and may require hospitalization, but respond to medical management without the need for surgery. The most serious, life-threatening Grade 3 complications require surgical intervention. Grade 4 complications are lethal.

In a retrospective analysis of 811 patients treated with radiation alone for carcinoma of the uterine cervix, Perez *et al.* (1984) correlated the frequency of Grade 2 and 3 complications with total dose delivered by external beam and intracavitary applications. They found the overall incidence of Grade 2 complications to be 10% and Grade 3, 8%. The total dose from both external beam and intracavitary irradiation delivered to the pelvic organs was the most significant factor, with the incidence of Grade 2 or 3 complications rising sharply with doses of over 80 Gy. This must be weighed against the greater likelihood of pelvic control and decreased metastatic rate achieved with increasing doses of radiation (Perez *et al.*, 1988).

In addition to the impact of total dose, techniques used in the delivery of radiation therapy also have an impact on complications. Complications from external beam therapy relate to beam energy, total dose, volume irradiated and daily fractionation. High-energy beams offer optimal dose distribution to deep pelvic tissues. AP/PA techniques employing low energy beams are to be avoided.

Table 42.1. Complications of radiation therapy of gynecologic malignancies.

	Grade 1	*Grade 2*	*Grade 3*
Bowel	Diarrhea Rectal irritation	Proctitis Sigmoiditis Rectal ulceration Small bowel obstruction	Perforation Obstruction Severe rectal ulceration
Bladder	Irritation	Chronic cystitis	Severe bladder ulceration Hemorrhagic cystitis
Ureter	Irritation	Partial stricture	Complete stricture
Vagina	Irritation	Stenosis Vault necrosis	Fistula: rectovaginal vesicovaginal ureterovaginal
Other			Pulmonary embolus

In designing external beam protocols, shaped fields will allow exclusion of considerable normal tissue, thereby decreasing the potential for late tissue damage. Small bowel contrast can help determine bowel position and motility and allow field or dose modification to avoid toxicity (Green, 1983). Techniques to push small bowel loops out of the pelvis have been described and include bladder distension and treatment in the prone position with upward external pelvic pressure or a 'false tabletop' for anterior displacement of the bowel (Gunderson *et al.*, 1985).

The volume of tissue irradiated is directly related to complication rate. Extended field irradiation has been advocated to include the paraaortic lymph nodes either prophylactically or therapeutically. Multiple field techniques and doses of 45–50 Gy have been advocated (Rotman *et al.*, 1979). Jolles *et al.* (1986) have reported results of 42 patients without previous surgery treated with extended field irradiation for carcinoma of the cervix and showed severe complications, particularly to the small intestine and sigmoid colon. The severity of complications increased when doses over 45 Gy were employed to boost gross disease. Russell *et al.* (1987) reported results of a technique for extended field irradiation to the pelvis and paraaortic nodes delivering 56–61 Gy to sites of known nodal involvement with acceptable acute and late morbidity.

Intracavitary applications may contribute to the development of late complications if careful attention is not paid to the applicator geometry, isotope loading, and bladder and rectal doses. Lee *et al.* (1976) reported on the incidence of severe complications to the bladder, rectum or vagina, and correlated this with the dose rates and total doses to these organs from intracavitary applications. Clark *et al.* (1994) reported on rectal complications of a Phase I/II trial of patients with carcinoma of the cervix treated with concomitant cisplatinum and radiation therapy consisting of external beam and three fractions of HDR brachytherapy. They found the rectal reference point defined by the ICRU to be a good prognostic indicator of late complications. The actuarial rate of Grade 3 or 4 rectal complications was 46% in patients whose rectal dose exceeded that received by Point A versus 14% where the rectal dose was less than the prescribed Point A dose.

Careful packing around the ovoids increases the source to mucosal distance, thus reducing the dose received by the bladder and rectum. The use of a protruding source at the external cervical os will increase bladder and rectal dose, leading to an increased complication risk. Good lateral separation of ovoids and the use of the largest ovoids that can be inserted for good geometry will optimize the dose to lateral pelvic structures without overdosing the bladder and rectum. Wherever possible, ovoids with shielding for the bladder and rectum should be employed. HDR ring applicators have been modified with the incorporation of tungsten for rectal shielding (Hetzel and McCoy, 1989), and a rectal retractor can be attached to the tandem/ring apparatus.

The type of applicator employed is important to the development of late tissue damage. Use of the rigid Ernst applicator has been related to excessive vaginal fistula formation (Rotman *et al.*, 1978). When patient anatomy was less than ideal, as with a small, atrophied or scarred vagina or with bulky tumor at the vaginal apex, bladder and rectal doses were increased. This occured because of downward displacement of the applicator system or poor lateral separation of the vaginal sources. Aristizabel *et al.* (1987) have reported a significantly higher complication rate for patients with Stage IIB carcinoma of the cervix treated with interstitial parametrial implants as opposed to conventional intracavitary irradiation, which resulted in no increase in pelvic control of disease.

Various high-risk factors are associated with an increased risk of late radiation complications, and when present may warrant a planned reduction in total dose. Advanced age, hypertension, anemia, poor nutritional status, diabetes mellitus and obesity have all been correlated with increased complications and poor outcome. A history of previous abdominal or pelvic surgery or of pelvic inflammatory disease, colitis or diverticulitis is likewise associated with an increase in complications (Unal *et al.*, 1981).

When surgery is employed in addition to radiation therapy, complication rates rise. Laparotomy causes an increased risk of bowel complications due to the development of adhesions that fix the bowel (Powel–Smith, 1965). Extent of surgery is also important. Radical hysterectomy with lymphadenectomy as opposed to simple extrafascial hysterectomy, in conjunction with radiation therapy, increases late complications (Rotman *et al.*, 1979). Paraaortic lymph node dissection, when employed, should be by the retroperitoneal approach. Biopsies performed because of suspicion of recurrent disease after definitive irradiation may lead to fistula formation and should be avoided wherever possible.

When chemotherapy is used in conjunction with radiation therapy, complications may occur earlier, with increased severity and at lower than expected radiation doses. Modifications in dose of radiation or chemotherapeutic agent may be necessary when these modalities are used together (Phillips and Fu, 1976).

The tumor grade and extent of disease are also major factors in determining the nature and degree of late complications (Nori *et al.*, 1987). Stage III or IV disease requires high-dose pelvic irradiation for control, and increasing doses correlate directly with complications (Barber, 1979). In recurrent disease, additional irradiation or surgical exenteration for attempted salvage is accomplished only with a very high morbidity risk, and the five-year survival statistics are poor for pelvic failures (local tumor recurrence) (Shingleton *et al.*, 1983).

It may be quite difficult to determine whether a complication is secondary to treatment or is a consequence of recurrent disease. In advanced disease, recurrent or persistent tumor is the more likely cause of post-treatment ureteral obstruction. In early-stage disease, radiation is implicated more often and is related to the total dose to Point A and the addition of surgery to the treatment regimen (Bahrassa and Ampil, 1987).

Future Prospects in Radiation Therapy

Three-Dimensional Treatment Planning and Conformal Dose Delivery

The use of 3D reconstructed images in radiation therapy treatment planning is a rapidly evolving new technology with the potential of significantly increasing the therapeutic ratio. The subject has recently been thoroughly reviewed by Lichter and Ten Haken (1994). The technique allows comprehensive visualization of the 3D anatomy of both tumor and normal tissue in terms of their extent, proximity and spatial relationships.

The traditional coplanar beam arrangements are dictated by treatment planning limited by the use of a single transaxial CT slice. Use of multiple noncoplanar crossfiring beams is possible only when 3D visualization is possible. Noncoplanar beams can then be directed so as to deliver a dose distribution that conforms to the shape of the target volume. The beam's eye view (BEV) feature of 3D planning systems allows one to view target and normal structures from any angle and to design customized blocking with much greater accuracy. Dosimetric calculations can now be performed in 3D, and the dose distributions molded by use of noncoplanar beams and customized blocking. This increased accuracy of dose delivery conforming to the target volume in 3D in turn should allow escalation of tumor doses with respect to surrounding normal tissue and also avoid geographic miss.

Technical improvements in block construction are now in progress with the development of multileaf collimator systems. These paired lead leaves located in the head of the treatment machine are directed by computer to assume the appropriate shape, and can alter their positions during treatment, eliminating the need for conventional block cutting or for treatment interruption for manual block changes.

3D treatment planning has been applied to intracavitary gynecologic implants employing a CT-compatible applicator and a CT-based treatment planning system with 3D capability (Schoeppel *et al.*, 1994). This technique demonstrated the delivery of much higher bladder and rectal doses than predicted by conventional dosimetry methods and the delivery of lower doses to the cervix than classically estimated by Point A dose.

There is no doubt that the advent of 3D treatment planning and conformal dose delivery has the potential of dramatically changing the field of radiation oncology. At this time, the technology is extremely labor intensive and time consuming, making the techniques currently available impractical for use in most patients. It still remains to be seen whether the theoretic improvement in therapeutic ratio is realized in clinical practice, justifying the expense and effort. The ultimate goal is the dynamic integration of computerized 3D treatment planning with computer-controlled conformal therapy. All manipulation of the treatment machine, collimator shape, beam energy, table and gantry angles, would be computer-driven in real time during delivery of treatment.

Hyperthermia

Much research effort has been directed at the use of hyperthermia in combination with radiation therapy to enhance cytotoxicity. Biolgoic evidence indicates that these modalities have synergistic and complementary effects on cell killing (Emami and Song, 1984; Kim, 1984). Cells in late S phase are most sensitive to heat-induced chromosome damage, while cells in G_1 phase are most resistant to heat damage (Dewey *et al.*, 1980). This is the opposite of the situation with conventional irradiation. Unlike radiation, the ability of hyperthermia to cause cell killing is not affected by hypoxia (Harisiadis *et al.*, 1975; Dewey *et al.*, 1980) and is enhanced by low pH (Gerweck, 1977) and nutritional deprivation. Hyperglycemia induction has been shown to lower tumor pH and may therefore offer a degree of tumor sensitization to hyperthermia (Thistlethwaite *et al.*, 1987). Lastly, hyperthermia enhances cell killing by radiation by inhibiting repair of sublethal damage (Ben–Hur *et al.*, 1974) and potentially lethal damage (Li *et al.*, 1976).

A minimum tumor temperature of 43°C appears optimal, and heating sessions of 30–90 minutes are employed in most trials. The development of thermal tolerance has prompted many trials designed to determine the best sequencing and treatment schedules of radiation therapy and hyperthermia sessions (Luk *et al.*, 1984). Radiation dose schedules have varied from daily to biweekly, and ongoing trials are under investigation. There have been several trials that looked at the optimal number of hyperthermia sessions. The randomized Radiation Therapy Oncology Group (RTOG) trial 81-04 showed no impact of number of hyperthermia treatment sessions on complete response rate in patients with superficial tumors treated with radiation alone versus radiation and hyperthermia (Perez *et al.*, 1989). Kapp *et al.* (1990) found no difference in outcome using two versus six hyperthermia treatment sessions, and Emami *et al.* (1992) found similar results comparing one versus two sessions.

Further research is being directed at the development of refined techniques for optimal temperature measurement and heat delivery. Microwave heating has been employed in multiple clinical trials using 433, 915 and 2450 MHz frequencies, but problems with poor tissue penetration have limited clinical application to superficial tumors. Efforts to develop deep heating microwave systems are continuing (Samulski *et al.*, 1987). Radiofrequency heating at 13.56 and 27.17 MHz, as well as ultrasound frequency heating at 0.5–3.0 MHz, have also been employed.

Research is also aimed at the integration of interstitial hyperthermia with brachytherapy (Prionas *et al.*, 1994). Hyperthermia can be delivered through the same catheters used for interstitial brachytherapy both immediately before insertion or after the removal of the radioactive sources. Continuous heating to 41°C with HDR brachytherapy appears to result in significant radiation sensitization and may further improve the therapeutic ratio in HDR treatments (Armour *et al.*, 1994).

As pointed out by Brady and Seegenschmiedt (1987), hyperthermia in addition to radiation has consistently resulted in improved response rates in clinical trials. This is seen in spite of numerous variables, including number of heating sessions per week, temperatures achieved, duration of heating, equipment employed, and time–dose–fractionation of the radiation therapy.

Altered Dose–Fractionation Schedules

Limitations in the radiocurability of tumors when conventional schedules of 1.8–2.0 Gy per fraction, five fractions per week, are employed has prompted investigation of altered fractionation schemes (Thames *et al.*, 1983; Fowler, 1984). Hyperfractionation refers to the delivery of multiple daily reduced-dose fractions with no change in overall treatment time, thus resulting in a greater total dose delivery. Accelerated fractionation reduces overall treatment time by delivering multiple daily fractions to conventional total doses. Hypofractionation employs higher than conventional doses per fraction at less frequent intervals.

Each schedule offers potential advantages and disadvantages. While hypofractionation may offer a more convenient treatment schedule, its use is limited because of increased late complications in normal tissues (Montague, 1968; Thames *et al.*, 1982). Furthermore, compromise in total dose delivered in an attempt to spare these tissues would likely result in decreased tumor control. Hypofractionation may, however, be an acceptable approach when used for palliation (Boulware *et al.*, 1979; Spanos *et al.*, 1987; Huilgol *et al.*, 1988).

Hyperfractionation or accelerated hyperfractionation schemes have gained more widespread acceptance and enthusiasm. They offer the theoretic advantages of allowing repair of normal tissue damage between fractions, while allowing tumor cell reoxygenation and redistribution. This would result in preferential tumor cell kill and lessen late tissue damage when smaller doses per fraction are employed. Hyperfractionation schemes therefore offer the potential of improved normal tissue tolerance, which is especially important in relapsed patients previously irradiated in whom additional radiation is contemplated or in patients who have had multiple surgical procedures or previous chemotherapy (Fein *et al.*, 1994).

Hyperfractionation additionally offers the potential advantage of allowing higher total doses of radiation therapy without increased normal tissue toxicity over conventional doses. This was recently the subject of a prospective Phase I/II study by the Radiation Therapy Oncology Group (Komaki *et al.*,

1994). This study delivered twice daily pelvic irradiation at 1.2 Gy per fraction followed by one or two intracavitary applications to patients with bulky carcinoma of the uterine cervix. Total parametrial doses 10% higher than those used in standard conventional once a day radiation therapy were tolerated and at least as effective as the standard regimen.

Optimizing the dose–fractionation schedule depending on tumor-associated factors and limiting normal tissue factors is the subject of ongoing trials. Cohen (1987) has attempted to employ computer-assisted planning strategies to determine the most effective treatment scheme by weighing all tumor-related and normal tissue variables.

Summary of Management Options

- It is essential that radiation oncologists have a full understanding of the anatomic relationships within the pelvis and are well-acquainted with the patterns of spread and failure of the tumor in question. Treatment should be directed to sites of known tumor extension with a margin of normal tissue, and may involve prophylactic irradiation of sites of potential subclinical nodal involvement.
- Ideal treatment employs megavoltage photon beams. Linear accelerators allow the treatment of deep pelvic structures with maximal sparing of skin and superficial tissue. With cobalt or linear accelerators in the low energy range of 4–10 MV, optimal dose distribution is usually attained by a four-field technique employing opposed anteroposterior and right and left lateral fields.
- Brachytherapy, or the placement of radioactive gamma-ray sources directly into or next to tumor-bearing structures, permits delivery of high doses of radiation over a short period of time to limited volumes of tissue.
- Brachytherapy may be the sole treatment mode for small carcinomas of the cervix that have little potential for nodal spread, or part of an integrated plan that includes external beam irradiation for more extensive disease.
- Interstitial implants, or radioactive material inserted directly into the vagina, cervix or parametria, are sometimes employed instead of or in addition to external beam or intracavitary techniques.
- High dose rate (HDR) remote afterloading brachytherapy systems are gaining wide acceptance and changing the traditional approach to gynecologic brachytherapy.
- Advantages of the HDR technique are many. There is complete elimination of radiation exposure to all personnel and short treatment time allows most patients to be treated on an outpatient basis.
- Various high-risk factors are associated with an increased risk of late radiation complications. Advanced age, hypertension, anemia, poor nutritional status, diabetes mellitus and obesity have all been correlated with increased complications and poor outcome.
- When surgery is used in addition to radiation therapy, complication rates rise. Laparotomy causes an increased risk of bowel complications due to the development of adhesions that fix the bowel. Extent of surgery is also important.
- When chemotherapy is used in conjunction with radiation therapy, complications may occur earlier, with increased severity and at lower than expected radiation doses.
- Limitations in the radiocurability of tumors when conventional schedules of 1.8–2.0 Gy per fraction, five fractions per week, are employed has promopted investigation of altered fractionation schemes.

References

■ Arai T, Hakano T, Morita S *et al.* (1992) High-dose-rate remote afterloading intracavitary radiation therapy for cancer of the uterine cervix: A 20-year experience. *Cancer* **69:** 75–179.

Aristizabel SA, Surwitt EA, Hevezi JM & Heusinkveld RS (1983) Treatment of advanced cancer of the cervix with transperineal interstitial irradiation. *Int. J. Radiat. Oncol. Biol. Phys.* **9:** 1013–1017.

■ Aristizabel SA, Woolfitt B, Valencia A, Ocampo G, Surwitt EA & Sim D (1987) Interstitial parametrial implants in carcinoma of the cervix stage II-B. *Int. J. Radiat. Oncol. Biol. Phys.* **13:** 445–450.

Armour EP, Wang Z, Corry PM, Chen PY & Martinez A (1994) Hyperthermic enhancement of high dose-rate irradiation in 9L gliosarcoma cell. *Int. J. Radiat. Oncol. Biol. Phys.* **28:** 171–177.

Bahrassa F & Ampil F (1987) Posttreatment ureteral obstruction in invasive carcinoma of the uterine cervix. *Int. J. Radiat. Oncol. Biol. Phys.* **13:** 23–28.

Barber HRK (1979) Management of failures and complications of cancer of the cervix. *Int. J. Radiat. Oncol. Biol. Phys.* **5:** 2143–2145.

Baud J (1948) Carcinoma of the cervix (Stage I) treated intracavitary with radium alone. *JAMA* **138:** 1138–1142.

Ben-Hur E, Elkind MM & Bronk BV (1974) Thermally enhanced radioresponse of cultured Chinese hamster cells. *Radiat. Res.* **58:** 38–51.

Boulware RJ, Caderao JB, Delclos L, Wharton JT & Peters LJ (1979) Whole pelvis megavoltage irradiation with single doses of 1000 rad to palliate advanced gynecologic cancers. *Int. J. Radiat. Oncol. Biol. Phys.* **5:** 333–338.

Brady LW & Seegenschmiedt HM (1987) Radiation therapy. *JAMA* **258:** 2285–2287.

Brady LW, Markow AM, DeEulis T & Lewis GC (1987a) Treatment of advanced and recurrent gynecologic cancer. *Cancer* **60:** 2081–2093.

■ Brady LW, Markoe AM, Micaily B, Damsker JI, Karlsson UL & Amendola BE (1987b) Clinical treatment planning in gynecologic cancer. *Front. Radiat. Ther. Onc.* **21:** 302–332.

Brenner DJ, Huang Y & Hall EJ (1991) Fractionated high dose-rate versus low dose-rate regimens for intracavitary brachytherapy of the cervix: Equivalent regimes for combined brachytherapy and external irradiation. *Int. J. Radiat. Oncol. Biol. Phys.* **21:** 1415–1423.

■ Chen M, Lin F, Hong C *et al.* (1991) High-dose-rate afterloading technique in the radiation treatment of uterine cervical cancer: 399 cases and 9 years experience in Taiwan. *Int. J. Radiat. Oncol. Biol. Phys.* **20:** 915–919.

Clark BG, Souhami L, Roman TN, Evans MD & Pla C (1994) Rectal complications in patients with carcinoma of the cervix treated with concomitant cisplatin and external beam irradiation with high dose rate brachytherapy: A dosimetric analysis. *Int. J. Radiat. Oncol. Biol. Phys.* **28:** 1243–1250.

Cohen L (1987) Optimization of dose-time factors for a tumor and multiple associated normal tissues. *Int. J. Radiat. Oncol. Biol. Phys.* **13:** 251–258.

Delclos L, Fletcher GH, Sampiere VS & Grant WH (1978) Can the Fletcher gamma ray colpostat system be extrapolated to other systems? *Cancer* **41:** 970–979.

Dewey WC, Freeman ML, Raaphorst GP *et al.* (1980) Cell biology of hyperthermia and radiation. In: Mayn RE & Withers HR (eds) *Radiation Biology in Cancer Research*, pp. 589–619. New York: Raven Press.

Emami B & Song CW (1984) Physiological mechanism in hyperthermia; a review. *Int. J. Radiat. Oncol. Biol. Phys.* **10:** 289–295.

Emami B, Myerson RJ, Cardenes H *et al.* (1992) Combined hyperthermia and irradiation in the treatment of superficial tumors: results of a prospective randomized trial of hyperthermia fractionation (1/wk vs 2/wk). *Int. J. Radiat. Oncol. Biol. Phys.* **24:** 145–152.

Fein DA, Morgan LS, Marcus RB Jr *et al.* (1994) Stage III ovarian carcinoma: An analysis of treatment results and complications following hyperfractionated abdominopelvic irradiation for salvage. *Int. J. Radiat. Oncol. Biol. Phys.* **29:** 169–176.

Fletcher GH (1980) Squamous cell carcinoma of the uterine cervix. In: Fletcher GH (ed) *Textbook of Radiotherapy*, pp. 720–733. Philadelphia: Lea & Febiger.

Fowler JF (1984) Nonstandard fractionation in radiotherapy. *Int. J. Radiat. Oncol. Biol. Phys.* **10:** 755–759.

Fowler JF (1990) The radiobiology of brachytherapy. In: Martinez AA, Orton CG & Mould F (eds) *Brachytherapy HDR and LDR*, pp. 121–135. Netherlands: Nucletron International BV.

Fu K & Phillips TL (1990) High-dose-rate intracavitary brachytherapy for carcinoma of the cervix. *Int. J. Radiat. Oncol. Biol. Phys.* **19:** 791–796.

Gerweck LE (1977) Modification of cell lethality at elevated temperatures: the pH effect. *Radiat. Res.* **70:** 224–235.

Green N (1983) The avoidance of small intestine injury in gynecologic cancer. *Int. J. Radiat. Oncol. Biol. Phys.* **9:** 1385–1390.

Grigsby PW, Perez CA, Eichling J, Purdy J & Slessinger E (1991) Reduction in radiation exposure to nursing personnel with the use of remote afterloading brachytherapy devices. *Int. J. Radiat. Oncol. Biol. Phys.* **20:** 627–629.

Gunderson LL, Russell AH, Llwellyn HJ, Doppke K & Tepper JE (1985) Treatment planning for colorectal cancer: Radiation and surgical techniques and value of small-bowel films. *Int. J. Radiat. Oncol. Biol. Phys.* **11:** 1379–1393.

Gupta BD, Ayyagari S, Sharma SC *et al.* (1989) Carcinoma of the cervix: Optimal time-dose fractionation of HDR brachytherapy and comparison with conventional dose-rate brachytherapy. In: Mould RF (ed) *Brachytherapy 2*, pp. 307–308. Netherlands: Nucletron International BV.

Haas JS, Dean RD & Mansfield CM (1985) Dosimetric comparison of the Fletcher family of gynecologic colpostats 1950–1980. *Int. J. Radiat. Oncol. Biol. Phys.* **11:** 1317–1321.

Harisiadis L, Hall EJ, Kraljevic U & Borek C (1975) Hyperthermia: biological studies at the cellular level. *Radiology* **117:** 447–452.

Henderson RH, Parsons JT, Morgan L & Million RR (1984) Elective ilioinguinal lymph node irradiation. *Int. J. Radiat. Oncol. Biol. Phys.* **10:** 811–819.

Hetzel H & McCoy M (1989) Rectal screens for the ring applicator for Selectron LDR/HDR afterloading system. In: Mould RF (ed) *Brachytherapy 2*, pp. 136–141. Netherlands: Nucletron International BV.

Heymàn J (1935) The so-called Stockholm method and the results of treatment of uterine cancer at the Radiumhemmet. *Acta Radiol.* **16:** 129–147.

Heyman J, Reuterwall O & Benner S (1941) The Radiumhemmet experience with radiotherapy in cancer of the corpus of the uterus; classification, method of treatment and results. *Acta Radiol.* **22:** 11–98.

Houdek PV, Schwade JG, Abitbol AA *et al.* (1991) Optimization of high dose-rate cervix brachytherapy; Part I: Dose distribution. *Int. J. Radiat. Oncol. Biol. Phys.* **21:** 1621–1625.

Huilgol NG, Mehta AR, Kulkarni V, Selvaraj N & Trivedi N (1988) Hypofractionated external radiation with high and low dose rates in the treatment of advanced cancer of the cervix. *Int. J. Radiat. Oncol. Biol. Phys.* **14:** 577–579.

International Commission on Radiation Units and Measurements (ICRU) Report #38 (1985) *Dose and Volume Specification for Reporting Intracavitary Therapy in Gynecology*, pp. 1–16. Bethesda, MD: ICRU.

Inoue T, Hori S, Miyata Y, Ozeki S & Shigematsu Y (1978) High versus low dose rate intracavitary irradiation of carcinoma of the uterine cervix – A preliminary report. *Acta Radiol. Oncol.* **17:** 277–282.

Jolles CJ, Freedman RS, Hamberger AD & Horbelt DV (1986) complications of extended-field therapy for cervical carcinoma without prior surgery. *Int. J. Radiat. Oncol. Biol. Phys.* **12:** 179–183.

Kapp DS, Peterson IA, Cox RS *et al.* (1990) Two or six hyperthermia treatments as an adjunct to radiation therapy yield similar tumor responses. Results of a randomized trial. *Int. J. Radiat. Oncol. Biol. Phys.* **19:** 1481–1495.

Kim JH (1984) Combined hyperthermia and radiation therapy in cancer treatment: Current status. *Cancer Invest.* **2(1):** 69–80.

■ Komaki R, Pajak TF, Marcial VA *et al.* (1994) Twice-daily fractionation of external irradiation with brachytherapy in bulky carcinoma of the cervix: Phase I/II study of the Radiation Therapy Oncology Group 88-05. *Cancer* **73:** 2619–2625.

Lee KH, Kagan AR, Nussbaum H, Wollin M, Winkley JH & Norman A (1976) Analysis of dose, dose-rate and treatment time in the production of injuries by radium treatment for cancer of the uterine cervix. *Br. J. Radiol.* **49:** 430–440.

Li CG, Evans RC & Hahn GM (1976) Modification and inhibition of repair of potentially lethal X-ray damage of hyperthermia. *Radiat. Res.* **67:** 491–501.

Lichter AS & Ten Haken RK (1994) Three-dimensional treatment planning and conformal radiation dose delivery. Principles & Practice of Oncology: PPO updates. **8:** 1–12.

Ling CC, Schell MC, Working KR *et al.* (1987) CT assisted assessment of bladder and rectum dose in gynecological implants. *Int. J. Radiat. Oncol. Biol. Phys.* **13:** 1577–1582.

Luk KH, Francis ME, Perez CA & Johnson RJ (1984) Combined radiation and hyperthermia: comparison of two treatment schedules based on data from a registry established by the Radiation Therapy Oncology Group (RTOG). *Int. J. Radiat. Oncol. Biol. Phys.* **10:** 801–809.

Martinez A, Edmundson GK, Cox RS, Gunderson LL & Howes AE (1985) Combination of external beam and multiple-site perineal applicator (MUPIT) for treatment of locally advanced or recurrent prostatic, anorectal and gynecologic malignancies. *Int. J. Radiat. Oncol. Biol. Phys.* **11:** 391–398.

Maruyama Y, Nagell JR, Wrede De *et al.* (1976) Approaches to optimization of dose in radiation therapy of cervix carcinoma. *Radiology* **120:** 389–398.

Montague ED (1968) Experience with altered fractionation in radiation therapy of breast cancer. *Radiology* **90:** 962–966.

■ Nag S, Abitbol AA, Anderson LL *et al.* (1993) Concensus guidelines for high dose rate remote brachytherapy in cervical, endometrial, and endobronchial tumors. *Int. J. Radiat. Oncol. Biol. Phys.* **27:** 1241–1244.

Nori D, Hilaris BS, Tome M, Lewis JL, Birnbaum S & Fuks Z (1987) Combined surgery and radiation in endometrial carcinoma: an analysis of prognostic factors. *Int. J. Radiat. Oncol. Biol. Phys.* **13:** 489–497.

■ Orton CG, Seyedsadr M & Somnay A (1991) Comparison of high and low dose rate remote afterloading for cervix cancer and the importance of fractionation. *Int. J. Radiat. Oncol. Biol. Phys.* **21:** 1425–1434.

Patel FD, Sharma SC, Negi PS *et al.* (1994) Low dose rate vs. high dose rate brachytherapy in the treatment of carcinoma of the uterine cervix: A clinical trial. *Int. J. Radiat. Oncol. Biol. Phys.* **28:** 335–341.

Perez CA, Breaux S, Bedwinek JM *et al.* (1984) Radiation therapy alone in the treatment of carcinoma of the uterine cervix. II. Analysis of complications. *Cancer* **54:** 235–246.

Perez CA, Kuske RR, Camel HM *et al.* (1988) Analysis of pelvic tumor control and impact on survival in carcinoma of the uterine cervix treated with radiation therapy alone. *Int. J. Radiat. Oncol. Biol. Phys.* **14:** 613–621.

Perez CA, Gillespie B, Pajak T, Hornback NB, Emami B & Rubin P (1989) Quality assurance problems in clinical hyperthermia and their impact on therapeutic outcome: A report by the RTOG. *Int. J. Radiat. Oncol. Biol. Phys.* **16:** 551–558.

Phillips TL & Fu K (1976) Quantification of combined radiation therapy and chemotherapy effects on critical normal tissues. *Cancer* **37:** 1186–1200.

Powel-Smith C (1965) Factors influencing the incidence of radiation injury in cancer of the cervix. *J. Can. Assoc. Radiol.* **16:** 132–137.

Prempree T (1983) Parametrial implant in stage IIIB cancer of the cervix: III. A five-year study. *Cancer* **52:** 748–750.

Prionas SD, Kapp DS, Goffinet CR, Ben-Yosef R, Fessenden P & Bagshaw MA (1994) Thermometry of interstitial hyperthermia given as an adjuvant to brachytherapy for the treatment of carcinoma of the prostate. *Int. J. Radiat. Oncol. Biol. Phys.* **28:** 151–162.

Roman TN, Souhami L, Freeman CR *et al.* (1991) High dose rate afterloading intracavitary therapy in carcinoma of the cervix. *Int. J. Radiat. Oncol. Biol. Phys.* **20:** 921–926.

Rotman M & John MJ (1979) Para-aortic irradiation in cervical carcinoma. *Int. J. Radiat. Oncol. Biol. Phys.* **5:** 2139–2141.

Rotman M, John MJ, Roussis K *et al.* (1978) The intracavitary applicator in relation to complications of pelvic radiation – the Ernst system. *Int. J. Radiat. Oncol. Biol. Phys.* **4:** 951–956.

Rotman M, John MJ, Moon SH *et al.* (1979) Limitations of adjunctive surgery in carcinoma of the cervix. *Int. J. Radiat. Oncol. Biol. Phys.* **5:** 327–332.

■ Russell AH, Jones DC, Russell KJ *et al.* (1987) High dose para-aortic lymph node irradiation for gynecologic cancer: Technique, toxicity, and results. *Int. J. Radiat. Oncol. Biol. Phys.* **13:** 267–271.

Samulski TV, Kapp DS, Fessenden P & Lohrbach A (1987) Heating deep seated eccentrically located tumors with an annular array system: a comparative clinical study using two annular array operating configurations. *Int. J. Radiat. Oncol. Biol. Phys.* **13:** 83–94.

Schoeppel SL, LaVigne ML, Martel MK *et al.* (1994) Three-dimensional treatment planning of intracavitary gynecologic implants: Analysis of ten cases and implications for dose specification. *Int. J. Radiat. Oncol. Biol. Phys.* **28:** 277–283.

Sewchand W, Prempree T, Patanaphan V, Whitley NO, Heidtman B & Scott R (1982) Value of multi-planar CT images in interactive dosimetry planning of intracavitary therapy. *Int. J. Radiat. Oncol. Biol. Phys.* **8:** 639–646.

Sherouse GW, Naves JL, Varia MA & Rosenman J (1987) A spreadsheet program for brachytherapy planning. *Int. J. Radiat. Oncol. Biol. Phys.* **13:** 639–646.

Shigematsu Y, Hishiyama K, Masaki N *et al.* (1983) Treatment of carcinoma of the uterine cervix by remotely controlled afterloading intracavitary radiotherapy with high-dose rate: A comparative study with a low-dose rate system. *Int. J. Radiat. Oncol. Biol. Phys.* **9:** 351–356.

Shingleton HM, Gore H, Soong SJ *et al.* (1983) Tumor

recurrence and survival in stage IB cancer of the cervix. *Am. J. Clin. Oncol.* **6:** 265–272.

Shu–Mo C, Xiang–E W & Qi W (1989) High dose-rate afterloading in the treatment of cervical cancer of the uterus. *Int. J. Radiat. Oncol. Biol. Phys.* **16:** 335–338.

Spanos WJ, Wasserman T, Meoz R, Sala J, Kong J & Stetz J (1987) Palliation of advanced pelvic malignant disease with large fraction pelvic radiation and misonidazole: Final report of RTOG phase I/II study. *Int. J. Radiat. Oncol. Biol. Phys.* **13:** 1479–1482.

■ Stitt JA, Fowler JF, Thomadsen BR *et al.* (1992) High dose rate intracavitary brachytherapy for carcinoma of the cervix: The Madison system: I. Clinical and radiobiological considerations. *Int. J. Radiat. Oncol. Biol. Phys.* **24:** 335–348.

■ Syed AMN & Puthwala AA (1987) Interstitial–intracavitary 'Syed Neblett' applicator in the treatment of carcinoma of the cervix. In: Nori D & Hilaris BS (eds) *Radiation Therapy of Gynecological Cancer*, pp. 297–301. New York: Alan R. Liss, Inc.

Teshima T, Chatani M, Hata K & Inoue T (1987) High-dose rate intracavitary therapy for carcinoma of the uterine cervix: I. General figures of survival and complication. *Int. J. Radiat. Oncol. Biol. Phys.* **13:** 1035–1041.

Thames HD, Withers HR, Peters LJ & Fletcher GH (1982) Changes in early and late radiation responses with altered dose fractionation: implications for dose–survival relationships. *Int. J. Radiat. Oncol. Biol. Phys.* **8:** 219–226.

Thames HD, Peters LJ, Withers HR & Fletcher GH (1983) Accelerated fractionation vs hyperfractionation: Rationales for several treatments per day. *Int. J. Radiat. Oncol. Biol. Phys.* **9:** 127–138.

Thistlethwaite AJ, Alexander GA, Moylan DJ & Leeper DB (1987) Modification of human tumor pH by elevation of blood glucose. *Int. J. Radiat. Oncol. Biol. Phys.* **13:** 610–613.

Thomadsen BR, Shahabi S, Stitt JA *et al.* (1992) High dose rate intracavitary brachytherapy for carcinoma of the cervix: II. Procedural and physical considerations. *Int. J. Radiat. Oncol. Biol. Phys.* **24:** 349–357.

Tod MC & Meredith WJ (1938) A dosage system for use in the treatment of cancer of the uterine cervix. *Br. J. Radiol.* **11:** 809–824.

Unal A, Hamburger AD, Seski JC & Fletcher GH (1981) An analysis of severe complications of irradiation of carcinoma of the uterine cervix: treatment with intracavitary radium and parametrial irradiation. *Int. J. Radiat. Oncol. Biol. Phys.* **7:** 999–1004.

Warmelink C, Ezzell G & Orton C (1989) Use of a time–dose–fractionation model to design high dose-rate fractionation schemes. In: Mould RF (ed) *Brachtherapy 2*, pp. 41–48. Netherlands: Nucletron International BV.

Wilson CS & Hall EJ (1971) On the advisability of treating all fields at each radiotherapy session. *Radiology* **98:** 419–424.

Yu WS, Sagerman RH, Chung CT *et al.* (1982) Anatomical relationships in intracavitary irradiation demonstrated by computed tomography. *Radiology* **143:** 537–541.

43 Fundamentals of Chemotherapy

N S A Stuart

Introduction

Since the discovery in the 1940s, of the first active drugs for the treatment of cancer there has been a role for chemotherapy in the treatment of gynecologic malignancy. This role is, however, an evolving one in which new drugs continue to develop and in which old drugs develop new applications. Given this constant evolution it is impractical to attempt a definitive account of chemotherapy practice. The role of this chapter is to outline the principles that guide chemotherapy usage and may apply whatever the particulars of the treatment.

In attempting to understand the fundamentals of chemotherapy it is important to realize that its practice is largely an empirical art. Our knowledge of how best to use chemotherapy is based, almost entirely, on observation and the principles for its use have developed from this. The more theoretic considerations may help our understanding of chemotherapy and may guide the use of cytotoxic drugs and our development of new regimens, but are often secondary to more practical considerations.

Practical Considerations

In defining how and when to use chemotherapy it must be placed in the clinical context of the patient and her malignancy. Consideration needs to be given to the balance between the side-effects of treatment, symptom relief from tumor shrinkage, the possibility of long-term survival and the need to find better ways of managing the cancer patient. These factors can be hard to quantify, but undoubtedly play the major part in defining the proper use of chemotherapy.

Aims of Chemotherapy

In any patient having chemotherapy the benefits and side-effects need to be balanced to ensure that the benefits predominate. The possible benefits of chemotherapy may range from a permanent cure, as in some non-epithelial ovarian cancers, through a probability of temporary tumor remission, as in advanced epithelial ovarian cancer, to only a possibility of transient tumor shrinkage, as in recurrent sarcoma. The degree of side-effects that is acceptable depends, to a great extent, on the expected benefits. If cure is the aim of treatment, considerable short-term toxicity, as produced by intensive combination chemotherapy, is likely to be acceptable. Where short-term palliation is the aim, few if any side-effects are acceptable. Therefore, before deciding on chemotherapy the clinician must be clear on what is likely to be achieved in each particular patient. It must also be remembered that what is achievable can change as the disease evolves. Initial therapy may be aimed at cure, but if relapse occurs, for most malignancies cure is not possible although further chemotherapy may achieve remission and may be indicated. Similarly second-line chemotherapy may achieve a worthwhile remission in a patient who has had a long remission following first-line therapy, but patients resistant to first-line therapy are unlikely to respond to second-line therapy (Blackledge *et al.*, 1989) and this should therefore be considered experimental, with major toxicity being unacceptable.

Assessment of Response

There is no disease in which chemotherapy inevitably gives a response and there will always be patients whose tumors fail to respond. It is essential that these are identified as soon as possible so that ineffective treatment is stopped and alternative therapy substituted. Standard methods of evaluating tumor response are also essential for reporting clinical trials so that like can be compared with like. Criteria for defining response have been drawn up by several groups, but all are based on the work of Miller *et al.* (1981) for the World Health Organization. These determine response by the accurate measurement of tumor dimensions expressed as a proportion of pre-treatment values. Complete remission (CR) is defined as 'complete disappearance of all clinically detectable malignant disease.' All abnormal tests and scans should return to normal and this should be maintained for at least four weeks. Partial remission (PR) is defined as 'a 50% reduction in tumor area' (product of maximum perpendicular diameters) or in the sum of such products when multiple lesions are being assessed. This should also be maintained for at least four weeks. Progressive disease occurs when there is a 25% increase in tumor area, either overall or at any one site, or when any new site of malignant disease is shown. Static disease is when neither progression or response is seen.

The criteria of Miller *et al.* (1981) also define the sites of tumor that can be assessed accurately enough for them to be considered indicative of the effect of therapy on the tumor as a whole. For instance the progress of ascites or a pleural effusion is sufficiently variable for it not to be a reliable index of tumor response.

The problems of imaging gynecologic tumors are discussed in more detail in Chapter 37, but the principles are the same for all tumors. Clinicians using chemotherapy should be familiar with the criteria for tumor response and should use them when assessing patients during treatment. The response of patients to therapy should ideally be assessed after each course and at least after every second course.

Toxicity of Chemotherapy

Many factors combine to determine the extent of toxicity experienced by patients having chemotherapy. Some of these are under the control of the clinician and include the nature of the drugs used, the dose prescribed, the route of administration and the skill with which antiemetics and other adjuncts to therapy are used. Other factors depend on the patient, for example the patient's renal and hepatic function and age, whether the patient has had previous therapy and the patient's psychologic condition during therapy. These complex interactions make it difficult to predict the extent of toxicity that will occur, but some side-effects, although not inevitable, are sufficiently common to be considered as the normal side-effects of chemotherapy. These are discussed in more detail below. Other side-effects of chemotherapy are less common, and are usually a feature of specific drugs. These are summarized in *Table 43.1*.

Myelosuppression

Myelosuppression is the dose-limiting toxicity of most cytotoxic drugs. Maximum effect is usually around ten days after treatment, with recovery occurring by day 21–28. Leucopenia is most common, but thrombocytopenia is a characteristic toxicity of some drugs, notably carboplatin. Anemia often develops as a chronic toxicity after several courses of therapy. Patients who are neutropenic (neutrophil count $< 1.0 \times 10^9\ l^{-1}$) are at risk of spontaneous septicemia. Such septicemias, if due to gram-negative organisms, can progress rapidly and become life-threatening within hours. Any patient who has recently had chemotherapy and is febrile or has other signs of infection should be assumed to be septicemic. They should be admitted for immediate complete blood count and blood cultures and to start-broad spectrum intravenous antibiotics. Standard antibiotic combinations for use in this situation include piperacillin, azlocillin, ticarcillin or ceftazidime, usually in combination with an aminoglycoside (Klastersky, 1993). Septicemias due to gram-positive organisms are increasingly common and may require different antibiotics. In some patients antifungal therapy is required.

The introduction of G-CSF (granulocyte colony stimulating factor) and GM-CSF (granulocyte/macrophage colony stimulating factor) into routine clinical practice has modified the importance of neutropenia as a side-effect of chemotherapy. These drugs can reduce the incidence and duration of neutropenia following chemotherapy and therefore reduce, though not abolish, the incidence of infections (American Society of Clinical Oncology, 1994). As a consequence the dose intensity of chemotherapy may be increased, though only to a modest degree before other dose-limiting toxicity supervenes. Whether such higher doses are more effective remains to be determined (see below).

The prolonged myelosuppression that follows very high doses of chemotherapy can not be prevented even by colony stimulating factors (CSFs). In such cases autologous bone marrow transplantation (ABMT) has been used. This technique is widely used in hematologic malignancy, but has only recently been introduced into the treatment of gynecologic tumors. Its use, even as an experimental technique, is limited by its cost and the prolonged period of hospitalization required. A more recent development has been peripheral blood stem cell (PBSC) harvesting in which the bone marrow progenitor cells are harvested from the peripheral blood (Gianni *et al.*, 1989). This technique avoids the need for procedures under general anesthetic and leads to more rapid engraftment. It is possible to repeat this procedure on several occasions and it can even be done as an outpatient. The lower cost of PBSC harvesting is likely to lead to greater use of high-dose chemotherapy, initially in an experimental setting, and in time in routine clinical practice.

Nausea and vomiting

Nausea and vomiting are common side-effects of cytotoxic drugs. Many of the most active drugs in gynecologic malignancy (cyclophosphamide, ifosfamide, cisplatin and doxorubicin) have significant potential for producing emesis. The degree of emesis experienced is, however, greatly influenced by the skill and interest of the clinician in preventing this side-effect. Control of emesis has improved greatly in recent years and the introduction of the $5HT_3$ (5-hydroxy-tryptamine type-3) receptor antagonists (ondansetron, granisetron, tropisetron) has been a significant advance. When combined with dexamethasone as many as 80% of patients receiving cisplatinum have complete absence of vomiting

(Smith *et al.*, 1991), a significant improvement over combinations of previous agents. This superiority does not, however, apply universally. Following moderately emetogenic outpatient chemotherapy, $5HT_3$ antiemetics seem no better that the combination of dexamethasone and metoclopramide (Jones *et al.*, 1991). $5HT_3$ antiemetics are also of little benefit in preventing the delayed emesis that occurs 1–7 days following chemotherapy and which is a particular problem following cisplatinum. Such delayed emesis seems to have a different mechanism from immediate emesis (within 24 hours of treatment) and is an

Table 43.1. Side-effects of specific cytotoxic drugs. (This is not a comprehensive list of reported side-effects. It summarizes the drug-specific adverse effects that are common or severe and that the clinician should be aware of.)

Drug	*Type of effect*	*Comments*
Bleomycin	Pulmonary fibrosis	Largely dose related. Can be exacerbated by high concentrations of oxygen or by previous radiotherapy. Irreversible. Rarely severe enough to cause symptoms, but occasional cases are fatal.
	Skin pigmentation	More marked in flexures. May be patchy and unsightly. Exacerbated by sunlight. Resolves slowly following treatment.
	Raynaud's phenomenon	Usually when given in combination with vinblastine and cisplatinum. Unavoidable, but not inevitable; may be permanent. May be severe and disabling, particularly if the patient has outdoor work.
	Pyrexia/rigors	Occurs during or immediately after therapy. Rarely severe, treat symptomatically. Preventable by concurrent administration of intravenous hydrocortisone.
Cisplatinum	Renal damage	Fall in creatinine clearance is common during therapy, but not usually sufficient to prevent therapy. Preventable by maintaining saline diuresis. Very rarely symptomatic. Irreversible.
	Renal tubular damage	Causes hypomagnesemia by preventing tubular re-uptake by Mg^{2+} ions. May be profound and persistent. Exacerbated by aminoglycoside antibiotics and by frusemide.
	Audiotoxicity	Dose-related high-tone hearing loss. Common, not always symptomatic. Possibly preventable by infusion rather than bolus injection. Irreversible.
	Peripheral neuropathy	Unpredictable and of late onset. Mainly sensory. Occasional case severe enough to cause marked disability. Largely irreversible.
Cyclophosphamide	Renal damage	More likely with high-dose therapy. Shown by falling creatinine clearance. Preventable by forced diuresis. Irreversible.
	Urothelial damage	Dose related. Shown by hematuria. May be marked; can potentially cause bladder necrosis. Preventable by concomitant administration of mesna and by forced diuresis.
Doxorubicin	Cardiotoxicity	Irreversible, dose-related cardiac damage causing congestive cardiac failure. Rare if cumulative dose less than 450 mg m^{-2}.
Ifosfamide	Renal damage	As for cyclophosphamide.
	Urothelial damage	As for cyclophosphamide; mesna required as a routine part of therapy.
	Encephalopathy	Reversible syndrome of disorientation/confusion/coma. More likely with short duration of therapy and in patients with high creatinine and low albumin.
Methotrexate	Mucositis	Dependent on dose and duration of exposure (half-life). Largely preventable by alkalinization of urine (to promote excretion) and by administration of folinic acid following therapy. These are essential with high-dose methotrexate therapy.
	Renal damage	Same as for mucositis.
	Liver damage	Unpredictable liver damage shown by abnormal liver function tests. Reversible on stopping therapy.
Vincristine	Neuropathy	Dose related, but more common in older patients. Usually mixed motor and sensory peripheral neuropathy. May be predominantly autonomic with severe constipation. Slowly reversible.
	Muscle pain	Uncommon. Usually occurs acutely 1–3 days following injection. Rarely severe; self-limiting.
Vinblastine	As for vincristine	More tendency to myelosuppression.

unsolved therapeutic problem. Of the antiemetics available, dexamethasone seems to give the best relief.

Clinicians should also be aware of the need to prevent emesis and of the impossibility of abolishing anticipatory vomiting once it is established. Antiemetics should therefore be an integral part of any chemotherapy regimen and antiemetics should never be prescribed on an 'as required' basis. Whenever possible antiemetic policies should be used with defined first- and second-line antiemetics.

Alopecia

Reversible alopecia is common with many regimens used in gynecologic malignancy, particularly those containing doxorubicin (Adriamycin) or cyclophosphamide. Hair loss can also occur with most other cytotoxic drugs. There is no universally effective way of preventing this and patients must be prepared to accept the possibility of hair loss and should be provided with a wig. Scalp cooling can prevent the alopecia that occurs following doxorubicin, but is less effective in preventing it after drugs with a longer half-life (e.g. cyclophosphamide). It is also time-consuming and may be uncomfortable for the patient. Hair regrowth is usually adequate by six months after finishing therapy.

Extravasation

Some cytotoxic drugs are chemically irritant and cause severe tissue necrosis if extravasated at the site of intravenous injection. This necrosis may be sufficient to require skin grafting or even amputation. There are antidotes to the extravasation of some cytotoxics (Cox *et al.*, 1988), but meticulous injection technique is required in all patients having chemotherapy and such treatment should be given by trained staff.

Infertility

Most intensive cytotoxic regimens can impair fertility, but this is only of consequence in younger patients with curable malignancy. Younger patients with non-epithelial ovarian cancer commonly retain fertility despite chemotherapy as long as extensive surgery has been avoided. The nature of the malignancies in older patients means that they are more likely to require radical surgery, and this, rather than the chemotherapy, will determine whether fertility is retained.

Psychologic

The psychologic effects of chemotherapy are hard to quantify and have received less attention than the physical effects. There is no doubt that many patients receiving chemotherapy are depressed or anxious and the clinician should be aware of this possibility (McGuire *et al.*, 1980; Lloyd *et al.*, 1984). Psychologic morbidity will be influenced by many factors, including the extent of family and social support, the degree of rapport with nursing and medical staff, and the patient's premorbid personality. It will also be greatly affected by the patient's appreciation of their prognosis.

Summary of side-effects

In summary, chemotherapy can produce side-effects in any of the body's systems. Some side-effects are avoidable and should not occur with the proper use of these drugs; the impact of others can be reduced and clinicians must be aware of how to manage them when they arise; others are inevitable and patients must be prepared for their occurrence. In all cases, following discussion with the patient, toxicity must be weighed against the expected benefits of treatment.

Duration of Therapy

Having decided to commence chemotherapy the question is immediately raised of when treatment should be stopped. When evaluable or measurable disease is present this can guide treatment. If at any time disease progression is seen, even if only after one course, this is indicative of treatment failure and alternative therapy should be considered. When there is a response therapy should normally continue at least until maximum tumor response is seen. If therapy is being given with curative intent then most clinicians would give two or three courses beyond the time complete remission is documented. When given for palliation there is probably no benefit to the patient from continuing chemotherapy beyond the point of maximum benefit as determined both by tumor response and by relief of symptoms. When disease remains stable a beneficial effect of therapy can not be excluded, but it is unlikely that survival will be increased. In such cases, if symptomatic relief is achieved, therapy should be continued to the point of maximum benefit, but in many, no such benefit is demonstrable and in order to avoid toxicity, therapy should be stopped once a reasonable therapeutic trial has been given (two or three courses). In many patients there is no way of accurately evaluating the disease progress either by tumor measurement or by symptom relief. Such patients should probably not receive chemotherapy unless it is of proven benefit in their tumor type.

Two randomized trials in ovarian cancer have addressed the duration of chemotherapy (Hakes *et al.*, 1992; Bertelsen *et al.*, 1989). These have suggested that five or six cycles of treatment are equivalent, in terms of survival, to 10 or 12 – a finding that is consistent with data in other tumor types (Bonadonna *et al.*, 1985). Numbers in these studies were, however, small and their conclusion has been disputed by some (Gershenson *et al.*, 1992). However, any benefit from prolonged chemotherapy would appear to be small and has to be weighed against the cumulative toxicity of chemotherapy. Most clinicians would therefore stop treatment after six cycles (Williams, 1992). Randomized trials have also shown that there is also no benefit from maintenance chemotherapy that may also compromise the administration of active second-line treatment.

Contraindications and Modifications to Chemotherapy

Perhaps the only absolute contraindication to chemotherapy is when the patient refuses to give consent or is unable to do so. There are, however, many relative contraindications. Patients whose disease is known not to benefit from chemotherapy should not be treated routinely, but may be considered for inclusion in a Phase I or Phase II study if they express this wish. Some patients may have contraindications to specific drugs, but these may be circumvented or in some cases may be ignored. Renal failure is a contraindication to cisplatinum and ifosfamide therapy, the two most active agents in cervical cancer, but it is not uncommon for patients with this disease to present with hydronephrosis. If hydronephrosis is unilateral, chemotherapy can often be given safely, perhaps at a reduced dose for the first course. If tumor response occurs then renal function may improve, allowing subsequent courses to be given at full dose. Bilateral hydronephrosis can be relieved by insertion of percutaneous nephrostomies, allowing definitive treatment to be given. Patients may present with impaired hepatic function, but where this is due to the malignancy, treatment should still be considered. Drugs excreted via the liver may need to be given at reduced doses to avoid severe toxicity, but if tumor response occurs, liver function may rapidly improve, allowing treatment to continue at full dose.

Many patients present in poor general condition either due to the effects of malignancy or to pre-existing conditions such as age or chronic disease and these patients are less able to tolerate the side-effects of chemotherapy. When malignancy is the cause of the patient's poor condition, and the tumor is known to be chemosensitive, the best course may be to give a trial of therapy. It is not necessarily the case though, that less intensive therapy is indicated. This is likely to have a lower response rate and a longer time to response. Patients in poor condition need to have a rapid tumor response and the best course may be to combine standard therapy with intensive supportive care. It is notable, for example in ovarian cancer, that performance status (as measured by the WHO or Karnofsky scales) is not of independent prognostic significance (Swenerton *et al.*, 1985; Creasman *et al.*, 1990). When the patient is in poor condition for other reasons no improvement can be expected as a result of chemotherapy and dose reduction, the use of a less toxic therapy, or a decision to withhold active treatment may be indicated.

Theoretic Considerations

The practical considerations discussed above should define 'what' we are aiming to achieve in any particular patient. In determining 'how' to achieve our aims there are a number of background principles regarding the action of chemotherapy, which although not in themselves defining which treatment to use, need to be taken into account.

Mechanisms of Cytotoxic Action

The ultimate effect of all cytotoxic drugs is to cause the death of malignant cells and as such they can be considered as nonspecific cell poisons. The mechanisms by which they achieve this end are, however, various and *Table 43.2* groups the common cytotoxic agents according to their mechanism of action. It must be borne in mind, however, that this continues to be an active area of research. The mechanism of action of even long-standing cytotoxic drugs such as 5-fluorouracil is not entirely clear. Some cytotoxics have multiple actions and new mechanisms continue to be identified.

Many cytotoxic drugs cause cell death by disrupting deoxyribonucleic acid (DNA) and ribonucleic acid (RNA) synthesis. The alkylating agents and cisplatinum form cross-links between the two strands of DNA, while others become intercalated between the strands of DNA, preventing transcription of RNA. Etoposide, doxorubicin, mitozantrone and possibly other agents, cause cell death by binding to a key enzyme involved in DNA synthesis, topoisomerase II. This allows DNA double strand breaks to occur and prevents their repair. Other drugs inhibit the production of DNA and RNA by interfering with nucleic acid synthesis. The vinca alkaloids and paclitaxel have tubulin as their target site, disrupting either its polymerization into microtubules (vincas) or its depolymerization (paclitaxel).

Despite much work into the actions of cytotoxic drugs this knowledge is of limited clinical application. It is, for example, impossible to predict which drugs might be active in a particular tumor type or in a particular patient. This can only be determined by clinical assessment. Similarly many theoretically

Table 43.2. Chemotherapeutic agents grouped according to site of action.

Group	*Site of action*	*Mechanism of action*	*Drugs*
Alkylating agents	DNA	Cross-linkage of DNA Prevent DNA replication	Cyclophosphamide Melphalan Lomustine (CCNU) Chlorambucil Ifosfamide
Platinum drugs	DNA	As for alkylating agents	Cisplatinum Carboplatin
Topoisomerase inhibitors	DNA	Intercalate between strands of DNA inhibiting topoisomerase II and inhibiting DNA and RNA synthesis	Doxorubicin Daunorubicin Etoposide
Vinca alkaloids	Mitotic spindles	Cause mitotic arrest, prevent cell division	Vincristine Vinblastine Vindesine
Antimetabolites		Inhibition of pyrimidine synthesis, disruption of DNA and RNA synthesis	5-Fluorouracil Hydroxyurea Methotrexate
		Inhibition of purine synthesis, as above	6-Thioguanine
Miscellaneous	DNA	DNA damage of various types	Bleomycin Procarbazine Mithramycin Mitomycin-C

better drugs or combinations have proved lacking when tested in the clinic. A knowledge of the mechanism of action of cytotoxic drugs is, however, of some relevance. Tumors resistant to one drug are usually resistant to others having a similar mechanism of action. Conversely a combination of drugs having different actions may have greater activity and most combinations select drugs from different groups.

Single Agent Versus Combination Therapy

Few malignancies show response rates over 50% when exposed to single cytotoxic agents, but those that are chemosensitive are often sensitive to a range of different agents. This raises the question of whether cytotoxic agents used in combination would increase the chances of obtaining complete remission or of cure. The knowledge that cytotoxic drugs act through different routes, that tumors may be resistant to one drug while retaining sensitivity to another and the theoretic work of Goldie and Coldman (1979) (see below) give additional support for this concept. In the more chemosensitive tumors such as germ cell tumors, lymphomas and leukemias, combination therapy has been shown to be essential if the majority of patients are to be cured. In the less chemosensitive tumors the position is less clear. There is no doubt that combination therapy produces an increased response rate in many tumors, including ovarian (Williams *et al.*, 1985; Aabo *et al.*, 1986) and cervical cancer (Buxton, 1992), but this is not always translated into an increased disease-free interval or improved survival. Using agents with different toxicities in combination allows a higher dose intensity to be achieved and this may also be important in determining the results achieved (see below). Only prospective randomized trials for each malignancy can answer the question of whether combination therapy gives better results than single agents and how increased activity balances against greater toxicity. Certainly combination therapy works best when active agents are available, and improved results should not be expected from combinations of relatively inactive agents.

Dose Intensity

In vitro work on single agents shows that some cytotoxic drugs have a steep dose–response curve, which extends beyond the normal level of *in vivo* exposure. In animal tumor models dose intensity is the most important factor in achieving cure, although only in chemosensitive tumors of small volume. In animals with a large burden of disease, dose has little effect on survival, even in chemoresponsive tumors. When temporary remission is all that is achieved, the duration of response and survival are more related to total dose given than to dose intensity (Ozols *et al.*, 1993).

The clinical dose–response relationship of chemotherapy in ovarian cancer has been assessed by Levin and Hryniuk (1987). This study analyzed 65 groups of patients treated with chemotherapy for Stage III or IV disease and calculated the relative dose intensity of therapy (as opposed to total dose). The study suggested that, for ovarian cancer, the use of combination chemotherapy and a higher cisplatinum dose intensity are associated with higher remission rates. The higher remission rates and greater dose intensity attributable to combination therapy are in turn correlated with a longer median survival.

Although thought-provoking, a number of points need to be taken into account when assessing the results of this and other dose intensity studies. Firstly the range of doses assessed is often modest, representing those used in standard clinical practice. Some studies have therefore essentially compared 'standard' doses with 'reduced' doses. Secondly some studies include groups of patients who from animal models would not be expected to benefit from higher doses, such as those with very bulky disease. Thirdly, a dose–response relationship may not apply to all drugs. In the Levin and Hryniuk study (1987), for example, the dose intensity of cyclophosphamide did not influence outcome. It should also be realized that a relationship between dose intensity and outcome at standard doses does not imply that even higher doses will produce even better survival. The dose–response curve may well plateau at some point and higher doses may produce side-effects that themselves impair outcome.

The difficulty of interpreting dose–response relationships is also illustrated by a study in cervical cancer by Bonomi *et al.* (1985). This showed a higher total response rate with greater doses of cisplatinum, but no increase in the complete remission rate. This might suggest that in some malignancies at least the small number of patients with highly chemosensitive disease is not increased by higher doses. An increase in the partial remission rate, although of interest and of relevance in palliation, is unlikely to increase the overall survival or cure rate.

Despite these reservations, the concept of dose intensity is rightly receiving much study. This has been helped by technical developments in supportive care, and in particular by improved hematologic support. Initial clinical studies in which a modest dose increase was achieved by using hematopoietic growth factors following chemotherapy have been superseded by studies in which five- or even ten-times standard dose is given with ABMT or PBSC support (see above). Although such regimens can produce remission in some patients, relapse is the rule. Attempts are now being made to build on this by repeating high-dose treatment on several occasions–an approach that was previously impossible due to the major toxicity of the treatment (Shea *et al.*, 1992). The rationale for this approach is the experience in curable tumors such as lymphoma, in which multiple timely courses of effective treatment are needed, to convert complete remission into cure.

Although high-dose treatment has no routine place in current clinical practice, it is likely that in due course it will play a part in the management of at least some patients with gynecologic malignancy.

Methods of Administration

Chemotherapy has traditionally been administered systemically by the oral or intravenous route. This exposes all tissues (except protected sites such as the central nervous system) to a broadly similar dose intensity. If the tumor could be selectively exposed to chemotherapy then either a higher dose intensity could be achieved for the same level of toxicity or a similar dose intensity could be given with less toxicity. Several experimental methods of administration have this aim. Intra-arterial chemotherapy has been studied in several tumors, but has been associated with increased toxicity without proven benefit. Many gynecologic malignancies are inappropriate for this approach because they are widely disseminated or do not have an anatomically well-defined arterial supply. Of more interest is intraperitoneal chemotherapy. This approach is of relevance for tumors that spread within the peritoneal cavity, but disseminate more widely only late in the disease course, as is typical of ovarian cancer. It is known that intraperitoneal administration leads to a peak local concentration of drug 20–1000 times that present in plasma (Dedrick *et al.*, 1978). This is of particular relevance for drugs that show a dose–response curve that continues above the levels attainable with the intravenous route. This is the case with cisplatinum and carboplatin, which are not chemically irritant and can be safely administered intraperitoneally. It has therefore received much attention for ovarian cancer. The major limitation to the action of intraperitoneal therapy is its inability to penetrate more than 1–2 mm into tumors (McVie *et al.*, 1985; Los *et al.*, 1990). Predictably therefore, major responses are rarely seen in tumor nodules above 1 cm in diameter. Similarly the pharmacokinetic advantage of intraperitoneal therapy (10–20-fold), although potentially significant in chemosensitive disease, is unlikely to be sufficient to overcome cisplatinum resistance. Although the true role of intraperitoneal chemotherapy is not yet defined, it is most likely to be helpful in patients with small-volume residual disease following a response to standard systemic therapy.

Mathematical Models of Chemotherapy

In recent years mathematical models of the action of chemotherapy have been devised (Birkhead *et al.*, 1986). These attempt to explain the effect of chemotherapy on the whole tumor and therefore suggest better ways of using these drugs. One of the most influential of these is the Goldie–Coldman hypothesis (1979), which arose out of work into the mechanism of antibiotic resistance in bacterial populations. The essential assumption of this hypothesis is that resistance to chemotherapeutic agents develops during tumor growth by means of random somatic mutation. Resistance to different drugs or classes of drugs is assumed to have different mechanisms and to develop independently. Tumors therefore comprise different populations of cells showing different levels of resistance to different groups of drugs. The overall level of resistance increases with time and therefore with the number of malignant cells and with the size of the tumor. The theory suggests that high levels of resistance develop quickly, during the early part of tumor growth.

When exposed to chemotherapeutic agents, the different populations of cells behave differently. Cells sensitive to the agents used undergo lysis, and if these represent the bulk of the malignant cell population, tumor shrinkage will occur ('clinical remission'). Cells resistant to the agents may represent a minority of the malignant population, but will continue to divide. In time these reach clinically measurable size and continue to increase despite further chemotherapy ('drug resistant relapse'). Complete tumor eradication only occurs if all populations of cells are exposed to cytotoxic agents to which they are sensitive. Exposure to a greater numbers of cytotoxic drugs should therefore increase the proportion of cells exposed to agents to which they are sensitive, increasing both the response rate and the chances of cure. The theory also implies that the chances of cytotoxic drug resistance being produced by somatic mutation will increase with time. Therefore early exposure to multiple active drugs should be superior to using some drugs first-line and reserving other active drugs for relapse.

The Goldie–Coldman hypothesis is in agreement with the general clinical experience of remission and drug-resistant relapse, and also agrees with the higher remission rates produced by combination chemotherapy compared to those produced by single agents. In Hodgkin's disease, for instance, the alternation of two non-cross resistant drug regimens seems to give superior results to the use of one regimen continuously. This finding is, however, in contrast to that in small cell lung cancer, a highly chemosensitive disease, in which combination chemotherapy may produce a greater response rate, but does not prevent drug-resistant relapse or substantially increase the small cure rate. The Goldie–Coldman hypothesis is therefore not a universal rule to be applied in all malignancies.

The Norton–Simon hypothesis (Norton and Simon, 1977) emphasizes the importance of tumor size on response to treatment and points out the inability of many regimens that are active in advanced malignancy, to influence remission duration when used in an adjuvant setting. They point out that *in vivo*, solid tumors do not grow exponentially, but rather follow a Gompertzian growth curve (i.e. growth slows as the tumor enlarges, with a plateau being reached). In this situation the maximum growth rate is seen in tumors of intermediate size. The Norton–Simon hypothesis assumes that the sensitivity of a tumor to chemotherapy is directly related to its growth rate. This is in contrast to the more simple log–kill hypothesis where a fixed proportion of cells are assumed to be killed at each exposure to chemotherapy. Based on these assumptions they devised a mathematical formula to represent the growth and regression of tumors. This formula gives results in close agreement with the observed growth patterns of a wide range of tumors, suggesting that it is indeed explaining the effect of chemotherapy on tumor growth.

The clinical corollary of the Norton–Simon hypothesis is that very large or very small tumors will have maximum resistance to therapy. Therefore as tumor size diminishes, rather than reducing the intensity of treatment, it should be increased. This is the basis for the use of late intensification in the treatment of leukemia and has implications for the use of chemotherapy in other settings. In particular, the tendency of ovarian cancer to relapse following surgically-documented complete remission indicates the inability of current therapy to eradicate microscopic disease. The hypothesis also explains the general finding that maintenance chemotherapy of equal or less intensity than the remission regimen is ineffective in preventing relapse. This hypothesis is not in conflict with ideas based on the development of drug resistance, but runs in parallel. That is, in some cases tumor relapse may be due to inappropriate scheduling of active drugs, while in others it may be due to acquired drug resistance.

These mathematical models of tumor growth and their response to therapy have undoubtedly increased our understanding of the effects of chemotherapy on malignancies. They are in agreement with many clinical findings and may give some guidance on the best way to use the active drugs that are available. It is, however, still the case that the biology of individual tumors, particularly their inherent sensitivity or otherwise to chemotherapy, has a greater influence on their curability than the scheduling or doses of drugs chosen. In the case of chemoresistant tumors such as endometrial carcinoma, the problem is not the best way to apply active agents, but simply the lack of any such drugs.

Acquired Drug Resistance

Many tumors are naturally resistant to some or all current cytotoxic agents – 'inherent drug resistance'. Other tumors are sensitive to chemotherapy, but can become resistant during the evolution of the disease. This acquired resistance has received much study because it is usually the final determinant of clinical outcome.

Broadly speaking three mechanisms of resistance have been described (Perez *et al.*, 1991). It may be due to decreased intracellular drug levels, to increased intracellular detoxification, or to an increased rate of repair of cellular damage. Each of these has been demonstrated *in vitro* and each can be overcome *in vitro*. The former is typified by the multidrug resistant phenotype (MDR) in which cells exposed to one cytotoxic drug develop cross-resistance to a wide range of other natural products and anticancer drugs. These include the anthracyclines, vinca alkaloids, podophyllotoxins and actinomycin-D. MDR is due to decreased intracellular drug accumulation, which in turn is due to increased drug efflux mediated by a membrane glycoprotein pump (p-glycoprotein). A wide range of drugs has been shown to inhibit the action of p-glycoprotein and thereby restore the sensitivity of p-glycoprotein-expressing cells to cytotoxic drugs.

Resistance to cyclophosphamide and other alkylating agents is more related to detoxification mechanisms. Cells can acquire resistance to these drugs by increasing their levels of glutathione-S-transferase (GST) or metallothionein, two key enzymes responsible for drug detoxification. Buthione sulfoximine (BSO) inhibits the action of GST and increases *in vitro* sensitivity to alkylating agents. In the case of nitrosoureas, resistance can be due to increased levels of O^6-methylguanine-DNA methyltransferase. This enzyme repairs the damaging alkylation of guanine bases in DNA produced by the drug. Streptozotocin depletes the methyl transferase enzyme and restores sensitivity to nitrosoureas *in vitro*.

Despite much work on the area of drug resistance and a huge increase in our understanding of mechanisms of resistance and of how to overcome them *in vitro*, clinical progress has been slight (Ozols *et al.*, 1987; Eder *et al.*, 1991). It is clear that multiple mechanisms of resistance exist and that different ones may apply in different tumors. While it is possible to overcome individual mechanisms of resistance *in vitro* it is much more difficult simultaneously to overcome all the mechanisms that apply *in vivo*.

Clinical Trials of Chemotherapy

Despite the general principles and practical considerations discussed above there are many unanswered questions regarding the best way to manage patients with malignancy. In many patients we simply do not know the best strategy for management and this uncertainty is exacerbated by the increasing number of new drugs and new approaches to treatment that need to be considered. Assessment of new therapies by individual clinical experience in a small number of patients may well be misleading and in most situations formal prospective studies are required. The stages whereby new therapies are assessed have traditionally been divided into three phases, each having a specific aim (Buyse *et al.*, 1984).

Following *in vivo*, animal or other background study, there must come a time when a new therapy is tried for the first time in patients. At this stage the effects on humans are uncertain and the first aim is to determine the nature and extent of any toxicity. Because of the uncertainty regarding toxicity and the probability that no benefit will accrue to the patient, these Phase I studies are usually confined to whose who have received all standard therapies, who are in the terminal stages of their illness, and who are aware that they are receiving a treatment with unknown effects. Patients with a wide range of malignancies are usually included. In the case of systemic therapy, dose escalation is used to define the safe dose for further study. Initial patients are treated at a fraction of the likely toxic dose (often one-tenth of the LD_{10} in mice), with subsequent patients receiving increasing doses until toxicity is noted. Patients in Phase I studies require frequent assessment of all systems in which toxicity might occur and clinicians should be alert to the possibility of unexpected effects. It is probable though, that less frequent side-effects will not be revealed.

The next step is to determine if the new treatment has any therapeutic activity. In some cases responses will have been seen in the Phase I study and this will give clues to possible diseases in which Phase II studies should be undertaken. For many drugs, however, this is not the case. Phase II studies are each confined to patients with one disease type and therefore many are required to define the spectrum of activity of a new agent. Phase II studies can be considered to have two stages. The first is to answer the question "Does the new therapy have any activity?" If it does, the second is to answer the question "What is the level of this activity?" In defining whether a new therapy has activity only a small number of patients is required (Gehan, 1961). A true response rate of less than 15% is considered to indicate a lack of activity. Therefore, if no responses are seen in 14 treated patients there is a less than 5% chance of the drug being active. If so, the new therapy will usually be dropped for that particular disease. If responses are seen in the first 15 patients, then many more patients are required to define the level of activity. If the new therapy shows a response rate of 30% in 30 patients then the

95% confidence interval extends from 16% (i.e. ineffective) to 46% (i.e. highly active). To reduce the confidence interval to ±10%., 85 patients would be needed. Many Phase II studies are smaller than this and the true level of activity only becomes apparent following the completion of several studies. The level of response seen in Phase II studies is partly determined by the type of patient treated. In malignancies where an active agent already exists most patients will have been exposed to chemotherapy before receiving the new agent. In this situation the response rate is often less than if the new agent had been used first (Bork *et al.*, 1986). Those patients, who have failed to respond to first-line therapy, are very unlikely to respond to any new therapy, regardless of its activity when used first-line, and these patients may be inappropriate for testing new therapies (Blackledge *et al.*, 1989).

The third stage of development is to compare the new treatment with the standard therapy to determine if the new therapy is an advance. This can only be done accurately in the context of a formal prospective randomized trial. Large numbers of patients are required to confirm therapeutic differences and such studies are a major undertaking. They are, however, the final determinant of therapeutic advances. The results of Phase III studies may, however, be compounded by a number of errors. The results of a trial are only applicable to patients having the same characteristics as those studied. Patients in the trial should therefore be representative of the total population having the disease under study. Ideally, all patients treated at the study center who are eligible for inclusion should be included. Secondly, random differences between the two arms in the distribution of patients with poor prognostic characteristics may bias the final results. Trials should be stratified for criteria of major prognostic significance such as stage. Thirdly, there is always the possibility of a type II error: that is, of falsely detecting no difference between the therapies. The likelihood of a type II error increases as the number of patients falls. A significant difference in results between the two arms of a trial is always of interest, but a lack of difference in a small study is to be expected and is of no relevance. Even in large studies, type II errors can occur by chance and usually more than one Phase III study is required to define an improvement in treatment. It must also be remembered that important subgroups of patients whose prognosis is improved by a new therapy may be obscured in clinical trials that include a wide range of patients. Finally, it is a general rule of assessing clinical trial results that the importance of the stated p-value alone can not be underestimated! The confidence interval of the result is of greater importance, and should always be quoted (Gardner and Altman, 1986).

New Therapies

The past 15 years have seen the introduction into clinical practice of a fourth arm of cancer therapy to supplement the three previously available (surgery, radiotherapy, chemotherapy). This has been the use of biologic products, which either have direct cytotoxicity or modulate the immune response to tumor cells thus producing an indirect cytotoxic effect. Several quite distinct avenues of research have been explored in detail both in the laboratory and more recently in the clinic and it is impossible for this section to give more than a brief mention of this rapidly developing field. It is clear that these are potent compounds that have the ability both to induce dramatic responses and to cause marked toxicity. However, initial clinical assessment of these compounds, although providing a lot of data about their toxicity and biologic effects, has shown no routine clinical role for them. Future studies will no doubt use more complex schedules and will assess specific subgroups of patients. The development of biologic therapies is therefore in its infancy.

Interferons

The interferons are a group of naturally occurring proteins with potent antiviral, antitumor and antiproliferative properties and were the first biologic response modifiers (BRMs) to be used in clinical trials. Assessment of studies using interferon is complicated by the range of different preparations used. Three interferon groups have been identified: interferons-α, -β and -γ, which are the products of leucocytes, fibroblasts and T cells respectively. These groups have different mechanisms of action and have been available in preparations of differing purity. Furthermore the biologic effects are greatly influenced by the route and schedule of administration and as the optimum approach is not known, several different schedules have been applied. What is known is that systemically administered α-interferon has produced responses in solid tumors such as those of the ovary, melanoma and renal cell carcinoma. Such responses have, however, been rare and sometimes at the expense of considerable toxicity such as fever, rigors, abnormal liver function tests and neutropenia. In ovarian cancer these compounds may be more active when given intraperitoneally (Berek, 1992), and this route is currently receiving much attention. Clear evidence of clinical benefit is, however, still lacking.

Interleukins

The interleukin-1s (IL-1s) are a group of polypeptides involved in the mediation of responses to infection, injury and neoplasia, many of which have been identified previously, but given other names such as endogenous pyrogen, mononuclear cell factor or catabolin. These molecules have complex biologic effects including direct and indirect cytotoxicity, radioprotection and induction of proliferation of B and T cells. Early clinical trials of IL-1s are underway.

Interleukin-2 (IL-2), previously called T cell growth factor, is a glycosylated protein essential for T cell growth. Among its actions is the induction of lymphokine-activated killer (LAK) cells, which have a broad spectrum of cytotoxicity towards tumor cells. This action is dependent on the presence of IL-2 receptors (IL-2R) on the resting T cells. The expression of IL-2R by circulating T cells is induced by interferon-γ, which therefore potentiates the effects of IL-2. It is probable that a positive feedback loop develops as IL-2 in turn stimulates release of interferon-γ. This is the rationale for combining these agents in clinical studies. When administered to patients, IL-2 has been associated with marked toxicity including hypotension, vascular leakiness, fluid retention, fever, nausea and vomiting. These may necessitate managing the patient in an intensive care unit and undoubtedly can be life-threatening. The fact that these side-effects begin some hours after starting treatment when IL-2 has a very short serum half-life suggests that they are indirectly mediated, perhaps via interferon-γ, and may therefore be preventable. The extent of toxicity associated with IL-2 therapy has led some clinicians to question whether such therapy is ethical either in the individual patient or in the wider context of competition for scarce health resources. Complete responses have, however, been seen in previously unresponsive tumors such as renal cell carcinoma and melanoma, and the results of further studies are awaited with interest.

Adoptive Cellular Therapy

In addition to the antigen-driven immune response, the body also has a range of nonspecific defence systems or natural immunity. These are mediated by a range of cells including polymorphonuclear cells, macrophages and monocytes, killer cells and natural killer cells. Some of these cells show cytotoxicity towards a broad range of tumors, which is not dependent on the presence of specific antigens. Attempts have been made to induce this phenomenon *in vivo* by extracting peripheral blood mononuclear cells and exposing them to IL-2. This induces proliferation of LAK cells, which can be re-infused into the patient in the hope that they will exert their cytotoxic effects on the host tumor. Such treatment is often combined with IL-2 therapy as described above and has a similar range of toxicities. LAK cell therapy produces a response rate of around 25% in melanoma and renal cell carcinoma and studies are in progress in other malignancies. These include studies of intraperitoneal therapy which has special attractions in the study of biologic response modifiers (BRMs). The large molecular interleukins and activated cells will be retained for a longer period with greater tumor exposure and less toxicity than if administered systemically. The LAK cells will also have direct access to the tumor, which is partially prevented with systemic administration because of cellular trapping in the lung, liver and spleen.

Monoclonal Antibodies and Immunoconjugates

The exquisite specificity of antibodies makes them attractive agents to explore in the search for a means of guiding therapeutic agents to their target, the cancer cell. Monoclonal antibodies have been produced to a number of cancer-associated antigens such as 17-1A and carcinoembryonic antigen (CEA) in colonic carcinoma and CA-125, OVLT3 and placental alkaline phosphate (PLAP) in ovarian cancer. These antibodies can be linked to a range of potent cytotoxic agents including toxins such as ricin, radionucleotides such as iodine-131 (^{131}I) and to drugs such as vindesine and doxorubicin. Again, clinical studies are underway focusing initially on the pharmacokinetics and pharmacodynamics of the compounds. Intravenous administration of such compounds has many problems, in particular poor antibody localization in the tumor and the induction of host neutralizing antibodies against the foreign monoclonal antibody. As with chemotherapy, an intraperitoneal approach is also being assessed in the hope of improving localization and encouraging results have been seen (Rosenblum *et al.*. 1991).

As yet, none of these interesting biological approaches to cancer has any proven role in clinical practice and it is likely to be several years before this will happen. Their clinical assessment is further complicated by the multiple interactions that can occur both among themselves and with standard therapies. For example, γ-interferon induces expression of tumor-associated antigens and may therefore make antibody-guided therapy more effective; it also induces expression of IL-2 receptors enhancing its effects and is synergistic, *in vitro*, with TNF; α-interferon both induces the expression of estrogen receptors on breast cancer cell lines, thus enhancing tamoxifen cytotoxicity, and also inhibits the growth-promoting effects of estrogen by binding to the estrogen receptor, raising the possibility of clinically active combinations of BRMs and hormone therapies; cisplatinum causes peritoneal macrophages to release IL-1 raising the possibility that this is its mode of action when administered intraperitoneally. Many other interactions have been described.

Whether these new therapies will represent an

advance over those currently available, and whether they will stand alone or will need to be used in conjunction with other therapies remains to be seen. There can be no doubt though, that they will continue to be areas of fruitful study well into the next century.

Summary of Core Information

- Chemotherapy is an important modality in the treatment of gynecologic cancers. Its use continues to evolve, guided by the results of clinical trials and as a result of introducing new agents.
- In deciding the appropriate use of chemotherapy the clinician must take account of the aims of treatment and the particular wishes and circumstances of the patient as well as the results of clinical research.
- Clinicians should be aware of the side-effects of treatment and how these can be best managed.
- The side-effects and benefits of treatment should be carefully monitored using standard criteria with the aim of determining whether it is being effective.
- Ineffective treatment should be stopped and if necessary the aim of the treatment changed.
- New therapies, in particular biologic therapy and high-dose chemotherapy, are the focus of much current research. At present, they remain experimental approaches.

References

Aabo D, Hald I, Horov S *et al.*(1986) A randomised study of single agent vs combination chemotherapy in FIGO stage IIb, III and IV ovarian adenocarcinoma. *Eur. J. Cancer Clin. Oncol.* **22:** 9.

American Society of Clinical Oncology (1994) American Society of Clinical Oncology recommendations for the use of hematopoietic colony-stimulating factors: evidence based, clinical practice guidelines. J. *Clin. Oncol.* **12:** 2471.

Berek JS (1992) Intraperitoneal immunotherapy for ovarian cancer with alpha interferon. *Eur. J. Cancer* **28A:** 719.

Bertelsen K, Jakobsen A, Kem Hansen M *et al.* (1989) A randomized trial of six cycles versus twelve cycles of cyclophosphamide, adriamycin and cisplatinum in advanced ovarian cancer. *Proc. Am. Soc. Clin. Oncol.* **8:** 150.

Birkhead BG, Gregory WM, Slevin ML & Harvey VJ (1986) Evaluating and designing cancer chemotherapy treatment using mathematical models. *Eur. J. Cancer Clin. Oncol.* **22:** 3.

Blackledge G, Lawton F, Redman C & Kelly K (1989) Response of patients in phase II studies of chemotherapy in ovarian cancer: implications for patient treatment and the design of phase II studies. *Br. J. Cancer* **59:** 650.

Bonadonna G, Valagussa P, Rossi A *et al.* (1985) Ten-year experience with CMF-based adjuvant chemotherapy in resectable breast cancer. *Br. Cancer Res. Treat.* **5:** 95.

Bonomi P, Blessing JA, Stehman FB *et al.* (1985) Randomised trial of three cisplatin dose schedules in squamous carcinoma of the cervix: a Gynaecologic Oncology Group study. *J. Clin. Oncol.* **3:** 1079.

Bork E, Hansen M, Dombernowsky P *et al.* (1986) Teniposide (VM-26) an overlooked highly active agent in small cell lung cancer: results of a phase II study in untreated patients. *J. Clin. Oncol.* **4:** 524.

Buxton EJ (1992) Experience with bleomycin, ifosfamide and cisplatin in primary and recurrent cervical cancer. *Semin. Oncol.* **19:** 9–17.

■ Buyse ME, Staquet MJ & Sylvester RJ (1984) *Cancer Clinical Trials: Methods and Practice.* Oxford: Oxford University Press.

Cox K, Stuart–Harris R, Abdini G *et al.* (1988) The management of cytotoxic drug extravasation – guidelines drawn up by a working party for the Clinical Oncological Society of Australia. *Med. J. Aus.* **148:** 185.

Creasman WT, Omura GA, Brady MF *et al.* (1990) A randomised trial of cyclophosphamide, doxorubicin, and cisplatin with or without Bacillus Calmette–Guerin in patients with suboptimal Stage III and IV ovarian cancer. A Gynaecologic Oncology Group study. *Obstet. Gynaecol.* **39:** 239.

Dedrick RL, Myers CE, Bungay PM *et al.* (1978) Pharmacokinetic rationale for peritoneal drug administration in the treatment of ovarian cancer. *Cancer Treat. Rep.* **62:** 1.

Eder JP, Wheeler CA, Teicher B, *et al.* (1991) A phase I clinical trial of novobiocin, a modulator of alkylating agent cytotoxicity. *Cancer Res.* **51:** 510.

Gardner MJ & Altman DG (1986) Confidence intervals rather than P values: estimation rather than hypothesis testing. *Br. Med. J.* **292:** 746.

Gehan EA (1961) The determination of the number of patients required in a preliminary and a follow-up trial of a new chemotherapeutic agent. *J. Chron. Dis.* **13:** 346.

Gershenson DM, Mitchell MF, Atkinson N *et al.* (1992) The effect of prolonged cisplatin-based chemotherapy on progression free survival in patients with optimal epithelial ovarian cancer: 'maintenance' therapy reconsidered. *Gynaecol. Oncol.* **47:** 7.

Gianni A, Bregni M, Stern A *et al.* (1989) Granulocyte–macrophage colony-stimulating factor to harvest circulating haematopoietic stem cells. *Lancet* **332:** 580.

Goldie JH & Coldman AJ (1979) A mathematical model for relating the drug sensitivity of tumours to their spontaneous mutation rate. *Cancer Treat. Rep.* **63:** 1727.

Hakes TB, Chalas E, Hoskins WJ *et al.* (1992) Randomized prospective trial of 5 versus 10 cycles of cyclophosphamide, doxorubicin and cisplatin in advanced ovarian cancer. *Gynecol. Oncol.* **45**(3): 284.

Jones AL, Hill AS, Soukop M *et al.* (1991) Comparison of dexamethasone and ondansetron in the prophylaxis of emesis induced by moderately emetogenic chemotherapy. *Lancet* **338:** 483.

Klastersky J (1993) Empirical antibiotic therapy in neutropenic cancer patients. *Eur. J. Cancer* **29A (suppl 1):** S6.

■ Levin L & Hryniuk WM (1987) Dose intensity analysis of chemotherapy regimens in ovarian carcinoma. *J. Clin. Oncol.* **5:** 756.

Lloyd GG, Parker AC, Ludlan CA & McGuire RJ (1984) Emotional impact of diagnosis and early treatment of lymphomas. *J. Psychosom. Res.* **28:** 157.

Los G, Mutsaers PHA, van der Vight WJF *et al.* (1990) Direct diffusion of cis-diamminedichloroplatinum(II) in intraperitoneal chemotherapy: a comparison with systemic chemotherapy. *Cancer Res.* **49:** 3380.

McGuire GP, Tait A, Brooke M *et al.* (1980) Psychiatric morbidity and physical toxicity associated with adjuvant chemotherapy after mastectomy. *Br. Med. J.* **1980:** 1179.

McVie JG, Dikhoff T, van der Heide J *et al.* (1985) Tissue concentration of platinum after intraperitoneal cisplatinum administration in patients. *Proc. Ann. Mtg Am. Assoc. Cancer Res.* **26:** 162.

■ Miller AB, Hoogstraten B, Staquet B & Winkler A (1981) Reporting results of cancer treatment. *Cancer* **47:** 207.

Norton L & Simon R (1977) Tumour size, sensitivity to therapy and design of treatment schedules. *Cancer Treat. Rep.* **61:** 1307.

Ozols RF, Cunnion RE, Klecker RW *et al.* (1987) Verapamil and Adriamycin in the treatment of drug-resistant. ovarian cancer patients. *J. Clin. Oncol.* **5:** 641.

■ Ozols RF, Thigpen JT, Dauplat J *et al.* (1993) Dose intensity. *Ann. Oncol.* **4 (suppl 4):** S49.

Perez RP, Godwin AK, Hamilton TC *et al.* (1991) Ovarian cancer biology. *Semin. Oncol.* **18:** 186.

Rosenblum MG, Kavanagh JJ, Burke TW *et al.* (1991) Clinical pharmacology, metabolism and tissue distribution of 90Y-labeled monoclonal antibody B72.3 after intraperitoneal administration. *J. Natl Cancer Inst.* **83:** 1629.

Shea T, Mason J, Storniolo AM *et al.* (1992) Sequential cycles of high-dose carboplatin administered with recombinant human granulocyte–macrophage colony stimulating factors and repeated infusions of autologous peripheral blood progenitor cells. A novel and effective method for delivering multiple courses of dose-intensive therapy. *J. Clin. Oncol.* **3:** 464.

Smith DB, Newlands ES, Rustin GJS *et al.* (1991) Comparison of ondansetron and ondansetron plus dexamethasone as antiemetic prophylaxis during cisplatin-containing chemotherapy. *Lancet* **338:** 487.

Swenerton KD, Hislop TG, Spinelli J *et al.* (1985) Ovarian carcinoma: a multivariate analysis of prognostic factors. *Obstet. Gynaecol.* **65:** 264.

Williams CJ, Mead GM, MacBeth FR *et al.* (1985) Cisplatin combination chemotherapy versus chlorambucil in advanced ovarian cancer: mature results of a randomised trial. *J. Clin. Oncol.* **3:** 1445.

Williams SD (1992) Chemotherapy for ovarian cancer: is longer better? *Gynaecol. Oncol.* **47:** 5–00.

44 Biostatistics for the Clinician

H L Weiss
S Soong

Introduction

This chapter is devoted to a discussion of the basic statistical methods applicable to clinical research. The main objective of this chapter is to present an array of basic statistical techniques that can assist clinicians in the conduct and evaluation of medical research. For ease of reference an appendix of key terms and definitions is supplied at the end of this chapter.

There are two main branches of statistics, descriptive statistics and inferential statistics. Descriptive statistics is discussed in the next section while inferential statistics is discussed later in the chapter.

In statistics, a 'population' is defined as the largest collection of subjects from which we have an interest in making conclusions about. A 'random sample' is a part or subset of the population such that each entity has an equal and independent chance of being drawn into the sample. A 'parameter' is a quantity that characterizes a population while a 'statistic' is a quantity that characterizes a sample. Thus, a parameter is constant while a statistic is a value that changes from one sample to the next.

Descriptive Statistics

'Descriptive statistics' includes methods for organizing and presenting a body of data into fewer values to represent them. There are two common sets of descriptive measures: measures of central tendency and measures of dispersion. Measures of central tendency characterize the central location of the data whereas measures of dispersion characterize the spread of the data. The most common measures of central tendency include the mean, median and mode.

- The 'mean' is defined to be the sum of all the data divided by the total number of observations in the data. The population mean is denoted by μ.
- The 'median' is defined to be the middle value when the data are arranged in ascending or descending order.
- The 'mode' is defined to be the most frequently occurring value in the data.

The mean as a measure of central tendency uses the most information from the data as compared to the median and mode. However, for a markedly skewed distribution, the mean is sensitive to extreme values. In such situations, the median would be a more appropriate measure of central tendency. The mode provides a crude measure of central tendency since it uses the least amount of information from the data.

The most common measures of dispersion are the range, variance and standard deviation.

- The 'range' is defined as the difference between the largest and the smallest value in the data.
- For a sample consisting of n observations, the sample 'variance' is defined as the sum of the squared deviations of each of the values from its sample mean, $\bar{x}$, divided by $n-1$. The sample variance is denoted by s^2.
- The 'standard deviation' is simply the square root of the variance, denoted as σ and s for a population and sample, respectively. The standard deviation provides a more intuitive interpretation of dispersion since it is expressed in the same units as the data as opposed to the variance, which is expressed in square units of the data. A large s implies a more dispersed distribution.

The range is a crude measure of dispersion since it only uses the largest and smallest value in the data. The 'standard error' refers to the standard deviation of a statistic, for example, the standard error of the sample mean. An estimate of the standard error of the sample mean is equal to $s/\sqrt{n}$ (i.e. the standard deviation divided by the square root of n, the number of observations in the sample).

Probability Distributions

A 'random variable' is a value that changes from one sample to the next. A random variable is 'discrete' if it represents counts, such as the number of patients diagnosed with cervical cancer, or 'continuous' if it represents measurements, such as a patient's weight, blood pressure or age. Usually a random variable is denoted by capital letters, say, X.

'Probability' gives a measure of how likely a specific value of a random variable is to occur. A probability lies between 0 and 1 with 1 representing a value of the random variable that is certain to occur. Probability distributions are classified into a discrete probability distribution or a continuous probability distribution.

- A 'discrete probability distribution' refers to the distribution of a discrete random variable. One of the most important discrete probability distributions encountered in medical research is the 'binomial distribution,' which refers to the probability distribution of a binomial random variable X, defined as the number of successes out of n trials when the probability of success in any one trial is equal to p. This distribution is applicable to random variables with dichotomous outcomes whereby one outcome is termed a 'success' and the other 'failure.' An example of a variable with dichotomous outcome is recurrence or non-recurrence of cancer of the cervix among patients treated with chemotherapy. The binomial random variable would then be the number of recurrences among n patients.
- A 'continuous probability distribution' refers to the distribution of a continuous random variable. The most important continuous distribution in statistics is the 'normal distribution' (*Figure 44.1*), which is completely determined by its parameters, μ and σ^2. Different values of μ and σ^2 give a different normal distribution. The 'standard normal distribution' is a special case of the normal distribution with mean 0 and variance 1. It gives the probability distribution of a standard normal random variable defined as $Z=(x-\mu)/\sigma$. The standard normal random variable is usually called a Z score. As such, any normally distributed random variable, X, can be transformed into a standard normal random variable. A table of the standard normal probability distribution is available in Mendenhall *et al.* (1990) and in most statistics texts. Such a table usually gives the probability that a standard normal random variable is between any two values z_1 and z_2, that is, $P(z_1 \leqslant Z \leqslant z_2)$.

Another important distribution is the 'Student's t-distribution,' which refers to the distribution of a t random variable defined as $t=(x-\mu)/s$. Normally distributed random variables with an unknown population standard deviation for small samples are transformed into the t random variable. The t distribution is completely determined by its parameter, called the 'degree-of-freedom' (df). There is a different t distribution for each value of its parameter. The t distribution approaches the normal distribution as n approaches ∞.

Another important continuous distribution is the 'chi-square (χ^2) distribution.' The χ^2 is a non-negative random variable ranging from 0 to ∞. Like the t distribution, the χ^2 distribution is a family of distributions, one for each value of its parameter, v, called the degrees-of-freedom (df). Interestingly, the square of the Z standard normal random variable

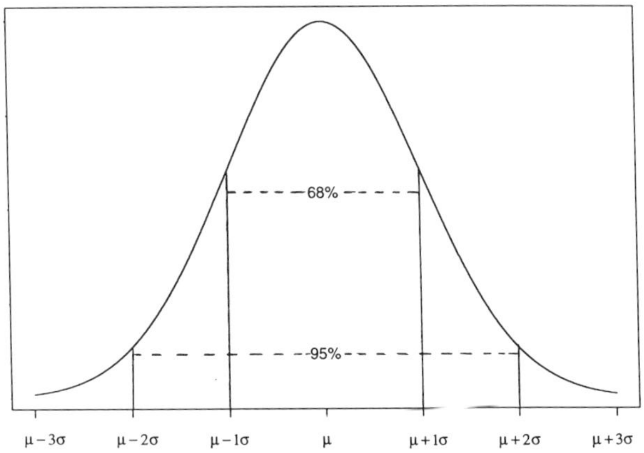

Figure 44.1. Normal distribution.

follows a χ^2 distribution with 1 degree-of-freedom. Tables of the t and χ^2 probability distributions are available in most statistics texts such as Daniel (1987).

Inferential Statistics

The second main branch of statistics is called 'inferential statistics.' It is concerned with making inferences about a population on the basis of sample observations drawn from that population. Inferential statistics can be further subdivided into two inference-making procedures: estimation and hypothesis-testing.

Estimation

'Estimation' is concerned with the calculation from the sample data of some statistic to estimate a population parameter. It answers the question "What is the value of the population parameter?" There are two types of estimation procedure, namely point estimation and interval estimation.

'Point estimation' gives a single value that is used to estimate the corresponding population parameter. For example, an estimator of the population mean μ would be the sample mean $\bar{x}$. The numerical value of an estimator is called an estimate.

'Interval estimation' gives two values defining an interval with an associated degree of confidence within which the parameter of interest would fall. This interval estimator is called a $100(1-\alpha)\%$ 'confidence interval' (CI) for a population parameter. Here, $1-\alpha$ is called the confidence coefficient and usually takes on the values 0.90, 0.95, 0.99. For example, we can calculate a 95% CI for the population mean. The lower value of the interval is called the lower confidence limit while the upper value of the interval is called the upper confidence limit. Suppose we want to calculate a 95% CI about the mean age of women with cervical intraepithelial neoplasia. Assuming that from a random sample of 20 women, the mean age, $\bar{x}$, was 31 years old and the standard deviation, s, was 4.0. Then a 95% CI about the population mean μ is given by $\bar{x} \pm t_{.025,19\text{df}}(s/\sqrt{n})$. Here $t_{.025,19\text{df}}$ refers to the value of the t random variable to the right of which lies 0.025 ($\alpha/2=0.05/2$) of the area under the curve. Based on the t distribution table with 19 degrees-of-freedom, this value equals 2.093. The 95% CI is then equal to (29.13, 32.87). This CI is interpreted as follows: we are 95% confident that the mean age of women with CIN lies between 29.13 and 32.87 years.

Hypothesis Testing

'Hypothesis-testing' is another statistical inference-making procedure. A hypothesis is a conjecture or an educated guess. Statistical hypothesis-testing answers the question "Is the parameter equal to a specific value?" It includes at least five steps:

- the null hypothesis (H_o);
- the alternative or research hypothesis (H_a);
- the test statistic;
- the rejection region;
- conclusion.

The 'null hypothesis' is a statement concerning the probability distribution of a random variable stated in terms of a specific value of a parameter of the distribution (e.g. H_o: $\mu=\mu_0$). The 'alternative' or 'research hypothesis' states alternative probability distributions of the random variable. An alternative hypothesis can be one-sided (i.e. H_a: $\mu>\mu_0$ or H_a: $\mu<\mu_0$) or it can be two-sided (i.e. H_a: $\mu\neq\mu_0$). A 'test statistic' is a random variable calculated from the sample that provides a measure to assess the null hypothesis in terms of a probability statement. A Z-score or a t random variable are examples of test statistics. The 'rejection region' consists of values of the test statistic that leads to the rejection of the null hypothesis. A one-sided alternative hypothesis leads to a one-sided test. This means that the rejection region is comprised of either the large or small extreme values of the test statistic. A two-sided alternative hypothesis leads to a two-sided test. This in turn means that the rejection region comprises both the large and small extreme values of the test statistic.

Table 44.1 shows the two types of error in hypothesis-testing – type I and type II errors. A 'type I error' is committed if we reject the null hypothesis when it is in fact true. The probability of a type I error is denoted as α. A 'type II error' is committed if we accept the null hypothesis when it is in fact false. The probability of a type II error is denoted as β. The 'power' of a test, denoted as $1-\beta$, is the probability of rejecting the null hypothesis when it is in fact false. That is, power is the probability of correctly detecting a difference when it truly exists. Thus, we always aim for high power in a statistical test. Another important concept is the 'p-value' of a test statistic, also called significance probability. Many times, the p-value of a test statistic is reported because it gives an idea of how consistent the sample data are with the null hypothesis. A p-value is defined as the probability of the observed value of a test statistic or its more extreme outcome under the null hypothesis.

Table 44.1. Type I and type II errors in hypothesis testing.

Decision	*H_o, null hypothesis.*	
	True	*False*
Reject H_o	Type I error α	Power $1-\beta$
Accept H_o	$1-\alpha$	Type II error β

Hypothesis-testing: Comparing Two Means

Suppose a study wishes to compare whether the mean age of patients with invasive cervical cancer differs between whites and non-whites. Here, the mean age for the white and non-white population will be denoted as μ_1 and μ_2, respectively. The test of hypothesis intends to compare the two population means. The null hypothesis will be H_o: $\mu_1-\mu_2=0$ versus the two-sided alternative H_a: $\mu_1-\mu_2\neq0$. When sampling is from two independent, normally distributed populations with an unknown, but equal, σ^2, then the test statistic is given by

$$t=\frac{(\bar{x}_1-\bar{x}_2)-(\mu_1-\mu_2)}{s\sqrt{\dfrac{1}{n_1}+\dfrac{1}{n_2}}}.$$

Here, s is the pooled sample standard deviation from the two random samples and n_1 and n_2 are the sample sizes for the first and second sample, respectively. A value of the test statistic that lies in the rejection region, or equivalently, a small p-value leads to the rejection of the null hypothesis. This is called a t-test. *Table 44.2* shows the steps for hypothesis testing for the example stated above based on hypothetic data. Assume that a random sample of 18 white and 18 non-white patients was drawn. The test statistic follows a t distribution with 34 degrees-of-freedom under the null hypothesis. For $\alpha=0.05$ and for a two-sided test, determine the value of the t random variable to the right of which lies

Table 44.2. Test of hypothesis: comparing two means.

1. H_o: $\mu_1-\mu_2=0$
2. H_a: $\mu_1-\mu_2\neq 0$
3. $t=\dfrac{(\bar{x}_1-\bar{x}_2)-0}{s\sqrt{\dfrac{1}{n_1}+\dfrac{1}{n_2}}}=\dfrac{(50-53)-0}{5\sqrt{\dfrac{1}{18}+\dfrac{1}{18}}}=-1.80$
4. For $\alpha=0.05$ and for a two-sided test, the rejection region includes values of $t\geqslant 2.032$ or $t\leqslant -2.032$.
5. Since the t statistic does not lie within the rejection region, we would accept the null hypothesis and conclude that white and non-white cervical cancer patients do not differ in age.
   p-value$=2\cdot P(t\geqslant|-1.80|)=0.081$

Table 44.3. Hypothetical example of a 2×2 contingency table.

Treatment	Outcome: Alive	Outcome: Dead	Total
Surgery	$n_{11}=66$	$n_{12}=16$	82
Surgery plus radiation	$n_{21}=67$	$n_{22}=36$	103
Total	133	52	$n=185$

$$\chi^2=\frac{n\left(|n_{11}n_{22}-n_{12}n_{21}|-\frac{1}{2}n\right)^2}{(n_{11}+n_{12})(n_{21}+n_{22})(n_{11}+n_{21})(n_{12}+n_{22})}$$

$$=\frac{185\left(|66\times 36-16\times 67|-\frac{185}{2}\right)^2}{82\times 103\times 133\times 52}=4.65$$

p-value$=0.031$

0.025 (0.05/2) of the area under the curve. Based on the t distribution table with 34 degrees-of-freedom, this is equal to 2.032. Thus, the rejection region for a two-sided test includes values of $t\geqslant 2.032$ or $t\leqslant -2.032$. Since our calculated test statistic does not lie within the rejection region, we would accept the null hypothesis. Equivalently, the p-value implies that we do not have enough evidence to conclude that white and non-white patients differ in age.

Depending on the study design, testing the equality of two population means can also be accomplished using two dependent samples. For example, each patient receives each of the two treatments under study at different time periods and is measured at both occasions. This is called a 'paired t-test' and it provides a way of controlling for heterogeneity among the subjects.

A comparison of more than two population means is achieved through the 'analysis of variance' method and is discussed in many statistics texts such as in Daniel (1987).

The test for equality of two proportions is discussed in the next section.

Chi-square Test for Two Proportions

Suppose we have two independent random samples, say, a random sample of patients who received surgery alone and a random sample of patients who received both surgery and radiation. The hypothesis of interest is whether the proportion of mortality after five years differs between these two treatment modalities (i.e. H_o: $p_1=p_2$ versus H_a: $p_1\neq p_2$). These two random samples will be represented horizontally in a contingency table with two rows (*Table 44.3*). Further, we classify patients as to whether they died or are alive after five years. These will be represented vertically in a contingency table with two columns. In this sampling plan, the row totals are considered to be fixed. The frequency of patients falling in each of the four cells is denoted as n_{11}, n_{12}, n_{21}, n_{22}. The appropriate test statistic for testing equality of two proportions is given by the χ^2 test statistic, which under the null hypothesis follows a χ^2 distribution with 1 degree-of-freedom. *Table 44.3* shows data for a 2 × 2 contingency table for the example stated above. Of 82 patients who had surgery alone, 16 died after five years while of 103 patients who had both surgery and radiation, 36 died. The χ^2 test compares equality of mortality rates between these two groups. As shown in *Table 44.3*, a large value of the χ^2-test statistic and therefore a small p-value leads to the rejection of the null hypothesis that the mortality rate is the same between the two populations.

Fleiss (1981) discusses comparison of more than two proportions as well as other computational forms of the χ^2-test statistic.

Regression and Correlation

'Regression analysis' is a statistical technique that models the relationship between a 'dependent' or 'response variable' Y and an 'independent' or 'predictor variable,' X. The main question addressed in regression analysis is "What happens to the dependent variable Y as the independent variable X changes?" For example, an investigator might be interested in determining what happens to blood pressure as dosage of a certain drug is increased. Regression analysis may include one or more independent variables. A regression model that contains only one independent variable is called a simple linear regression model.

We will begin with a discussion of the simple

linear regression model. The 'simple linear regression model' is written as $Y=\beta_0+\beta_1X+\varepsilon$ where Y is the dependent variable, β_0 is the intercept of the line, β_1 is the slope of the line, and ε is the random error term. The parameters β_0 and β_1 are called the regression coefficients. The above model is said to be simple because there is only one independent variable, and linear in the parameters because no parameter is expressed as an exponent or is multiplied or divided by another parameter.

Regression analysis begins with the estimation of the regression coefficients in order to obtain a regression equation or prediction equation given by $\hat{Y}=\hat{\beta}_0+\hat{\beta}_1X$. Here the hats ($\hat{}$) are used to denote estimates of the parameters. The estimation of the regression coefficients is achieved through the method of least squares. The least squares estimates, $\hat{\beta}_0$ and $\hat{\beta}_1$, are then used to obtain a regression equation or prediction line. For example, we might be interested in modelling systolic blood pressure as a function of age. *Figure 44.2* shows a scatter-plot of age with systolic blood pressure. After fitting a simple linear regression model, the least squares estimates were equal to 100.76 and 0.59 for the intercept and slope, respectively. The fitted least squares regression line based on these estimates is also shown in *Figure 44.2*. We can perform a test hypothesis on the regression parameter, specifically, on the β_1. The hypothesis generally of interest is given by H_o: $\beta_1=0$, that is whether the slope is equal to zero. One way to test the null hypothesis that the slope is equal to zero is with the t-test statistic given by $t=(\hat{\beta}_1-0)/s_{\beta_1}$ with $n-2$ degrees-of-freedom and where s_{β_1} is the standard error of the sample slope. If we accept the null hypothesis, then the regression equation is of little use in predicting values of Y, otherwise the regression equation is useful in predicting values of Y. Using the sample example

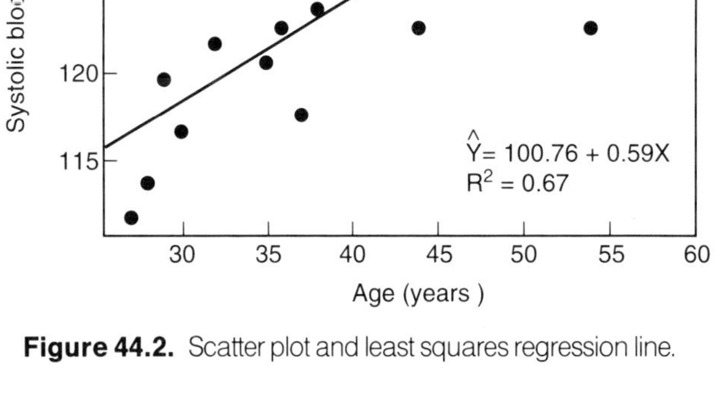

Figure 44.2. Scatter plot and least squares regression line.

above, the t statistic was equal to 7.18 and the corresponding p-value was <0.01. Thus, age, in this example, was an important predictor of a person's systolic blood pressure.

One important concept in regression analysis is the 'coefficient of determination,' denoted as R^2. It is the proportion of the total variation in Y that is explained or accounted for by the regression equation. R^2 ranges from 0–1 with a value close to one implying a close fit of the prediction line to the sample observations. The corresponding R^2 of the least squares regression line for the age and blood pressure example was 0.67. Thus, the regression equation accounts for only 67% of the variation in systolic blood pressure. Indeed, the graph in *Figure 44.2* shows some data points that are widely scattered about the regression line.

Two important limitations that should be kept in mind in regression analysis is that first, the prediction of Y is applicable only within the range of values of the independent variable X in the data. Secondly, the adequacy of the linear fit should be examined in detail. Myers (1986) and Neter *et al.* (1990) discuss a number of regression diagnostics to examine the adequacy of the fit of a regression model.

Extension of simple linear regression into 'multiple linear regression' is possible in different ways. One way is called 'polynomial regression,' which includes higher-order terms of the same independent variable (e.g. $Y=\beta_0+\beta_1X_1+\beta_2X_1^2+\beta_3X_1^3+\varepsilon$). Another would be the inclusion of more than one independent variable in the model, X_1, X_2, ..., X_p, where p refers to the number of independent variables. The latter is a common extension of the simple linear regression model. In many applications, a single independent variable in a regression model provides an inadequate prediction of the dependent variable. Multiple linear regression with additional independent variables is typically more helpful in providing better predictions of the response variable. Again, β_0, β_1, ..., β_p, are the partial regression coefficients that need to be estimated in the model. Glantz and Slinker (1990) provide extensive discussion of applied linear regression.

'Correlation analysis' is concerned with the quantification of the degree to which two variables tend to correlate. Here, both the variables X and Y are viewed as dependent, as opposed to regression analysis where Y is considered as a dependent variable and X as the independent variable. Correlation analysis addresses the question "Do X and Y tend to be related?" The 'Pearson correlation coefficient,' ρ, describes the degree of linear relationship between X and Y. The sample correlation coefficient, r, provides an estimate of the population correlation coefficient. The range of all possible values of r is from -1 to $+1$, with values close to one (positive or negative) implying a strong linear relationship, while values close to zero imply

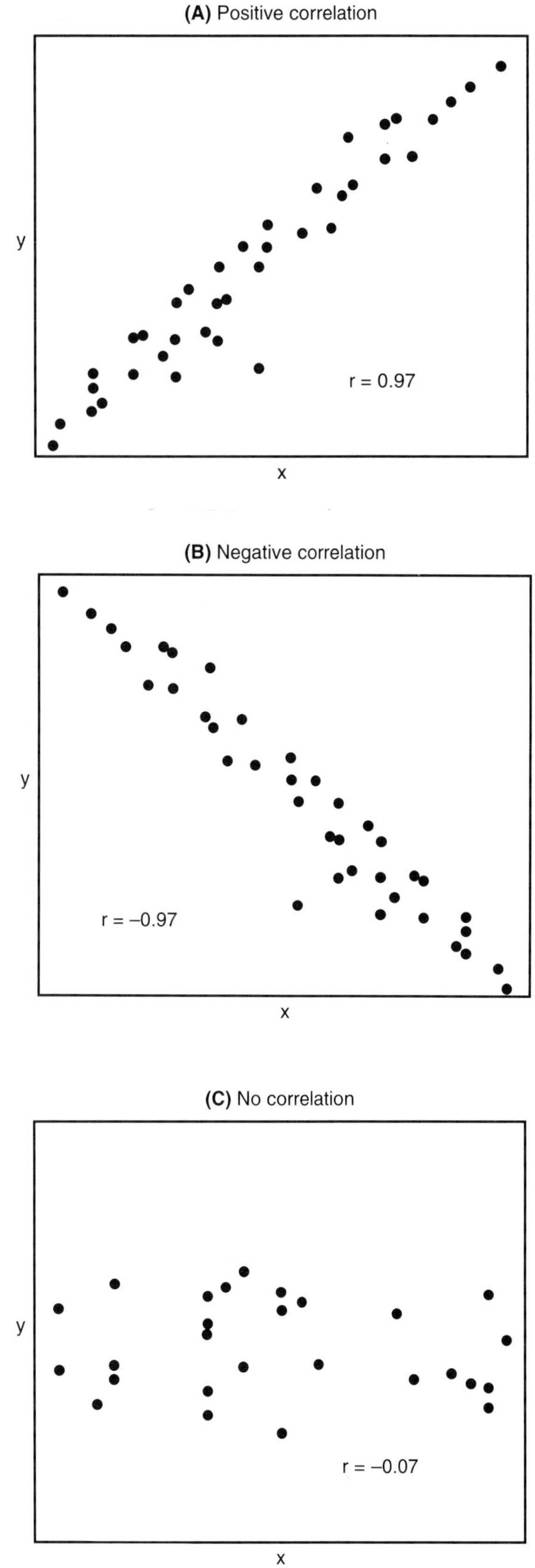

Figure 44.3A–C. Correlation plots.

a weak relationship between *X* and *Y*. *Figure 44.3* shows a scatter plot of points indicating a positive (a), negative (b) and no correlation (c), between variables *X* and *Y*. Test of hypothesis on whether the population correlation coefficient is equal to zero (i.e. H_o: $\rho=0$) can be performed using the *t*-test statistic.

Other methods for calculating a correlation coefficient can be found in most statistics texts, for example Fleiss (1981).

Planning Clinical Trials

A 'clinical trial' is a prospective study designed to determine the effectiveness and/or efficacy of a preventive or therapeutic regimen. Clinical trials are usually divided into three phases namely, Phase I, Phase II, and Phase III trials. 'Phase I' trials are designed to establish safety and toxicity profiles as well as the pharmacologic effects of a regimen.

'Phase II' trials are designed to demonstrate the effectiveness of a therapeutic regimen administered at safe doses during the Phase I trials. Phase II trials are sometimes divided into two sub-phases: 'Phase IIA' called preliminary trials, and 'Phase IIB' called follow-up trial.

The objective of a Phase IIA trial is to decide if a therapeutic regimen is effective enough to warrant further study. More specifically the preliminary trial determines, for a given treatment effectiveness level of say, 30%, the minimum number of consecutive failures to be observed before terminating a study (Gehan, 1961). For example, if treatment effectiveness is assumed to be 30%, then for nine consecutive patients, there would be more than a 95% ($1-0.70^9=0.9596$) chance that one or more treatment successes would be obtained. If nine consecutive failures are observed, the treatment is unlikely to be effective in 30% of the patients. If a regimen has passed the Phase IIA preliminary trial or has been sufficiently effective in a Phase I trial, the Phase IIB trial is performed. The objective of the Phase IIB trial is to provide a precise estimate of the effectiveness of the regimen. An estimate of the true effectiveness is the proportion of patients in the sample who are treated successfully. Gehan (1961) studied the number of patients required, in addition to the number of patients in the Phase IIA trial, to get an estimate of the true percentage of treatment effectiveness for a specified level of precision (standard error).

'Phase III' trials or comparative clinical trials are designed to compare the effectiveness of a new treatment with a standard or control treatment. Some of the important considerations in planning and designing Phase III trials include randomization of subjects to treatments, issues relating to design, monitoring, and analysis of the clinical trial, and the number of patients to be entered into the trial (i.e. sample size) in order to obtain sufficient power of the test. Lee (1992) discusses the issues related to the conduct of Phase III trials in detail.

'Randomization' refers to the allocation of subjects to treatments by a random process such that each subject has an equal and independent chance of receiving any of the treatments. Randomization helps ensure there is no bias in the assignment of patients to the treatments.

Clinical trial designs can be classified into two general groupings: fixed sample designs and sequential designs. Fixed sample design includes completely randomized design, stratified randomized design, crossover design and factorial design. Sequential designs include open sequential and closed sequential designs. The choice of an appropriate design to be used in a clinical trial is crucial in making valid comparisons of the treatment effects and in achieving a powerful test.

An important aspect in the planning of a Phase III trial is the determination of the sample size needed in the study. The calculation of 'sample size' required for a comparative clinical trial requires, at a minimum the following information:

- level of significance, α;
- the value of the desired power;
- the minimum amount of difference, d, between two treatments that it is important to detect.

Additional information must be specified such as the smaller of the two response rates, p_s, for testing equality of proportions. *Table 44.4* gives the number of patients required in each treatment group for different combinations of d and p_s. For example, it is of interest to compare the recurrence rate of endometrial cancer among patients receiving a hormonal therapy versus those receiving placebo. Assume that the amount of difference to be detected of interest to the investigators, was 30% and that the hypothesized proportion of recurrence (p_s) among those receiving hormonal therapy is 0.20. Using *Table 44.4*, for $\alpha=0.05$, power of 90%, and based on a two-sided test, 57 subjects will be required in each treatment group. A more detailed table on the number of samples required for testing equality of two proportions is available in Fleiss (1981).

The calculation of sample size when testing two population means requires information on the amount of variation, σ^2, of the outcome variable. Hulley and Cummings (1988) present a table on the sample size requirements for testing equality of two means.

Often, multiple testing is needed during the course of the trial to allow early termination of the trial if one treatment performs markedly better than the other. 'Group sequential methods' are designed for such planned interim analyses. It entails determination of the maximum number of repeated testing to be done and the number of patients needed in each testing for a given overall significance level α, power, and true difference, d, to be detected. Geller and Pocock (1987) compare several group sequential methods for two treatments.

Other important considerations that need to be addressed in the conduct of comparative clinical trials include the number of treatment groups to be compared, selection of the appropriate control group, comparability among treatment groups with respect to prognostic factors and blinding.

Table 44.4. Number of patients required in each treatment group.

	Two-sided test			*One-sided test*		
	Difference to be detected Larger minus smaller proportion $(P_l-P_s)=d$					
Smaller proportion (P_s)	*0.20*	*0.25*	*0.30*	*0.20*	*0.25*	*0.30*
0.20	91	62	45	74	50	37
	118	79	57	98	66	49
0.25	98	65	47	79	53	38
	127	85	60	106	71	51
0.30	103	68	48	83	55	39
	134	88	62	111	73	53

(Upper figure: test of significance at $\alpha=0.05$, power=0.80. Lower figure: test of significance at $\alpha=0.05$, power=0.90.)

Evaluation of Diagnostic Tests

A 'diagnostic test' is a procedure used to identify the presence or absence of disease. When evaluating a diagnostic test, the results are compared with an outcome variable, which is the presence or absence of a disease. *Table 44.5* shows four different situations that can occur: a true positive (TP) result; a false positive (FP) result; a true negative (TN) result; and a false negative (FN) result. The validity of a diagnostic test is usually evaluated by calculating its sensitivity and specificity.

'Sensitivity' is the probability of correctly classifying those with the disease and it indicates how good a test is at classifying those with the disease. It is calculated as the ratio of the TPs over all those who have the disease. 'Specificity' is the probability of correctly classifying those without the disease and it indicates how good a test is at identifying those without the disease. It is calculated as the ratio of those who are TNs over all those free of the disease. Simply put, sensitivity is the ability to detect cases, while specificity is the ability to screen out non-cases.

Table 44.5. Sensitivity and specificity. (TP, true positive result; FP, false positive; FN, false negative; TN, true negative.)

Endometrial biopsy result	Disease status Cancer	No cancer
Positive	TP (105)	FP (45)
Negative	FN (13)	TN (87)

$$\text{Sensitivity} = \frac{TP}{TP+FN} = \frac{105}{105+13} = 90\%$$

$$\text{Specificity} = \frac{TN}{TN+FP} = \frac{87}{87+45} = 66\%$$

Table 44.5 also gives hypothetical data on the results of biopsy in the diagnosis of endometrial cancer. The sensitivity of the endometrial biopsy was high at 90%, while its ability to screen out non-cases was only 66%.

The 'predictive value of a positive test (PPV)' is the probability that a person with a positive test result actually has the disease. It is calculated as PPV=TP/(TP+FP). The 'predictive value of a negative test (NPV)' is the probability that a person with a negative test result does not have the disease. It is calculated as NPV= TN/(TN+FN). 'Prevalence' of a disease in a population is the number of existing cases of a disease. Unlike sensitivity and specificity, the predictive value is dependent on the prevalence of the disease in a particular population. Hulley and Cummings (1988) and Hennekens and Buring (1987) present a more detailed description of procedures for evaluating diagnostic tests.

Survival Data Analysis

The response recorded in many medical research is often some measure of time, such as survival time. 'Survival time' can be defined, in various ways:

- length of life from onset of disease;
- time free of disease following treatment;
- time to recovery from start of a specified treatment.

In all of these situations, the response variable of interest is time until an event occurs. Subjects are followed-up prospectively over time. Unfortunately, a portion of the patients may be lost to follow-up because the investigator cannot find the patient for follow-up. And for some patients, the event of interest did not occur during the duration of the study. A survival time is 'censored' when the patient did not experience the event of interest at the end of the study or is lost to follow-up. Survival data analysis accounts for censored observations.

Survival data analysis proceeds with the estimation of survival curves or survival function denoted as $S(t)$. 'Survival curves' show the proportion of subjects free of the event of interest at a given time t. The 'Kaplan–Meier product limit' method is often used to estimate survival curves. This procedure does not require any assumptions about the form of the survival function that is being estimated. For example, consider a study where cervical cancer patients who have undergone anterior exenteration are followed to death. Thus, survival time, t_1, t_2, $\ldots$, t_n, for n patients are recorded. This may include both censored and uncensored observations. *Figure 44.4* shows the Kaplan–Meier estimate of survival curve among patients with a lesion of 3 cm or less and patients with lesions larger than 3 cm. It can be seen from the graph that among those with lesions of 3 cm or less, 74% are surviving in five years' time. Further, an estimate of median survival time (i.e. the time at which 50% of the patients are surviving) is equal to 5.4 years among those with these lesions.

Other methods of estimating survival curves involved fitting a distribution to survival times. Some well-known survival distributions include exponential, weibull, lognormal, gamma and gompertz distribution.

The comparison of different survival distributions is often of interest to a researcher. Using the same example above, an oncologist may be further interested in comparing survival between those with lesions of 3 cm or less versus those with lesions larger than 3 cm. A statistical test is necessary to determine whether the difference in survival curves between the two groups are significant or merely chance variations. Two commonly used tests for comparing

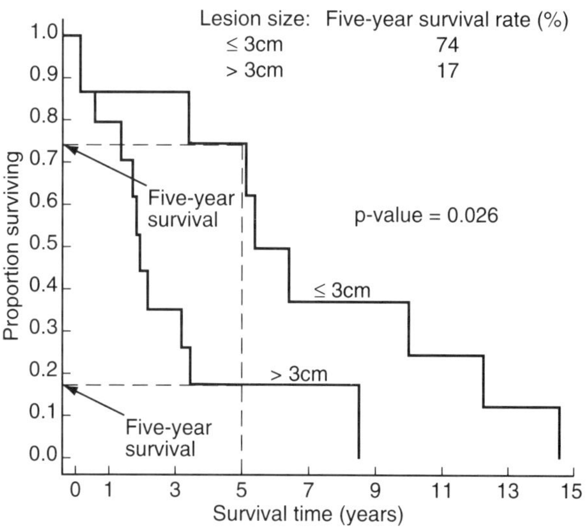

Figure 44.4. Kaplan–Meier estimate of survival curves by lesion size.

survival curves are the 'log-rank' and 'Gehan's generalized wilcoxon test.'

Figure 44.4 shows the Kaplan–Meier estimate of survival curves for the two groups. As can be expected, patients with smaller lesions have a better survival experience compared to those with a bigger lesion size. At five years time, 74% of the patients with a smaller lesion size are surviving compared to only 17% of those with a bigger lesion.

Using the log-rank test to compare these two survival curves, the log-rank test statistic yielded a p-value of 0.026 indicating a statistically significant difference in survival experience between the two groups.

Often, aside from investigating the relationship of a main independent variable with a dependent variable, it is important to incorporate multiple independent variables or 'prognostic factors,' X_1, X_2, ..., X_p, in the model. The 'Cox proportional hazards' model and the 'logistic regression' model are two such methods that address this issue. The dependent variable in Cox model is survival time. Logistic regression, on the other hand, models a dichotomous dependent variable (e.g. disease or no disease, remission or no remission). In these models, we are able to:

- model the dependent variable adjusting for the presence of confounding variables;
- identify a subset of variables that relate significantly to the dependent variable;
- compare relative risks for patients with different values of the prognostic factors.

Summary of Core Information

- Statistics is composed of two branches: descriptive and inferential. Descriptive statistics is concerned with summarizing and presenting a body of data into a few meaningful values. Inferential statistics is concerned with making inferences about a population on the basis of sample observations.
- Two sample t-test, chi-square test, regression and correlation analysis, and survival analysis are some of the more common statistical methods used in the analyses of medical data.
- The choice of study design, number of subjects required, study monitoring, and analysis are some of the important issues in the conduct of clinical trials.
- Test statistics, p-values, and confidence intervals determine the statistical significance of the observed differences. However, considerations on the clinical significance of the data (i.e. whether data represent differences that impact health) is equally as important in making medical decisions.

References

Daniel WW (1987) Biostatistics: *A Foundation for Analysis in the Health Sciences,* 4th ed, New York: John Wiley & Sons, Inc.

Fleiss JL (1981) *Statistical Methods for Rates and Proportions,* 2nd ed, pp. 321. New York: John Wiley & Sons, Inc.

■ Gehan A (1961) The determination of the number of patients required in a follow-up trial of a new chemotherapeutic agent. *J. Chron. Dis.* **13:** 346–353.

■ Geller NL (1987) Planned interim analyses and its role in cancer clinical trials. *J. Clin. Oncol.* **5:** 1485–1490.

■ Geller NL & Pocock SJ (1987) Interim analyses in randomized clinical trials: ramifications and guidelines for practictioners. *Biometrics* **43:** 213–223.

Glantz SA & Slinker BK (1990) Primer of applied regression and analysis of variance, pp. 776. New York: McGraw–Hill, Inc.

Hennekens CH & Buring JE (1987) *Epidemiology in Medicine,* pp. 383. Boston: Little, Brown, and Company.

Hulley SB & Cummings SR (1988) *Designing Clinical Research: An Epidemiologic Approach,* pp. 247. Baltimore: Williams and Wilkins.

Lee ET (1992) *Statistical Methods for Survival Data Analysis,* 2nd ed, pp. 482. New York: John Wiley & Sons, Inc.

Mendenhall W, Wackerly DD & Scheaffer RL (1990) *Mathematical Statistics with Applications,* 4th ed, pp. 818. Boston: PWS–Kent Publishing Company.

Myers RH (1986) *Classical and Modern Regression with Applications,* pp. 359. Boston: Duxbury Press.

Neter J, Wasserman W & Kutner MH (1990) *Applied Linear Statistical Models,* 3rd ed, pp. 1181. Homewood: Irwin.

Appendix: Key Terms and Definitions in Biostatistics

Alternative hypothesis (H_a) A statement asserting that differences exist among study treatments or that associations exist between a response variable and prognostic variable.

Analysis of variance (ANOVA) A statistical method that compares equality of more than two independent populations. This is accomplished by partitioning the total variation of a response variable into different component parts, where each component represents an identified source of variation.

Binomial distribution A distribution of a discrete random variable defined as the number of successes out of n independent trials.

Censored data This refers to data for those subjects who are lost to follow-up or who did not experience the event of interest up to the end of the study period.

χ^2-test A statistical test used to determine whether two or more proportions are significantly different from each other.

Clinical trials A prospective study on subjects designed to determine the effectiveness and/or efficacy of a preventive or therapeutic regimen.

Coefficient of variation A measure of dispersion independent of the unit of measurement. It is the ratio of the standard deviation over the mean.

Confidence interval This refers to two estimator values defining an interval with an associated degree of confidence within which the population parameter will fall.

Correlation analysis A statistical method that determines the linear relationship between two variables.

Correlation coefficient A measure of the strength of linear relationship between two variables.

Covariate A characteristic of subjects hypothesized to be associated with the response variable. Also called prognostic factors.

Cox regression model A statistical technique that models survival time with a set of prognostic variables. It assumes proportionality of hazards across different levels of a covariate over time.

2 × 2 Contingency table A four-fold table cross-classifying data into four subcategories. One variable with two levels is represented horizontally (row) and the other variable, also with two levels, is represented vertically (column). Each of the four cells in the table contains frequencies or proportions of subjects falling into a particular subcategory.

Diagnostic test A procedure employed to identify presence or absence of a disease.

Estimation This is concerned with the use of a sample to get an accurate and precise estimate of an unknown population parameter.

Fisher's exact test A method for calculating exact p-values for small samples in a contingency table. The p-value is the sum of the probabilities or outcomes at least as favorable to the alternative hypothesis as the observed outcome.

Hypothesis-testing A statistical technique to determine whether or not the null hypothesis is compatible with observed data.

Interim analysis An analysis performed during the course of a trial to determine the possibility of early termination of a trial resulting from a statistically significant evidence of superiority of one treatment over the other.

Kaplan–Meier estimate A method of estimating survival curves based on individual survival times.

Logistic regression A statistical technique that models a binary response variable with a set of prognostic variables.

Log-rank test A nonparametric test for comparing survival curves among different levels of a covariate.

Mean A measure of central tendency. It is the average of all the values of a variable in a population or sample. Population mean is denoted as μ and sample mean is denoted as $\bar{x}$.

Median A measure of central tendency. It is defined as the middle value when data are arranged in ascending or descending order.

Mode A measure of central tendency. It represents the most frequently occurring value in the data.

Normal distribution A continuous frequency distribution of a random variable characterized as being symmetric about its mean and that one, two and three standard deviations from the mean in both directions gives 68%, 95% and 99.7%, respectively of the total area under the curve.

Null hypothesis (H_o) A statement asserting that no differences exist among study treatments or that no associations exist between a response variable and prognostic variable. Acceptance of the null hypothesis asserts that the observed deviation is due to chance alone.

Paired *t*-test A statistical test used to determine the equality of two normally distributed populations from related observations resulting from non-independent samples.

Parameter A value (usually unknown) that defines a population. A parameter is a constant.

Phase I trials Trials designed to establish safety and toxicity profiles as well as the pharmacologic effects of a new regimen on a small group of subjects.

Phase II trials Trials designed to demonstrate the effectiveness and efficacy of a new treatment administered at safe doses established during Phase I trials.

Phase III trials Trials designed to determine the relative merit of a new treatment with a standard treatment. Also called comparative clinical trials.

Population The largest collection of subjects from which the sample is drawn.

Power The probability of rejecting the null hypothesis when it is in fact false. Or the probability of detecting a difference when it truly exists. It is denoted as $1-\beta$.

Predictive value The probability that a person with a positive (negative) diagnostic test is truly positive (negative).

Probability A value between 0 and 1 that gives a measure of the likelihood of occurrence of a specific value of a random variable.

***p*-value** A probability that gives a measure of how likely an observed difference or association is due to chance.

The smaller the p-value, the more we can exclude chance as an explanation for an observed difference.

Randomization This is concerned with the allocation of subjects into two or more treatment groups to ensure that each subject has an equal and independent chance of receiving any of the treatments.
Random sample A part or subset of the population such that each entity has an equal and independent chance of being selected into the sample.
Random variable A variable that occurs due to chance.

Sample size The number of subjects necessary for a given study to enable it to detect differences when they truly exist for a given significance level and power.
Sensitivity The probability of correctly classifying those with the disease. It is the ratio of true positives over all those who have the disease.
Significance level The probability of rejecting the null hypothesis when it is in fact true. Also called the type I error in hypothesis-testing and is denoted as α.
Specificity The probability of correctly classifying those without the disease. It is the ratio of true negatives over all those without the disease.
Standard deviation This is the square root of the variance expressed in the same unit of measurement as the variable.
Standard error The standard deviation of a statistic. For example, standard error of the sample mean, $\bar{x}$.
Statistic A value that defines a sample. A statistic is a variable.
Survival analysis A statistical method for analyzing survival time data where survival time is defined as time until an event of interest occurs.
Survival function A function defined as the probability that an individual survives longer than a given time, t. It is denoted as $S(t)$.

Type I error The probability of rejecting the null hypothesis when it is in fact true. It is denoted as α.
Type II error The probability of accepting the null hypothesis given that it is in fact false. It is denoted as β.

Unpaired *t*-test A statistical test used to determine the equality of two independent, normally distributed populations.

Variable A characteristic or measurement that varies from one sample to the next.
Variance A measure of dispersion. It is the average of the squared deviations of all the observations from its mean.

45 Oncogenes and Tumor Suppressor Genes

H H Gallion

Introduction

Although the concept of cancer as a genetic disease originated in the early part of this century, there was little in the way of supporting evidence until the 1950s when early cytogenetic studies uncovered the presence of numeric and structural chromosome abnormalities in malignant ascites. Soon thereafter, the first human tumor-specific genetic abnormality, the Philadelphia chromosome, was identified in the lymphocytes of patients with chronic myeloid leukemia (CML) (Nowell and Hungerford, 1960). Although this was an intriguing finding, the biologic significance of this acquired chromosome abnormality was uncertain. Did the Philadelphia chromosome represent a direct factor in the carcinogenesis of CML or was it simply an incidental byproduct of tumor progression with little or no biologic significance?

With the advent of chromosome banding techniques in 1970, precise identification of each individual chromosome based on unique banding patterns could be done. Using this technique, specific chromosome aberrations were soon identified in most hematologic malignancies and even some solid tumors. The Philadelphia chromosome, whose origin was previously unknown, was found to be the result of a reciprocal translocation between chromosomes 9 and 22. When modern molecular biological techniques became available in the 1980s it was discovered that the abl (Abelson Murine leukemia virus) proto-oncogene on chromosome 9 was translocated to the Philadelphia chromosome, suggesting abl may have been activated by transloca-tion. This hypothesis was confirmed by additional analysis of translocation breakpoints and studies of abl gene expression. On chromosome 22, most of the breakpoints fell within a 6 kb region, referred to as the breakpoint cluster region (bcr). The juxtaposi-tion of these two genes, abl and ber, resulted in a fusion gene consisting of the s' portion of bcr and abl. The resultant bcr/abl MRNA transcript, which contained sequences from both genes, encoded an aberrant protein product with enhanced tyrosine kinase activity. Although the exact role of the Philadelphia chromosome in the pathogenesis of CML has yet to be defined, tyrosine protein kinases such as that coded by the c-abl oncogene, are known to be important signal mediators that send growth stimulatory messages to the nucleus in response to growth factors.

A decade after the initial identification of oncogenes, a second class of cancer regulatory genes, the tumor suppressor genes, were discovered. Although, both are normal cellular genes with critical roles in the regulation of cell proliferation and differentiation, proto-oncogenes act to stimulate cellular proliferation, whereas tumor suppressor genes code for proteins that inhibit cell growth (*Figure 45.1*). Alteration of only a single allele or copy of a proto-oncogene by point mutation, translocation or amplification can 'activate' the gene, converting it to an oncogene with enhanced growth stimulatory activity. Because activation of only a single allele is required to transform a cell, oncogenes are considered to be 'dominant transforming genes.' In contrast, inactivation of both copies of a tumor suppressor gene is needed to remove the normal constraints to cell proliferation. Tumor suppressor genes are therefore generally considered as 'recessive transforming genes.'

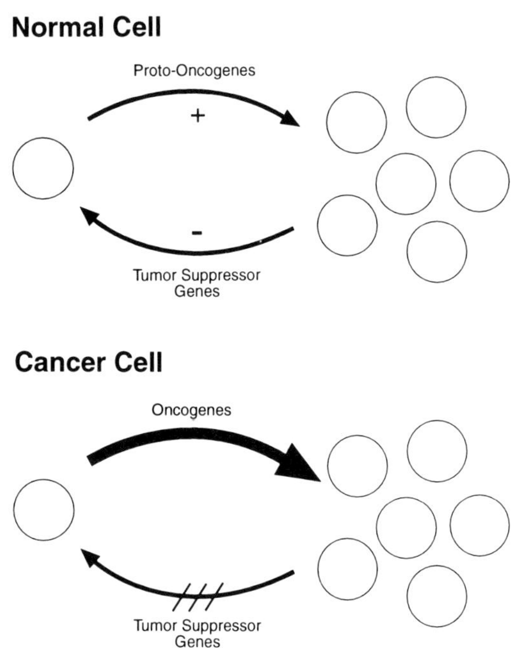

Figure 45.1. Activation of oncogenes and inactivation of tumor suppressor genes can lead to conversion of a normal cell to its malignant counterpart.

Oncogenes

Discovery

The first oncogenes were identified in the 1970s through the study of ribonucleic acid (RNA) tumor viruses. These retroviruses, which infect a number of animals including chickens, rodents, cats and monkeys, carry a unique enzyme known as reverse transcriptase. This enzyme allows the virus to transcribe its own RNA into single-strand deoxyribonucleic acid (DNA), which can then be incorporated into the host cell's genome. Certain retroviruses are capable of efficiently transforming cells in culture and rapidly inducing tumors in the host animal, hence, their name, acute transforming retroviruses. These retroviruses, contained one or more genes which were not involved in viral replication but were directly responsible for the transforming potential of these viruses, the retroviral oncogenes. Although these tumor producing genes were originally thought to be of viral origin, they are actually mutated forms of cellular genes. For example, the Rous sarcoma virus, which induces tumors in chickens soon after infection, was found to contain a single gene which was not necessary for viral replication, but was responsible for the transforming potential of the virus. This gene, the v-src oncogene, is a mutated form of a normal vertebrate gene important in growth regulation which had been acquired by the virus from an earlier animal host through a process known as transduction (Stehelin *et al.*, 1976). When integrated into the host cell genome following viral infection, the v-src oncogene possesses potent transforming activity (*Figure 45.2*). To date, over two dozen different oncogenes have been identified in the genomes of acute transforming retroviruses. Although retroviral infection *per se* has not been found to be a primary cause of cancer in humans, this Nobel Prize winning work provided clear proof that alteration of a single gene present in normal vertebrate cellular DNA could result in tumorigenesis.

Work with another type of RNA virus, the leukemia or leukosis virus led to the identification of additional cellular oncogenes. These viruses induce tumors in the animal host after a relatively long latent time. In contrast to the acute transforming retrovrus model, the leukemia viruses do not carry oncogenes, but rather result in malignant transformation by a process known as insertional mutagenesis. That is, by integrating into the host cell genome either close to or within a normal host cell proto-oncogene, the virus enhances that gene's activity (see *Figure 45.2*). As viral insertion into the human genome occurs randomly, and as insertion must be in close proximity to a proto-oncogene to have an effect, there is a relatively long latent period between infection and tumor formation. At least a dozen proto-oncogenes were discovered through

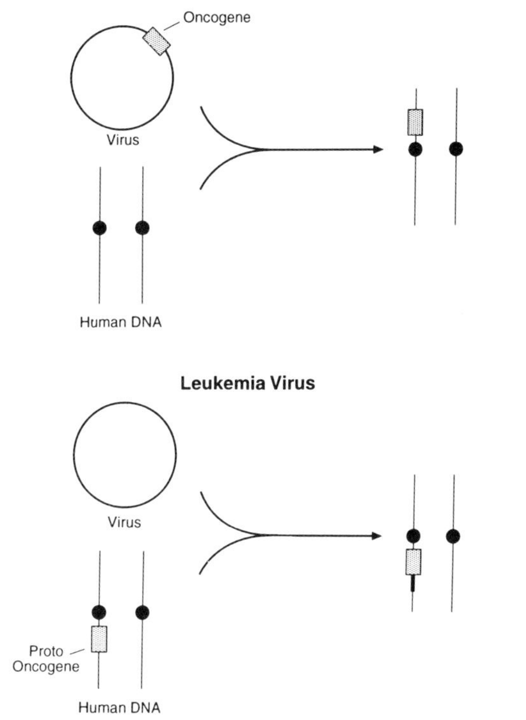

Figure 45.2. Oncogene activation by RNA tumor viruses. Acute transforming retroviruses result in oncogene activation by insertion of a mutated oncogene that had been acquired from an earlier animal host into the host cell DNA. With the leukemia viruses, oncogene activation is the result of viral insertion close to a host cell oncogene.

work with retroviruses, and each is named after the virus in which it was discovered (i.e. ras, rat sarcoma virus; myc, avian myelocytomatosis virus; and abl, Abelson murine leukemia virus).

Finally, a novel group of cellular oncogenes were identified by DNA transfection assays. In these experiments, fragments of genomic DNA isolated from human tumors were found to be capable of transforming non-tumorigenic mouse cell lines in culture. The presence of human repetitive DNA segments were then used to isolate the specific human DNA segment responsible for malignant transformation from the hybrid cell line. Of note, many of the transfectable human transforming genes were found to be related to the ras family of oncogenes, and clearly established their importance in human tumorigenesis.

As mentioned earlier, many cellular oncogenes important in malignant transformation were localized because they mapped to the sites of consistent chromosome breakpoints seen in human malignancies. For example, the c-myc and the c-mos oncogenes were localized to the specific chromosomal breakpoints seen in Burkitt's lymphoma and acute myeloblastic leukemia, respectively. Cytogenetically detectable homogeneous staining regions

Table 45.1. Oncogenes: detection methods and examples.

Method	*Examples*
Acute transforming retrovirus	v-Hras, v-fos
Leukemia retrovirus	v-abl, v-ets
Chromosome translocation	c-abl, c-myc, c-mos
Chromosome amplification	N-myc, L-myc, her-2-neu
Deoxyribonucleic acid (DNA) transfection	neu, met, N-ras, mas

(HSRS) and small accessory chromosomes known as double minutes (DMS) have also been helpful in identifying and localizing oncogenes important in human malignancies. These chromosome regions contain multiple copies of the same gene, a process known as gene amplification. In human neuroblastoma, HSRS were found to contain up to as many as 700 copies of the n-myc oncogene, and the severity of this disease is directly related to the number of copies present. Similarly, in human breast and ovarian cancer, amplification of the her-2-neu oncogene has been associated with a poor prognosis (Slamon *et al.*, 1989).

To date, over 50 oncogenes have been identified (*Table 45.1*). Functionally, oncogenes all have one thing in common; they are able to cause phenotypic changes consistent with malignancy when introduced into a normal cell (Bishop, 1983). Each proto-oncogene in the human genome has been highly conserved through evolution and plays an essential role in normal cell growth. Oncogene activation results from genetic alterations that result in either unregulated or over-expression of the normal product or mutations within the gene itself with a resultant abnormal product with enhanced activity. These genetic alterations range from single point mutations as seen in the ras family of oncogenes to chromosome translocation or gene amplification as observed with c-abl and n-myc, respectively. Although the total number of proto-oncogenes fulfilling the functional definition is much larger, only about 20 have actually been found to be mutated in human tumors (Weinberg, 1994).

Function

The discovery that some oncogenes were homologs of growth factors or growth factor receptors provided a direct link between oncogenes themselves and their transforming capability (*Figure 45.3*). In order to understand their function, some basic knowledge regarding the growth characteristics of normal cells is required (Weinberg, 1994). Cell growth and division is closely regulated by its surroundings. That is, a normal cell will not proliferate unless instructed to do so by messages originating from neighboring tissues. These messages can be either growth stimulatory or growth inhibitory and are generally carried by glycoprotein growth factors, which are released into the local environment. These growth factors can be secreted directly by the cell to influence itself (autocrine), by a neighboring cell of a different cell type (paracrine), or by growth factors from immediately adjacent cells (juxtacrine). Each cell possesses complex mechanisms to receive and process such growth-activating signals. These include:

- growth factors;
- cell surface receptors, which bind growth factors and transmit their signal into the cell;
- a cascade of cytoplasmic signal mediators, which receive the message and transmit it further into the cell;
- transcription factors within the nucleus, which activate cellular genes.

Proto-oncogenes code for many of the components of this complex signal pathway and alterations at any level can lead to unregulated cell proliferation.

It was the v-sis oncogene that provided the initial correlation between oncogenes and growth factors. This gene codes for one of the polypeptide chains of platelet-derived growth factor (PDGF), which is critical for wound healing. PDGF is normally released by thrombocytes in response to cell injury and stimulates neighboring fibroblastic cells to proliferate. Activation of this gene in the fibroblast itself leads to continuous production of PDGF by the fibroblast and inappropriate autocrine proliferation. Like PDGF, other transforming growth factors may function in an autocrine fashion to stimulate cell proliferation. For example, tumor cells frequently express the transforming growth factor

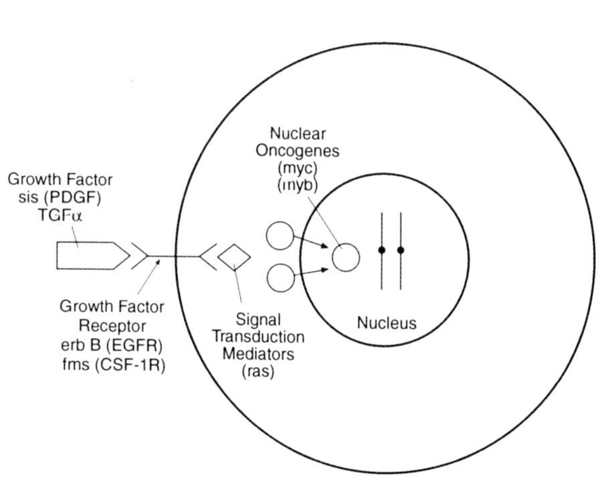

Figure 45.3. Proto-oncogenes code for many of the components involved in the growth factor/growth factor receptor signal cascade.

TGF-α into the local environment. TGF-α, which is highly homologous to epidermal growth factor (EGF), can bind to the EGF receptor (EGFR) and activate growth stimulating pathways in an autocrine fashion.

Most of the growth factor receptors important in cancer are composed of an extracellular ligand-binding domain, a membrane-spanning region, and an inner tyrosine kinase domain. Activating mutations in these receptors enhance their kinase activity and result in continuous activation of receptors despite the absence of a growth factor message. For example, v-erbB, an oncogene of avian erythroblastosis virus, encodes a protein tyrosine kinase which is a truncated form of epidermal growth factor receptor (EGFR). This protein contains the tyrosine kinase and the transmembrane domain but not the extracellular ligand binding domain which normally binds EGF. This deletion leads to a constitutively active protein–tyrosine kinase which continuously floods the cell with growth stimulatory messages, independent of EGF binding, leading to unregulated cell proliferation. This mechanism of oncogene activation appears to be responsible for the transforming activity of a number of other important oncogenes including erbB-2, ret and trk. Additional molecular mechanisms, such as mutation in the transmembrane domain and overexpression of the normal product can also convert normal receptor protein-tyrosine kinases. For example, in human tumors, mutations in the erbB-2 oncogene also known as her-2/neu for human epidermal growth factor, which is related to but distinct from erbB have nor been identified. However, amplification and overexpression of the normal her-2/neu gene product is a common fnding in both human breast and ovarian cancers (Slamon *et al.*, 1989). In these tumors, her-2/neu overexpression is correlated with clinical behavior, with overexpression being associated with poor prognosis.

Although cytoplasmic signal transduction from the surface receptors to the interior of the cell is poorly understood, the ras family of G proteins is known to be involved. The normal ras protein rests on the cytoplasmic surface of the cell membrane and only sends stimulatory signals into the cell when instructed to do so by binding of growth factor to receptor tyrosine kinases. A single point mutation in the ras proto-oncogene results in production of an abnormal ras protein, which is constitutively activated, continually sending growth stimulatory messages into the cell.

Finally, in response to the proliferation pathway initiated by the growth factors, each cell possesses a family of genes whose protein products bind DNA directly, thereby regulating the expression of genes that induce DNA synthesis and cell division. Enhanced activity of these nuclear transcription factors may result from inappropriate stimulation by any component of the growth factor–receptor-mediated signal cascade. Alternatively, they may become constitutively activated by a mutation within the nuclear gene itself as is observed in the myc family of nuclear oncogenes.

Tumor Suppressor Genes

The first evidence for the existence of tumor suppressor genes came from somatic cell hybridization studies (Harris *et al.*, 1969). Fusion of a normal cell with a malignant cell almost always yielded a non-tumorigenic hybrid. This implied that a gene or genes present in the normal cell was capable of suppressing oncogenic mutations in the malignant cell. Of note, reversion of the hybrid cell to a malignant phenotype frequently occurred following loss of certain chromosomes. For example, when normal fibroblasts are fused with HeLa cells, a human cervical cancer cell line, the resultant hybrid cell is non-tumorigenic. However, following loss of chromosome 11, the hybrid cell reverts to a malignant phenotype. Moreover, reintroduction of a normal chromosome 11 into the hybrid cell results in loss of tumorigenicity (Harris, 1988). These fusion studies clearly demonstrated that oncogenic mutations in malignant cells could be suppressed by genetic material present in normal cells, providing clear laboratory evidence for the pressure of tumor suppressor genes.

It was through the study of the rare childhood malignancy, retinoblastoma, that the essential role of tumor suppressor genes in human malignancies was established. In 1971, Knudson formulated his 'two hit' theory of tumorigenesis based on observations of the familial and sporadic forms of retinoblastoma (Knudson, 1971). He noted that in the hereditary form of this disease, tumors were typically bilateral, multifocal and had an early age of onset. Whereas, in the sporadic form of the diseases, tumors tended to be unilateral single tumors with a late age of onset. According to his hypothesis, these observed differences could be explained by the presence of an inherited germline mutation, the so-called 'first hit,' which would be present in all somatic cells of individuals with the hereditary form of the disease. A tumor would develop in these individuals only when a second mutation or 'second hit' occurred somatically in the rapidly dividing retinoblast. In the sporadic form of the disease, he postulated that both mutations must occur somatically in a single retinoblast before a tumor could develop. The low probability of two independent mutations occurring somatically in the same retinoblast explained the observed clinical differences in the sporadic retinoblastoma.

The clue to the first mutational event came from cytogenetic studies, which revealed visible deletions of chromosome 13q in the lymphocytes of patients with inherited retinoblastoma (Yunis and Ramsay,

1978). Similar losses of the 13q14 region were also observed in both sporadic and inherited tumors, suggesting that deletions of the same locus were involved in both forms of the disease (Godbout *et al.*, 1983). Familial linkage studies with the esterase D gene, which is located in the same region of 13q, were integral in identifying inherited mutations in the Rb gene in familial patients without cytogenically detectable 13q deletions. Molecular genetic analysis of retinoblastomas using restriction fragment length polymorphism analysis (RFLP), which demonstrated submicroscopic deletions of the 13q14 region in retinoblastoma tumors, provided the site of the second mutation (Cavanee *et al.*, 1983, 1985). In inherited retinoblastoma, the copy of chromosome 13 lost in the tumor was always the normal wildtype allele, which had been inherited from the unaffected parent (*Figure 45.4*). These tumor cells had therefore lost the wild-type copy of the Rb gene inherited from the unaffected parent leaving only the mutated Rb copy with resultant complete loss of gene function.

These studies clearly established that retinoblastoma involved the inactivation or loss of both copies of the Rb gene and led to the identification and cloning of this gene. The early age of onset and presence of multifocal bilateral tumors observed in patients with the hereditary form of the disease is a direct result of the presence of a pre-existing inherited germline deletion or mutation of Rb alleles in patients with the familial form of the disease. A cancer does not develop until the second copy becomes inactivated, usually by deletion, in the retinoblast itself. Although the disease is clinically transmitted in an autosomal dominant fashion, as two mutations must occur for a tumor to develop, it is recessive at the cellular level. Additional tumor suppressor genes have been identified in a number of other Mendelian dominant forms of cancer (*Table 45.2*). They are important not only in inherited cancers, but also in many sporadic human tumors. Indeed, mutation in the p53 tumor suppressor gene is the most common genetic abnormality detected in human tumors.

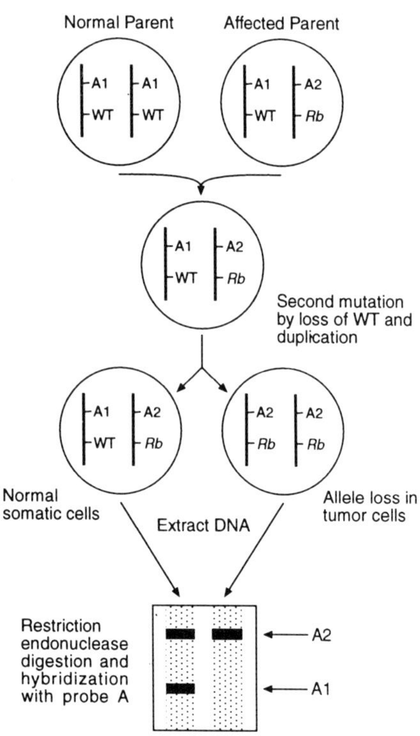

Figure 45.4. Restriction fragment length polymorphism analysis of the 13q14 region in a patient with hereditary retinoblastoma demonstrates loss of heterozygosity in the tumor DNA compared to normal somatic cell DNA from the same patient. This is consistent with retention of the mutant Rb allele (A2), which had been inherited from the affected parent, and loss of the wild-type (WT) Rb allele (A1) leading to functional loss of both copies of the Rb gene in the tumor cell.

Function

Loss of tumor suppressor gene function may occur by a number of inactivating mechanisms including complete deletion of the gene mutations, which result in a non-functional product, lack of gene transcription or inactivation of the functional gene product. In the case of retinoblastoma, loss of both functional copies of the gene is most commonly the result of a mutation in one copy of the Rb gene and deletion of the remaining copy, leading to total loss of Rb function in the cell. Although less is known about tumor suppressor gene function than oncogene function, these negative regulatory genes appear to code either directly for growth inhibitory messages or for the proteins involved in processing these messages. TGF-β has been identified as a growth inhibiting message that may be important in Rb gene function. Cells without an active Rb gene product become unresponsive to TGF-β and proliferate despite the presence of this growth inhibitory factor. So, although TGF-β is not the

Table 45.2. Tumor suppressor genes.

Syndrome	*Gene*	*Chromosome*
Retinoblastoma	Rb	13q
Wilms' tumor	WT1	11p
Colon carcinoma	DCC	18q
Familial adenomatous polyposis	APC	5
Hereditary nonpolyposis colon cancer	hMSH2 MLH1	2p 3p
Neurofibromatosis	NF1	17q
Breast–ovarian cancer	BrCa1 BrCa2	17q 13q

direct product of the Rb gene, the protein coded by Rb must be important in allowing a cell to respond to this message.

In the case of the p53 tumor suppressor gene, which is the most common genetic abnormality in human tumors, the situation is more complex. The normal or wild-type p53 gene product inhibits cell division by directly binding nuclear transcription factors. As in retinoblastoma, inactivation of both copies of the p53 tumor suppressor gene removes the normal constraints to cell proliferation. The mutated p53 gene product is an abnormal protein, which lacks its normal growth suppressive activity. However, in many human cancers, mutation in only one copy of the p53 gene is observed. The mutant p53 gene product can complex with wild-type p53 protein, thereby inhibiting the suppressive effect of the remaining wild-type allele. Hence, although a normal gene and gene product exists in the cell, its message is hampered by the mutant p53 protein and confers a growth advantage to the cell. This is referred to as a 'dominant negative' mode of action, compared to the 'simple recessive' loss of both copies of a tumor suppressor gene seen in retinoblastoma.

Hereditary Ovarian Cancer

It has been estimated that an inherited predisposition to hereditary overian cancer may be responsible for as many as 5–10% of all ovarian cancer cases. In these women, the susceptibility to ovarian cancer appears to be inherited in three distinct patterns (Lynch *et al.*, 1981). The most common of these is the breast–ovarian cancer syndrome in which the excess cancer cases are ovarian and early age of onset (<50 years) breast cancer. The second most common syndrome is known as Lynch syndrome II or hereditary nonpolyposis colorectal cancer (HNPCC). In HNPCC families, the most common cancers occur in the proximal colon and endometrium, but excess cases of ovarian, pancreatic and breast cancer are also seen. In the least common site-specific ovarian cancer families the excess cancer cases are strictly ovarian. In each of these families, susceptibility to cancer is transmitted as an autosomal dominant trait. Accordingly, the children of an affected individual have a 50% risk of inheriting the disease gene.

In 1990, a susceptibility gene for breast and ovarian cancer was linked to the long arm of chromosome 17 (Hall, *et al.,* 1990). This gene, which has become known as BrCa1, representing the first breast cancer gene, appears to be responsible for the majority of breast ovarian and site-specific ovarian cancer families (Easton *et al.,* 1993, Steichen–Gersdorf *et al.*, 1994). In these families, the lifetime risk for breast or ovarian cancer in BrCa1 carries approaches 100%. Using genetic linkage analysis, the search for BrCa1 further localized this gene to a 2 megabase region on chromosome 17q21-12 (*Figure* 45.5) (Smith *et al.* 1994, Goldgar *et al.* 1994). Intensive international efforts resulted in the identification of the BrCa1 gene in 1994 when Miki and colleagues identified germline BrCa1 mutations in 5 of 6 breast cancer families which

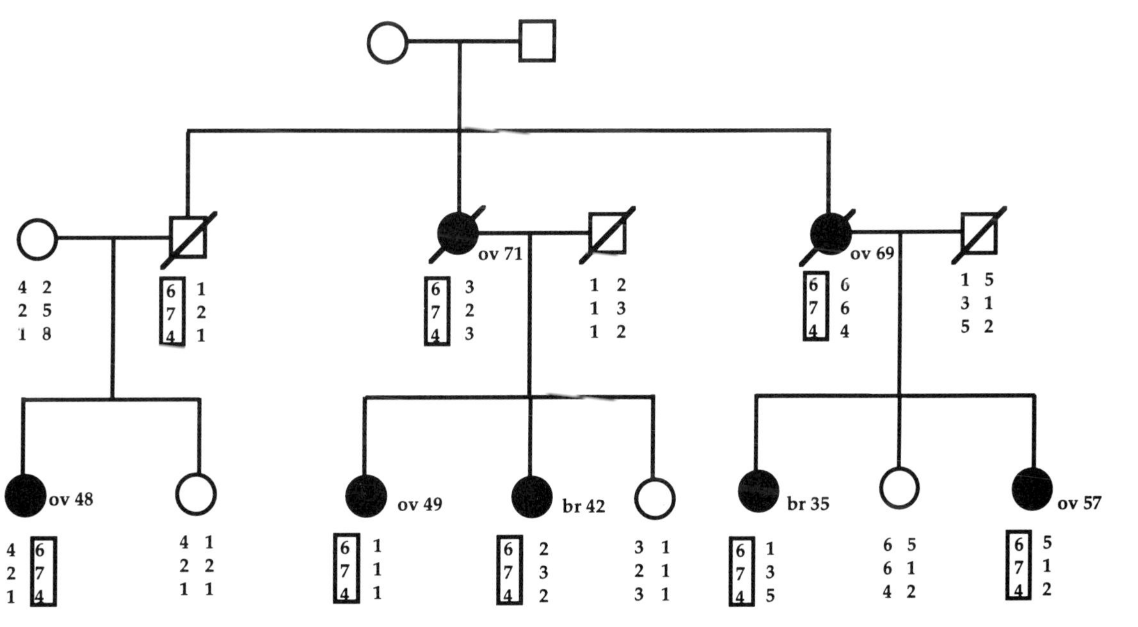

Figure 45.5. Pedigree and haplotype for markers spanning the BRCA1 region in a 17q-linked breast–ovarian cancer family. Marker order from centromere to telomere is Mfd 15, Mfd 188 and 42D6. Females are represented by circles and males by squares. Blackened symbols represent ovarian or breast cancer. Type of cancer and age at diagnosis is indicated under the symbol. The boxed haplotype indicates the linked chromosome carrying the predisposition to cancer.

showed linkage to the BrCa1 region on chromosome 17q. The BrCa1 gene consists of 22 coding exons spread over 100 kilobases. Although the function of the BrCa1 protein is unknown, it appears to contain a ring finger motif which is characteristic of proteins which regulate gene transcription. Since the initial identification of the BrCa1 gene, 80 different predisposing mutations scattered throughout the gene have been identified (Shattuck–Eidens *et al.* 1994). The majority of these mutations are frameshift, nonsense and regulatory mutations which are predicted to result in a truncated protein product.

Allele losses in tumors from 17q-linked families suggest BrCa1 is a classic tumor suppressor gene (Smith *et al.*, 1992). Accordingly, women in these families inherit a mutant BrCa1 allele and a malignancy occurs only when the normal remaining wild-type allele is lost in the breast or ovarian epithelium. Why the same gene gives rise to phenotypically different familial syndromes (i.e. breast only, breast- ovarian and site-specific ovarian cancer) is unknown. Easton and co-workers have recently suggested that this apparent genetic heterogeneity may result from the presence of two different BrCa1 alleles (Easton *et al.*, 1995). One conferring a breast cancer risk of 62% and an ovarian cancer risk of 11% by age 60 years and the other conferring a breast cancer risk of 39% and an ovarian cancer risk of 42%, with the first allele accounting for the majority of BrCa1 mutations. It is hoped that when clinical BrCa1 mutation testing becomes feasible, individuals at high risk can be identified and women who have inherited the disease gene can be offered appropriate screening measures or prophylactic oophorectomy. It is possible, that once the protein product of the BrCa1 gene is known, it may be useful in preventing disease in these women.

Recently, similar genetic linkage analysis identified a susceptibility locus on chromosome 2 in HNPCC families (Peltomaki *et al.*, 1993; Aaltonen *et al.*, 1993). At about the same time, a critical observation was made in tumors from HNPCC families. That is, somatic alterations in the size of repetitive microsatellite polymorphisms throughout the genome were identified, suggesting the presence of a defect in DNA mismatch repair enzymes (Thibodeau *et al.*, 1993). A human homolog of such a DNA mismatch repair enzyme, MSH2, was known to reside on the linked region of chromosome 2. Subsequent mutation analysis revealed germline mutations in this gene in a proportion of HNPCC families (Leach *et al.*, 1993). More recently, germline mutations in another mismatch repair gene, MLH1 on chromosome 3p, has been identified in some HNPCC families (Lindblom *et al.*, 1993; Bronner, 1994). These data indicate that mutations in mismatch repair genes are responsible for the spectrum of mutations identified in these families. As such, they represent an entirely new class of cancer-related genes. Although the precise mechanism of carcinogenesis is unknown, it is thought that replication errors caused by deficiencies in these genes may result in the activation of oncogenes and inactivation of tumor suppressor genes.

Conclusion

With the exception of some hereditary forms of cancer, tumorigenesis is rarely the result of mutation in a single gene. Instead, most human tumors result from a complex process involving a succession of genetic changes in multiple cancer-related genes (Vogelstein *et al.*, 1988). To date, these cancer-related genes include oncogenes, tumor suppressor genes and the newly identified mismatch repair genes. Most assuredly in the future, novel cancer-related genes will be identified.

It is hoped that the continued elucidation of the underlying genetic mechanisms responsible for human tumorigenesis will lead to clinically useful information. Already, genetic aberrations provide diagnostic and prognostically useful information in hematologic malignancies, breast cancer and neuroblastoma. Moreover, individuals at high risk for a number of hereditary forms of malignancies including retinoblastoma, Wilms' tumor, familial adenomatosis polyposis and now HNPCC can be identified by germline mutation analysis for the associated genes. In the future, it is hoped that as the mechanisms of tumor suppressor gene function are determined, these genes or their products may be useful not only in treating established malignancies, but perhaps more importantly, in preventing the development of cancer.

Summary of Core Information

- Most human tumors result from an accumulation of genetic changes in cancer-related genes, including oncogenes and tumor suppressor genes, which are normal cellular genes with critical roles in the regulation of cell growth and differentiation.
- Oncogenes normally act to stimulate cell proliferation. Alteration of a single allele by point mutation, translocation or amplification can 'activate' an oncogene leading to enhanced growth stimulatory activity.
- Many oncogenes code for components of the growth factor–growth factor receptor signal pathway.
- Tumor suppressor genes code for proteins that inhibit cell proliferation. Inactivation of both alleles of a tumor suppressor gene is needed to remove the normal constraints to cell proliferation.
- Loss of tumor suppressor gene function characteristically occurs by deletion of one copy with mutational inactivation of the remaining copy. This can be detected by the presence of loss of heterozygosity in tumor cells compared to normal cells.
- Many hereditary human cancers (i.e. retinoblastoma, Wilms' tumor) are the result of an inherited germline mutation in a tumor suppressor gene and somatic inactivation of the remaining normal copy.
- Recently, a new class of cancer-related genes has been identified. Defects in mismatch repair genes lead to DNA transcription errors and widespread microsatellite instability.

References

Aaltonen LA, Peltomaki P, Leach FS *et al.* (1993) Clues to the pathogenesis of familial colorectal cancer. *Science* **260:** 812–816.

Bishop JM (1983) Cellular oncogenes and retroviruses. *Annu. Rev. Biochem.* **52:** 301–354.

Cavanee WK, Dryja TP, Phillips RA *et al.* (1983) Expression of recessive alleles by chromosomal mechanisms in retinoblastoma. *Nature* **305:** 779–784.

Cavanee WK, Hansen MF, Nordenskjold M *et al.* (1985) Genetic origin of mutations predisposing to retinoblastoma. *Science* **228:** 501–503.

■ Easton DF, Bishop DT, Ford D & Crockford GP (1993) Genetic linkage analysis in familial breast and ovarian cancer: Results from 214 families. *Am. J. Hum. Genet.* **52:** 678–701.

Godbout R, Dryja TP, Squire J, Gallie BL & Phillips RA (1983) Somatic inactivation of genes on chromosome 13 is a common event in retinoblastoma. *Nature* **304:** 451–453.

Goldgar DE, Fields P, Lewis CM *et al.* (1994) A large kindred with 17q-linked breast and ovarian cancer: Genetic phenotypic and genealogical analysis. *J. Natl. Cancer Inst.* **86:** 200–209.

Hall JM, Lee MK, Morrow J *et al.* (1990) Linkage analysis of early onset familial breast cancer to chromosome 17q21. *Science* **250:** 1684–1689.

Harris H, Miller OJ, Klein G, Worst P & Tachibana T (1969) Suppression of malignancy by cell fusion. *Nature* **223:** 363–368.

Harris H (1988) The analysis of malignancy by cell fusion: the position in 1988. *Cancer Res.* **48:** 3302–3306.

■ Knudson AG (1971) Mutation and cancer: statistical study of retinoblastoma. *Proc. Natl. Acad. Sci.* **68:** 820–823.

Leach FS, Nicolaides NC, Papadopoulos N *et al.* (1993) Mutations of a MutS homolog in hereditary non polyposis colorectal cancer. *Cell* **75:** 1215–1225.

Lindblom A, Tannergard P, Werelius B *et al.* (1993) Genetic mapping of a second locus predisposing to hereditary non-polyposis colon cancer. *Nature Genet.* **5:** 279–282.

Lynch HT, Albana W, Black L *et al.* (1981) Familial excess of cancer of the ovary and other anatomic sites. *J. Am. Med. Assoc.* **245:** 261–264.

Nowell PC & Hungerford DA (1960) A minute chromosome in human chronic granulocytic leukemia. *Science* **132:** 1497.

Peltomaki P, Aaltonen LA, Sistonen P *et al.* (1993) Genetic mapping of a locus predisposing to human colorectal cancer. *Science* **260:** 810–812.

Slamon DJ, Godolphin W, Jones LA *et al.* (1989) Studies of the HER2/neu protooncogene in human breast and ovarian cancer. *Science* **244:** 707–712.

Smith SA, Easton DF, Evans DGR *et al.* (1992) Allele losses in the region 17q-21 in familial breast and ovarian cancer involve the wild-type chromosome. *Nature Genet.* **2:** 128–131.

Smith SA, DiCioccio RA, Struewing JP *et al.* (1994) Localisation of the breast–ovarian cancer susceptibility gene (BRCA1) on 17q12-21 to an interval of ⩽1cM. *Genes Chrom. Cancer* **10:** 71–76.

Steichen-Gersdof E, Gallion HH, Ford D *et al.* (1994) Familial site-specific ovarian cancer is linked to BRCA1 on 17q12-21. *Am. J. Hum. Genet.* **55:** 870–875.

Stehelin D, Varmus HE, Bishop JM & Vogt PK (1976) DNA related to the transforming genes(s) of avian sarcoma viruses is present in normal avian DNA. *Nature* **260:** 170–173.

Thibodeau SN, Bren G & Schaid D (1993) Microsatellite instability in cancer of the proximal colon. *Science* **260:** 816–819.

■ Vogelstein B, Fearon ER, Hamilton SR *et al.* (1988) Genetic alterations during colorectal-tumor development. *New Engl. J. Med.* **319:** 525–532.

■ Weinberg RA (1994) Oncogenes and tumor suppressor genes. *CA Cancer J. Clin.* **44:** 160–170.

Yunis JJ & Ramsay N (1978) Retinoblastoma and subband deletion of chromosome 13. *Am. J. Dis. Child* **132:** 161–163.

46 Tumor Markers in Gynecologic Cancers

N J Finkler

Introduction

The use of tumor markers in gynecologic cancers has become an area of wide interest and intense research over the past several years. The ability to detect or follow patients with gynecologic cancers through serum or urine tests has major potential benefits to patients and physicians and may provide avenues to accurately diagnose disease without the use of expensive time-consuming tests. To this end, our knowledge of potential tumor markers has blossomed with the development of newer testing techniques, mostly aided through the development of monoclonal antibody technology.

Before discussing tumor markers available today and their specific application to gynecologic disease, it is important to recognize potential drawbacks to our reliance on such tests. Most importantly, the ideal tumor markers should have the following characteristics: secretion specifically by a specific tumor; secretion under all circumstances when tumor is present; no detection or secretion in benign disease; and accurately reflect tumor status at all times. Unfortunately, the ideal tumor marker has not yet been identified. Rather, we have learned to rely on a group of oncofetal, hormonal and tumor-associated antigen markers. A number of generalized markers also exist, with descriptions of new nonspecific markers occurring with great frequency.

In this chapter, the role of commonly used tumor markers will be discussed and related to the diagnosis and follow-up of patients with gynecologic disease. For detailed discussion of the markers used within a specific gynecologic cancer diagnosis, the reader is referred to the chapters discussing individual disease processes.

Oncofetal Tumor Markers

Carcinoembryonic antigen (CEA) and alpha feto-protein (AFP) are the two most commonly used oncofetal tumor markers in gynecologic cancers. Although the clinical use of AFP is restricted to ovarian endodermal sinus tumors, embryonal cell carcinomas and mixed germ cell tumors containing these two elements, CEA determinations may be useful in patients with a variety of gynecologic cancers.

CEA is a glycoprotein with a molecular weight of approximately 200,000 daltons. Although originally described as a tumor-specific antigen for colonic adenocarcinomas, CEA levels can be elevated in up to 50% of patients with gynecologic cancers (Van Nagell *et al.*, 1978). CEA levels may be useful in patients with mucinous cystadenocarcinomas, with mean CEA levels much higher than in patients with serous tumors. CEA levels may also be useful in patients with endocervical adenocarcinomas and keratinizing squamous cell carcinoma.

Interestingly, CEA-positive staining of tissue samples demonstrates that CEA can be detected in up to 80% of endocervical adenocarcinomas as opposed to less than 10% of endometrial adenocarcinomas. Occasionally, this differential staining pattern may be most useful to the clinician in determining whether a lesion is endocervical or endometrial in origin (Wahlstrom *et al.*, 1979).

Despite its widespread use in colon cancer, CEA has limited use in gynecologic cancer because of its lack of specificity. Furthermore, benign hepatic disease as well as benign gynecologic and non-gynecologic disease can cause elevations in serum CEA levels.

AFP is a glycoprotein with a molecular weight of 10,000 daltons. It is produced by embryonic hepatic and yolk sac cells and the highest concentrations of AFP are produced by hepatocellular carcinomas and malignant germ cell tumors of the ovary and testis.

AFP is elevated in patients with both endodermal sinus tumors and embryonal cell carcinomas, as well as mixed germ cell tumors containing one of these elements. AFP levels can be monitored in patients undergoing therapy for germ cell tumors, with AFP levels correlating well with tumor progression or regression in the majority of cases reported to date (Sell *et al.*, 1976).

Hormonal Markers

The most widely used hormonal marker available is human chorionic gonadotropin (HCG), a trophoblastic glycoprotein with a molecular weight of 39,000. This glycoprotein is comprised of two dissimilar subunits, A and B, joined non-covalently.

Recently, a fragment of HCG-b-subunit has been identified in the urine of patients with gynecologic tumors and is under investigation as a potential marker of various gynecologic cancers. This urinary gonadotropin fragment (UGF) is produced through cleavage of the B-subunit in non-trophoblastic cancers (Cole *et al.*, 1988).

Early observations in patients with choriocarcinoma demonstrated the clinical use of HCG. HCG concentrations are known to be elevated in patients with gestational trophoblastic noeplasia (GTN) and concentrations can accurately predict tumor response. The increased sensitivity of the β subunit assay for HCG has greatly aided both diagnosis and management of patients with GTN. Elevated levels of serum β HCG are also found in patients with non-trophoblastic tumors, notably non-gestational choriocarcinomas of the ovary, and to some degree, cervical and ovarian malignancies. The greatest clinical use has come from the management of GTN and germ cell tumors with choriocarcinoma.

As previously outlined, the development of UGF has added some excitement to the possibility of using hormonal markers in the evaluation of gynecologic cancers. Since the original description in 1988 of the sensitivity and specificity of UGF in gynecologic cancer patients many articles have appeared describing the potential role of this marker. UGF levels may be elevated in all gynecologic cancers, with sensitivities approaching 75%. The sensitivity for UGF in cervical (73%), ovarian (83%) and endometrial (65%) cancers exceeded that of CA-125 as a single test. Furthermore, serial UGF levels have been shown to accurately reflect disease status in patients undergoing therapy for carcinomas of the ovary (Cole *et al.*, 1984).

UGF levels have also been examined in a large group of women with benign and malignant disease in order to establish sensitivities and specificities. Using a cut-off level of over 3 fmol ml^{-1}, UGF sensitivity and specificity were 90% and 66%, respectively. Levels exceeded 3 fmol ml^{-1} in 76% of women with recurrent disease (Wang *et al.*, 1988). For screening purposes, it was felt that a level of 8 fmol ml^{-1} was indicated, with this level providing a specificity and sensitivity of 99% and 46%, respectively. Whether UGF can provide screening capabilities remains to be documented because there remain serious concerns with the number of false positive and false negatives generated using an individual screening test.

The efficacy of UGF in discriminating benign from malignant pelvic masses has been examined. Using a cut-off of over 8 fmol ml^{-1}, the combination of CA-125 and UGF appeared to have increased sensitivity (86%) when compared to each test performed alone. Importantly, this schema had minimal false detection of benign disease (1.2%) (Nam *et al.*, 1990). Elevated levels of UGF may be clinically useful in endometrial cancer. Elevated levels of UGF may indicate extrauterine disease, specifically lymph node involvement. Unfortunately, UGF does not appear to be of great clinical benefit in patients with cervical or vulvar carcinomas (Nam *et al.*, 19??).

As more experience is gained with UGF, we will begin to better understand the role of this new hormonal tumor marker in gynecologic cancers. In the interim, more data should be obtained and more clinical trials completed to properly place this marker in our antitumor armory.

Tumor-associated Antigens

The refinement of techniques for antigen isolation and the development of monoclonal antibody technology has resulted in an ever increasing number of tumor-associated antigens available to gynecologic oncologists. These tumor-associated antigens can be expressed at the time of malignant transformation or they may represent normal tissue antigens that are quantitively increased through enhanced production by tumor cells. Rather than attempting to define each antigen or monoclonal antibody available, discussion will be limited to antigens most commonly used in gynecologic cancers.

The best known antigen in squamous cell carcinoma is the SCC antigen, a glycoprotein originally described by Kato and Torigoe (1977) as a byproduct of the original TA-4 antigen. SCC antigen levels may be useful in monitoring patients with locally advanced disease, with serial measurements having the potential to accurately reflect disease status. Unfortunately, the majority of patients with small volume tumors have undetectable levels of SCC antigen.

Ovarian carcinomas pose a particular problem best suited for tumor-associated antigens: difficulty in diagnosis; difficulty in monitoring disease status during therapy; difficulty in assessing tumor response at completion of therapy; predicting tumor recurrence; and discriminating benign from malignant disease. The ideal tumor marker for ovarian cancer would help in alleviating many of these problems. As previously stated, the ideal tumor marker has not yet been described, although a number of tumor-associated antigens may help in the problems outlined.

The best suited and most widely published tumor-associated antigen is CA-125. Originally described by Bast and Knapp, this tumor-associated antigen remains the only Food and Drug Administration (FDA)-approved tumor-associated antigen for patients with ovarian cancer (Bast *et al.*, 1981) CA-125 levels are elevated in a majority of patients with serous carcinomas of the ovary (approximately 80%), but can also be falsely elevated by a number of benign gynecologic and other malignant conditions including endometriosis, pelvic inflammatory disease, fibroids, peritonitis, pancreatic cancer, liver failure and pericarditis (Finkler *et al.*, 1987). The landmark paper on CA-125 outlined the use of this marker in predicting response to primary therapy in patients with known ovarian cancer undergoing chemotherapy (Bast *et al.*, 1983). Correlation between rising CA-125 levels and progressive disease was shown, as well as correlation between falling CA-125 levels and disease regression. CA-125 levels were also examined as a potential marker for tumor status at the completion of primary chemotherapy. If CA-125 was higher than 35 u ml^{-1} at completion of therapy, persistent disease was identified in 100% of patients including those with negative radiographic studies. If CA-125 was less than 35 u ml^{-1}, however, up to 40% of patients were found to have persistent disease at second-look (Berek *et al.*, 1986).

Many data have also been collected on the ability of CA-125 to predict recurrences. It appears as though an elevated CA-125 level in a patient with a history of ovarian carcinoma can predict tumor recurrence several months before clinical or radiographic detection. Whether this early identification of tumor recurrence can translate into prolonged survival, however, remains to be demonstrated.

An obvious potential role for CA-125 is in the preoperative evaluation of pelvic masses. Determining if a mass is benign or malignant preoperatively would be of great clinical use. A multitude of studies has demonstrated relatively poor sensitivity and specificity of CA-125 in the premenopausal population with pelvic masses. In postmenopausal patients, however, sensitivities and specificities were found to be 84% and 92%, respectively. The addition of CA-125 to ultrasound or clinical impression may provide statistically significant increases in positive and negative predictive values in the postmenopausal group (Finkler *et al.*, 1988). As shown in *Table 46.1*, predictive values increase significantly in the postmenopausal population with the use of CA-125. Again, the major benefit appears to be in the positive predictive value. Negative predictive values of only 80% are achieved in the postmenopausal population by adding CA-125 to either ultrasound or clinical impression.

One of the great hopes for CA-125 has been the ability to detect early ovarian cancer and CA-125's potential role as a screening tool. Data to date suggest that the sensitivity and specificity for CA-125 is too low to use as a single screening test. Whether CA-125 has any role in screening remains to be documented.

Table 46.1. Impact of adding CA-125 to ultrasound or clinical impression (adapted from Finkler *et al.* 1988).

Predictive value (%)	**Premenopausal**		**Postmenopausal**	
	No CA-125	*With CA-125*	*No CA-125*	*With CA-125*
Positive	26	36	92	100
Negative	74	80	41	80

Another tumor-associated antigen that has gained use in ovarian cancer is NB/70K, originally described by Knauf *et al.* (1984). NB/70K measures a different antigen than CA-125 and data on its use suggest a high sensitivity in patients with epithelial cancer of the ovary. In addition, elevated levels of NB/70K have been found in all stages, grades and histologic types of ovarian cancer.

Whether or not NB/70K can add significant complementary information to CA-125 levels is an area of great interest and must await clinical trials of large numbers of patients (Petru *et al.*, 1990).

Hormonal Receptors

A discussion of gynecologic cancers and tumor markers would not be complete without a brief discussion on estrogen receptor and progesterone receptor proteins (ERP, PRP) and their relationship to endometrial adenocarcinomas.

The clinical usefulness of ERP and PRP is in the identification of biologic behavior and tumor responsiveness. Cytosol ERP and PRP are found in higher concentration in early-stage endometrial cancer compared with more widely disseminated or recurrent disease (Kauppila *et al.*, 1982). Both receptors are present more commonly and in higher concentration in better differentiated tumors. However, even well differentiated tumors may be receptor poor (Gurpide, 1981).

Receptor-rich neoplasms have higher response rates than receptor-poor neoplasms and receptor-poor neoplasms behave more aggressively than those that are receptor-rich (Creasman *et al.*, 1980).

Because of the potential role in predicting response to progestational agents, ERP and PRP should be measured in endometrial cancers and, if possible, in recurrent tumors.

Future Directions

The ideal markers for gynecologic cancers have not yet been identified. Oncofetal markers, tumor-associated antigens and hormonal receptors can aid the clinician greatly, yet each tool has its limitations.

Two new directions are developing in the field of tumor markers. First is the identification of site-nonspecific markers that will indicate an ongoing malignant process without identifying the primary.

An example of such an approach is cancer procoagulant (CP) (Gordon and Cross, 1990), a cysteine proteinase capable of activating coagulation factor X directly that is only found in malignant cells. CP is produced by a wide variety of malignant cells, but not normal tissue, with the exception of amniochorion. Preliminary data suggest that CP may be detected in a variety of tumors, including those of the genitourinary tract.

The second approach in tumor marker research is the identification of genetic probes used for diagnostic and therapeutic purposes. Examples of genetic probes exist with other malignancies such as CML (BCR–ABBL translocation, i.e. Philadelphia chromosome) and AML (t15:17). Identification of genetic probes in gynecologic cancers will be an important step in the application of tumor markers in gynecologic cancers.

Summary of Core Information

- The ideal markers for gynecologic cancers have not yet been identified. Oncofetal markers, tumor-associated antigens and hormonal receptors can aid the clinician greatly, yet each tool has its limitations.
- The clinical use of alpha fetoprotein (AFP) is restricted to ovarian endodermal sinus tumors, embryonal cell carcinomas and mixed germ cell tumors containing these two elements.
- Despite its widespread use in colon cancer, carcinoembryonic antigen (CEA) has limited use in gynecologic cancer because of its lack of specificity. Furthermore, benign hepatic disease as well as benign gynecologic and non-gynecologic disease can cause elevations in serum CEA levels.
- The most widely used hormonal marker available is human chorionic gonadotropin (HCG). The increased sensitivity of the beta subunit assay for HCG has greatly aided both diagnosis and management of patients with gestational trophoblastic tumors.
- The sensitivity of the urinary gonadotropin fragment (UGF) in cervical (73%), ovarian (83%) and endometrial (65%) cancers exceeds that of CA-125 as a single test. Furthermore, serial UGF levels have been shown to accurately reflect disease status in patients undergoing therapy for carcinomas of the ovary.
- Elevated levels of UGF may have a clinical use in endometrial cancer. Unfortunately, UGF does not appear to be of great clinical benefit in patients with cervical or vulvar carcinomas.
- The best-known antigen in squamous cell carcinoma is the SCC antigen, a byproduct of the TA-4 antigen. SCC levels may be useful in monitoring patients with locally advanced disease. Unfortunately, the majority of patients with small volume tumor have undetectable levels of SCC antigen.
- The tumor-associated antigen CA-125 remains the only Food and Drug Administration (FDA)-approved tumor-associated antigen for patients with ovarian cancer. Data to date suggest that the sensitivity and specificity for CA-125 is too low to use as a single screening test.
- If CA-125 is higher than 35 u ml^{-1} at completion of therapy, persistent disease will be identified in 100% of patients including those with negative radiographic studies. If CA-125 is 35 u ml^{-1} or less, up to 40% of patients are still found to have persistent disease at second-look.
- With regard to estrogen and progesterone receptors in endometrial cancer, receptor-rich neoplasms have higher response rates than receptor-poor neoplasms and receptor-poor neoplasms behave more aggressively than those that are receptor rich.

References

Bast RC Jr, Feeney M, Lazarus H *et al.* (1981) Reactivity of a monoclonal antibody with human ovarian carcinoma. *J. Clin. Invest.* **68:** 1331–1334.

■ Bast RC Jr, Klug TC *et al.* (1983) A radioimmunoassay using a monoclonal antibody to monitor the course of epithelial ovarian cancer. *New Engl. J. Med.* **309:** 883–887.

Berek JS, Knapp RC, Malkasian GD *et al.* (1986) CA 125 serum levels correlated with second look operations among ovarian cancer patients. *Obstet. Gynecol.* **67:** 685–689.

Cole LA, Kroll TG, Ruddon RW & Hussa RO (1984) Differential occurrence of free (A) and free (D) subunits of human chorionic gonadotropin in pregnancy sera. *J. Clin. Endocrinol. Metab.* **58:** 1200–1202.

■ Cole LA, Schwartz PE & Wang Y (1988) Urinary gonadotropin fragments (UGF) in cancers of the female reproductive system. I. Sensitivity and specificity, comparison with other markers. *Gynecol. Oncol.* **31:** 82–90.

Creasman WT, McCarty KS, Barten TK *et al.* (1980) Clinical correlates of estrogen and progesterone binding proteins in human endometrial adenocarcinoma. *Obstet. Gynecol.* **55:** 363–370.

Finkler NJ, Bast RC & Knapp RC (1987) Monoclonal antibodies in ovarian cancer. In: Kupchick HZ (ed) In Vitro *Diagnosis of Human Tumors Using Monoclonal Antibodies*, pp. 141–167. New York, NY: Marcel Dekker, Inc.

Finkler NJ, Benacerraf B, Lavin PT *et al.* (1988) Comparison of serum CA 125, clinical impression and ultrasound in the preoperative evaluation of ovarian masses. *Obstet. Gynecol.* **72:** 659–664.

Gordon SG & Cross BA (1990) An enzyme-linked immunosorbent assay for cancer procoagulant and its potential as a new tumor marker. *Cancer Res.* **50,** 6229–6234.

Gurpide E (1981) Hormone receptors in endometrial cancer. *Cancer* **48:** 638–641.

Kato H & Torgoie T (1977) Radioimmunoassay for tumor antigen of human cervical squamous cell carcinoma. *Cancer* **40:** 16–1628.

■ Kauppila A, Kujansuu E & Vihko R (1982) Cytosol estrogen and progesterone receptors in endometrial carcinoma of patients treated with surgery, radiotherapy and progestin. *Cancer* **50:** 2157–2162.

Knauf S, Taillon–Miller P, Helkamp BF *et al.* (1984) Selectivity for ovarian cancer of an improved serum radioimmunoassay for human ovarian tumor-associated antigen NB/70K. *Gynecol. Oncol.* **17:** 349–355.

Nam JH, Cole LA, Chambers JT & Schwartz PE (1989) Urinary gonadotropin fragment, a new tumor marker. I. Assay development and cancer-specificity. *Gynecol. Oncol.* **36:**

Nam JH, Cole LA, Chambers JT & Schwatz PE (1989) Urinary gonadotropin fragment, a new tumor marker, II. For differentiating a benign from a malignant pelvic mass. *Gynecol. Oncol.* **36:** 391–394.

Petru F, Sevin BU, Averette HF *et al.* (1990) Comparison of three tumor markers – CA 125, lipid associated sialic acid (LASA), and NB/70K in monitoring ovarian cancer. *Gynecol. Oncol.* **38:** 181–186.

Sell A, Sogaard H & Horgaard–Pedersen B (1976) Serum alpha feto-protein as a marker for the effect of post-operative radiation or chemotherapy in eight cases of ovarian endodermal sinus tumor. *Int. J. Cancer* **18:** 574–580.

Van Nagell Jr, Donaldson ES, Wood EC *et al.* (1978) The clinical significance of carcinoembryonic antigen in the plasma and tumors of patients with gynecologic malignancies. *Cancer* **42:** 1527–1532.

Wahlstrom T, Lindgren J, Korhonen M *et al.* (1979) Distinction between endocervical and endometrial adenocarcinoma with immunoperoxidase staining of carcinoembryonic antigen in routine histologic tissue specimens. *Lancet* **24:** 1159–1160.

Wang Y, Schwartz PE, Chambers JT & Cole LA (1988) Urinary gonadotropin fragments (UGF) in cancers of female reproductive system. II. Initial serial studies. *Gynecol. Oncol.* **31:** 91.

47 Current Staging Classifications

M B Dinerman
H M Shingleton

Summary of Contents

Overview

All staging systems are designed to describe the primary tumor location, local or regional spread, and the presence or absence of metastatic tumor. Cancer staging is fundamental to treatment and management planning, evaluating results and offering prognostic information to supply the patient. Moreover, staging systems are an internationally accepted and standardized means of communication between cancer care providers allowing comparability of results of clinical trials, quality assurance programs, cancer surveillance and tumor registry statistics. A systematic and universal classification allows the clinician to contribute to the ongoing investigation of cancer and to objectively convey clinical experience without ambiguity.

Clinical staging is based on evidence acquired before treatment. Presently, the most widely accepted staging system for gynecologic tumors is the classification of the *Fédération internationale gynécologie et d'obstétrique* (FIGO). The preferred method for most other solid tumors, including breast cancer, is the TNM classification of *Union internationale contre le cancer* (UICC) and the American Joint Committee on Cancer (AJCC).

General Rules of TNM Staging

TNM staging relates to three primary areas: T, the extent of the primary *tumor*; N, the regional lymph *node* status; and M, the presence or absence of distant *metastases*. This system is modified further by the addition of numbers; for example, T0, no evidence of primary tumor; Tis, carcinoma *in situ*; T1, T2, T3, and T4, increase in size and/or local extent of the primary tumor. TX represents a primary tumor that cannot be assessed. Multiple synchronous tumors should be classified with the highest T number; for example 2.5 cm and 0.5 cm carcinomas occurring in the same breast would be classified as T2(M), where M designates multiple. Bilateral synchronous tumors in paired organs should be independently classified.

Regional lymph nodes are classified as follows: NX, regional lymph nodes cannot be assessed; N0, no regional lymph node metastasis; N1, N2, N3, increasing involvement of regional lymph nodes. Metastasis in a lymph node distant from the primary tumor is classified as a distant metastasis. A distant metastasis is assessed as follows: M0, no distant metastasis; M1, distant metastasis.

The clinical stage is critical for the selection of initial therapy, whereas the pathologic stage provides more accurate information for the estimation of prognosis. The pathologic stage, or pTNM, is formulated on the basis of histopathologic information derived by the pathologist for the primary tumor, regional lymph nodes and/or histologic examination of a distant metastasis following surgery or invasive biopsies. The pathologic stage is based on the evidence acquired before treatment, during surgery and during pathologic examination. Ordinarily, for pathologic staging, either all or sufficient tissue from the primary cancer and regional lymph nodes is excised to enable one to determine the greatest extent of the cancer (such as T4 and

N3). Two other less frequently used stage groupings in the TNM system are retreatment for recurrence (rTNM) and autopsy classification (aTNM).

General Rules for FIGO Staging

Clinical FIGO staging should be based on careful examination and performed before any definitive therapy. It is desirable that the examination be performed by an experienced examiner and under anesthesia when appropriate. Surgical–pathologic findings are adapted for staging of corpus, ovary, fallopian tube, vulvar cancer and trophoblastic disease. The clinical stage must under no circumstances be changed on the basis of subsequent findings. When it is doubtful to which stage a particular case should be allotted, the case must be referred to the earlier stage.

For clinical FIGO staging purposes, the following examination methods are permitted before the first definitive treatment: palpation, inspection, colposcopy, endocervical curettage, hysteroscopy, cystoscopy, proctoscopy, intravenous urography, and X-ray examination of the lungs and skeleton. Suspected bladder or rectal involvement should be confirmed by biopsy and histologic evidence.

Findings by examinations such as computed tomography (CT), magnetic resonance imaging (MRI), lymphangiography, arteriography, venography and laparoscopy are of value for the planning of therapy, but because these are not yet generally available and the interpretation of results is variable, the findings of such studies should not be the basis for changing the clinical staging.

Only if the rules of staging are strictly observed will it be possible to compare results among clinics and by differing modes of therapy. Perspectives on the advantages and limitations of current staging classifications are provided following the staging systems for each tumor site by experienced clinicians in the disciplines of gynecologic oncology, medical oncology, and radiation therapy.

Cervical Cancer

The staging classification adopted by the International Federation of Gynecology and Obstetrics (FIGO) is based on clinical findings as shown in *Table 47.1*. This classification system is intended to standardize the reporting of treatment results, to group patients into similar prognostic categories, and to further universal acceptance of methodology.

Studies accepted by FIGO for staging purposes include: examination under anesthesia, chest radiography, bone radiography, intravenous urogram, cystoscopy and proctoscopy. Studies such as lymphangiography, CT and laparoscopy are performed for patients and can alter their therapy. However, the results of these studies should not be used to change the clinical stage. This can result in stage migration (especially when assigning patients with positive paraaortic lymph nodes to Stage IVB) and a lack of standardization of reporting results.

The use of prognostic factors for stage groupings for cervical cancer has not been adequately addressed. Tumor size and lymph node status are two dominant prognostic factors. Tumor size can vary greatly between Stage IB, IIA, IIB, IIIA and IIIB. Tumor diameter should be recorded whenever possible. Other indicators of tumor size that can be recorded are medial versus lateral parametrial extension and fixation to one or both pelvic side-walls. Lymph node status is not addressed in the current FIGO system.

Universal acceptance and ease of use of a staging system are necessary for successful implementation. A patient's treatment should be individualized based upon all available information. However, the current FIGO clinical staging system can be improved to include such factors as tumor size and lymph node status. Staging rules should be strictly interpreted and used when results of therapy are reported.

Treatment modalities for cervical cancer have been, and still are, radical surgery for early disease and radiation for more advanced disease. Past attempts to classify the disease extent of an individual patient have been affected by this dichotomy in management (Christopherson, 1992). The German Gynecological Society (GSS) first staged cervical cancer in 1923, differentiating between operable and nonoperable cases. In 1929, and later in 1937, the League of Nations (LON) defined the clinical parameters that correlated with operability: Stage I, tumor growth confined to the cervix, which was clearly operable; Stage II, tumor infiltrates the parametrium, upper two-thirds of the vagina and/or corpus and was doubtfully operable; Stage III, invasion of the pelvic side-wall with no free space on rectal examination and/or involvement of lower third of vagina, which was inoperable; Stage IV, involvement of bladder, rectum and/or tumor outside the pelvis, which was considered hopeless.

FIGO first formulated a staging classification in 1950, accepting most of the LON clinical criteria, but adding carcinoma *in situ* as Stage 0. Since then, several modifications have been introduced (in 1961, 1971, 1974, 1985), based on surgical–pathologic studies of cervical carcinoma. The concept of microinvasive carcinoma was introduced in 1961 as Stage IA (early stromal invasion), which was not further defined. In 1988, a further subdivision of Stage IA was introduced to separate very minimal, microscopic invasion (IA-1) from 'microcarcinoma,' a superficial lesion, but a definitely measurable invasive tumor mass (IA-2). For the first time, actual microscopic dimensions, up to a size of 5 mm deep and 7 mm lateral extension for Stage IA-2 were

Table 47.1. FIGO staging of carcinoma of the cervix uteri (1995).

TNM[1]	*FIGO*[2]	*Definition*
Primary tumor (T)		
TX	—	Primary tumor cannot be assessed
T0	—	No evidence of primary tumor
Tis	0	Carcinoma *in situ*, intraepithelial carcinoma
T1	I	Cervical carcinoma confined to cervix (extension to the corpus should be disregarded)
T1a	IA	Invasive carcinoma, diagnosed microscopically only. All gross lesions even with superficial invasion are Stage IB cancers. Invasion is limited to measured stromal invasion with maximum depth of 5.0 mm* and no wider than 7.0 mm
T1a1	IA-1	Minimal microscopically evident stromal invasion. Measured invasion of stroma no greater than 3.0 mm in depth and no wider than 7.0 mm
T1a2	IA-2	Measured invasion of stroma greater than 3 mm and no greater than 5 mm,* and no wider than 7 mm
		*The depth of invasion should not be more than 5 mm taken from the base of the epithelium, either surface or glandular, from which it originates. Vascular space involvement either venous or lymphatic should not alter the staging
T1b	IB	Clinical lesions confined to the cervix or preclinical lesions greater than Stage IA
	IB-1	Clinical lesions no greater than 4.0 cm in size
	IB-2	Clinical lesions greater than 4.0 cm in size
T2	II	Cervical carcinoma invades beyond the uterus, but not to the pelvic wall or to the lower third of the vagina
T2a	IIA	No obvious parametrial invasion
T2b	IIB	Obvious parametrial invasion
T3	III	Extends to the pelvic wall and/or involves lower third of the vagina and/or causes hydronephrosis or nonfunctioning kidney
T3a	IIIA	Tumor involves the lower third of the vagina; no extension to the pelvic wall
T3b	IIIB	Tumor extends to the pelvic wall and/or causes hydronephrosis or nonfunctioning kidney
T4	IV	The carcinoma has extended beyond the true pelvis or has clinically involved the mucosa of the bladder or rectum. A bullous edema as such does not permit a case to be allotted to Stage IV
	IVA	Tumor invades mucosa of bladder or rectum and/or extends beyond true pelvis
M1	IVB	Distant metastasis

[1]AJCC/UICC, 1992.
[2]Society of Gynecologic Oncologists (1994) *Handbook: Staging of Gynecologic Malignancies* 1st ed, Chicago: Society of Gynecologic Oncologists.

given. Data from pretherapeutic surgical staging, including pelvic–aortic lymph node dissection and evaluation of direct tumor extension into the parametria, added to the understanding of spread patterns of cervical cancer, but also added confusion in terminologies and international communication.

In addition, two other staging systems were introduced (Beahrs *et al.*, 1988). In 1964, the AJCC adopted the TNM classification, developed by the UICC, which attempted to better differentiate the extent of the primary tumor from regional and metastatic tumor spread. This was widely applied by radiation oncologists and tumor registries. These systems have the advantage of separating pretherapeutic clinical staging (cTNM) from pathologic staging (pTNM), which includes surgical–pathologic evidence of tumor spread of the primary tumor and metastatic sites (e.g. lymph nodes). The FIGO staging system for cervical cancer remains largely clinical, but an ever increasing array of imaging techniques is now widely available and may provide more accurate information on the extent of disease. In addition, pretreatment surgical staging, including laparoscopic biopsy of the retroperitoneal nodes, has been more widely used (Delgado *et al.*, 1990; Kamura *et al.*, 1992). However, none of these additional studies are accepted to define the clinical FIGO stage.

The current definition of microinvasive carcinoma (MIC) includes FIGO Stages IA-1, defined as "minimal microscopic invasion," which is not further specified, and a IA-2, "tumor with invasive component 5 mm or less from the base of the epithelium and 7 mm in horizontal spread." This definition represents a compromise of volumetric studies based on pathologic giant sections of the cervix done by only a few pathologists in Europe (Burghardt *et al.*, 1991).

In the United States and Japan, a different definition of Stage IA, proposed by the Society of Gynecologic Oncologists (SGO), has been widely used. In 1974, the Committee on Staging and Nomenclature of the SGO proposed the following definition: "A microinvasive lesion is one in which the neoplastic epithelium invades the stroma in one or more places to a depth of 3 mm or less below the base of the epithelium, and in which lymphatic or blood vessel involvement is not demonstrated" (Seski *et al.*, 1977). The pathologic assessment of these parameters can be applied to all methods of tissue preparation and can therefore be used worldwide. Patients with such a lesion have a very low risk of nodal spread, and it is generally agreed that they can be treated by simple hysterectomy, or in some cases, even by a large cone biopsy (Kolstad, 1989). Recent data support the validity of this 'treatment-oriented' definition, which permits conservative management of patients with MIC (e.g. conization or hysterectomy) (Sevin *et al.*, 1992).

Thus the definition of Stage IA cervical cancer remains extremely controversial with no widespread agreement concerning depth of invasion, involvement of lymph–vascular spaces, or presence of confluent tongues of invasion. Nodal metastases and parametrial spread are clearly related to tumor volume, but what are reasonable practical histopathologic parameters for evaluating tumor volume? Are they the number of cone biopsy sections or one or two dimension tumor measurements? (Editor's Note: FIGO staging has been amended in 1995 to re-define Stage IA and also to change the definition of Stage IB, see *Table 47.1*).

Some clinicians have observed that bulky or 'barrel-shaped' cervical cancers 5 cm or greater in diameter, but without parametrial invasion, have a worse prognosis and may benefit from adjunctive hysterectomy after radiation (Gallion *et al.*, 1985; Weems *et al.*, 1985). Such patients have been stated as 'IC' by some centers. Although involvement of the uterine corpus by extension of cervical cancer may decrease survival, no practical way to accurately stage such patients has been available. Although involvement of the uterine corpus by extension of cervical cancer may decrease survival, upstaging of such patients was dropped from the staging classification years ago because accurate methods of evaluating such patients were not available (Perez *et al.*, 1981). However, new imaging techniques may provide this information and might be reconsidered in the future.

There is a discrepancy between the FIGO and TNM system in assessing disease extending beyond the cervix. For example, Stage IIIB based on rectovaginal examination or intravenous pyelogram, can be the result of direct continuous tumor extension from the cervix to the pelvic side-wall or large metastasis to pelvic lymph nodes. The AJCC/UICC staging system reflects these differences, while the FIGO does not. Parametrial lymph node metastasis poses a similar problem. In this regard, international reports on radical hysterectomy for Stage IIB disease frequently lack a clear separation between surgical and clinical findings. Only a dual staging system like the cTNM and pTNM would be able to resolve these areas of controversy.

The various prognostic indicators as well as the practical histopathologic study of cone biopsy specimens will need to be evaluated still further in an attempt to reach an agreement for staging IA or 'microinvasive' cervical cancer. At the moment, the disagreement is based largely on the differences in the perception of a staging system as either a prognostic classification only or as a guideline for therapy.

The newer imaging techniques, which may provide additional information on the extent of disease, need to be investigated since this equipment now is more widely available for clinical staging. In addition, minimally invasive surgical techniques may provide an opportunity for surgical staging even when the primary method of treatment is radiation therapy.

Vaginal Cancer

Carcinoma of the vagina is a rare cancer made even rarer by the strict diagnostic rules that apply: if a cancer involves the cervix or vulva in addition to the vagina, then the primary is assumed not to have arisen in the vagina. Since most patients are treated with radiotherapy, a clinical staging system is appropriate.

The FIGO staging is as shown in *Table 47.2*. Although the staging system does in general divide patients into broad groups with different outcome (Manetta *et al.*, 1988), stage definition is inaccurate in some circumstances. In differentiating Stage I from Stage II, it may be difficult to clinically determine Stage II subvaginal spread and particularly with large lesions, surrounding inflammation, and those adjacent to the bladder and rectum (Ball and Berman, 1982). The overall five-year survival for patients with Stage I disease, based on international figures, is only 53.4% (FIGO, 1989), although figures from smaller series are better (Al-Kurdi and Monaghan, 1981; Manetta *et al.*, 1988; Eddy *et al.*, 1991; Kucera and Vaura, 1991). As with other gynecologic cancers, it would be helpful to divide this stage to differentiate groups with very good outcomes from those that do poorly.

Within Stage II, there exists a clear difference in outcome between tumors with and without parametrial involvement. Consequently, it has been suggested that Stage II be divided into IIa with

Table 47.2. Staging of carcinoma of the vagina.

TNM[1]	*FIGO*[2]	*Definition*
Tis	0	Carcinoma *in situ*, intraepithelial carcinoma
T1	I	Carcinoma limited to the vaginal wall
T2	II	Carcinoma has involved the subvaginal tissue, but has not extended to the pelvic wall
T3	III	Carcinoma has extended to the pelvic wall
T4	IV	Carcinoma has extended beyond the true pelvis or has clinically involved the mucosa of the bladder or rectum. Bullous edema as such does not permit a case to be allotted to Stage IV
	IVa	Spread to adjacent organs and/or direct extension beyond the true pelvis
M1	IVb	Spread to distant organs

[1]AJCC/UICC, 1992.
[2]Society of Gynecologic Oncologists (1994) *Handbook: Staging of Gynecologic Malignancies*, 1st ed, Chicago: Society of Gynecologic Oncologists.

subvaginal infiltration not into the parametrium, and IIb with parametrial infiltration not extending to the pelvic wall (Perez *et al.*, 1974).

The incorporation of other prognostic factors might provide for improvements in the future. Other factors not currently included in the FIGO system include clinical inguinal node involvement, surgically-determined inguinal and pelvic node involvement, tumor site in the vagina, histologic subtype, grade, depth of invasion, and patient age (Al-Kurdi and Monaghan, 1981; Eddy *et al.*, 1991; Kucera and Vavra, 1991).

Cancer of the vagina remains a problem in gynecologic oncology for many reasons. It occurs rarely, accounting for only 1–2% of all gynecologic cancers. Because of the abundant lymphatic drainage present within a millimeter of the basement membrane of the surface epithelium, these cancers are usually extensive at the time of initial presentation, and often have lymphatic metastases. Early invasion on the anterior vaginal wall can disrupt the bladder, just as tumor on the posterior wall can affect the rectum.

Because of the location adjacent to the cervix and similar spread patterns, the staging of vaginal cancer is akin to that of the cervix. But since this is an uncommon lesion, the actual prognostic factors have not been well studied. One of the most important tumor characteristics in regard to selection of treatment is tumor location. Lesions in the vaginal fornices and those just inside the introitus are sometimes suitable for radical surgery, while those in the middle vagina are usually treated with radiation. It is unknown whether the tumor location is an independent prognostic variable. If this is so, it might be a factor to consider in staging. As with cervical cancer, newer imaging techniques and minimally invasive surgery may provide avenues for more accurate staging and a study of the spread patterns of this uncommon cancer. (Hoskins *et al.*, 1992; DiSaia and Creasman, 1993; Morrow *et al.*, 1993)

Endometrial Cancer

At the 1988 meeting of the FIGO Cancer Committee, major revisions were made for staging of endometrial cancer. Clinical evaluation (*Table 47.3 and 47.3A*), which had been in place since 1971 was replaced with surgical staging.

The basic prerequisites of a cancer staging system are universal application, standardization for reporting of results, and grouping patients in comparable categories. The adoption of an endometrial cancer surgical staging system does not lead to universal applicability since many centers have a philosophic resistance to pelvic node dissection. At some centers, there may not be the surgical expertise available to perform both pelvic and periaortic selective node sampling. Nevertheless, standardization is best achieved with surgical staging for the reporting of results and grouping of patients in comparable risk categories. Treatment comparisons and assessment of surgical morbidity can best be evaluated through reporting of results in a standardized fashion.

Because of difficulties of universal applicability, there is a recommendation that the 1971 FIGO clinical staging is used in situations in which the patient is inoperable or complete surgical staging is not performed. There are other difficulties in a surgical staging system, including treatment by radiation therapy alone, preoperative radium and preoperative external radiation therapy.

In the 1971 clinical staging system, nearly all patients were unfortunately allotted to Stage I (Homesley *et al.*, 1976; Homesley *et al.*, 1977). There was no differentiation between low- and high-risk patients by sounding of the uterus by determining endometrial cavity size using a calibrated sound. Additionally, there was no segregation into low- and high-risk by depth of myometrial penetration, especially in Grade 3 tumors. Depth of myometrial penetration and grade, which can change once the operative specimen is evaluated by the pathologist, both lend themselves well to a surgical staging system

Table 47.3. Staging of carcinoma of the corpus uteri.

TNM[1]	*FIGO*[2]	*Definition*
TX	—	Primary tumor cannot be assessed
T0	—	No evidence of primary tumor
Tis	—	Carcinoma *in situ*
T1	I	Tumor confined to corpus uteri
T1a	1AG123	Tumor limited to endometrium
T1b	IBG123	Tumor invades up to one-half of the myometrium
T1c	ICG123	Tumor invades more than one-half of the myometrium
T2	II	Tumor invades cervix, but does not extend beyond uterus
T2a	IIA	Endocervical glandular involvement only
T2b	IIB	Cervical stromal invasion
T3 and/or N1	III	Local and/or regional spread as specified in T3a, T3b, N1 and FIGO IIIA, B and C below
T3a	IIIA	Tumor involves serosa and/or adnex a (direct extension or metastasis) and/or cancer cells in ascites or peritoneal washings
T3b	IIIB	Vaginal involvement (direct extension or metastasis)
N1	IIIC	Metastasis to the pelvic and/or paraaortic lymph nodes
T4	IVA	Tumor invades bladder mucosa and/or bowel mucosa
M1	IVB	Distant metastasis (excluding metastasis to vagina, pelvic serosa, or adenexa; including metastasis to intra-abdominal lymph nodes other than paraaortic, and/or inguinal lymph nodes)

[1]AJCC/UICC (1992).
[2]Homesley HD (1992) Revised 1988 International Federation of Gynecology and Obstetrics staging systems for endometrial and vulvar cancer: an assessment. *Clin. Obstet. Gynecol.* **35:** 89–94.

Table 47.3A. Histopathology – degree of differentiation. Grading and staging notes (Annual report, FIGO, 1989).

Cases of carcinoma of the corpus should be classified (or graded) according to the degree of histologic differentiation, as follows.

- Grade 1: 5% or less of a nonsquamous or nonmorular solid growth pattern.
- Grade 2: 6–50% of a nonsquamous or nonmorular solid growth pattern.
- Grade 3: more than 50% of a nonsquamous or nonmorular solid growth pattern.

Notes on pathologic grading

- Notable nuclear atypia, inappropriate for the architectural grade, raises the grade of a Grade 1 or Grade 2 tumor by 1.
- In serous adenocarcinomas, clear-cell adenocarcinomas and squamous cell carcinoma, nuclear grading takes precedence.
- Adenocarcinomas with squamous differentiation are graded according to the nuclear grade of the glandular component.

Rules related to staging

- Because corpus cancer is now staged surgically, procedures previously used for determination of stages are no longer applicable such as the findings from fractional dilatation and curettage to differentiate between Stage I and Stage II.
- It is appreciated that there may be a small number of patients with corpus cancer who will be treated primarily with radiation therapy. If that is the case, the clinical staging adopted by FIGO in 1971 would still apply, but designation of that staging system would be noted.
- Ideally, width of the myometrium should be measured along with the width of tumor invasion.

(Creasman *et al.*, 1987). The operative stage of disease is also important in assessing the true extent of cervical involvement since there is a substantial difference in outcome related to glandular or stromal cervical involvement. The distinction must be made between the two. Cervical glandular or stromal invasion can be accurately assessed only post-operatively. Finally, patients with extensive disease beyond the uterus are unrecognized before surgical exploration (Homesley, 1994). Beforehand, evidence of advanced spread is not readily apparent.

A major advantage of the 1988 endometrial cancer staging system is the categorization of grade and myometrial invasion into three categories for disease confined to the uterus. The categories are no invasion, less than one-half myometrial invasion, and greater than one-half myometrial invasion. There are significant treatment implications if the patient has no invasion or minimal early invasion compared to patients with anaplastic tumors and deep invasion (Morrow *et al.*, 1991; Kadar *et al.*, 1992).

The other important independent prognostic factors relating to Stage II–IV disease need to be assessed, particularly the status of pelvic and periaortic lymph nodes (Creasman, 1994). A patient with negative nodes in surgical Stage I disease has a very different prognosis to one with the same intrauterine findings, but with positive pelvic or periaortic lymph nodes. The staging system allows for reporting by the 1971 clinical staging system for patients treated primarily with radiation therapy. For patients not undergoing full surgical staging, either the 1971 clinical staging or the 1988 surgical reporting with the surgeon denoting lack of full surgical staging can be applied. Debate will continue on the ideal system for endometrial cancer and whether or not there should be any treatment implications (Burke and Wolfson, 1994).

Recently, the value of nuclear grading has been reviewed by the Gynecologic Oncology Group (GOG) pathologists. Nuclear grading has validity in predicting outcome in that a higher nuclear grade can predict a more ominous outcome than lower architectural grading. Both architectural and nuclear grading should therefore be recorded prospectively so that they can be analyzed in the future.

The essential goal of surgical staging is to discover the actual extent of disease in appropriate but not all patients. There are advocates for pelvic and periaortic lymphadenectomy as opposed to the selective lymph node dissection as used by the GOG. Indeed there may be an increased incidence of positive nodes found when lymphadenectomy is performed, particularly in patients with anaplastic or deep invasive lesions. On the other hand, in patients with Grade 1 minimally invasive lesions, the likelihood of node metastasis will be less than 5%.

Staging for endometrial cancer as proposed by FIGO has been used worldwide for several decades. The staging has changed over the years to take into consideration changing conditions and new information. Before 1971, FIGO included a category within Stage I cancers for the patient that was medically inoperable. As management of older and sicker patients improved fewer patients fell into this category, and it was therefore dropped from the FIGO classification since it affected only a small subset of patients. In 1971, FIGO, appreciating that clinical and histologic prognostic factors were important, included these parameters in its staging criteria for corpus cancer. Stage I cancers were divided into six substages based on the size of the uterus and grade of the tumor. Using these criteria, prognosis correlated with this subclassification.

During the 1970s and early 1980s, several large worldwide studies suggested that clinical staging carried a large margin of error compared with the true extent of disease. Since at that time many institutions routinely used preoperative irradiation before surgery, it became apparent that a significant number of patients were overtreated with irradiation and others treated inappropriately (disease was present outside the treatment field). Several studies indicated that as many as 25% of clinical Stage I cancer patients had disease outside the uterus at the time of surgery (Creasman *et al.*, 1987). In patients with clinical Stage II disease there may have been a greater than 50% margin of error with regard to the actual extent of the tumor. In many instances, the disease process was overdiagnosed and excess treatment was given, resulting in unnecessary expense and potential morbidity. Since multiple prognostic factors were identified for this malignancy and only one, grade of tumor, could be determined preoperatively, it was felt that surgical staging, as had been accepted for other cancers, would give the clinician a more accurate method of determining the true extent of disease. More appropriately determined optimal therapy could then hopefully be given to the individual patient. Prognostic factors such as depth of invasion, extent of the disease in the uterus (endocervix), nodal involvement and other extrauterine extent such as adenexal metastases, intraabdominal disease and peritoneal cytology, could only be accurately determined with surgical staging. Because of this information, in 1988 FIGO changed endometrial carcinoma to a surgically-staged disease.

Although it is generally agreed that surgical staging of endometrial cancer is preferable to clinical staging, the extent of appropriate staging surgery remains controversial (Homesley *et al.*, 1992; Larson *et al.*, 1992). Obesity, age and medical complications render extensive lymph node dissection difficult. Although it is clear that patients proven to have nodal metastasis have a decreased survival rate, the results of a change in therapy in order to produce an improvement in survival are mixed. The value of this staging procedure has been questioned (Candiani *et al.*, 1990; Belinson *et al.*, 1992; Kim and Niloff, 1993). It must be remembered that FIGO has specifically stated that staging is to determine the extent of the disease and not to be used for treatment protocols.

The need and extent of the lymphadenectomy and biopsy as part of the surgical staging continues to be debated. The more extensive the lymphadenectomy, the greater the incidence of lymph node metastasis. Unfortunately, terms such as 'partial,' 'selective' and 'simple' to describe the extent of lymphadenectomy have crept into the literature without definition. Some investigators feel some patients do not require lymphadenectomy (e.g. Grade I, without significant invasion) because of the low incidence of node metastasis. Others would not dissect pelvic nodes if they are going to irradiate the patient because of other prognostic factors (e.g. Grade III or deep invasion). However, there is no data to suggest that irradiation in that group of patients without extrauterine disease is beneficial. There is no doubt that adequate surgical staging will optimally define the extent of disease. Risks and benefits as well as clinical judgement should be considered in regard to determining the extent of surgery.

Ovarian Cancer

The reasons for staging ovarian cancer are to direct treatment planning, prognosticate and compare results. The modern staging is a relatively recent development. Before the 1960s, there was surprisingly little agreement or emphasis on a systematic approach. The sixth edition of Novak's *Textbook of Gynecology* (1961) mentions that the classification usually employed is that of Hesel: Group I, involvement of one ovary; Group II, bilateral involvement or a removable local extension; Group III, locally irremovable extension or metastasis; and Group IV, a frozen pelvis or distant metastasis.

In 1964, FIGO accepted its first version of the now familiar FIGO stage grouping. A decade later, a revised classification provided clarification about ascites in Stage II, retroperitoneal nodes in Stage III, and malignant pleural effusion in Stage IV. In addition, there was an attempt to prognosticate better in Stage I with regard to capsular rupture and the presence or absence of tumor on the external surface of the ovary. In 1985, the special category was eliminated, the five substages of Stage I were condensed into three, Stage IIC was expanded to recognize surface tumor or capsular rupture, and three substages of Stage III were defined, based mainly on the tumor volume found at surgery. Current staging as determined at surgery is as shown in *Table 47.4.*

It is understandable that the special category 'unexplored cases' was removed, presumably because such cases are of uncertain relevance to ovarian cancer. Yet there is another special category which might have been substituted; namely, cases where the cancer does not appear to arise histologically in the ovary (Omura, 1981). Although it might seem obvious to exclude such cases, it is unclear whether that always happens. If such a special category were to exist, it would be interesting to see how often pathologists empty it. Since pathology is an integral part of the FIGO staging system, it is unfortunate that grade and cell type are not included. Well-defined and reproducible information with regard to pathology would enhance prognostication.

Better prognostication in Stage I is especially important since there is a wide range of outcomes, chemotherapy is still unproven in this stage, and some patients are adequately treated with surgery and meticulous abdominal exploration. Does a patient having only positive retroperitoneal nodes, which otherwise would be Stage I, have the same prognosis as another IIIC case? Does a patient with only omental spread have the same outcome as one with diaphragmatic involvement? It is surprising that malignant pleural effusion does not have a better prognosis than parenchymal liver involvement. Further refinements in prognostication may be possible using such tools as deoxyribonucleic acid (DNA) ploidy and oncogene expression. However, unless they were to be widely available, they might not be practical for an international system used by many countries, even if the prognostic value of such tools is well established.

In the 1994 Society of Gynecologic Oncologists Staging Handbook, Partridge (1994) points out that the independent prognostic value of capsular rupture, tumor excrescences or bilaterality as assessed by FIGO has not been confirmed by several reports in the literature that use multivariate techniques. A landmark paper on statistical techniques for considering multiple prognostic factors in the same analysis was published by Cox (1972) but not widely employed until later in the decade. Therefore, the first two versions of the FIGO system were presumably based on univariate comparisons. The extent to which Cox modeling was used in developing the 1985 versions is unclear.

Since the ultimate focus is on cure, especially in Stage I, one would especially appreciate some consideration of ten-year survival figures rather than five-year figures alone. Recurrence between five and ten years is not a rarity. The incorporation of residual tumor volume into the FIGO system is problematic because the prognostic importance of cytoreductive surgery remains controversial (Hoskins *et al.*, 1992).

The current FIGO stage grouping represents an evolutionary improvement over earlier versions. Further refinements are expected from the use of improved statistical techniques, more reliance on histopathology, and perhaps tumor biology.

There are two major points of controversy with regard to ovarian cancer staging. The major issue is whether the paraaortic nodes should be sampled at every ovarian cancer operation. It is reasonable to have some form of assessment of the nodes, but this can be carried out in retrospect by CT scanning. Although generalists worldwide operate on the vast majority of ovarian cancer, the idea of general obstetricians and gynecologists sampling nodes or

Table 47.4. Staging of carcinoma of the ovary.

TNM[1]	*FIGO*[2,3]	*Description*
T1	I	Growth limited to the ovaries
T1a	IA	Growth limited to one ovary; no ascites present containing malignant cells; no tumor on the external surface; capsule intact
T1b	IB	Growth limited to both ovaries; no ascites present containing malignant cells; no tumor on the external surfaces; capsules intact
T1c	IC	Tumor either Stage IA or IB, but with tumor on the surface of one or both ovaries; or with capsule ruptured; or with ascites present containing malignant cells or with positive peritoneal washings
T2	II	Growth involving one or both ovaries with pelvic extension
T2a	IIA	Extension and/or metastases to the uterus and/or tubes
T2b	IIB	Extension to other pelvic tissues
T2c	IIC	Tumor either Stage IIA or IIB, but with tumor on the surface of one or both ovaries; or with capsule(s) ruptured; or with ascites present containing malignant cells or with positive peritoneal washings
T3 and/or N1	III	Tumor involving one or both ovaries with peritoneal implants outside the pelvis and/or positive retroperitoneal or inguinal nodes. Superficial liver or metastases equals Stage III. Tumor is limited to true pelvis, but with histologically verified malignant extension to small bowel or omentum
T3a	IIIA	Tumor grossly limited to the true pelvis with negative nodes, but with histologically-confirmed microscopic seeding of abdominal peritoneal surfaces
T3b	IIIB	Tumor involving one or both ovaries with histologically-confirmed implants of abdominal peritoneal surfaces, none exceeding 2 cm in diameter; nodes are negative
T3c and/or N1	IIIC	Abdominal implants greater than 2 cm in diameter and/or positive retroperitoneal or inguinal nodes
M1	IV	Growth involving one or both ovaries with distant metastases. If pleural effusion is present there must be positive cytology to allot a case to Stage IV; parenchymal liver metastasis equals Stage IV

[1]AJCC/UICC.
[2]International Federation of Gynecology and Obstetrics (1987) Changes in definitions of clinical staging for carcinoma of the cervix and ovary. *Am. J. Obstet. Gynecol.* **156:** 246
[3]International Federation of Gynecology and Obstetrics (1989) Annual report on the results of treatment in gynecologic cancer. *Int. J. Gynecol. Oncol.* **29:** 189–190.

passing judgement on them is a cause for concern. Nevertheless, a thorough laparotomy is essential.

The other point of controversy is whether a total omentectomy is necessary in all patients with Stage I disease. Although an adequate sampling and assessment is essential, the author believes that a total omentectomy is not. The omentum, after all, is a source of pathology and has useful physiologic roles.

Fallopian Tube Cancer

Primary carcinoma of the fallopian tube is one of the rarest gynecologic malignancies and limited understanding of the disease led to a disagreement between authors regarding staging. A system introduced by Erez *et al.* (1967) based on the degree of tumor penetration and similar to the familiar Duke's system for rectal cancer was later modified by Schiller and Silverberg (1971). In the early 1980s, most centers used a fallopian tube malignancy staging by Dodson *et al.* (1970) similar to the FIGO ovarian cancer staging. It was only at the Singapore Meeting in 1991 that FIGO provided a standardized staging system for primary tubal carcinoma. The system, largely based on ovarian cancer staging with components of Schiller and Silverberg's classification (Petterson, 1992), uses the tumor nodule size at the time of entry before debulking and after careful evaluation of the upper abdomen. This includes the diaphragm, liver, omentum, bowel, mesentery and retroperitoneal nodes. Extension into the submucosa and/or muscularis, or onto tubal serosa is considered in Stage I disease. Differentiation between primary tubal cancer and tumors arising from the uterus or ovaries will remain difficult.

The staging system of both ovarian and tubal carcinoma assumes unproven and similar clinical, therapeutic and prognostic indicators. The current classification, as shown in *Table 47.5*, enables reliable comparisons between studies. Many

Table 47.5. FIGO staging of carcinoma of the fallopian tube.[1] (Staging for fallopian tube carcinoma is by the surgical-pathologic system. Operative findings designating stage are determined before tumor debulking.)

FIGO[1]		*Definition*
0		Carcinoma *in situ* (limited to tubal mucosa)
I		Growth limited to fallopian tubes
	IA	Growth limited to one tube with extension into submucosa and/or muscularis, but not penetrating serosal surface; no ascites
	IB	Growth limited to both tubes with extension into submucosa and/or muscularis, but not penetrating serosal surface; no ascites
	IC	Tumor either Stage IA or Stage IB, but with extension through or onto tubal serosa, or with ascites containing malignant cells, or with positive peritoneal washings
II		Growth involving one or both fallopian tubes with pelvic extension
	IIA	Extension and/or metastasis to uterus and/or ovaries
	IIB	Extension to other pelvic tissues
	IIC	Tumor either Stage IIA or IIB and with ascites containing malignant cells or with positive peritoneal washings
III		Tumor involving one or both fallopian tubes with peritoneal implants outside pelvis and/or positive retroperitoneal or inguinal nodes. Superficial liver metastasis equals Stage III. Tumor appears limited to true pelvis, but with histologically-confirmed malignant extension to small bowel or omentum
	IIIA	Tumor grossly limited to true pelvis with negative nodes, but with histologically-confirmed microscopic seeding of abdominal peritoneal surfaces
	IIIB	Tumor involving one or both tubes with histologically-confirmed implants of abdominal peritoneal surfaces, none exceeding 2 cm in diameter. Lymph nodes are negative
	IIIC	Abdominal implants larger than 2 cm in diameter and/or positive retroperitoneal or inguinal nodes
IV		Growth involving one or both fallopian tubes with distant metastases. If there is pleural effusion, cytologic fluid must be positive for malignant cells to be Stage IV. Parenchymal liver metastasis equals Stage IV

[1]FIGO staging adapted from the ovarian schema; current classification since 1991.

questions will be difficult to answer regarding molecular, morphologic and anatomic factors; for example, the significance of residual disease volume following initial surgery, and histologic grade, cytogenetics and tumor ploidy. However, the rarity of tubal cancer limits randomized prospective clinical trials.

It is obvious that the lack of specific symptoms of fallopian tube cancer is primarily responsible for a delay in diagnosis and therapy. Moreover, primary malignant tumor of the tubes has to be considered a pathologic rarity, while secondary involvement of the tube from tumors arising in the adjacent fundus or ovaries is much more common. In the literature, cancer involving the fallopian tube is secondary in 75–88% of cases. It is obvious, however, that in advanced disease, the differentiation between primary and secondary tubal cancer is increasingly difficult, if not impossible. The difficulties in determining the origins of tubal cancer have led in some instances to the formulation of macroscopic and microscopic criteria for primary tubal malignancies, as proposed by some authors. The following guidelines are given by Sedlis.

Macroscopic criteria

- The main tumor, presenting itself as papillary growth, is found in the endosalpinx.
- The uterus and ovaries are normal or present lesions other than carcinoma.

Microscopic criteria

- Carcinoma arises in the mucosa or endosalpinx and shows a papillary pattern and histologic characteristics of endosalpinx.
- The transition between benign and malignant tubal epithelium is demonstrable.
- The endometrium and ovaries are normal or present a benign lesion or are involved in a malignant lesion, which by its smaller size, distribution and histologic characteristics, is assumed to be metastatic from the tube.

There are some similarities between primary tubal carcinoma and endometrial cancer. Both are contiguous structures with the same embryonic origin, both respond clinically to steroid hormones, and both are found in the same age group and are more common among the nulliparous. However, in practice, a comparison with ovarian cancer seems highly preferable because of the clinical, therapeutic and prognostic similarities between the neoplasms. Therefore the FIGO ovarian carcinoma staging seems appropriate and less complex, even if true difficulties arise in the diagnosis of advanced disease.

The new FIGO classification should provide a common tool in order to combine case lists and to study the spread and prognostic factors, at least in early-stage disease. At present, carcinoma of the fallopian tube is treated similarly to ovarian cancer, but future research will determine if these two malignancies respond in a similar fashion. Although there may be consensus on most disseminations of tubal cancer, the true incidence of pelvic and paraaortic lymph node metastasis in various stages of the disease is a question that remains unanswered.

Vulvar Cancer

The FIGO staging system (*Table 47.6*) attempts to classify patients to reflect prognosis in an accurate, practical and uniformly applicable manner. Staging was changed most recently in 1988 (Committee on Gynecologic Oncology, 1989). Before this time, the main determinants of stage were tumor size, site and the clinical impression of nodal status.

The major changes adopted at the 1988 FIGO meeting included the following.

- Lymph node status was to be determined by histologic examination: Stage I and Stage II, negative nodes; Stage III, unilateral positive nodes; Stage IV, bilateral positive nodes.
- Involvement of the perineum, previously Stage III, was removed from the system.
- Involvement of the lower urethra was downstaged from Stage IV to Stage III.
- Stage IV was subdivided into IVA and IVB to differentiate patients with advanced local spread, including groin nodes, from patients with distant metastases, including pelvic lymph nodes.

Overall, the new system showed statistically significant differences between all stages and a better differentiation between Stage III and Stage IV than previously (Hopkins *et al.*, 1992).

Clinical assessment of nodal status has been reported to be inaccurate (Sedlis *et al.*, 1987; Shanbour *et al.*, 1992), and since lymph node status is one of the major determinants of outcome (Homesley *et al.*, 1991), the change to allow histologic examination of lymph nodes was a significant improvement.

There are areas of the 1988 system that could still be refined. In both Stage III and Stage IV, large lesions with two or more positive nodes or bilaterally positive nodes have an especially high risk, but not characterized separately (Homesley *et al.*, 1991). Within Stage III, there is a wide range of survival varying from 34–100%, and a modification of this stage has been proposed based on tumor size, the number of positive nodes, and whether the positive nodes are unilateral or bilateral (Homesley *et al.*, 1991). Although Stage I clearly identifies patients at low risk, the five-year survival varies from 94–100% (Homesley *et al.*, 1991; Hopkins *et al.*, 1992; Shanbour *et al.*, 1992). It might be beneficial to identify a group of patients with an extremely good prognosis within Stage I, possibly by using depth of invasion less than 1 mm.

Some prognostic factors are still not part of FIGO staging, including the number of positive nodes (Curry *et al.*, 1980; Hoffman *et al.*, 1985), the degree of involvement of the node (Origoni *et al.*, 1992),

Table 47.6. Staging of carcinoma of the vulva (from International Federation of Gynecology and Obstetrics (1989) Annual report on the results of treatment in gynecological cancer (1989) *Int. J. Gynecol. Oncol.* **28:** 189–190.)

TNM	*FIGO*	*Definition*
Tis	0	Carcinoma *in situ*, intraepithelial carcinoma
T1	I	Tumor confined to the vulva and/or perineum and 2 cm or less in greatest dimension; nodes are negative
T2	II	Tumor confined to the vulva and/or perineum and more than 2 cm in greatest dimension; nodes are negative
T3N0M0	III	Tumor of any size with any of the following
T3N1M0	III	Adjacent spread to the lower urethra and/or vagina, or anus
T1N1M0	III	Unilateral regional lymph node metastasis
T2N1M0	III	
T1N2M0	IVA	Tumor invades any of the following:
T2N2M0	IVA	Upper urethra, bladder mucosa, rectal mucosa and pelvic bone, and/or bilateral regional node metastasis
T3N2M0	IVA	
T4 any N M0	IVA	
Any T	IVB	Any distant metastasis including the following:
Any N, M1	IVB	Pelvic lymph nodes

the degree of increasing tumor size (Homesley *et al.*, 1991), and the depth of invasion in early-stage disease (Wilkinson, 1985). These may be considered for the future.

The staging system for vulvar cancer was previously based on tumor size, location and the examiner's clinical evaluation of the lymph node status. Before the new staging system, enlarged lymph nodes that were clinically suspicious or clinically positive were incorporated into the staging system, regardless of the actual disease status. Alternatively, if clinically negative lymph nodes were found to be positive at the time of groin node dissection, this would not change the stage. The groin lymph node status is known with certainty when almost all patients undergo radical vulvectomy and bilateral groin dissection. The staging system was therefore changed to a surgical system, which incorporates the actual pathologic status of the lymph nodes. The other change was the elimination of perineal involvement, which previously classified patients as Stage III. The new system incorporates accepted prognostic variables for carcinoma of the vulva. These include positive unilateral (Stage III) versus positive bilateral groin nodes (Stage IVA) versus positive pelvic lymph nodes (Stage IVB).

When using the clinical staging system, there is very little survival difference between patients with Stage I or II disease and those patients with Stage III or IV disease. In the new system, the only difference between Stage I and II is the lesion size, and this difference alone produces little difference in survival. Patients with Stage III disease in the earlier staging system had a marked decrease in survival because patients with bilateral positive groin nodes were included. Under the new system there are more pronounced survival differences between Stages IIIA, IVA and IVB. Patients with Stage III disease have a better prognosis in the new system because patients with bilateral positive groin nodes are now classified as Stage IVA. When using the new staging system, authors have reported that survival for Stage III is in the range of 50–75%, while survival for Stage IVA is approximately 30%, and for Stage IVB, 15%.

There is a difference in survival of almost 40% between Stage III and IVA; therefore, other known risk factors will be needed to predict survival. The clinical impression of the lymph node status may indicate a worse prognosis for these patients with clinically suspicious nodes (Homesley *et al.*, 1991), but in a large review of the Gynecology Oncology Group data base, only two independent factors related to survival were reported: lesion size and number of positive nodes. Location, including bilaterality, was not a significant prognostic indicator. There are five independent factors that predict an increased risk for nodal metastases: tumor grade; lymphovascular invasion; clinically suspicious, fixed or ulcerated nodes; tumor thickness and age (Homesley *et al.*, 1993).

Because the pelvic node dissection for vulvar cancer has in large part been eliminated, the pelvic lymph node status will rarely be known. The presence of metastatic disease to pelvic lymph nodes is a highly significant predictor of survival, decreasing survival to approximately 15%. Most patients with positive groin nodes will be classified as Stage IVA because the pelvic lymph nodes will not be known. Thus, over time, the reported survival for Stage IVA may decrease when compared to studies in which the pelvic lymph node status is determined surgically. Studies addressing the significance of a positive Cloquet's node without the knowledge of the pelvic lymph nodes would be useful.

Breast Cancer

Modifications in the staging of breast carcinoma have evolved since its conception at the turn of the twentieth century. A staging system should be designed so that data can be easily compiled, analyzed and transmitted from one physician or institution to another for purposes of outcome analysis and use in prospectively randomized multi-institutional trials. Consistent application of staging criteria is possible only through adjunctive use of universally accepted staging systems that permit accurate and objective comparisons between groups of patients. Moreover, the staging system must be flexible and revisable. Such is the case with the AJCC TNM system for breast cancer. This system offers the most universally applied system because former clinical staging methods (e.g. Manchester System, Columbia Clinical Classification) often failed to recognize tumor size and nodal characteristics as essential criteria of staging. The TNM system for breast cancer was first introduced in 1943. In 1958, the UICC described the first recommendations for staging that have evolved into the present TNM classification as shown in *Table 47.7*. Current UICC and AJCC staging systems for breast cancer are now identical (*Table 47.8*).

The current AJCC staging system for breast cancer based on the TNM classification is the most commonly used system for the staging of breast cancer. The advantages of the TNM system are its simplicity – it does not require complex technical support or expensive equipment – and its applicability to the many types of human solid tumors. However, for breast cancer, it does not take into account the role of other well-defined prognostic factors that are related to survival. This is of greatest concern in those patients with early-stage breast cancer where adjuvant systemic therapy with tamoxifen or chemotherapy or both has been shown

Table 47.7. TNM staging of carcinoma of the breast.

Stage	*Definition*
Primary tumor (T)	
TX	Primary tumor cannot be assessed
T0	No evidence of primary tumor
Tis	Carcinoma *in situ*: intraductal carcinoma, lobular carcinoma *in situ*, or Paget's disease of the nipple with no tumor
T1	Tumor ≤2 cm in greatest dimension
T1a	Tumor ≤0.5 cm in greatest dimension
T1b	Tumor 0.5–1 cm in greatest dimension
T1c	Tumor 1–2 cm in greatest dimension
T2	Tumor 2–5 cm in greatest dimension
T3	Tumor >5 cm in greatest dimension
T4	Tumor of any size with direct extension to chest wall or skin[1]
T4a	Extension to chest wall[2]
T4b	Edema (including peau d'orange) or ulceration of the skin of the breast or satellite skin nodules confined to the same breast
T4c	Both of the above (T4a and T4b)
T4d	Inflammatory carcinoma
Regional lymph nodes (N) (clinical)	
NX	Regional lymph nodes cannot be assessed (e.g. previously removed or not removed for pathologic study)
N0	No regional lymph node metastasis
N1	Metastasis to movable ipsilateral axillary lymph node(s)
N2	Metastases to ipsilateral axillary lymph node(s) fixed to one another or to other structures
N3	Metastases to ipsilateral internal mammary lymph node(s)
Distant metastasis (M)	
MX	Presence of distant metastases cannot be assessed
M0	No evidence of distant metastasis
M1	Distant metastasis (including metastases to ipsilateral supraclavicular lymph node(s))

[1]Paget's disease associated with a tumor is classified according to the size of tumor.
[2]Chest wall includes ribs, intercostal muscles and serratus anterior muscle, but not pectoral muscle.

to significantly improve overall survival (Early Breast Cancer Trialists' Collaborative Group, 1992).

In patients with 'node-negative' invasive breast cancer there is a wide range in survival probability, even for patients with small (T1; ≤2 cm) tumors. Changes in tumor size as small as 1 cm may result in major differences in survival, with tumors less than or equal to 1 cm and tumors 1–3 cm having 18-year survival rates of 86% and 70% respectively (Rosen *et al.*, 1993). Moreover, as many as one-quarter of the relapses in node-negative patients may occur more than ten years after diagnosis (Rosen *et al.*, 1993). Perhaps in no other malignancy has there been such an array of potentially helpful prognostic factors as in breast cancer. Tumor grade, estrogen and progesterone receptor status, and the extent of tumor proliferation (e.g. S-phase activity as measured by flow cytometry) have all been shown to be important in helping refine survival probability (McGuire and Clark, 1992) and in the selection of systemic therapy (Glick *et al.*, 1992). Moreover, prognostic factors such as estrogen and progesterone receptors are also 'predictive factors' in that they predict the response to treatment.

For patients with node-positive breast cancer, the probability of survival is inversely related to the number of positive nodes found during axillary dissection. The differences in survival can be substantial; patients with 1–3 positive nodes have a ten-year survival of about 40–50%, while patients with four or more positive nodes have a ten-year survival of only 10%. Also, adjuvant systemic therapy has the greatest impact for improving survival for patients with positive nodes (Early Breast Cancer Trialists' Collaborative Group, 1992). The current TNM system accounts for these distinctions in the N1b category.

In spite of these caveats, the AJCC staging criteria remain the benchmark for cancer staging worldwide. Patient records, clinical trials data and all scientific studies related to human breast cancer should use the AJCC staging system. Other well-defined

Table 47.8. American Joint Committee on Cancer (AJCC)/International Union Against Cancer (UICC) stage grouping for breast cancer (from American Joint Committee on Cancer (AJCC)/International Union Against Cancer (UICC), 1992.)

Cancer stage	*Tumor (T)*	*Node (N)*	*Metastasis (M)*
0	Tis	N0	M0
I	T1	N0	M0
IIA	T0	N1	M0
	T1	N1*	M0
	T2	N0	M0
IIB	T2	N1	M0
	T3	N0	M0
IIIA	T0	N2	M0
	T1	N2	M0
	T2	N2	M0
	T3	N1	M0
	T3	N2	M0
IIIB	T4	Any N	M0
	Any T	N3	M0
IV	Any T	Any N	M1

*The prognosis of patients with pN1a is similar to that of patients with pN0.

prognostic factors, when available, should be used in concert with the AJCC data to more precisely define prognosis.

Gestational Trophoblastic Neoplasms

The current FIGO staging system for gestational trophoblastic neoplasms (GTN) (*Table 47.9*), although relatively simple, provides for reliable comparisons of treatment results in centers throughout the world. The vast majority of Stage I disease (that confined to the uterus) is persistent hydatidiform mole, documented by plateauing or rising human chorionic gonadotropin (HCG) titers after evacuation of either complete or partial mole. Some clinicians prefer to further document disease histologically by repeat curettage, although this may be fraught with complications such as uterine perforation. The concept of debulking has no real meaning in GTN, as sensitivity to chemotherapy is usually exquisite. Stage II GTN comprises disease confined to the pelvis, usually vaginal metastasis, but also including rare GTN after tubal, ovarian or abdominal pregnancy. Documentation of Stage II disease requires imaging confirmation in addition to elevated HCG titers. However, biopsy of obvious vaginal metastasis merely to confirm is ill-advised because these can bleed briskly and hemorrhagic control can be difficult. Stage II GTN occurs when lung metastasis is present, with or without pelvic disease. The diagnosis is usually rendered on plain chest radiography, although computerized tomography (CT) or magnetic resonance imaging (MRI) may be necessary in difficult cases. Finally, Stage IV disease exists when GTN is metastatic to sites other than the pelvis or lung, including the gastrointestinal tract, kidney or other abdominal sites, or more ominously, metastasis to the liver or brain.

Most clinicians treating patients with GTN use one of two systems for planning therapy: the simplified categorization system popularized by Hammond or the more complex prognostic scoring system originally proposed by Bagshawe and more recently adopted by the World Health Organization (WHO) (*Table 47.10*). The former divides GTN into either non-metastatic, confined to the uterus, or metastatic disease. When confined to the uterus, GTN may be histologically persistent mole, invasive mole (chorioadenoma destruens), or the pure epithelial tumor, choriocarcinoma. Regardless, treat-

Table 47.9. FIGO staging of gestational trophoblastic neoplasms. (From Society of Gynecologic Oncologists (1994) SGO Handbook: Staging of Gynecologic Malignancies, 1st ed, Chicago: Society of Gynecologic Oncologists) (Risk factors affecting staging include the following: serum human chorionic gonadotropin >100,000 mIU ml^{-1}; duration of disease >six months from termination of antecedent pregnancy.)

Stage	*Definition*
I	Disease confined to uterus
IA	No risk factors
IB	One risk factor
IC	Two risk factors
II	Disease confined to uterus and pelvis
IIA	Involves genital structures without risk factors
IIB	Extends outside uterus, but limited to genital structures with one risk factor
IIC	Extends outside uterus, but limited to genital structures with two risk factors
III	Extends to lungs with or without known genital tract involvement
IIIA	Extends to lung with or without genital tract involvement and with no risk factors
IIIB	Extends to lungs with or without genital tract involvement and with one risk factor
IIIC	Extends to lungs with or without genital tract involvement and with two risk factors
IV	All other metastatic sites
IVA	Without risk factor
IVB	One risk factor
IVC	Two risk factors

Table 47.10. World Health Organization scoring system for gestational trophoblastic neoplasms based on prognostic factors (from Lewis JL (1993) Diagnosis and management of gestational trophoblastic disease. *Cancer* **71(4) (Suppl.):** 1639–1647).

Prognostic factor	*Score*[1] *1*	*2*	*3*	*4*
Age (yrs)	⩾39	>39		
Antecedent pregnancy	Hydatiform mole	Abortion	Term	
Interval (months)	4	4–6	7–12	12
Human chorionic gonadotropin (IU l^{-1})	1000	1000–10,000	10,000–100,000	100,000
ABO groups (female × male)		O × A A × O	B AB	
Largest tumor		3–5 cm	5 cm	
Site of metastases		Spleen, kidney	Gastrointestinal tract, liver	Brain
Number of metastases		1–4	4–8	8
Previous chemotherapy			Single drug	Two or more drugs

[1]Total score for a patient determines risk category. It is derived by adding individual scores in each prognostic category: low risk ⩽4; medium risk 5–7; high risk ⩾8.

ment for non-metastatic disease involves single-agent therapy, regardless of uterine size of the HCG titer. Metastatic disease is further divided into two subgroups based on the presence or absence of simple criteria. Good-prognosis, low-risk disease is present when the HCG titer is less than 40,000 mIU ml^{-1}, there are no brain or liver metastases, the duration of disease is less than four months, and there has been no previous chemotherapy. On the contrary, poor-prognosis, high-risk disease is present when the HCG titer at diagnosis is higher than 40,000 mIU ml^{-1}, liver or brain metastases are present, the duration of disease is greater than four months, previous chemotherapy has been administered, or GTN develops after a term pregnancy. Usually, single-agent chemotherapy is appropriate for good-prognosis disease, and if properly administered in sufficiently dose-intense regimens, the outlook for such patients is excellent. For patients with poor-prognosis disease, combination chemotherapy is almost always mandatory to avoid disastrous results. Even with intensive chemotherapy, those patients with high-risk disease may not be cured, especially if advanced liver or brain metastases are present.

The more complex prognostic scoring system is preferred by some clinicians since it offers certain advantages over the simplified system. When analyzed, it is apparent that there is further dissection and weighting of the same prognostic variables in the simplified system, giving credence to the theory that not all prognostic variables are created equal. For instance, previous chemotherapy is clearly of high-risk significance, but the scoring system differentiates between prophylactic chemotherapy, usually single agent, and the therapeutic chemotherapy, possibly combination treatment. Similarly, the scoring system gives more importance to brain/liver metastasis than gastrointestinal or kidney spread, although there is variation in some versions of the system. Further, volume of disease is stratified not only by HCG titer, with increasing score for logarithmic increments, but also by the number of metastases, as well as the size of metastatic deposits. Some authorities also include ABO blood grouping and the age of the patient as additional factors. Although quite complex, the prognostic scoring system offers certain advantages. Most importantly, it allows the establishment of a middle-risk group that may need less intensive chemotherapy. The system also allows retrospective analysis of large groups of patients to ferret out different categories and to assist in the formulation of future treatment regimens. However, when cumulative series treated under the auspices of the simplified classification system are reanalyzed using the more complex scoring system, the treatment results predicted compared to actual are remarkably similar.

The physician treating GTN must adhere to strict treatment parameters that are time-honored and well established, whether the FIGO staging, the simplified classification, or the more complex scoring system is employed. The treatment parameters include accurate diagnosis, compulsive timing of appropriate dose intensive chemotherapy, and periodic monitoring of serum HCG. Patients with GTN should never be managed casually, and those suffering from high-risk disease must be treated by physicians with special expertise.

There are currently several different classification systems being used to stage GTN. These include the FIGO system (see *Table 47.9*), the WHO scheme

Table 47.11. NIH classification of gestational trophoblastic neoplasms (GTN).

Stage	Definition
I	Benign GTN
A	Complete hydatidiform mole
B	Partial hydatidiform mole
II	Malignant GTN
A	Nonmetastatic GTN
B	Metastatic GTN
1	Good prognosis, low risk – absence of any risk factor
2	Poor prognosis, high risk – presence of any risk factor
a	Duration >four months
b	Pretherapy level of β-human chorionic gonodotropin in serum >40,000 mIU ml^{-1}
c	Brain or liver metastases
d	GTN after term gestation
e	Previous to failed therapy

(see *Table 47.10*), and a clinical National Institutes of Health (NIH) system (*Table 47.11*), as well as others that are less widely used. None of the currently used systems has achieved universal acceptance, which reflects inadequacies present in each method of classification. The recent change in the FIGO staging of trophoblastic tumors is an attempt to address the deficiencies of the old FIGO staging system. If the new FIGO system or any other current system is to be generally accepted, several objectives will have to be satisfied. The first major objective of any staging system for this disease should be to place untreated patients into distinct prognostic categories so that treatment results may be objectively compared. The second major objective should be to aid multiple agent or investigational regimens for those at high risk for treatment failure with standard combination regimens.

The WHO system (World Health Organization Scientific Group, 1983) was derived from a prognostic scoring system used by Bagshawe. In this scheme, multiple prognostic factors are assigned a score, and patients are categorized into low-, middle- and high-risk score groups based on scores of 1–4, 5–7 or 8 and over, respectively. Because both the WHO and the earlier NIH systems accept previously treated patients, they are not pure staging systems *per se,* but rather patient assignment into prognostic categories when they present for therapy. Patients with low-risk scores are treated with single-agent regimens, while those with middle- or high-risk scores receive combination chemotherapy. Virtually all deaths occur in the high-risk score group. Critics of the WHO scheme point to its complexity and to the inclusion of several prognostic factors that have not been generally recognized, such as the number and size of metastases. In a large multivariant analysis, Azab (Azab *et al.*, 1988) have failed to document the prognostic significance of β-HCG levels, although most other investigators consider them important. Nevertheless, the quantitative nature of this system has been used by several investigators (Dubeshter *et al.*, 1987; Gordon *et al.*, 1989; Dubuc–Lissoir *et al.*, 1992) to identify patients likely to fail conventional combination chemotherapy with methotrexate, dactinomycin, cyclophosphamide (MAC), and who therefore should be treated with new and more intensive regimens. The WHO system has not been superior to others in selecting single versus combination chemotherapy for patients with low-risk metastatic disease (NIH system), as a similar percentage of patients classified as low-risk by either system eventually need treatment with combination chemotherapy (Soper *et al.*, 1988).

The earlier FIGO system based solely on the anatomic distribution of disease has not been widely used despite its elegant simplicity. This classification was deficient because it failed to account for a number of accepted prognostic factors such as the type of antecedent pregnancy, HCG level and previous failed chemotherapy. Therefore, patients with both low- and high-risk metastatic disease were included among Stage III patients, making this stage grouping indistinct both in terms of prognosis and treatment. The new FIGO system will address these deficiencies, although the type of antecedent pregnancy has still been omitted from this classification. Stage III now has three subcategories: patients with lung metastases and without any high-risk factors are assigned to substage A; those with one or more risk factors are grouped in substages B and C, respectively. Treatment results will have to be reported according to the new FIGO system in order to determine how well this system separates patients into different prognostic categories and whether the substages as currently defined (Creasman, 1992), are useful in determining the appropriate type of therapy that should be employed.

The clinical classification system (NIH) has until recently been the most widely used staging system for GTN in the USA. The logical grouping of patients into non-metastatic, low-risk metastatic, and high-risk metastatic disease is certainly useful for determining therapy, although non-metastatic and low-risk patients both have an excellent outlook and are treated similarly with single-agent chemotherapy. The recently recognized disadvantage of this system is that it might not be helpful in selecting those patients who are likely to fail combination chemotherapy with MAC. The quantitative nature of the WHO system has been useful in identifying these ultra high-risk patients although opinions differ on the exact WHO score necessary for a patient to achieve ultra high-risk status. In most centers, the chemotherapy regimen EMA–CO (etoposide, methotrexate, dactinomycin, cyclophosphamide and viricristine (ONCOVIN) has now replaced MAC as the preferred therapy of all patients with high-risk metastatic GTN.

Future study should examine whether the WHO system or the new FIGO system is helpful in identifying patients likely to fail combination chemotherapy with EMA–CO, and new innovative regimens should be explored for this subgroup of patients. In addition, investigation of the therapeutic index of widely used single-agent regimens with methotrexate or dactinomycin versus combination therapy in patients with one or more risk factors according to the new FIGO scheme is needed. Perhaps the duration of therapy can be decreased using alternating single-agent treatment or combination chemotherapy. Further scrutiny of prognostic factors using current therapy will be necessary to reach accord on the best method of GTN classification.

References

Cervical cancer

Beahrs OH, Henson DE, Hutter RVP & Myers MH (1988) *Manual for Staging of Cancer*, pp. 151–156. Philadelphia: JB Lippincott.

Burghardt E, Girardi F, Lahousen M, Pickel H & Tamussino K (1991) Microinvasive carcinoma of the uterine cervix (FIGO Stage IA). *Cancer* **67:** 1037.

Christopherson WA (1992) The Spread and Staging of Cervical Cancer. In: Sciarra JJ (ed) *Gynecology and Obstetrics*, vol. 4, pp. 1–14.

Delgado G, Bundy B, Zaino R, Sevin BU, Creasman WT & Major F (1990) Prospective surgical–pathological study of disease-free interval in patients with Stage IB squamous cell carcinoma of the cervix: a Gynecologic Oncology Group study. *Gynecol. Oncol.* **38:** 352–357.

Gallion HH, von Nagell JR *et al.* (1985) Combined radiation therapy and extrafascial hysterectomy in the treatment of Stage IB barrel-shaped cervical cancer. *Cancer* **56:** 262.

Kamura T, Tsukamoto N, Tsuruchi N *et al.* (1992) Multivariate analysis of the histopathologic prognostic factors of cervical cancer in patients undergoing radical hysterectomy. *Cancer* **69:** 181.

Kolstad P (1989) Follow-up study of 232 patients with Stage IA1 and 411 patients with Stage IA2 squamous cell carcinoma of the cervix (microinvasive carcinoma). *Gynecol. Oncol.* **33:** 265–272.

Perez CA, Camel HM, Askin F & Breaux S (1981) Endometrial extension of carcinoma of the uterine cervix: a prognostic factor that may modify staging. *Cancer* **48:** 170–180.

Seski JC, Murray RA & Morley G (1977) Microinvasive squamous carcinoma of the cervix. Definition, histologic analysis, late results of treatment. *Obstet. Gynecol.* **50:** 410.

Sevin BU, Nadji M, Averette HE, Hilsenbeck S, Smith D & Lampe B (1992) Microinvasive carcinoma of the cervix. *Cancer* **70:** 2118.

Weems DH, Mendelhall WM, Bova FJ, Marcus RB, Morgan LS & Million RM (1985) Carcinoma of the intact uterine cervix, IB-IIA-B ⩾6 cm in diameter: irradiation alone vs preoperative irradiation and surgery. *Int. J. Rad. Oncol. Biol. Phys.* **11:** 1911.

Vaginal cancer

Al-Kurdi M & Monaghan JM (1981) Thirty-two years experience in management of primary tumours of the vagina. *Brit. J. Obstet. Gynecol.* **88:** 1145–1150.

Ball HG & Berman ML (1982) Management of primary vaginal carcinoma. *Gynecol. Oncol.* **14:** 154–163.

DiSaia PJ & Creasman WT (1993) *Clinical Gynecologic Oncology*. St Louis: Mosby–Year Book.

Eddy GL, Marks RD, Miller MC & Underwood PB (1991) Primary invasive vaginal carcinoma. *Am. J. Obstet. Gynecol.* **165:** 292–298.

FIGO (1989) Annual report on the results of treatment in gynecological cancer **20:** 175.

Hoskins WJ, Perez CA & Young RC (1992) *Principles and Practice of Gynecologic Oncology*. Philadelphia: JP Lippincott.

Kucera H & Vavra (1991) Radiation management of primary carcinoma of the vagina: clinical and histopathological variables associated with survival. *Gynecol. Oncol.* **40:** 12–16.

Manetta A, Pintol JL, Larson JE, Stevens CW, Pinto JS & Podczaski ES (1988) Primary invasive carcinoma of the vagina. *Obstet. Gynecol.* **72:** 77–81.

Morrow CP, Curtin JP & Townsend DE (1993) *Synopsis of Gynecologic Oncology*. New York: Churchill Livingstone.

Perez CA, Arneson AN, Dehner LP & Galakatos A (1974) Radiation therapy in carcinoma of the vagina. *Obstet. Gynecol.* **44:** 862–872.

Endometrial cancer

Belinson JL, Lee KR, Badger GJ, Pretorius RG & Jarrell MA (1992) Clinical Stage I adenocarcinoma of the endometrium – Analysis of recurrences and potential benefits of staging lymphadenectomy. *Gynecol. Oncol.* **44:** 17–23.

Burke TW & Wolfson AH (1994) Limited endometrial carcinoma: adjuvant therapy. *Sem. Oncol.* **21:** 84–90

Candiani GB, Belloni C, Maggi R, Colombo G, Frigoli A & Carinelli SG (1990) Evaluation of different surgical approaches in the treatment of endometrial cancer at FIGO Stage I. *Gynecol. Oncol.* **37:** 6 8.

Creasman WT (1994) Limited disease: role of surgery. *Sem. Oncol.* **21:** 79–83.

Creasman WT, Morrow CP, Bundy BN, Homesley ND, Graham JE & Heller SP (1987) Surgical pathologic spread patterns of endometrial cancer: a Gynecologic Oncology Group study. *Cancer* **60:** 2035–2041.

Homesley HD (1994) Endometrial cancer: prognostic factors. *Sem. Oncol.* **21:** 71–78.

Homesley HD, Boronow RC & Lewis JL Jr (1976) Treatment of adenocarcinoma of the endometrium. Memorial–James Erving Hospitals, 1949–1965. *Obstet. Gynecol.* **47:** 100.

Homesley HD, Boronow RC & Lewis JL Jr (1977) Stage II endometrial adenocarcinoma. Memorial Hospital for Cancer 1949–1955. *Obstet. Gynecol.* **49:** 604.

Homesley HD, Kadar N, Barrett RJ & Lentz SS (1992) Selective pelvic and periaortic lymphademectomy does

not increase morbidity in surgical staging of endometrial carcinoma. *Am. J. Obstet. Gynecol.* **167**: 1225–1230.
International Federation of Gynecology and Obstetrics (1989) Annual report on the results of gynecological cancer. *Int. J. Gynecol. Obstet.* **28**: 189–190.
Kadar N, Malfetano JH & Homesley HD (1992) Determinants of survival of surgically staged patients with endometrial carcinoma histologically confined to the uterus: implications for therapy. *Obstet. Gynecol.* **8**: 655–659.
Kim YB & Niloff JM (1992) Endometrial carcinoma: analysis of recurrence in patients treated with a strategy minimizing lymph node sampling and radiation therapy. *Obstet. Gynecol.* **82**: 175–180.
Larson DM, Johnson K & Olson KA (1992) Pelvic and para-aortic lymphadenectomy for surgical staging of endometrial cancer: morbidity and mortality. *Obstet. Gynecol.* **79**: 998–1001.
Morrow CP, Bundy BN, Kurman RJ *et al.* (1991) Relationship between surgical–pathological risk factors and outcome in clinical stage I and II carcinoma of the endometrium: a Gynecologic Oncology Group study. *Gynecol. Oncol.* **40**: 55–65.

Ovarian cancer

Cox DR (1972) Regression models and life tables. *J. R. Stat. Soc.* **34**: 187–220.
Hoskins WJ, Bundy BN, Thigpen JT & Omura GA (1992) The influence of cytoreductive surgery on recurrence-free interval and survival in small-volume stage III epithelial ovarian cancer: a Gynecologic Oncology Group study. *Gynecol. Oncol.* **47**: 159–166.
Omura GA (1981) Are all stage III cancers of the ovary really cancers of the ovary? *Cancer Clin. Trials* **4**: 219–220.
Partridge EE (1994) Carcinoma of the ovary. In: *SGO Handbook: Staging of Gynecologic Malignancies*, pp. 31–35. Chicago: Society of Gynecologic Oncologists.

Fallopian tube cancer

Dodson MI, Ford JH & Averette HE (1970) Clinical aspects of fallopian tube carcinoma. *Obstet. Gynecol.* **36**: 935.
Erez S, Kaplan AL & Wall JA (1967) Clinical staging of carcinoma of the uterine tube. *Obstet. Gynecol.* **30**: 547.
Petterson F (1992) Staging rules for gestational trophoblastic tumors and fallopian tube cancer. *Acta Obstet. Gynecol. Scand.* **71**: 224.
Schiller HM & Silverberg SG (1971) Staging and prognosis in primary carcinoma of the fallopian tube. *Cancer* **28**: 389.

Vulvar cancer

Committee on Gynecologic Oncology, International Federation of Gynecology and Obstetrics (1989) Annual report on the results of gynecological cancer. *Int. J. Gynecol. Oncol.* **28**: 189–193.
Curry SL, Wharton JT & Rutledge F (1980) Positive lymph nodes in vulvar squamous carcinoma. *Gynecol. Oncol.* **9**: 63–67.
Friedrich EG & Di Paola GR (1977) Postoperative staging of vulvar carcinoma: a retrospective study. *Int. J. Gynecol. Oncol.* **15**: 270–274.
Hoffman JS, Kumar NB & Morley GW (1985) Prognostic significance of groin lymph node metastases in squamous carcinoma of the vulva. *Obstet. Gynecol.* **66**: 402–405.
Homesley HD, Bundy BN, Sedlis *et al.* (1991) Assessment of current International Federation of Gynecology and Obstetrics staging of vulvar carcinoma relative to prognostic factors for survival. *Am. J. Obstet. Gynecol.* **164**: 997–1004.
Homesley HD, Bundy BN, Sedlis A *et al.* (1993) Prognostic factors for groin node metastasis in squamous cell carcinoma of the vulva (a Gynecologic Oncology Group study). *Gynecol. Oncol.* **49**: 279–283.
Hopkins MP, Reid GC, Johnston CM & Morley GW (1991) A comparison of staging systems for squamous cell carcinoma of the vulva. *Gynecol. Oncol.* **47**: 34–37.
International Federation of Gynecology and Obstetrics (1989) Annual report on the results of treatment in gynecological cancer. *Int. J. Gynecol. Oncol.* **28**: 189–190.
Iversen T (1981) The value of groin palpation in epidermoid carcinoma of the vulva. *Gynecol. Oncol.* **12**: 291–295.
Origoni M, Sideri M, Garsia S, Carinelli SG & Ferrari AG (1992) Prognostic value of pathological patterns of lymph node positivity in squamous cell carcinoma of the vulva stage III and IVA FIGO. *Gynecol. Oncol.* **45**: 313–316.
Sedlis A, Homesley H, Bundy BN *et al.* (1987) Positive groin lymph nodes in superficial squamous cell vulvar cancer. *Am. J. Obstet. Gynecol.* **156**: 1159–1164.
Shanbour KA, Mannel RS, Morris PC, Yadack A & Walker JL (1992) Comparison of clinical versus surgical staging systems in vulvar cancer. *Obstet. Gynecol.* **80**: 927–930.
Wilkinson EJ (1985) Superficial invasive carcinoma of the vulva. *Clin. Obstet. Gynecol.* **28**: 188–195.

Breast cancer

Early Breast Cancer Trialists' Collaborative Group (1992) Systemic treatment of early breast cancer by hormonal, cytotoxic, or immune therapy. 133 randomized trials involving 31,000 recurrences and 24,000 deaths among 75,000 women. *Lancet* **339**: 1–15, 71–85.
Glick JH, Gelber RD, Goldhirsch A & Senn H (1992) Meeting highlights: Adjuvant therapy for primary breast cancer. *J. Natl. Cancer Inst.* **84**: 1479–1485.
McGuire WL & Clark GM (1992) Prognostic factors and treatment decisions in axillary-node-negative breast cancer [see comments]. *New Engl. J. Med.* **326**: 1756–1761.
Rosen PP, Groshen S, Kinne DW & Norton L (1993) Factors influencing prognosis in node-negative breast carcinoma: analysis of 767 T1N0M0/T2N0M0 patients with long-term follow-up. *J. Clin. Oncol.* **11**: 2090–2100.

Gestational trophoblastic neoplasms

Azab MB, Pejovic MH, Theodore C *et al.* (1988) Prognostic factors in gestational trophoblastic tumors. A multivariate analysis. *Cancer* **62(3)**: 585–592.
Creasman WT (1992) Revision in classification by International Federation of Gynecology and Obstetrics. *Am. J. Obstet. Gynecol.* **167**: 857.
Currie JL (1991) Gestational trophoblastic neoplasia. In: Blackledge *et al.* (eds) *Textbook of Gynecology*. WB Saunders.
Dubeshter B, Berkowitz RS, Goldstein DP, Cramer DW & Bernstein MR (1987) Metastatic gestational trophoblastic disease: experience at the New England Trophoblastic

Disease Center, 1965 to 1985. *Obstet. Gynecol.* **69:** 390–395.

Dubuc–Lissoir J, Sweizig S, Schlaerth JB & Morrow CP (1992) Metastatic gestational trophoblastic disease: a comparison of prognostic classification systems. *Gynecol. Oncol.* **45:** 40–45.

Gordon AN, Gershenson DM, Copeland LJ, Stringer CA, Morris M & Wharton JT (1989) High-risk metastatic gestational trophoblastic disease: further stratification into two clinical entities. *Gynecol. Oncol.* **34:** 54–56.

Soper JT, Clarke–Pearson D & Hammond CB (1988) Metastatic gestational trophoblastic disease: prognostic factors in previously untreated patients. *Obstet. Gynecol.* **71:** 338–343.

Index